THIRD EDITION
PULMONARY REHABILITATION
Guidelines to Success

EDITED BY

John E. Hodgkin, MD
Clinical Professor of Medicine
University of California, Davis
Davis, California
Medical Director, Respiratory Care and Pulmonary Rehabilitation
St. Helena Hospital
Deer Park, California

Bartolome R. Celli, MD
Chief, Pulmonary and Critical Care Medicine
St. Elizabeth's Medical Center
Professor of Medicine
Tufts University
Boston, Massachusetts

Gerilynn L. Connors, BS, RCP, RRT
Adjunct Faculty, Respiratory Therapy Program
Northern Virginia Community College
Annandale, Virginia

With 53 contributors

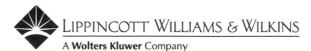
LIPPINCOTT WILLIAMS & WILKINS
A **Wolters Kluwer** Company
Philadelphia • Baltimore • New York • London
Buenos Aires • Hong Kong • Sydney • Tokyo

THIRD EDITION
PULMONARY REHABILITATION
Guidelines to Success

To my family—Jeanie, Steven, Kathryn, Carolyn, Jonathan, and Jamie—which has allowed me to spend so much time focusing on Pulmonary Rehabilitation, *and to all the individuals participating in our rehabilitation programs through the years who have been such an inspiration to me.*

John E. Hodgkin

To all the trainees from the United States and around the world who have made my professional life so enjoyable; to all the members of my family who have supported my academic dreams; and to my co-editors who have put so much work into this book.

Bartolome R. Celli

To my husband, Frank, for his support and understanding; to my daughter, Shannon Mae, for her laughter and smiles; to my parents, Barbara and Erwin, for their encouragement; to my mentor, Dr. Hodgkin, for his vision; to my colleagues for their passion; and to our patients and their families for their strength.

Gerilynn L. Connors

Contributors

Nicolino Ambrosino, MD
Head, Lung Function and Pulmonary
  Rehabilitation Unit
Fondazione Salvatore Maugeri
Medical Center of Gussago
Gussago, Italy

John R. Bach, MD, FCCP, FAAPMR
Professor and Vice Chairman, Physical
  Medicine and Rehabilitation
Department of Physical Medicine and
  Rehabilitation
Professor of Neurosciences, Department of
  Neurosciences
UMDNJ–New Jersey Medical School
Newark, New Jersey

Kathy Lee Bishop-Lindsay, MS, PT, CCS
Manager, Emory HeartWise Risk Reduction
  Program
The Emory Clinic
Atlanta, Georgia

Dina Brooks, PhD, MSc, BSc (PT)
Assistant Professor of Physical Therapy
Department of Physical Therapy
University of Toronto
Research Associate
Department of Respiratory Medicine
West Park Hospital
Toronto, Ontario, Canada

Mary R. Burns, RN, BS
Executive Vice President
Pulmonary Education and Research
  Foundation
Lomita, California

Aquiles A. Camelier, MD
Associate Physician
Pulmonary Rehabilitation Center
Federal University of São Paulo (UNIFESP)
São Paulo, Brazil

Brian W. Carlin, MD
Assistant Professor of Medicine and
  Anesthesiology
MCP-Hahnemann University School of
  Medicine
Medical Director, Pulmonary Rehabilitation
Division of Pulmonary and Critical Care
  Medicine
Allegheny General Hospital
Pittsburgh, Pennsylvania

**Virginia Carrieri-Kohlman, RN, DNSc,
  FAAN**
Professor of Nursing
Department of Physiological Nursing
University of California, San Francisco
San Francisco, California

Bartolome R. Celli, MD
Chief, Pulmonary and Critical Care Medicine
St. Elizabeth's Medical Center
Professor of Medicine
Tufts University
Boston, Massachusetts

Roberta N. Clarke, PhD
Associate Professor of Marketing
Boston University Health Care Management
  Program
Boston University
Boston, Massachusetts

Gerilynn Long Connors, BS, RCP, RRT
Adjunct Faculty, Respiratory Therapy Program
Northern Virginia Community College
Annandale, Virginia

Susan Coppola, MS, OTR/L
Clinical Assistant Professor
Department of Allied Health Sciences
Division of Occupational Science
University of North Carolina at Chapel Hill
Chapel Hill, North Carolina

Philip R. Corsello, MD, MHA, FCCP
Medical Director, National Jewish Disease
  Management Programs
Department of Medicine
National Jewish Medical Research Center
Denver, Colorado

James I. Couser Jr., MD
Medical Director, Pulmonary Rehabilitation
St. Mary's Hospital Medical Center
Madison, Wisconsin

Rebecca H. Crouch, MS, PT, FAACVPR
Clinical Associate Professor of Physical
  Therapy
Director of Pulmonary Rehabilitation
Duke University Medical Center
Durham, North Carolina

Patrick J. Dunne, MEd, RRT
Regional President
Southwest HomeTech
Fullerton, California

Charles F. Emery, PhD
Associate Professor of Psychology
Department of Psychology
Director, Cardiopulmonary Behavioral
    Medicine Program
Center for Wellness and Prevention
Ohio State University
Columbus, Ohio

Roger S. Goldstein, MD, ChB, FRCP(C)
Professor of Medicine and Physical Therapy
University of Toronto
Toronto, Ontario, Canada

John E. Heffner, MD
Professor of Medicine and Associate Dean
College of Medicine
Medical University of South Carolina
Charleston, South Carolina

John E. Hodgkin, MD
Clinical Professor of Medicine
University of California, Davis
Davis, California
Medical Director, Respiratory Care and
    Pulmonary Rehabilitation
St. Helena Hospital
Deer Park, California

Kathleen Collins Insel, PhD, RN
Assistant Professor of Nursing
School of Nursing
University of Texas Health Science Center at
    San Antonio
San Antonio, Texas

José R. Jardim, MD
Associate Professor of Respiratory Diseases,
    Respiratory Division
Director, Pulmonary Rehabilitation Center
Federal University of São Paulo (UNIFESP)
São Paulo, Brazil

Douglas C. Johnson, MD
Assistant Professor of Medicine, Harvard
    Medical School
Associate Physician, Pulmonary and Critical
    Care Unit
Department of Medicine
Massachusetts General Hospital
Boston, Massachusetts

Robert M. Kacmarek, PhD, RRT
Associate Professor
Department of Anesthesia and Critical Care
Harvard Medical School
Director, Respiratory Care
Massachusetts General Hospital
Boston, Massachusetts

Robert M. Kaplan, PhD
Professor of Family and Preventive Medicine
    and Chair
Department of Family and Preventive
    Medicine
University of California, San Diego
San Diego, California

Kozui Kida, MD, PhD, FCCP
Director, Pulmonary Division
Tokyo Metropolitan Geriatric Hospital
Tokyo, Japan

Bruce P. Krieger, MD
Professor of Medicine
Division of Pulmonary Diseases
University of Miami School of Medicine
Director, Medical Intensive Care
Mount Sinai Medical Center
Miami Beach, Florida

Suzanne C. Lareau, RN, MS
Pulmonary Clinical Nurse Specialist
Department of Veterans Affairs
Jerry L. Pettis Memorial VA Medical Center
Assistant Clinical Professor of Nursing
School of Nursing
Loma Linda University
Loma Linda, California

G. Scott Lea, BS, RRT
Senior Vice President
Alpine Medical
Bensalem, Pennsylvania

Kim R. Lebowitz, MA
Graduate Research Assistant
Department of Psychology and Center for
    Wellness and Prevention
Ohio State University
Columbus, Ohio

Marie Lingat, MD
Fellow, Division of Pulmonary Medicine
Allegheny General Hospital
Pittsburgh, Pennsylvania

Donald A. Mahler, MD
Professor of Medicine
Dartmouth Medical School
Director, Pulmonary Function and
  Cardiopulmonary Exercise Laboratories
Dartmouth-Hitchcock Medical Center
Lebanon, New Hampshire

Fernando J. Martinez, MD
Associate Professor of Medicine
Division of Pulmonary and Critical Care
  Medicine
Department of Internal Medicine
University of Michigan School of
  Medicine
Ann Arbor, Michigan

Susan L. McInturff, RCP, RRT
Staff Respiratory Care Practitioner
Farrell's Home Health
Bremerton, Washington

Denise Miki, MD
Associate Physician
Pulmonary Rehabilitation Center
Federal University of São Paulo
  (UNIFESP)
São Paulo, Brazil

Lia Shaw Miller, BS, RCP
Senior Health Insurance Consultant
Temecula, California

William F. Miller, MD, FACP, FACCP
Clinical Professor, Internal Medicine
Pulmonary Division
University of Texas Southwestern Medical
  Center, Dallas
Medical Director, Home Care Program,
  Parkland Hospital
Dallas, Texas

Jean-François Muir, MD
Head and Professor of Pulmonology
Pulmonary Division and Respiratory Intensive
  Care Unit
Service de Pneumologie
Centre Hospitalier Universitaire de Rouen
Rouen, France

Richard S. Novitch, MD
Director, Pulmonary Rehabilitation
Burke Rehabilitation Hospital
White Plains, New York
Assistant Professor of Medicine
Division of Pulmonary and Critical Care
  Medicine
New York Presbyterian Hospital
Weill College of Medicine of Cornell
  University
New York, New York

Walter J. O'Donohue Jr., MD
Associate Dean, Graduate Medical Education
Creighton University School of Medicine
Omaha, Nebraska

Percival A. Punzal, MD
Program Director, Pulmonary Rehabilitation
  Section
Pulmonary and Critical Care Division
Philippine Heart Center
Quezon City, Philippines

Andrew L. Ries, MD, MPH
Professor and Director, Pulmonary
  Rehabilitation Program
Department of Medicine
University of California, San Diego
San Diego, California

Daniel O. Rodenstein, MD
Chief, Pulmonary Division
Cliniques Universitaires Saint Luc
Université Catholique de Louvain
Brussels, Belgium

Jeanne F. Ruff, MS, FAACVPR
Director, Cardiovascular and Pulmonary
  Rehabilitation and Health Promotion
Peninsula Regional Medical Center
Salisbury, Maryland

Kevin Ryan, BS, RRT, FAACVPR
Director, Pulmonary Rehabilitation
St. Helena Hospital
Deer Park, California

David P.L. Sachs, MD
Director
Palo Alto Center for Pulmonary Disease
  Prevention
Palo Alto, California
Clinical Associate Professor of Medicine
Division of Pulmonary and Critical Care
  Medicine
Stanford University School of Medicine
Stanford, California

A.M.W.J. Schols, PhD
Associate Professor
Department of Pulmonology
University Hospital Maastricht
Maastricht, The Netherlands

David R. Schwartz, MD
Pulmonary and Critical Care Fellow
Department of Medicine
Massachusetts General Hospital
Boston, Massachusetts

Paul A. Selecky, MD, FACP, FCCP
Medical Director, Pulmonary Department
Hoag Memorial Hospital
Newport Beach, California
Clinical Professor of Medicine
School of Medicine
University of California, Los Angeles
Los Angeles, California

Michael S. Stulbarg, MD
Professor of Clinical Medicine
School of Medicine
University of California, San Francisco
San Francisco, California

Wendy Wood, PhD, OTR/L, FAOTA
Assistant Professor of Occupational Science,
Department of Allied Health Sciences
Division of Occupational Science
University of North Carolina at Chapel Hill
Chapel Hill, North Carolina

Emiel F.M. Wouters, MD
Professor of Pulmonology and Chairman
Department of Pulmonology
University Hospital Maastricht
Maastricht, The Netherlands

Richard ZuWallack, MD
Professor of Clinical Medicine
University of Connecticut School of Medicine
Associate Chief, Pulmonary and Critical Care
  Medicine
St. Francis Hospital and Medical Center
Hartford, Connecticut

Preface

It seems fitting as we start a new millennium that the state-of-the-art of pulmonary rehabilitation be described in the new edition of this book. The first edition of *Pulmonary Rehabilitation: Guidelines to Success* was published in 1984, and the second edition in 1993. The prefaces to the first two editions have also been included in this book.

Pulmonary rehabilitation has become increasingly accepted during the past 2 decades as a standard of care for patients with chronic lung disease. In 1994, a group of experts, under the auspices of the National Heart, Lung, and Blood Institute, published a report with recommendations about areas of investigation that could further the science of pulmonary rehabilitation.[1] In 1996, the Medical Advisory Panel of the National Blue Cross Blue Shield Association issued a report stating that pulmonary rehabilitation is a reasonable technology for individuals with chronic obstructive pulmonary disease (COPD). A joint committee representing the American College of Chest Physicians and the American Association of Cardiovascular and Pulmonary Rehabilitation produced an evidence-based guidelines statement, in 1997, reporting on the scientific evidence supporting pulmonary rehabilitation.[2] Also in 1997, the Rehabilitation and Chronic Care Scientific Group of the European Respiratory Society published a position paper on the selection criteria and programs for pulmonary rehabilitation in COPD patients.[3] In 1999, the American Thoracic Society (ATS) published a new position statement supporting pulmonary rehabilitation[4]; the previous, and initial, ATS position statement on pulmonary rehabilitation was published in 1981.[5]

Chronic lung disease continues to be an important cause of suffering and premature death. Since the previous edition of this book was published, COPD has moved from fifth place to fourth place as a leading cause of death in the United States.

All of the chapters in this new edition of *Pulmonary Rehabilitation: Guidelines to Success* have been extensively revised or are entirely new. We are particularly pleased that this edition of the book has incorporated input from international experts, with seven chapters written by authorities from outside the United States. Through international collaboration, we can more effectively improve the standard of care for individuals with chronic lung disease worldwide.

The first two editions of the book emphasized the importance of an interdisciplinary team of health care providers working together in the assessment, education, and training of patients with chronic lung disease. As in the previous editions, we have selected experts representing the variety of health professionals that make up pulmonary rehabilitation teams to author chapters.

We thank all the authors who took time out of their busy schedules to contribute to this book. Their willingness to share their knowledge will help to make this book a valuable resource for those who are helping to care for individuals with chronic lung disease.

We also express our appreciation to Holly Chapman, Frank Musick, Debby Hartman, Angela Heubeck, Shannon Benner, Jacquelyn Merrell, and Lawrence McGrew from Lippincott Williams & Wilkins for their assistance with the production of the book and to Pat Jones, Bridgitte MacDonnell, and Robin Powell for their assistance with the clerical challenges of multiple drafts of chapters.

John E. Hodgkin, MD
Bartolome R. Celli, MD
Gerilynn L. Connors, BS, RCP, RRT

References

1. Fishman AP. Pulmonary rehabilitation research: NIH workshop summary. Am J Respir Crit Care Med 1994;149:825–833.
2. ACCP/AACVPR Pulmonary Rehabilitation Guidelines Panel. Pulmonary rehabilitation evidence-based guidelines. J Cardiopulm Rehabil 1997;17:371–405.
3. Donner CF, Muir JF. Rehabilitation and Chronic Care Scientific Group of the European Respiratory Society: ERS Task Force position paper: selection criteria and programmes for pulmonary rehabilitation in COPD patients. Eur Respir J 1997;10:744–757.
4. Pulmonary rehabilitation—1999: official statement of the American Thoracic Society. Am J Respir Crit Care Med 1999;159:1666–1682.
5. Pulmonary rehabilitation: official statement of the American Thoracic Society. Am Rev Respir Dis 1981;124:663–666.

Preface to the Second Edition

The approach to caring for patients with chronic lung disease has evolved through the years from an attempt to improve their level of comfort with simple medications to the science of pulmonary rehabilitation. In 1942 the Council on Rehabilitation defined rehabilitation as "the restoration of the individual to the fullest medical, mental, emotional, social, and vocational potential of which he or she is capable." The principles of rehabilitation have been used widely for decades for individuals with neurologic and musculoskeletal disorders. Recently some patients with cardiovascular or pulmonary impairment have been offered the advantages of rehabilitation.

In 1984 the first edition of this book was published by Butterworths. In that edition the importance of using a team of health care professionals to improve the quality of care of patients with lung disease was emphasized. Support has continued to grow for the concepts presented in the first edition of this book. It is time to update our knowledge of this process for enhancing the ability to function of individuals with chronic lung disease.

In 1989 11.6 million people in the United States reported that they had asthma, 12 million reported that they had chronic bronchitis, and 2 million reported that they had emphysema. While individuals with a variety of pulmonary disorders can benefit from pulmonary rehabilitation, most patients participating in these programs have chronic obstructive pulmonary disease (COPD). The term COPD is best reserved for those individuals with chronic bronchitis or emphysema who have obstruction to airflow on a spirogram. Patients with COPD may also have a component of bronchial asthma.

COPD is a major source of morbidity and is the fifth leading cause of death in the United States. Between 1969 and 1989 there was a 54% increase in the age-adjusted death rate for COPD, compared to a 49% decrease for coronary artery disease.

The cost of health care in 1991 in the US was estimated to be approximately 740 billion dollars. In 1988 the estimated expenditure for COPD, including direct expenses and costs related to morbidity and mortality, was 13.2 billion dollars. This does not take into account the cost in terms of human suffering. Pulmonary rehabilitation can not only result in many benefits to patients and their families, but also can provide significant economic benefits (e.g., reducing the need for hospitalization).

This second edition of *Pulmonary Rehabilitation: Guidelines to Success* presents information which is crucial to those delivering pulmonary rehabilitation, including new knowledge which has become available since the first edition was published: the latest concepts regarding smoking cessation, pharmacologic therapy, aerosol therapy, oxygen therapy, nutrition support, and exercise training; the newest technology for providing out-of-hospital ventilator assistance; current concepts about marketing the program; and important advice regarding reimbursement. All the chapters from the first edition have been revised, and new chapters have been added, dealing with the history of pulmonary rehabilitation, biofeedback, respiratory muscle training, laughter as therapy, respiratory physiology, rehabilitation of the pediatric patient, and dyspnea.

One of the great challenges of the future is to acquaint primary care providers and third-party payors with the benefits of pulmonary rehabilitation, so more individuals with pulmonary impairment and their families can take advantage of these programs. All patients with COPD should be considered as candidates for pulmonary rehabilitation.

We would like to thank all of those individuals who shared their knowledge with us by contributing chapters. We also want to express our gratitude to Carol Lewis and Debra Duckett who assisted with the clerical challenges of multiple drafts of chapters, and to Wendy Greenberger of J.B. Lippincott Company who assisted with the production of this book.

Preface to the First Edition

One of the handicaps of patients with chronic disease is the fact that many health care professionals prefer to take care of patients who get well quickly. The field of rehabilitation developed as an attempt to deal with those individuals who have disorders resulting in long-term impairment or disability. Rehabilitation specialists first focused on patients with musculoskeletal or neurologic ailments, with the goal being to restore them to the highest level of functioning possible. Subsequently, those with cardiac or pulmonary disorders were also considered as candidates for the rehabilitation process.

There is no better area than pulmonary rehabilitation to demonstrate the value of team care. Patients with respiratory disorders can benefit from the talents of many health care disciplines in both the assessment of the individual and the development of a treatment plan.

It was this recognition of the importance of multiple disciplines in evaluating and caring for patients with pulmonary disease that led us to develop this book. The chapters in this book deal with the many disciplines that constitute good comprehensive respiratory care, i.e., pulmonary rehabilitation for patients with lung disorders. We recognize that every hospital or outpatient rehabilitation facility may not have a health professional trained to deal with pulmonary patients from each of the disciplines covered in this book. This problem, however, can often be alleviated by one health professional providing the services from more than one discipline.

The major goal of this book is to help physicians and allied health professionals as they attempt to outline a care program for patients with chronic lung disease. We feel that the material presented throughout the book can help health professionals develop pulmonary rehabilitation teams that will result in improved care for their patients. If the quality of care for these patients is enhanced by the efforts of the many authors in this book, we will be gratified that the long hours spent in compiling the book will have been well worthwhile.

We would like to acknowledge the inspiration that Thomas L. Petty has been to us, as well as to countless others who have taken care of patients with respiratory disorders. We feel honored that Dr. Petty was willing to write the Foreword for this book.

The many authors who contributed their time and expertise to the content of the book deserve a special note of thanks. We also want to express our gratitude to Carol Lewis and Donna Littlefield who assisted with the clerical challenges of typing multiple drafts of chapters, and to Kathleen Benn and Julie Stillman of Butterworths who assisted with the copyediting and structuring of the book. Without their contributions, there would be no book.

Contents

IV.   Special Considerations in Pulmonary Rehabilitation

V.   Pulmonary Rehabilitation for Miscellaneous Disorders

VI.   International Approach to Pulmonary Rehabilitation

1

Historical Perspective of Pulmonary Rehabilitation

William F. Miller

⟩ Professional Skills

Upon completion of this chapter, the reader will:

- Identify early workers who defined the concepts of rehabilitation
- Describe the events involved in development of pulmonary rehabilitation
- Indicate the smoking behavior factors that determine the amount of smoke consumed
- Know the role of the U.S. Surgeon General in education; health effects of tobacco
- Identify Drs. Alvan Barach, Lucien Dautrebande, and George Thorn
- Briefly trace three key elements recognized early in the development of the principles of physical rehabilitation for patients with chronic obstructive pulmonary disease (COPD)

HISTORICAL PERSPECTIVE OF PULMONARY REHABILITATION

The concept of rehabilitation, involving organized holistic efforts to restore patients with debilitating and disabling disease to an optimally functioning state, is not new. However, application to patients with chronic pulmonary disease is a relatively recent practice. Before 1950, our understanding of pulmonary physiology and the nature of functional impairment was limited. Thus, it would have been difficult to formulate a physiologic approach to treatment. While preparing this chapter for the previous edition of this book it was decided that anything written on this subject before 1970 would be considered history. In preparing for this edition it was clear after perusal of current literature on COPD that material written since 1985 dominates the references used and that most of what was written before 1970 is ancient history. The exception is noted if the author of a current writing is a part of the history, then the number of references to works appearing before 1985 increases strikingly, especially if the article is a review. Therefore, this chapter will be extended to include works published before 1985.

PHILOSOPHIC CONCEPT OF REHABILITATION

The American Medical Association Council on Rehabilitation in 1942 defined rehabilitation as "the restoration of the individual to the fullest medical, mental, emotional, social and vocational potential of which the person is capable." These principles gained prompt acceptance for treatment of patients with neuromuscular and metabolic disorders. Later, programs emerged for rehabilitation of patients with other debilitating diseases, including heart and lung disease. Some have noted that rehabilitation for patients with heart disease started in the early 1960s, whereas rehabilitation for patients with pulmonary disease emerged in the 1970s. This experience varied in different regions of the country because our work was started in the early 1950s and our first publications appeared in the latter part of that decade and the early years of the next decade. Cardiac rehabilitation was not being practiced in our region until the mid-1970s. Certainly, the prevailing attitude in most of the country was that patients with debilitating pulmonary disease had little or no potential for rehabilitation.

Charles G. Eustace presented a pertinent and concise philosophic review of general rehabilitation in 1966.[1] He emphasized the importance of a historical perspective to the understanding of where we are today and where we hope to be in the future. Eustace defined rehabilitation as a process that demonstrates the impulse of people of goodwill to make other people whole. He noted that many different types of health care providers are involved with rehabilitation activities, and each group thinks their contribution is the most important. Thus, interdisciplinary rivalries often result in a shift of control, away from the physician. Eustace found this to be a deplorable situation based on ethical and practical considerations. Successful rehabilitation requires teamwork. The nonmedical components of rehabilitation are not primarily the responsibility of the physician, except as the director of the overall program.

Eustace emphasized that all handicapped persons do not have the same potential or motivation for rehabilitation. He states, "We cannot escape the fact that the quality of the finished product will depend on the quality of the raw material that went into it." Eustace cites Dr. Howard Sprague of Boston, who noted that the greatest resource for help to the patient involved in rehabilitation is *self-help*. An appropriate goal of the rehabilitation effort is to return the patient to a state of *self-help*. Eustace cites a warning by Sprague, "The greatest danger the disabled patient faces is not necessarily the loss of earning power but boredom, apathy and despair wherein an awareness of self-worth and dignity are lost."

While emphasizing the virtues of humility, tolerance, and compassion, Eustace urges all to heed the advice of another medical giant from the past, Sir William Osler. He reminds us that some patients never have been and never will be able to stand entirely on their own feet. Therefore, when careful evaluation of the patient indicates a lack of potential for rehabilitation, the inappropriate use of valuable personnel time and talent as well as money and facilities "merely indicates an absence of clinical intelligence and personal courage," according to Osler. On the other hand, when patients are properly selected, no doubt exists that pulmonary rehabilitation is, in an economic and practical sense, valuable.

DEVELOPMENT OF THE MODERN CONCEPTS

Rehabilitation methods, as part of a holistic approach to treatment of patients with pulmonary disease, were slow to be accepted. Rehabilitation was thought of as an optional therapeutic "add on," an activity in which few physicians had much knowledge or interest. A prevalent attitude was that after known medical treatment was in place and acceptable benefit achieved, the restoration of a patient's physical well-being was the responsibility of the individual. If the patient's rehabilitation succeeded, motivation was usually a product of economic necessity or personal desire. The patient seldom received any suggestions or encouragement and certainly no specific directives from most physicians. As a student and intern before 1945 I was told that chronic bronchitis was not a medically recognized condition and that pulmonary emphysema and its concomitants were untreatable. Patients were routinely told that they could only "learn to live with it," but they were given no direction regarding how they would accomplish this. Moreover, physicians generally were not prepared to provide any direction to patients.

As interest in physical restoration was revived, it was difficult to get physicians' attention so they could function as effective therapists to improve the quality of life for their patients. In retrospect, the present level of physicians' involvement has been achieved, it seems inadvertently, by applying the principle of incorporating rehabilitation into those components of therapy that were easily accepted. Thus, the message was being disseminated that rehabilitation begins with initial symptomatic treatment. In this way it was made an essential part of acute and subacute care, not to be ignored until after all medical and pharmacologic measures have been used to fullest advantage or just completely avoiding it as an exercise in futility.

In the early 1970s the Human Interaction Research Institute (HIRI), under the leadership of E.M. Glaser, found that physicians generally were not aware of all the known modalities available for the treatment of COPD. Moreover, even if they were aware they seldom made appropriate use of known methods (EM Glaser, Strategies for Facilitating Knowledge Utilization in the Biomedical Field, Report to the National Science Foundation, grant DAR 73-07767 A06, Washington, DC, 1975).

Under the auspices of the HIRI, many physicians with an expressed interest in the field of pulmonary rehabilitation were brought together with the goal of formulating a document that would represent the current state of the art with respect to the diagnosis and treatment of COPD. This report was published in the *Journal of the American Medical Association* in 1975[2] with the added intent to disseminate this widely for review to several hundreds of health care providers who treat patients with COPD. The responses were collated and analyzed to provide the basis for a monograph published by the American College of Chest Physicians in 1979.[3]

In 1974 a committee of the American College of Chest Physicians developed the following definition: Pulmonary rehabilitation is "an art of medical practice wherein an individually tailored, multidisciplinary program is formulated which through accurate diagnosis, therapy, emotional support and education stabilizes or reverses both physio*pathological* and psychopathological *manifestations* of pulmonary diseases and attempts to return the patient to the highest possible functional capacity allowed by his handicap and overall life situation" (italics added for accuracy and clarity). This was adopted by an American Thoracic Society (ATS) committee and in 1975[4] was published in the ATS newsletter, *Basics of RD*. Based on this definition, the ATS in 1981[5] published a comprehensive official position statement on pulmonary rehabilitation that has been reprinted several times in various documents but is too lengthy to include in this chapter.

The goals of rehabilitation programs have been clear from the beginning and have been related by many in various ways and include the following: (*a*) to decrease and control respiratory symptoms, (*b*) to increase physical efficiency and capacity, (*c*) to improve quality of life, (*d*) to reduce the psychologic impact of physical impairment and disability, (*e*) to decrease the number of critical care days, and (*f*) to prolong life in selected patients.

The background of a definition of pulmonary rehabilitation is presented in Chapter 2. I will discuss early developments in the processes of treatment.

PATIENT AND FAMILY EDUCATION

In early days, patient and family education were given some attention because the physician had limited therapeutic options aside from being able to provide counsel and reassurance to the patients. Ironically, with the advent of improved technology, emphasis on patient and family education waned. Moreover, an attitude of negativism toward patient education emerged when it became apparent that although use of therapeutic products might help symptoms, the disease process seemed inexorably progressive. New and better agents—such as selective, longer-acting β-agonist bronchodilators; anticholinergic bronchodilators; and anti-inflammatory drugs—brought new interest and hope.

Education of the patient and significant others as an essential part of treatment of all chronic diseases progressively gained attention. Although the importance of patient motivation and commitment to the success of the rehabilitation process of chronic disease was well recognized, the patient's innate intelligence may determine the number of times the education process will need to be repeated. For most patients the process needs to be repeated many times, including reminders about the nature of the disease process and the role of all medications and other elements of treatment. This is usually a demanding requirement because of the complexity of the problem in which at times more than one disease process may be involved. The patience and persistence required from all caregivers is often underestimated and has resulted in less than optimal success and frustration for many.

Numerous reviews and monographs have appeared that introduced new technical advances that involved patient and family in self-help procedures. Notable among these were Barach's[6] 1948 book titled *Physiologic Therapy in Respiratory Diseases;* Barach and Bickerman's[7] 1956 book titled *Pulmonary Emphysema;* and Miller's reviews of 1954,[8] 1958,[9] and 1967.[10] Petty and Nett[11] wrote the first comprehensive monograph for patients in 1967 titled *For Those Who Live and Breathe.*

SMOKING CESSATION

Today, smoking cessation is accepted universally for management of these patients. However, because Barach was a cigarette smoker, as were many physicians in the 1940s and 1950s, smoking cessation was seldom mentioned by Barach in discussions of therapy. Moreover, Barach and others were critical of the antismoking programs for patients with COPD. Barach always emphasized that he felt that smoking had great psychologic benefit and did little or no harm as long as the patient did not inhale. He always reminded those who criticized his smoking that he did not inhale, and I noted that he puffed gently on the cigarette and blew the smoke out quickly.

I recall this was long after A.C. Hilding[12] published his classic studies on the effects of smoking behavior on the quantity of tobacco smoke consumed. The factors demonstrated to be determinants include the following: *(a)* The force used to draw on the cigarette determines the temperature at which the tobacco burns and the number of toxic chemicals released. *(b)* The volume of air and smoke inhaled determines the distribution of smoke in the total lung volume. *(c)* The duration of time the smoke is held in the lung determines the completeness of the deposition of the smoke. *(d)* The length of each cigarette smoked determines the amount of filtering action by the smoked portion of the cigarette. *(e)* The number of cigarettes smoked. Contrary to popular opinion, the latter is not the most important factor but often the least important, especially if the other factors are maximized. Every health care worker should be aware of these studies because aside from genetic factors that determine individual resistance to the irritant chemicals, the above factors demonstrated by Hilding account for much of the variability in individual responses in relation to the number of cigarettes used. Somewhat surprising is the fact that, to my knowledge, this aspect of smoking has been largely ignored and no one has explored this further. The self-evident danger in tobacco smoking of any sort makes this a moot point.

Animal studies dating back to the 1850s by Van Praeg and Claude Bernard, as well as studies on humans in the early 1900s, proclaimed the toxic consequences of tobacco use. Two particularly important early works were the epidemiologic study by Anderson and Ferris[13] in 1962 and the pathophysiologic study by Thurlbeck[14] in 1963. After the Surgeon General's first report on the health aspects of tobacco smoke in 1964,[15] arguments against cigarette smoking generally were accepted. There followed an intense focus on factors related to why people smoke, how to achieve cessation, and definition of factors involved in success or failure of cessation as well as more on the health consequences of cigarette smoking. This period is detailed in a state-of-the-art review by Edwin B. Fisher, Jr, and his colleagues.[16]

Since that time a huge body of literature on the adverse health effects of tobacco use, as well as studies on smoking cessation techniques, has accumulated. Regular reports from the Surgeon General's office have sustained the initiatives to eliminate tobacco smoking. A coalition of major voluntary health agencies brought together by the Surgeon General in 1964 was named the Interagency Council on Smoking and Health. In 1969, Diehl[17] reviewed the early objectives and accomplishments of this group.

Dr. Norman Hepper and colleagues at the Mayo Clinic were pioneers in the antismoking endeavors.[18a,18b] The state of Minnesota was the world leader, followed closely by California, in developing aggressive programs to eliminate smoking in the general population. Since 1970, many people and agencies have been engaged actively in education of the public concerning the adverse effects of tobacco use. They are also aggressively promoting smoking cessation programs. J.L. Swartz was an early dominant figure in this activity.[19] David Sachs, S.M. Hall, and associates subsequently contributed much to the study and evaluation of smoking cessation techniques.[20a-20d] They found the *rapid smoking method* to be an effective approach to producing an aversion to smoking and smoking cessation; however, it has not been used widely.

PSYCHOSOCIAL CONSIDERATIONS

Psychosocial aspects of chronic disabling lung disease usually have been discussed as an afterthought in presentations on rehabilitation. Experience has taught us to consider these matters at the outset if other therapy is to be effective.

In 1950, Hurst et al.[21] noted that early workers—Binger, Christie, Alexander, and Faulkner—recognized the influence of psychologic factors on breathing. The results of the first systematic studies were published by Dudley, a psychiatrist, and Martin, a pulmonary physiologist, in 1969.[22] At about the same time, DeCencio and the Leshners[23] defined the personality characteristics of COPD patients. Agle and associates[24] reiterated and expanded on the observation of Sprague, cited by Eustace.[1] They stated that the greatest danger the candidate for pulmonary rehabilitation faces is a feeling of helplessness and a lack of self-worth that can, and often does, lead to depression, hopelessness, and suicide.[24] Prompt help to restore the patient's courage and dignity is crucial to successful rehabilitation. The most comprehensive summary of psychosocial considerations, in this early period, was presented by Dudley et al.[25] They stated: "The best thing to do with these patients is to treat their depression or anxiety or anger in a subtle way—that is with medication. At the same time give them emotional support and be the good listener they need." In addition they stated, "emphysema patients generally can't tolerate insight-oriented group therapy; they feel more comfortable as loners." This is ignored by most proponents of group therapy, but I feel it is a recommendation that should be given careful consideration. He also emphasized honesty in dealing with disabled patients. Certain personality traits that are important in therapists and physicians are confidence, humility, courage, tolerance, compassion, and an optimistic casual sense of humor. It is essential to convince the patient that although the road to success is not always smooth or predictable, experience has taught us that often great things come out of adversity.

MEDICAL TREATMENT

The unquestioned pioneer of physiologic treatment of chronic pulmonary disease was Alvan L. Barach (Fig. 1-1). He began his career, after graduating in 1919 from the College of Physicians and Surgeons in New York, at Massachusetts General Hospital in Boston under the sponsorship of Dr. James H. Means studying oxygen therapy and pulmonary physiology. He published his first reports with Dr. Margaret N. Woodwell, a series of three papers on oxygen therapy in the *Archives of Internal Medicine*.[26a–26c] In 1922 he returned to New York, to stay, and he started working at Presbyterian Hospital under the sponsorship of Drs. Walter W. Palmer and Robert F. Loeb. The same year he published his first solo report on the therapeutic use of oxygen in the *Journal of the American Medical Association*.[26d] He wrote his first review article on physiologic methods of diagnosis and treatment in 1938.[26e] This was followed by a monograph titled *Principles and Practice of Inhalation Therapy* in 1944.[27] In 1948 he revised and renamed the monograph *Physiological Therapy in Respiratory Diseases*.[28]

Bronchodilator Therapy

Bronchodilator therapy was variably effective in the early days because little was known about the pharmacodynamics of the limited agents available. Ephedrine and aminophylline have been used orally since the early 1930s. In most instances ephedrine was a poor bronchodilator and caused side effects, especially in elderly men, who would develop urinary retention as well as nervousness, insomnia, and tachyarrythmia. The only available theophylline preparation, aminophylline, because of its propensity for causing gastrointestinal distress as well as nervousness and increased cardiac irritability, usually was given in doses inadequate to achieve therapeutic blood levels. Epinephrine by subcutaneous injection was effective but, like ephedrine, frequently caused side effects, including trophic changes at the sites of injection.

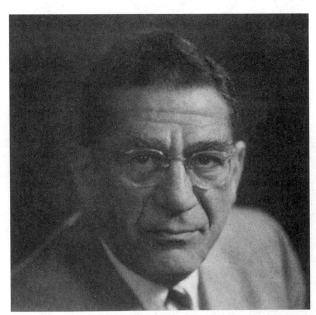

Figure 1-1. Alvan L. Barach, MD, "father" of modern-day physiologic therapy of COPD.

Aerosol Sympathomimetics

In 1935 Graeser and Rowe[29] introduced to the United States the aerosol inhalation of 1:100 epinephrine for relief of bronchospasm and bronchial congestion. This had been introduced in Germany in 1919 by Heubner.[30] Barach promptly adopted this great technologic advance and, subsequently, promoted its use.[31] He also aerosolized into the airways 1% phenylephrine (Neo-Synephrine), a sympathetic agonist decongestant originally used as an atomized spray or drops for nasal congestion. This was not an effective bronchodilator, but it helped in those instances in which bronchial edema was a factor.

Lucien Dautrebande, a French physiologist, first published studies on aerosols in 1941.[32] He became the world authority on microaerosols. The results of his years of work, which include more than 100 papers, are summarized in his monograph, Microaerosols, published in 1962.[33] By using systematic, carefully conducted studies he produced what became the best bronchodilator solution at the time. This consisted of 0.25% isoproterenol, a nonselective β-adrenergic agonist; 0.5% cyclopentamine, a superior adrenergic agonist decongestant; and 0.1% atropine, an anticholinergic agent. Cyclopentamine was considered superior to both phenylephrine and ephedrine because of fewer side effects and longer duration of action. It is intriguing that this agent was never used subsequently as a mucous membrane decongestant. It was not until oxymetazoline appeared that a long-acting decongestant was available. To my knowledge, long-acting decongestants have not been evaluated as adjuncts to bronchodilators in selected patients with bronchial inflammatory disease since Dautrebande did his studies. Later, atropine was removed from this combination because of rare serious cardiogenic side effects and because incidental deposition of aerosol in the eyes caused profound dilation and fixation of pupils. This was most often unilateral and led to clinical confusion, suggesting the presence of a focal central nervous system problem. Today the cogener ipratropium bromide (Atrovent) is used. For a long time, isoproterenol was the standard aerosol bronchodilator. It is a potent bronchodilator, but often its brief duration of action was not appreciated; hence, when patients routinely received two to four doses daily, they were often undertreated.

In 1958, Lands et al.[34] introduced the concept of β-2-bronchoselective adrenergic agonists as opposed to β-1-cardioselective agents for bronchodilator therapy. Isoetherine, a somewhat more selective bronchodilator, was a product of this early work. Its principal disadvantage, similar to isoproterenol, was a short duration of action. Only a few workers in the field recognized this shortcoming and adjusted the dosage and frequency to provide adequate bronchodilator action for patients with chronic recurring airway obstruction.

Ariens[35] in 1964 demonstrated that it was the deposition and absorption of large droplets in the mouth that was responsible for the side effects. Superior microaerosol nebulizers and tube extenders were used to control this problem. In the late 1970s and early 1980s we learned that extenders and reservoirs also enhanced the deposition of fine-particle aerosol.

Only two small-jet nebulizers were available in the United States in the 1940s: the Vaponephrin and DeVilbiss hand-held glass units. Wilson and LaMer[36] indicated that the Vaponephrin device was more efficient because of more consistent small particles in the size (median, 5.2 μm). Most European workers, as reflected best by Dautrebande's work, found that pulmonary deposition required a preponderance of particles in the 1-μm or smaller range. Small-particle nebulizers did not become standard until about 1989, following which a progressive development of more bronchoselective sympathomimetic agents occurred. These new agents had not only fewer side effects but also a longer duration of effectiveness. Thus, they could be given in larger doses. As a result, control of airway obstruction moved into a new age.

Methylxanthines

Theophylline was introduced as a bronchodilator in the 1930s with varying success because it was not until 1972 that Jenne et al.[37] clarified the clinical pharmacology of this substance. Then the introduction of sustained-release agents, which allowed once- or twice-daily treatment with sustained blood levels of drug, revolutionized treatment with this substance. This improved especially the control of nocturnal symptoms in some patients. For a period before 1975 theophylline preparations were administered rectally as suppositories or solutions. This was an effective method of administration for some patients but often resulted in both local and systemic undesirable side effects. This method is no longer recommended.

Theophylline preparations were occasionally used in aerosol form by some physicians. They were irritating to the airways but, in some cases, probably had a favorable effect by promoting bronchial evacuations of thick secretions. This approach was never widely appreciated or carefully evaluated.

Alternative preparations of theophylline, such as oxytriphylline, glyphylline, diphylline, dynophylline, and aminophylline, were generally unsatisfactory and more unpredictable than theophylline. Of these, aminophylline, which per milligram is equivalent to 0.8 mg of anhydrous theophylline, was the most widely used. It is a short-acting, rapidly absorbed agent that for oral use was in most cases administered in subtherapeutic doses. As a result, its value was often debated, and it was replaced by the sustained-release theophylline preparations. Aminophylline has been and still is used intravenously in acutely distressed patients.

Owing to the potential for side effects and toxic effects, as well as the need to monitor blood levels, use of theophylline has decreased. The advent of new, apparently safe and long-acting aerosol agents has contributed much to the decline in the use of theophylline. This complex problem was reviewed by Miller and Geumei.[38]

Anticholinergics

Atropine, stramonium, and belladonna were introduced to the Western world in the early 1900s in the form of atropine-medicated tobacco cigarettes. A complete historical review was written by C.W. Hertz,[39] who noted that the first writings of the use of anticholinergics (Datur) was in 1807 by Thomas Christie. He made reference to yet another reference by Brian Gandevia,[40] who noted that the use of Datura smoke inhalation to treat asthma was actually first recorded in the Ayurvedic literature in the 17th century.

The first real attempt at investigation was by Herxheimer[41] in 1959. He used specially prepared cigarettes from which the usual irritants were removed. Atropine was added at two dose levels: 0.5 and 1.45 mg. It was estimated that 80% was delivered to the patient. He found this method effective in patients with COPD, without significant side effects. He commented that other investigators had not found larger doses of atropine administered by aerosol methods to be effective. Moreover, the aerosol method was plagued by a high incidence of side effects, such as dryness of the mucous membranes, tachycardia, urinary retention, and mental confusion. He felt that this was a result of the much larger droplets delivered by standard nebulizer methods compared with the microaerosol from the cigarette. We confirmed these observations and suggestions by giving 1% atropine solutions in doses of 0.05 to 0.1 mg/kg body weight in 2 to 4 mL of water by an ultramicronebulizer designed by Dautrebande, with which we observed no untoward side effects. Lowell[42] also demonstrated that the side effects were caused by the large droplets delivered by the standard nebulizers, leading to significant systemic absorption. However, neither the special atropine cigarette nor the special nebulizers were available in this country for clinical use, and it was not until the late 1970s that similar nebulizers were commercially available.

An effective and safer anticholinergic, ipratropium bromide, an atropine congener, was first described in 1975, identified as Sch 1000.[43,44] It was not available until the mid-1980s for clinical use as the metered-dose inhaler Atrovent. It is now known to be a most effective agent in patients with COPD, and the combination of albuterol and ipratropium is more effective than either agent alone.

Assessing bronchodilator response in the usual way, by the improvement of the forced expiratory volume in 1 second (FEV_1), is disadvantaged in patients with emphysema in whom the mechanical defect of loss of lung elasticity dominates the character of forced expiratory flow, causing premature closure of the airways. However, it has long been known that these patients may experience significant decreased airway resistance measured during nonforced breathing, despite little or no change in the FEV_1.[45-48]

Anti-Inflammatory Agents

Hench and colleagues[49] first introduced corticotropin (ACTH) and corticosteroid therapy for treatment of the inflammatory component of rheumatoid arthritis. Bordley et al.[50] and Randolph and Rollins[51] in 1949 reported use of these agents in the treatment of inflammatory bronchial disease, especially allergic asthma. The first definitive study was by Carryer et al.[52] in 1955. Rose[53] provided the first authoritative review in 1954. Barach and associates[54] reviewed their large experience in 1955. It is important to appreciate that most of what is known about the pharmacology of corticosteroids was described by Thorn and his associates,[55] 1953 to 1955. Nevertheless, therapy with these agents, to this day, is largely empirical. George Thorn and his colleagues are responsible for most major developments in the use of corticosteroids. These included the recommendation of a single daily early-morning dose rather than multiple doses throughout the day for the stable patient and the use of alternate-day doses to reduce adrenal suppressive side effects to systemic therapy.[56] Many workers have verified these observations, but these principles often are still ignored in current clinical practice.

Cromolyn Sodium

Roger Altounyan discovered the prophylactic effect of cromolyn sodium in the mid-1960s. The first report of a controlled evaluation in patients with asthma was by Howell and Altounyan[57] in 1967. Cromolyn sodium for many years was considered to be of value only in young asthmatics. The mechanism seemed to be the inhibition of degranulation of sensitized mast cells when exposed to a substance that is capable of causing the release of chemical mediators. As the true nature of this agent became better understood, it was apparent that prolonged use in patients with chronic nonspecific bronchial inflammatory disease exhibited decreased reactivity of the airways. The result was improved control of obstructive disease symptoms and decreased dependence on corticosteroid therapy. Similar agents, such as neodocromil, have and undoubtedly will continue to become available. Patient selection remains to be clarified, and the value of prolonged use in patients with COPD remains to be proven.

Bronchopulmonary Clearance

The effects of viscid bronchial secretions and exudates in causing aggravated breathing difficulties and fatiguing cough have been recognized since antiquity. In the 1940s through the 1970s this was a major factor in the natural character of COPD. Inhalations have been used, especially hot vapors of saltwater, often with a variety of volatile substances added such as eucalyptus, menthol, creosote, ammonium chloride, and calcium salts, with varying degrees of enthusiasm and often questionable results. None of these substances were ever evaluated in controlled studies, but the one consistent component of most techniques was hot water vapor, which has withstood the test of time. Today we still use the steam vaporizer.

From the 1940s through the 1970s a variety of agents, such as hyaluronidase, trypsin, pancreatic dornase, and acetylcysteine, were used as aerosols to help mobilize obstructing viscid secretions. Segal and his associates were active in evaluating some of these agents. They were also enthusiastic promoters of (intermittent) *inspiratory* positive-pressure breathing (IPPB) as an adjunct for the delivery of aerosols to promote bronchial evacuation. Much of their interesting work is reviewed in the book by Segal and Dulfano.[58]

Because chronic productive bronchitis was such a common manifestation of patients with chronic airflow limitation, good methods of bronchial clearance were a major concern. The advent of more effective bronchodilators, antibiotics, corticosteroids, and other agents to improve airway function and control inflammation has drastically reduced the frequency of this problem. Occasionally, mucous plugging still occurs and often goes unrecognized. In some patients with chronic asthma, an unexpectedly low arterial oxygen tension in relation to ventilatory function may be the only clue, especially if cough is a major symptom.

The pattern of breathing during aerosol administration was first emphasized by Stalport[59] and later reaffirmed by Dautrebande.[60] They found that slow, deep breathing with an inspiratory pause was optimal for deposition of microaerosols in the lower airways. Simple relaxed normal-pattern breathing results in less than 40% deposition, whereas slow exhalation, followed by slow inhalation to near total lung capacity, followed by an inspiratory pause of 15 seconds could result in up to 85% deposition of aerosol.[60]

In 1954, the first paper I published was a clinical evaluation of these principles of aerosol administration.[61] Using the Oxygen Equipment Manufacturers mask, recommended by Barach, I demonstrated the superiority of an expiratory-inspiratory-pause method compared with conventional methods of breathing bronchodilator aerosols. Surprisingly, it was not until many more recent workers repeated the deposition studies with radioactive-labeled aerosols and metered-dose inhalers that these important considerations were more widely adopted. Education of patients to consistently employ these controlled patterns of breathing is still a major challenge.

Mist Therapy

Patients who demonstrated gas exchange impairment and volume limitation proportionate to flow impairment and cough as a prominent symptom were suspected of having a bronchial plugging problem and were subjected to aggressive bronchial hygiene therapy. In 1955 we adopted an idea that we had learned from Jack Emerson, who had heated the water reservoir of oxygen gas humidifiers to improve their efficiency. I also was aware of the claims in the writings from the early and mid-1800s for heated inhalations, so we started by using a small laboratory heater to heat water in a stainless steel bucket into which we placed the nebulizer reservoir jar. This system was reported in *Anesthesiology* in 1957,[62] and it was later revised to be heated by an immersion-type element, first made by Mist O-2 Gen Corp and later adopted by Puritan-Bennett and others.

As soon as we began using the reservoir nebulizers (1953–1954), we began finding an increased frequency of pulmonary infections caused by Gram-negative rods. I was convinced that this was related to contamination of the nebulizer systems, but I could not convince the hospital administration that added personnel was necessary to maintain and change the equipment every 12 to 24 hours, especially because many infectious disease investigators at that time did not consider these common environmental contaminants as serious pathogens, although they may be resistant to most antibiotics. However, when some of these patients developed fatal Gram-negative pneumonia, I was able to convince my colleagues Alan K. Pierce and Jay P. Stanford to study this problem. The results of those studies were published by Reinarz and colleagues[63] in 1965. We found high-density mist therapy to be effective in achieving good bronchial clearance, even in patients with severe ventilatory insufficiency, if we provided ventilatory assistance.[64] Subsequent reports have confirmed that in patients who have adequate function, clearance can be affected with aerosols, voluntary augmented breathing, and chest physiotherapy.[65] Unfortunately, reactionary rejection of this mode of treatment occurred for many years. It now seems to be returning to use as an aid to bronchial clearance on a more selective and rational basis, with appropriate precautions to prevent nosocomial infection.[66]

Much research needs to be done in the area of bronchial clearance to determine the role of evacuant aerosols and pharmacologic expectorants in the treatment of chronic bronchitic and bronchiectatic syndromes. Other agents that have been used were reviewed previously by Miller and Geumei.[38]

Pressure-Breathing Methods

Welch,[67] in 1878, reported the use of IPPB to successfully treat acute pulmonary edema. Norton[68] reported use of IPPB to treat acute toxic pulmonary edema in 1896, and Emerson in 1909[69] again treated pulmonary edema with IPPB. It was not until 1936 that the next report by Poulton[70] appeared. From that point on, Barach focused a great deal of attention on various modes of pressure breathing. In 1935, he introduced continuous positive-pressure breathing (CPPB), which he defined as 4 to 20 cm of water during both inspiration and expiration.[71] This technique was used at first with helium and oxygen to treat obstructive dyspnea and later, in 1937, with high oxygen mixtures to treat acute pulmonary edema of various causes.[72] These observations were verified by Segal[73] in 1943 and Segal and Aisner in 1944,[74] and then by Ansbro[75] in 1945 and Barach and associates[76] in 1947. This modality, CPPB, was often combined with inspiratory positive-pressure mechanical ventilation (IPPV). Thus, when Ashbaugh et al.,[77] in 1969, added positive expiratory pressure (PEP) with inspiratory positive-pressure ventilators to treat adult respiratory distress syndrome, they called it CPPB. In a subsequent article, they revised the terminology and introduced the terms IPPV with positive end-expiratory pressure (PEEP).[78]

Gregory and coworkers,[79] apparently unaware of the previous publications on CPPB, described a method, similar to Barach's, that they used to treat infant respiratory distress syndrome. They called it continuous positive airway pressure (CPAP). This term has been popularized and widely accepted. As a result, few people realize that Barach first described the method. When CPAP is modified to provide greater pressure assistance during inspiration, IPAP, compared with expiration, EPAP, this technique is called BiPAP.[80] The terminology has been confusing because each author applies a personal selective term to the method being used. I will not attempt to clarify this here because I am sure that most readers are well aware of the problem.

In the interim, IPPB became known after Segal as *intermittent* inspiratory positive pressure breathing (I/IPPB), which subsequently gave way to *intermittent* positive-pressure breathing (IPPB) when administered by a portable device on a short-term basis. This method was first used in clinical medicine as recommended by physiologists to ventilate patients with acute ventilatory failure and carbon dioxide retention.[81,82] The approach lost popularity as aggressive endotracheal intubation and mechanical volume ventilation gained interest as a quick, easy, often effective solution to the management of respiratory failure. However, this approach was often made without consideration of the likelihood that the patient could recover stability without continued ventilatory support. This experience has led to a resurgence of interest in noninvasive methods of ventilatory assistance for COPD patients.

Motley et al.[83] popularized IPPB as a method of administering bronchodilator aerosols. The unwarranted overuse of this method in patients who clearly demonstrated no indication of a need for ventilatory assistance occurred as a result of a combination of several factors: *(a)* a general lack of knowledge, among clinicians, about pulmonary physiology as it relates to treatment of respiratory failure in COPD patients; *(b)* third-party payers, including Medicare, employing a liberal payment policy for use of these devices despite a lack of evidence to support the widespread use without established criteria; and *(c)* vigorous promotion of IPPB use by multiple manufacturers and distributors, especially to respiratory therapy technologists, general physicians, and surgeons who for the most part were unable to critically assess the message at that time.

As a result, the use of IPPB was seriously challenged. It is not my intent to review the controversy that followed but rather to suggest studies that revealed the essence of the physiologic and clinical basis for the use of mechanically assisted breathing. Three early studies were attempts to do just that.[84–86] These studies have a double message. The first and most frequently cited message is that for stable patients, especially those with emphysema, using ventilatory assistance to administer bronchodilator aerosols offers no advantage. The second message is that in patients with ventilatory failure and ineffective cough with abundant tenacious secretions, often a better response to aerosol bronchodilator treatments was observed with ventilatory assistance. Much later two review papers summarized the controversy.[87,88] To my knowledge, a long-term study has never been done wherein patients were selected on the basis of clinical and physiologic indicators for ventilatory assistance. Such patients were specifically excluded in other short-term[89] and long-term[90,91] studies, including the elaborate multicenter clinical trial reported in 1983.[92]

PHYSICAL REHABILITATION

The principal components of physical rehabilitation for patients with clinical pulmonary disease include stress control, breathing control training, and physical conditioning. Optimal medical control of the inflammatory components of the process, proper nutritional adjustments, and supplemental oxygen where indicated are addressed first. Certain therapy procedures such as pneumoperitoneum, emphysema belts, thoracoabdominal compressors, and exsufflation with negative pressure are of only historical interest largely because none of the devices are available and no one has explored any of these with current methods.

Relaxation, Stress Control, and Biofeedback

From 1935 to 1948 many writings of a descriptive nature appeared concerning psychologic factors in relation to breathing. Jacobson[93] described classic relaxation techniques in 1938. Some of these were modified by Fink,[94] who first wrote his book *Release From Nervous Tension* in 1943. This became a paperback in its third expanded edition in 1962. Both authors used patients with asthma and breathing difficulty as examples for application of their techniques. It was not until 1976, when Vachon and Rich[95] did their formal studies on visceral learning in asthma, that methods of objective assessment were applied to this area. The term "biofeedback" was not in use until the 1970s, although the concepts of self-awareness, mind–body interrelations, and physiologic self-regulation existed long before. The term "autogenic training" was first used as early as 1959 by Schultz and Luthe.[96] Recognition of the role of both conscious and subconscious feedback to the process led to the term "autogenic feedback training." It was later shortened to "biofeedback." The development of this field is best and most colorfully reviewed by Elmer and Alyce Green.[97] They cite reasons for proposing the concepts that go back to ancient times and were aggressively pursued by the yogis.

Pursed-lips breathing is a form of biofeedback that helps the patient with emphysema to moderate expiratory effort, thereby reducing the transairway pressure gradient and the tendency for the airways to close, which exaggerates flow obstruction. In an effort to standardize the expiratory resistance that can be appreciated by the patient as a feedback signal, we used mouthpieces with selected small orifices. The resistance that the patient senses causes them to control their expiratory effort to optimize the expiratory flow. These simple devices were inexpensive, and we found them to be just as effective as the more expensive spring-loaded constant resistances. It is necessary to use larger orifices for the higher levels of ventilation associated with exercise. We always ask the patient to inhale through the nose. Ideally, the level of resistance needs to be defined in relation to the nature and degree of airway obstruction, a study that needs to be done. Biofeedback means the subjects are receiving immediate ongoing physiologic information about their own biologic processes, with the intent of using that information to control or change function in a desirable way. We most often used a visual form of feedback[8–10] to help patients control breathing and reduce dyspnea. Patients monitored their own volume versus time breathing tracing and could see how increasing the frequency of breathing caused air trapping, with an increase in the functional residual capacity. They also saw how forced exhalation caused a slowing of the emptying rate owing to airway closure.

They learned that less forceful exhalation with pursed lips actually led to increased flow. Others used the visual image of the flow–volume tracing on a video screen or plotter. Patients are taught to reproduce an ideal frequency or flow pattern.

Yet another approach was to use a simulated audible breathing signal. The specific characteristics of the signal were selected to optimize the patient's breathing, with the least effort for each patient. These and even more sophisticated approaches to control of breathing frequency, pattern, and effort as adjuncts to breathing retraining have never been fully investigated. Clinical experience with nonsophisticated patients clearly demonstrated that simply controlling breathing frequency was the most direct and most simple solution to breathing control and retraining. An example of observations we made during studies on exercise training is presented in the Exercise Reconditioning section.

The literature on biofeedback is vast, with well-controlled studies in many areas, but little has been published on its use in treatment of pulmonary problems. Relaxation techniques seem to be helpful in teaching breathing and dyspnea control.

Breathing Control Training

The principal aim of breath control techniques is to help the patient learn to breathe with the least expenditure of effort compatible with adequate alveolar ventilation for any given level of physical activity.[10] The physiologic basis for breathing control training was elucidated in part by many,[98,99] including Hofbauer,[100] 1925. Methods were first described by Schutz[101] and Livingston.[102] Barach modified and popularized "breathing exercises" in 1944[27] and 1948.[28] I preferred the designation breathing control training because the goal is to teach a slow, relaxed form of breathing. The term "exercise" implies a vigorously aggressive form of breathing. Barach did not believe that patients could be taught slow, relaxed breathing.

Our data on the physiologic assessment of the training was published in 1954.[8] The small group of patients showed the desired reduction in ventilation and breathing frequency with an increase in tidal volume. They also showed some improvement in ventilatory and gas exchange functions at rest and exercise. The magnitude of the changes were small but were consistently found, so statistical significance was achieved. The essence of our favorable effects was confirmed by Bolton and associates[103] and Dayman[104] in 1956. Howard Dayman was one of my contemporaries from whom I learned much. His 1951 paper is a classic,[99] then in 1956[104] he stated most succinctly, "In this disease (emphysema) expiration is fixed by the check valve mechanism (airway collapse) and inspiration by the hyperinflated condition of the thorax. The purpose of therapy is to enhance the efficiency of breathing within these fixed limits."

Following our study, several reports appeared that did not find measured improvement with breathing training. The key point here is that our goal was to train the patients to use a slow, deep pattern of breathing. This, in fact, was achieved, as demonstrated by the data. If the patient cannot be trained, no benefit will be observed. In the negative studies, evidence that training had been accomplished in most of their patients did not exist. An additional consideration is that our patients were active and showed signs of increased strength as reflected by the increased maximum expiratory pressure (MEP) and forced vital capacity (FVC). This suggests that the patients achieved an element of physical conditioning. This is an effect not specifically attributable to training in breathing control, but as they learned breathing control they were able to resume their more important activities. It is also possible that our patients achieved some clinical improvements in their bronchitis. This also is an effect not specifically a consequence of the breathing control training but coincidental to improved quality of the regular bronchodilator and bronchial hygiene therapy. In retrospect, these factors are difficult to control in a variable disease condition.

Even more impressive were some brief observations reported 13 years later.[10] In that investigation we studied three persons with stable pulmonary emphysema of a severe degree. In all, the FEV_1 values were less than 1 L/sec. None of these persons had any previous instruction in breathing control, and none had discovered pursed-lips breathing. They were asked to walk on a motor-driven treadmill at 2.5 mph for as long as they could. None of the patients were able to walk for more that 2 minutes, and one was able to walk for only 30 seconds. Breathing frequencies ranged from 37 to 44 breaths/min, with marked air trapping. The patients showed increased hypoxemia and carbon dioxide retention during the walks. After the first walk, the patients were allowed 30 to 45 minutes of rest. During that time they were advised to note that they were comfortable at rest breathing slowly. They were asked to observe their spirometer tracing during the walk to note how when they were breathing fast their tidal volume got progressively smaller and they trapped air as their lungs became more overdistended. They were asked to try to keep their breathing rate as slow as they could when the exercise was repeated. The breathing frequencies varied from 24 to 34 breaths/min and, in every instance, the duration of walking increased twice the initial time or more. This sequence was repeated two more times the same day, and each time the duration of walking increased strikingly. For the last two periods of walk we used taped signals from a breathing simulator[105] to facilitate breathing control. The magnitude of the increase in walking tolerance was proportional to the slowing of the breathing frequency. In two patients the arterial oxygen saturation and arterial partial pressure of carbon dioxide improved strikingly, although the patients were walking longer. The maximum increase in duration of walking was five to eight times above the initial duration. We also have noted patients who demonstrate exaggerated hypoxemia and carbon dioxide retention as a result of resting hyperpnea and air trapping, precipitated by a variety of circumstances other than exercise. This also could be corrected with control of breathing frequency alone. These observations have been confirmed by others.[105-109] It is important to note that achieving slow, controllable, deep breathing, by whatever method available, is essential to optimal gas exchange and activity tolerance. Thoman and coauthors[108] and Meuller and associates[109] have confirmed the immediate effects of slow pursed-lips breathing. These included a decrease of required minute ventilation, a slowing of breathing frequency, and increasing tidal volume. The pursed-lip maneuver, which produces PEP, prevents premature airway collapse.

Other adjuncts to breathing control training were described. Barach[110] emphasized use of a 20 to 30° head-down position with added weights (up to 15 lb) on the abdomen in conjunction with expiratory pursed-lips breathing. This has the same inspiratory muscle training effect as inspiratory resistors. Emphysema belts[110,111] and therapeutic pneumoperitoneum are now only of historical interest.[112-114] Abdominal muscle-strengthening exercises are a much more cost-effective approach and have fewer potential side effects. There probably are occasional patients, with very relaxed abdominal walls, who would benefit from an abdominal support if muscle strengthening is not feasible.

I believe confusion often exists about the objectives of the various approaches to breathing maneuvers. Barach and others who use the term ''breathing exercises'' are actually trying to strengthen the diaphragm and other respiratory muscles, which is a separate objective from what is usually meant by the terms ''breathing retraining'' or ''breathing control training,'' in which the objective is to teach the patient to recognize the limitation of forced breathing as an approach to alleviating dyspnea. Forced breathing at rapid frequencies simply leads to air trapping, impaired gas exchange, and worsened dyspnea. In some cases both respiratory muscle strengthening and breathing control may be necessary. We must be clear about the objectives of our exercise or training efforts.

Assessment of therapeutic benefit on the basis of subjective dyspnea is not necessarily the most appropriate indicator of what is beneficial for the patient. Patients exercising with controlled breathing may say that they have no improvement in their dyspnea although they are capable of performing more work even with improved gas exchange. I suspect that in those patients the fact that they are focusing more attention to their breathing sensitizes their awareness of the sensations related to breathing. I have observed that patients who are more relaxed and tend not to focus on somatic sensations achieve breathing control with greater ease and experience more subjective benefit.

Exercise Reconditioning

The concept of therapeutic exercise is not new. Cristobal Mendez in 1553 wrote a monograph titled *Book of Bodily Exercise*.[115] The modern era of therapeutic exercise for pulmonary disease was initiated by Barach.[6,7] On many occasions Barach was known to state, "I am of the opinion that a program generally dedicated to physical and mental rest is fraught with hazard!" He also stated, "Measures which have as their purpose an expansion of the life of the patient as much as may be feasible is to my mind a proper objective. We should encourage these stimulating activities not simply because our patients deserve to live fully as human beings, but also because constricting their activities for the sake of conserving their energies leads to psychosomatic disturbances that impair respiratory function itself. The heart of the matter is the physicians attitude."

Our first studies were reported in 1962[116] and 1963[117] and were followed by more extensive observations by Pierce and others[118] in our laboratory in 1964. The details of our techniques, summarized in 1967,[10] were independently developed but embody many of the principles of Donaldson and colleagues[119,120] in Australia. Oxygen-supported exercise was first described by Barach in 1938.[26] The first physiologic evaluation was undertaken by Cotes and Gilson[121] in 1956. Pierce and coworkers[122] demonstrated the same training effects with oxygen-supported exercise as with exercise at ambient oxygen levels. Paez and associates[123] in 1967 demonstrated that in short-term exercise training, the major element accounting for the improvement was a specific learning effect for the particular activity used for training. Training effects were not transferred from the treadmill to the bicycle. The learning effect was predominantly a lengthening of stride and improved posture on the treadmill so that the patient performed more efficiently. I suspect that if the patients had trained for a longer period, to a stable optimum degree of conditioning on the treadmill, more evidence of training effect transference would exist.

Finally, Pierce et al.[124] in 1968 found that patients with moderate to severe chronic airway obstruction were able to achieve significantly greater flow during both inspiration and expiration on exercise than they achieved during forced spirometry maneuvers.[118] This effect was accomplished as a result of modulation of the respiratory efforts during exhalation to minimize the airway's closure, which is demonstrated on maximal forced exhalation in the patients. Again, this becomes a function of a slow respiratory frequency, as emphasized previously in the section on breathing control.

Once patients were able to exercise or work in a regimented program, it was usually possible with reassurance for patients to apply the approach of slowly progressive intensity to other activities of interest. These ranged from work functions to pleasurable pursuits, such as dancing or sexual intercourse. In our opinion, the secret to success is an interested and enthusiastic physician coupled with a motivated patient who has achieved effective breathing control. We always saw our primary objective as improvement in quality of life.

ADDED PERSPECTIVE

The year 1970 marked the beginning of a new era for rehabilitation of patients with COPD. Since that time, the number of publications has increased immensely. After 1985 a further marked increase in rehabilitation research occurred, and the application of rehabilitation procedures has become fairly widespread but is not universal in clinical practice. It is now recognized that patients with COPD are not considered stable for purposes of evaluating new therapeutic procedures such as lung volume reduction surgery and transplantation unless the patient has achieved a stable optimal level of improvement by all therapeutic procedures including rehabilitation. Every established rehabilitation program has had some patients who have made incredible levels of improvement sometimes requiring several years of comprehensive rehabilitation care. The following chapters in this text deal with how continued advances in our knowledge have brought rehabilitation for patients with COPD to its current level of acceptance.

I have made several observations that did not fit easily into the context of this chapter. During the many years that I have been involved in the study and treatment of COPD, I have felt that the following considerations are important to this perspective. If we are to move forward in the process of learning more than the fact that if we apply some combination of therapies to a group of patients with chronic respiratory disease, they will exhibit certain desirable outcomes, we will need to define the character of the individuals that make up the study groups more precisely than has been the custom in the past.

Many investigators tend to ignore the precise anatomic, physiologic, personal, and regional differences of individual patients in relation to the natural history of the chronic airflow limitation. In so doing, they lump cases of a heterogeneous population that are classified on the basis of some arbitrary factor such as the FEV_1 value. Any given FEV_1 value may have significantly different meaning depending on the factors that are responsible for the airflow limitation. One example of this is presented in the Anticholinergics section. It is also common practice in many laboratories around the country to record only the expiratory flow volume tracing instead of the complete loop, thus neglecting precise characterization of inspiratory flow. Most computerized systems do not have standards for inspiratory flow values. As a result, most interpretations ignore the values. It seems clear that this is a situation that calls for better definition of inspiratory flow in health and disease, and which certainly needs definition for purposes of patient selection in evaluations of therapeutic procedures.

When patients with severe emphysema who are receiving home oxygen therapy are presented for a blood gases study on room air breathing, it is often not recognized that because of the reservoir effect of poorly perfused areas of emphysema it may take 45 minutes or longer to wash the excess oxygen out of the slowly ventilated spaces. This was first described by Dr. Julius Comroe.[125] After these patients are taken off oxygen, they should be monitored with an oximeter, and the arterial sample is not drawn until the arterial oxygen percent saturation reaches a plateau at its lowest level. Comroe found that failure to do this could result in a false high arterial partial pressure of oxygen being reported for room air breathing.

Now a few words about exacerbations in patients with COPD. Much of the literature addresses exacerbations as if they were virtually identical events from a pathophysiologic perspective. However, what is an exacerbation in one person may be a far different phenomenon in another. Each individual's exacerbation, whatever its proximate cause, starts from that person's specific background of anatomic changes, functional reactions, and constitutional nature. The primary cause itself is often an important determinant of the nature and severity of the event. The precipitating circumstances always should be sought not only from the standpoint of affecting the immediate therapeutic approach but also for purposes of patient and family education about how behavior needs to be modified, hopefully to prevent the next exacerbation. The following list includes the principal factors recognized as being associated with exacerbations from my perspective: (*a*) virus infection; (*b*) failure of bronchial hygiene with bacterial infection; (*c*) chemical inflammation of the airways resulting from personal, local, general, or occupational air pollution or from gastroesophageal reflux with aspiration; (*d*) allergic inflammation, or nonspecific vasomotor reactions to temperature and humidity changes; and (*e*) severe physical or emotional stress setting the stage for a vicious cycle of events including vasomotor responses, rapid breathing, air trapping, gas exchange impairment, and all the far-reaching consequences. I invite the reader to note the editorial by Anthonisen[126] in 1997.

Finally, owing to the limitations imposed on each chapter, I offer my sincere apology to the many workers who contributed sometimes in very significant ways to the historical development of pulmonary rehabilitation but who were not mentioned here. It was not always easy to know where to draw the line. I appreciate what you and your colleagues have done and I hope that the recognition due you will be forthcoming in the many chapters that follow.

REFERENCES

1. Eustace CG. Rehabilitation: an evolving concept. JAMA 1966;195:1129.
2. Hodgkin JE, Balchum OJ, Kass I, et al. Chronic obstructive airway diseases: current concepts in diagnosis and comprehensive care. JAMA 1975;232:1243.
3. Hodgkin JE, ed. Chronic Obstructive Pulmonary Disease: Current Concepts in Diagnosis and Comprehensive Care. Park Ridge, IL: American College of Chest Physicians, 1979.
4. Petty TL. Pulmonary rehabilitation. In: Basics of RD. New York: American Thoracic Society, 1975.
5. American Thoracic Society. Pulmonary rehabilitation: Official American Thoracic Society Position Statement. Am Rev Respir Dis 1981;124:663.
6. Barach AL. Physiologic Therapy in Respiratory Diseases. Philadelphia: JB Lippincott, 1948.
7. Barach AL, Bickerman HA. Pulmonary Emphysema. Baltimore: Williams & Wilkins, 1956.
8. Miller WF. A physiologic evaluation of the effects of diaphragmatic breathing training in patients with chronic pulmonary emphysema. Am J Med 1954;17:471.
9. Miller WF. Physical therapeutic measures in the treatment of chronic bronchopulmonary disorders: methods for breathing training. Am J Med 1958;24:929.
10. Miller WF. Rehabilitation of patients with chronic obstructive lung disease. Med Clin North Am 1967;51:349.
11. Petty TL, Nett LM. For Those Who Live and Breathe: A Manual for Patients With Emphysema and Chronic Bronchitis. Springfield, IL: Charles C Thomas, 1967.
12. Hilding AC. On cigarette smoking: smoking habits and measurements of smoking intake. N Engl J Med 1956;254:775.
13. Anderson DO, Ferris BG Jr. Role of tobacco smoking in the causation of chronic respiratory disease. N Engl J Med 1962;267:787.
14. Thurlbeck WM. The incidence of pulmonary emphysema, with observations on the relative incidence and spatial distribution of various types of emphysema. Am Rev Respir Dis 1963;87:206.
15. Smoking and health: a report of the Advisory Committee to the Surgeon General. US Department of Health, Education and Welfare, 1964. PHS publication 1103.
16. Fisher EB Jr., Haire-Joshu D, Morgan GD, et al. Smoking and smoking cessation, state of the art. Am Rev Respir Dis 1990,142:702.
17. Diehl HS. Tobacco and health: the controversy. New York: McGraw-Hill, 1969.
18. [a]Hepper NGG. Cigarette smoking and chronic respiratory disease. Minn Med 1969;52:1373.
    [b]Hepper NGG, Carr DT, Anderson HA, et al. Anitsmoking clinic: report of an experience and comparison with published results. Mayo Clin Proc 1970;45:189.
19. Swartz JL. A critical review and evaluation of smoking control methods. Public Health Rep 1969;84:483.
20. [a]Sachs DPL, Hall RG, Hall SM. Effects of rapid smoking: physiological evaluation of a smoking cessation therapy. AMN Intern Med 1978;88:634.
    [b]Sachs DPL, Hall RG, Hall SM. Two years efficacy and safety of rapid smoking therapy in patients with cardiac and pulmonary disease. J Consult Clin Psychol 1984;52:874.
    [c]Sachs DPL. Office strategies to help your patients stop smoking. J Respir Dis 1984;5(2):35.
    [d]Sachs DPL. Smoking cessation: what are your referral options? J Respir Dis 1984;5(2):49.
21. Hurst A, Henkin R, Lustig GL. Some psychosomatic aspects of respiratory disease. Am Practitioner 1950;1:486.
22. Dudley DL, Martin CJ, Masuda M, et al. The Psychophysiology of Respiration in Health and Disease. New York: Appleton Century Crofts, 1969.
23. De Cencio DV, Leshner M, Leshner B. Personality characteristics of patients with chronic obstructive pulmonary emphysema. Arch Phys Med 1968;49:471.
24. Agle DP, Baum GL, Chester EH, et al. Multidiscipline treatment of chronic pulmonary insufficiency, I: psychological aspects of rehabilitation. Psychosom Med 1973;35:41.
25. Dudley DL, Glaser EM, Jorgenson MSW, et al. Psychosocial concomitants to rehabilitation in chronic obstructive pulmonary disease. Part I–III. Chest 1980;77:413.
26. [a]Barach AL, Woodwell MN. Studies in oxygen therapy with determination of the blood gases, I. In Cardiac insufficiency and related conditions. Arch Intern Med 1921;28:367.
    [b]Barach AL, Woodwell MN. Studies in oxygen therapy with determination of the blood gases, II. In Pneumonia and it's complications: Arch Intern Med 1921;28:394.
    [c]Barach AL, Woodwell MN. Studies in oxygen therapy with determination of the blood gases, III. In An extreme type of shallow breathing occurring in encephalitis: Arch Intern Med 1921;28:421.
    [d]Barach AL. The therapeutic use of oxygen. JAMA 1922;79:693.
    [e]Barach AL. Physiological methods in diagnosis and treatment of asthma and emphysema. Ann Intern Med 1938;12:454.
27. Barach AL. Principles and Practice of Inhalation Therapy. Philadelphia: JB Lippincott, 1944.
28. Barach AL. Physiological Therapy in Respiratory Diseases. Philadelphia: JB Lippincott, 1948.
29. Graescr JB, Rowe AH. Inhalation of epinephrine. J Allergy 1935;6:415.
30. Heubner W. Uber inhalation zerstaubter flussigkeiten. Z Gesamte Exp Med 1919;10:269.
31. Barach AL. Physiological methods in the diagnosis and treatment of asthma and emphysema. Ann Intern Med 1938;12:454.
32. Dautrebande L. Aerosols medicamenteux, III: possibites de traitment des etats asthmatiformes par aerosols de substances dites bronchodilatrices. Arch Intern Pharmacodyn 1941;66:379.

33. Dautrebande L. Microaerosols. New York: Academic Press, 1962.

34. Lands AM, Luduena FP, Hoppe JO, et al. The pharmacologic actions of the bronchodilator drug isoetherine. J Am Pharm Assoc 1958;47:744.

35. Ariens EJ. Pharmacology of bronchodilating and bronchoconstricting drugs. In: Orie NGM, Sluiter HJ, eds. Bronchitis II. Assen, The Netherlands: Royal Van Gorcum, 1964:209.

36. Wilson IB, LaMer VK. The retention of aerosol particles in the human respiratory tract as a function of particle radius. J Ind Hyg Toxicol 1948;30:265.

37. Jenne JW, Wyze E, Rood FS, et al. Pharmacokinetics of theophylline: application to adjustment of the clinical dose of aminophylline. Clin Pharmacol Ther 1972;13:349.

38. Miller WF, Geumei AM. Respiratory and pharmacological therapy in COPD: lung biology in health and disease. In: Petty TL, editor. Chronic Obstructive Pulmonary Disease. 2nd ed. New York: Marcel Dekker, 1985;28:205–338.

39. Hertz CW. Historical aspects of anticholinergic treatment of obstructive airways disease: Scandinavian Symposium on Chronic Obstructive Airways Disease, Stockholm. Scand J Respir Dis 1979;60(Suppl 103):105.

40. Gandevia B. Historical review of the use of parasympatholytic agents in the treatment of respiratory disorders. Postgrad Med J 1975;51(Suppl 7):13.

41. Herxheimer H. Atropine cigarettes in asthma and emphysema. Br Med J 1959;2:167.

42. Lowell FC. Experimentally induced asthma in man. Proceedings of the 4th Conference on Respiration in Emphysema, Aspen, 1961.

43. Storms WW, Dopico GA, Reed CE. Aerosol Sch 1000, an anticholinergic bronchodilator. Am Rev Respir Dis 1975;11:419.

44. Gross NJ. Sch 1000: a new anticholinergic bronchodilator. Am Rev Respir Dis 1975;112:823.

45. Stead WW, Fry DL, Ebert RV. The elastic properties of the lung in normal subjects and in patients with emphysema. J Lab Clin Med 1952;40:674.

46. Miller WF, Johnson RL Jr, Cushing IE. Mechanics of breathing. In: Gordon BL, Kory RL, eds. Clinical Cardiopulmonary Physiology. New York: Grune & Stratton, 1960.

47. Johnson RL Jr, Miller WF, Wu N. Timed forced expiratory volumes and pulmonary conductance. Am Rev Respir Dis 1962;86:228–237.

48. Miller WF, Paez PN. Physiological alterations in emphysema. In: Gordon BL, ed. Clinical Cardiopulmonary Physiology. New York: Grune & Stratton, 1969.

49. Hench PS, Ward LE. Luken's medical uses of cortisone. In: Rheumatoid Arthritis and Other Rheumatic or Articular Diseases. New York: Blakiston, 1954:177.

50. Bordley JE, Harvey AMCG, Howard JE, et al. Preliminary report on the use of ACTH. Proc Clin ACTH Conf 1949;1:469.

51. Randolph TG, Rollins JP. Relief of allergic diseases by ACTH therapy. Proc Clin ACTH Conf 1949;1:479.

52. Carryer HM, Koelsche GA, Prickman LE, et al. The effect of cortisone on bronchial asthma and hay fever occurring in subjects sensitive to ragweed pollen. J Allergy 1955;21:282.

53. Rose B. Asthma and rhinitis. In: Luken's Medical Uses of Cortisone. New York: Blakiston, 1954:326.

54. Barach AL, Bickerman HA, Beck GJ. Clinical and physiological studies on the use of metacortandracin in respiratory disease. Bronchial Asthma Dis Chest 1955;28:515.

55. Thorn GW, Jenkins D, Laidlaw JC, et al. Pharmacologic aspects of adrenocortical steroids and ACTH in man. N Engl J Med 1953;248:414, 588.

56. Harter JC, Reddy WJ, Thorn GW. Studies on an intermittent corticosteroid dosage regimen. N Engl J Med. 1963;269:591.

57. Howell JB, Altounyan RE. A double-blind trial of disodium cromoglycate in the treatment of allergic bronchial asthma. Lancet 1967;2:539.

58. Segal MS, Dulfano MJ. Chronic pulmonary emphysema: physiopathology and treatment. New York: Grune & Stratton, 1953.

59. Stalport J. Aerosols medicamenteux, VII: nouvelles reserches sur quelues characteristiques physiochimques des aerosols: estude de leur absorption par les porimons: actin chez l'hormone d'aerosols formes a partir de substances diuritiques. Arch Intern Pharmacodyn 1958;71:248.

60. Dautrebande L. Physiological and pharmacological characteristics of liquid aerosols. Physiol Rev 1952;32:214.

61. Miller WF. A consideration of improved methods of nebulization therapy. N Engl J Med 1954;251:589.

62. Miller WF, Cade JR, Crusing IE. Preoperative recognition and treatment of bronchopulmonary disease. Anesthesiology 1957;18:483.

63. Reinarz JA, Pierce AK, Mays BB, et al. The potential role of inhalation therapy equipment in nosocomial pulmonary infections. J Clin Invest 1965;44:831.

64. Miller WF, Johnston FF, Tarkoff MP. Use of ultrasonic aerosols with ventilatory assistors. J Asthma Res 1968;5:335.

65. Sutton PP. Chest physiotherapy and cough. In: Clarke SW, Pavia D, eds. Aerosols and the Lung: Clinical and Experimental Aspects. London: Butterworths, 1984:156.

66. Wanner A, Ras A. Clinical indicators for and effects of bland, mucolytic and antimicrobial aerosols. Am Rev Respir Dis 1968;122:79.

67. Welch WH. Zur pathologie des lungenodems. Virchows Arch [A] 1878;72:375.

68. Norton NR. Forced respiration in a case of carbolic acid poisoning. Med Surg Rep Presby Hosp N Y 1896;1:127.

69. Emerson H. Artificial respiration in the treatment of edema of the lungs. Arch Intern Med 1909;3:368.

70. Poulton EP. Left-sided heart failure with pulmonary edema treated with the pulmonary plus pressure machine. Lancet 1936;2:283.

71. Barach AL. The use of helium in the treatment of asthma and obstructive lesions of larynx and trachea. Ann Intern Med 1935;9:739.

72. Barach AL, Martin S, Eckman M. Positive pressure respiration and its application to the treatment of acute pulmonary edema and respiratory obstruction. Proc Am Soc Clin Invest 1937; 6:664.

73. Segal MS. Inhalation therapy in the treatment of serious respiratory disease. N Engl J Med 1943;229:235.

74. Segal MS, Aisner M. Management of certain aspects of gas poisoning with particular reference to shock and pulmonary complications. Ann Intern Med 1944;20:219.

75. Ansbro FP. Positive pressure respiration in treatment of acute pulmonary edema. Am J Surg 1945;68:185.

76. Barach AL, Fenn WO, Ferris EB, et al. The physiology of pressure breathing: a brief view of its status. J Aviat Med 1947;18:73.

77. Ashbaugh DG, Petty TL, Bigelow DB, Levine BE. Continuous positive pressure breathing (CPPB) in adult respiratory distress syndrome. J Thorac Cardiovasc Surg 1969;57:31.

78. Petty TL, Nett LM, Ashbaugh DG. Improvement in oxygenation in the adult respiratory distress syndrome by positive end expiratory pressure (PEEP). Resp Care 1971;16:173.

79. Gregory GA, Kitterman JA, Phibbs RH, et al. The treatment of the idiopathic respiratory distress syndrome with continuous positive airway pressure. N Engl J Med 1971;284:1333.

80. Strumpf DA, Charlisle CC, Millman RP, et al. An evaluation of the Respironics BiPAP Bi-Level CPAP device for delivery of assisted ventilation. Respir Care 1990;35:415–422.

81. Courand A, Motley HL, Werko L, et al. Physiolological studies of effects of intermittent position pressure breathing on cardiac output in man. Am J Physiol 1948;152:163.

82. Bourtourline-Young HJ, Whittenberger JL. Use of artificial respiration in pulmonary emphysema accompanied by high carbon dioxide levels. J Clin Invest 1951;30:838.

83. Motley HL, Lang LP, Gordon B. Use of intermittent positive pressure breathing combined with nebulization in pulmonary disease. Am J Med 1948;5:853.

84. Fowler WS, Helmholtz HF, Miller RD. Treatment of emphysema with aerosolized bronchodilator drugs and intermittent positive pressure breathing. Proc Staff Mayo Clin 1953;28:741.

85. Wu N, Miller WF, Cade RF, et al. Intermittent positive pressure breathing in patients with chronic bronchopulmonary disease. Am Rev Tuberc 1955;71:693.

86. Chester EH, Racz I, Barlow PB, et al. Bronchodilator therapy: comparison of acute response to three methods of administration. Chest 1972; 62:394.

87. Demers RR. IPPB treatments: indications and alternatives. Respir Care 1978;23:758–759.

88. Miller WF. Inspiratory positive pressure breathing. In: Kacmarek RM, Stroller JF, eds. Current Respiratory Care Techniques and Therapy. Philadelphia: BC Dekker, 1988.

89. Goldberg I, Cherniack RM. The effects of nebulized bronchodilator delivered with and without IPPB on ventilatory function in obstructive emphysema. Am Rev Respir Dis 1965;91:13.

90. Curtis JK, Rasmussen HK, Cree EM. IPPB therapy in chronic airway obstructive pulmonary disease. JAMA 1968;206:1037.

91. Cherniack RM, Svanhill E. Long-term use of intermittent positive pressure breathing (IPPB) in chronic obstructive pulmonary disease. Am Rev Respir Dis 1976;113:721.

92. Intermittent Positive Pressure Breathing Trial Group. Intermittent positive pressure breathing therapy of chronic obstructive pulmonary disease. Ann Intern Med 1983;99:612.

93. Jacobson E. Progressive Relaxation: A Physiological and Clinical Investigation of Muscular States and Their Significance in Psychology and Medical Practice. 2nd ed. Chicago University Press, 1938.

94. Fink DH. Release From Nervous Tension. New York: Simon & Schuster, 1943.

95. Vachon L, Rich ES Jr. Visceral learning in asthma. Psychosom Med 1976;38:12.

96. Schultz J, Luthe W. Autogenic Training: A Psychophysiological Approach in Psychotherapy. New York: Grune & Stratton, 1959.

97. Green E, Green A. Beyond Biofeedback. New York: Dell, 1977.

98. Cournard A, Brock HJ, Rappaport I, et al. Disturbance of the respiratory muscles as contributing cause of dyspnea. Arch Intern Med 1936;57:1008.

99. Dayman HG. Mechanics of airflow in health and emphysema. J Clin Invest 1951;30:1175.

100. Hofbauer L. Pathologische physiologie der atmung. In: Bethe A, Bergmann G, Emden G, et al., eds. Handbuch der Normalen und Pathologischen Physiologie. Berlin: Julius Springer, 1925:337.

101. Schutz K. Respiratory and physical exercises. Wien Klin Wochenschr 1935;48:392.

102. Livingston JL, Gillespie M. The value of breathing exercises in asthma. Lancet 1935;2:705.

103. Bolton JH, Gandevia B, Ross M. Rationale and results of breathing exercises in asthma. J Aust 1956;2:675.

104. Dayman HG. Management of dyspnea in emphysema. N Y J Med 1956;56:1585.

105. Williams MH Jr, Kane C. Effects of simulated breath sounds on ventilation. J Appl Physiol 1964;19:233.

106. Motley HL. Effects of slow deep breathing on the blood gas exchange in emphysema. Am Rev Respir Dis 1963;88:485.

107. Pfeffer VR, Wilson RL. Breathing patterns and gas mixing. J Am Phys Ther [A] 1964;44:331.

108. Thoman RL, Stoken GL, Ross JC. Efficacy of pursed-lips breathing in patients with chronic obstructive pulmonary disease. Am Rev Respir Dis 1966;93:100.

109. Meuller RE, Petty TL, Filley GF. Ventilation and arterial blood gas exchanges induced by

pursed lips breathing. J Appl Physiol 1970; 28:784.

110. Barach AL. Breathing exercises in pulmonary emphysema and allied chronic respiratory disease. Arch Phys Med Rehabil 1955;36:379.

111. Barach AL. Breathing exercises and allied aids to breathing in the treatment of emphysema. Med Res Ann 1952;46:323.

112. Reich L. Der einfluss des pneumoperitoneum auf das lungen emphysema. Wien Arch Inn Med 1924;8:245.

113. Gaensler EA, Carter MG. Ventilation measurements in pulmonary emphysema treated with pneumoperitoneum. J Lab Clin Med 1950; 35:945.

114. Beck GJ, Eastlake C Jr, Barach AL. Venous pressure as a guide to pneumoperitoneum therapy in pulmonary emphysema. Dis Chest 1952;22:130.

115. Mendez C. Book of bodily exercise, 1553. Guerra F, trans. Kilgore FG, ed., 1953 and 1960. New Haven: Elizabeth Glick.

116. Miller WF, Taylor HD, Jasper L. Exercise training in the rehabilitation of patients with obstructive lung disease: the role of oxygen breathing. South Med J 1962;55:1216.

117. Miller WF, Taylor HD, Pierce AK. Rehabilitation of the disabled patient with chronic bronchitis and pulmonary emphysema. Am J Public Health 1963;53:18.

118. Pierce AK, Taylor HF, Archer RK, et al. Response to exercise training in patients with emphysema. Arch Intern Med 1964;113:28.

119. Donaldson A, Gandevia B. The physiotherapy of emphysema. Aust J Physiother 1962;8:55.

120. White A, Donaldson A, Gandevia B. A therapeutic regimen for the emphysematous patient in hospital. Aust J Physiother 1963;9:68.

121. Cotes JE, Gilson JC. Effect of oxygen on exercise ability in chronic respiratory insufficiency: use of portable apparatus. Lancet 1956;1:872.

122. Pierce AK, Paez PN, Miller WF. Exercise training with the aid of portable oxygen supply patients with emphysema. Am Rev Respir Dis 1965; 91:653.

123. Paez PN, Phillipson EA, Masangkay M, et al. The physiologic basis of training patients with emphysema. Am Rev Respir Dis 1967;95:944.

124. Pierce AK, Luterman D, Loudermilk J, et al. Exercise ventilatory patterns in normal subjects and patients with airway obstruction. J Appl Physiol 1968;25:249.

125. Comroe JH Jr, Forster RE, Dubois AB, et al. The Lung: Clinical Physiology and Pulmonary Function Tests. Chicago: Year Book Publishers Inc, 1955.

126. Anthonisen NR. Editorial OM-85 BV for COPD. Am J Respir Crit Care Med 1997; 156:1713.

BASIC CONCEPTS OF PULMONARY REHABILITATION

2 Pulmonary Rehabilitation: Definition and Characteristics

John E. Hodgkin

▷ Professional Skills

Upon completion of this chapter, the reader will:

- State the prevalence of asthma and chronic obstructive pulmonary disease (COPD)
- Discuss morbidity and mortality information for asthma and COPD
- Discuss the economic consequences of chronic lung disease
- Define pulmonary rehabilitation
- List disease states that should be considered as appropriate for pulmonary rehabilitation
- Review characteristics of pulmonary rehabilitation programs

---

INTRODUCTION

Although rehabilitation has been practiced for several decades, its application to patients with pulmonary disorders is relatively recent. In 1942, the Council on Rehabilitation defined *rehabilitation* as the restoration of the individual to the fullest medical, mental, emotional, social, and vocational potential of which he or she is capable.

This process has found widespread acceptance throughout the medical profession for patients with musculoskeletal and neuromuscular disorders. Even rehabilitation programs for cardiac patients have become common. Despite initial articles[1-7] reporting that pulmonary rehabilitation programs result in benefits for patients with COPD, it is only within the past 2 decades that such programs have become common.

In the mid-1970s, a study by the Human Interaction Research Institute (HIRI) in Los Angeles, Calif, showed that many physicians in the United States either were not aware of or were not using various facets of care for patients with pulmonary disease that had been shown previously to be useful.[8] As part of this HIRI project, which was funded by the National Science Foundation, a state-of-the-art paper on the diagnosis and treatment of COPD was developed and published in the *Journal of the American Medical Association* in 1975.[9] Hundreds of physicians and allied health personnel around the country were invited to critique this paper, following which the article was modified, expanded, and published in 1979 as a book by the American College of Chest Physicians.[10] It was the goal of those involved in this project to disseminate widely to physicians and allied health professionals those principles of care that had been demonstrated to produce both subjective and objective benefits in respiratory patients. Although this goal, in large part, has been realized, many primary care physicians still seem unaware of the benefits of pulmonary rehabilitation.

IMPACT OF CHRONIC PULMONARY DISEASE

The term *chronic obstructive pulmonary disease* (COPD) is best reserved for those individuals with chronic bronchitis or emphysema who have obstruction to airflow on a spirogram. It should be recognized that those with COPD may also have a component of bronchial asthma.

It is estimated that 14.9 million individuals in the United States have bronchial asthma and that 15.7 million have COPD (chronic bronchitis and/or emphysema).[11] Of individuals with COPD, it has been estimated that 14.5 million have chronic bronchitis and 1.9 million have emphysema. Most individuals with emphysema also have chronic bronchitis, whereas most people with chronic bronchitis do not have concomitant emphysema. This compares with an estimated 58.8 million individuals in the United States with cardiovascular disease (50 million with hypertension, 12 million with coronary heart disease, 4.6 million with congestive heart failure, and 4.4 million with stroke).[11] Whereas emphysema is more common in males, chronic bronchitis and asthma are more common in females (see Table 2-1).

Bronchial asthma, chronic bronchitis, and emphysema are among the leading chronic conditions in the United States (see Fig. 2-1 and Table 2-2).

In 1995, COPD was the first-listed discharge diagnosis for 553,000 hospitalizations and 16,087,000 physician office visits.[11] This compares with asthma as the first-listed discharge diagnosis for 511,000 hospitalizations and 9,026,000 physician office visits.[12] Asthma was also reported to cause more than 1.5 million emergency department visits.[12]

Although death rates peaked in 1950 for total cardiovascular disease and in 1963 for coronary heart disease, death rates for lung cancer and COPD have steadily increased during the same period (see Fig. 2-2).[11] Asthma mortality declined between 1968 and 1978 but has increased since then.[11,12] COPD and allied conditions constitute the fourth leading cause of death in the United States (see Table 2-3).[13]

The death rate for total cardiovascular disease has decreased 60% since its peak in 1950 and for coronary heart disease has decreased 60% since its peak in 1963.[11] In

Table 2-1. Prevalence Data for Obstructive Airway Disease in the United States

Disease	Number (per 1000)	
	Males	Females
Bronchial asthma	52.6	61.0
Chronic bronchitis	44.5	63.1
Emphysema	9.7	6.0

From Morbidity and mortality: 1998 chartbook on cardiovascular, lung and blood diseases. US Department of Health and Human Services, National Institutes of Health, National Heart, Lung, and Blood Institute, 1998.

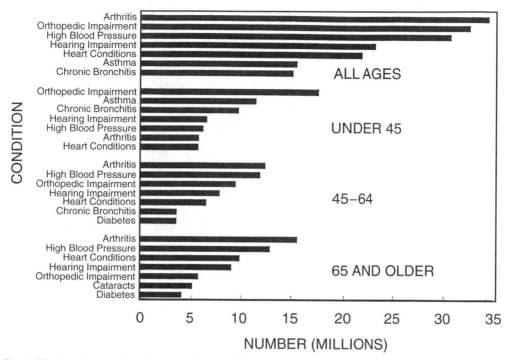

Figure 2-1. Prevalence of leading chronic conditions by age, United States, 1995. (From Morbidity and mortality: 1998 chartbook on cardiovascular, lung, and blood diseases. Bethesda, MD: US Department of Health and Human Services, Public Health Service, National Institutes of Health, National Heart, Lung, and Blood Institute, 1998.)

comparison, between 1979 and 1995 the death rate from COPD increased 40%. The mortality rate from COPD, between 1979 and 1995, increased by 3.6% in white males, 124% in white females, 27% in black males, and 132% in black females.[11]

Although cardiovascular disease is the leading contributor to the economic burden of health care in the United States, chronic lung disease also is a significant factor (see Table 2-4).[11] Most patients with COPD develop the problem as a direct result of smoking cigarettes. Although progress has been made in reducing the number of persons who smoke in the United States, efforts to help individuals avoid or cease smoking must be intensified. In 1965, 40% of individuals (52% of men and 34% of women) 18 years and older in the United States smoked cigarettes compared with approximately 25% (26% of men and 23% of women) currently.[14,15] The decline began in the late 1960s for men and a decade later for women, whose rate of decrease has been much more gradual. Despite this decline in smoking in the United States, it is still estimated that more than 400,000 individuals in the United States die each year as a result of smoking cigarettes.[16]

Some data related to cigarette smoking in the United States is troubling. From 1988 to 1996, among persons aged 12 to 17 years, the incidence of initiation of first use increased by 30% and of first daily use increased by 50%.[17] Data indicated that current smoking increased 26.5% from 1991 to 1995 among high school students in the United States, with one-third of ninth-grade students and 38.2% of twelfth-grade students reporting current smoking in 1995.[18] Smoking has also increased among college-aged students.[19] Between 1993 and 1997 the prevalence of current (30-day) cigarette smoking among college students rose by 23.8% (from 22.3% to 28.5%). Eleven percent of college smokers had their first cigarette and 28% began to smoke regularly at or after age 19 years, by which time most were already in college. Cigarette use is increasing in high schools and colleges nationwide.

Whereas the prevalence of cigarette smoking among U.S. adults (18 years or older)

Table 2-2. Prevalence of Leading Chronic Conditions Causing Limitation of Activity, United States, 1990–1992

Chronic Condition	Prevalence (in millions)
Orthopedic impairments	8.8
Arthritis	6.7
Heart disease	5.4
Hypertension	2.9
Asthma	2.5
Diabetes	2.4
Intervertebral disc disorders	1.8
Mental retardation	1.4
Hearing impairments	1.3
Visual impairments	1.3
Cerebrovascular disease	1.1
Paralysis	1.1
Emphysema	0.8

From Morbidity and mortality: 1998 chartbook on cardiovascular, lung and blood diseases. US Department of Health and Human Services, National Institutes of Health, National Heart, Lung, and Blood Institute, 1998.

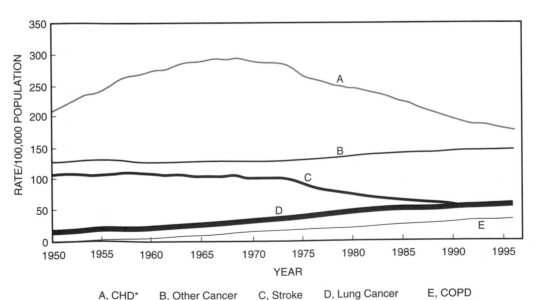

A, CHD*   B, Other Cancer   C, Stroke   D, Lung Cancer   E, COPD

Figure 2-2. Crude death rates for selected causes, United States, 1950–1996. *Comparability ratio applied to rates for years 1968–1978. (From Morbidity and mortality: 1998 chartbook on cardiovascular, lung, and blood diseases. Bethesda, MD: US Department of Health and Human Services, Public Health Service, National Institutes of Health, National Heart, Lung, and Blood Institute, 1998.)

Table 2-3. Deaths and Death Rates for the 12 Months Ending June 1998 for the 15 Leading Causes of Death: United States[a]

Rank	Causes of Death[b]	Number of Deaths	Death Rate (per 100,000 population)
	All causes	2,329,520	865.8
1	Diseases of the heart (390–398, 402, 404–409)	727,624	270.4
2	Malignant neoplasms, including neoplasms of lymphatic and hematopoietic tissues (140–208)	540,702	201.0
3	Cerebrovascular diseases (430–438)	159,059	59.1
4	Chronic obstructive pulmonary diseases and allied conditions (490–496)	111,823	41.6
5	Accidents and adverse effects (E800–E949)	94,266	35.0
	Motor vehicle accidents (E810–E825)	42,693	15.9
	All other accidents and adverse effects (E800–E807, E826–E949)	51,572	19.2
6	Pneumonia and influenza (480–487)	92,048	34.2
7	Diabetes mellitus (250)	63,813	23.7
8	Suicide (E950–E969)	29,732	11.1
9	Nephritis, nephrotic syndrome, and nephrosis (580–589)	25,755	9.6
10	Chronic liver disease and cirrhosis (571)	24,981	9.3
11	Septicemia (038)	22,817	8.5
12	Alzheimer's disease (331.0)	22,467	8.3
13	Homicide and legal intervention (E960–E978)	18,890	7.0
14	Atherosclerosis (440)	15,563	5.8
15	Human immunodeficiency virus infection (042–044)	13,930	5.2
	All other causes	366,050	136.0

Reprinted with permission from National Vital Statistics Reports: Centers for Disease Control and Prevention, National Center for Health Statistics. Hyattsville, MD: US Department of Health and Human Services, Public Health Service, 1999.
[a] Data are based on a continuous file of records received from the states.
[b] Based on the *Ninth Revision, International Classification of Diseases,* 1975.

fell steadily from 1965 to 1990, data for the 1990s suggest that the smoking initiation rate is increasing and that the decline in the prevalence of smoking may have stalled.[14] It has been estimated, however, that if current initiation and cessation behaviors persist, the prevalence of smoking among adults will decline from its current level of 25% to 15 to 16% by 2025.[14] Even so, cigarette smoking is expected to remain the United States' leading cause of premature death. It is estimated that one in every five deaths in the United States is smoking related.[20]

Cigarette smoking continues to be a serious problem worldwide. The number of adult smokers in the world is estimated to rise by a third during the next 20 years, from 1.2 to 1.6 billion adults. It is estimated that nearly half of the world's children, more than 700 million, live with a smoker. Worldwide, cigarettes will cause about 4 million deaths in the year 2000. If current smoking trends continue, the total will be 10 million deaths per year by 2030, with 70% coming from developing nations. China makes up 20% of the world's population but smokes 30% of the world's cigarettes. Two-thirds of the men become smokers before age 25 years. This means that tobacco will kill 100 million of the

Table 2-4. Economic Cost of Cardiovascular, Lung, and Blood Diseases in Billions of Dollars, United States, 1998

Disease	Total	Direct[a]	Indirect[b] Morbidity	Indirect[b] Mortality
Total cardiovascular disease	274.2	171.1	25.2	77.9
Heart disease	175.3	97.9	15.7	61.7
Coronary	95.6	51.1	6.6	37.9
Congestive heart failure	20.2	18.8	[c]	1.3
Stroke	43.3	28.3	5.1	9.9
Hypertensive disease[d]	31.7	23.3	4.8	3.6
Selected lung disease	121.9	84.6	20.9	16.4
Chronic obstructive pulmonary disease	26.0	13.6	6.0	6.4
Asthma	11.3	7.5	2.4	1.4
Selected blood disease	7.8	5.8	0.6	1.4
Anemias	4.0	2.8	0.5	0.7

From Morbidity and mortality: 1998 chartbook on cardiovascular, lung and blood diseases. US Department of Health and Human Services, National Institutes of Health, National Heart, Lung, and Blood Institute, 1998.
[a] Direct costs are expenditures for hospital care, physician and other professional care, home care, nursing home care, and drugs.
[b] Indirect morbidity costs represent lost earnings because of illness. Indirect mortality costs represent lost future earnings by those who died of the given disease in 1998.
[c] No estimate was made for indirect morbidity costs.
[d] Most costs for hypertensive disease are included in total heart disease.

300 million males now younger than 30 years.[20,21] Surprisingly, smoking is decreasing among Chinese women, having dropped from 10% before 1950 to 1% today. China now logs the highest number of deaths from smoking of any country, having recently overtaken the United States.[20,21]

DEFINITION OF PULMONARY REHABILITATION

Attempts have been made to define *pulmonary rehabilitation*. In 1974, a committee of the American College of Chest Physicians developed the following definition[22]:

> *Pulmonary rehabilitation may be defined as an art of medical practice wherein an individually tailored, multi-disciplinary program is formulated which through accurate diagnosis, therapy, emotional support, and education, stabilizes or reverses both the physio- and psychopathology of pulmonary disease and attempts to return the patient to the highest possible functional capacity allowed by his pulmonary handicap and overall life situation.*

In the late 1970s, pulmonary rehabilitation programs began to spring up around the country. Because of a growing recognition that the term *pulmonary rehabilitation* was defined differently by many pulmonary specialists, in 1979 an ad hoc committee of the Scientific Assembly on Clinical Problems of the American Thoracic Society (ATS) was delegated the responsibility of defining pulmonary rehabilitation. This committee developed a statement that not only defined pulmonary rehabilitation but also listed the essential components of such a program.

The ATS statement[23] listed the two principal objectives of pulmonary rehabilitation as *(a)* to control and alleviate as much as possible the symptoms and pathophysiologic complications of respiratory impairment and *(b)* to teach the patient how to achieve optimal capability for carrying out his or her activities of daily living. This 1981 statement also stated that:

> *In the broadest sense, pulmonary rehabilitation means providing good, comprehensive respiratory care for patients with pulmonary disease.*

A logical sequence for an individual participating in a pulmonary rehabilitation program is as follows[23]: *(a)* select the individual, *(b)* evaluate the individual to determine his or her needs, *(c)* develop goals, *(d)* determine components of care, *(e)* assess the individual's progress, and *(f)* arrange for long-term follow-up. See Box 2-1 for a list of services required for pulmonary rehabilitation.

Several principles from the 1981 ATS statement[23] are worth repeating:

1. A physician knowledgeable about respiratory disease should perform the initial complete examination and assist in outlining a proper regimen of treatment.
2. The specific provider for the program's services may vary from program to program. A large, multidisciplinary team is appropriate for settings where large numbers of patients are referred and for teaching or research purposes. However, in other settings, it may be possible to provide similar services with fewer individuals if they are highly qualified and specially trained in evaluation and management of the patient.

In 1987, the ATS published a statement dealing with standards for the diagnosis and care of patients with COPD and asthma.[24] Many of the components of care used in pulmonary rehabilitation programs were discussed in this statement.

In 1994, the National Heart, Lung, and Blood Institute published the results of a consensus conference on pulmonary rehabilitation.[25] The individuals participating in this conference developed the following definition of pulmonary rehabilitation:

> *A multidimensional continuum of services directed to persons with pulmonary disease and their families, usually by an interdisciplinary team of specialists, with a goal of achieving and maintaining the individual's maximum level of independence and functioning in the community.*

Box 2-1. Services Required for Pulmonary Rehabilitation

Initial medical evaluation and care plan
Patient education, evaluation, and program coordination
Respiratory therapy techniques
Chest physiotherapy
Daily performance evaluation
Social service evaluation
Exercise conditioning
Nutritional assessment
Psychological evaluation

In 1995, an update on the diagnosis and care of patients with COPD was published by the ATS.[26] This new statement included pulmonary rehabilitation in the algorithm of care for patients with COPD.

The ATS published a new official statement on pulmonary rehabilitation in 1999.[27] The following definition was developed and included in this statement:

> *Pulmonary rehabilitation is a multidisciplinary program of care for patients with chronic respiratory impairment that is individually tailored and designed to optimize physical and social performance and autonomy.*

CANDIDATES FOR PULMONARY REHABILITATION

Pulmonary rehabilitation is most commonly used for individuals with COPD; however, patients with other diseases leading to chronic respiratory impairment can also benefit from this process. The following quotations comment on when pulmonary rehabilitation should be considered:

> *Any patient whose breathlessness from COPD has resulted in functional limitations that affect his or her quality of life should be considered a candidate for pulmonary rehabilitation.[28]*

> *Historically, pulmonary rehabilitation has been used primarily for patients with COPD. However, it has also been applied successfully to patients with other chronic lung conditions such as interstitial diseases, cystic fibrosis, bronchiectasis, thoracic cage abnormalities, and neuromuscular disorders as well as part of the evaluation, preparation for, and recovery from surgical interventions such as lung transplantation and lung volume reduction surgery. Pulmonary rehabilitation is appropriate for any patient with stable disease of the respiratory system and disabling symptoms.[29]*

> *Pulmonary rehabilitation for interstitial lung diseases [ILD] and for other nonobstructive lung diseases has been reported to be beneficial, but has received little attention in the literature. To a large extent, this lack of attention is due to the low frequency of nonobstructive diseases relative to chronic obstructive pulmonary disease (COPD). In the United States, the prevalence of COPD is 53.5 cases per 1000 men and 63.5 cases per 1000 women. In contrast, Coultas and associates, gathering epidemiological data from Bernalillo County, New Mexico, found that the combined prevalence of ILD was only 0.8 cases per 1000 men and 0.67 cases per 1000 women. Thus, it is no surprise that the most common diagnosis in any pulmonary rehabilitation program is COPD.[30]*

> *Foster and Thomas reported that approximately 10% (37/354) of the patients admitted to their institution for inpatient pulmonary rehabilitation in the mid-1980's had pathophysiological mechanisms other than airway obstruction as the cause of ventilatory limitation. These patients improved with rehabilitation to a degree similar to that of patients with COPD.[30]*

> *The precepts of pulmonary rehabilitation that have traditionally been applied to patients with chronic obstructive pulmonary disease (COPD) apply equally well to patients with neuromuscular or paralytic/restrictive conditions.[31]*

> *Pulmonary rehabilitation is indicated for patients with chronic respiratory impairment who, despite optimal medical management, are dyspneic, have reduced exercise tolerance, or experience a restriction in activities. It should be emphasized that symptoms, disability, and handicap, not the severity of physiologic impairment of the*

lungs, dictate the need for pulmonary rehabilitation. Thus, no specific pulmonary function criteria exist to indicate the need for pulmonary rehabilitation.[27]

CHARACTERISTICS OF PULMONARY REHABILITATION

Characteristics of pulmonary rehabilitation programs in the United States have been gathered through two national surveys, with the results of the first survey published in 1988[32] and of the second survey in 1995.[33] The first survey reported on responses received from 150 pulmonary rehabilitation programs in 37 states, and the second survey reported on responses received from 283 programs in 44 states. The more recent survey reported that, on the average, pulmonary rehabilitation programs enrolled nine patients at a given time and that the average program was presented for 2 hours per day, 2.5 days per week, for 9 weeks. The main program length was 45 hours. Ninety-four percent of the programs reported that they worked with outpatients, whereas 27% reported that they also included inpatients. Ninety-nine percent of the programs reporting included patients with COPD, 94% included adults with asthma, 92% included individuals with restrictive diseases, 37% included patients undergoing lung transplantation, 34% included patients with cystic fibrosis, and 13% included children with asthma. Seventy-eight percent of the programs reported that a physician was a member of the pulmonary rehabilitation team. The most common program director was a Respiratory Care Practitioner. The program director's credentials were as follows: Registered Respiratory Therapist, 38%; Registered Nurse, 24%; Exercise Physiologist, 12%; Certified Respiratory Therapy Technician, 12%; Physical Therapist, 3%; and another credential, 11%. Four percent of the programs had a director with both respiratory therapy and nursing credentials.

Pulmonary rehabilitation programs bill for their services in different ways: 99 programs reported using only one billing code for all services, whereas 147 programs reported using multiple codes to bill for their program services.

Pulmonary rehabilitation programs reported an average of 2.5 paid full-time employees (range, 0.1–21.6).

Guidelines that describe the needed characteristics of pulmonary rehabilitation programs are available.[34]

SUMMARY

Pulmonary rehabilitation programs may vary in size and configuration. All allied health professions may not be represented on every team in every hospital; however, all the services needed must be available and provided by someone. Although every patient with chronic lung disease does not need all these services, many patients need them all.

Although most patients participating in pulmonary rehabilitation programs have COPD, these programs may also be helpful for patients with other types of pulmonary dysfunction. Fortunately, pulmonary rehabilitation is more widely accepted now than in 1984, when the first edition of this book was published.[35] The remainder of this book is devoted to describing the components of pulmonary rehabilitation and providing guidelines that can lead to the successful rehabilitation of patients with pulmonary impairment.

REFERENCES

1. Barach AL. The treatment of pulmonary emphysema in the elderly. J Am Geriatr Soc 1956;4:884.

2. Miller WF. Rehabilitation of patients with chronic obstructive lung disease. Med Clin North Am 1967;51:349.

3. Balchum OJ. Rehabilitation in chronic obstructive pulmonary disease. Arch Environ Health 1968;16:614.

4. Haas A, Cardon H. Rehabilitation in chronic obstructive pulmonary disease: a five-year study of 252 male patients. Med Clin North Am 1969; 53:593.

5. Cherniack RM, Handford RG, Svanhill E. Home care of chronic respiratory disease. JAMA 1969; 208:821.

6. Petty TL. Ambulatory care for emphysema and chronic bronchitis. Chest 1970;58:441.

7. Kimbel P, Kaplan AS, Alkalay I, et al. An in-hospital program for rehabilitation of patients with chronic obstructive pulmonary disease. Chest 1971;60(Suppl):6s.

8. Glaser EM. Strategies for facilitating knowledge utilization in the biomedical field: final report to the National Science Foundation, grant No. DAR 73-07767 A06. Washington, DC: National Science Foundation, 1975.

9. Hodgkin JE, Balchum OJ, Kass I, et al. Chronic obstructive airway disease: current concepts in diagnosis and comprehensive care. JAMA 1975; 232:1243.

10. Hodgkin JE, ed. Chronic Obstructive Pulmonary Disease: Current Concepts in Diagnosis and Comprehensive Care. Park Ridge, IL: American College of Chest Physicians, 1979.

11. Morbidity and mortality: 1998 chartbook on cardiovascular, lung, and blood diseases. Bethesda, MD: US Department of Health and Human Services, Public Health Service, National Institutes of Health, National Heart, Lung, and Blood Institute, 1998.

12. National Heart, Lung, and Blood Institute data fact sheet: asthma statistics. Bethesda, MD: US Department of Health and Human Services, Public Health Service, National Institutes of Health, 1999.

13. National Vital Statistics Reports: Centers for Disease Control and Prevention, National Center for Health Statistics. Hyattsville, MD: US Department of Health and Human Services, Public Health Service, 1999.

14. Mendez D, Warner KE, Courant PN. Has smoking cessation ceased? expected trends in the prevalence of smoking in the United States. Am J Epidemiol 1998;148:249–258.

15. Zang EA, Wynder EL. Smoking trends in the United States between 1969 and 1995 based on patients hospitalized with non-smoking related diseases. Prev Med 1998;27:854–861.

16. National Center for Health Statistics. Health, United States, 1998 with socioeconomic status and health chartbook. Hyattsville, MD: US Department of Health and Human Services, Centers for Disease Control and Prevention, 1998.

17. Incidence of initiation of cigarette smoking— United States, 1965-1996. MMWR Morb Mortal Wkly Rep 1998;47:837–840.

18. Everett SA, Husten CG, Warren CW, et al. Trends in tobacco use among high school students in the United States, 1991-1995. J Sch Health 1998; 68:137–140.

19. Wechsler H, Rigotti NA, Gledhill-Hoyt J, et al. Increased levels of cigarette use among college students: a cause for national concern. JAMA 1998;280:1673–1678.

20. Liu BQ, Peto R, Chen AM, et al. Emerging tobacco hazards in China: 1, retrospective proportional mortality study of one million deaths. Br Med J 1998;317:1411–1422.

21. Niu SR, Yang GH, Chen ZM, et al. Emerging tobacco hazards in China: 2, early mortality results from a prospective study. Br Med J 1998;317: 1423–1424.

22. Petty TL. Pulmonary rehabilitation. In: Basics of RD. New York: American Thoracic Society, 1975.

23. American Thoracic Society. Position statement on pulmonary rehabilitation. Am Rev Respir Dis 1981;124:663.

24. American Thoracic Society. Standards for the diagnosis and care of patients with chronic obstructive pulmonary disease (COPD) and asthma. Am Rev Respir Dis 1987;136:225.

25. Fishman AP. Pulmonary rehabilitation research: NIH workshop summary. Am J Respir Crit Care Med 1994;149:825–833.

26. ATS statement: standards for the diagnosis and care of patients with chronic obstructive pulmonary disease. Am J Respir Crit Care Med 1995; 152:S84–S113 (part 2 of 2).

27. Pulmonary rehabilitation—1999: Official Statement of the American Thoracic Society. Am J Respir Crit Care Med 1999;159:1666–1682.

28. Staats BA, Simon PM. Comprehensive pulmonary rehabilitation in chronic obstructive pulmonary disease. In: Fishman AP, ed. Pulmonary Rehabilitation. New York: Marcel Dekker, 1996:651– 681.

29. ACCP/AACVPR Pulmonary Rehabilitation Guidelines Panel. Pulmonary rehabilitation: evidence-based guidelines. J Cardiopulm Rehabil 1997;17:371–405.

30. Novitch RS, Thomas HM III. Pulmonary rehabilitation in chronic pulmonary interstitial disease. In: Fishman AP, ed. Pulmonary Rehabilitation. New York: Marcel Dekker, 1996:683– 700.

31. Bach JR. Pulmonary rehabilitation in musculoskeletal disorders. In: Fishman AP, ed. Pulmonary Rehabilitation. New York: Marcel Dekker, 1996: 701–723.

32. Bickford LS, Hodgkin JE. National pulmonary rehabilitation survey. In: Hodgkin JE, guest ed. Pulmonary rehabilitation symposium. J Cardiopulm Rehabil 1988;8:473.

33. Bickford LS, Hodgkin JE, McInturff SL. National pulmonary rehabilitation survey: update. J Cardiopulm Rehabil 1995;15:406–411.

34. Connors G, Hilling L, eds. AACVPR Guidelines for Pulmonary Rehabilitation Programs. 2nd ed. Champaign, IL: Human Kinetics, 1998.

35. Hodgkin JE, Zorn EG, Connors GL, eds. Pulmonary Rehabilitation: Guidelines to Success. Boston: Butterworths, 1984.

3 Selection and Assessment of the Chronic Respiratory Disease Patient for Pulmonary Rehabilitation

Philip R. Corsello

▷ Professional Skills

Upon completion of this chapter, the reader will:

- Understand the importance of early identification of the patient with chronic respiratory disease who can benefit from pulmonary rehabilitation
- Understand why early detection and intervention is so important for patients with chronic respiratory disease and why clinical screening for lung disease is a component of total health care
- Appreciate why simple spirometry should be done on all cigarette smokers
- Know why pulmonary rehabilitation is interdisciplinary and individualized to the patient's needs
- Be able to explain why every patient who is functionally limited by symptomatic, stable, chronic lung disease is a candidate for pulmonary rehabilitation
- Know the *non*–chronic obstructive pulmonary disease (non-COPD) indications for pulmonary rehabilitation
- Know why generally accepted "exclusion criteria" may only be impediments to rehabilitation
- Be sensitive to the high incidence of depression in the chronic lung disease population and the relevance of this to pulmonary rehabilitation efforts
- Understand the three-step enrollment process for pulmonary rehabilitation
- Explain how the patient selection criteria may also include patients whose impediments are correctable
- Understand the multiple functions served by the initial interview
- Explain why the assessment is an ongoing process not just one performed at the time of the initial evaluation
- Understand the concept of *benefit without physiologic change*—the essence of pulmonary rehabilitation

Chronic respiratory disease, when severe, can be devastating. It destroys the body and dampens the spirits of both patient and spouse. Until the 1960s and the independent reports of benefit from pulmonary rehabilitation by Drs. Alvan Barach,[1] Albert Haas,[2] William Miller,[3] Tom Petty,[4] and Reuben Cherniak,[5] it was widely held that efforts to treat COPD/emphysema were futile. It was believed that the irreversibility of airway obstruction, the often unremitting dyspnea, the muscular wasting, and the downward spiral characterized by recurrent bouts of respiratory failure and ending in death by suffocation were not amenable to therapeutic intervention.

A period of much enthusiasm for the alleged benefits of pulmonary rehabilitation ensued in the 1970s, followed by increased skepticism in the face of repeated failure to demonstrate significant physiologic change. And it was only in the early 1990s that attitudes and beliefs began to change again, fueled by the emergence of evidence-based medicine, meta-analysis, and the understanding that benefit was not to be found in statistically significant physiologic change. Rather, it was to be demonstrated by what had previously been held to be a nonobjective outcome: enhanced quality of life. It is ironic that the early critics of pulmonary rehabilitation focused their scorn on reports of improved patient attitudes, improved functional capacity, and improved quality of life, the very measures we now take for granted as legitimate outcomes. It is now easy to be critical of those who questioned the efficacy of pulmonary rehabilitation, but it must be remembered that the 1960s and 1970s were the golden age of pulmonary physiology, exemplified by the pioneering work of Drs. Andre Cournand, David Bates, Peter Macklem, Giles Filley, and Julius Comroe. Their contributions were followed by those of Tom Petty, Nicholas Anthonisen, Ben Branscomb, David Flenley, and others who brought this new knowledge to the clinical pulmonary function laboratory and the bedside. Is it any wonder, then, that clinical research, on the alleged benefits of pulmonary rehabilitation, looked primarily for evidence of measurable physiologic change. That they should have chosen this approach at that time is understandable, however, for only in retrospect does this focus on objective measurements, rather than our present focus on *improvements in patient well-being*, seem strange.

THE PROPER CANDIDATE

Yet, even now, with the issue of efficacy having been resolved by a plethora of evidence-based studies,[6–10] questions remain about how we might best identify and engage those who will benefit from pulmonary rehabilitation. I discuss proposed approaches to this question, including measures to objectify the process.

As with many new therapeutic modalities, the initial offering is often to those with the most severe disease, be that chronic respiratory disease or, as was the case in the not too distant past, valvular heart disease. There is reason to believe, however, that just as the early identification of patients with chronic respiratory disease is important, so may their early participation in pulmonary rehabilitation prove to be equally important.[11] Pulmonary rehabilitation is not a single, uniform, "one size fits all" approach but is composed of a variety of interventions, some specific, others more globally beneficial, for example, exercise, resulting in improved muscle strength and endurance but also in mood elevation and higher self-esteem. Our task then is to identify, assess, select, and enroll patients in individualized pulmonary rehabilitation programs according to their needs.

This process can be initiated by assessing either deficits or desired outcomes. In either event, a comprehensive pulmonary rehabilitation program must encompass optimum medical therapy, smoking cessation efforts, attention to psychosocial needs, exercise and physical reconditioning, nutritional support, education, and follow-up. Although chronic respiratory disease is intrinsically a disease of the lungs, it is akin to a clinical syndrome to the extent that the patient with advanced or severe chronic respiratory disease will always exhibit one or more of the following, to varying degrees and in various combinations:

shortness of breath, cough, disturbances of sleep and/or mood, generalized weakness and loss of energy, muscle wasting with reduced muscle strength and endurance, diminished self-esteem, loss of independence with increased dependence on others, hypoxemia, increased feelings of hopelessness, and progressive isolation. Some of these features are signs, some symptoms, some perceptions, and some emotions/behaviors. In contrast to those features of a syndrome, however, a single therapy does not alleviate all; that is, each feature, although partially responsive to general therapeutic measures, invariably requires specific therapy, be that feature malnutrition or dyspnea, depression or muscle weakness. Thus, the need exists for comprehensive multispecialty therapy in the treatment of chronic respiratory disease.

I firmly believe that all patients with incapacitating chronic respiratory disease, COPD first and foremost, are *potential candidates* for pulmonary rehabilitation, and I agree with Andrew Ries[12] who asserts that

> *Any patient with symptomatic, stable chronic lung disease who is disabled either by the underlying disease or by related therapy or complications, is a candidate for pulmonary rehabilitation.*

I also agree with the official American Thoracic Society (ATS) Statement[13]:

> *Pulmonary rehabilitation is indicated for patients with chronic respiratory impairment who, despite optimal medical management, are dyspneic, have reduced exercise tolerance, or experience a restriction in activities.*

And further, with the European Respiratory Society Task Force Position Paper[14] on pulmonary rehabilitation that

> *Pulmonary rehabilitation is a process which systematically uses scientifically based diagnostic management and evaluation options to achieve the optimal daily functioning and health-related quality of life of individual patients suffering from impairment and disability due to chronic respiratory disease, as measured by clinically and/or physiologically relevant outcome measures.*
>
> *Since the requirements of individual patients vary with time and in relation to other individuals, programs must be comprehensive and flexible enough to address each patient's needs, and also to advance the health care provision for the entire population with chronic respiratory disease.*

Ries[12] succinctly defines the ideal candidate as:

> *one with functional limitation from moderate to severe lung disease who is stable with standard therapy, not distracted or limited by other serious or unstable medical conditions, willing and able to learn about his disease and motivated to devote the time and effort necessary to benefit from a comprehensive care program.*

Although we welcome the ideal patient, we must often settle for less than the ideal, and we should, for it is the rare patient who does not benefit from some component of the rehabilitative process. And to reiterate, it is not only patients with COPD who stand to benefit from rehabilitation, but all equally disabled patients with a variety of other chronic pulmonary diseases (Box 3-1).

It is reasonable to adopt selection criteria for the enrollment of those most likely to benefit, but we must take care to not establish criteria so stringent as to exclude patients who, like the ideal candidates, might also benefit from pulmonary rehabilitation. The danger is that a rigid application of selection criteria[12,13] may result in the permanent exclusion of candidates who fail to satisfy the criteria and thereby lose the opportunity to benefit from pulmonary rehabilitation.

Box 3-1. Non-COPD Indications for Pulmonary Rehabilitation

Asthma
Chest wall disease
Cystic fibrosis
Interstitial lung disease, including post-ARDS pulmonary fibrosis
Lung cancer
Selected neuromuscular diseases
Perioperative states (e.g., thoracic, abdominal surgery)
Postpolio syndrome
Prelung and postlung transplantation
Prelung and postlung volume reduction surgery

With permission from Pulmonary rehabilitation—1999: the official statement of the American Thoracic Society, adopted by the ATS Board of Directors, November 1998. Am J Respir Crit Care Med 1999;159:1670.
COPD, chronic obstructive pulmonary disease; ARDS, adult respiratory distress syndrome.

The ATS Statement[13] recognizes two types of exclusion criteria: *(a)* those that may interfere with participation and *(b)* those that may place the patient at undue risk during exercise training. The latter is tempered by the acknowledgment that patients who are unable to exercise may still benefit from educational, psychosocial, and/or nutritional activities alone, and clearly they may. The ATS Statement also suggests that "patients who are poorly motivated are not ideal candidates," followed by the caveat that "their level of motivation may change if they attend rehabilitation sessions." That assertion may have some validity, but I believe that the more common scenario for motivational change occurs in response to *the recognition and treatment of clinically significant depression* that is so highly prevalent in this population. Motivation, like noncompliance, is a complex process influenced by multiple variables—physical, emotional, financial, and situational. It is entwined with one's lifelong beliefs and with one's current sense of hope or hopelessness and *is often a temporary, reversible state.* A highly motivated patient is more likely to benefit from pulmonary rehabilitation than is a less motivated one, but, before we exclude the less-than-ideal patients on the basis of their motivation, we must seek to identify and address the cause(s) of their diminished motivation before enrollment.

Absolute contraindications or obstacles to participation in *all components* of pulmonary rehabilitation exist. *But these are relatively rare.* Examples include dementia; severe, virtually untreatable mental illness; advanced neurologic disease; and, perhaps, intractable congestive heart failure or cor pulmonale. But, I would prefer to define as *impediments* other factors often cited as contraindications or exclusionary criteria, such as suboptimally treated ischemic heart disease or congestive heart failure, severe arthritis, or poor motivation. Alleged poor motivation (see the previous paragraph) is especially problematic as an exclusionary criterion given the factors that contribute to it that may be reversible with appropriate therapy. I deem the distinction to be important, for whereas contraindications or exclusionary criteria prohibit participation, impediments can and should be overcome before active participation in a rehabilitation program.

ENROLLMENT: A THREE-STEP PROCESS

The first step is identification of the patient with severe, moderate, or even mild (yet clinically manifest) respiratory disease, guided by the defining characteristics set forth by Ries[12] and the ATS.[13] In any chronically ill population, a wide range of coping skills exist that are closely linked to personal health belief systems and feelings of self-efficacy and mastery, or the lack thereof. It is not surprising, therefore, that some patients, even those with physiologically severe disease, may not require pulmonary rehabilitation, in accordance with the above-mentioned criteria. But, these individuals are a decided minority of all patients with respiratory disease, and we should assume that every patient with moderate to severe disease will benefit from participation in pulmonary rehabilitation.

The second step is identification of relative and absolute contraindications and impediments to participation. The rationale for defining impediments is that corrective action may be taken to overcome or neutralize them and that although this may require substantial time and effort, the patient will eventually meet the established selection criteria. Consider, for example, the following selection criteria: motivation; being under the care of a primary care physician; and the absence of other uncompensated medical conditions, advanced arthritis, unstable angina or recent myocardial infarction, and depression. All of these preclude uninhibited, effective, and/or safe participation in pulmonary rehabilitation. Yet, all of these are potentially reversible or eradicable. Motivation, akin to compliance, especially warrants careful investigation because it may emanate from fear, worry, depression, or a sense of hopelessness; financial worries; domestic turmoil; lack of confidence in one's physician; an entrenched pattern of dependency; a lack of self-esteem; or a lack of understanding. The importance of defining these impediments is twofold: first, the avoidance of failure of the rehabilitative effort, occasioned by seriously compromised participation and, second, defining them so that they can be addressed in a comprehensive manner in preparation for later enrollment. Failure of the rehabilitative effort is discouraging to the staff but may be devastating for the patient, who may not have the strength or energy to mount another effort. Every problem that, alone or in combination with others, could sabotage the patient's participation must be recognized and addressed.

The third step is either enrollment in the program or initiation of the actions required to alleviate the diagnosed obstacles to enrollment. To engage in pulmonary rehabilitation requires energy, both physical and emotional. Depression, for example, attenuates both and must be treated effectively before a patient can be expected to participate. The advantage of evaluating patients for rehabilitation is that the assessment may unearth diagnoses (pulmonary and nonpulmonary) that might otherwise remain hidden. With alleviation of the aforementioned impediments, many patients who at first evaluation were deemed to be inappropriate candidates may on reevaluation meet the selection criteria (see Ries, Box 3-2).

It should be clear, then, that a comprehensive assessment must proceed in a systematic fashion, with attention to both physical and emotional domains and with the understanding that the patient may not require all rehabilitation modalities or, because of handicaps, may not be able to engage in one or more of them. An individualized plan of care should be developed for each patient based on the assessment. This plan of care must specify the necessary interventions and the *mutually agreed on, reality-based, desired outcomes.* Most

Box 3-2 Patient Selection Criteria Used in the Pulmonary Rehabilitation Program at UCSD[a]

Symptomatic chronic lung disease
Stable with standard therapy
Functional limitation from the chronic lung disease
In the care of a primary care provider
Motivated to be involved in and responsible for own health care
No other interfering or unstable medical conditions

[a]We avoid using the patient's age and lung function alone in the selection process.
Reprinted with permission from Ries AL. What pulmonary rehab can do for your patients. J Respir Dis 1995;16(8):R16–R24.
USCD, University of California, San Diego

anticipated outcomes will relate directly to the patient but, not uncommonly, may include the outcome of interventions on the patient's spouse and other family members.

PATIENT SELECTION AND ASSESSMENT

Selection begins with identification of patients with chronic respiratory disease. Failure to identify patients with chronic respiratory disease in the early to middle stages of their disease, for example, remains problematic because evidence suggests that they too may benefit, perhaps even more than patients with severe, end-stage disease and/or disqualifying comorbid states. The reasons for this failure to make the diagnosis reside with both patients and physicians. Physicians may not routinely inquire about shortness of breath or cough, and patients, all too often, accept a chronic, morning "smoker's" cough as normal. Progressive shortness of breath with exertion is insidious, especially for sedentary individuals, and all too often attributed to aging, being overweight, or being deconditioned. In addition, as shortness of breath worsens, patients unconsciously reduce their physical activities so as to not experience the discomfort of dyspnea. Thus, the establishment of a negative feedback loop is inapparent to all until the person begins to experience dyspnea with the activities of daily living (ADLs). Other reinforcing feedback loops are established as well. Reduced physical activity leads to one's feeling less healthy, reduced self-esteem, and weight gain, and with these one is less likely to exercise, leading to more of the same. We must be aware that patient *self-identification is insensitive and unreliable* and that physicians must be more probing with questions about respiratory symptoms.

It is estimated that more than 15 to 20% of all smokers develop clinically significant COPD. This is, at once, a small fraction of all smokers but a large number of individuals, worthy of our attention. If primary care physicians were to *screen all cigarette smokers* under their care, either clinically and/or with simple spirometry, it is a near certainty that the age at which the diagnosis of COPD is made would be dramatically lowered. Earlier identification would then lead to earlier intervention, with more vigorous smoking cessation efforts, and could lead to enhanced quality of life as a byproduct of pulmonary rehabilitation.

Clinical screening for chronic respiratory disease, especially for those with a history of smoking, should be a component of all total health care. A careful history, including family history of respiratory disease (with the use of health screening questionnaires) and physical examination can raise suspicion of the diagnosis. But even more sensitive is screening spirometry, not only for the diagnosis of chronic respiratory disease but as a predictor of cardiac failure and premature death.[15,16] Heightened awareness of the importance of early identification has led to the National Lung Health Education Program (NLHEP),[17] cosponsored by the National Cancer Institute and the Lung Division of the National Heart, Lung, and Blood Institute. The Lung Health Study,[18] an impetus to establishment of the NLHEP, showed that middle-aged (average, 48.4 years) patients with a smoking history of greater than 10 years (mean, 30 pack-years [pack-years = number of packs smoked/day × number of years smoked]) already exhibited mild airflow abnormalities (average $FEV_1/FVC = 63.5\%$).

Many of the patients in this study were asymptomatic. Early identification of the person whose lungs are vulnerable to the damaging effects of cigarette smoke has been deemed to be of the utmost importance by the NLHEP. It is anticipated that great benefit will accrue to those patients thus identified, who will then be recruited for smoking cessation efforts as part of total pulmonary rehabilitation.

It is important to assess not just the existence of pulmonary function impairment but the severity of it as well. Having heretofore stressed the importance of loss of functional capacity, as opposed to absolute loss of measured lung function, one might question why quantification of severity of chronic respiratory disease is desirable. It is as it enables physicians to assess the urgency of smoking cessation efforts and as a guide to the establishment of realistic goals for the patient, particularly physical rehabilitation goals.

Because pulmonary rehabilitation encompasses many modalities, so must the assessment look to those deficits characteristic of COPD and other chronic respiratory disease, addressed by each: physical, emotional, knowledge of disease, health belief systems, cognitive function, nutritional status, etc. The rehabilitation staff must have an acute understanding of all aspects of the candidate's function so that all disabilities will be addressed, especially those that might directly limit full, enthusiastic, effective participation.

THE INTERVIEW

The care and professionalism with which the initial interview is conducted is of the utmost importance. The interviewer should be a mature individual, a good listener and communicator who is knowledgeable about all aspects of the rehabilitation process and sensitive to nuances of patient–spouse interactions.

The spouse or a surrogate should be in attendance for most of the interview, but the patient should also have the opportunity to share personal or confidential information, fears or concerns, one on one with the interviewer.

The careful observer can learn a great deal about the patient: mental state, the presence of depression, motivation and health belief systems, history of compliance/noncompliance with previous medical regimens, and knowledge of the treatment and prognosis of the respiratory illness.

The interview is also an opportunity to assess memory, short-term retention of information, and overall cognitive function. Finally, it affords us a grand opportunity to assess the spouse with respect to his or her love, caring, empathy, concern, respect and, most important, willingness to actively participate in and provide both emotional support and support of the rehabilitation process.

The interview serves not only to gather information about the patient but also as an opportunity for the staff member to favorably present himself or herself and the program, allay patient fears, identify misconceptions about the disease and rehabilitation, provide information about what pulmonary rehabilitation entails, discuss realistic patient expectations, and establish a climate of concern and mutual respect. It is an opportunity for the interviewer to convey competence and empathy and thus set the stage for a working partnership.

PHYSICAL EXAMINATION AND MEDICAL RECORD REVIEW

Physical examination and review of previous medical records is important for what can be learned about the onset, severity, response to therapy, and progression of chronic respiratory disease. Of equal importance is what is gleaned from the records about uncompensated comorbidities and other previously undiagnosed or inadequately treated diseases, history of patient adherence, and patient response to illness. The physical examination provides information about vital signs, especially respiratory rate and pulse rate at rest and with mild exertion; pulmonary hypertension and cor pulmonale (possible contraindications to exercise training); nutritional state; and patient state of mind.

The medical record review and physical examination will often reveal significant comorbid states frequently associated with chronic respiratory disease, including but not limited to the following: osteoporosis, cardiovascular disease, gastroesophageal reflux disease, sinusitis, sleep disturbances, and musculoskeletal disorders, any of which could be impediments to optimum patient participation.

EXERCISE ASSESSMENT

Because exercise training is at the core of all rehabilitation, careful assessment of baseline exercise capacity is crucial. This need not entail sophisticated testing. It can be performed with a treadmill or a 6-minute walk but must permit evaluation of cardiac arrhythmias and oxygen status. Undetected hypoxemia will undermine not just exercise training but the entire rehabilitative effort. A history of cardiac disease should be clarified with the patient's primary care physician (PCP) or cardiologist to confirm the safety of contemplated exercise. The physical evaluation should also include assessment of muscle strength, joint mobility, coordination and gait stability, and ability to perform ADLs. Frequently of great value to both patient and staff is the demonstration to each (in a safe environment) that the patient is capable of greater exertion than either might have expected. With this, also, is the demonstration to the patient that dyspnea is a normal response to exercise, for all of us, and need be neither feared nor necessarily seen as a signal to cease exercising.

COGNITIVE AND PSYCHOSOCIAL EVALUATION

Concerns may arise, either during the interview or following entry and initial participation in the program, about cognitive deficits or emotional disturbances. The incidence of each of these is high in this population, and either one can compromise the patient's comprehension and/or memory. The seriousness of this relates closely to the importance of education and understanding, without which effective participation may be seriously compromised. Patients with chronic respiratory disease are, by and large, an older population with a high incidence of sleep disorders and recurrent hypoxemia, which, together or separately, can precipitate or potentiate cognitive or emotional problems. Such concerns, arising from clinical observations, should be pursued with formal cognitive testing by a clinical psychologist and/or the administration of one of the many available depression scales/inventories. Any suggestion of clinically significant anxiety or depression should result in referral to a mental health professional, preferably before entry into the program, but actually at any time, to forestall failure of the rehabilitation. Consultation with the patient's PCP is mandatory in this circumstance. The PCP may be able to shed light on the issues of concern and should be a party to the process of referral, testing, and the provision of encouragement and emotional support. In some instances, PCP knowledge of the patient's cognitive function and mental status may obviate the need for further assessment because the PCP can provide or arrange for proper treatment.

NUTRITIONAL ASSESSMENT

Malnutrition is common in patients with chronic pulmonary disease[19] secondary to the disease state and to psychosocial and financial problems. Nutritional problems occur in more than 50% of patients with severe COPD.[20] Proper nutritional assessment should include not only objective testing and monitoring of weight but a history of the time of onset and the magnitude of weight loss, circumstances of meal preparation and frequency, drug/nutrient interactions, and the presence of financial or logistic constraints on food availability. Nutritionist consultation is appropriate for every candidate who demonstrates excessive weight gain or loss. Decreased weight is associated with decreased exercise performance and increased mortality.[21] It correlates with disease severity[22] and is characterized by decreased fat-free body mass.[23] When extreme, some weight correction may need to occur before the patient will be able to safely or effectively participate in pulmonary rehabilitation.

ASSESSMENT OF ACTIVITIES OF DAILY LIVING

Few things are as important to the patient and his or her family as the ability to freely engage in ADLs. Lacking this capacity, the patient must increasingly rely on friends, family, physicians, and others. Independence is highly treasured by all of us. And the loss of independence, so characteristic of severe respiratory disease, superimposed as it is all too frequently on the loss of job and the inability to engage in leisure activities, can be devastating. On this basis alone, life can seem "to be not worth living."

The ADL assessment should include energy conservation techniques, upper extremity strength, proper breathing techniques with activity, and the need for adaptive equipment.[24] Functional task performance and work environment demands should also be assessed, as should food procurement and preparation.[25] Sexual function is, too frequently, ignored for complex reasons related to both patient and health care provider apprehension. It should be addressed, without embarrassment, by a mature, knowledgeable member of the team who should stress that the preservation of intimacy, not sexual performance, must be the first priority.

CONCLUSIONS

Identification of the chronic respiratory disease candidate for pulmonary rehabilitation should proceed on the basis of identified deficits and needs. Enrollment follows, on the basis of a match between needs and program components and the absence of mitigating factors that would preclude participation. Patient need is the overriding driving force, and pulmonary rehabilitation is so valuable that an initial decision to not enroll, for failure to meet selection criteria, should not be final. Instead, it should lead to initiation of measures to address the presently limiting impediments to participation, with the intent to *reconsider the patient's candidacy* after these impediments have been neutralized or corrected.

Finally, *assessment must be an ongoing process*, not a one-time event at the moment of enrollment. Staff must remain sensitive to patient fears and misgivings about this dramatic change in lifestyle and must continue to be empathetic and encouraging to both patient and spouse. Early identification of an emotional state or behavior that could be detrimental to the rehabilitation process is crucial. Goals must be mutually agreed on by patient and staff and must be realistic so as to avoid failure of the rehabilitative effort and the terrible disappointment and loss of hope attendant to that failure.

SELECTED READING

American Association of Cardiovascular & Pulmonary Rehabilitation. Guidelines for Pulmonary Rehabilitation Programs. 2nd ed. Champaign, IL: Human Kinetics Press, 1998.

REFERENCES

1. Barach AL. Principles and practices of inhalation therapy. Philadelphia: JB Lippincott, 1944.
2. Haas A, Cardon H. Rehabilitation in chronic obstructive pulmonary disease: a five-year study of 252 male patients. Med Clin North Am 1969;53: 593–606.
3. Miller WF. Rehabilitation of patients with chronic obstructive lung disease. Med Clin North Am 1967;51:349–361.
4. Petty TL, Nett LM, Finigan MM, et al. A comprehensive care program for chronic airway obstruction: methods and preliminary evaluation of symptomatic and functional improvement. Ann Intern Med 1969;70:1109–1113.
5. Lertzman MM, Cherniak RM. Rehabilitation of patients with chronic obstructive pulmonary disease. Am Rev Respir Dis 1976;114:1145–1165.
6. Lacasse Y, Wong E, Guyatt GH, et al. Meta-analysis of respiratory rehabilitation in chronic obstructive pulmonary disease. Lancet 1996;348:1115–1119.
7. Sacks HS, Berrier J, Reitman D, et al. Meta-analyses of randomized controlled trials. N Engl J Med 1987;316:450–455.
8. Guyatt GH, Townsend M, Berman LB, et al.

Quality of life in patients with chronic airflow limitation. Br J Dis Chest 1987;81:45–54.

9. Lacasse Y, Guyatt GH, Goldstein RS. Is there really a controversy surrounding the effectiveness of respiratory rehabilitation in COPD? Chest 1998;114(1):1–4.

10. ACCP/AACVPR Pulmonary Rehabilitation Guideline Panel. Pulmonary rehabilitation evidence-based guidelines. J Cardiopulm Rehabil 1997;17:371–405.

11. Murray JF, Petty TL, et al. Frontline treatment of COPD: a monograph for primary care physicians. Hackettstown, NJ: Snowdrift Pulmonary Foundation, Inc.:74.

12. Ries AL. What pulmonary rehab can do for your patients. J Respir Dis 1995;16(8):R16–R24.

13. Pulmonary rehabilitation—1999: the official statement of the American Thoracic Society, adopted by the ATS Board of Directors, November 1998. Am J Respir Crit Care Med 1999;159: 1666–1682.

14. Donner CF, Muir JF. Rehabilitation and Chronic Care Scientific Group of the European Respiratory Society: ERS Task Force position paper selection criteria and programmes for pulmonary rehabilitation in COPD patients. Eur Respir J 1997;10: 744–757.

15. Sorlie P, Lakatos E, Kannel WB, et al. Influence of cigarette smoking on lung function at baseline and at follow-up in 14 years: the Framingham Study. J Chronic Dis 1987;40:849–856.

16. Tockman MS, Pearson JD, Fleg JL, et al. Rapid decline in FEV$_1$: a new risk factor for coronary disease mortality. Am J Respir Crit Care Med 1995;151:390–398.

17. The National Lung Health Education Program (NLHEP). Executive Committee. Strategies in preserving lung health and preventing COPD and associated diseases. Chest 1998;113(2 Suppl): 123S–155S.

18. Anthonisen NR, Connett JE, Kiley JP, et al: Effects of smoking intervention and the use of an inhaled anticholinergic bronchodilator on the rate of decline of FEV$_1$: the Lung Health Study. JAMA 1994;272:1497–1505.

19. Schols A, Soeters P, Dingemans A, et al. Prevalence and characteristics of nutritional depletion in patients with stable COPD eligible for pulmonary rehabilitation. Am Rev Respir Dis 1993;147: 1151–1156.

20. Wilson DO, Rogers RM, Openbrier D. Nutritional aspects of chronic obstructive pulmonary disease. Clin Chest Med 1986;7:643–656.

21. Gray-Donald K, Gibbons L, Shapiro SH, et al. Nutritional status and mortality in chronic obstructive pulmonary disease. Am J Respir Crit Care Med 1996;153:961–966.

22. Belman MJ. Exercise in patients with chronic obstructive pulmonary disease. Thorax 1993;48: 936–946.

23. Jones PW, Baveystock CM, Littlejohns P. Relationship between general health measured with the sickness impact profile and respiratory symptoms, physiologic measures, and mood in patients with chronic airflow obstruction. Am Rev Respir Dis 1989;140:1538–1543.

24. Schols AMWJ, Soeters PB, Dingemans ANC, et al. Prevalence and characteristics of nutritional depletion in patients with COPD eligible for pulmonary rehabilitation. Am Rev Respir Dis 1993; 147:1151–1156.

25. Reed KL. Cardiopulmonary disorders. In: Quick Reference to Occupational Therapy. Gaithersburg, MD: Aspen, 1991:195–209.

4 Pathophysiology of Chronic Obstructive Pulmonary Disease

Bartolome R. Celli

▷ Professional Skills

Upon completion of this chapter, the reader will:

- Gain insight about the anatomic and pathologic lung abnormalities leading to airflow obstruction
- Understand the physiologic changes associated with the development of COPD
- Relate the pathophysiologic changes to the cardinal symptom of dyspnea
- Review the consequence of exercise and increased ventilatory demands on pulmonary mechanics
- Better comprehend the rationale behind some of the possible forms of treatment of COPD

Chronic obstructive pulmonary disease (COPD) currently ranks as the fourth cause of death in the United States.[1] Its prevalence has increased as overall mortality from myocardial infarction and cerebrovascular accident, the two organ systems affected by the same risk factor (namely, cigarette smoking), have decreased. Once diagnosed, COPD is progressive and leads to disability usually owing to dyspnea at a relatively early age (sixth or seventh decade). Limitation to airflow occurs as a consequence of destruction of lung parenchyma or to alterations in the airway itself. This chapter integrates the pathologic changes of COPD with the known adaptive and maladaptive consequences of those changes. Knowledge of these factors should help us understand the rationale behind the different therapeutic strategies aimed at decreasing the symptoms and improving the well-being of patients with COPD.

DEFINITION

COPD is a disease state characterized by the presence of airflow obstruction owing to emphysema or intrinsic airway disease classically typified by chronic bronchitis. The airflow limitation is generally progressive, may be accompanied by airway hyperactivity, and may be partially reversible. Emphysema is defined pathologically as an abnormal permanent enlargement of the air spaces distal to the terminal bronchioles, accompanied by destruction of their walls, without fibrosis. Enlargement of the air space to a large diameter (>1 cm) is defined as a bullae. The pathologic spectrum of bullae is large, ranging from asymptomatic subpleural lesions to giant ones that may compress otherwise normal parenchyma. In most patients with emphysema, the air space enlargement is variable, with uneven distribution in the site and extent of these bullous changes.[2,3] On the other hand, chronic bronchitis is defined clinically as the presence of chronic predictive cough for 3 months in each of

2 successive years in patients in whom other causes of chronic cough have been excluded. Most patients have a variable degree of airway inflammation and mucous gland hypertrophy, and up to 30% have airway hyperreactivity. In most patients both processes coexist. The disease does not affect all portions of the lung to the same degree. This uneven distribution influences the physiologic behavior of different parts of the lung.

PATHOPHYSIOLOGY

Biopsy studies from the large airways of patients with COPD reveal the presence of a large number of neutrophils.[4] This neutrophilic predominance is more manifest in smoking patients who develop airflow obstruction compared with smoking patients without airflow limitation.[5] Interestingly, biopsy samples of smaller bronchi reveal the presence of a large number of lymphocytes, especially of the CD8+ type.[6] The same type of cells, as well as macrophages, have been shown to increase in biopsy samples that include lung parenchyma.[6,7] Taken together, these findings suggest that cigarette smoking induces an inflammatory process characterized by intense interaction and accumulation of cells, which are capable of releasing many cytokines and enzymes that may cause injury. Indeed, the level of interleukin 8 is increased in the secretions of patients with COPD.[8] This is also true for tumor necrosis factor[9] and markers of oxidative stress.[10] In addition, the release of enzymes known to be capable of destroying lung parenchyma, such as neutrophilic elastase and metalloproteinases, by many of these activated cells has been documented in patients with COPD.[11,12] Therefore, an increasing body of evidence indicates that the anatomic alterations of COPD, such as airway inflammation and dysfunction as well as parenchymal destruction, could result from altered cellular interactions triggered by external agents such as cigarette or environmental smoke. A schematic representation of these events is shown in Figure 4-1. Whatever the mechanisms, the disease distribution is not uniform, so in a single patient areas of the lung with severe destruction may coexist with less affected areas.

Functionally, COPD is characterized by a decrease in airflow, which is more prominent on maximal efforts. Like the pathologic distribution, the airflow limitation is not uniform in nature. This causes uneven distribution of ventilation and also of blood perfusion.[13,14] This in turn results in arterial hypoxemia (decreased arterial partial pressure of oxygen [PaO_2]) and, if overall ventilation is decreased, in hypercarbia (increased arterial partial pressure of carbon dioxide [$PaCO_2$]). In patients with an important component of emphysema or bullous disease, total lung volume increases, resulting in hyperinflation. Each of these interrelated elements is important in the adaptive changes observed in patients with COPD and helps explain the clinical manifestations of the disease.

The relationship between structure and function in COPD is not well understood. Whether owing to loss of attachments or tethering forces and/or owing to inflammation and mucous secretion, patients with COPD have decreased airflow. Despite this, no good correlation exists between the currently used scoring system of either emphysematous or bronchitic changes and the degree of airflow obstruction. Therefore, it is practical to describe the patient by the degree of physiologically determined airflow limitation. At present, the best predictor of morbidity and mortality in COPD is the value of postbronchodilator forced expiratory volume in one second (FEV_1).[15] Because we define the obstruction as being only minimally reversible (if airflow limitation is highly reversible we speak of asthma), it seems desirable to develop a more comprehensive staging system that would allow categorization of the heterogeneous population of patients with COPD for epidemiologic and clinical studies, health resource planning, and prognosis. Such a system would also greatly simplify and facilitate the application of clinical information and recommendations.

The literature on factors that affect mortality in COPD is extensive. The principal variables are age and FEV_1.[15,16] The data are relatively old and by and large precede the

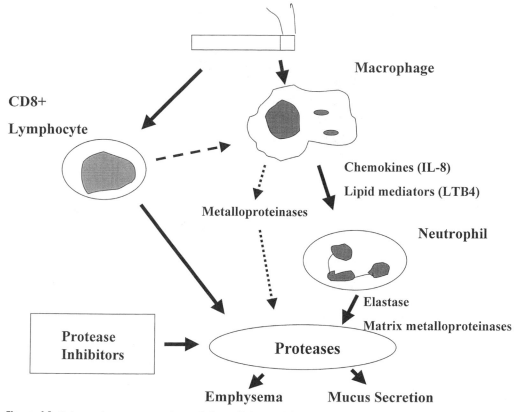

Figure 4-1. Schematic representation of the cellular and biologic response to inhalation of noxious agents, such as cigarette smoke. Similar events could occur after inhalation of environmental smoke. The *intermittent lines* represent potentially important interactions.

advent of low-flow oxygen and mechanical ventilation. The presence of hypoxemia and hypercapnia is also important in that they are predictive of mortality once the patient has moderate to severe airflow limitation. Conversely, death is not the only outcome attributable to COPD, and the impact of COPD on the ability of patients to perform the normal activities of a vocation or daily living are incompletely described by the FEV_1 and arterial blood gases.

A comprehensive dynamic staging system can be construed based on available information.

The first element should be the postbronchodilator FEV_1 as a percentage of its predicted value. This value is the best single predictor of mortality in COPD. However, it is not until values fall below 50% of predicted that mortality begins to increase.[16] Once patients reach very low values of FEV_1, this measurement has little predictive value, but no other measurements have been thoroughly validated.

The severity of gas exchange derangement obtained in the upright, sitting position while breathing room air is easily categorized as to the presence or absence of significant hypoxemia (or evidence of hypoxic and organ injury) and hypercarbia. Although the degree of hypoxemia has been correlated with mortality in COPD, this relationship is obviated by chronic domiciliary use of supplemental oxygen. Nonetheless, a patient with significant hypoxemia represents a complicated medical problem and one likely to require more resources. Similarly, the presence of hypercarbia is recognized as a significant correlate of mortality and a marker of advanced, complicated disease.[17]

Box 4-1. Variables That Could Be Included
in a New Staging System for
Patients With COPD

Forced expiratory volume in 1 second
Arterial blood gases
Timed walked distance
Dyspnea rating
Nutrition

COPD, chronic obstructive pulmonary disease.

The cardinal symptom of COPD is dyspnea.[1,18] This sensation is the consequence of the interaction between cognitive and nonvolitional neural processes and respiratory mechanics including airway obstruction. Dyspnea often limits functional activity and frequently causes the patient to seek medical attention.[19] Because COPD is a chronic disorder that limits a patient's ability to work and, in severe cases, impairs the activities of daily living, a monitoring system that includes some attribute of this limitation is highly desirable. Furthermore, in at least one study, dyspnea was an independent predictor of survival.[20] A practical, simple, and validated instrument to measure dyspnea is the Medical Research Council scale, which in its modified version is readily accessible.[1]

As stated previously, spirometric measurements and arterial blood gases are the best predictors of mortality but provide an incomplete picture of all the other elements that are important for patients. Little has been done to evaluate the use of other instruments that evaluate the patient's function or performance. One study recently evaluated a large number of patients with symptomatic severe COPD who had a uniformly low FEV_1. In this rather homogeneous population, FEV_1 failed to predict survival, whereas the 6-minute walk test was the single most important predictor of mortality in this population.[21] Recent data from our group[22] and one of the lung volume reduction programs[23] supports the predictive value of the 6-minute walking distance. Inclusion of this component is therefore desirable and justified.

Perhaps the time has come to integrate our newly acquired knowledge into a more comprehensive monitoring. A new classification system that monitors lung function, arterial blood gases, dyspnea, and functional status is likely to provide a more comprehensive picture of the disease. The information required for such a system is readily and inexpensively obtained: a simple questionnaire, a walking test, spirometry, and arterial blood gases. This new staging system should be helpful in several areas. The first is to adequately stratify patients. As clinicians we are familiar with patients with similar degrees of airflow obstruction but different functional capacities, gas exchanges, and perceptions of dyspnea. A second area is that of evaluating therapeutic interventions. Until now, we have traditionally tested efficacy of treatment by its impact on lung function (FEV_1). This seems paradoxical because we have defined the airflow limitation of COPD as being relatively "fixed" in nature. Under this new staging system it is easy to see how patients who receive therapy that does not alter lung function, such as supplemental oxygen, pulmonary rehabilitation, and noninvasive mechanical ventilation, may improve in this clinical stage. Finally, with this new staging system we will shed the constant nihilism that is associated with a disease that is staged with an irreversible "marker." Perhaps we will find out that we are doing better than we thought for our patients. The elements of a potential staging system are shown in Box 4-1.

AIRFLOW LIMITATION

To move air in and out of the lungs, the bellows must force air through the conducting airways. The resistance to flow is given by the interaction of air molecules with each other

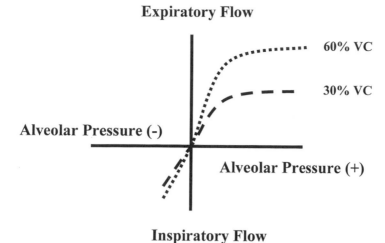

Figure 4-2. At a given lung volume (expressed as percent vital capacity [*VC*]), inspiratory flow is proportional to inspiratory pressure. In contrast, expiratory flow does not increase with increased expiratory pressure as the airways are dynamically compressed by the increased pressure.

and with the internal surface of the airways. Therefore, airflow resistance depends on the physical property of the gas and the length and diameter of the airways. For a constant diameter, flow is proportional to the applied pressure. This relationship holds true in healthy individuals for inspiratory flow measured at fixed lung volume, as shown in Figure 4-2. In contrast, expiratory flow is linearly related to the applied pressure only during the early portion of the maneuver. Beyond a certain point, flow does not increase despite further increase in driving pressure. This flow limitation is caused by the dynamic compression of airways as force is applied around them during forced expirations. This can be readily understood in the commonly determined flow–volume expression of the vital capacity. Figure 4-3 shows the flow–volume loop of a healthy individual. It is clear that as effort increases, expiratory flow increases up to a certain point (outer envelope), beyond which further efforts result in no further increase in airflow. During tidal breathing (inner tracing)

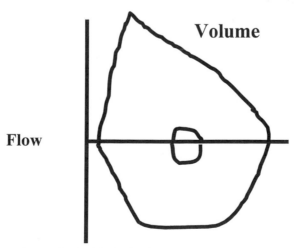

Figure 4-3. Flow–volume loop of a healthy individual. Ample flow reserve exists between tidal and forced breathing.

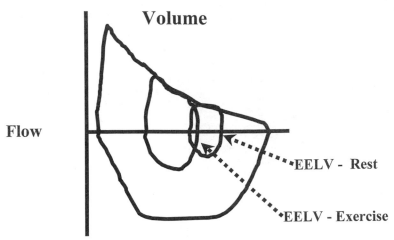

Figure 4-4. Flow–volume loop of a patient with COPD. These patients may reach airflow limitation even during tidal breathing.

only a small fraction of the maximal flow is used, and therefore flow is not limited under these circumstances.

In contrast, the flow–volume loop of patients with COPD is significantly different, as shown in Figure 4-4. The expiratory portion of the curve is caved out. This shape is caused by the smaller diameter of the intrathoracic airways, which decreases even more as pressure is applied around them. The flow limitation can be severe enough that maximal flow may be reached even during tidal breathing, as represented in this diagram. A patient with this degree of obstruction (a not uncommon finding in clinical practice) cannot increase flow with increased ventilatory demand. As we shall review later, increased demands can only be met by increasing respiratory rate, which in turn is detrimental to the expiratory time, a significant problem in patients with COPD.

The precise reason for the development of airflow obstruction in COPD is not entirely clear, but it may likely be multifactorial. In pure emphysema, destruction of the tissue around the airways will decrease the forces that act to keep the airways open.[24] In patients with a component of airway inflammation, the problem is compounded by intrinsic narrowing of the airways.[25]

Because airflow obstruction is physiologically evident during exhalation, COPD has been thought to be a problem of "expiration." Unfortunately, inspiration is also affected because inspiratory resistance is also increased and, more important, the inability to expel the inhaled air, coupled with parenchymal destruction, leads to hyperinflation.[26]

HYPERINFLATION

As the parenchymal destruction of many patients with COPD progresses, the distal air spaces enlarge. The loss of the lung elastic recoil resulting from this destruction increases resting lung volume. In a pervasive way, the loss of elastic recoil and airway attachments narrows even more the already constricted airways. The decrease in airway diameter increases resistance to airflow and worsens the obstruction. Decreased lung elastic recoil therefore is a major contributor of airway narrowing in emphysema.[26–28] Because in most patients the distribution of emphysema is not uniform, portions of lung with low elastic recoil may coexist with portions with more normal elastic recoil property. It follows that ventilation to each one of those portions will not be uniform. This helps explain some of the differences in gas exchange. It also explains why reduction of the uneven distribution of recoil pressures by procedures that resect more afflicted lung areas results in better ventilation of the remainder of the lung and improved gas exchange.

Increased breathing frequency worsens hyperinflation[29,30] because the expiratory time decreases, even if patients simultaneously shorten their inspiratory time. The resulting "dynamic" hyperinflation is detrimental to lung mechanics and helps explain many of the findings associated with higher ventilatory demand, such as exercise or acute exacerbation.

ALTERATION IN GAS EXCHANGE

The uneven distribution of airway disease and emphysema helps explain the change in blood gases. The lungs of patients with COPD can be considered as consisting of two portions: one more emphysematous and the other one more normal. The pressure volume curve of the emphysematous portion is displaced up and to the left compared with that of the more normal lung (Fig. 4-5). At low lung volume the emphysematous (more compliant) portion undergoes greater volume changes than does the more healthy lung. In contrast, at higher lung volume the emphysematous lung is overinflated and accepts less volume change, per unit of pressure change, than does the healthy lung. Therefore, the distribution of ventilation is nonuniform, and, overall, the emphysematous areas of the lung are underventilated compared with the more normal lung. Because perfusion is even more compromised than ventilation in the emphysematous areas, they have a high ventilation:perfusion ratio and behave as dead space. Indeed, this wasted portion of ventilation (VD/VT), corresponding to approximately 0.3 to 0.4 of the tidal breath of a healthy person, has been measured to be much higher in patients with severe emphysema.[31] At the same time, narrower bronchi in other areas may not allow appropriate ventilation to reach relatively well-perfused areas of the lung. This low ventilation perfusion ratio will contribute to venous admixture (V/Q) and hypoxemia.[32,33] The overall result is the simulta-

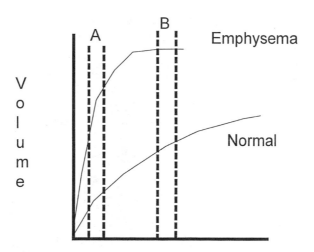

Figure 4-5. Volume–pressure relationship in portions of lung with "normal" and "emphysematous" behavior. At low volume (*A*), a small change in pressure results in a larger volume increase in the emphysematous portion. At higher lung volume (*B*), a similar change in pressure results in minimal change in volume in the emphysematous portion, which now behaves as a "stiff" lung. See text for details.

neous coexistence of high VD/VT regions with regions of low V/Q match. Both increase the ventilatory demand, thereby taxing even more the respiratory system of these patients.

As ventilatory demand increases, so does the work of breathing, so the patient with COPD must attempt to increase ventilation to maintain an adequate delivery of oxygen. Alveolar ventilation must also be sufficient to eliminate the produced carbon dioxide (CO_2). If this does not occur, $PaCO_2$ will increase. Indeed, the arterial blood gas changes over time in patients with COPD parallel this sequence. Initially PaO_2 progressively decreases, but it is compensated by increased ventilation. When the ventilation is insufficient, the $PaCO_2$ rises.[34,35] This is consistent with the observation that patients with COPD who develop severe hypoxemia and hypercarbia have a poor prognosis.[16]

CONTROL OF VENTILATION

For gas exchange to occur, it is necessary to move air in and out of the lung. This is achieved by the respiratory pump, which is composed of the respiratory centers; the nerves that carry the signals from those centers; the respiratory muscles, which are the pressure-generating structures; and the rib cage and abdomen. These components are linked and ordinarily function in a well-orchestrated manner whereby ventilation goes unnoticed and uses little energy.[36,37]

The central controller or respiratory center is located in the upper medulla and integrates input from the periphery and other parts of the nervous system.[38] The output of this generator is not only modulated by mechanical, cortical, and sensory input but also by the state of oxygenation (PaO_2), CO_2 concentration ($PaCO_2$), and acid base status (pH). Once generated, the output is distributed by the conducting nerves to the respiratory muscles, which shorten, deform the rib cage and abdomen, and generate intrathoracic pressures. These pressure changes displace volume and air moves in and out depending on the direction of the pressure changes.

The relation between "drive" and inspiratory pressure or volume is referred to as "coupling." Coupling is usually smooth and occurs with minimal effort. That is the reason breathing is perceived as effortless. Whenever the act of breathing requires effort this effort is perceived as "work," which we define as the unpleasant sensation of dyspnea. The interaction between the central drive (controller output) and the final output (ventilation) is complex and involves many components.[39,40] This complexity renders it difficult to ascribe dyspnea to a dysfunction in any individual portion of the system. The ventilatory control can be assessed at different levels. The simplest is the minute ventilation (VE), which reflects the final effectiveness of the ventilatory drive. Further insight can be obtained by measuring the two contributors to VE: tidal volume (VT), represented by the volume of air inhaled in a breath, and respiratory frequency.

Analysis of these variables in COPD reveals that as the disease progresses, VE increases.[40] This is expected because the need to keep oxygen uptake and CO_2 removal constant is challenged by the changes in lung mechanics and ventilation perfusion. The increase in VE is achieved first by an increase in VT, but as the resistive work owing to airflow obstruction worsens, VT decreases (Fig. 4-6). The respiratory rate responds in a more linear fashion, increasing as the obstruction progresses (Fig. 4-7).[41] The VE can also be expressed in terms of the mean inspiratory flow rate. This is obtained by relating the VT to the inspiratory time (VT/Ti) and the fractional duration of inspiration (Ti/Tot). VT/Ti reflects drive and Ti/Ttot reflects timing. In COPD, both are altered by the need to increase VE. The Ti/Ttot, which normally has values of close to 0.38, shortens somewhat and the VT/Ti increases more to accommodate the increase in respiratory rate and shortened Ti/Ttot.

A relatively noninvasive way to measure central drive is the mouth occlusion pressure measured 0.1 seconds after the onset of inspiration (P0.1).[42] With increased central drive, the increase in P0.1 is higher than that of VT/Ti[43] owing to airflow impedance that

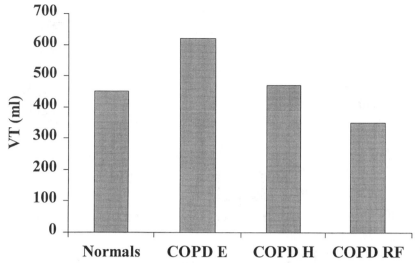

Figure 4-6. With progression of airflow limitation, work of breathing increases. To provide the increased oxygen demanded by the breathing pump, tidal volume (*VT*) increases in eucapnic (*E*) patients, begins to decrease as the response fails with hypercapnia (*H*), and falls even below the value in normals in patients with chronic obstructive pulmonary disease (*COPD*) and respiratory failure (*RF*).

decreases mean inspiratory flow measured at the mouth while air is moving. The P0.1 is much less affected in COPD because it is measured in conditions of no airflow because the airway is temporarily obstructed. Mouth occlusion pressure or P0.1 has been shown to increase as the degree of obstruction worsens irrespective of the alteration in arterial blood gases. As shown in Figure 4-8, the central drive increases as the degree of airflow obstruction progresses, reaching its maximum in patients in respiratory failure.[35,44] The drive is effectively "coupled" to increased VT in the early stages of obstruction, but VT actually drops as the work to move air becomes very high. The only alternative is to increase

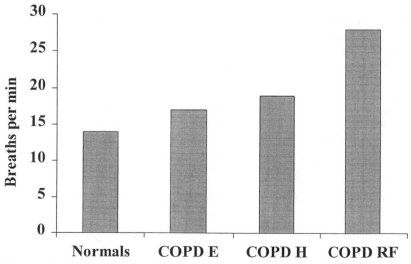

Figure 4-7. In patients with chronic obstructive pulmonary disease (*COPD*), respiratory rate (in breaths per minute) increases as airflow progresses from eucapnia (*E*) to hypercapnia (*H*), reaching the highest value in patients in respiratory failure (*RF*).

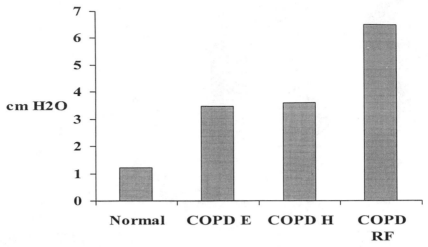

Figure 4-8. Mouth occlusion pressure in centimeters of water at 0.1 seconds of an occluded tidal breath. This value increases as a function of the progression of airflow limitation and is lower in normals than in eucapnic (*E*) and hypercapnic (*H*) individuals and highest in patients with chronic obstructive pulmonary disease (*COPD*) and respiratory failure (*RF*).

respiratory rate. This also occurs, but as determined by the flow limitation characteristics of these patients, this adaptive phenomena may result in further hyperinflation. As described earlier, hyperinflation displaces diseased portions of lung higher in their pressure–volume relationship. This effectively turns many portions of the lung into "restrictive" tissue. At this point, respiration is less demanding (in terms of work or pressure changes) when a fast and shallower ventilatory pattern is adopted. Indeed, this is the observed breathing strategy in patients with the most severe COPD.[45]

RESPIRATORY MUSCLES

As noted previously, breathing depends on the coordinated action of different groups of muscles. The respiratory muscles can be divided into those that help inflate the lungs (inspiratory) and those that have an expiratory action. In addition, there are upper airway muscles (tongue and muscles of the palate, of the pharynx, and of the vocal cords), the function of which is to contract at the beginning of inspiration and hold the upper airways open throughout inhalation. Although important in normal function, they play a limited role in pure COPD and are not discussed further in this chapter.

The diaphragm and the other inspiratory muscles are innervated by a wide array of motor neurons that range from cranial nerve 11 (C-11), which provides neuronal input to the sternomastoid, to lumbar roots L2-L3, which innervate abdominal muscles. The respiratory cycle is regulated by a complex series of centrally organized neurons, which maintain rhythmic breathing that usually goes unnoticed and that can be voluntarily overridden by the cortex.

The most important inspiratory muscle is the diaphragm.[46] It is well suited to perform its work because of its anatomic arrangement and histochemical composition. Its long fibers extend from the noncontractile central tendon and are directed down and outward to insert circumferentially in the lower ribs and upper lumbar spine. This concave shape allows the muscle its lifting action as it contracts. The diaphragm can shorten up to 40% between full expiration and end inspiration.[47] During quiet breathing, it accounts for most of the force needed to displace the rib cage. Other inspiratory muscles are also agonists during quiet breathing and contribute to inspiratory effort: the scalene and parasternal intercostal. Yet other muscles (truly accessory in nature) are not active during quiet breathing in healthy individuals but may contribute to ventilation in situations of increased demand. Muscles such as the sternomastoid, pectoralis minor, latissimus dorsi, and trapezius are some of these truly "accessory" muscles.[36,41] The abdominal muscles are expiratory in action because their contractions decrease lung volume.[48] Inasmuch as they provide tone to the abdominal wall, they help the diaphragm because they contribute to the generation of the gastric pressure needed for diaphragmatic contraction to be effective.

It has been postulated that the automatic and voluntary ventilatory pathways are different and that the respiratory and tonic functions of these muscles are driven from different central nervous areas and integrated at the spinal level. In patients in whom some of these muscles are participating in respiration, to perform nonventilatory work they must maintain a high degree of coordination. Either because of the load or because of competing central integration, muscle function may become dyscoordinated and result in dysfunction. We have shown this to occur in patients with COPD who perform unsupported arm exercise. This type of exercise leads to early fatigue of the muscles involved in arm positioning and to dyssynchrony between the rib cage and the diaphragm–abdomen. This could also be caused by competing outputs of the various driving centers that control rhythmic respiratory and tonic activities of the accessory ventilatory muscles and the diaphragm. This dyssynchrony may be perceived as dyspnea. Its occurrence has been observed in healthy individuals breathing against resistive loads and in patients with COPD breathing during voluntary hyperventilation.[49,50] Likewise, it has been observed in patients immediately after disconnection from ventilators but before evidence of contractile fatigue, which suggests that dyssynchrony is a consequence of the load and not an indication of fatigue itself. Whatever the reason, this breathing pattern is ineffective and is associated with respiratory muscle dysfunction.[40,49]

DYSPNEA

Many patients with COPD stop exercising because of dyspnea, and dyspnea is the dominant symptom during acute exacerbations of the disease.[31,50–52] Recent studies have shown that in COPD, dyspnea with exercise correlates better with the degree of dynamic hyperinflation[51–54] than with changes in airflow indices or blood gas exchange. Dyspnea also correlates better to respiratory muscle function than to airflow obstruction.[21,39] Studies in healthy individuals have shown that dyspnea increases as the ratio between the pressure needed to ventilate and the maximal pressure that the muscles can generate. Dyspnea also worsens in proportion to the duration of the inspiratory contraction (Ti/Ttot) and respiratory frequency. These are also the factors that are associated with electromyographic evidence of respiratory muscle fatigue.[55] Therefore, it has been suggested that patients with COPD develop dynamic hyperinflation that compromises ventilatory muscle function and that this is the main determinant of dyspnea in these patients. Although respiratory muscle fatigue has been reasonably well documented in patients with COPD suffering from acute decompensation,[56] its presence in stable patients remains in doubt. It is fair to state that the respiratory muscles of patients with severe COPD are functioning at a level closer to the fatigue threshold but are not fatigued. It is possible that restoration of the respiratory muscles to a better contractile state could improve the dyspnea of these patients. Indeed, Martinez et al.[57] observed that the factor that best predicted the improvement in dyspnea reported by COPD patients after lung volume reduction surgery was the lesser dynamic hyperinflation seen during exercise after the procedure. This is consistent with similar reports from other groups[58–60] and the close association between decreased dynamic hyperinflation and dyspnea in patents treated with bronchodilators.[30,51]

Dyspnea in patients with severe COPD may also be owing to the level of resting respiratory drive and the individual's response of the central output to different stimuli. In other words, at similar mechanical load and similar levels of respiratory muscle dysfunction, dyspnea may result from an individual's response of the central motor output. This hypothesis is supported by work from Marin et al.,[62] who demonstrated that the most important predictor of dyspnea with exercise was the baseline central drive response to CO_2. The importance of this observation lies in the possibility that a group of patients with COPD may manifest increased central drive, and adequate manipulation of this drive may result in decreased dyspnea. Until further studies are completed, this remains just an interesting hypothesis.

PERIPHERAL MUSCLE FUNCTION

Many patients with COPD will stop exercising because of leg fatigue rather than dyspnea. This observation has prompted renewed interest in the function of limb muscles in these patients. Perhaps the most important of these studies are those reported by Maltais et al.,[63,64] who performed biopsies of the vastus lateralis before and after lower extremity exercise training in patients with severe COPD. At baseline, patients with COPD have lower levels of the oxidative enzymes citric synthase and 3-hydroxy-acyl-CoA-hydrogenase than do healthy individuals. After exercise, the mitochondrial content of these enzymes increased. This was associated with an improvement in exercise endurance and decreased lactic acid production at peak exercise. These biochemical changes are in line with the observation of several groups that have suggested the presence of a dysfunctional myopathy in patients with COPD. The importance of deconditioning, peripheral muscle dysfunction, and training in COPD is addressed in a different chapter in this book.

INTEGRATIVE APPROACH

The overall function of the respiratory system in COPD can be represented by the model shown in Figure 4-9. Central to the model is the problem of airway narrowing and

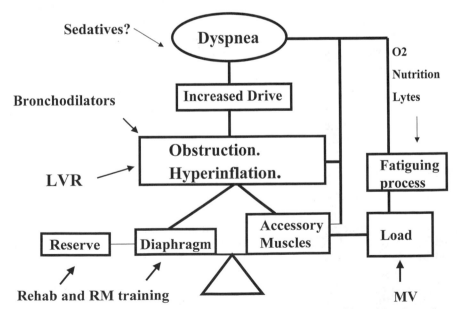

Figure 4-9. Schematic model that integrates the different components of breathing in patients with COPD. Based on this model, several interventions may be beneficial. See text for details.

hyperinflation. To reverse the model to a normal state, it is necessary to resolve those two problems. Efforts to prevent the disease from developing (smoking cessation) must be associated with methods aimed at reversing airflow obstruction. Indeed, pharmacotherapy, including bronchodilators, antibiotics, and corticosteroids, is given to improve airflow. If this is effective, hyperinflation should consequently decrease. One alternative is to resect the portion of the lungs that are severely diseased, such as has been done in cases of large bullae.[65] Partial resection of lesser evident emphysematous areas (lung volume reduction surgery) seems effective for a few patients. From a strict pathophysiologic point of view, lung resection in patients with COPD whose main problem is inflammatory airway disease does not seem justifiable. For this large majority, pulmonary rehabilitation through improvement in peripheral muscle function and nutrition and implementation of adequate coping mechanisms remains the best available option.

REFERENCES

1. Standards for the diagnosis and care of patients with chronic obstructive pulmonary disease (COPD). Am J Respir Crit Care Med 1995;154: 1–120.
2. Mitchell RS, Stanford RE, Johnson JM, et al. The morphologic features of the bronchi, bronchioles and alveoli in chronic airway obstruction. Am Rev Respir Dis 1976;114:137–145.
3. Thurlbeck WM. Pathophysiology of chronic obstructive pulmonary disease. Clin Chest Med 1990;11:389–403.
4. Jeffrey PK. Structural and inflammatory changes in COPD: a comparison with asthma. Thorax 1998;53:129–136.
5. Keatings VM, Barnes PJ. Granulocyte activation markers in induced sputum: comparison between chronic obstructive pulmonary disease, asthma and normal subjects. Am J Respir Crit Care Med 1997;155:449–453.
6. Saetta M, Di Stefano A, Turato G. CD8+ T-lymphocytes in peripheral airways of smokers with chronic obstructive pulmonary disease. Am J Respir Crit Care Med 1998;157:822–826.
7. Finkelstein R, Fraser RS, Ghezzo H, et al. Alveolar inflammation and its relation to emphysema in smokers. Am J Respir Crit Care Med 1995;152: 1666–1672.
8. Yamamoto C, Yoneda T, Yoshikawa M, et al. Airway inflammation in COPD assessed by sputum level of interleukin-8. Chest 1997;112:505–510.
9. Barnes PJ. New therapies for chronic obstructive pulmonary disease. Thorax 1998;53:137–147.
10. Pratico D, Basili S, Vieri M, et al. Chronic obstructive pulmonary disease is associated with an increase in urinary levels of isoprostane F_{2a}-111, an index of oxidant stress. Am J Respir Crit Care Med 1998;158:1709–1714.
11. Finlay GA, O'Driscoll LR, Russell KJ, et al. Matrix-metalloproteinase expression and production by alveolar macrophages in emphysema. Am J Respir Crit Care Med 1997;156:240–247.
12. Vignole AM, Riccobono L, Mirabella A, et al. Sputum metalloprotinase-9/tissue inhibitor of metalloprotinase-1 ratio correlates with airflow obstruction in asthma and chronic bronchitis. Am J Respir Crit Care Med 1998;158:1945–1950.
13. Berend N, Woolcock AJ, Marlin GE. Correlation between the function and the structure of the lung in smokers. Am Rev Respir Dis 1979;119:695–702.
14. Buist AS, Van Fleet DL, Ross BB. A comparison of conventional spirometric tests and the tests of closing volume in one emphysema screening center. Am Rev Respir Dis 1973;107:735–740.
15. Fletcher C, Peto R. The natural history of chronic airflow obstruction. BMJ 1977;1:1645–1648.
16. Anthonisen NR. Prognosis in chronic obstructive pulmonary disease: results from multicenter clinical trials. Am Rev Respir Dis 1989;133:95–99.
17. Hodgkin JE. Prognosis in chronic obstructive pulmonary disease. Clin Chest Med 1990;11:555–569.
18. Sweer L, Zwillich CW. Dyspnea in the patient with chronic obstructive pulmonary disease. Clin Chest Med 1990;11(3):417–455.
19. Mahler DA, Weinburg DH, Wells CK, et al. The measurement of dyspnea: contents, interobserver agreement, and physiologic correlates of two new clinical indexes. Chest 1984;85:751–758.
20. Ries A, Kaplan R, Limberg T, et al. Effects of pulmonary rehabilitation on physiologic and psychosocial outcomes inpatients with COPD. Ann Intern Med 1995;122:823–832.
21. Gerardi D, Lovett L, Benoit-Connors J, et al. Variables related to increased mortality following outpatient pulmonary rehabilitation. Eur Respir J 1996;9:431–435.
22. Pinto-Plata V, Girish M, Taylor J, et al. Natural decline in the six minute walking distance (6 MWD) in COPD. Am J Respir Crit Care Med 1998;157:20A.
23. Szekely L, Oelberg D, Wright C, et al. Preoperative predictors of operative mortality in COPD patients undergoing bilateral lung volume reduction surgery. Chest 1997;111:550–558.
24. Nagai A, Yamawaki I, Takizawa T, et al. Alveolar attachments in emphysema of human lungs. Am Rev Respir Dis 1991;144:888–891.
25. Postma DS, Slinter HJ. Prognosis of chronic obstructive pulmonary disease: the Dutch experience. Am Rev Respir Dis 1989;140:100–105.
26. Bates DV. Respiratory Function in Disease. 3rd ed. Philadelphia: WB Saunders, 1989:172–187.
27. Greaves IA, Colebatch HJ. Elastic behavior and

structure of normal and emphysematous lungs postmortem. Am Rev Respir Dis 1980;121:127–128.

28. Hogg JC, Macklem PT, Thurlbeck WA. Site and nature of airways obstruction in chronic obstructive lung disease. N Engl J Med 1968;278:1355–1359.

29. O'Donnell SE, Sanil R, Anthonisen NR, et al. Effect of dynamic airway compression on breathing pattern and respiratory sensation in severe chronic obstructive pulmonary disease. Am Rev Respir Dis 1987;135:912–918.

30. O'Donnell D, Lam M, Webb K. Measurement of symptoms, lung hyperinflation and endurance during exercise in COPD. Am J Respir Crit Care Med 1998;158:1557–1565.

31. Javahari S, Blum J, Kazemi H. Pattern of breathing and carbon dioxide retention in chronic obstructive lung disease. Am J Med 1981;71:228–234.

32. Rodriguez-Roisin R, Roca J. Pulmonary gas exchange. In: Calverly PM, Pride NB, eds. Chronic Obstructive Pulmonary Disease. London: Chapman & Hall, 1995:167–184.

33. Parot S, Miara B, Milic-Emili J, et al. Hypoxemia, hypercapnia and breathing patterns in patients with chronic obstructive pulmonary disease. Am Rev Respir Dis 1982;126:882–886.

34. Begin P, Grassino A. Inspiratory muscle dysfunction and chronic hypercapnia in chronic obstructive pulmonary disease. Am Rev Respir Dis 1991;143:905–912.

35. Montes de Oca M, Celli BR. Mouth occlusion pressure, CO_2 response and hypercapnia in severe obstructive pulmonary disease. Eur Respir J 1998;12:666–671.

36. Celli BR. Respiratory muscle function. Clin Chest Med 1986;7:567–584.

37. Roussos CH, Macklem PT. The respiratory muscles. N Engl J Med 1982;307:786–797.

38. VonEuler C. On the central pattern generator for the basic breathing rhythmicity. J Appl Physiol 1983;55:1647–1659.

39. Derenne JP, Macklem PT, Roussos CH. The respiratory muscles: mechanics, control and pathophysiology. Am Rev Respir Dis 1978;119:119–133, 373–390.

40. Sears TA. Central rhythm and pattern generation. Chest 1990;97:45–47.

41. Martinez FJ, Couser JI, Celli BR. Factors influencing ventilatory muscle recruitment in patients with chronic airflow obstruction. Am Rev Respir Dis 1990;142:276–282.

42. Murciano D, Broczkowski J, Lecocguic M, et al. Tracheal occlusion pressure: a simple index to monitor respiratory muscle fatigue during acute respiratory failure in patients with chronic obstructive pulmonary disease. Ann Intern Med 1988;108:800–805.

43. Milic-Emili J, Grassino AE, Whitelaw WA. Measurement and testing of respiratory drive. In: Horbein TF, ed. Regulation of Breathing: Lung Biology in Health and Disease. New York: Marcel Dekker, 1981:675–743.

44. Sasoon CS, Te TT, Mahutte CR, et al. Airway occlusion pressure: an important indicator for successful weaning in patients with chronic obstructive pulmonary disease. Am Rev Respir Dis 1987;135:107–113.

45. Loveridge B, West P, Anthonisen NR, et al. Breathing patterns in patients with chronic obstructive pulmonary disease. Am Rev Respir Dis 1984;130:730–733.

46. Rochester DF. The diaphragm contractile properties and fatigue. J Clin Invest 1985;75:1397–1402.

47. Braun NM, Arora NS, Rochester DF. The force-length relationship of the normal human diaphragm. J Appl Physiol 1982;53:405–412.

48. DeTroyer A, Estenne M. Functional anatomy of the respiratory muscles. Clin Chest Med 1988;9:175–193.

49. Sharp JT. The respiratory muscles in emphysema. Clin Chest Med 1983;4:421–432.

50. Killian K, Jones N. Respiratory muscle and dyspnea. Clin Chest Med 1988;9:237–248.

51. LeBlanc P, Bowie DM, Summers E, et al. Breathlessness and exercise in patients with cardiorespiratory disease. Am Rev Respir Dis 1986;133:21–25.

52. Girish M, Pinto V, Kenney L, et al. Dyspnea in acute exacerbation of COPD is associated with increase in ventilatory demand and not with worsened airflow obstruction. Chest 1998;114:266S.

53. Marin J, Carrizo S, Gallego B, et al. Walk distance and exertional dyspnea is better predicted by dynamic hyperinflation than FEV_1 in COPD. Am J Respir Crit Care Med 1999;159:A476.

54. Killian K, Jones N. Respiratory muscle and dyspnea. Clin Chest Med 1988;9:237–248.

55. Bellemare F, Grassino A. Forces reserve of the diaphragm in patients with chronic obstructive pulmonary disease. J Appl Physiol 1983;55:8–15.

56. Cohen C, Zagelbaum G, Gross D, et al. Clinical manifestations of inspiratory muscle fatigue. Am J Med 1982;73:308–316.

57. Martinez F, Montes de Oca M, Whyte R, et al. Lung-volume reduction surgery improves dyspnea, dynamic hyperinflation and respiratory muscle function. Am J Respir Crit Care Med 1997;155:2018–2023.

58. Brantigan OC, Mueller E, Kress MB. A surgical approach to pulmonary emphysema. Am Rev Respir Dis 1959;80:194–202.

59. Cooper JD, Trulock ER, Triantafillou AN, et al. Bilateral pneumonectomy (volume reduction) for chronic obstructive pulmonary disease. J Thorac Cardiovasc Surg 1995;109:116–119.

60. Knudson RJ, Gaensler E. Surgery for emphysema. Ann Thorac Surg 1965;1:332–362.

61. Belman M, Botnick W, Shin W. Inhaled bronchodilators reduce dynamic hyperinflation during exercise in patients with chronic obstructive pulmonary disease. Am J Respir Crit Care Med 1996;53:967–975.

62. Marin J, Montes De Oca M, Rassulo J, et al. Ventilatory drive at rest and perception of exertional dyspnea in severe COPD. Chest 1999;115:1293–1300.

63. Maltais F, Simard A, Simard J, et al. Oxidative

capacity of the skeletal muscle and lactic acid kinetics during exercise in normal subjects and in patients with COPD. Am J Respir Crit Care Med 1995;153:288–293.

64. Maltais F, LeBlanc P, Simard C, et al. Skeletal muscle adaptation of endurance training in patients with chronic obstructive pulmonary disease. Am J Respir Crit Care Med 1996;154:442–447.

65. Fitzgerald MX, Keelan PJ, Cugel DW, et al. Long-term results of surgery for bullous emphysema. J Thorac Cardiovasc Surg 1974;68:566–587.

5 Dyspnea: Assessment and Management

Virginia Carrieri-Kohlman
Michael S. Stulbarg

⏵ Professional Skills

Upon completion of this chapter, the reader will:

- Define dyspnea
- Identify components of the patient history and physical examination that can be used to differentiate the diagnostic cause(s) of dyspnea
- Describe two methods to measure dyspnea, including one method that can be used during exercise and one method to determine dyspnea with activities of daily living (ADLs)
- State two possible physiologic and/or psychologic causes of dyspnea and two strategies that can be targeted toward these mechanisms
- Describe a program of strategies that could be used to assist patients in managing the symptom of dyspnea

WHAT IS DYSPNEA?

Dyspnea is a clinical term for shortness of breath or breathlessness, that is, the discomfort associated with effort in breathing or the urge to breathe. Dyspnea may be considered part of the warning system for human beings to know when they are at risk of receiving inadequate ventilation. For example, asthmatics with a blunted perception of dyspnea may be at greater risk for near-fatal attacks.[1]

Although this symptom has challenged clinicians for years, only relatively recently has it been the subject of both scientific and clinical investigation.[2] Dyspnea is an important outcome measure in studies of interventions for chronic lung disease and in the evaluation of pulmonary rehabilitation programs. Dyspnea occurs in healthy individuals with exercise and/or altitude, but it is experienced by patients with a variety of diseases at lower levels of physical exercise or altitude. Shortness of breath becomes especially important when it interferes with ADLs. As with other sensations, heterogeneity is great in reporting of shortness of breath.[3]

A recent consensus statement from the American Thoracic Society[4] offered the following definition of dyspnea:

"Dyspnea is a term used to characterize a subjective experience of breathing discomfort that is comprised of qualitatively distinct sensations that vary in intensity. The experience derives from interactions among multiple physiological, psychological, social and environmental factors, and may induce secondary physiological and behavioral responses."

Although dyspnea is a common complaint in the general population, little data exists on the prevalence of the symptom. It is a frequent cause of emergency department visits.[5] Dyspnea is an independent predictor of cardiovascular mortality and has been found to be more related to quality of life than pulmonary function.[6,7] Because many diseases in which dyspnea occurs are not reversible, management of the symptom of dyspnea per se is a desirable therapeutic goal. Unfortunately, dyspnea is more difficult than pain for health care providers to treat, perhaps because the underlying basis of it is less well understood than is that of pain. This is especially true in the chronically ill and terminally ill patient where the control of pain is generally effective but control of dyspnea is not.[8,9]

MECHANISMS OF DYSPNEA

Although the physiologic and psychosocial mechanisms of dyspnea are still poorly understood, numerous investigations have shed light on this complex symptom. As with other sensations, the experience of dyspnea results from neural activity within the part of the cerebral cortex responsible for sensory perception. Unlike localized sensations, such as touch or pain, which arise from peripheral stimulation, dyspnea is a visceral sensation somewhat analogous to hunger or nausea, sensations that are experienced as a result of central neural activity. Dyspnea requires perception and must therefore be studied in humans. Dyspnea arises from stimuli (e.g., exercise, breathholding, hypoxia) that do not have a common neurophysiologic pathway of peripheral receptor stimulation. Recent studies in normal subjects have shown that the sensations associated with voluntary respiratory effort are perceived in the primary sensory cortex,[10] whereas the feeling of an urge to breathe (as during breathholding) activates the limbic structures of the brain.[11]

Except in patients with advanced disease who are dyspneic at rest, dyspnea usually does not occur unless breathing is actively stimulated (e.g., by exercise, hypoxia, hypercapnia, or metabolic acidosis).[12-15] In contrast to stimulation of breathing, voluntary increases in ventilation induce little or no dyspnea.[16-18] These observations lead to the key concept in understanding the mechanisms of dyspnea: it is not just increased effort or movement of the chest wall that results in dyspnea, but rather the respiratory center must be stimulated for dyspnea to occur.

Dyspnea Is Multifactorial

Many factors interact to determine the ultimate central experience of dyspnea after ventilation is stimulated. For example, if a patient is bronchoconstricted, dyspnea will be greater for any given level of ventilation than when the patient has received bronchodilators.[19] This is because a greater "signal" or "command" to breathe will be required to overcome the resistance, and this will be experienced centrally as greater dyspnea. However, the simple relationship between ventilatory stimulation and dyspnea is not maintained in all circumstances. Exercising while breathing through an inspiratory resistor dampens the subsequent relationship between ventilation and dyspnea during exercise.[20] Similarly, spending prolonged time at high altitude decreases dyspnea in relation to ventilation during exercise, and this effect lasts for at least 6 weeks.[21]

Evidence shows that other factors may modify the central experience of dyspnea. For example, in asthmatic patients, dyspnea is greater when bronchospasm occurs naturally than when it is chemically induced,[22] and treatment of asthma may improve dyspnea even in the absence of improvement in airflow.[23] Evidence also shows that airway inflammation may affect the dyspnea of asthmatics.[24] External factors, such as cold air blowing on the face, may also affect the rating of dyspnea,[25] as many patients discover on their own.

Dyspnea is also modulated by significant cognitive, psychosocial, and behavioral factors. Dyspnea is worse when it is unexpected, when it occurs in inappropriate situations, and when it is perceived as dangerous.[26] Reporting of dyspnea may be affected by an individual's age,[27,28] emotional state (e.g., depression and anxiety[29-31]), personality, previous experience with the symptom,[28] cognitive function, fatigue,[32-34] self-efficacy,[35] and mood.[20,36,37] Physical fitness results in less dyspnea for a given exercise stimulus.[3] Whether this is related to the frequency of dyspnea experiences with exercise or other psychologic effects of regular exercise is unknown.

Physiologic Mechanisms

Respiratory Muscles and Chest Wall

It is also clear that the respiratory muscles and chest wall play an important role in dyspnea. Early studies on the dyspnea of breathholding showed that the respiratory discomfort could be relieved by allowing the chest to move or by partial paralysis of the respiratory muscles.[38] The mechanisms by which these maneuvers relieve dyspnea is unclear. More recent work has shown that dyspnea can be experienced even in the absence of signals coming from the respiratory muscles. For example, carbon dioxide breathing can elicit dyspnea in experimentally paralyzed normal subjects[39,40] or in individuals with high-level spinal cord transection.[41] Evidence shows that stimulation of mechanoreceptors in the respiratory muscles and/or chest wall may modify dyspnea. Stimulation of the chest wall with external vibration can lessen experimentally induced dyspnea.[42,43]

Parenchymal Lung Receptors

Evidence shows that stimulation of lung receptors can either decrease or increase dyspnea, but the fact that lung transplant recipients experience dyspnea fairly normally[44] suggests that such receptors are not important. Acute pneumothorax may cause severe dyspnea, probably related to stimulation of rapidly adapting stretch receptors. Stimulation of pulmonary C-fibers may contribute to breathlessness conditions, such as pulmonary hypertension, pneumonia, and pulmonary embolism.[45]

Airway Receptors

If airway receptors were important for dyspnea, blocking them with an inhaled anesthetic might change the experience of dyspnea; however, in one study, inhaled bupivacaine had no effect on dyspnea during exercise in patients with restrictive lung disease.[46] In sum, these studies do not suggest that afferent activity from pulmonary receptors is a major source of the neural information that leads to exercise-induced dyspnea.

Awareness of Motor Command

Some investigators have likened dyspnea to the sense of effort in peripheral muscles, that is, the awareness of a "motor command." As applied to dyspnea, these ideas have developed from studies involving constraints to breathing such as breathing through external resistors, breathing at high lung volume (i.e., hyperinflation), and induction of respiratory muscle weakness (i.e., partial curarization).[47-50] Dyspnea in these studies is better understood in terms of differences in the outgoing command to breathe rather than afferent feedback from respiratory muscles. The literature in this area is confusing, in part because the questions that patients are asked are not uniform. Patients with mechanically impaired lungs complain of the excessive effort of breathing, but it is not clear to what extent this sensation as opposed to that of "unsatisfied" breathing or urge to breathe is contributing to their global perception of shortness of breath. In most physiologic and clinical situations, sensations of "effort" and "urge to breathe" increase together, but experimentally they can be separated.[51] This separation implies that the feeling of an urge to breathe is more directly related to reflex stimulation of the respiratory system than to the external work of breathing performed by the respiratory muscles.

Summary of Mechanisms

In sum, dyspnea in patients with lung disease is multifactorial and is the result of one or more physiologic and/or psychologic mechanisms: (*a*) increased central respiratory drive because of either an excessive stimulus (e.g., hypoxemia, acidosis, anxiety) or the need to overcome constraints on the respiratory system (e.g., obstruction, stiff lungs, chest wall problems); (b) weakness of the muscles of respiration presenting as either relative weakness, as in hyperinflation, or as absolute weakness, as in myopathy; and (c) abnormal central perception of dyspnea, for example, in anxiety or hyperventilation syndrome.

Several authors have expanded the sole physiologic approach to multifactorial models conceptualizing dyspnea, similar to pain, with a cognitive-motivational-affective dimension in addition to a sensory dimension. The models incorporate antecedent biopsychosocial factors that affect the perception of dyspnea, such as personal, illness, or environmental factors; cognitive-behavioral strategies to treat the symptom; and outcomes affected by the symptom, including physical performance, functional status, and quality of life.[52–56]

These conceptual models provide the clinician with theoretical propositions that go beyond physiologic mechanisms and propose related personal and environmental factors and consequences that may be used to guide patient teaching about triggers for dyspnea and daily management of this chronic, debilitating symptom.

MEASUREMENT OF DYSPNEA

What Is the Value of Measuring Dyspnea?

The outcomes committee of the American Association of Cardiovascular and Pulmonary Rehabilitation has endorsed the recommendation that dyspnea be one of the three important outcome measures included in the evaluation of pulmonary rehabilitation programs.[57] Five primary reasons for quantifying the intensity of shortness of breath are as follows: (a) clinical ratings of dyspnea provide a different dimension not provided by pulmonary function tests; (b) clinical measurements of dyspnea influence and predict general health status to a greater extent than do physiologic measurements; (c) dyspnea during daily activities and after a paced walk test relates well to quality of life measurements[7,29]; (d) a baseline rating of dyspnea can be used to determine the type and intensity of exercise treatments and as a guide for determining an exercise prescription; and (e) dyspnea is important to measure as a response to therapies within a rehabilitation program.[58]

When Should Dyspnea Be Measured?

An initial interview with one of the staff of the rehabilitation program to determine the "dimensions" of the symptom, including persistence or variability of the symptom, what it feels like, location, aggravating factors or triggers, individual strategies, and medications for alleviating the symptom, helps the clinician understand the meaning of the symptom for the individual patient and heightens the awareness of triggers and reinforces strategies patients have been using to manage their shortness of breath.[32] The patient may be unaware of factors that precipitate dyspnea (e.g., cigarettes, foods, medications, allergens, obesity, or severe weight loss) or relieve dyspnea (e.g., position, medications) for them. An initial interview is an excellent time to determine the extent of the consequences of the symptom on functional status, social and role relationships, and quality of life. This knowledge about the symptom can assist the health care provider in formulating an individual treatment plan. The treatment program, including type and modality of exercise, frequency, and level of intensity of exercise, is, in part, determined by the severity of the symptom.

Ideally, dyspnea should be measured during baseline and outcome exercise testing with an incremental or endurance test and/or the 6-minute or shuttle walk to classify the symptom severity and the level of dyspnea the patient experiences with a certain amount of exercise (work). This measurement provides a baseline of symptom severity that can be used to evaluate the patient's progress through the intensive and maintenance phases of the program. When symptom reduction is a goal and an expected outcome of the pulmonary rehabilitation program, dyspnea also should be considered an outcome of pulmonary rehabilitation. In that context, dyspnea can be measured during preexercise and postexercise tests using incremental, endurance stress tests, 6-minute or shuttle walk tests. This knowledge about the symptom can assist the health care provider in formulating an individual treatment plan for each patient. The individualized treatment program, including type and modality of exercise, frequency, and level of intensity of exercise, in part, can be determined by the severity of the symptom.

In addition, during the rehabilitation program, dyspnea is monitored during exercise treatments to aid in the monitoring and coaching of patients to increasing levels of exercise or after the institution of a new therapy to measure the efficacy of a specific therapy. Dyspnea with ADLs at home can be measured at the beginning and as an outcome of pulmonary rehabilitation.

METHODS TO MEASURE DYSPNEA

Specific instruments that are commonly used in the clinical setting to measure dyspnea are briefly described. Extensive descriptions and the psychometric testing of these instruments are published elsewhere.[4,57,59,60]

Early attempts to evaluate the severity of dyspnea involved patient assessments of their own exercise tolerance (the Medical Research Council Scale, the American Thoracic Society Grade of Breathlessness Scale, and the Oxygen Cost Diagram).[61] Although such scales have been used in the past to define or characterize a patient sample and are simple to use, they require individuals to make comparisons to others, including items that measure more than one variable and have not been used recently to measure changes with therapeutic interventions. Therefore, they are not recommended for use in pulmonary rehabilitation programs.

Unidimensional Scales to Measure Dyspnea During Exercise

Either the visual analog scale (VAS) or the Modified Borg Scale for Breathlessness (Borg) can be used to measure dyspnea intensity during exercise stress tests before and after the program, during exercise treatments, and at home in a daily log of symptoms. Patients are asked to rate their shortness of breath at maximum exercise and at specific times during the exercise test. The patient can practice using the scale and should be given specific instructions regarding the exact sensation to be rated, such as shortness of breath, effort of breathing, etc.

It is important to determine the words that the individual patient uses to describe his or her dyspnea or shortness of breath before having him or her rate the dyspnea. Recently, words used to describe shortness of breath have been found to vary with different disease groups and different cultures.[62–66] With exercise, most patients reported increased "effort" and "heaviness" in breathing. Patients with chronic obstructive or interstitial lung disease were more likely to choose "increased inspiratory difficulty" and "unsatisfied inspiratory effort"; obstructed patients further identified "shallow breathing," and those with interstitial lung disease reported "rapid breathing."[67,68]

Visual Analog Scale (VAS)

The VAS is a vertical or horizontal line with anchors to indicate extremes of the sensation (Fig. 5-1). The VAS is most commonly 100 cm long. Patients indicate their dyspnea intensity by marking a line at the level of their dyspnea with their finger or a pencil. Anchors at the bottom and top should be no breathlessness and worst imaginable breathlessness. Concurrent validity with the Borg scale is high ($r = .90$), indicating that either of these rating scales can be used to rate the patient's dyspnea in your program and have the ability to compare these findings with those of others.[14,69] The VAS is reproducible at the same level of exercise and at maximal exercise.[70,71] It has demonstrated sensitivity to treatment effects.[72] Although most clinicians use the vertical VAS, the correlation between a horizontal and vertical VAS is reported at $r = .97$.[73]

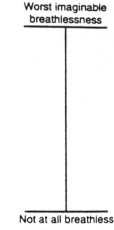

Figure 5-1. Visual analog scale.

Modified Borg Scale for Breathlessness (Borg)

The Borg scale to measure breathlessness is a 10-point scale with a nonlinear scaling scheme using descriptive terms to anchor responses.[74] This scale has strong and significant correlations with the VAS in patients with chronic obstructive pulmonary disease (COPD) ($r = .99$),[69] with minute ventilation ($r = .98$), and with oxygen consumption during exercise ($r = .95$).[13] Advantages of the Borg scale are that the scale is "open ended," the descriptors may help patients in selecting the sensation intensity, facilitate more absolute responses to stimuli, and allow direct comparisons between individuals. This scale also seems to be conceptually easier to use for older patients for exercise prescriptions than the VAS. Disadvantages are that the sensitivity of the scale may be blunted by "ceiling effects" triggered by the verbal descriptors and that patients may tend to only choose the numbers by the descriptors.

Numeric Rating Scale

Recently the Numeric Rating Scale, a 0 to 10 scale, has been shown to correlate well with the VAS and the Borg scale.[75] If the rehabilitation team or the patients prefer this type of scale it could be used; however, the lack of testing or ability to compare outcomes with other programs makes this scale less desirable at this time for measuring dyspnea during exercise.

Measurement of the Affective Responses to Dyspnea

We believe that the affective responses to dyspnea, for example, distress and anxiety related to dyspnea, also should be measured within a pulmonary rehabilitation program. Both healthy subjects[76] and patients with COPD[77] can distinguish the intensity of their shortness of breath from the anxiety and distress it is causing them while exercising. After a pulmonary rehabilitation program, some patients may not perceive a decrease in their intensity of the shortness of breath, especially if they are doing a higher level of exercise (working harder) with the same amount of dyspnea. In addition, dyspnea intensity has been found *not* to change over time with worsening physiologic changes.[78] Even in end-stage pulmonary disease, patients have been found to decrease their activity, essentially to almost immobility, while still rating their level of perceived dyspnea at the same intensity. Apparently patients tend to choose to decrease their level of activity rather than tolerating greater breathlessness. However, affective responses to dyspnea, such as anxiety or distress with the symptom, may decrease after pulmonary rehabilitation or exercise training.[77] In our research studies, patients have frequently commented that their shortness of breath may be at the same level after pulmonary rehabilitation, but they can do more activity with the same level of symptom, they are less anxious about the symptom, and they feel more in control of the symptom. The same amount of shortness of breath is less distressing for them.

The VAS or Borg scale can be used to measure the "distress" of the symptom for the patient with different instructions. Patients are asked to rate their response to the following questions on a Borg scale or VAS: "How anxious are you about your shortness of breath?" or "How bothersome or distressing is your shortness of breath to you?"

Multidimensional Indirect Measures of Dyspnea Targeted to Activities

Recently, investigators have used psychometrically tested instruments to gain a more comprehensive evaluation of dyspnea with activities. Instruments that can be used are the Baseline/Transitional Dyspnea Index (BDI/TDI), the dyspnea with activity scale of the Chronic Respiratory Questionnaire (CRQ), the University of California at San Diego Shortness of Breath Questionnaire (UCSDQ), and the Pulmonary Functional Status and Dyspnea Questionnaire (PFSDQ).

Daily logs can be used to monitor dyspnea with prescribed walking regimens or to demonstrate the impact on ADLs. The decision to use one or several of these instruments will depend on the outcome you wish to measure, the time available for administration, and the frequency with which the team is able and needs to measure the symptom and quality of life.

Baseline/Transitional Dyspnea Index

BDI/TDI measures functional impairment (the degree to which ADLs are impaired), magnitude of effort (the overall effort exerted to perform activities), and the magnitude of task that provokes the breathing difficulty. The focus is on the activity consequences of the individual's breathlessness. Content validity was established by correlation of scores of the BDI with the Medical Research Council Scale ($r = -.70, P < .01$) and the Oxygen Cost Diagram ($r = -0.54, P < .01$).[23,24] Interobserver agreement (interrater reliability) between physician and pulmonary technician has been evaluated by weighted percentages and weighted kappa. The results demonstrated a range across dimensions of 91 to 93 weighted percent agreement and a weighted kappa ranging from 0.66 to 0.73, demonstrating creditable agreement of the two observers.[79] The TDI measures the change in dyspnea from the baseline state to another point in time; typically after an intervention, such as pulmonary rehabilitation or pharmacologic therapy.[80,81]

Several randomized trials measuring effects of exercise training and rehabilitation programs,[80,81] inspiratory muscle training,[82] or theophylline therapy[83] have found significant reductions in dyspnea measured by the BDI/TDI after the interventions. The TDI also has been reported to correlate with changes in the Medical Outcomes Study Short-Form 36 Quality of Life domains of physical and social function, mental health, and general health perceptions.[84] Advantages include extensive testing and extensive use in research studies; therefore, you are able to compare your outcomes with those of other studies. A disadvantage of this instrument is that although dyspnea is a subjective sensation, the health care provider rates the functional consequences of dyspnea for the patient.

Pulmonary Functional Status and Dyspnea Questionnaire (PFSDQ)

The PFSDQ elicits rating of 79 activities in 6 categories: self-care (15 activities), mobility (14 activities), eating (8 activities), home management (22 activities), social (10 activities), and recreational (10 activities). The activities are independently evaluated for performance, as well as in association with dyspnea. Internal consistency of the activity and dyspnea components was 0.91 with high test–retest.[85,86] The level of dyspnea for many activities can be monitored over time, and the instrument is sensitive to small changes in dyspnea with activities.

The University of California at San Diego Shortness of Breath Questionnaire (UCSDQ)

The UCSDQ measures shortness of breath with daily activities before and after a rehabilitation program or therapy, is easy for the patient to understand, and does not take long to administer. Patients rate on a 6-point scale how frequently in the past week they had experienced shortness of breath during 21 ADLs associated with varying levels of exertion. Three additional questions ask about limitations caused by shortness of breath, fear of harm from overexertion, and fear of shortness of breath. Reliability and validity are reported.[87,88]

Disease-Specific Quality of Life Instruments: Instruments That Measure Dyspnea With Activities and Other Components of Quality of Life

Chronic Respiratory Questionnaire (CRQ)

The CRQ is a 20-item self-report questionnaire administered by an interviewer that measures four dimensions: dyspnea, fatigue, emotional function, and mastery of breathing.[34] The patient rates the level of dyspnea he or she has with five usual individual activities. The instrument requires a 15-minute interview; however, less time is required for repeated administrations. An advantage of this questionnaire is that many researchers have used it. Therefore, outcomes from one program can be compared with those from others, the instrument is responsive to therapy, and a level of change that can be used to judge a clinically significant change has been reported.[89] Reliability and responsiveness of the instrument have also been reported. Because the ratings for the dyspnea with activities scale are individualized, this dimension was found to have lower reliability in one study[90]; however, other investigators have found high reliability.[34]

St. George's Respiratory Questionnaire

The St. George's Respiratory Questionnaire is a disease-specific quality of life self-administered questionnaire listing 53 questions measuring three areas of illness: symptoms, activity, and impact of disease on daily life. The symptom category elicits information about cough, sputum, wheeze, and dyspnea. Test–retest reliability of the questionnaire in COPD patients is $r = .92$.[91] The instrument has been found to be responsive to treatments.[92] Thresholds of significant clinical change also are reported.[93] Advantages of this instrument are that it is self-administered, has computerized scoring, and has extensive psychometric testing. One disadvantage of this instrument is that dyspnea is not measured as a separate symptom; therefore, the dyspnea response to therapy cannot be measured separately.

DIAGNOSTIC APPROACH TO THE PATIENT WITH DYSPNEA: PROCEDURES AND METHODS

Diseases and Clinical States Presenting With Dyspnea

From the point of view of a pulmonary rehabilitation program, it is crucial to be sure that the patient has been properly diagnosed before beginning rehabilitation. Input from the rehabilitation team may play a major role in ensuring that adequate diagnostic studies have been done. Although patients with almost any disease may benefit from rehabilitation, it is important to be sure that they have received appropriate care for their underlying disease.

Any disease involving the respiratory system can present with dyspnea. Although the differential diagnosis usually focuses on diseases of the respiratory and cardiovascular systems, diseases of many other organ systems (e.g., neuromuscular, skeletal, renal, endocrine [including pregnancy[94]]), rheumatologic, hematologic, and psychiatric may affect the respiratory system and present with dyspnea.[95] A detailed description of the features that distinguish these disorders is beyond the scope of this chapter. The initial approach is greatly affected by whether this is an acute, subacute, or chronic problem. The differential diagnosis is relatively narrow for acute dyspnea (e.g., pneumonia, pulmonary embolism, congestive heart failure, myocardial infarction).[96] The differential diagnosis for chronic dyspnea is much broader.

The diagnostic approach to dyspnea may be thought of in terms of disease with mechanical limitations on the respiratory system, diseases with increased drive to breathe, and diseases affecting the central perception of the symptom. Many diseases (e.g., asthma) fall into more than one category. In search for a diagnosis, one may eventually perform tests to look for evidence of disease affecting all three. Diseases that mechanically interfere with ventilation result in increases in the work and effort of breathing, whether because of narrowing of the airways or changes in the elasticity of the lungs or chest wall. If the respiratory muscles are weakened, then the effort of breathing seems greater and this is experienced as greater dyspnea. If respiration is stimulated (e.g., by acidosis, hypoxia), the increased drive is perceived centrally as dyspnea. Abnormalities of ventilation–perfusion matching (e.g., pulmonary emboli) cause dyspnea directly through their secondary physiologic effects (e.g., hypoxemia, bronchospasm, or fall in cardiac output). Psychologic problems may exaggerate dyspnea of any cause, as well as cause dyspnea primarily.[97]

History

A comprehensive history and physical examination are required for the diagnosis of dyspnea. It is important to identify activities that provoke or relieve it. Input from family members or close acquaintances may clarify how limited a patient really is. It is worth noting that lung disease patients may report that they are more limited by "fatigue" or "leg fatigue" than by dyspnea. Key questions relate to persistence or variability of the symptom, aggravating factors (e.g., ambulation, eating, position, exposures), and medications or activities that help relieve the symptoms. For example, intermittent dyspnea is likely caused by asthma or heart failure, whereas persistent or progressive dyspnea suggests more chronic conditions (e.g., COPD, interstitial fibrosis, pulmonary hypertension). Dyspnea may occur in conditions where ventilation is stimulated by lactic acid production at relatively low levels of exercise (e.g., deconditioning, anemia, low cardiac output states). Nocturnal dyspnea is typical of asthma, congestive heart failure, gastroesophageal reflux, or even nasal obstruction.[98] As activity generally accentuates dyspnea of physiologic origin, dyspnea occurring independent of physical activity suggests allergic or psychologic problems. Dyspnea coming on after exercise suggests exercise-induced asthma. Although emotions may affect dyspnea of any cause, psychogenic dyspnea should be suspected when dyspnea varies greatly and is unrelated to physical activity,[97] or if an individual is involved in a lawsuit.[99]

Review of factors that may affect breathlessness (e.g., cigarettes, foods, medications, allergens) or relieve breathlessness (e.g., position, medications) is helpful. Obesity may aggravate dyspnea because of the effort of moving the extra weight and the increased metabolic demand. Cachexia may be associated with respiratory muscle weakness.[100] Sleep-disordered breathing may interact with other problems to increase dyspnea. Symptoms of systemic congestion (e.g., pitting edema, abdominal swelling) may suggest right ventricular failure of any cause (e.g., pulmonary hypertension, obstructive sleep apnea, left ventricular failure). Raynaud's phenomenon as well as skin, joint, or swallowing problems may suggest collagen vascular disease.

Physical Examination

Physical examination may provide vital clues to diagnosis: respiratory rate, body habitus (e.g., cachexia, obesity), posture, use of pursed lips, use of accessory muscles, and emotional state. Abnormal chest expansion may suggest restriction or severe hyperinflation. Cough on inspiration or expiration may suggest obstructive or interstitial lung disease, and a decrease in the intensity of the breath sounds may suggest emphysema, pneumothorax, or pleural effusion. Forced expiration may uncover focal or diffuse wheezing. The cardiac examination may suggest pulmonary hypertension (e.g., right ventricular heave, increased pulmonic sound) or right ventricular failure (e.g., jugular venous distention, hepatojugular reflux, pedal edema). Clubbing may be associated with many processes, notably cancer. Lower extremity edema suggests congestive failure if symmetrical and thromboembolic disease if asymmetrical.

Laboratory Evaluation

The laboratory is often not helpful in the diagnosis of dyspnea. Anemia may be a clue to occult bleeding or serious systemic problems. Polycythemia may suggest chronic hypoxemia. Elevation of the sedimentation rate may suggest occult inflammation in the lungs but is insensitive for inflammatory disease of the interstitium.[101] Laboratory testing may reveal unsuspected renal disease, metabolic acidosis, or thyroid disease.

The database should include chest radiographs, spirometry, and an electrocardiogram. Classic findings that are of help include hyperinflation, parenchymal infiltration, and pleural disease. Less obvious findings may include early findings of interstitial lung disease (e.g., decreases in lung volume or subtle increases in lung density). Though the yield of "routine" electrocardiography is low, it may reveal previously unsuspected coronary artery disease or even pulmonary hypertension (i.e., signs of right ventricular hypertrophy or strain).

Special Studies (Including Pulmonary Function)

Although pulmonary function tests are critical for the diagnosis of dyspnea, the degree of abnormality in tests of respiratory function correlates only moderately with severity of dyspnea.[102] Spirometry, including forced expiratory volume in 1 second (FEV_1) and forced vital capacity, are excellent screening tests for both obstructive and restrictive disease, though both may be normal despite significant asthma or interstitial fibrosis. As airway obstruction in asthma may be intermittent, peak flow monitoring with a portable meter at times of dyspnea in the home or in the workplace may be more useful. Arterial blood gases may reveal unexpected hypoxemia or hypercapnia.[103]

Cardiopulmonary exercise testing helps in determining whether exercise is limited by the pulmonary or cardiovascular system (or even some unrelated problem such as leg pain or fatigue). The breathing reserve (fraction of maximal ventilation not used at peak exercise) is useful in distinguishing obstructive disease from cardiac disease, even when cardiac response is similar (49.7% in the chronic heart failure group vs. 8.4% in the COPD group [$P < .01$] in one study).[104]

Unfortunately, exercise testing is insensitive for distinguishing cardiac disease from deconditioning.[105] If these studies are not sufficient for diagnosis, a broad array of other studies may be helpful. Spiral CT scanning of the chest with iodinated contrast is gradually replacing ventilation–perfusion lung scanning as the screening procedure of choice for the diagnosis of pulmonary embolic disease.[106,107] Gallium and high-resolution CT scanning are sensitive but not specific for occult infectious (e.g., *Pneumocystis carinii*) and inflammatory (e.g., interstitial pneumonitis) lung disease.[108,109] If exercise testing suggests cardiac dysfunction, echocardiography, radionuclide scanning, or even cardiac catheterization (preferably combined with supine exercise) may identify unsuspected wall motion abnormalities, valvular disease, or pulmonary hypertension.[110,111] An echocardiogram may reveal mitral valve prolapse, a rare cause of occult dyspnea, even with normal hemodynamics.[112]

If dyspnea is clearly unrelated to exercise, and especially if it increases with medical attention or emotional distress, psychologic consultation should be sought.[97,113] Patients with chronic lung disease are prone to anxiety and symptoms of panic, and patients with panic disorder may present with dyspnea as a primary symptom. Because the symptoms of panic attacks and lung disease may overlap, determination of the primary disorder may not always be easy.[114]

SYMPTOMATIC TREATMENTS FOR DYSPNEA

In some patients, dyspnea may remain an incapacitating symptom after traditional treatment strategies have been exhausted. At this point, treatment should focus on the symptom rather than on the disease. Ideally, treatment would focus on the specific mechanisms contributing to an individual's dyspnea (e.g., respiratory muscle dysfunction, hypoxemia, anxiety).[4] Unfortunately, it is difficult to be sure which factors are primarily responsible for the symptom in an individual patient, and the tests one might use (e.g., muscle testing, exercise testing with and without oxygen supplementation, psychometrics) are imprecise and time-consuming. A recent American Thoracic Society Position Statement[4] recommended whenever possible to attempt to target the therapeutic interventions to the physiologic or psychologic mechanism. This categorization of the physiologic mechanisms and appropriate therapeutic interventions is shown in (Table 5-1) and will be used to discuss alternative treatments for dyspnea. Until guidelines for specific therapy for dyspnea are established, a generic approach to treatment must be used, with focus on *(a)* reducing ventilatory demand, *(b)* reducing ventilatory impedance, *(c)* improving muscle function, and/or *(d)* altering the central perception of dyspnea.

Reduce Ventilatory Demand

Reduce Metabolic Load

Multicomponent Pulmonary Rehabilitation
Comprehensive pulmonary rehabilitation programs typically include many or all of the therapeutic interventions listed in Table 5-1. This combination of interventions within a comprehensive pulmonary rehabilitation program has been shown in *all* randomized clinical trials to result in improvement in dyspnea during laboratory exercise and with ADLs.[80,81,115–118] Evidence also suggests that this reduction in symptoms is maintained if reinforcement of education and a maintenance exercise program exist.[116]

The committee of the American College of Chest Physicians/American Association of Cardiovascular and Pulmonary Rehabilitation reviewed the research studies that have measured dyspnea as an outcome measure after pulmonary rehabilitation. Nine scientific studies measured dyspnea before and after an inpatient, outpatient, or home comprehensive pulmonary rehabilitation program. Five studies were randomized controlled trials,[80,81,115–117] one was a nonrandomized trial,[80] and two were observational studies.[119,120]

Every published study has shown an improvement in dyspnea following pulmonary rehabilitation. Using recently developed valid and reliable measurements of dyspnea, three randomized studies[81,115,116] and one nonrandomized study[80] found significant decreases in dyspnea during laboratory exercise testing for the group that had completed comprehensive pulmonary rehabilitation compared with a control group. One of these studies was longitudinal and reported that the decrease in dyspnea during laboratory exercise extended 24 months.[116]

Exercise Training Is Critical
Exercise training seems to be critical for the decrease in dyspnea during and after pulmonary rehabilitation programs. Exercise training alone also has been shown to decrease dyspnea.[121,122] Though most exercise studies have used treadmills or cycles, weight training of upper and lower limb muscles may also improve exercise performance and dyspnea.[123] Because upper extremity activity may be particularly troublesome for patients with COPD, training of these muscles may have an important impact on dyspnea.[124,125]

Table 5-1. Therapeutic Interventions for Dyspnea Targeted
to Pathophysiologic Mechanisms

Pathophysiologic Mechanisms	Therapeutic Intervention
Reduce ventilatory demand	
Reduce metabolic load	Exercise training—improve efficiency of carbon dioxide elimination
	Supplemental oxygen therapy
Decrease central drive	Supplemental oxygen therapy
	Pharmacologic therapy
	Opiate therapy
	Anxiolytic therapy
	Alter pulmonary afferent information: vibration, ventilator settings, inhaled pharmacologic therapy, fans
	Improve efficiency of carbon dioxide elimination: alter breathing pattern
Reduce ventilatory impedance	
Reduce/counterbalance lung hyperinflation	Surgical volume reduction: continuous positive airway pressure
Reduce resistive load	Pharmacologic therapy
Improve inspiratory muscle function	Nutrition
	Inspiratory muscle training
	Positioning
	Partial ventilatory support
	Minimizing use of steroids
Alter central perception	Education
	Cognitive-behavioral approaches
	Desensitization
	Pharmacologic therapy

With permission from American Thoracic Society. Dyspnea: mechanisms, assessment, and management: a consensus statement. Am J Respir Crit Care Med 1999;159(1):321–340.

Exercise training may improve dyspnea by many mechanisms. Most authors have reported improvement in neither pulmonary mechanics nor respiratory muscle strength.[126] Exercise training may result in true conditioning with decreased lactate production and thereby decreased stimulation of ventilation.[127] Increased mechanical efficiency (e.g., longer stride length)[128] may lower oxygen consumption and ventilation for a given activity.[116] Subtle changes in peripheral muscles as a result of training may result in decreased dyspnea, though the mechanisms are still being elucidated,[129] or through a process of desensitization defined as less perceived dyspnea for the same ventilation.[121] In addition, changes in mediating cognitive, emotional, sensory, and behavioral factors, such as self-efficacy, self-confidence, or anxiety with the symptom, may enhance the improvement in dyspnea.[35,130]

Exercise Prescription and "Dose"
It remains unclear how intense and how many sessions of exercise training are necessary to achieve improvement in dyspnea, with programs varying from 12 outpatient sessions in 4 weeks[121] to intense inpatient programs.[115] Although some have suggested "high-

intensity" training, approximately 80% of peak oxygen consumption to promote "conditioning,"[127,131] others have found improvement in dyspnea and exercise performance with lower levels of intensity of exercise training.[81,121,132] Findings of a meta-analysis of 14 clinical trials strongly supported pulmonary rehabilitation programs that include at least 4 weeks of exercise training for clinically statistically significant improvements in the dyspnea, with activities and mastery of breathing scales measured by the CRQ.[133]

Patients with symptomatic COPD can be taught to use both heart rate and dyspnea to monitor their level and length of daily exercise. In several studies, Mahler and colleagues[134–136] have shown that patients with COPD were able to use dyspnea ratings and heart rate to accurately and reliably produce an expected exercise intensity.

Activity Modification and Energy Conservation

Metabolic load can also be reduced by decreasing respiratory effort. Patients can learn energy conservation techniques that reduce physical effort so that less ventilatory effort is necessary. Dyspnea and fatigue are related to each other and are highly related to activity level.[32,33] Conservation of energy, activity modification, and advanced planning of activities decrease the amount of respiratory effort or minute ventilation and most probably fatigue, and, therefore, may decrease dyspnea.

Most of the information known about the relationship between energy conservation and dyspnea has been reported in descriptive studies.[32,137,138] A recent randomized study instructed one group in energy conservation techniques as part of a dyspnea management program and found minimal differences in dyspnea compared with a control health education group.[139] No randomized studies have examined the effect of teaching or using energy conservation techniques on dyspnea.

People with chronic shortness of breath describe complex planning to be able to carry out even ADLs, but especially sporadic vacations and adventures out of their daily environment. For people with chronic shortness of breath, some of the most difficult tasks are to learn to pace their activities, to slow down, and to conserve energy.[140] (Energy conservation is discussed in Chapter 13.) People can be taught to sit when possible while completing chores, avoid unnecessary motions, break the job down into steps, minimize steps in any task, avoid overreaching and bending by arranging equipment closely, use good posture and body mechanics, and use breathing techniques in performing any task.[141] Activities can be substituted that are pleasurable yet require less effort. For example, a hobby such as playing cards can be suggested as a less strenuous activity to replace the weekly golf game.

Patients need help with planning in advance for almost any activity. Trips should be organized early to allow time to anticipate the availability of oxygen, the altitude, the potential for triggers/irritants, the amount of energy needed, and the scheduling of rest periods. Daily walks, restaurant lunches, and activities need to be planned ahead of time to anticipate "breathing stations." Most clinicians suggest a "daily outline," dividing the day into morning, afternoon, late afternoon, and early evening, with exact activities and scheduled rests. Rest periods need to be a high priority.

Patients should be instructed that a crucial balance exists between pacing or resting and appropriate exercise. Graduated exercise and activity to stay physically conditioned has to be stressed while at the same time emphasizing the need for a slower pace. Teaching can include contrasting energy used for tasks that are unnecessary with energy used for leisure activities and daily exercises that will enhance the efficiency of the muscles and the body. It is important that teaching be individual, according to the intensity of the symptom, functional ability, daily routine, and home environment.

It is important to provide patients with guidelines for strategies for managing their shortness of breath during each of their daily activities. Management strategies targeted to the symptom of shortness of breath that might be included in teaching patients[130] include strategies for decreasing shortness of breath with dressing and bathing, homemaking, cooking, and meal preparation. The following are examples.

Strategies for Decreasing Dyspnea With Eating or Meal Preparation

Approximately one-third of patients with COPD are underweight. Dyspnea may be increased during meal preparation and eating because of energy requirements for chewing and arm movements, the reduction in airflow while swallowing, and oxygen desaturation.[142] In addition, many patients who are chronically short of breath often lose their appetite and desire to eat. Self-care strategies that can be taught to the patient to decrease dyspnea during eating are listed in Table 5-2.

In contrast, for some patients, obesity may contribute to shortness of breath. Patients may be motivated to lose weight if they understand that obesity restricts breathing volume and increases work of breathing; therefore, if they successfully lose weight, they most likely will have less shortness of breath. Helping patients to plan meals, constant encouragement, weighing the patient, and referral to a weight loss program and/or dietitian can help patients lose weight.

Strategies for Decreasing Dyspnea During Sexual Activity

Patients who are comfortable confiding in a health professional frequently complain of experiencing dyspnea during sexual activity. Strategies to decrease energy expenditure and dyspnea during sexual activity include planning a rest period and inhaled bronchodilators before sexual relations, use of supplemental oxygen, appropriate timing of sexual relations before meals and after resting, avoiding positions that require supporting body weight or that increase pressure on the chest, and choosing less active positions for the partner with lung disease.[143] Patients should be reminded of alternative expressions of love, including holding hands, caressing, sharing favorite times, and conversation. (See Chapter 17 for a complete discussion of this topic.)

Decrease Central Drive

Supplemental Oxygen Therapy

Because dyspnea is so closely related to respiratory drive, treatments that can reduce the drive (e.g., oxygen, opiates) may reduce dyspnea. Oxygen can reduce carotid body output[144] and the ventilatory response to exercise[145-147] Conflicting evidence exists about whether oxygen has a direct central effect on dyspnea apart from its effect on ventilation mediated through the carotid bodies.[13,18,148-150] Beneficial effects of oxygen on dyspnea that are unrelated to reduction in respiratory drive include effects on ventilatory muscle function[151] and pulmonary artery pressure[152]; these might explain improvement in dyspnea apart from effects on respiratory drive.

The dose of oxygen should be titrated to prevent desaturation,[153] though higher doses may be more beneficial for dyspnea during exercise.[147,152] Though patients believe that oxygen after exercise will speed recovery, a randomized blinded trial did not find that postexercise oxygen supplementation affected dyspnea recovery time after a submaximal treadmill test.[154] The value of oxygen solely for treatment of dyspnea (i.e., without hyp-

Table 5-2. Self-Care Strategies for Decreasing Dyspnea During Eating

Preparing meals in advance, allowing rest time before eating
Eating smaller portions more frequently
Avoiding high carbohydrate and gas-forming foods
Assuming a body position that minimizes perceived work of breathing and using pursed-lips breathing
Using oxygen during meals
Using liquid supplements between meals to provide nutrition without the work of chewing
Eating with significant others in a pleasing environment

oxemia), even if its value is shown during blinded testing, remains controversial and may not be reimbursed by third-party payers.[152,155]

Treatment aimed specifically at receptors or reflex pathways have been investigated. Topical anesthetics aimed at airway receptors that might mediate dyspnea have not been able to affect either ventilatory responses or dyspnea.[46,156] In experimental studies, stimulation of the nasal mucosa with oxygen cannulae,[155] facial stimulation with cold air,[25] and in-phase chest vibration[42,43] have all been shown to reduce dyspnea. Although the mechanisms of these interventions are uncertain, they might stimulate peripheral receptors whose activation might inhibit dyspnea, offering hope for treatment of dyspnea with therapy directed at peripheral receptors. The clinical relevance of these interventions is uncertain at present.

Pharmacologic Therapy

Opiate Therapy. Although opiates do have pharmacologic effects that might modulate dyspnea (e.g., reduce ventilation at rest, with exercise, and with hypoxia[12,157–160]), fear of respiratory depression has discouraged their therapeutic use.[161] Opiates have been enthusiastically recommended for clinical treatment of dyspnea in uncontrolled trials[159]; however, longitudinal placebo-controlled outpatient studies have shown inconsistent benefits and frequent side effects.[162–165] A recent controlled 14-week crossover study with 16 patients with severe stable COPD looked at the value of long-acting morphine for treatment of dyspnea and improvement in quality of life.[166] Exercise performance measured by 6-minute walks, dyspnea, and mastery (measured by the CRQ) were not improved or actually deteriorated. Almost all of the subjects experienced significant, though not life-threatening, side effects.

Although results of controlled studies discourage routine use of opiates for stable outpatients with COPD, they may still be appropriate for treatment of dyspnea in a carefully selected individual patient with far-advanced but not yet terminal disease.[167] In such patients, it is important to educate them about the risks and side effects that they may encounter so that they may make informed decisions. Although constipation and nausea can usually be controlled, central nervous side effects may be limiting. Regular medical use of opiates may result in physiologic dependence, but this is not unexpected and is clearly distinct from opiate addiction, which is a behavioral syndrome involving drug seeking for nonmedical purposes.

Anxiolytic Therapy. Centrally acting pharmacologic agents have a limited role in the treatment of dyspnea. Although controlled studies of unselected COPD patients have shown no benefit of anxiolytics,[165,168–170] they may still be useful in controlling dyspnea in carefully selected patients when anxiety is known to trigger their dyspnea.[171,172] It is important to determine by asking the patient whether anxiety or dyspnea is the primary symptom. Which sensation do they feel first or which sensation triggers the other?

Antidepressant Therapy. Little information is available on antidepressants and dyspnea, but a recent small case series suggested that sertraline, a serotonin reuptake inhibitor, in doses of 25 to 100 mg/d may be useful in treatment of dyspnea even in patients who are not otherwise considered candidates for antidepressant therapy.[173] The mechanism of improvement was uncertain but was thought possibly to be related to impact on mood or anxiety. In two cases of dyspnea caused by fibromyalgia, a multisystemic illness of controversial origin, an antidepressant, amitriptyline, was found to be remarkably effective for both dyspnea and other symptoms of the disease.[174]

Alter Pulmonary Afferent Information

Vibration. Stimulation of the chest wall with external vibration can lessen experimentally induced dyspnea.[42,43] The vibration must be given in phase with inspiration. This form of vibration was found to reduce the breathing discomfort of breathholding but not that of exercise. The value in clinical practice of applying in phase vibration to the chest wall is unknown. To the authors' knowledge this approach is not currently being utilized in any rehabilitation program.

Inhaled Opiate Therapy. Based on the concept of opiate receptors in the airways, inhalation of opiates has been examined as a way of relieving dyspnea without the side effects of systemic administration. Although earlier studies showed positive results[175,176]; subsequent controlled studies have shown disappointing results for exercise performance and dyspnea.[177–179] The findings are contradictory at best, but anecdotal reports are sufficient to justify a trial in patients with terminal illness and intolerance of oral or transcutaneous delivery.[180] As optimal doses are uncertain, individual titration to symptom relief without unacceptable side effects is required.

Fans. People with chronic dyspnea have described their use of fans or fresh air as one strategy for managing their dyspnea[32] In the laboratory, cool air on the face has decreased dyspnea in normal volunteers in response to hypercapnia and inspiratory resistive loads.[25] Although this modality has not been tested in pulmonary patients, cool air or a fan can be suggested as strategies for managing dyspnea.

Improve Efficiency of Carbon Dioxide Elimination: Altered Breathing Pattern

Breathing Retraining and Pursed-Lips Breathing. Clinically we observe and patients report that using pursed-lips breathing (PLB) during periods of acute dyspnea or during ADLs is the most important strategy they have for decreasing shortness of breath. The exact reason for this decrease in dyspnea for some patients during PLB is still unknown. Some have suggested that PLB provides distraction and that this enables the patient to slow breathing. Investigators have found a slowing of respiratory rate; a substantial increase in tidal volume; increased rib cage, accessory, and abdominal muscle recruitment; less recruitment and resting of the diaphragm; and improved oxygen saturation. All of these changes in pattern of breathing and oxygenation may reduce the respiratory effort and decrease dyspnea for an individual patient.[181–183] Education about these techniques is a fundamental part of pulmonary rehabilitation programs (see Chapter 6).

To date, only physiologic measures have been used in earlier studies to investigate the effect of diaphragmatic and abdominal breathing techniques on pulmonary function. The duration of treatment, type of technique, and length of measurement time varied considerably. Collectively, these studies found an increase in tidal volume and vital capacity and a decrease in respiratory rate, functional residual capacity, and oxygen consumption.[184,185]

Presumably these changes in lung function would result in a concomitant decrease in dyspnea. However, different investigators have studied the effect of diaphragmatic breathing on thoracoabdominal motion and found that this technique increases asynchronous and paradoxic breathing in COPD patients.[186,187] Therefore, the true effect of abdominal and diaphragmatic breathing on ventilatory function or dyspnea is unknown.

Reduce Ventilatory Impedance

Reduce/Counterbalance Lung Hyperinflation

Lung Volume Reduction Surgery
The advent of lung volume reduction surgery for relief of dyspnea in advanced emphysema deserves special mention.[188,189] Removal of multiple bullous or emphysematous portions of the lungs reduces the size of the lungs and improves lung recoil. Though a large multicenter controlled trial is currently under way to define the indications and benefits of this expensive and risky procedure, numerous reports have highlighted the potentially dramatic improvement in pulmonary function and dyspnea that may occur. Improvement in dyspnea may be explained by the combination of the decreased end-expiratory lung volume relative to total lung capacity, decreased respiratory rate, and the ability to increase

tidal volume.[190,191] Pulmonary rehabilitation is considered a vital part of the preparation for this potentially dramatic surgical procedure.

Continuous Positive Airway Pressure

Continuous positive airway pressure during exercise alleviates dyspnea provoked by exercise or by weaning from the ventilator by the addition of partial ventilatory support, which reduces the effort required to breathe.[192–194] Nasal pressure support ventilation for 2 hours for 5 consecutive days also decreased dyspnea at rest in nonintubated COPD patients.[195] Currently, no studies have examined the long-term effect of partial ventilatory support on dyspnea.

Reduce Resistive Load

Pharmacologic Therapy

Inhaled β_2-adrenergic agonists, inhaled anticholinergics, and sustained-release theophylline have all been shown in randomized clinical trials to improve dyspnea in patients with stable COPD. It has been suggested that this improvement may be related to reduced operational lung volumes associated with an increase in FEV_1.[4] These bronchodilators are expected usual medical therapy and provide an initial minimal, yet important, decrease in dyspnea. In fact, we have observed that frequently after learning to correctly administer their medications with a metered dose inhaler and spacer, patients will report a good deal of relief from their unrelenting dyspnea.

Improve Inspiratory Muscle Function

Nutrition

Nutritional repletion can improve respiratory muscle function[196,197] and decrease dyspnea in cachectic patients with COPD.[100] One randomized clinical trial that examined the effects of a 4-month nutrition supplementation program on dyspnea, measured with the VAS and Oxygen Cost Diagram, showed no significant improvement.[198]

Ventilatory Muscle Training

If ventilation limits exercise tolerance, then strengthening the respiratory muscles should improve maximal ventilation, and exercise performance and dyspnea should decrease.[199] Although strength training of the inspiratory muscles remains somewhat controversial,[200] a few studies have reported significant reductions in dyspnea.[82,201,202] Significant correlations occurred between changes in maximum inspiratory pressure and changes in dyspnea ratings.

Positioning

Patients with COPD have described the importance of "breathing stations" or places where they can rest when they are short of breath in their attempts to carry out normal activities like shopping or doing housework.[203] Adults and children with chronic lung disease have described standing still, being "motionless," "keeping still," "staying quiet," or finding a "breathing station to sit or lean on during acute dyspnea."[32,204] Studies have shown a decrease in dyspnea with the leaning forward position and a reduction in respiratory effort and the use of accessory muscles in the head-down position.[205,206] The important principle for the health care provider working in pulmonary rehabilitation is to allow the patient to assume the position in which he or she feels more breathing comfort and less shortness of breath. The patient's awareness of this position can be heightened, and the use of this position as a dyspnea management strategy in daily activities should be reinforced.

Partial Ventilatory Support

Although it is intuitively appealing to "rest" respiratory muscles (e.g., with nasal ventilation) that are chronically "fatigued" so that they will perform better with less dyspnea,[207,208] the value of doing so has not been established.[209–212] Patient tolerance of the available devices is a major problem.[211,213]

Minimizing Use of Steroids

Steroids can be used to reduce ventilatory impedance from airway inflammation and to increase vital capacity in interstitial diseases. However, the deleterious effects of muscle wasting and weakness must be considered when prescribing steroids for the symptom of dyspnea.[4] Steroid-dependent patients need to be monitored for reductions in muscle strength and function.

Medications That Increase Muscle Strength

Medications that improve muscle contractility might also affect dyspnea.[34,214,215] The value of theophylline for augmenting inspiratory muscle function remains controversial,[216–220] but the data are sufficient[83] to justify a cautious therapeutic trial in the persistently dyspneic COPD patient.

Alter Central Perception

Cognitive Behavioral Approaches

Benefits of Distraction Versus Attention Strategies

If a stressful life occurrence is acute, relatively brief, and has no serious consequences, distraction can be a useful means with which to cope.[221] Avoiding the noxious stimulus may provide more benefits than attention strategies if used early after a crisis or upset. However, when the noxious stimuli continues and is experienced chronically, attention strategies are associated with more positive outcomes.[221] Attention becomes more beneficial over time, when the individual may be more able to actively and successfully confront the situation. In general, research findings suggest that using attentional coping strategies (e.g., symptom monitoring, information seeking) to cope with chronic problems such as pain or arthritis is associated with better illness adjustment, whereas using coping strategies that avoid the problem (e.g., hoping, praying, ignoring, denial, attention diversion) results in higher levels of physical and psychologic disability and poorer adjustment to illness.[222,223]

Self-Care Strategies Described by Patients

Self-care strategies learned and used by patients themselves to cope with chronic dyspnea have been described and compared across different pulmonary diseases.[137,138,140] They span every category of intervention that is listed in Table 5-1. Environmental and social strategies included postponing, prioritizing, and careful planning; "breathing stations"; avoiding precipitants; and making environmental alterations. Taking medications and using breathing strategies are examples of physiologic strategies. Cognitive–behavioral strategies included focusing on the positive aspects of life, normalization or minimization, pacing activities, reminiscing and reflecting, and problem solving.

People with chronic shortness of breath become excellent "symptom managers." They develop a "repertoire" of management strategies for dyspnea. The patient in a rehabilitation program can be asked to describe or list the strategies he or she typically use at home to decrease their shortness of breath. These strategies should be practiced and reinforced during the program. People with chronic dyspnea become skilled in knowing their exercise tolerance relative to the amount of exposure for infection and the level of tolerable dyspnea and learn to regulate their activity accordingly.

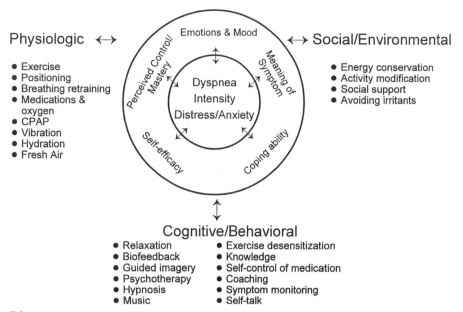

Figure 5-2. Strategies to modulate dyspnea perception and interpretation. (Reprinted with permission from Carrieri-Kohlman V, Gormley J. Coping strategies for dyspnea. In: Mahler D, ed. Dyspnea, Lung Biology in Health and Disease. New York: Marcel Dekker, 1998:287–313.)

Attention Strategies

Education. Few patients living with chronic dyspnea care about physiologic changes in their lungs, that is, the severity of FEV_1 or their hypoxemia. They are more interested in learning about strategies to manage symptoms on a day-to-day basis so they can keep their activity level the same or greater. Education should focus on symptom management versus the disease process. Teaching sessions provide patients with coping and self-care strategies that can be used in the future and enhance their feeling of control and mastery over their shortness of breath.[141,224–226] Learning new strategies for managing dyspnea has been found to enhance cognitive variables, such as the perception of self-efficacy and control over the symptom. Pulmonary rehabilitation increases self-efficacy for managing dyspnea in varied situations[227] and increases the feeling of mastery or control of difficulty breathing.[133] These cognitive perceptions may have an indirect effect on the perception of dyspnea intensity or distress, as shown in Figure 5-2.[130] The belief of patients that they have behavioral strategies to cope with a symptom decreases the distress of the symptom in other illnesses.[228] Patients can be taught the principles of self-care for both acute and chronic dyspnea described in Tables 5-3 and 5-4.

The positive effects of education programs on patients with asthma has been established.[229] However, in patients with COPD, education alone has not been systematically evaluated apart from other components of pulmonary rehabilitation. One exception was the study of Sassi-Dambron and coworkers,[139] which compared education and practice about dyspnea management strategies with general health education lectures. The experimental treatment group did not differ in dyspnea measures or 6-minute walking distance from the control group; however, it has been suggested that the investigators did not control for knowledge level or application of the dyspnea management strategies.[4]

A recent study showed that treadmill exercise training with and without nurse coaching is equally effective in reducing dyspnea during exercise testing and with ADLs.[121] In that study, nurse coaching involved teaching dyspnea management strategies, goal setting, relaxation, and PLB, all of which are common elements of rehabilitation programs. It is proposed that the group without nurse coaching consisted of patients with chronic pulmonary disease who already had developed a repertoire of dyspnea management skills and with supervised exercise were able to use these skills.

Two earlier studies contradict the above findings of Sassi-Dambron and colleagues. One study using teaching and counseling by a nurse compared to three other groups (nonspecific surveillance with psychotherapy, analytic psychotherapy from experienced psychotherapists, and supportive psychotherapy from experienced psychotherapists) found that the group treated by the nurse was the only one that experienced a "sustained relief in breathlessness."[230] In addition, more recently, eight interactive small-group education-only sessions did significantly decrease dyspnea with activity, measured by the CRQ, compared with untreated controls. No associated changes occurred in the 12-minute walk or pulmonary function variables.[231]

Self-Management of Medication Regimens. Clinically and in research studies we observed that just teaching the patient to correctly use their metered dose inhaler to deliver medications may decrease reported dyspnea and increase their exercise performance. Therefore, all patients should be taught the correct use of the inhaler with return demonstration. Management of dyspnea in the face of severe episodic or continuous symptoms may require that patients learn to manipulate complex medication regimens. Patients can be taught early symptom recognition and awareness of signs and symptoms of infection so that the dose or type of medications can be altered by the patient before later contact with the physician. This early recognition of increasing dyspnea and cough may prevent exacerbation of acute illness.

Monitoring Triggers and Intensity of Shortness of Breath. Patients can be taught different factors that may make their dyspnea worse or better by discussing the list of factors illustrated in Table 5-5 to individualize the experience. Recording the intensity and the timing of dyspnea in daily logs or health diaries can be useful for both the patient and the health care provider to identify a baseline level of the symptom, triggers, patterns, and timing of the symptom, as well as providing a measure of effectiveness for treatments. Monitoring of other symptoms has been reported to help patients and providers understand the contribution of other cognitive and emotional factors and improve adherence to a treatment regimen. Daily symptom monitoring also provides more accurate reflection of symptoms than does recall during maintenance phases.[232,233]

Social Support
Although clinical observations suggest that sharing experiences and strategies for dealing with dyspnea with others may reduce the intensity of dyspnea and distress associated with

Table 5-3. Tips for Coping with Acute Episodes of Dyspnea

1. Assess severity of the episode by rating how short of breath you feel on a scale of 1 to 10.
2. Monitor changes in your body that alert you to increased shortness of breath. Call health-care provider if shortness of breath changes in frequency or intensity. If you have asthma, measure peak flow rate with a peak flow meter. If the value is lower than your baseline, use a metered-dose inhaler with sustained inspiration and breath-holding. Take a second puff and then measure peak flow rate again. Tell your health-care provider the values you have recorded when you call.
3. Use all the techniques you have learned to decrease your shortness of breath: pursed-lip breathing, relaxation, abdominal breathing, position, fluids, fans, and medication, including those delivered by nebulizer. Simple relaxation or meditation strategies may relax you and permit slower, deeper breathing, thus allowing a sense of control over breathing.
4. Evaluate your response to the strategies and medications you have tried. If symptoms have not markedly improved, proceed to the clinic, doctor's office, or emergency room without delay.

Reprinted with permission from Carrieri-Kohlman V, Janson-Bjerklie S. Coping and self-care strategies. In: Dyspnea. Mahler DA, ed. Mount Kisco, NY: Futura, 1990:220.

Table 5-4. Tips for Coping with Chronic Dyspnea

1. Know your own pattern of episodes. Monitor your shortness of breath. Know what brings your attacks on or makes them worse. Make it predictable! Evaluate severity of episodes by rating how short of breath you feel on a scale of 1 to 10. Monitor signs of infection such as tightness, changes in sputum, fatigue, and increased cough; start medication, oxygen, etc., as necessary.

2. If you have asthma, measure peak flow at least daily in the early morning upon arising, before medications. Know your normal baseline peak flow. Measure twice daily before medications in the early morning and at bedtime, if possible. If peak flow drops in the A.M. to 50% of the P.M. value or 50% of previous known value for 2 days, seek help from health-care provider. Keep a record of your peak flow. When you have an altered pattern, know what your baseline is and how far you have deviated from your normal baseline.

3. Identify and prioritize strategies that work for you to reduce the intensity and distress of your symptoms. Use any techniques that decrease your shortness of breath in the order that works best for you. Try to exercise every day and "move through" graduated levels of shortness of breath so you can tolerate more shortness of breath.

4. Have a crisis plan. Know what you will do in the event of a severe episode that does not get better with medications that you carry with you. Know how to get to medical help quickly. Have a partner or friend that you can call for help to get to the emergency room or the clinic quickly.

5. Plan ahead. Before going into a new situation, think of what you will do if you become short of breath. Keep resources and medications handy. Don't get caught without your medicine and other resources that help you get through a situation. Anticipate activities, plan far ahead so you can conserve energy and make arrangements, and determine "breathing stations."

6. Get the information and the data that you need to cope with shortness of breath by forming a partnership in self-management with your health-care provider. Prepare a list of questions you want answered before you go to your clinic appointments. Ask for resources and help, including phone numbers to use when you need advice and support. Ask your health-care provider what the medications that are ordered are supposed to do for you and what you can reasonably expect. Teach other people, including physicians, nurses, and family, the strategies that you have learned so they can help you use them during acute shortness of breath.

Reprinted with permission from Carrieri-Kohlman V, Janson-Bjerklie S. Coping and self-care strategies. In: Dyspnea. Mahler DA, ed. Mount Kisco, NY: Futura, 1990:221.

Table 5-5. Factors Related to Shortness of Breath

1. Irritants (smoke, smog)
2. Altitude
3. Living situations/stairs
4. Ventilation/air conditioning
5. Humidity/weather
6. Distractions like music, TV
7. Infections
8. Other illnesses
9. Congestion
10. Breathing pattern (rate and depth of breath)
11. Exercise/activity
12. Mood (depression, anxiety)
13. Social support (friends/community/financial resources)
14. Stress
15. Lack of understanding (lung problem, medications, treatments)

it,[26,234] no controlled trials show the effect of support groups on the symptom. In one study, the level of dyspnea was related to the number of persons in the social support network, amount of material aid, affirmation, and affection. The frequency of contact with others was also positively related to the intensity of dyspnea.[32] However, evidence also suggests that some patients need to be alone when they are experiencing extreme dyspnea.[26,235] The key issues for relating social support and symptom outcomes are the timing and matching of the type, amount, and source of social support to the person's needs. If the dyspnea is escalated by anxiety and/or depression, formal or informal psycho-therapy or counseling may be helpful.[236,237]

Distraction Strategies

Active distraction, or removing oneself from a noxious physical sensation or from one's own reaction to it, can increase physical tolerance and modify both physiologic arousal and psychologic distress. This often facilitates tolerance of and adaptation to the physical stressor.[226] During acute dyspnea, distraction is often effective in the short term because it is difficult to focus on two demands at once. Adults with asthma report using television, distancing themselves from a trigger, and other stimuli to distract themselves.[32] Children report various types of distraction, including music and "walking anywhere and looking at things that are good, like flowers and trees."[204]

Relaxation Techniques. It has long been observed clinically that dyspnea and anxiety increase in a summative fashion. Two controlled studies have shown this relationship to be true. In a small sample of asthmatic patients, anxiety was higher during high levels of dyspnea in an emergency department.[238] In another study, patients rated their anxiety related to dyspnea greater as their intensity of dyspnea increased during treadmill stress testing.[121] If dyspnea is increased by anxiety or panic, relaxation that is presumed to decrease anxiety would be expected to decrease dyspnea. This has been true during the actual relaxation sessions; however, in the two available studies the effect of relaxation treatments on subsequent dyspnea was not maintained.[239,240] Although the long-term effects with small samples are questionable, relaxation is clinically observed to provide a response that is incompatible with anxiety and muscle tension and may help escalating dyspnea in panic situations. Patients report more feeling of control of their breathing, slow their respiratory rate, and increase their volume of breaths, all of which have been shown to be related to dyspnea in the laboratory.

Relaxation can take many forms depending on which method works for the patient. Most relaxation methods include the use of a quiet environment, a comfortable position, loose clothing, some type of word or imagery repeated in a systematic fashion, slow abdominal breathing with deep breaths and slow expirations, and systematic tensing or relaxing of muscles, including concentrating on the muscles. Various "relaxation" tapes are available, and individualized tape recordings with a therapist can be used to coach patients throughout a session in the home.[241]

Biofeedback. Using patients' own respiratory parameters to help chronic pulmonary patients change their breathing pattern, biofeedback has been shown to reduce the respiratory rate and paradoxical breathing, increase tidal volume, and decrease weaning time.[242,243] However, to date the effect of biofeedback on dyspnea has not been reported.

Music. Listening to music impacts cognitive and emotional processes, which can distract people sufficiently so that they do not attend to internal sensory information to the same extent.[244] Thornby and colleagues[245] found that at every level of treadmill exercise, perceived "respiratory effort" was lower in patients with COPD while listening to music than while listening to gray noise or silence. Patients also performed significantly more exercise while listening to music. The gray noise was not as effective as music, indicating that the content of the distracting stimulus is important in determining its distractive power. The authors interpreted these findings as evidence that music allows a person to exercise more by decreasing the discomfort of breathing.

Hypnosis. Hypnosis is a trance state that combines a heightened inner awareness with a diminished awareness of one's surroundings. It has been suggested that hypnosis may bring about a type of "desensitization" by modifying the cortical centers. Grading dyspnea as severe, moderate, slight, or none, 16 patients with asthma had a decrease in their dyspnea from prehypnosis to immediately posthypnosis. The decrease in dyspnea was sustained at 30 minutes after hypnosis.[246]

More recently, in one patient with severe COPD, hypnotically induced relaxation and biofeedback with peak expiratory flow rate was measured in an attempt to reduce dyspnea during periods of anxiety. Respiratory rate and anxiety decreased and oxygen saturation and peak expiratory flow rate increased. The author infers that hypnotic relaxation and peak flow feedback may increase tolerance for chronic dyspnea.[247]

Guided Imagery. Guided imagery is another method of distraction that can be used in a comfortable position or while exercising. Patients are asked to allow their minds to take them to a desirable scene and focus on something other than their uncomfortable breathing. It can be a structured method with tapes or used in an informal way while the patient is exercising. In one uncontrolled study of the effect of guided imagery on dyspnea, depression, quality of life, anxiety, and functional status, 19 patients with COPD met weekly for 4 weeks for 1 hour of practice with guided imagery. As a standard guided imagery script was read, patients were asked to visualize the scene described. Audiotapes of the script were provided for twice daily patient practice.[248] Dyspnea did not change significantly in this uncontrolled study.

Self-talk. Self-talk is a form of cognitive restructuring. It can be used by patients to "think positively" not only in acute dyspnea but also to maintain daily self-management skills. This strategy was included in a cognitive–behavioral exercise program tested for its effect on exercise adherence in COPD patients; however, it is not possible to separate the individual effect of this strategy from other strategies in the program.[249]

Graduated Levels of Dyspnea or "Exercise Desensitization"

Clinically, one approach to decreasing a patient's perceived dyspnea for a certain activity level has been to encourage exercise to the point that moderate to severe dyspnea occurs, while coaching the patient to use breathing strategies such as PLB. If this procedure is performed in a supportive environment with someone the patient trusts, the patient's fear of dyspnea may decrease while confidence is gained in the ability to control the symptom. This empiric observation was first reported for patients with COPD after participation in research protocols when the investigators observed that even control subjects described less fear and anxiety with dyspnea at home after participating in exercise testing.[234,237] The investigators suggested that this decrease in the anxiety associated with dyspnea was caused by a type of "systematic desensitization" that occurred because of a decrease in dyspnea as a result of exposure to a greater-than-usual level of exercise in a safe, monitored environment. These authors seemed to suggest that this process of desensitization was a decrease in the fear accompanying the breathlessness rather than a decrease in dyspnea, per se.

Based on findings from the study of social learning theory, we proposed a dyspnea management model in which we hypothesized that similar to phobias and other symptoms, repeated exposure to dyspnea in a safe, monitored environment would result in increased and more effective coping skills, a change in the appraisal of the symptom, and decreased anxiety and distress about the dyspnea, therefore, an increased tolerance for the symptom (Fig. 5-3).[250] Other investigators have measured patients' ratings of the intensity of dyspnea itself and reported that repeated exercise may result in desensitization to the symptom (i.e., where the same ventilatory stimulus results in less dyspnea so that patients tolerate more exercise before reaching their maximal levels of dyspnea).[80,81,251] We subsequently showed that this experience increases their control or self-efficacy of coping with the

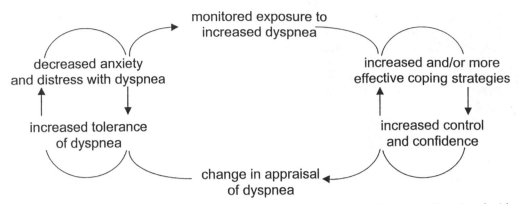

Figure 5-3. A suggested mechanism to decrease the anxiety and distress of dyspnea. (Reprinted with permission from Carrieri KV, Douglas MK, Gormley JM, et al. Desensitization and guided mastery: treatment approaches for the management of dyspnea. Heart Lung 1993;22[3]:226–234.)

symptom and changes the appraisal of dyspnea or heightens the "perceptual threshold" for dyspnea so that the dyspnea intensity is less for a given level of work.[121] Desensitization may be especially important because it may occur regardless of the ability to improve physical exercise performance.[121,126,252] The precise mechanism of a decrease in dyspnea relative to ventilation after exercise is unknown. Exercise has been suggested as the strongest treatment to bring about desensitization to dyspnea.[244] In any one patient it is difficult to know which of these many mechanisms is operant, but for clinical purposes it may not be very important.

Treatment programs for other symptoms, such as pain, place emphasis on how the treatment affects an individual's confidence and ability to cope with specific threats or sense of control over that symptom. Components of these programs may include *(a)* mastery of graduated small subtasks, *(b)* construction of short-term goals, *(c)* physical support and protective aids, *(d)* modeling of activities and coping strategies by the therapist, *(e)* elimination of defensive maneuvers, *(f)* varied performance of the task, and *(g)* gradual increase in time with the feared stimulus.[253] These components are not unlike strategies that should be used while patients are exercising in pulmonary rehabilitation programs or at home to increase their tolerance for shortness of breath. Typical "coaching" maneuvers while patients are exercising in a pulmonary rehabilitation program might include development of short-term goals, modeling of breathing strategies and relaxation techniques, small increases in work load and duration of exercise, distraction, encouragement, and feedback of physiologic parameters.

SUMMARY

Dyspnea is a complex symptom that arises from the central processing of information relayed from the respiratory center and integrated within the psychologic and intellectual makeup of the individual. It is still unclear whether a final common pathway exists for the sensation, but much is being learned from studying dyspnea both in normal volunteers in the laboratory with induced dyspnea (e.g., with exercise or gas mixtures) and in patients with spontaneous or induced dyspnea. It is clear that dyspnea is not one sensation but many, and that nuances of it relate to some extent to the stimulus (i.e., the nature of the physiologic dysfunction). It is exacerbated by stimuli to ventilation, but correlation with physiologic dysfunction is moderate at best.

Dyspnea may be caused by diseases in virtually any organ system, whether owing to

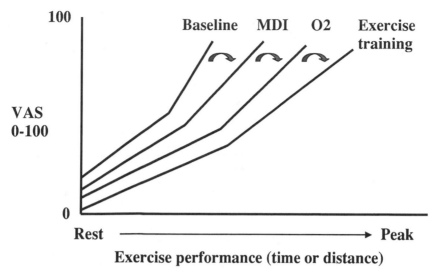

Figure 5-4. Potentially additive effects of different dyspnea treatments on the response to exercise. Bronchodilators, oxygen, and exercise training can each increase the amount of work or exercise individuals can do before reaching their maximum tolerable level of dyspnea. The relative benefit of each of these treatments would vary from individual to individual. Note that the maximum tolerable level of dyspnea tends to stay about the same. (Adapted with permission from American Thoracic Society. Dyspnea: mechanisms, assessment, and management: a consensus statement. Am J Respir Crit Care Med 1999;159[1]:321–340.)

interference with breathing, increased demand for breathing, or effective weakening of the respiratory pump. Diagnosis of dyspnea requires a comprehensive database that will uncover many of the causes. When the cause is not obvious, a series of studies assessing cardiopulmonary function at rest and with exercise will usually uncover a specific diagnosis. Sophisticated studies of the heart, pulmonary vascular bed, lung parenchyma, and even esophagus may be necessary. Psychogenic or behavioral dyspnea should usually be a diagnosis of exclusion after detailed clinical and physiologic evaluation.

Treatment of dyspnea is most effective when based on a specific diagnosis. When treatment of the underlying disease is inadequate, treatment focused on the symptom per se is appropriate. A combination of education, medications, exercise training, oxygen, and muscle strengthening will help most patients control and/or increase their tolerance for this disabling chronic symptom (Fig. 5-4).

As with other symptoms, the experience of dyspnea is affected by many factors, including education, cultural background, knowledge of the disease, emotional state, bodily preoccupation, previous experience with illness, judgment about the intensity of the activity that brings it on, and involvement in litigation (e.g., alleged industrial injury). Altering the central experience of dyspnea may be the focus of treatment even when physiologic approaches have proven inadequate.

REFERENCES

1. Kikuchi Y, Okabe S, Tamura G, et al. Chemosensitivity and perception of dyspnea in patients with a history of near-fatal asthma [see comments]. N Engl J Med 1994;330(19):1329–1334.
2. Mahler D. Dyspnea, Lung Biology in Health and Disease. New York: Marcel Dekker, 1998.
3. Adams L, Chronos N, Lane R, et al. The measurement of breathlessness induced in normal subjects: individual differences. Clin Sci 1986; 70:131–140.
4. American Thoracic Society. Dyspnea: mechanisms, assessment, and management: a consensus statement. Am J Respir Crit Care Med 1999; 159(1):321–340.
5. Fedullo AJ, Swinburne AJ, McGuire-Dunn C.

Complaints of breathlessness in the emergency department. N Y State J Med 1986;86:4–6.

6. O'Connor GT, Anderson KM, Kannel WB, et al. Prevalence and prognosis of dyspnea in the Framingham Study. Chest 1987;92:90S.

7. Curtis JR, Deyo RA, Hudson LD. Pulmonary rehabilitation in chronic respiratory insufficiency, 7: health-related quality of life among patients with chronic obstructive pulmonary disease. Thorax 1994;49(2):162–170.

8. Hinton JM. The physical and mental stress of dying. Q J Med 1963;32:1–21.

9. Ripamonti C, Bruera E. Dyspnea: pathophysiology and assessment. J Pain Symptom Manage 1997;13(4):220–232.

10. Fink GR, Corfield DR, Murphy K, et al. Human cerebral activity with increasing inspiratory force: a study using positron emission tomography. J Appl Physiol 1996;81(3):1295–1305.

11. Mulnier H, Adams L, Murphy K, et al. Areas of human cerebral cortex activated by dyspnoea. Neuroimage 1998;7:S30.

12. Stark RD, Gambles SA, Lewis JA. Methods to assess breathlessness in healthy subjects: a critical evaluation and application to analyze the acute effects of diazepam and promethazine on breathlessness induced by exercise or by exposure to raised levels of carbon dioxide. Clin Sci 1981; 61:429–439.

13. Adams L, Chronos N, Lane R, et al. The measurement of breathlessness induced in normal subjects: validity of two scaling techniques. Clin Sci 1985;69(1):7–16.

14. Wilson RC, Jones PW. A comparison of the visual analogue scale and modified Borg scale for the measurement of dyspnoea during exercise. Clin Sci 1989;76:277–282.

15. Lane R, Adams L. Metabolic acidosis and breathlessness during exercise and hypercapnia in man. J Physiol (Lond) 1993;461(47):47–61.

16. Adams L, Lane R, Shea SA, et al. Breathlessness during different forms of ventilatory stimulation: a study of mechanisms in normal subjects and respiratory patients. Clin Sci 1985;69:663–672.

17. Lane R, Cockcroft A, Guz A. Voluntary isocapnic hyperventilation and breathlessness during exercise in normal subjects. Clin Sci 1987; 73(5):519–523.

18. Lane R, Cockcroft A, Adams L, et al. Arterial oxygen saturation and breathlessness in patients with chronic obstructive airways disease. Clin Sci 1987;72(6):693–698.

19. Stark RD, Gambles SA, Chatterjee SS. An exercise test to assess clinical dyspnoea: estimation of reproducibility and sensitivity. Br J Dis Chest 1982;76:269–278.

20. Wilson RC, Jones PW. Influence of prior ventilatory experience on the estimation of breathlessness during exercise. Clin Sci (Colch) 1990; 78(2):149–153.

21. Wilson RC, Oldfield WL, Jones PW. Effect of residence at altitude on the perception of breathlessness on return to sea level in normal subjects. Clin Sci (Colch) 1993;84(2):159–167.

22. Boudreau D, Styhler A, Gray DK, et al. A comparison of breathlessness during spontaneous

asthma and histamine-induced bronchoconstriction. Clin Invest Med 1995;18(1):25–32.

23. Moy ML, Lantin ML, Harver A, et al. Language of dyspnea in assessment of patients with acute asthma treated with nebulized albuterol. Am J Respir Crit Care Med 1998;158(3):749–753.

24. Veen JC, Smits HH, Ravensberg AJ, et al. Impaired perception of dyspnea in patients with severe asthma: relation to sputum eosinophils. Am J Respir Crit Care Med 1998;158(4):1134–1141.

25. Schwartzstein RM, Lahive K, Pope A, et al. Cold facial stimulation reduces breathlessness induced in normal subjects. Am Rev Respir Dis 1987; 136(1):58–61.

26. Dudley DL, Glaser, Jorgenson BN, et al. Psychosocial concomitants to rehabilitation in chronic obstructive pulmonary disease, part 1: psychosocial and psychological considerations. Chest 1980;77:413–420.

27. Manning H, Harver A, Mahler D. Dyspnea in the elderly. In: Mahler D, ed. Pulmonary Disease in the Elderly Patient. New York: Marcel Dekker, 1993;81–111.

28. Janson-Bjerklie S, Ruma SS, Stulbarg M, et al. Predictors of dyspnea intensity in asthma. Nurs Res 1987;36(3):179–183.

29. Jones PW, Baveystock CM, Littlejohns P. Relationships between general health measured with the sickness impact profile and respiratory symptoms, physiological measures, and mood in patients with chronic airflow limitation. Am Rev Respir Dis 1989;140(6):1538–1543.

30. Gift AG, Cahill CA. Psychophysiologic aspects of dyspnea in chronic obstructive pulmonary disease: a pilot study. Heart Lung 1990;19(3): 252–257.

31. Janson C, Bjornsson E, Hetta J, et al. Anxiety and depression in relation to respiratory symptoms and asthma. Am J Respir Crit Care Med 1994;149(4 Pt 1):930–934.

32. Janson-Bjerklie S, Carrieri VK, Hudes M. The sensations of pulmonary dyspnea. Nurs Res 1986;35:154–159.

33. Gift AG, Pugh LC. Dyspnea and fatigue. Nurs Clin North Am 1993;28(2):373–384.

34. Guyatt GH, Berman LB, Townsend M, et al. A measure of quality of life for clinical trials in chronic lung disease. Thorax 1987;42(10): 773–778.

35. Gormley J, Carrieri-Kohlman V, Douglas M, et al. Patients with COPD increase their self-efficacy and performance during an exercise program. Am Rev Respir Dis 1992;145:A477.

36. Chetta A, Gerra G, Foresi A, et al. Personality profiles and breathlessness perception in outpatients with different gradings of asthma. Am J Respir Crit Care Med 1998;157(1):116–122.

37. Jones PW, Oldfield WLG, Wilson RC. Reduction in breathlessness during exercise at sea level after 4 weeks at an altitude of 4000 metres. J Physiol 1990;422:105P.

38. Campbell EJ, Freedman S, Clark TJ, et al. The effect of muscular paralysis induced by tubocurarine on the duration and sensation of breathholding. Clin Sci 1967;32(3):425–432.

39. Banzett RB, Lansing RW, Brown R, et al. "Air hunger" from increased PCO_2 persists after complete neuromuscular block in humans. Respir Physiol 1990;81:1–18.
40. Gandevia SC, Killian K, McKenzie DK, et al. Respiratory sensations, cardiovascular control, kinaesthesia and transcranial stimulation during paralysis in humans. J Physiol (Lond) 1993; 470(85):85–107.
41. Banzett RB, Lansing RW, Reid MG, et al. "Air hunger" arising from increased PCO_2 in mechanically ventilated quadriplegics. Respir Physiol 1989;76:53–68.
42. Nakayama H, Shibuya M, Yamada M, et al. In-phase chest wall vibration decreases dyspnea during arm elevation in chronic obstructive pulmonary disease patients [see comments]. Intern Med 1998;37(10):831–835.
43. Cristiano LM, Schwartzstein RM. Effect of chest wall vibration on dyspnea during hypercapnia and exercise in chronic obstructive pulmonary disease. Am J Respir Crit Care Med 1997; 155(5):1552–1559.
44. Banner NR, Lloyd MH, Hamilton RD, et al. Cardiopulmonary response to dynamic exercise after heart and combined heart-lung transplantation. Br Heart J 1989;61:215–223.
45. Guz A. Brain, breathing and breathlessness. Respir Physiol 1997;109(3):197–204.
46. Winning AJ, Hamilton RD, Guz A. Ventilation and breathlessness on maximal exercise in patients with interstitial lung disease after local anaesthetic aerosol inhalation. Clin Sci 1988; 74(3):275–281.
47. Gandevia SL, Killian KJ, Campbell EJM. The effect of respiratory muscle fatigue on respiratory sensations. Clin Sci 1981;60:463–466.
48. Killian KJ, Gandevia S, Summers E, et al. Effect of increased lung volume on perception of breathlessness, effort and tension. J Appl Physiol 1984;57:686–691.
49. El-manshawi A, Killian KJ, Summers E, et al. Breathlessness during exercise with and without resistive loading. J Appl Physiol 1986;61:896–905.
50. Leblanc P, Bowie DM, Summers E, et al. Breathlessness and exercise in patients with cardiorespiratory disease. Am Rev Respir Dis 1986;133: 21–25.
51. Demediuk BH, Manning H, Lilly J, et al. Dissociation between dyspnea and respiratory effort. Am Rev Respir Dis 1992:1222–1225.
52. Steele B, Shaver J. The dyspnea experience: nociceptive properties and a model for research and practice. ANS Adv Nurs Sci 1992;15(1):64–76.
53. Lenz ER, Pugh LC, Milligan RA, et al. The middle-range theory of unpleasant symptoms: an update. ANS Adv Nurs Sci 1997;19(3):14–27.
54. Breslin EH, Roy C, Robinson CR. Physiological nursing research in dyspnea: a paradigm shift and a metaparadigm exemplar. Sch Inq Nurs Pract 1992;6(2):81–104; discussion 105–109.
55. Harver A, Mahler D. Dyspnea: sensation, symptom and illness. In: Mahler D, ed. Dyspnea, Lung Biology in Health and Disease. New York: Marcel Dekker, 1998;1–34.
56. Carrieri-Kohlman V, Janson S. Managing dyspnea. In: Hinshaw AS, Feetham SL, Shaver JLF, eds. Handbook of Clinical Nursing Research. Thousand Oaks, CA: Sage Publications, 1999: 379–393.
57. Pashkow P, Ades PA, Emery CF, et al. Outcome measurement in cardiac and pulmonary rehabilitation: AACVPR Outcomes Committee, American Association of Cardiovascular and Pulmonary Rehabilitation. J Cardiopulm Rehabil 1995;15(6):394–405.
58. Mahler D. Breathlessness in chronic obstructive pulmonary disease. In: Adams L, Guz A, eds. Respiratory Sensation. New York: Marcel Dekker, 1996:242.
59. ACCP/AACVPR Pulmonary Rehabilitation Guidelines Panel. Pulmonary rehabilitation: joint ACCP/AACVPR evidence-based guidelines [see comments]. Chest 1997;112(5): 1363–1396.
60. Mahler D, Guyatt G, Jones P. Clinical measurement of dyspnea. In: Mahler D, ed. Dyspnea, Lung Biology in Health and Disease. New York: Marcel Dekker, 1998:149–189.
61. Mahler DA, ed. Dyspnea. Mount Kisco, NY: Futura, 1990.
62. Simon PM, Schwartzstein RM, Weiss JW, et al. Distinguishable types of dyspnea in patients with shortness of breath. Am Rev Respir Dis 1990; 142(5):1009–1014.
63. Simon PM, Schwartzstein RM, Weiss JW, et al. Distinguishable sensations of breathlessness induced in normal volunteers. Am Rev Respir Dis 1989;140(4):1021–1027.
64. Elliott MW, Adams L, Cockcroft A, et al. The language of breathlessness: use of verbal descriptors by patients with cardiopulmonary disease. Am Rev Respir Dis 1991;144(4):826–832.
65. Jones PW. Dyspnea and quality of life in chronic obstructive pulmonary disease. In: Mahler D, ed. Dyspnea, Lung Biology in Health and Disease. New York: Marcel Dekker, 1998:199–220.
66. Hardie GE, Janson S, Boushey HA, et al. Ethnic differences in the language of breathlessness used by African American and Caucasian asthmatics. Am Rev Respir Crit Care Med 1998;157(Part 2 of 2):A631.
67. O'Donnell DE, Bertley JC, Chau LK, et al. Qualitative aspects of exertional breathlessness in chronic airflow limitation: pathophysiologic mechanisms. Am J Respir Crit Care Med 1997; 155(1):109–115.
68. O'Donnell DE, Chau L, Webb KA. Qualitative aspects of exertional dyspnea in patients with interstitial lung disease. J Appl Physiol 1998; 84(6):2000–2009.
69. Lush MT, Janson BS, Carrieri VK, et al. Dyspnea in the ventilator-assisted patient. Heart Lung 1988;17(5):528–535.
70. Muza SR, Silverman MT, Gilmore GC, et al. Comparison of scales used to quantitate the sense of effort to breathe in patients with chronic obstructive pulmonary disease. Am Rev Respir Dis 1990;141:909–913.
71. Mador MJ, Rodis A, Magalang UJ. Reproducibility of Borg scale measurements of dyspnea

during exercise in patients with COPD. Chest 1995;107(6):1590–1597.

72. Mahler DA, Faryniarz K, Lentine T, et al. Measurement of breathlessness during exercise in asthmatics: predictor variables, reliability, and responsiveness. Am Rev Respir Dis 1991;144(1): 39–44.

73. Gift AG. Validation of a vertical visual analogue scale as a measure of clinical dyspnea. Rehabil Nurs 1989;14(6):323–325.

74. Burdon JGW, Juniper EF, Killian KJ, et al. The perception of breathlessness in asthma. Am Rev Respir Dis 1982;126:825–828.

75. Gift AG, Narsavage G. Validity of the numeric rating scale as a measure of dyspnea. Am J Crit Care 1998;7(3):200–204.

76. Wilson RC, Jones PW. Differentiation between the intensity of breathlessness and the distress it evokes in normal subjects during exercise. Clin Sci 1991;80(1):65–70.

77. Carrieri-Kohlman V, Gormley JM, Douglas MK, et al. Differentiation between dyspnea and its affective components. West J Nurs Res 1996; 18(6):626–642.

78. Lareau SC, Meek PM, Press D, et al. Dyspnea in patients with chronic obstructive pulmonary disease: does dyspnea worsen longitudinally in the presence of declining lung function? Heart Lung 1999;28(1):65–73.

79. Mahler DA, Weinberg DH, Wells CK, et al. The measurement of dyspnea: contents, interobserver agreement and physiological correlates of two new clinical indexes. Chest 1984;85:751–758.

80. O'Donnell DE, McGuire M, Samis L, et al. The impact of exercise reconditioning on breathlessness in severe chronic airflow limitation. Am J Respir Crit Care Med 1995;152:2005–2013.

81. Reardon J, Awad E, Normandin E, et al. The effect of comprehensive outpatient pulmonary rehabilitation on dyspnea. Chest 1994;105(4): 1046–1052.

82. Harver A, Mahler DA, Daubenspeck JA. Targeted inspiratory muscle training improves respiratory muscle function and reduces dyspnea in patients with chronic obstructive pulmonary disease. Ann Intern Med 1989;111(2):117–124.

83. Mahler DA, Matthay RA, Snyder PE, et al. Sustained-release theophylline reduces dyspnea in nonreversible obstructive airway disease. Am Rev Respir Dis 1985;131:22–25.

84. Mahler DA, Tomlinson D, Olmstead EM, et al. Changes in dyspnea, health status, and lung function in chronic airway disease. Am J Respir Crit Care Med 1995;151(1):61–65.

85. Lareau SC, Carrieri-Kohlman V, Janson-Bjerklie S, et al. Development and testing of the Pulmonary Functional Status and Dyspnea Questionnaire (PFSDQ). Heart Lung 1994;23(3):242–250.

86. Lareau SC, Meek PM, Roos PJ. Development and testing of the modified version of the pulmonary functional status and dyspnea questionnaire (PFSDQ-M). Heart Lung 1998;27(3):159–168.

87. Eakin EG, Resnikoff PM, Prewitt LM, et al. Validation of a new dyspnea measure: the UCSD Shortness of Breath Questionnaire: University of California, San Diego. Chest 1998;113(3):619–624.

88. Eakin E, Sassi-Dambron D, Ries A, et al. Reliability and validity of dyspnea measures in patients with obstructive lung disease. Int J Behav Med 1995;2:118–134.

89. Jaeschke R, Singer J, Guyatt GH. Measurement of health status: ascertaining the minimal clinically important difference. Control Clin Trials 1989;10(4):407–415.

90. Wijkstra PJ, TenVergert EM, Van Altena R, et al. Reliability and validity of the Chronic Respiratory Questionnaire (CRQ). Thorax 1994;49(5): 465–467.

91. Jones PW, Quirk FH, Baveystock CM, et al. A self-complete measure of health status for chronic airflow limitation: the St. George's Respiratory Questionnaire. Am Rev Respir Dis 1992;145(6):1321–1327.

92. Jones PW, Bosh TK. Quality of life changes in COPD patients treated with salmeterol. Am J Respir Crit Care Med 1997;155(4):1283–1289.

93. Jones PW, Quirk FH, Baveystock CM. The St George's Respiratory Questionnaire. Respir Med 1991;85(Suppl B):25–31; discussion 33–37.

94. Tenholder MF, South PJ. Dyspnea in pregnancy [clinical conference]. Chest 1989;96(2):381–388.

95. Tobin MJ. Dyspnea: pathophysiologic basis, clinical presentation, and management. Arch Intern Med 1990;150(8):1604–1613.

96. Marantz PR, Kaplan MC, Alderman MH. Clinical diagnosis of congestive heart failure in patients with acute dyspnea [see comments]. Chest 1990;97(4):776–781.

97. Howell JB. Behavioural breathlessness. Thorax 1990;45(4):287–292.

98. Togawa K, Konno A, Miyazaki S, et al. Obstructive sleep dyspnea: diagnosis and treatment. Acta Otolaryngol Suppl (Stockh) 1988;458(167): 167–173.

99. Morgan WKC, Lapp L, Seaton R. Respiratory disability in coal miners. JAMA 1980;243:2401–2404.

100. Efthimiou J, Fleming J, Gomes C, et al. The effect of supplementary oral nutrition in poorly nourished patients with chronic obstructive pulmonary disease. Am Rev Respir Dis 1988; 137(5):1075–1082.

101. Turner-Warwick M, Burrows B, Johnson A. Cryptogenic fibrosing alveolitis: clinical features and their influence on survival. Thorax 1980; 35:171–180.

102. Killian KJ, Campbell EJ. Dyspnea and exercise. Ann Rev Physiol 1983;45:465–479.

103. Strunk BL, Cheitlin MD, Stulbarg MS, et al. Right-to-left interatrial shunting through a patent foramen ovale despite normal intracardiac pressures. Am J Cardiol 1987;60:413–415.

104. Messner-Pellenc P, Ximenes C, Brasileiro CF, et al. Cardiopulmonary exercise testing: determinants of dyspnea due to cardiac or pulmonary limitation. Chest 1994;106(2):354–360.

105. Martinez F, Stanopoulos I, Acero R, et al. Graded comprehensive cardiopulmonary exercise testing in the evaluation of dyspnea unexplained by routine evaluation. Chest 1994; 105:168–174.

106. Cross JJ, Kemp PM, Walsh CG, et al. A randomized trial of spiral CT and ventilation perfusion scintigraphy for the diagnosis of pulmonary embolism. Clin Radiol 1998;53(3):177–182.

107. Mayo JR, Remy-Jardin M, Möller NL, et al. Pulmonary embolism: prospective comparison of spiral CT with ventilation-perfusion scintigraphy. Radiology 1997;205(2):447–452.

108. Santín M, Podzamczer D, Ricart I, et al. Utility of the gallium-67 citrate scan for the early diagnosis of tuberculosis in patients infected with the human immunodeficiency virus. Clin Infect Dis 1995;20(3):652–656.

109. Witt C, Dörner T, Hiepe F, et al. Diagnosis of alveolitis in interstitial lung manifestation in connective tissue diseases: importance of late inspiratory crackles, 67 gallium scan and bronchoalveolar lavage. Lupus 1996;5(6):606–612.

110. Caidahl K, Svardsudd K, Eriksson H, et al. Relation of dyspnea to left ventricular wall motion disturbances in a population of 67-year-old men. Am J Cardiol 1987;59(15):1277–1282.

111. Himelman RB, Stulbarg MS, Kircher B, et al. Non-invasive evaluation of pulmonary pressure with exercise by Doppler echocardiography in chronic pulmonary disease. Circulation 1989; 79:863–871.

112. Vavuranakis M, Kolibash AJ, Wooley CF, et al. Mitral valve prolapse: left ventricular hemodynamics in patients with chest pain, dyspnea or both. J Heart Valve Dis 1993;2(5):544–549.

113. Bass C. Unexplained chest pain and breathlessness. Med Clin North Am 1991;75(5):1157–1173.

114. Smoller JW, Pollack MH, Otto MW, et al. Panic anxiety, dyspnea, and respiratory disease: theoretical and clinical considerations. Am J Respir Crit Care Med 1996;154(1):6–17.

115. Goldstein RS, Gort EH, Stubbing D, et al. Randomised controlled trial of respiratory rehabilitation. Lancet 1994;344(8934):1394–1397.

116. Ries AL, Kaplan RM, Limberg TM, et al. Effects of pulmonary rehabilitation on physiologic and psychosocial outcomes in patients with chronic obstructive pulmonary disease. Ann Intern Med 1995;122(11):823–832.

117. Strijbos JW, Sluiter HJ, Postma DS, et al. Objective and subjective performance indicators in COPD. Eur Respir J 1989;2:666–669.

118. Wijkstra PJ, Van AR, Kraan J, et al. Quality of life in patients with chronic obstructive pulmonary disease improves after rehabilitation at home. Eur Respir J 1994;7(2):269–273.

119. Cockcroft AE, Saunders MJ, Berry G. Randomized controlled trial of rehabilitation in chronic respiratory disability. Thorax 1981;36:200–203.

120. Mall RW, Medeiros M. Objective evaluation of results of a pulmonary rehabilitation program in a community hospital. Chest 1988;94:1156–1160.

121. Carrieri-Kohlman V, Gormley JM, Douglas MK, et al. Exercise training decreases dyspnea and the distress and anxiety associated with it: monitoring alone may be as effective as coaching. Chest 1996;110(6):1526–1535.

122. Lake FR, Henderson K, Briffa T, et al. Upper-limb and lower-limb exercise training in patients with chronic airflow obstruction. Chest 1990; 97(5):1077–1082.

123. Simpson K, Killian K, McCartney N, et al. Randomised controlled trial of weightlifting exercise in patients with chronic airflow limitation. Thorax 1992;47(2):70–75.

124. Ries AL, Ellis B, Hawkins RW. Upper extremity exercise training in chronic obstructive pulmonary disease. Chest 1988;93(4):688–692.

125. Celli BR, Rassulo J, Make BJ. Dyssynchronous breathing during arm but not leg exercise in patients with chronic airflow obstruction. N Engl J Med 1986;138:856–861.

126. Ramirez-Venegas A, Ward JL, Olmstead EM, et al. Effect of exercise training on dyspnea measures in patients with chronic obstructive pulmonary disease. J Cardpulm Rehabil 1997;17(2): 103–109.

127. Casaburi R, Patessio A, Ioli F, et al. Reductions in exercise lactic acidosis and ventilation as a result of exercise training in patients with obstructive lung disease. Am Rev Respir Dis 1991; 143(1):9–18.

128. McGavin CR, Gupta SP, Lloyd EL, et al. Physical rehabilitation for the chronic bronchitic: results of a controlled trial of exercises in the home. Thorax 1977;32(3):307–311.

129. Clark CJ, Cochrane L, Mackay E. Low intensity peripheral muscle conditioning improves exercise tolerance and breathlessness in COPD. Eur Respir J 1996;9(12):2590–2596.

130. Carrieri-Kohlman V, Gormley J. Coping strategies for dyspnea. In: Mahler D, ed. Dyspnea, Lung Biology in Health and Disease. New York: Marcel Dekker, 1998:287–313.

131. Punzal PA, Ries AL, Kaplan RM, et al. Maximum intensity exercise training in patients with chronic obstructive pulmonary disease. Chest 1991;100(3):618–623.

132. Niederman MS, Clemente PH, Fein AM, et al. Benefits of a multidisciplinary pulmonary rehabilitation program: improvements are independent of lung function. Chest 1991;99(4):798–804.

133. Lacasse Y, Wong E, Guyatt GH, et al. Meta-analysis of respiratory rehabilitation in chronic obstructive pulmonary disease [see comments]. Lancet 1996;348(9035):1115–1119.

134. Horowitz MB, Littenberg B, Mahler DA. Dyspnea ratings for prescribing exercise intensity in patients with COPD. Chest 1996;109(5):1169–1175.

135. Horowitz MB, Mahler DA. Dyspnea ratings for prescription of cross-modal exercise in patients with COPD. Chest 1998;113(1):60–64.

136. Mejia R, Ward J, Lentine T, et al. Target dyspnea ratings predict expected oxygen consumption as well as target heart rate values. Am J Respir Crit Care Med 1999;159(5 Pt 1):1485–1489.

137. Brown ML, Carrieri V, Janson B, et al. Lung cancer and dyspnea: the patient's perception. Oncol Nurs Forum 1986;13(5):19–24.

138. Janson-Bjerklie S, Ferketich S, Benner P, et al. Clinical markers of asthma severity and risk: importance of subjective as well as objective factors. Heart Lung 1992;21(3):265–272.

139. Sassi-Dambron DE, Eakin EG, Ries AL, et al. Treatment of dyspnea in COPD: a controlled clinical trial of dyspnea management strategies [see comments]. Chest 1995;107(3):724–729.

140. Carrieri VJ, Janson-Bjerklie S. Strategies patients use to manage the sensation of dyspnea. West J Nurs Res 1986;8:284–305.

141. Kohlman-Carrieri V, Janson-Bjerklie S. Coping and self-care strategies. In: Mahler DA, ed. Dyspnea. Mount Kisco, NY: Futura, 1990:201–230.

142. Hodgkin JE, Connors GL, Bell CW, eds. Pulmonary Rehabilitation: Guidelines to Success. 2nd ed. Philadelphia: JB Lippincott, 1993.

143. Kravetz H, Pheatt N. Sexuality in the pulmonary patient. In: Hodgkin JE, Connors GL, Bell CW, eds. Pulmonary Rehabilitation: Guidelines to Success. 2nd ed. Philadelphia: JB Lippincott, 1993:293–310.

144. Davidson JT, Whipp BJ, Wasserman K, et al. Role of the carotid bodies in breath-holding. N Engl J Med 1974;290:819–822.

145. Stein DA, Bradley BL, Miller W. Mechanisms of oxygen effects on exercise patients with chronic obstructive pulmonary disease. Chest 1982;81: 6–10.

146. Swinburn CR, Wakefield JM, Jones PW. Relationship between ventilation and breathlessness during exercise in chronic obstructive airways disease is not altered by prevention of hypoxemia. Clin Sci 1984;67:515–519.

147. O'Donnell DE, Bain DJ, Webb KA. Factors contributing to relief of exertional breathlessness during hyperoxia in chronic airflow limitation. Am J Respir Crit Care Med 1997;155(2): 530–535.

148. Lane R, Adams L, Guz A. The effects of hypoxia and hypercapnia on perceived breathlessness during exercise in humans. J Physiol (Lond) 1990;428(579):579–593.

149. Chronos N, Adams L, Guz A. Effect of hyperoxia and hypoxia on exercise-induced breathlessness in normal subjects. Clin Sci 1988;74(5):531–537.

150. Ward SA, Whipp BJ. Effects of peripheral and central chemoreflex activation on the isopnoeic rating of breathing in exercising humans [published erratum appears in J Physiol (Lond) 1990;420:489]. J Physiol 1989;411(4):27–43.

151. Bye PTP, Esau SA, Levy RD, et al. Ventilatory muscle function during exercise in air and oxygen in patients with chronic air-flow limitation. Am Rev Respir Dis 1985;132:236–240.

152. Dean NC, Brown JK, Himelman RB, et al. Oxygen may improve dyspnea and endurance in patients with chronic obstructive pulmonary disease and only mild hypoxemia. Am Rev Respir Dis 1992;146(4):941–945.

153. Tiep BL. Long-term home oxygen therapy. Clin Chest Med 1990;11(3):505–521.

154. Marques MJ, Storer TW, Cooper CB. Treadmill exercise duration and dyspnea recovery time in chronic obstructive pulmonary disease: effects of oxygen breathing and repeated testing. Respir Med 1998;92(5):735–738.

155. Liss HP, Grant BJ. The effect of nasal flow on breathlessness in patients with chronic obstructive pulmonary disease. Am Rev Respir Dis 1988;137(6):1285–1288.

156. Stark RD, O'Neill PA, Russell NJW, et al. Effects of small-particle aerosols of local anaesthetic on dyspnoea in patients with respiratory disease. Clin Sci 1985;69:29–36.

157. Santiago TV, Johnson J, Riley DJ, et al. Effects of morphine on ventilatory response to exercise. J Appl Physiol 1979;47:112–118.

158. Weil JV, McCullough RE, Kline JS, et al. Diminished ventilatory response to hypoxia and hypercapnia after morphine in normal man. N Engl J Med 1975;292:1103–1106.

159. Sackner MA. Effects of hydrocodone bitartrate on breathing pattern of patients with chronic obstructive pulmonary disease and restrictive lung disease. Mt Sinai Med J 1984;51:222–226.

160. Kryger MH, Yacoub O, Dosman J, et al. Effect of meperidine on occlusion pressure response to hypercapnia and hypoxia with and without external inspiratory resistance. Am Rev Respir Dis 1976;114:333–340.

161. Wilson RH, Hoseth W, Dempsey ME. Respiratory acidosis: effects of decreasing respiratory minute volume in patients with severe chronic pulmonary emphysema, with specific reference to oxygen, morphine and barbiturates. Am J Med 1954;17:464–470.

162. Woodcock AA, Johnson MA, Geddes DM. Breathlessness, alcohol and opiates. N Engl J Med 1982;306:1363–1364.

163. Johnson MA, Woodcock AA. Dihydrocodeine for breathlessness in "pink puffers." BMJ 1983; 286:675–677.

164. Eisner N, Luce P, Denman W, et al. Effect of oral diamorphine on dyspnea in chronic obstructive pulmonary disease (COPD). Am Rev Respir Dis 1990;141:A323.

165. Rice KL, Kronenberg RS, Hedemark LL, et al. Effects of chronic administration of codeine and promethazine on breathlessness and exercise tolerance in patients with chronic airflow obstruction. Br J Dis Chest 1987;81(3):287–292.

166. Poole PJ, Veale AG, Black PN. The effect of sustained-release morphine on breathlessness and quality of life in severe chronic obstructive pulmonary disease. Am J Respir Crit Care Med 1998;157:1877–1880.

167. Robin ED, Burke CM. Single-patient randomized clinical trial: opiates for intractable dyspnea. Chest 1986;90:888–892.

168. Woodcock AA, Gross ER, Geddes DM. Drug treatment of breathlessness: contrasting effects of diazepam and promethazine in pink puffers. BMJ 1981;283:343–346.

169. Man GCW, Hsu K, Sproule BJ. Effect of alprazolam on exercise and dyspnea in patients with chronic obstructive pulmonary disease. Chest 1986;90:832–836.

170. Eimer M, Cable T, Gal P, et al. Effects of clorazepate on breathlessness and exercise tolerance in patients with chronic airflow obstruction. J Fam Pract 1985;21:359–362.

171. Mitchell-Heggs P, Murphy K, Minty K, et al. Diazepam in the treatment of dyspnoea in the 'Pink Puffer' syndrome. Q J Med 1980; 49(193):9–20.

172. Greene JG, Pucino F, Carlson JD, et al. Effects of alprazolam on respiratory drive, anxiety, and dyspnea in chronic airflow obstruction: a case study. Pharmacotherapy 1989;9(1):34–38.

173. Smoller JW, Pollack MH, Systrom D, et al. Sertraline effects on dyspnea in patients with obstructive airways disease. Psychosomatics 1998; 39(1):24–29.

174. Weiss DJ, Kreck T, Albert RK. Dyspnea resulting from fibromyalgia. Chest 1998;113(1):246–249.

175. Young IH, Daviskas E, Keena VA. Effect of low dose nebulised morphine on exercise endurance in patients with chronic lung disease. Thorax 1989;44(5):387–390.

176. Farncombe M, Chater S, Gillin A. The use of nebulized opioids for breathlessness: a chart review. Palliat Med 1994;8(4):306–312.

177. Noseda A, Carpiaux JP, Markstein C, et al. Disabling dyspnoea in patients with advanced disease: lack of effect of nebulized morphine. Eur Respir J 1997;10(5):1079–1083.

178. Masood AR, Subhan MM, Reed JW, et al. Effects of inhaled nebulized morphine on ventilation and breathlessness during exercise in healthy man. Clin Sci (Colch) 1995;88(4):447–452.

179. Leung R, Hill P, Burdon J. Effect of inhaled morphine on the development of breathlessness during exercise in patients with chronic lung disease. Thorax 1996;51(6):596–600.

180. Chandler S. Nebulized opioids to treat dyspnea [see comments]. Am J Hospice Palliative Care 1999;16(1):418–422.

181. Tiep BL, Burns M, Kao D, et al. Pursed lips breathing training using ear oximetry. Chest 1986;90(2):218–221.

182. Tiep BL. Reversing disability of irreversible lung disease. West J Med 1991;154(5):591–597.

183. Breslin EH. The pattern of respiratory muscle recruitment during pursed-lip breathing. Chest 1992;101(1):75–78.

184. Miller WF. A physiologic evaluation of the effects of diaphragmatic breathing training in patients with chronic pulmonary emphysema. Am J Med 1954;17:471–477.

185. Campbell E, Friend J. Action of breathing exercises in pulmonary emphysema. Lancet 1955;1: 325–329.

186. Sackner MA, Gonzalez HF, Jenouri G, et al. Effects of abdominal and thoracic breathing on breathing pattern components in normal subjects and in patients with chronic obstructive pulmonary disease. Am Rev Respir Dis 1984; 130(4):584–587.

187. Willeput R, Sergysels R. Respiratory patterns induced by bent posture in COPD patients. Rev Mal Respir 1991;8(6):577–582.

188. Keller CA, Ruppel G, Hibbett A, et al. Thoracoscopic lung volume reduction surgery reduces dyspnea and improves exercise capacity in patients with emphysema. Am J Respir Crit Care Med 1997;156(1):60–67.

189. Brenner M, McKenna RJ, Gelb AF, et al. Dyspnea response following bilateral thoracoscopic staple lung volume reduction surgery. Chest 1997;112(4):916–923.

190. O'Donnell DE, Webb KA, Bertley JC, et al. Mechanisms of relief of exertional breathlessness following unilateral bullectomy and lung volume reduction surgery in emphysema. Chest 1996; 110(1):18–27.

191. Martinez FJ, de Oca MM, Whyte RI, et al. Lung-volume reduction improves dyspnea, dynamic hyperinflation, and respiratory muscle function. Am J Respir Crit Care Med 1997;155(6):1984–1990.

192. Petrof BJ, Legare M, Goldberg P, et al. Continuous positive airway pressure reduces work of breathing and dyspnea during weaning from mechanical ventilation in severe chronic obstructive pulmonary disease. Am Rev Respir Dis 1990; 141(2):281–289.

193. Petrof BJ, Calderini E, Gottfried SB. Effect of CPAP on respiratory effort and dyspnea during exercise in severe COPD. J Appl Physiol 1990; 69(1):179–188.

194. Maltais F, Reissmann H, Gottfried SB. Pressure support reduces inspiratory effort and dyspnea during exercise in chronic airflow obstruction. Am J Respir Crit Care Med 1995;151(4):1027–1033.

195. Renston JP, DiMarco AF, Supinski GS. Respiratory muscle rest using nasal BiPAP ventilation in patients with stable severe COPD. Chest 1994;105(4):1053–1060.

196. Arora NS, Rochester DF. Effect of body weight and muscularity on human diaphragm muscle mass, thickness and area. J Appl Physiol 1982; 52:64–70.

197. Arora NS, Rochester DF. Respiratory muscle strength and maximal voluntary ventilation in undernourished patients. Am Rev Respir Dis 1982;126:5–8.

198. Goldstein SA, Thomashow B, Askanazi J. Functional changes during nutritional repletion in patients with lung disease. Clin Chest Med 1986; 7(1):141–151.

199. Gandevia SC. Neural mechanisms underlying the sensation of breathlessness: kinesthetic parallels between respiratory and limb muscles. Aust N Z J Med 1988;18(1):83–91.

200. Smith K, Cook D, Guyatt GH, et al. Respiratory muscle training in chronic airflow limitation: a meta-analysis. Am Rev Respir Dis 1992;145(3): 533–539.

201. Lisboa C, Munoz V, Beroiza T, et al. Inspiratory muscle training in chronic airflow limitation: comparison of two different training loads with a threshold device. Eur Respir J 1994;7(7): 1266–1274.

202. Lisboa C, Villafranca C, Leiva A, et al. Inspiratory muscle training in chronic airflow limitation: effect on exercise performance. Eur Respir J 1997;10(3):537–542.

203. Fagerhaugh SY. Getting around with emphysema. Am J Nurs 1973;73(1):94–99.

204. Carrieri VK, Kieckhefer G, Janson-Bjerklie S, et al. The sensation of pulmonary dyspnea in school-age children. Nurs Res 1991;40(2):81–85.

205. Barach A, Beck G. The ventilatory effects of head-down position in pulmonary emphysema. Am J Med 1954;16:55–60.

206. Faling LJ. Pulmonary rehabilitation: physical modalities. Clin Chest Med 1986;7(4):599–618.

207. Nava S, Ambrosino N, Zocchi L, et al. Diaphragmatic rest during negative pressure ventilation by pneumowrap: assessment in normal and COPD patients. Chest 1990;98(4):857–865.

208. Belman MJ, Soo HG, Kuei JH, et al. Efficacy of positive vs negative pressure ventilation in unloading the respiratory muscles. Chest 1990; 98(4):850–856.

209. Levine S, Henson D, Levy S. Respiratory muscle rest therapy. Clin Chest Med 1988;9(2):297–309.

210. Green M. Respiratory muscle rest. Eur Respir J 1989;2(Suppl 7):578s–580s.

211. Zibrak JD, Hill NS, Federman EC, et al. Evaluation of intermittent long-term negative-pressure ventilation in patients with severe chronic obstructive pulmonary disease. Am Rev Respir Dis 1988;138(6):1515–1518.

212. Celli B, Lee H, Criner G, et al. Controlled trial of external negative pressure ventilation in patients with severe chronic airflow obstruction. Am Rev Respir Dis 1989;140(5):1251–1256.

213. Strumpf DA, Millman RP, Carlisle CC, et al. Nocturnal positive-pressure ventilation via nasal mask in patients with severe chronic obstructive pulmonary disease. Am Rev Respir Dis 1991; 144(6):1234–1239.

214. Murciano D, Auclair M-H, Pariente R, et al. A randomized, controlled trial of theophylline in patients with severe chronic obstructive pulmonary disease. N Engl J Med 1989;320:1521–1525.

215. Eaton ML, MacDonald FM, Church TR, et al. Effects of theophylline on breathlessness and exercise tolerance in patients with chronic airflow obstruction. Chest 1982;82:538–542.

216. Foxworth JW, Reisz GR, Knudson SM, et al. Theophylline and diaphragmatic contractility: investigation of a dose-response relationship. Am Rev Respir Dis 1988;138(6):1532–1534.

217. Moxham J. Aminophylline and the respiratory muscles: an alternative view. Clin Chest Med 1988;9(2):325–336.

218. Aubier M. Pharmacotherapy of respiratory muscles. Clin Chest Med 1988;9(2):311–324.

219. Aubier M, Murciano D, Viires N, et al. Effects of digoxin on diaphragmatic strength generation in patients with chronic obstructive pulmonary disease during acute respiratory failure. Am Rev Respir Dis 1987;135(3):544–548.

220. Chrystyn H, Mulley BA, Peake MD. Dose response relation to oral theophylline in severe chronic obstructive airways disease. BMJ 1988; 297(6662):1506–1510.

221. Suls J, Fletcher B. The relative efficacy of avoidant and nonavoidant coping strategies: a meta-analysis. Health Psychol 1985;4(3):249–288.

222. Keefe FJ, Dunsmore J, Burnett R. Behavioral and cognitive-behavioral approaches to chronic pain: recent advances and future directions. J Consult Clin Psychol 1992;60(4):528–536.

223. Lazarus RS. The costs and benefits of denial. In: Breznitz S, ed. The Denial of Stress. New York: International Universities Press, 1983:1–30.

224. Hunter SM, Hall SS. The effect of an educational support program on dyspnea and the emotional status of COPD clients. Rehabil Nurs 1989; 14(4):200–202.

225. Strijbos JH, Koeter GH, Meinesz AF. Home care rehabilitation and perception of dyspnea in chronic obstructive pulmonary disease (COPD) patients. Chest 1990.

226. Cioffi D. Beyond attentional strategies: cognitive-perceptual model of somatic interpretation. Psychol Bull 1991;109(1):25–41.

227. Scherer YK, Schmieder LE. The effect of a pulmonary rehabilitation program on self-efficacy, perception of dyspnea, and physical endurance. Heart Lung 1997;26(1):15–22.

228. Thompson SC. Will it hurt less if I can control it? a complex answer to a simple question. Psychol Bull 1981;90(1):89–101.

229. Devine EC, Pearcy J. Meta-analysis of the effects of psychoeducational care in adults with chronic obstructive pulmonary disease. Patient Educ Counsel 1996;29(2):167–178.

230. Rosser R, Denford J, Heslop A, et al. Breathlessness and psychiatric morbidity in chronic bronchitis and emphysema: a study of psychotherapeutic management. Psychol Med 1983; 13:93–110.

231. Ashikaga T, Vacek PM, Lewis SO. Evaluation of a community-based education program for individuals with chronic obstructive pulmonary disease. J Rehabil 1980;46(2):23–27.

232. Verbrugge LM. Health diaries. Med Care 1980; 18(1):73–95.

233. Burman ME. Health diaries in nursing research and practice. Image J Nurs Sch 1995;27(2):147–152.

234. Levine S, Weiser P, Gillen J. Evaluation of a ventilatory muscle endurance training program in the rehabilitation of patients with chronic obstructive pulmonary disease. Am Rev Respir Dis 1986;133:400–406.

235. DeVito AJ. Dyspnea during hospitalizations for acute phase of illness as recalled by patients with chronic obstructive pulmonary disease. Heart Lung 1990;19(2):186–191.

236. Emery CF, Leatherman NE, Burker EJ, et al. Psychological outcomes of a pulmonary rehabilitation program. Chest 1991;100(3):613–617.

237. Agle DP, Baum GL, Chester EH, et al. Multidiscipline treatment of chronic pulmonary insufficiency, 1: psychologic aspects of rehabilitation. Psychosom Med 1973;35:41–49.

238. Gift AG. Psychologic and physiologic aspects of acute dyspnea in asthmatics. Nurs Res 1991; 40(4):196–199.

239. Gift AG, Moore T, Soeken K. Relaxation to reduce dyspnea and anxiety in COPD patients. Nurs Res 1992;41(4):242–246.

240. Renfroe KL. Effect of progressive relaxation on dyspnea and state anxiety in patients with chronic obstructive pulmonary disease. Heart Lung 1988;17(4):408–413.

241. Horsman J. Using tape recordings to overcome panic during dyspnea. Respir. Care 1978;23:767–768.

242. Sitzman J, Kamiya J, Johnson J. Biofeedback training for reduced respiratory rate in chronic obstructive disease: a preliminary study. Nurs Res 1987;32:218–223.

243. Holliday JE, Hyers TM. The reduction of weaning time from mechanical ventilation using tidal volume and relaxation biofeedback. Am Rev Respir Dis 1990;141(5 Pt 1):1214–1220.

244. Haas F, Salazar-Schicchi J, Axen K. Desensitization to dyspnea in chronic obstructive pulmonary disease. In: Casaburi R, Petty T, eds. Principles and Practice of Pulmonary Rehabilitation. Philadelphia: WB Saunders, 1993:241–251.

245. Thornby MA, Haas F, Axen K. Effect of distractive auditory stimuli on exercise tolerance in patients with COPD. Chest 1995;107(5):1213–1217.

246. Aronoff GM, Aronoff S, Peck LW. Hypnotherapy in the treatment of bronchial asthma. Ann Allergy 1975;34(6):356–362.

247. Acosta AF. Tolerance of chronic dyspnea using a hypnoeducational approach: a case report. Am J Clin Hypn 1991;33(4):272–277.

248. Moody LE, Fraser M, Yarandi H. Effects of guided imagery in patients with chronic bronchitis and emphysema. Clin Nurs Res 1993;2(4):478–486.

249. Atkins CJ, Kaplan RM, Timms RM, et al. Behavioral exercise programs in the management of chronic obstructive pulmonary disease. J Consult Clin Psychol 1984;52:591–603.

250. Carrieri KV, Douglas MK, Gormley JM, et al. Desensitization and guided mastery: treatment approaches for the management of dyspnea. Heart Lung 1993;22(3):226–234.

251. Belman MJ, Brooks LR, Ross DJ, et al. Variability of breathlessness measurement in patients with chronic obstructive pulmonary disease. Chest 1991;99(3):566–571.

252. Belman M. Exercise in chronic obstructive pulmonary disease. Clin Chest Med 1986;7:585–597.

253. Bandura A. Sources of self-efficacy. In: Bandura A, ed. Self Efficacy: The Exercise of Control. New York: W.H. Freeman, 1997:79–113.

6 Patient and Family Education

Suzanne C. Lareau
Kathleen C. Insel

◈ Professional Skills

Upon completion of this chapter, the reader will:

- Identify the goals of the educational portion of a program in pulmonary rehabilitation as they direct efforts toward assisting the patient (and family) to perform self-care
- Cite the foundational aspects of educational theories that can be used to enhance the design and implementation of a program in pulmonary rehabilitation
- Describe client characteristics that may affect the educational plan, including cognitive, emotional, and physical characteristics
- Suggest memory strategies that may enhance remembering to promote adherence to prescribed treatments and medicines
- List strategies to assist with learning problems for patients with cognitive deficits or mood disorders
- Outline the standard educational content of a pulmonary rehabilitation program, including building knowledge and self-management skills

"Knowing is not enough; we must apply. Willing is not enough; we must do."
Johann Goethe 1749–1832

INTRODUCTION

The educational component of a pulmonary rehabilitation program has multiple goals, which include assisting the patient (and family) to perform self-care by (*a*) increasing knowledge of the patient's health status; (*b*) applying this information to monitor, modify, treat, and seek assistance appropriately; (*c*) becoming better partners in their health care by communicating more effectively with health care providers; and (*d*) preparing for the end of life. Education supports the secondary benefits of pulmonary rehabilitation: to improve health-related quality of life, reduce symptoms, decrease disability, and increase participation in physical and social activities.[1] Improved self-care through education is particularly important for those with chronic diseases because dependence on others for day-to-day activities can result in depression and impact the quality of life for both the patient and his or her family. However, although the benefits of education are considered obvious, it is not clear what parts of the educational process are critical or in what contexts education is most effective for this patient population. Programs must therefore integrate known educational theories and findings with clinical experience in designing the educational intervention that best fits their clientele.

This chapter begins to organize thinking about (*a*) the educational intervention as a part of pulmonary rehabilitation, (*b*) how client characteristics and settings may interact, and (*c*) how instructional strategies may be modified. First, learning theories that support the development of an educational program in pulmonary rehabilitation are offered. Next, client characteristics that amend the nature of the educational intervention are discussed, followed by learning strategies, including memory strategies that help patients apply their learning and remembering, for example, to perform treatments such as taking medications. These strategies are offered because so many of those in need of pulmonary rehabilitation are older adults and have hypoxemia related to compromised pulmonary function, both of which have been demonstrated to affect thinking and remembering.[2,3] Finally, an overview of educational content in a typical pulmonary rehabilitation program is offered.

EDUCATIONAL THEORIES

Because most of the chronic pulmonary diseases are irreversible, interventions are often directed toward improving the individual's quality of life through strategies of self-care. Education is only one of many planned interventions geared toward optimizing health and mobility for this group; however, in some ways it is the most important intervention. The goal of an educational program in a pulmonary rehabilitation setting is the promotion of self-care. This goal can best be accomplished if the patient has the tools to make informed and appropriate decisions about his or her health care. Education provides a vehicle by which patients can learn about their disease process, its symptoms, and decisions regarding treatment. Second, education is assumed to affect how patients interpret their illness, which in turn influences adherence to prescribed regimens.[4,5] With knowledge, patients will be able to make appropriate ongoing decisions concerning their care and recognize the importance of preventive care to avert avoidable illness.

Educating patients and families involves a process of changing behavior and is multidirectional. Although teaching is directed toward educating by presenting information that is meaningfully integrated into previous knowledge structures, it is unfortunately often assumed to be unidirectional. However, the difference between an effective and an ineffective teacher is that the effective teacher encourages feedback, thereby allowing modification of the educational plan. In this way, education is more than advising. Advising is merely the transmission of information, whereas education takes the learner where they are and reveals options of where they can go. This basic premise, "educating" versus "advising," should underlie both the development and the implementation of educational programs in pulmonary rehabilitation.

Educational theories forming the basis of an educational program include those that emphasize the importance of the relationship between teacher and learner. The interaction between educator (teacher) and patient (learner) often provides an opportunity for patients to relate unique experiences, discuss confusion regarding prescribed regimens, and communicate day-to-day variations in functioning. This interaction begins with an adequate understanding of the patient's problems and the mechanisms by which the prescribed interventions are intended to work. This includes the level and intensity of disease and the manner in which the patient reacts to the prescribed regimen. This often underrated relationship can be pivotal, increasing the potential for the patient to learn and thereby impact health outcomes. The pulmonary rehabilitation educator is in a key position to provide this education. Rehabilitation staff must be well equipped with both the knowledge of pulmonary disease and the desire to understand the unique situations of patients.

Interactional Theories

A theoretical framework, defining the interaction between teacher and learner as paramount to learning, comes from a social constructivist's perspective. Social constructivists view social and individual processes as interdependent.[6] In keeping with this view, social interactions promote learning and are by nature culturally bound. Understanding cultural differences, therefore, is an essential aspect of the context of teaching and learning. Given the diversity of backgrounds of individuals enrolled in programs, awareness of the cultural implications of respiratory conditions and their treatment is imperative. Within the social constructivist framework, a joint construction of meaning between the teacher and the learner develops. This joint construction of meaning evolves from a commitment to find a common ground on which to build shared understanding.[6] The perspective offered by this view is consistent with Kleinman's[7] use of explanatory models. Explanatory models are used to make the initial assessment, the first step in determining the educational plan.[7] Within this framework, the meaning to the patient of the disease process and treatment plan is assessed. The initial assessment must consider the patient's cultural context and the influence culture may have on readiness to learn as well as the compatibility of the intended educational plan with the patient's expectations. Finding common ground and establishing goals that build on shared meaning, when undertaken at the beginning of the relationship, can save time in the end by enhancing the patient's personal involvement and motivation. In addition, this process may reduce potential frustration to both the educator and the patient later in the program.

Assessment is considered an ongoing activity and is therefore dynamic. Dynamic assessment provides a prospective measure of performance so that future needs are anticipated and guidance is offered. "The (educator) must not limit his analysis to functions that have matured; he must consider those that are in the process of maturation."[8] Innovative ways of continuing this assessment, as well as modeling problem-solving skills for the patient, can include the use of "think-alouds." Think-alouds make use of public modeling, with the educator actively and openly problem-solving with the learner.[9] This technique can be applied when the patient seems to be confused or when the patient does not apply strategies that have been discussed. For example, if the pursed-lips breathing (PLB) technique has been discussed in class and the patient subsequently demonstrates altered breathing during exercise, one might question why the patient does not apply PLB during exercise. Stating, "I wonder if pursed-lips breathing would help you right now?" can generate a discussion of the technique. Explore whether the patient has tried PLB, what his or her experience has been, and whether the patient may benefit from its use. Patients are likely to recall more information and be more aware of why particular information is important with this strategy. Furthermore, when the role is reversed, that is, when the learner shares his or her thinking with the educator, deeper cognitive processing occurs.[10]

Finally, important to the social constructivist framework, the teacher and the learner are not always defined as the educator and the patient. Educators are sometimes learners, and patients can be teachers. Often, when individual responses to situations, or unique approaches to problems, are shared by patients, the educator realizes possibilities that may enhance his or her ability to influence others. So, when an individual with long-standing chronic pulmonary disease offers a method that he or she has used to recall whether the evening's inhaler dosage was taken, the educator adds one more possible way to help others confronting the same problem. In addition, the patient's and family members' knowledge of situations in which symptoms occur, and the exact triggers (what makes symptoms better or worse), is often superior to the experts' and has been found to be the key ingredient to the patient seeking health care.[11] Therefore, it is important to listen to what the patient and his or her family members are saying to have an adequate understanding about how the disease is affecting the patient, his or her interests in life, and the compromises made in relation to activities.

Social Learning Theory

Similar to the social constructivists view of learning as a social endeavor, Bandura's[12,13] work on social learning theory is used to enlighten development of educational programs for pulmonary rehabilitation. Social learning theory offers that patients learn through the observation of models.[12,13] According to this theory, learning can occur by observing another person making skilled responses (or reading about it or viewing pictures), followed by imitating the responses of the model. Learning is facilitated if the information is distinct, can be identified with the other person's experience, and is relevant. The rehabilitation program provides numerous opportunities to observe modeling by peers with similar conditions.

Learned Resourcefulness

The theory of learned resourcefulness offers another guiding framework for the development of educational programs.[14] The basic premise of learned resourcefulness is that behavior is owing not only to external forces (e.g., the diagnosis of chronic obstructive pulmonary disease [COPD]) but also to internal forces. Learned resourcefulness is based on the perception that we can do something about our particular situation and that this change occurs through education. The implication of emphasizing personal mastery over inherent problems is that the response to the circumstance is largely within the patient's control. Therefore, education can influence the way people see themselves in relationship to their illness by changing the way people approach and deal with chronic illness. Education can arm the person with the tools to control their illness.

Consistent with theories of learned resourcefulness are empiric findings on learned helplessness, claiming that depression will result when individuals expect that bad events will occur and anticipate that they can do nothing about it.[15] The focus in learned resourcefulness is on behaviors that keep people healthy rather than on what makes them sick.[14]

Cognitive Learning Theories

Principles from cognitive learning theories also enrich education when these premises are incorporated into a program for pulmonary rehabilitation. First, learning is an active and constructive process in which meaning is derived and information, when meaningful to the patient and his or her family, is more likely to be remembered. The plans and goals of the learner influence acquiring and retaining new knowledge; therefore, it is important to take the time to listen to the expectations and goals of the patient and family members. Using the patient's goals when introducing a new strategy can be reinforcing to learning educational content. Second, higher-level processes play a role in learning, with meaningful information undergoing "deeper" processing.[16] Again, this principle reinforces the importance of meaningfulness to the learner and the role of meaning in enhancing memory. Third, learning is cumulative and is influenced by previous knowledge. Learners attempt to interpret new information in relationship to their personal skills and experiences. If something is perceived as not relevant, or does not "ring true" based on previous experience, it is unlikely to be remembered. The patient's experiences and interactions with other health care providers therefore shape the educational intervention because previous learning will speed the intake of related but new information. Conversely, old information or beliefs that contradict information being taught will slow acquisition. Fourth, cognitive theories are concerned about the way knowledge is represented and organized in memory. Therefore, analyzing learning tasks to reflect logical presentation of new learning should proceed in a hierarchical fashion.[17] Finally, metacognitive strategies can be used to encourage learning. Metacognition is knowing about one's own knowing. These strategies ask learners to reflect on their learning. Allowing the patient and family members to reflect on their learning also provides an opportunity for confusion to be clarified or questions to be answered. This gives the educator an opportunity for ongoing assessment for the purpose of making alterations in the education plan. Metacognitive strategies include setting goals with the learner, who is actively selecting stimuli to be attended to. Open discussion of the learning process with the educator is part of making use of metacognitive strategies.

Box 6-1. Key Points From Learning Theories

Understand the patient's culture because information that is meaningful is more likely to be remembered
Determine the significance of the disease and treatment to the patient—find a common ground
Build on previous learning
Plan educational material logically—build information from simple to complex
Clarify information
Assess the patient's unique learning needs
Be open and willing to learn from the patient
Empower the patient to take control of his or her illness

In summary, learning is active, constructive, and goal oriented. It is critically important to understand how the patient defines the problem and what they perceive to be the desirable outcome. *Learners seek meaning, not just performance.* Understanding why an intervention is planned and how it will help their breathing is important. Acquiring and remembering new information requires that the learner actively construct new knowledge and strategies. New knowledge and strategies are easier to build when based on previous knowledge and experience because higher-level processes are implicated in learning and learning is cumulative. Whenever possible, connect new learning to the patient's view, use the patient's words, work from his or her experiences, and use rich examples with familiar contexts. Also, present other ways of dealing with situations and ways of preventing problems. The educational plan needs to proceed logically. In fact, learners attempt to organize stimuli even when there is no apparent organization. In addition, previous knowledge influences new learning both positively and negatively. Therefore, the educator needs to be aware of barriers to new learning based on previously learned misconceptions. The overall approach to providing an educational intervention should acknowledge the importance of an environment that is conducive to learning, using the educator/client relationship to facilitate learning. Finally, educational programs must be evaluated. Evaluation asks whether the outcomes of interest were achieved, including did learning occur and did the learning result in transfer of new information to real world problems (Box 6-1).

CLIENT CHARACTERISTICS—UNIQUE NEEDS OF PULMONARY PATIENTS

Patient characteristics alter the educational plan. These characteristics can be cognitive, emotional, or physical. Cognitive characteristics include the previous educational level of the patient and family members as well as current cognitive ability. When someone has a medical background, certain vocabulary may be familiar and require less explanation. More likely, however, medical terminology needs to be explained and treatment discussed in terms and phrases that can be understood by the patient and family members. Rehabilitation staff need to take care that terms such as dyspnea, alveoli, and congestive heart failure are clearly understood by the patient. When potentially confusing terms like dyspnea are used, the staff may wish to first present alternate terms (e.g., shortness of breath, uncomfortable breathing), followed by asking the patient what term they usually use to describe the experience. Variations in cognitive, emotional, and physical client characteristics influence educational interventions.

Cognitive

In planning an educational program, the pulmonary rehabilitation team must take into consideration cognitive changes occurring in their patient population. Cognitive changes can affect memory and retention of information and subsequently interfere with the patient obtaining full benefit from the program. Cognitive changes have been measured with hypoxemia, aging, depression, and anxiety.

Hypoxemia is a known complication of pulmonary disease. It has been well established that patients with hypoxemia experience greater neurophysiologic deficits than do others. In a study of 203 patients with COPD, more than 75% showed neurophysiologic deficits, with 40% measuring moderate to severe deficits.[18] In these patients, the ability to think abstractly, perform simple motor tasks, analyze, and integrate perceptual information was affected. More recently, significant deterioration in verbal and verbal memory tasks have been measured in hypoxic–hypercapnic patients.[19,20] These findings among hypoxemic patients reinforce the need for presentation of frequent, simple instructions combined with written instructions. Evaluation of the patient's ability to perform motor skills, such as measuring the required amount of medication or calculating variable dosages of steroids (e.g., prednisone), may also be necessary. The rehabilitation setting provides an opportunity to evaluate the patient for these limitations and work on techniques to overcome these deficits.

Age is considered a strong predictor of cognitive function, but great diversity exists among older adults in their ability to think and remember. Therefore, although some older adults are compromised on tasks requiring thinking and remembering, others are no different than their young counterparts. However, because laboratory evidence documents the tendency for older adults to experience age-related cognitive changes, educators in pulmonary rehabilitation programs need to be aware of these potential changes and the implication of these changes for learning and remembering.

First, decline in the ability to learn and retain new information has been demonstrated in investigations showing impaired recall among older, in contrast to young, adults.[21] Allowing more time for learning and creating linkages to previous learning may overcome these changes. Second, decline is also demonstrated in tasks hypothesized to reflect working memory, usually considered the simultaneous retention and manipulation of information.[22] Older adults benefit from clearly and logically presented information. Furthermore, as a group, older adults exhibit less inhibitory control over processes that are irrelevant to the task at hand.[23] It follows that older adults learn better in an environment where distractions are limited. Older adults are also slower at both information processing and perceptual speed.[24] Therefore, slowing the presentation of new information may be beneficial. The effects of age-related cognitive change need to be considered in amending the program to meet the needs of patients.

Emotional

In addition to cognitive deficits, pulmonary patients may experience emotional changes requiring modification of the educational plan (Box 6-2). Depression and anxiety affect cognitive performance and therefore learning and remembering. The prevalence of clinically significant depression and anxiety in this population is approximately 20%.[25–27] Clinically significant depression or anxiety may result in difficulty with the educational compo-

Box 6-2. Strategies to Overcome Learning Problems in Patients With Cognitive Deficits or Mood Disorder

Make verbal instructions simple and clear
Write instructions simply
Obtain return demonstration or verbal instructions
Observe for motor coordination

nents of rehabilitation because memory and attention are affected by these disorders.[28] Mood disorders may also affect motivation or exercise performance.

Physical

Many individuals in need of pulmonary rehabilitation programs are older than 65 years and have been ill for a long time. These two factors combine to suggest a picture of increasing physical frailty. Patients need comprehensive assessment with coordinated planning to address the additional stresses that occur through declining physical abilities. Physical frailty may impact both the design and the implementation of the educational plan. For example, sensory changes may make hearing more difficult and visualizing information on a board, or physical demonstration, blurry and difficult to see. Changes in motor coordination owing to the effects of medication (e.g., tremors secondary to β-agonist use), arthritis, or nervous system disorders stress the importance of repeat demonstrations to enable the educator to identify needs for adapting procedures. What works for one patient does not always meet the needs of another.

MEMORY STRATEGIES

Memory strategies[29,30] are used to heighten retention of information while in the rehabilitation program and for application on completion of the program. Many previously mentioned learning strategies, such as increasing the relevance of the intended content and building on previous knowledge, are strategies for enhancing retention. Memory strategies may also be shared with patients for their use in the home setting.

Memory strategies can make use of external cues (clocks, alarms, calendars, lists, etc.) or internal cues (focusing attention, association, elaboration). Patients use external cues by placing to-be-remembered medications in areas that are consistently viewed at the time of day when the medicine needs to be taken. For example, placing inhalers scheduled for evening use on the end table when the evening routine is consistently oriented to a specific television program, or placing the medications by the coffee pot if the morning ritual is connected to making coffee. In addition, charts can be designed that allow the patient to mark off the day and time when the inhaler has been used. Medication dispensers can help when multiple medications are needed. This also may require a routine such as filling the dispenser each Sunday morning after church. This assumes of course that the patient is capable of properly filling the dispenser. The rehabilitation setting offers the opportunity to observe the patient to ensure that he or she can safely and accurately perform this activity.

Creating salient visual cues to enhance recognition of the appropriate inhaler further encourages clear recognition even when distracted. Using active alarms, found now in many memory-assist devices, including wristwatches, can also be used to assist patients to remember to take their nebulizer treatment or other medications or to perform other needed treatments. Discussion of ways to assist recall can precipitate lively discussion in rehabilitation groups whereby patients share innovative ways of dealing with their problems.

Internal cues are signs patients can use to encourage remembering. Many instances of forgetting are not instances of forgetting at all, rather failing to encode information (learn) to begin with. Focusing attention on the to-be-remembered item as well as actively associating the to-be-remembered item with something known enhances retention. In a similar way, elaborating on to-be-remembered information encourages later recall. This occurs when stories of experiences are used as a teaching strategy. The story is more often remembered than a series of abstract facts. Memory strategies are helpful both in the educational program and later for use at home to recall needed treatments and medications as well as follow-up appointments.

EDUCATIONAL CONTENT OF PROGRAMS

Education has become such an integral part of pulmonary rehabilitation programs that it is difficult to measure the precise impact of education alone. Controlled studies of patients receiving education versus those with no education have not been done. Neither have studies of the specific content of programs or topics most effective. At the same time, health care providers and the media are providing an increasing amount of health-related information to patients, much of which may or may not be clear to the patient or consistent with the teachings of the program. Most clinicians believe education is critical to proper self-management because lack of knowledge about one's chronic respiratory disease is likely to result in inappropriate health management.

Programs commonly offer 1- to 2-hour weekly blocks devoted to educational content. The content of rehabilitation programs has become standard,[1,31] and topics are typically aimed to aid patients in their understanding of how the lungs normally work (anatomy and physiology of the lung) and how the lungs are affected by chronic lung disease (pathophysiology). Communicating this information serves to provide a foundation whereby patients should be better able to comprehend why medications are required on a routine basis and how various medications work to provide bronchodilation or decrease inflammation, etc. Medications discussed include bronchodilators (β-agonists, anticholinergics, and theophylline), anti-inflammatory agents, antibiotics, mucolytics, and diuretics. Because most pulmonary medications are administered by metered dose inhalers, heavy emphasis is placed on inhaler technique and indications for "as needed" inhaler use. The program environment provides an excellent opportunity to observe the patient self-administer medications and to monitor their activities. Training in the action, side effects, dosage, frequency, and correct administration of all oral and inhaled respiratory medications is provided. Instruction in metered dose inhaler technique is particularly important because deficiencies in technique in individuals with lung disease are common.[32-34] In addition, as new vehicles for administering inhalers are introduced (solutions, powders, inhaler activated versus finger activated, etc.), education and re-education is required on a regular basis (e.g., annually). Oxygen may be discussed as part of the medication content or as a section on respiratory equipment, depending on the group's needs (Box 6-3).

Most patients with chronic pulmonary disease misinterpret the symptom of dyspnea, for hypoxemia. The significance of dyspnea can be discussed as a separate section or incorporated into other sections such as activity modification. Dyspnea is often the motivation to both seek care and pursue a rehabilitation program. In addition to exercise, dyspnea improves significantly after rehabilitation.[35-38] Patients are assisted in differentiating dyspnea as a symptom (signaling pathophysiologic changes) from a symptom of deconditioning.

Box 6-3. Educational Content of Pulmonary Rehabilitation Programs

Anatomy and physiology of the lung
Pathophysiology of chronic lung disease
Medications, oxygen use, and cleaning of equipment
Symptom management
Energy conservation and activity modification techniques
Exercise
Respiratory and chest physiotherapy techniques
Psychologic adjustment to changes in health
Nutrition
Preventive measures
Advanced directives

Symptom monitoring is described, as well as energy conservation techniques. Techniques include pacing techniques, PLB, advanced planning of activities, and learning to prioritize activities.

The rehabilitation setting provides a unique opportunity to capitalize on the learning behavior of patients. Although programs are often designed with formal classes, the exercise component of the program provides the opportunity to observe patients and reinforce information. For example, during the course of exercise sessions, patient technique in the use of inhalers can be observed and immediate feedback provided by the health care team.

Exercise is a major component of pulmonary rehabilitation programs, and exercise tolerance has been found to be the major outcome that improves (in addition to dyspnea) after pulmonary rehabilitation.[39] Exercise is a treatment modality available in all rehabilitation programs. Unfortunately, convincing patients to continue exercising at home is a challenge. Patients often find it difficult to maintain the same degree of discipline to exercise in their home as they did during the program. Maintenance programs, if available, often fill this need after formalized rehabilitation.

Respiratory and chest therapy techniques are included as indicated. Although most programs include discussion of techniques to enhance bronchial hygiene and aid mucociliary clearance, additional emphasis may be placed on these techniques, depending on the population. For example, rehabilitation groups composed of patients with cystic fibrosis will emphasize techniques for mucous clearance, which may include controlled cough, postural drainage, percussion, vibration, and use of positive expiratory pressure or flutter devices.

Anxiety frequently accompanies chronic respiratory disorders, and the fear of dyspnea may limit the patient's ability to participate in activities of daily living. Instruction in progressive muscle relaxation, stress reduction, and panic control may help reduce dyspnea and anxiety.[40] Given the high incidence of depressive symptoms in COPD patients, the rehabilitation team may discuss the effect of chronic illness on mood.

The nutritional content of programs will vary with the composition of each rehabilitation group. Smaller programs may find that some groups of patients are all under ideal body weight, over ideal body weight, or a mixture. Smaller programs then are more likely to need to adapt to each patient group than are larger programs. Patients who are under ideal body weight will need information and guidance on options to increase body weight, whereas those who are overweight will require assistance with weight reduction. Maintaining ideal body weight, eating frequent small meals, and paying attention to adequate fluid intake are important factors in nutritional counseling.

The importance of preventive measures should also be addressed. Topics covered may include smoking cessation, avoidance of smoking exposure, immunizations, and early recognition of infection. Although some programs will not enroll current smokers, others believe that the rehabilitation setting is a supportive environment, conducive to assisting with smoking cessation. Although many patients understand the dangers of smoking, many do not wish to confront the fact that exposure to smoke may also adversely affect their health. Second-hand smoke not only has potential carcinogenic effects on the lungs but may chronically irritate those with bronchial hyperresponsiveness, resulting in unstable breathing. The area of prevention includes discussion of the need for pneumonia and influenza vaccination. In keeping with the philosophy of empowering the patient to provide self-care, many clinicians prescribe antibiotics to be taken in the event of infection. The rehabilitation staff can discuss the signs and symptoms of recognizing infection and the appropriate use of antibiotics. Given the classroom environment, many of the issues related to preventive measures and treatment, can be addressed in the less stressful environment of the program.

Education and discussion about end-of-life planning is becoming more commonplace in pulmonary rehabilitation programs. In addition, patients indicate a desire for information on end-of-life planning.[41] The rehabilitation staff have been viewed by patients as useful sources of information regarding end-of-life issues.[41] End-of-life planning includes a discussion of making known one's preference for life-sustaining interventions as well as planning for the well-being of family members. The pulmonary rehabilitation environment provides an ideal setting to discuss end-of-life issues because patients are medically stable, in a supportive environment, and with others with similar questions and needs.

SUMMARY

As health care changes occur, patients and their loved ones will be required to take on more responsibility for their health and care. This includes becoming better diagnosticians of changes in their health status and knowing when seeking help is needed on an emergency basis. Although the educational content of programs is standard (see Box 6-3), each program should evaluate and adjust to the educational needs of their patients given variations in the geographic, cultural, and pulmonary conditions affecting their population.

"When we treat man as he is we make him worse than he is, When we treat man as if he already were what he potentially could be, We make him what he should be."

Johann Goethe 1749–1832

REFERENCES

1. American Thoracic Society. Official statement: pulmonary rehabilitation—1999. Am J Respir Crit Care Med 1999;159:1666–1682.
2. Incalzi RA, Gemma A, Marra C, et al. Chronic obstructive pulmonary disease: an original model of cognitive decline. Am Rev Respir Dis 1993; 148:418–424.
3. Craik FIM, Jennings JM. Human memory. In: Craik FIM, Salthouse TA, eds. The Handbook of Aging. Hillsdale, NJ: Lawrence Erlbaum, 1992: 51–110.
4. Leventhal H, Meyer DE, Nerenz D. The common sense representation of illness danger. In: Rachman S, ed. Contributions to Medical Psychology. New York: Pergamon, 1980:7–30.
5. Leventhal H, Diefenbach M. The active side of illness cognition. In: Skelton JA, Croyle RT, eds. Mental Representation in Health and Illness. New York: Springer-Verlag, 1991:247–272.
6. Palinscar AS. Social constructivist perspectives on teaching and learning. Annu Rev Psychol 1998;49:345–375.
7. Kleinman A. Patients and Healers in the Context of Culture. Berkeley: University of California Press, 1980.
8. Vygotsky L. Thought and language. In: Kozulin A, ed. Thought and Language 1934. Cambridge, MA: MIT Press, 1986.
9. Duffy GG, Rochler L, Meloth MS, et al. The relationship between explicit verbal explanations during reading skill instruction and student awareness and achievement: a study of reading teacher effects. Read Res Q 1986;22:347–368.
10. Scardamalia M, Bereiter C. Intentional learning as a goal of instruction. In: Knowing, Learning and Instruction. Resnick LB, ed. Hillsdale, NJ: Lawrence Erlbaum, 1989:361–392.
11. Cameron L, Leventhal E, Leventhal H. Symptom representations and affect as determinants of care seeking in a community-dwelling adult sample population. Health Psychol 1993;12:171–179.
12. Bandura A. Social Learning Theory. New York: General Learning Press, 1971.
13. Bandura A. 1977. Social Learning Theory. Englewood Cliffs, NJ: Prentice-Hall.
14. Rosenblaum M. Introduction: from helplessness to resourcefulness. In: Learned Resourcefulness on Coping Skills, Self-Control, and Adaptive Behavior. Rosenbaum M, ed. New York: Springer Publishing, 1990:25–35.
15. Abramson LY, Seligman MEP, Teasdale J. Learned helplessness in humans: critique and reformulation. J Abnorm Psychol 1978;87:49–74.
16. Craik FIM, Lockhardt RS. Levels of processing: a framework for memory research. J Verbal Learn Verbal Behav 1972;11:671–684.
17. Shuell TJ. Cognitive conceptions of learning. Rev Ed Res 1996;56:411–436.
18. Grant I, Heaton RK, McSweeny AJ, et al. Neuropsychologic findings in hypoxemic chronic obstructive pulmonary disease. Arch Intern Med 1982;142:1470–1476.
19. Incalzi RA, Gemma A, Marra C, et al. Chronic obstructive pulmonary disease. An original model of cognitive decline. Am Rev Respir Dis 1993; 148:418–424.
20. Incalzi RA, Gemma A, Marra C, et al. Verbal memory impairment in COPD. Chest 1997;112: 1506–1513.
21. Light LL. The organization of memory in old age. In: Craik FIM, Salthouse TA, eds. The Handbook of Aging and Cognition. Hillsdale, NJ: Lawrence Erlbaum, 1992:111–165.
22. Salthouse TA, Babcock RL, Shaw RJ. Effects of adult age on structural and operational capacities in working memory. Psychol Aging 1991;1: 118–127.
23. Hasher L, Zacks RT. Working memory, comprehension and aging: a review and a new view. In:

Bower GH, ed. The Psychology of Learning and Motivation. New York: Academic Press, 1998; 22:193–225.

24. Cerella J. Information processing rates in the elderly. Psychol Bull 1985;98:67–83.

25. Borson S, Barnes RA, Kukull WA, et al. Symptomatic depression in elderly medical outpatients. J Am Geriatr Soc 1986;34:341–347.

26. Kukull WA, Koepsell TD, Unui TS, et al. Depression and physical illness among elderly general medical clinic patients. J Affect Dis 1986;10: 153–162.

27. Karajgi B, Rifkin A, Doddi S, et al. The prevalence of anxiety disorders in patients with chronic obstructive pulmonary disease. Am J Psychiatry 1990;147:200–201.

28. Emery CF. Cognitive functioning among patients in cardiopulmonary rehabilitation. J Cardiopulm Rehabil 1997;17:407–410.

29. Verhaeghen P, Marcoen KA, Goossens L. Improving memory performance in the aged through mnemonic training: a meta-analytic study. Psychol Aging 1992;7:242–251.

30. West RL. Compensatory strategies for age-associated memory impairment. In: Baddeley AD, Wilson BA, eds. Handbook of Memory Disorders. Chichester, England: John Wiley & Sons, 1995: 481–500.

31. American Association of Cardiovascular & Pulmonary Rehabilitation. Patient training. In: Guidelines for Pulmonary Rehabilitation. Champaign, IL: Human Kinetics, 1998:37–50.

32. De Blaquiere P, Christensen DB, Carter WB, et al. Use and misuse of metered-dose inhalers by patients with chronic lung disease: a controlled randomized trial of two instruction methods. Am Rev Respir Dis 1989;140:910–916.

33. Thompson J, Irvine T, Grathwohl K. Misuse of metered-dose inhalers in hospitalized patients. Chest 1994;105:715–717.

34. Braunstein GL, Trinquet G, Harper AE, et al. Compliance with nedocromil sodium and a nedocromil sodium/salbutamol combination. Eur Respir J 1996;9:893–898.

35. Goldstein RS, Gort EH, Stubbing D, et al. Randomised controlled trial of respiratory rehabilitation. Lancet 1994;344:1394–1397.

36. Reardon J, Awad E, Normandin E, et al. The effect of comprehensive outpatient pulmonary rehabilitation on dyspnea. Chest 1994;105:1046–1052.

37. Wijkstra PJ, Van der Mark TW, Kraan J, et al. Effects of home rehabilitation on physical performance in patients with chronic obstructive pulmonary disease (COPD). Eur Respir J 1996;9: 104–110.

38. Strijbos JH, Postma DS, Van Altena R, et al. A comparison between an outpatient hospital-based pulmonary rehabilitation program and a home-care pulmonary rehabilitation program in patients with COPD. Chest 1996;109:366–372.

39. Lacasse Y, Wong E, Guyatt GH, et al. Meta-analysis of respiratory rehabilitation in chronic obstructive pulmonary disease. Lancet 1996;348:1115–1119.

40. Renfroe KL. Effect of progressive relaxation on dyspnea and state anxiety in patients with chronic obstructive pulmonary disease. Heart Lung 1988; 17:408–413.

41. Heffner JE, Fahy B, Hilling L, et al. Attitudes regarding advanced directives among patients in pulmonary rehabilitation. Am Rev Respir Crit Care Med 1996;154:1735–1740.

THERAPEUTIC INTERVENTION IN PULMONARY REHABILITATION

Pharmacologic Therapy

James I. Couser Jr.

◗ Professional Skills

Upon completion of this chapter, the reader will:

- Understand the mechanism of action of each class of drug used to treat patients with chronic obstructive pulmonary disease (COPD)
- Recognize the risks associated with the use of pharmacologic agents in patients with COPD
- Have a framework for clinical pharmacologic management of symptomatic patients with COPD

The goal of pharmacologic management for patients with COPD is to improve activities of daily living and quality of life by preventing symptoms and preserving optimal lung function. Ideally, patients referred to pulmonary rehabilitation programs have already been placed on optimal medical therapy.[1] Appropriate drug treatment depends on an understanding of the pathophysiology of airflow obstruction and the mechanisms of action of the various bronchodilators and anti-inflammatory agents. This chapter focuses on pharmacologic treatment of individuals with COPD and reviews recent guidelines for appropriate outpatient management.

BRONCHODILATORS

One of the proposed mechanisms for airflow obstruction in COPD is bronchoconstriction.[1] Up to one-third of patients with COPD will demonstrate significant increases in forced expiratory volume in 1 second (FEV_1) after a single inhalation of bronchodilators; with repeated testing, this proportion increases to two-thirds.[2] The first line of medical therapy for COPD is the inhalation of bronchodilator aerosols. Symptomatic benefit may be achieved even in the absence of significant spirometric improvement.

Anticholinergic Agents

Anticholinergic agents now play an integral part in COPD therapy, and ipratropium bromide is considered by some to be the drug of first choice in the medical treatment of moderate to severe disease.[3] It is a quaternary anticholinergic agent that is poorly absorbed and does not usually cause significant atropine-like side effects. Although its onset of action is slower than that of β_2-adrenergic agonists, ipratropium provides greater peak bronchodilator effect and a more sustained duration of action.[4] Anticholinergics may produce bronchodilation in some COPD patients who have no response to β_2-agonists.[5] Therapy with ipratropium bromide for 90 days was associated with improved baseline FEV_1 compared with albuterol[6]; however, when used for 5 years, it does not seem to retard disease progression.[7] Ipratropium has also been shown to reduce sputum volume without changing sputum viscosity.[5]

The recommended dosage for ipratropium bromide is 2 puffs by metered dose inhaler (MDI) every 6 hours; however, this dose may be safely doubled or tripled for maximal benefit in severely obstructed patients. For acute exacerbation, or for patients with ineffective MDI technique, 0.5 mg of nebulized solution may be given up to every 4 to 6 hours.

β_2-Adrenergic Agonists

β_2-Agonists have the most rapid onset of action of all bronchodilators and have long been the mainstays of COPD management. They produce bronchial smooth muscle relaxation by stimulating adenyl cyclase, reducing bronchomotor tone and airway resistance in patients with COPD. In addition, mucociliary clearance and diaphragmatic contractility may be enhanced by these agents. A variety of formulations are available (Table 7-1), including MDIs and dry powder inhalers, inhalant solutions for nebulization, and oral preparations. Because of their rapid onset of action, short-acting β_2-agonists are the preferred method for treating acute symptoms of COPD, and in patients with mild intermittent disease, they can be used as needed.[1] Regular use of β_2-agonists by patients with COPD does not seem to be harmful; however, some studies in patients with asthma have suggested that it may contribute to a slow decline in FEV_1.[8] Recommended doses of short-acting β_2-agonists in patients with COPD are 1 to 2 puffs every 2 to 6 hours for mild symptoms, 1 to 4 puffs as needed 4 times daily for mild to moderate ongoing symptoms, and up to 6 to 8 puffs every 1/2 to 2 hours in severe exacerbations.[1]

Long-acting β_2-agonists have been used extensively as maintenance treatment for patients with asthma. Limited data are available on the efficacy of these agents in patients with COPD; however, recent studies have shown that use of long-acting β_2-

Table 7-1. Selected β_2-Agonists

Agent	Delivery System	Duration of Action (h)	Dose
Metaproterenol	MDI	3–4	2–4 puffs every 3–4 h
	Nebulized solution	3–4	0.3 mL every 3–4 h
	Tablets, syrup	6–8	20 mg every 6–8 h
Albuterol	MDI	4–6	2–4 puffs every 4–6 h
	Nebulized solution	4–6	2.5 mg every 4–6 h
	Dry powder inhaler	4–6	200 μg every 4–6 h
	Tablets, syrup	6–8	2–4 mg every 6–8 h
	Extended-release tablets	12	8 mg every 12 h
Terbutaline	MDI	4–6	1–2 puffs every 4–6 h
	Subcutaneous	6–8	0.5 mg every 6–8 h
	Tablets	6–8	2.5–5 mg every 6–8 h
Pirbuterol	MDI (breath actuated)	4–6	2 puffs every 4–6 h
Salmeterol	MDI	10–12	2 puffs every 12 h
	Dry powder inhaler	10–12	1 inhalation (50 μg) every 12 h

Reprinted with permission from American Thoracic Society. Standards for the diagnosis and care of patients with chronic obstructive pulmonary disease. Am J Respir Crit Care Med 1995;152(Suppl):S77–S120.
MDI, metered dose inhaler.

agonists can reduce dyspnea,[9,10] improve spirometry,[9,11] increase exercise capacity,[11] and improve health-related quality of life[12] in patients with COPD. These drugs may be particularly effective in patients with nocturnal symptoms, and the longer dosing intervals may enhance compliance. In the United States, the only available long-acting agent is salmeterol xinafoate (Serevent). The recommended dose is 2 puffs twice daily.

Oral β_2-agonists are less effective, produce more adverse effects, and have a slower onset of action than the same drugs given by inhalation, but their ease of use may improve compliance. Evidence to support the regular use of these agents is lacking, so they should be used only in patients who are unable to use inhaled therapy. Adverse effects of β_2-agonists include tachycardia, arrhythmias, palpitations, and tremor. Hypokalemia has been reported in patients taking high doses.

Combination Therapy

Combination therapy with inhaled ipratropium bromide and β_2-agonists is potentially more effective and safer than use of maximal doses of either agent alone. Combination therapy provides the rapid onset of action of the adrenergic agent and prolonged duration of action of the anticholinergic. Most short-term studies have demonstrated that at approved doses delivered by MDI, combination therapy results in improved pulmonary function over either component used alone.[13] Two long-term studies, one using MDIs and the other using nebulized therapy, have shown that maintenance combination therapy with ipratropium bromide and albuterol sulfate provides better bronchodilation than does either therapy alone without increasing side effects.[14,15] It has also been suggested that combination therapy is associated with fewer exacerbations of COPD than is monotherapy with albuterol alone.[16] Compliance with combination therapy may be enhanced by the use of Combivent, an MDI that combines ipratropium bromide and albuterol sulfate in one inhaler. Each inhalation delivers 18 μg of ipratropium bromide and 103 μg of albuterol sulfate. The recommended dose of Combivent is 2 inhalations 4 times daily.

Theophylline

Oral theophylline is a less effective bronchodilator than inhaled anticholinergics and β_2-agonists, and it has a slower onset of action. Its mechanism of action is poorly understood. Potentially beneficial nonbronchodilator effects in COPD include improved strength and effectiveness of respiratory muscles,[17] augmentation of respiratory drive, and anti-inflammatory activity.[18] When used with either ipratropium bromide[19] or a β_2-agonist,[20] theophylline seems to have an additive bronchodilator effect. Combining theophylline with albuterol and ipratropium together may provide additional benefit in stable patients with COPD.[21] Use of long-acting theophylline preparations has been shown to reduce overnight declines in FEV_1 and morning respiratory symptoms in patients with COPD.[22]

The therapeutic index of theophylline is narrow, and some patients experience side effects even when blood levels are in the therapeutic range. Smoking, infection, hypoxia, and other drugs may affect theophylline clearance. It is generally recommended that a low dose of long-acting theophylline (200–400 mg/d) be initiated and then adjusted after a few days based on plasma theophylline levels,[1,23] aiming for a therapeutic blood level of 8 to 12 μg/mL. Serum levels should be checked when symptoms change, acute illness develops, new drugs are added, or symptoms suggestive of toxicity develop.[1] Early side effects include gastrointestinal tract symptoms, tremulousness, headache, and insomnia. At high serum concentrations, vomiting, hypokalemia, hyperglycemia, tachycardia, cardiac arrhythmias, neuromuscular irritability, and seizures may develop.

The risk-benefit ratio of theophylline should be weighed carefully in each patient. It should be considered when inhaled medication has failed to provide adequate symptom relief and when patients cannot use aerosol therapy optimally.[23]

CORTICOSTEROIDS

Inflammatory changes in the airways associated with airway narrowing have been noted in patients with COPD,[24] although the mechanisms for inflammation in COPD may not be the same as those seen in patients with asthma.[5] The presence of inflammation provides a rationale for the use of corticosteroids in COPD; however, their role is still controversial. Side effects of corticosteroids, both inhaled and systemic, may be significant and are probably underappreciated. A recent critical review of adverse effects in patients with COPD suggests that these drugs may contribute to development of osteoporosis, myopathy, adverse psychiatric events, lethal and nonlethal infection, diabetes, and skin changes.[25] Vertebral compression fractures are common in older men with COPD who use continuous systemic corticosteroids.[26]

Systemic Corticosteroids

Oral corticosteroids have been used with success to treat outpatients with acute exacerbations of COPD, improving dyspnea, lung function tests, and oxygenation and reducing treatment failure rates.[27] They have also been shown to reduce relapses in a minority of patients with a history of frequent exacerbations.[5] Short bursts of corticosteroids should be considered during acute exacerbations in COPD patients who have failed to respond to aggressive bronchodilator therapy. These patients should be tapered off the drugs rapidly because of the potential side effects mentioned previously.[1,26]

The role of systemic steroids in the management of stable outpatients is controversial. High doses given over the short term have been shown to cause a small increase in mean FEV_1 of patients with stable COPD,[28] and long-term use of low-dose oral corticosteroids has been shown to slow the rate of decline of FEV_1.[29] Most studies suggest that only a minority of patients will benefit,[1] and it is difficult to predict which patients will respond. A recent study reported that the presence of sputum eosinophilia predicts a beneficial effect of prednisone treatment in patients with severe obstructive bronchitis.[30] Guidelines have recommended a carefully monitored 2-week trial of up to 40 mg/d of oral prednisone in patients with persistent limiting symptoms despite maximal bronchodilator therapy.[1,3,5,31] Only those patients with significant documented physiologic improvement should be considered for long-term therapy, with the goal of reducing dosage to the lowest possible.

Inhaled Corticosteroids

The use of inhaled steroids in COPD has become widespread in North America even in the absence of clear-cut benefit.[32,33] Moderate doses of inhaled steroids have generally not been effective,[34,35] and results of studies in patients with COPD using higher doses of inhaled corticosteroids have been inconsistent. One recent study using 1 mg of fluticasone daily for 6 months suggested that frequency of exacerbations decreased and that small improvements in lung function and cough and sputum production, but not dyspnea, occurred.[36] A Canadian study using budesonide in a group of patients with stable COPD who had not responded to systemic corticosteroids failed to show improvement in lung function, exercise capacity, and respiratory symptoms compared with placebo.[37] In a small study of stable COPD patients using 3 mg/d of beclomethasone diproprionate, a Japanese group demonstrated improvements in FEV_1, wheezing, and dyspnea in a minority of patients, but these investigators felt that the outcome did not justify the widespread use of this treatment.[38]

Several long-term studies are underway that may help establish definitive treatment recommendations for inhaled corticosteroids in COPD.[32] Current guidelines recommend use of inhaled corticosteroids only in patients who show objective benefit during a steroid trial, either inhaled or systemic.[1,23] Inhaled steroids are generally safe, although some mild cosmetic and upper airway effects may be seen, and dermal thinning, easy bruisability, and other skin abnormalities are associated with higher doses.[25] Recent data also suggest that use of inhaled corticosteroids is associated with the development of cataracts.[39]

ANTIBIOTICS

Chronic infection or colonization of the lower airways is common in patients with COPD. Although evidence is lacking to support the use of prophylactic antibiotics in stable COPD patients, these drugs are often used to treat acute exacerbations. The most common organisms recovered from the lower airways are *Streptococcus pneumoniae, Haemophilus influenzae,* and *Moraxella catarrhalis.* During acute exacerbations, these organisms may be present in increasing numbers, although some studies have shown that up to one-third to one-half of patients will have no growth.[40] Antibiotic choice must take into account local resistance patterns, the ability of an agent to penetrate into respiratory tract tissues and secretions, and patient sensitivities. Sputum culture has not been shown to be cost effective but probably should be obtained in patients who are sick enough to be hospitalized.[1]

The use of antibiotics in acute exacerbations of COPD is supported by the results of a meta-analysis showing that patients who received oral antibiotic therapy had a small but clinically significant improvement in peak expiratory flow rates and more rapid resolution of symptoms.[41] One study demonstrated that patients receiving amoxicillin, trimethoprim-sulfamethoxazole, or doxycycline experienced a more rapid recovery in FEV_1 after an acute exacerbation of chronic bronchitis than did patients receiving placebo.[42] Patients whose exacerbations were characterized by two of the following benefited most from antibiotic treatment: increases in dyspnea, sputum production, and sputum purulence.

The most widely used agents in the management of acute exacerbations of chronic bronchitis are ampicillin, amoxicillin, trimethoprim-sulfamethoxazole, and tetracyclines. If resistant organisms are suspected, amoxicillin-clavulanic acid, a newer macrolide such as clarithromycin or azithromycin, or a fluoroquinolone may be considered, although these agents are considerably more expensive. The fluoroquinolones are more potent than β-lactams and other traditional agents against *H. influenzae* and *M. catarrhalis.*

If acute exacerbation of COPD is believed to be caused by acute influenza A infection, amantidine or rimantidine therapy should be considered in unimmunized patients if started within 48 hours of infection.[43] In stable patients with COPD and chronic bronchiectasis or immunodeficiency, courses of one antibiotic for 2 to 3 weeks followed by another antibiotic for a few weeks may be justified.[5]

MUCOLYTIC AGENTS

Clearance of thick, tenacious secretions is difficult for many patients with COPD, but little evidence exists that thinning of secretions or improving sputum clearance rates produces any clinical improvements.[1] The oral agent acetylcysteine has been widely used in Europe; however, clinical trials of its effectiveness have produced variable results.[44,45] The oral agent is not readily available in the United States, and the aerosolized drug can induce significant bronchoconstriction.[5] Iodinated glycerol has been shown to improve cough and chest discomfort in some patients with chronic bronchitis,[46] but this drug is no longer marketed owing to lack of objective evidence of benefit. Guaifenesin is often prescribed in the United States for its mucoactive effect; however, efficacy has not been demonstrated in controlled trials.[47]

Use of aerosolized recombinant human DNAse (rhDNAse) has been shown to reduce exacerbations of respiratory symptoms and improve pulmonary function in patients with cystic fibrosis.[48] Viscous lung secretions are often present in patients with COPD and consist of mucus-derived glycoproteins and leukocyte-derived DNA, thus providing a rationale for the use of rhDNAse in these patients. No data are yet available regarding the efficacy of rhDNAse in chronic bronchitis, but the results of its use in idiopathic bronchiectasis were disappointing. Use of rhDNAse was ineffective and potentially harmful in that group of patients.[49]

The American Thoracic Society (ATS) recommends that a mucokinetic agent be considered for symptomatic patients receiving maximal inhaled bronchodilator treatment and for severe exacerbation if sputum is very viscous[1]; however, they do not say which drug to use. The British Thoracic Society suggests further study before these drugs can be recommended.[23]

OTHER PHARMACOLOGIC THERAPY

Annual vaccine prophylaxis against influenza is recommended for all patients with COPD.[43,50] The vaccine formulation and potency are revised yearly. Vaccination can reduce the morbidity and mortality associated with influenza infections.[50] Chemoprophylaxis with amantidine or rimantidine should be considered in unimmunized patients with COPD who are at high risk for influenza infection if adequate time is not available for immunization to become effective or in patients in whom immunization is contraindicated. Amantidine and rimantidine may be given in doses of 200 mg daily until immunization is accomplished (6 weeks after vaccination) or the high-risk period is over.

Pneumococcal vaccination is currently recommended for COPD patients, with revaccination to be considered every 6 years in patients at high risk for significant reduction in immune function.[51] Routine revaccination is not recommended for all patients. Both influenza and pneumococcal vaccines are thought to be underused.[51]

Replacement therapy with α_1-antitrypsin is available for emphysema patients with documented deficiency in this protein. Intravenous therapy is able to produce appropriate levels of α_1-protease inhibitor in the blood and alveolar fluid.[52,53] Recent nonrandomized studies have shown that augmentation therapy can slow the rate of decline of FEV_1 and improve survival in selected patients with α_1-antitrypsin deficiency.[54,55] Despite increasing awareness of the role of protease/antiprotease imbalance in the pathogenesis of COPD, α_1-antitrypsin replacement is not indicated in the usual forms of COPD.

A variety of respiratory stimulants have been studied as a means of increasing ventilation, reducing hypercapnea, and improving oxygenation in patients with COPD. These drugs include medroxyprogesterone, acetazolamide, and doxapram in the United States and almitrine in Europe. The beneficial effects of these agents are often short lived, and they have significant associated side effects; therefore, they are not recommended.

Patients with severe COPD may develop pulmonary hypertension and cor pulmonale, conditions associated with a poor prognosis.[56] Although oxygen remains the primary therapy for hypoxemic COPD patients with pulmonary hypertension, a variety of other agents should be considered in these patients. Unfortunately, studies examining the benefits of vasodilators have yielded disappointing results because these drugs often cause limiting side effects, including systemic hypotension and worsening hypoxemia.[56]

Digoxin may be used for rate control in patients with atrial fibrillation and may also be helpful in COPD patients with cor pulmonale if associated left-sided congestive heart failure is present.[57] Diuretics may be used in patients with biventricular heart failure, but these patients should be observed carefully for hypotension and electrolyte imbalance.

Depression and anxiety are common in COPD patients.[58] Pharmacologic therapy is complicated in these patients by limited respiratory reserve and potential for adverse drug interactions. Drug treatment should be considered if anxiety and depression worsen symptoms or contribute to functional impairment.[59] Tricyclic antidepressants can be safely used in patients with COPD,[60] but the newer selective serotonin reuptake inhibitors have not been systematically studied. These agents have a low side effect profile and are considered by some to be first-line therapy for depressed patients with COPD. These drugs are also considered to be effective for treating anxiety and panic disorders in COPD patients.[59] Benzodiazepines should be used with caution in patients with severe COPD because of potential depressant effects on the respiratory centers. Buspirone is an antianxiety medication that does not depress respiratory drive[61]; however, it may be less effective than benzodiazepines.[59]

The importance of nutritional status in COPD has been emphasized in recent reviews[1,3,23] and is discussed elsewhere in this book (Chapter 14). Weight loss is common in COPD patients and is associated with reduced respiratory muscle function and increased mortality.[62] A recent study examined the effects of 6 months of oral anabolic steroid use in undernourished patients with COPD. Although lean body mass increased in this group, no significant changes in exercise capacity were observed.[63] Recombinant human growth hormone has also been proposed as a treatment to improve nitrogen balance and to increase muscle strength in underweight COPD patients. A recent controlled, randomized study showed that growth hormone also increases lean body mass without improving symptoms, muscle strength, or exercise tolerance.[64]

MANAGEMENT OF COPD: AN INCREMENTAL APPROACH

Several incremental approaches to outpatient management of COPD have been proposed in recent years.[1,3,23,65] From a pharmacologic treatment perspective, each has advocated the use of inhaled quaternary anticholinergic agents plus β_2-agonists in the early stages, with the addition of theophylline and corticosteroids for worsening symptoms. Dosages may be titrated upward until an optimal outcome is achieved.

Box 7-1 summarizes the ATS recommendations for step-by-step management of COPD.[1] Inhaled β_2-agonists, used as needed, may be initiated in mildly to moderately obstructed patients with intermittent symptoms. For patients with persistent symptoms, ipratropium bromide is the drug of first choice. β_2-Agonists may be added to ipratropium on an as needed basis if more rapid relief is sought or as a regular supplement if symptoms are not controlled using the anticholinergic alone at the highest recommended doses. For worsening symptoms, theophylline may be started and consideration given to the addition of sustained-release albuterol and/or a mucokinetic agent. If control of symptoms is still considered to be unacceptable, a 10- to 14-day trial of systemic steroids is recommended. For patients with objective benefit from oral steroid use, doses should be decreased as tolerated and a trial of inhaled corticosteroids is warranted. For those patients who do not benefit, use of oral steroids should be discontinued abruptly.

For acute severe exacerbations of COPD, patients must often be hospitalized. Doses and frequency of inhaled or nebulized bronchodilators are increased, and intravenous theophylline and methylprednisolone are added. Antibiotics are often used in this setting, and mucokinetic agents may be added if sputum is very viscous and difficult to clear.

Box 7-1. Step-by-Step Pharmacologic Therapy for COPD

1. For mild, variable symptoms
   - Selective β_2-agonist MDI aerosol, 1–2 puffs every 2–6 h as needed, not to exceed 8–12 puffs per 24 h
2. For mild to moderate continuing symptoms
   - Ipratropium MDI aerosol, 2–6 puffs every 6–8 h; not to be used more frequently

   plus
   - Selective β_2-agonist MDI aerosol, 1–4 puffs as required 4 times daily for rapid relief, when needed, or as regular supplement
3. If response to step 2 is unsatisfactory or a mild to moderate increase in symptoms occurs
   - Add sustained-release theophylline, 200–400 mg twice daily or 400–800 mg at bedtime for nocturnal bronchospasm

   and/or
   - Consider use of sustained-release albuterol, 4–8 mg twice daily, or at night only

   and/or
   - Consider use of a mucokinetic agent
4. If control of symptoms is suboptimal
   - Consider a course of oral steroids (e.g., prednisone), up to 40 mg/d for 10–14 d

     If improvement occurs, wean to low daily or alternate-day dose, e.g., 7.5 mg

     If no improvement occurs, stop abruptly

     If steroid seems to help, consider possible use of aerosol MDI, particularly if patient has evidence of bronchial hyperreactivity
5. For severe exacerbation
   - Increase β_2-agonist dosage, e.g., MDI with spacer, 6–8 puffs every 1/2–2 h, or inhalant solution, unit dose every 1/2–2 h, or subcutaneous administration of epinephrine or terbutaline, 0.1–0.5 mL

   and/or
   - Increase ipratropium dosage, e.g., MDI with spacer every 3–4 h, or inhalant solution of ipratropium, 0.5 mg every 4–8 h

   and
   - Provide theophylline dosage intravenously with calculated amount to bring serum level to 10–12 μg/mL

   and
   - Provide methylprednisolone dosage intravenously, giving 50–100 mg immediately, then every 6–8 h; taper as soon as possible

   and add
   - An antibiotic, if indicated
   - A mucokinetic agent if sputum is very viscous

From American Thoracic Society. Standards for the diagnosis and care of patients with chronic obstructive pulmonary disease (COPD): official statement of the American Thoracic Society. Am J Respir Crit Care Med 1995;152:S77. With permission.
COPD, chronic obstructive pulmonary disease; MDI, metered dose inhaler.

REFERENCES

1. American Thoracic Society. Standards for the diagnosis and care of patients with chronic obstructive pulmonary disease (COPD): official statement of the American Thoracic Society. Am J Respir Crit Care Med 1995;152:S77.
2. Anthonisen NR, Wright EC, the IPPB Trial Group. Bronchodilator response in chronic obstructive pulmonary diseases. Am Rev Respir Dis 1986;132:814.
3. Ferguson GT, Cherniak RM. Management of chronic obstructive pulmonary disease. N Engl J Med 1993;328:1017.
4. Braun SR, McKenzie WN, Copeland C, et al. A comparison of the effect of ipratropium and albuterol in the treatment of chronic obstructive airway disease. Arch Intern Med 1989;149:544.
5. The National Lung Health Education Program (NLHEP). Strategies in preserving lung health and preventing COPD and associated diseases. Chest 1998;113:123S.
6. Rennard SI, Serby CW. Extended therapy with ipratropium is associated with improved lung function in patients with COPD: a retrospective analysis of data from seven clinical trials. Chest 1996;110:62.
7. Anthonison NR, Connett JE, Kiley JP, et al. Effects of smoking intervention and the use of inhaled anticholinergic bronchodilator on the rate of decline of FEV_1: the Lung Health Study. JAMA 1994;272:1497.
8. Van Schayck CP, Dompeling E, van Herwaarden CLA, et al. Bronchodilator treatment in moderate asthma or chronic bronchitis: continuous or on demand. BMJ 1991;303:1426.
9. Boyd G, Morice AH, Pounsford JC, et al. An evaluation of salmeterol in the treatment of chronic obstructive pulmonary disease (COPD). Eur Respir J 1997;10:815.
10. Ulrik CS. Efficacy of inhaled salmeterol in the management of smokers with chronic obstructive pulmonary disease: a single centre randomised, double blind, placebo controlled, crossover study. Thorax 1995;50:750.
11. Grove A, Lipworth BI, Smith RP, et al. Effects of regular salmeterol on lung function and exercise capacity in patients with chronic obstructive airways disease. Thorax 1996;51:689.
12. Jones PW, Bosh TK. Quality of life changes in COPD patients treated with salmeterol. Am J Respir Crit Care Med 1997;155:1283.
13. Ikeda A, Nishimura K, Koyama H, et al. Bronchodilating effects of combined therapy with clinical dosages of ipratropium bromide and salbutamol for stable COPD: comparison with ipratropium bromide alone. Chest 1995;107:401.
14. Combivent Inhalation Aerosol Study Group. In chronic obstructive pulmonary disease, a combination of ipratropium and albuterol is more effective than either agent alone: an 85-day multicenter trial. Chest 1994;105:1411.
15. Combivent Inhalation Aerosol Study Group. Routine nebulized ipratropium and albuterol together are better than either alone in COPD. Chest 1997;112:1514.
16. Friedman M, Witek TJ, Serby CW, et al. Combination bronchodilator therapy is associated with a reduction in exacerbations of COPD. Am J Respir Crit Care Med 1996;153:A126.
17. Murciano D, Auclair M-H, Pariente R, et al. A randomised controlled trial of theophylline in patients with severe chronic obstructive pulmonary disease. N Engl J Med 1989;320:1521.
18. Weinberger M, Hendeles L. Theophylline in asthma. N Engl J Med 1996;334:1380.
19. Chapman KR. Therapeutic algorithm for chronic obstructive pulmonary disease. Am J Med 1991; 91(Suppl 4A):17S.
20. Filuk RB, Easton PA, Anthonison NR. Responses to large doses of salbutamol and theophylline in patients with chronic obstructive pulmonary disease. Am Rev Respir Dis 1985;132:871.
21. Karpel JP, Kotch A, Zinny M, et al. A comparison of inhaled ipratropium, oral theophylline plus inhaled β-agonist, and the combination of all three in patients with COPD. Chest 1994;105:1089.
22. Martin RJ, Pak J. Overnight theophylline concentrations and effects on sleep and lung function in chronic obstructive pulmonary disease. Am Rev Respir Dis 1992;145:540.
23. British Thoracic Society. BTS guidelines for the management of chronic obstructive pulmonary disease. Thorax 1997;52:S1.
24. Cosio M, Ghezzo H, Hogg JC, et al. The relations between structural changes in small airways and pulmonary function tests. N Engl J Med 1978; 298:1277.
25. McEvoy CE, Niewoehner DE. Adverse effects of corticosteroid therapy for COPD. Chest 1997; 111:732.
26. McEvoy CE, Ensrud KE, Bender E, et al. Association between corticosteroid use and vertebral fractures in older men with chronic obstructive pulmonary disease. Am J Respir Crit Care Med 1998;157:704.
27. Thompson WH, Nielson CP, Carvalho P, et al. Controlled trial of oral prednisone in outpatients with acute COPD exacerbation. Am J Respir Crit Care Med 1996;154:407.
28. Callahan C, Dittus R, Katz B. Oral corticosteroid therapy for patients with stable chronic obstructive pulmonary disease: a meta-analysis. Ann Intern Med 1991;114:216.
29. Postma DS, Peters I, Steenhuis EJ, et al. Moderately severe airflow obstruction: can corticosteroids slow down obstruction? Eur Respir J 1988;1:22.
30. Pizzichini E, Pizzichini MMM, Gibson P, et al. Sputum eosinophilia predicts benefit from prednisone in smokers with chronic obstructive bronchitis. Am J Respir Crit Care Med 1998;158:1511.
31. Siafakas NM, Vermeire P, Pride NB, et al. Optimal assessment and management of chronic obstructive pulmonary disease (COPD). Eur Respir J 1995;8:1398.
32. Anthonisen NR. Steroids in COPD: the nearly eternal question. Chest 1999;115:3.

33. Jackevicius C, Joyce DP, Kesten S, et al. Prehospitalization inhaled corticosteroid use in patients with COPD or asthma. Chest 1997;111:296.

34. Shim CS, Williams MH. Aerosol beclomethasone in patients with steroid-responsive chronic obstructive pulmonary disease. Am J Med 1985; 78:655.

35. Engel T, Heinig JH, Madsen O, et al. A trial of inhaled budesonide on airway responsiveness in smokers with chronic bronchitis. Eur Respir J 1989;2:935.

36. Paggiaro PL, Dahle R, Bakran I, et al. Multicentre randomized placebo controlled trial of inhaled fluticasone propionate in patients with chronic obstructive pulmonary disease. Lancet 1998;351: 773.

37. Bourbou J, Rouleau MY, Boucher S. Randomised controlled trial of inhaled corticosteroids in patients with chronic obstructive pulmonary disease. Thorax 1998;53:477.

38. Nishimura K, Koyama H, Ikeda A, et al. The effect of high-dose inhaled beclomethasone dipropionate in patients with stable COPD. Chest 1999; 115:31.

39. Cumming RG, Mitchell P, Leeder SR. Use of inhaled corticosteroids and the risk of cataracts. N Engl J Med 1997;337:8.

40. Balter MS, Hyland RH, Low DE, et al. Recommendations on the management of chronic bronchitis: a practical guide for Canadian physicians. CMAJ 1994;151(Suppl):5.

41. Saint S, Bent S, Vittinghoff, et al. Antibiotics in chronic obstructive disease exacerbations: a meta-analysis. JAMA 1995;273:957.

42. Anthonisen NR, Manfreda J, Warren CPW. Antibiotic therapy in exacerbations of chronic obstructive pulmonary disease. Ann Intern Med 1987; 106:196.

43. Recommendations of the Immunization Practices Advisory Committee, Centers for Disease Control. Ann Intern Med 1987;107:521–525.

44. Bowman G, Backer U, Larsson S, et al. Oral acetylcysteine reduces exacerbation rate in chronic bronchitis: report of a trial organized by the Swedish Society for Pulmonary Diseases. Eur J Respir Dis 1983;64:405.

45. British Thoracic Society Research Committee. Oral N-acetylcysteine and exacerbation rates in patients with chronic bronchitis and severe airways obstruction. Thorax 1985;40:832.

46. Petty TL. The National Mucolytic Study: results of a randomized, double-blind, placebo-controlled study of iodinated glycerol in chronic obstructive bronchitis. Chest 1990;97:75.

47. Hirsch SR, Vierns PF, Kory RC. The expectorant effect of glycerol guaiacolate in patients with chronic bronchitis. Chest 1973;63:9.

48. Fuchs HJ, Borowitz DS, Christiansen DH, et al. Effect of aerosolized recombinant human DNAse on exacerbations of respiratory symptoms and on pulmonary function in patients with cystic fibrosis. N Engl J Med 1994;331:637.

49. O'Donnell AE, Barker AF, Ilowite JS, et al. Treatment of idiopathic bronchiectasis with aerosolized recombinant human DNAse. Chest 1998;113: 1329.

50. Fiebach N, Beckett W. Prevention of respiratory infections in adults: influenza and pneumococcal vaccines. Arch Intern Med 1994;154:2545.

51. Mostow SR, Cate TR, Ruben FL. Prevention of influenza and pneumonia. Am Rev Respir Dis 1990;142:487.

52. Wewers MD, Casalaro MA, Sellers SE, et al. Replacement therapy for alpha$_1$-antitrypsin deficiency associated with emphysema. N Engl J Med 1987;316:1055.

53. Hubbard RC, Sellers S, Czerski D, et al. Biochemical efficacy and safety of monthly augmentation therapy for alpha$_1$-antitrypsin deficiency. JAMA 1988;260:1259.

54. Seersholm N, Wencker M, Banik N, et al. Does alpha$_1$-antitrypsin augmentation therapy slow the annual decline in FEV$_1$ in patients with severe hereditary alpha$_1$-antitrypsin deficiency? Eur Respir J 1997;10:2260.

55. The Alpha$_1$-antitrypsin Deficiency Registry Study Group. Survival and FEV$_1$ decline in individuals with severe deficiency of alpha$_1$-antitrypsin. Am J Respir Crit Care Med 1998;158:49.

56. MacNee W. State of the art: pathophysiology of cor pulmonale in chronic obstructive pulmonary disease. Am J Respir Crit Care Med 1994;150:pt I-II:833, 1158.

57. Mathur PN, Powles ACP, Pugsley SO, et al. Effect of digoxin on right ventricular function in severe chronic airflow obstruction. Ann Intern Med 1981;95:283.

58. Light RW, Merrill EJ, Despars JA, et al. Prevalence of depression and anxiety in patients with COPD: relationship to functional capacity. Chest 1985; 87:35.

59. Wingate BJ, Hansen-Flaschen J. Anxiety and depression in advanced lung disease. Clin Chest Med 1997;18:495.

60. McDonald G, Borson S, Gayle T, et al. Nortriptyline effectively treats depression in COPD. Am Rev Respir Dis 1989;139:4.

61. Garner SJF, Eldridge PG, et al. Buspirone, an anxiolytic drug that stimulates respiration. Am Rev Respir Dis 1989;139:946.

62. Wilson DO, Rogers RM, Wright EC, et al. Body weight in chronic obstructive pulmonary disease: the National Institutes of Health Intermittent Positive Pressure Breathing Trial. Am Rev Respir Dis 1989;139:1435.

63. Ferreira IM, Verreschi IT, Nery LE, et al. The influence of 6 months of oral anabolic steroids on body mass and respiratory muscles in undernourished COPD patients. Chest 1998;114:19.

64. Burdet L, de Muralt B, Schutz Y, et al. Administration of growth hormone to underweight patients with chronic obstructive pulmonary disease: a prospective, randomized, controlled study. Am J Respir Crit Care Med 1997;156:1800.

65. Canadian Thoracic Society Workshop Group. Guidelines for the assessment and management of chronic obstructive pulmonary disease. CMAJ 1992;147:420.

8 Aerosol Therapy

Robert M. Kacmarek
David R. Schwartz

⟫ Professional Skills

Upon completion of this chapter, the reader will:

- Identify the various bronchodilator compounds available and classify their mode of action
- Discuss the appropriate use of corticosteroids in the management of patients with COPD
- Describe concerns and indications for the use of mucokinetic agents in COPD patients
- Discuss the appropriate use of antibiotics in this population of patients
- Identify the components of a small-volume nebulizer and discuss its proper use
- Define when spacers and holding chambers should be used and discuss the operation of metered dose inhalers
- Describe the proper use of dry powder inhalers and outline the settings where they may be employed
- Contrast the advantages and disadvantages of small-volume nebulizers, metered dose inhalers, and dry powder inhalers

Aerosolization of medications in lung disease provides an opportunity to deliver high concentrations of a therapeutic agent to its target while minimizing systemic effects. For this reason, an explosion occurred in research and development of drugs that may be aerosolized and of techniques designed to improve drug delivery. Though bronchodilators remain the most important class of aerosolized medications, delivery of anti-inflammatory agents, antibiotics, mucolytics, and immunomodulators directly to the airway all have a role in specific instances.

In chronic obstructive pulmonary disease (COPD) patients, airway mucosal edema, glandular hypertrophy, and airway secretions combine with a loss of airway "tethering" resulting from the parenchymal destruction of emphysema to produce chronic airflow obstruction. In addition, at least two-thirds of these patients have bronchoconstriction contributing to obstructive disease.[1] Increasing obstruction—measured by the drop in forced expiratory volume in 1 second (FEV_1)—disordered ventilatory mechanics, and gas exchange abnormalities result in decreased functional capacity. The course of the illness is often punctuated by periodic acute exacerbations resulting in significant morbidity and mortality. Short of providing long-term oxygen therapy to patients with severe hypoxemia, and promoting smoking cessation, nothing else has been shown to alter the disease course. Therefore, chronic medical therapy of these patients centers around improving functional capacity through medications designed to relieve airflow obstruction. This chapter concentrates on the use of aerosolized medications in COPD. Although focusing on patients with "COPD" as defined by the American Thoracic Society,[2] that is, patients with chronic bronchitis/emphysema, we briefly touch on aerosol therapy in other chronic airway diseases, such as asthma, bronchiectasis, and cystic fibrosis.

BRONCHODILATORS

Aerosolized bronchodilators are considered a first-line therapy in both the acute and the chronic setting for patients with asthma and COPD, though significant differences exist. In general, asthmatics are believed to respond better to bronchodilators. Differentiating these diseases in adult smokers with obstructive lung disease can be difficult. At least one-third of COPD patients have a significant bronchodilator response when tested once, whereas more than two-thirds will show a bronchodilator response with serial testing.[1] In addition, inhaled bronchodilators may provide substantial subjective benefits in COPD in the absence of significant changes in expiratory flows. This may be related to reduction of hyperinflation and improved lung mechanics that may be independent of large airway tone. For these reasons, all patients with COPD should receive bronchodilator therapy. Although β-agonists are the most potent bronchodilators in asthmatic patients, anticholinergic agents may be better bronchodilators in COPD. In addition, COPD patients, as a group, are older, have more comorbidity, and may be less able to tolerate adverse systemic effects.[2] In both diseases, bronchodilation is used for symptom control and does not positively affect the course of the underlying process.[3]

Anticholinergic Therapy

Anticholinergic agents are recommended for all patients with COPD and daily symptoms; they are considered the bronchodilators of choice in this disease by many (Table 8-1). Parasympathetic innervation of the airways via branches of the vagus nerve is the primary determinant of resting airway smooth muscle tone. Activation of muscarinic receptors on effector cells, such as airway smooth muscle, submucosal glands, and postsynaptic nerves, by acetylcholine released from presynaptic nerve terminals results in bronchoconstriction and an increase in airway secretions. Parasympathetic innervation predominates in large airways and contributes to the bronchoconstriction produced by diverse stimuli. Cholinergic tone has a circadian rhythm, peaking during the night, and likely contributing to the worsened airflow and oxygen desaturation during sleep that is often seen in chronic obstructive lung disease.[4] Atropine, the tertiary ammonium alkaloid derived from the Belladonna plant, is the classic anticholinergic bronchodilator. In addition to bronchodila-

Table 8-1. Quaternary Ammonium Anticholinergic Agents for Inhalation

Drug	Formulation	Adult Dosage	Peak/Total Duration of Action (hr)
Ipratropium (Atrovent)	MDI (18 μg/puff)	2 puffs every 6–8 hr	1–2/3–8
	Nebulized (.02%)	500 mg every 6–8 hr	
Ipratropium/albuterol[a] (Combivent)	MDI (18 μg/103 μg/puff)	2 puffs every 6–8 hr	1–2/3–8
Glycopyrrolate (Robinul)	Nebulized (.2 mg/cc)[b]	1–2 mg every 2–6 hr	1/2–6

[a]Combivent is a combination metered dose inhaler (see page 115 for details).
[b]Glycopyrrolate (Robinul) solution can be used off label for nebulization.

tion and reduction of all upper and lower airway secretions, atropine can also cause antimuscarinic side effects such as sedation, tachycardia, ileus, bladder dysfunction, and elevated intraocular pressure. Because it is lipid soluble, it is well absorbed through the airway and oral mucosa, and systemic side effects limit aerosolized use of the drug. Ipratropium bromide, the synthetic N-isopropyl derivative of atropine, is the main anticholinergic medicine used for aerosolization in the United States, and the only one available as a metered dose inhaler (MDI). Because it is a quaternary ammonium ion, it is poorly absorbed through mucus membranes, and when aerosolized, it is remarkably free of systemic adverse effects. Because its peak effect is delayed compared with the intermediate-acting β_2-agonist bronchodilators (90 to 120 minutes), it is inappropriate for use as a "rescue" medication. Peak bronchodilation and length of effect are greater than with intermediate-acting β_2-agonists in patients with COPD.[5] Ipratropium may be nebulized as a 0.02% solution. The standard dose is 500 μg (2.5 cc) usually given three or four times a day. Each canister of MDI carries 200 inhalations of 18 μg each. Although the American Thoracic Society recommends a starting dose of 2 to 4 puffs with a spacer three to four times a day, its safety profile allows for up to 8 puffs three or four times a day to be given in patients with chronically severe airflow obstruction or during an exacerbation. Tolerance to the bronchodilator effects of this medication has not been an issue. Ipratropium decreases airway mucus secretion but does not impair ciliary function or have adverse effects on secretion viscosity.[6] Its use relieves dyspnea, improves exercise tolerance, and improves sleep quality in patients with COPD. It does not alter the natural history of the disease and has no role in asymptomatic patients. Several other synthetic quaternary ammonium anticholinergic agents are available for use around the world, and more selective and longer-acting agents are being studied. In the United States, glycopyrrolate is available for nebulization (off label). This agent, like atropine, is often used to decrease airway or pharyngeal secretions before surgery or endoscopy. Its bronchodilator effect has not been compared directly with that of ipratropium bromide.

The combination of ipratropium and albuterol in an MDI is available in the United States.[7] In addition, ipratropium 0.02% solution is often combined with one of the β_2-agonist solutions for nebulization for acute and chronic therapy in COPD and asthma.[8,9] Combinations may provide additive bronchodilation and are easier to use. For acute exacerbations of COPD or asthma, they have become the standard of care in many institutions. In COPD patients with adrenergic side effects such as ectopy or tremor, we prefer to limit β_2-agonists to "rescue" therapy, though the combination inhaler is useful in patients desiring simplification of their medication regimen.

β_2-Agonists

β_2-Agonists are potent bronchodilators that interact with the β_2-receptors that are most dense on airway smooth muscle cells of the smaller airways (Table 8-2). The activation of adenylate cyclase results in a cyclic adenosine monophosphate–dependent decrease in cytosolic calcium that relaxes airway smooth muscle. In the United States, short-acting (isoproterenol), intermediate-acting (terbutaline, albuterol, bitolterol, pirbuterol), and long-acting (salmeterol) agents are available. β-Agonists also increase mucociliary transport and may decrease airway edema.[6] Intermediate-acting β-agonists are the drugs of choice for acute, symptomatic relief of bronchospasm in all obstructive lung diseases owing to their rapid peak effect (5–15 minutes). Significant side effects of these agents include tremor, palpitations, and anxiety. The cardiac, β_1 effects, are dose dependent and are decreased with the β_2-selective agents (all except isoproterenol, metaproterenol). Fine tremor is probably a β_2 effect.[6] Hypokalemia and hyperglycemia may also occur. As with anticholinergic agents, no evidence exists that bronchodilator therapy with β_2-agonists will alter the natural history of COPD. Intermediate-acting β_2-agonists are recommended for symptomatic relief of bronchospasm in COPD patients with variable symptoms or during an acute exacerbation. In patients with continuing symptoms, intermediate-acting,

Table 8-2. Inhaled β_2-Agonists, Intermediate and Long Acting[a]

Drug	Formulation	Adult Dosage	Peak/Total Duration of Action (hr)
Albuterol			0.5–2/0.5–2
Proventil/Ventolin	MDI (90 μg/puff)	2 puffs every 4–6 hr PRN	—
Ventolin Rotacaps	DPI (200 μg/inhalation)	1–2 capsules every 4–6 hr PRN	—
Albuterol sulfate	Nebulized (5 mg/mL)	2.5 mg every 4–6 hr PRN	—
Pirbuterol			0.5–2/4–6
Maxair	MDI (200 μg/puff)	2 puffs every 4–6 hr PRN	—
Maxair Autohaler	MDI (breath actuated)		—
Bitolterol mesylate			0.5–2/4–6
Tornalate	MDI (370 μg/puff)	2 puffs every 4–6 hr PRN	—
	Nebulized (2 mg/mL)	1.5–3.5 mg two or four times daily PRN	—
Terbutaline	MDI (200 μg/puff)	2 puffs every 4–6 hr PRN	0.5–2/4–6
Metaproterenol			Within 1/1–5
Alupent, Metaprel	MDI (.65 mg/puff)	2–3 puffs every 4–6 hr PRN	—
Alupent	Nebulized (50 mg/cc)	15 mg every 4–6 hr PRN	—
Isoetharine			5–15 min/ 1–4
Bronkometer	MDI (340 μg/spray)	1–2 sprays every 4–6 hr PRN	—
Isoetharine hydro-chloride	Nebulized (0.1, 0.125, 0.2%)	3–5 mg every 2–4 hr PRN	—
Salmeterol			2–4/≤12
Serevent	MDI (21 μg/puff)	2 puffs every 12 hr	—
Serevent Diskus	DPI (50 μg/inhalation)	1 inhalation every 12 hr	—

MDI, metered dose inhaler; PRN, as needed; DPI, dry powder inhaler.

[a]Listed dose schedule is for daily, "maintenance," or PRN use. All the intermediate-acting drugs may be used more frequently PRN for acute bronchospasm. Metaproterenol and bitolterol have a slightly longer time to action than the other intermediate-acting drugs, which have an initial bronchodilating effect in 5–15 minutes (bitolterol is a prodrug metabolized to the active bronchodilator colterol in the liver). Salmeterol, the only long-acting β_2-agonist currently approved in the United States, is inappropriate for use as a "rescue" inhaler and should be used twice daily, not PRN.

β_2-agonists are recommended either for daily use up to four times a day or as needed.[2] In asthma, β_2-agonists are clearly the most potent bronchodilators, though much controversy surrounds their use. It has been suggested that chronic use of β-agonists in asthma may result in tolerance to the medication and worsened asthma control.[10] The best study to date found no significant difference in subjective or objective asthma control in mild asthmatics treated with either four times daily inhaled albuterol or albuterol as needed.[11] We agree with the recommendation of the authors of this study to use the intermediate-acting drugs as needed in asthma and have adopted this strategy in COPD patients as well. The higher systemic doses of nebulized versus inhaled β-agonists may place patients at risk for atrial or ventricular arrhythmias or coronary ischemia. In addition, the pulmonary vasodilator effects of these agents may worsen ventilation/perfusion ratio ($\dot{V}/\dot{Q}$) matching and worsen hypoxemia in asthma or COPD. We try to limit nebulized β_2-agonist use to significant acute exacerbations of COPD presenting with bronchospasm.

In the patient with COPD and airway hyperresponsiveness, exercise-induced broncho-constriction (seen in up to 80% of asthmatics) may limit strenuous exercise in the rehabilitation setting. Cool, dry ambient air will worsen this response. Use of 2 puffs of an intermediate-acting β_2-agonist 5 to 10 minutes before beginning exercise should be the treatment of choice in these patients.

The long-acting β_2-agonist salmeterol (lasts up to 12 hours) is becoming increasingly important in the management of chronic asthma and is beginning to find a role in COPD as well. In asthma, multiple studies have shown that the addition of 2 puffs twice daily of salmeterol provides better results than doubling the dose of inhaled corticosteroids in patients with suboptimal control.[12,13] In COPD, a body of evidence is accumulating to suggest that long-acting β_2-agonists are safe and effective bronchodilators and may be useful even in patients without a short-term bronchodilator response.[14,15] One recent, well-designed study suggested improved lung function with the use of salmeterol compared with low-dose ipratropium bromide (2 puffs four times a day) in moderate COPD.[15] In COPD patients requiring multiple daily treatments with intermediate-acting β_2-agonists for symptomatic bronchospasm, the addition of salmeterol to ipratropium bromide is a rational choice.

Levalbuterol, the R-isomer of racemic albuterol, has recently become available as a solution for nebulization in asthma. Whereas this isomer is responsible for β_2-mediated bronchodilation, the longer-lasting S-isomer has no intrinsic bronchodilator activity and may be responsible for the tolerance sometimes seen with use of β_2-agonists in asthmatics.[16] Initial studies comparing this agent to racemic albuterol show a modest increase in bronchodilation, and mild reduction in tremor and heart rate increase.[17] Further studies are needed to show whether use of levalbuterol will result in clinically significant improvement. The drug has not been studied in COPD.

CORTICOSTEROIDS

Inhaled corticosteroids are the mainstay of therapy in patients with persistent asthma and have revolutionized treatment of this disease (Table 8-3). Full discussion of the benefits and side effects of corticosteroids in asthma is beyond the scope of this discussion; it has been the subject of many excellent reviews.[18,19] Several points, however, are worth making: (a) Inhaled corticosteroids decrease airway inflammation in asthma, reducing bronchial hyperresponsiveness, improving airflow and overall disease control. (b) Current recommendations are to begin therapy with a relatively high dose of one of the available steroids (see Table 8-3) to achieve control and then slowly taper to the lowest possible dose maintaining control; any change in dose should be made at intervals of 3 months or more. (c) As the dose-response curve of the airway effect of inhaled corticosteroids is relatively flat, the addition of other drugs, including salmeterol (see above), theophylline prepara-

Table 8-3. Inhaled Corticosteroids

Drug	Formulation	Adult Dosage
Beclomethasone dipropionate		
Beclovent/Vanceril	MDI (42 μg/puff)	4–8 puffs BID
Vanceril Double-Strength	MDI (84 μg/puff)	2–4 puffs BID
Budesonide		
Pulmicort Turuhaler	DPI (200 or 400 μg/inhalation)	1–2 inhalations BID
Flunisolide		
Aerobid	MDI (250 μg/puff)	2–4 puffs BID
Fluticasone propionate		
Flovent	MDI (44, 110, 220 μg/puff)	2–4 puffs BID
Flovent rotadisk	DPI (50, 100, 250 μg/inhalation)	1 inhalation BID
Triamcinalone acetonide		
Azmacort	MDI (100 μg/puff)	2 puffs TID–QID

MDI, metered dose inhaler; BID, twice daily; DPI, dry powder inhaler; TID, three times daily; QID, four times daily.

tions, and leukotriene inhibitors, to a suboptimal regimen may be preferable to doubling the dose of inhaled steroid. *(d)* Systemic manifestations of inhaled corticosteroids are dose related; because of the flat dose-response for efficacy, chronic doses above 2000 μg should be avoided. The higher-potency inhaled steroids, budesonide and fluticasone propionate, have extensive first-pass metabolism and may be preferable. Further comparative studies are needed.[18]

In patients with COPD, a clear-cut beneficial effect of inhaled corticosteroids is lacking. Two recent, large studies document the lack of efficacy of long-term, inhaled budesonide on pulmonary function in these patients.[20,21] Generalization to the broad COPD population is limited by the careful screening out of COPD patients with an asthmatic phenotype by history and failure to show an acute bronchodilator response to β_2-agonists during pulmonary function testing. Several studies suggest that a subgroup of COPD patients with significant airway eosinophilic inflammation may be inhaled steroid "responders," but further studies are needed to determine how to identify this group.[22,23] Currently, inhaled steroids are not routinely recommended in COPD.

MUCOKINETIC AGENTS

Retained tracheobronchial mucus contributes to the airflow obstruction of COPD, but large quantities of mucus secretion are uncommon in this disease.[2] Whereas copious sputum production is characteristic of diseases with predominant bronchiectasis, such as cystic fibrosis, COPD patients rarely cough up more than 60 mL of mucoid sputum per day. Aerosol delivery of agents to enhance mucociliary clearance by reducing mucus viscosity (mucokinetic agents) should provide symptomatic relief of airflow obstruction and could theoretically have a positive effect on the degree of chronic airway inflammation and remodeling by limiting contact of infected, inflammatory secretions with the airway mucosa. Trials of mucokinetic therapy in COPD patients has traditionally been disappointing, although a recent meta-analysis of oral agents showed a modest beneficial effect on COPD exacerbations.[24] Mucokinetic agents that are delivered directly to the airway include bland aerosols and various drugs and enzymes that interfere with mucus structure (mucolytics).

Bland Aerosols

Little clinical evidence suggests that simple humidification, aerosolized water (i.e., mist) or isotonic saline, can significantly "hydrate" respiratory secretions and reduce secretion viscosity.[25] Conversely, the use of bland aerosols or humidification to prevent further desiccation of the airway mucosal surface during administration of aerosolized drugs or high-flow oxygen is clearly warranted.[6] Nebulized hypertonic saline (1.8–20%) is an airway irritant that causes cough and mucus hypersecretion; it may be used to facilitate acquisition of sputum specimens for microbiologic tests such as acid-fast smears for tuberculosis or staining for pneumocystis organisms. Again, little evidence suggests that the hypertonic fluid can promote dilution of the airway secretions. Reflex cough and bronchospasm limit its use in obstructive lung disease, although data suggest improved sputum rheology and transiently improved sputum clearance in cystic fibrosis patients treated with hypertonic saline aerosols.[26,27]

Alkalinization of mucus may weaken strand cross-linking and improve mucus viscosity.[6] Aerosolization of a 2% sodium bicarbonate solution has been tried in this regard. Although reported to be safe, bronchospasm and cough produced by the irritant require concurrent β_2-agonist use (must be mixed fresh and used immediately to prevent breakdown of β_2-agonist). No good data support use of alkaline aerosols in COPD.

Mucolytics

Much clinical experience has been had with drugs containing reactive sulfhydryl groups that disrupt disulfide links in mucus proteins and reduce sputum viscosity. Topical acetylcysteine (N-acetyl-L-cysteine) rapidly liquefies sputum (maximal at 5 to 10 minutes) when instilled down endotracheal or tracheal tubes or bronchoscopically instilled in patients with tenacious mucus plugs (5 to 10 cc of 10 to 20% solution). Again, induced bronchoconstriction, severe at times, limits the use of acetylcysteine in patients with obstructive lung disease. In rare cases, we have found it more helpful and bronchospasm less troublesome when the agent is directly instilled through the bronchoscope. We do not recommend its routine use or its use as an aerosol.

Aerosolized recombinant human DNase I (rhDNase) has found a role as a mucolytic in patients with cystic fibrosis, where the significantly increased sputum viscosity is largely a function of excessive amounts of leukocyte and bacterial DNA.[28] DNase I is given daily or twice daily in 2.5-mg doses. Despite initial hope, DNase has not had a beneficial effect in either chronic bronchitis or bronchiectasis other than cystic fibrosis.[29]

ANTIBIOTICS

As with other aerosolized drugs, direct delivery of antibiotics to the respiratory tract in patients with suppurative lung infection has the theoretical advantage of delivering high local doses of the drug while avoiding systemic toxicity. Aerosol delivery of antibiotics has been limited by fear of inducing antibiotic resistance. Although aerosolization of β-lactam antibiotics, aminoglycosides, and colistin can decrease the bacterial burden in the airways, controlled outcome trials have been positive only in patients with cystic fibrosis.[30] In these patients, chronically colonized with multiresistant pseudomonal species, aerosolized tobramycin has been most extensively studied. In a 24-week, randomized, controlled trial, the use of the tobramycin inhalational formulation via a jet ventilator (300 mg twice daily) resulted in significant clinical improvement without substantial toxic effects.[31] Although there was a trend toward an increase in aminoglycoside resistance of the airway flora, this will need to be followed closely in longer-term studies. Though the role of chronic and acute infection in the pathogenesis of COPD/COPD exacerbations is unclear, and many flares resolve without systemic antibiotics, treatment of acute exacerbations of COPD with antibiotics directed against the classic colonizing flora—*Streptococcus pneumoniae, Haemophilus influenzae,* and *Moraxella catarrhalis*—remains the standard of care. New data suggest that isolates in patients with severe COPD or exacerbations requiring hospitalization are predominantly enteric Gram-negative bacteria and pseudomonas species.[32,33] With widespread bacterial antibiotic resistance growing, aerosolization of potent antibiotics with systemic toxicity may eventually be considered in COPD exacerbations. At present, we occasionally use aerosolized aminoglycosides or colistin (150 mg twice daily) in chronically ventilated patients with persistent, symptomatic pseudomonal infection unresponsive to systemic therapy or highly resistant to other available agents.

MODES OF AEROSOL DELIVERY

Aerosolized pharmacologic agents can be delivered to the lower respiratory tract of spontaneously breathing patients by the use of small-volume nebulizers (SVN), MDIs without or with a spacer or holding chamber (MDIh), and dry powdered inhalers (DPIs).[34] SVNs and MDI/MDIhs have been readily available for use in the home for years. More recently, DPIs have gained popularity for aerosol administration in the home as a result of international agreements to eliminate the use of chlorofluorocarbons in the next few years.[35] Recent data,[34] as illustrated in Figure 8-1, indicates that patient response to these three approaches are similar. All three result in approximately 8 to 12% of delivered drug depositing in the lower respiratory tract.[36] However, the distribution of the remainder of the delivered drug differs among approaches.[35] With SVNs, most of the delivered drug deposits in the apparatus itself, with little drug depositing in the oropharynx and about 20% of the drug lost to the atmosphere.[37] MDIs result in little loss of the drug to the atmosphere; however, about 80% of the drug deposits in the oropharynx.[38] The use of a spacer essentially moves the 80% oropharyngeal deposition to deposition in the spacer.[38] With DPIs, little drug is lost to the atmosphere or deposited in the oropharynx, but about 80% of the drug is deposited in the apparatus.[39] It should be emphasized that these data greatly depend on technique. Poor technique with any of these devices can result in marked changes in deposition within the respiratory tract. When a particular drug is available for delivery by all three techniques, at least theoretically patient response can be expected to be similar with each technique.[39] However, specific issues associated with use of each of these techniques can direct the clinician to choose a particular device for a specific patient.

SMALL-VOLUME NEBULIZERS

A typical SVN is illustrated in Figure 8-2.[40] All of these devices operate by use of the jet drag effect. That is, the high velocity of a rapidly flowing gas moving through the narrow outlet of the compressed gas inlet port draws fluid from the liquid reservoir by establishing a subatmospheric pressure lateral to the high-velocity flow. Fluid as a result is drawn up in front of the gas flow. When the gas strikes the fluid it aerosolizes the liquid. The large particles are removed from the aerosol by striking the baffle, the walls, and the cap of the SVN.[41] These particles are in turn renebulizied. Despite the fact that all SVNs function in this manner, their performance is clearly different. Figure 8-3 illustrates the respirable mass of aerosol produced by 17 different SVNs.[42] In addition, performance of a particular model SVN from the same company may vary from year to year as a result of changes in overall design features. Because of this variability in performance of SNVs, many newer drugs, especially antibiotics, indicate the precise nebulizer that should be used to deliver the drug.[41] SVNs are the only delivery devices that do not come packaged with the specific

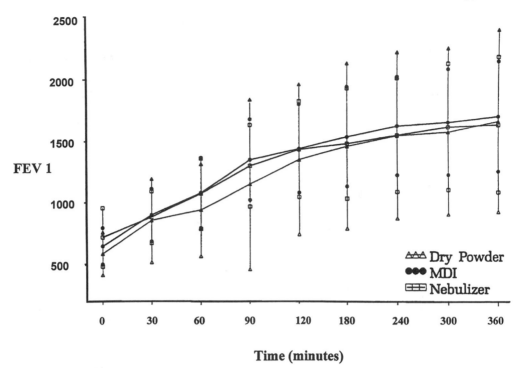

Time (minutes)

Figure 8-1. Absolute changes in forced expiratory volume in 1 second (FEV_1) (mean ± SD) following cumulative doses of inhaled albuterol in the 27 patients in the emergency department with an FEV_1 of less than 30% predicted. Patients (9 in each group) were treated with albuterol via nebulizer (5 mg), metered dose inhaler (*MDI*) with a spacer or holding chamber (400 μg), and DPI (Rotohaler, 400 μg). All groups received the respective treatments on arrival in the emergency department, every 30 minutes during the first 2 hours, and then hourly until the sixth hour. The total dose of inhaled albuterol administered during the 6-hour treatment was 45 mg of nebulized solution or 3600 μg via MDI and DPI. All groups improved compared with baseline, with no difference between groups. (Reprinted from Raimondi AC, Schottlender J, Lombardi D, et al. Treatment of acute severe asthma with inhaled albuterol delivered via jet nebulizer, metered dose inhaler with spacer, or dry powder. Chest 1997;97[1]:24–28.)

drug to deliver. MDIs and DPIs are designed specifically for the drug they deliver. As a result, efficacy of a drug delivered by SVN may depend on the SVN used to aerosolize it.

Factors Affecting SVN Function

In addition to the design of the SVN, several other factors affect the quantity of drug delivered, including gas flow powering the SVN,[42,43] diluent volume,[42,44] the drug solution to be nebulized,[45] the gas used to power the unit,[46] and the temperature of the solution being nebulizied.[41]

All SVNs have a dead volume, that is, a volume of fluid that will never be nebulized regardless of the solution used, the volume of solution nebulized, or the driving gas flow.[42] Generally, this volume varies between about 1 and 1.5 mL. As a result, the smaller the actual volume of solution the greater the percentage of "drug" remaining in the dead volume. In general, about 25 to 30% of the drug placed in the nebulizer remains in the dead volume even if optimal solution volume is used.[42] As nebulization time continues,

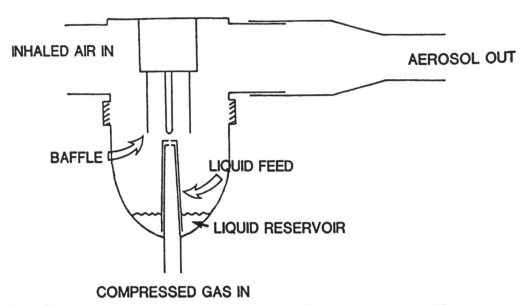

Figure 8-2. Schematic drawing of an SVN. See page 120 for discussion. (Reprinted from Newman SP. Aerosol generators and delivery systems. Respir Care 1991;36:939–951.)

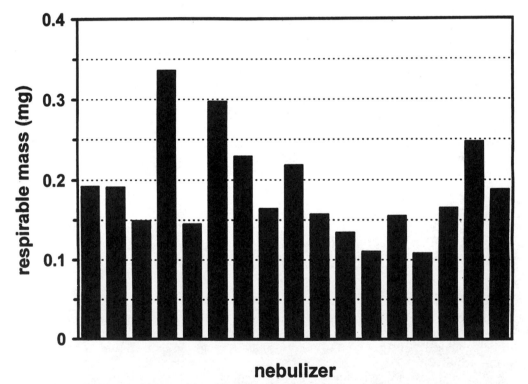

Figure 8-3. Respirable mass delivered from 17 SVNs. Respirable mass represents the particles measuring 1 to 5 μm in size delivered to the mouthpiece with simulated spontaneous breathing and 2.5 mg of albuterol in 4 mL of volume placed in the SVN. (Reprinted from Hess D, Fisher D, Williams P, et al. Medication nebulizer performance: effects of diluent volume, nebulizer flow and nebulizer brand. Chest 1996;110:498–505.)

the drug tends to concentrate in the dead volume. Increasing driving gas flow decreases the dead volume and also increases the percentage of aerosol particles in the therapeutic range (1 to 5 μm). However, from a practical perspective, the greater the solution volume the longer the treatment time, the greater the delivered flow the greater the drug volume lost to the room. As a result, based on current data,[42,46] we recommend that the total drug volume be 4 mL and the driving gas flow be 6 to 8 L/min. This results in a total treatment time of about 8 to 12 minutes.

Because SVNs are designed to be used with oxygen/nitrogen mixtures, the use of a less dense driving gas (heliox) decreases delivered mass at the specific driving gas flow rate. If heliox is used to power the SVN, driving gas flow should be increased 30 to 40% or set at 8 to 11 L/min.[46]

Temperature and humidity of the nebulized solution and driving gas can affect the size of particles delivered by SVNs and the concentration of the drug in the dead volume.[47,48] Evaporation of water and adiabatic expansion of the driving gas reduces the temperature of the aerosol solution to about 8 to 12°F below atmospheric. The evaporation of water increases the concentration of the drug in the nebulizer solution. Because gas temperature increases once the aerosol leaves the nebulizer, particle size of the aerosol is reduced. Therefore, ideally nebulizer driving gas should be at room temperature and saturated with water vapor. This, of course, is impractical; however, use of a gas compressor instead of compressed gas increases the temperature and humidity of the driving gas. The aerosol solution temperature can be kept more constant by the patient grasping the SVN in the hand during treatment.[42]

SVN Delivery Technique

Box 8-1 outlines the procedure for using an SVN. As indicated earlier, all nebulizers have a dead volume that affects drug delivery. As a result, nebulization should continue until no aerosol is produced. This may require tapping of the sides of the aerosol to force large drops of solution to fall to the bottom of the device. Some have recommended placing a Y piece in the gas delivery tubing so that the patient can control when the drug is nebulized.[42] This markedly reduces the volume of drug lost to the environment but increases nebulization time two- to three-fold and requires significant patient coordination. Patients should be instructed to inspire normally to avoid hyperventilation. However, a periodic deep breath with an inflation hold does increase retention of the drug in the lower respiratory tract.

Advantages/Disadvantages

The major advantages of SVNs are their ability to deliver large quantities of drugs without patients having to coordinate aerosol delivery for optimal effect. In addition, nebulization

Box 8-1. Technique for Use of a Small-Volume Nebulizer (SVN)

Place drug in nebulizer, total solution volume 4 mL
Set driving flow to 6–8 L/min
Connect patient to SVN via mouthpiece or mask (in some a nose clip may be necessary)
Instruct patient to inspire through an open mouth if using a mask or to close lips around mouthpiece
Have patient hold nebulizer upright
Have patient inhale slowly (0.5 L/sec) at normal tidal volumes
Continue treatment until no aerosol is produced

can be performed continuously, they do not release environmental contaminants, and any drug conceivable can theoretically be delivered by SVNs. However, important disadvantages of these devices are as follows: a pressurized gas source is required to operate the device, the drug must be mixed before administration, contamination is highly likely if the device is not cleaned properly, drug is wasted, SVNs are expensive, and a lengthy administration time (8–12 min) is required.[42] Of these, the lack of portability (high-pressure gas source) and the need for drug preparation make this approach undesirable for use outside the hospital.

METERED DOSE INHALERS

Figure 8-4 illustrates the basic operation of a typical MDI.[49] All MDIs are constructed and operate in a similar manner. On actuating the MDI, drug stored in the metering chamber is released as an aerosol through the valve stem. When the metering chamber empties, solution from the tank retaining cup enters the metering chamber and solution from the main reservoir enters the tank retaining cup. All of this can take time and requires the stimulation of vigorous shaking. As a result, all manufacturers recommend waiting at least 10 to 20 seconds before a second actuation and shaking vigorously before every actuation.[49,50] Vigorous shaking also ensures that the drug is evenly mixed with propellant/surfactant solution.[51]

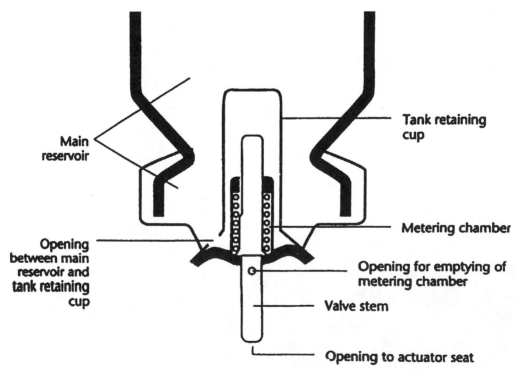

Figure 8-4. Metering chamber of an MDI. See above for discussion. (Reprinted from Byron RR. Performance characteristics of pressurized metered dose inhalers in vitro. J Aerosol Med 1997;10: S3–S6.)

Box 8-2. Technique for Use of Metered Dose Inhaler (MDI)

Warm MDI to body temperature
Assemble apparatus
Shake canister vigorously
Hold canister upright
Place mouthpiece at mouth opening
(If using a spacer, tightly seal lips around mouthpiece)
Begin to inhale slowly at <0.5 L/min
Actuate MDI (if using a spacer, actuate first then begin to slowly inhale at <0.5
  L/min)[a]
Continue to inspire to total lung capacity
Hold breath for 4–10 sec
Wait 10–20 sec before repeating above sequence for additional actuations

[a]Some spacers have unit-specific instructions.

Inspiring With MDI

To maximize drug delivery with an MDI, proper technique must be used. Following vigorous shaking of the canister, the patient should be instructed to exhale to functional residual capacity, place the MDI mouthpiece between open lips, and begin to inhale slowly with inspiratory flows less than 30 L/min.[52] Immediately after the onset of inspiration, the MDI should be actuated while the patient continues to inhale to total lung capacity.[53] After completing a maximal inspiration, patients ideally should hold their breath for about 4 to 10 seconds (Box 8-2).

Other issues with the use of MDIs that patients should be aware of are loss of prime and identification of quantity of drug within the canister.[42,52] If an MDI has been sitting for a few days, solution in the metering chamber can either evaporate or drain from it,[54,55] resulting in inadequate dose of the drug being delivered in the first one to two actuations. As a result, with all new MDIs or an MDI that has not been used for longer than 48 hours, two actuations should be wasted to the room to ensure consistent dosing on every actuation the patient receives.

Most MDIs, when full, can deliver about 200 actuations. Unfortunately, it is impossible to look at the MDI and determine whether 10 or 190 actuations are left in the device. One useful method of estimating the number of actuations left is placing the device in a pot of water.[50] A full MDI sinks to the bottom, an empty MDI floats flat on the surface of the water, and partially filled MDIs float or sink to various levels.

Advantages and Disadvantages of MDIs

Use of MDIs has several compelling advantages.[50,52,53] They are convenient, small, lightweight, portable, difficult to contaminate, and inexpensive and do not require any drug preparation. However, the patient must coordinate actuation of the MDI with inspiration, and a high level of pharyngeal deposition of the drug occurs with MDIs.[50,52,53] It is also easy to increase dosing with MDIs but difficult to deliver large quantities of the drug; not all medications are available by MDIs, and drugs cannot be mixed.

Spacers/Holding Chambers

The two most important disadvantages to the use of MDIs, coordination and pharyngeal deposition of the drug, can be overcome by the use of spacers or holding chambers.[56] However, it is important to note that no physiologic benefit has been found for the use of spacers/holding chambers. Figure 8-5 illustrates several different types of these devices. Some are small and compact (OptiHaler, Heathscan, Cedar Grove,NJ), others are large (InspirEase, Schering Plough, Kenilworth, NJ); most have one-way valves and require less coordination than a simple MDI.[42,50] These devices are designed to allow actuation of the drug into the device before the patient inspires. As a result, patients can simply inspire without coordinating actuation during inspiration, and, most importantly, large aerosol particles deposit in the spacer not in the oral pharynx. Spacers should always be used when steroids are administered.

Spacer-specific instructions should be followed. However, with most of these devices, after the drug is actuated, the patient should immediately inspire from the chamber.[57] The longer the wait, the smaller the respirable mass. In addition, multiple actuation into the spacer should be avoided.[57] More than one actuation into the spacer results in diminished drug delivery.[57]

Breath-Actuated MDIs

At least one company manufactures a breath-actuated MDI (Figure 8-6).[58] With this device, the patient must generate enough flow to trigger the device. If the patient cannot

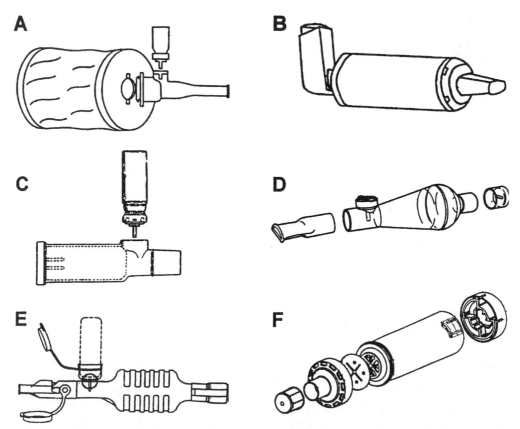

Figure 8-5. MDI spacers/holding chambers. **A.** InspirEase (Schering Plough, Kenilworth, NJ). **B.** Aerochamber (Monaghan, Plattsburgh, NY). **C.** Optihaler (Heathscan, Cedar Grove, NJ). **D.** Aerosol Cloud Chamber (ACE) (DHD, Canasta, NY). **E.** MidSpacer (Baxter, Deerfield, IL). **F.** OptiChamber (Healthscan, Cedar Grove, NJ). (Reprinted from Hess DR. Aerosolized medication delivery. In: Branson RD, Hess DR, Chatburn RL, eds. Respiratory Care Equipment, 2nd edition. Philadelphia: Lippincott Williams & Wilkins, 1999:147.)

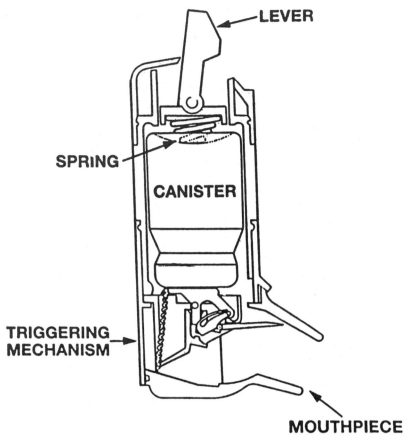

Figure 8-6. Schematic illustration of the breath-actuated autohaler. (Reprinted from Newman DP, Weisz AWB, Talau N, et al. Improvement of drug delivery with a breath activated pressurized aerosol for patients with poor inhaler technique. Thorax 1991;46:712–716.)

generate sufficient flow, the device will not actuate. In addition, this device is only available with pirbuterol and cannot be used with other MDIs.[50]

DRY POWDER INHALERS

During the past decade, DPIs have been increasingly available and used in the ambulatory setting, where DPIs have been shown to be comparable to SVNs and MDIs.[35,41,52] DPIs create drug aerosols by drawing room air through the powdered drug preparation. The powder contains either micronized (<5 μm in diameter) drug particles bound into loose aggregates or micronized drug particles that are loosely bound to large (>30 μm in diameter) lactose or glucose particles.[59] Because micronized particles adhere to each other and to most surfaces, the addition of larger carrier particles decreases interparticular forces so that the powder separates into individual respirable particles more readily.[59] That is, the carrier particles aid flow of the drug from the device and act as fillers by adding bulk to the powder when the drug dose is very small. Usually the drug is stripped from the carrier particles[60] by the energy of the patient's inhalation (Fig. 8-7).[61] As a result, release of respirable particles of the drug requires inspiration at relatively high flow rates (>30

L/min).[62,63] In general, drug particles of 1 to 2 μm are delivered along with large carrier particles (>30 μm) that impact in the pharynx.

Factors Affecting Drug Delivery

Several factors influence drug delivery from DPIs, including manufacturer's design, resistance to airflow, proper assembly of components (loading of drug), and accumulation of powder within the device.[35] Particle deposition in the device is influenced by electrostatic charge on the particles in the powder and the materials of the DPI device. The overall internal design of the device influences the resistance to gas flow (Fig. 8-8)[64] and, as a result, the peak flow required during inhalation. Of primary concern for patients is the correct assembly and priming of the DPI. It is critical for the patient to correctly set up the DPI for use to ensure consistent dosing.

High environmental humidity can be extremely problematic for DPIs.[65] The high humidity produces clumping of the dry powder, creating larger particles that are not effectively aerosolized and therefore less likely to reach the lung. Devices that contain a single large reservoir of the drug rather than individually packaged doses generally contain a desiccant to prevent clumping by ambient humidity. Use of a desiccant minimizes but does not eliminate the problems of humidity.

Technique for Use of DPI

Box 8-3 lists the steps for use of a DPI. First and most important, the DPI must be correctly assembled and primed. As with MDIs, inspiration through a DPI should be from resting functional residual capacity level. The device needs to be placed between the patient's lips and a tight seal created. For most effective use, all inspired gas should move through the device. Because these devices are patient activated, the patient's inspiration produces aerosolization. As discussed, a rapid inspiratory flow of greater than 30 L/min is required. Generally, the greater the flow the greater the percentage of particles in the respirable range. Breath holding after inhalation allows greater time for drug particles to deposit by sedimentation in the airways[35]; however, the need for a breath hold is controversial.[66] It is also important to ensure that patients do not exhale back through the DPI. Exhalation through the device blows drug from the device and adds humidity, reducing the amount of aerosol produced.

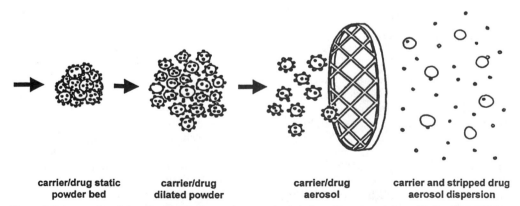

| carrier/drug static powder bed | carrier/drug dilated powder | carrier/drug aerosol | carrier and stripped drug aerosol dispersion |

Figure 8-7. Aerosolization of a drug using a dry powder inhaler. (Reprinted from Dalby RN, Hickey AJ, Tiano SL. Medical devices for the delivery of therapeutic aerosols to the lungs. In: Hickey AJ, ed. Inhalation Aerosols: Physical and Biological Basis for Therapy: Lung Biology in Health and Disease. New York: Marcel Dekker, 1996;94:441–473.)

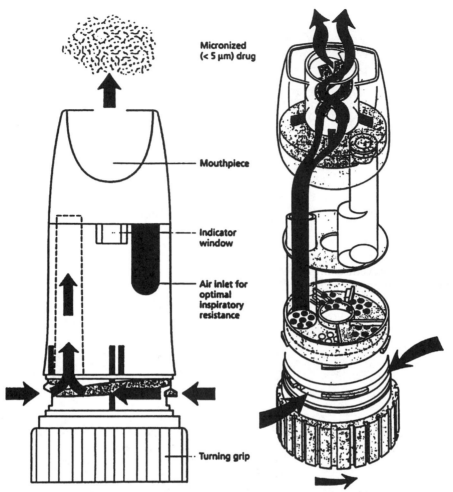

Figure 8-8. Components and airflow of the Turbuhaler (Astra US Inc, Wesborough, MA). The inhaler contains up to 200 doses in its reservoir. A rotating disc below the reservoir has a series of clusters of conical cavities. Turning the grip at the bottom of the device rotates the disc, and plastic scrapers above the closing unit load the dose into a group of conical holes. The inhaler must be held upright during this operation so that a reproducible quantity of drug is fed, by gravity, into the conical cavities. A desiccant in the device protects the drug from moisture. The powder used in this device consists of micronized drug particles, without carrier particles. Because a minute amount of powder is inhaled, the patient may not experience any sensation of receiving a dose. The Turbuhaler does not have a dose counter, but a red sign appears in the dose indicator window when 20 doses remain in the device. When the patient inhales, air enters through channels at the base of the operating unit, passes through the pressure plate, through the cavities in the dosing unit, and into the inhalation channel. Turbulent airflow in the spiral channels deaggregates the particles. The twisting channels cause resistance to inhalation, so inspiratory airflow greater than 30 L/min is needed to obtain an adequate dose. Particles that are poorly entrained are retained in the channels and become reentrained as smaller particles during subsequent inhalations. (Reprinted from Crompton GK. Delivery systems. In: Kay AB, ed. Allergy and Allergic Diseases. London: Blackwell Science, 1997:1440–1450.)

Box 8-3. Technique for Use of a DPI

Assemble apparatus
Open capsule (technique specific for each device)
Exhale normally to functional residual capacity
Place device mouthpiece in mouth and seal lips around mouthpiece
Inhale rapidly (>30 L/min) through device
Hold breath for 4–10 sec
Repeat process until capsule is empty
Rinse mouth after use if inhaling steroids

Box 8-4. Comparision of Advantages and Disadvantages Among SVN, MDI, and DPI

SVN

Advantages	*Disadvantages*
No patient coordination required	Compressed gas source required
No chlorofluorocarbon release	Easily contaminated
Able to easily mix drugs	Treatment time lengthy
Easy to administer high doses	Drug preparation required
Can administer drugs continuously	Expensive
Little pharyngeal deposition of drug	Lacks portability

MDI

Advantages	*Disadvantages*
No drug preparation required	Significant patient coordination required
Difficult to contaminate	Patient actuation required
Easily portable	High pharyngeal deposition
Convenient	Difficult to deliver high doses
	Not all medications available
	Many are chlorofluorocarbon driven

MDI With Spacer/Holding Chamber

Advantages	*Disadvantages*
No drug preparation required	Patient actuation required
Difficult to contaminate	Difficult to deliver high doses
Convenient	Not all medications available
No coordination required	Many are chlorofluorocarbon driven
Little pharyngeal deposition	Some are large and bulky

DPI

Advantages	*Disadvantages*
Little coordination required	Some assembly and priming required
Difficult to contaminate	Patient actuation required
Convenient	High inspiratory flow needed
Little pharyngeal deposition	Not many medications available
No chlorofluorocarbons	Difficult to deliver high doses
Highly portable	

SVN, small-volume nebulizer; MDI, metered dose inhaler; DPI, dry powder inhaler.

Advantages and Disadvantages

DPIs are small, portable, and lightweight drug delivery devices. In addition, DPIs do not contain chlorofluorocarbons and do not require patient coordination during inspiration. However, a great deal of patient coordination may be required to set up and prime DPIs. In addition, very high sustained peak flow rates are required for correct use. The presence of high humidity is a clear problem with these devices that can markedly limit their use in certain seasons in parts of the country.

SVN VS. MDI VS. MDIh VS. DPI

Comparison among SVNs, MDIs, MDIhs, and DPIs is provided in Box 8-4. As noted, each of these devices has several advantages and disadvantages. Based on these ratings, we recommend use of MDIs or MDIhs when available. However, because of legislation regarding chlorofluorocarbons, it can be expected that increasing use of DPIs will occur, unless alternate propellants (Hydrofluoroalkane) for MDIs become widely available.

REFERENCES

1. Anthonisen NR, Wright EC. Bronchodilator response in chronic obstructive pulmonary disease. Am Rev Respir Dis 1986;133:814–819.
2. American Thoracic Society. ATS statement: standards for the diagnosis and care of patients with chronic obstructive lung disease. Am J Respir Crit Care Med 1995;152:78–121.
3. Anthonisen NR, Connett JE, Kiley JP, et al. Effects of smoking intervention and the use of an inhaled anticholinergic bronchodilator on the rate of decline of FEV_1: the Lung Health Study. JAMA 1994;272:1497–1505.
4. Martin RJ, Bartelson BL, Smith P, et al. Effect of ipratropium bromide treatment on oxygen saturation and sleep quality in COPD. Chest 1999; 115:1338–1345.
5. Tashkin DP, Ashutosh K, Bleecker ER, et al. Comparison of the anticholinergic bronchodilator ipratropium bromide with metaproterenol in chronic obstructive pulmonary disease: a 90-day multi-center study. Am J Med 1986;81:81–90.
6. Chernow B. The Pharmacologic Approach to the Critically Ill Patient. 3rd ed. Baltimore: Williams & Wilkins, 1994.
7. COMBIVENT Inhalation Aerosol Study Group. In chronic obstructive pulmonary disease, a combination of ipratropium and albuterol is more effective than either agent alone: an 85-day multicenter trial. Chest 1994;105:1411–1419.
8. The COMBIVENT Inhalation Solution Study Group. Routine nebulized ipratropium and albuterol together are better than either alone in COPD. Chest 1997;112:1514–1521.
9. Gross N, Tashkin D, Miller R, et al. Inhalation by nebulization of albuterol-ipratropium combination (Dey combination) is superior to either agent alone in the treatment of chronic obstructive pulmonary disease. Respiration 1998;65:354–362.
10. Johnson M. The beta-adrenoceptor. Am J Respir Crit Care Med 1998;158:146–153.
11. Drazen JM, Israel E, Boushey HA, et al. Comparison of regularly scheduled with as-needed use of albuterol in mild asthma: Asthma Clinical Research Network. N Engl J Med 1996;335:841–847.
12. van Noord JA, Schreurs AJ, Mol SJ, et al. Addition of salmeterol versus doubling the dose of fluticasone propionate in patients with mild to moderate asthma. Thorax 1999;54:207–212.
13. Condemi JJ, Goldstein S, Kalberg C, et al. The addition of salmeterol to fluticasone propionate versus increasing the dose of fluticasone propionate in patients with persistent asthma: Salmeterol Study Group. Ann Allergy Asthma Immunol 1999;82:383–389.
14. Cazzola M, Matera M. Should long-acting beta 2-agonists be considered an alternative first choice option for the treatment of stable COPD? Respir Med 1999;93:227–229.
15. Mahler DA, Donohue JF, Barbee RA, et al. Efficacy of salmeterol xinafoate in the treatment of COPD. Chest 1999;115:957–965.
16. Nelson HS, Bensch G, Pleskow WW, et al. Improved bronchodilation with levalbuterol compared with racemic albuterol in patients with asthma. J Allergy Clin Immunol 1998;102:943–952.
17. Levalbuterol for asthma. Med Lett 1999;11:51–53.
18. Barnes PJ. Efficacy of inhaled corticosteroids in asthma. J Allergy Clin Immunol 1998;102:531–538.
19. Kamada AK, Szefler SJ, Martin RJ, et al. Issues in the use of inhaled glucocorticoids: The Asthma Clinical Research Network. Am J Respir Crit Care Med 1996;153:1739–1748.
20. Pauwels RA, Lofdahl CG, Laitinen LA, et al. Long-term treatment with inhaled budesonide in persons with mild chronic obstructive pulmonary disease who continue smoking: European Respira-

tory Society Study on Chronic Obstructive Pulmonary Disease. N Engl J Med 1999;340:1948–1953.

21. Vestbo J, Sorensen T, Lange P, et al. Long-term effect of inhaled budesonide in mild and moderate chronic obstructive pulmonary disease: a randomised controlled trial. Lancet 1999;353:1819–1823.

22. Fujimoto K, Kubo K, Yamamoto H, et al. Eosinophilic inflammation in the airway is related to glucocorticoid reversibility in patients with pulmonary emphysema. Chest 1999;115:697–702.

23. Pizzichini E, Pizzichini MM, Gibson P, et al. Sputum eosinophilia predicts benefit from prednisone in smokers with chronic obstructive bronchitis. Am J Respir Crit Care Med 1998;158:1511–1517.

24. Poole PJ, Black PN. Mucolytic agents for chronic bronchitis. Oxford: The Cochrane Library, 1999.

25. Ziment I. Pharmacologic therapy of obstructive airway disease. Clin Chest Med 1990;11:461–486.

26. Robinson M, Hemming Al, Regnis JA, et al. Effect of increasing doses of hypertonic saline on mucociliary clearance in patients with cystic fibrosis. Thorax 1997;52:900–903.

27. King M, Hemming AL, Regnis JA, et al. Rheology of cystic fibrosis sputum after in vitro treatment with hypertonic saline alone and in combination with recombinant human deoxyribonuclease I. Am J Respir Crit Care Med 1997;156:173–177.

28. Fuchs HJ, Borowitz DS, Christiansen DH, et al. Effect of aerosolized recombinant human DNase on exacerbations of respiratory symptoms and on pulmonary function in patients with cystic fibrosis: The Pulmozyme Study Group. N Engl J Med 1994;331:637–642.

29. Wills PJ, Wodehouse T, Corkery K, et al. Short-term recombinant human DNase in bronchiectasis: effect on clinical state and in vitro sputum transportability. Am J Respir Crit Care Med 1996; 154:413–417.

30. Itozaku G, Weinstein R. Aerosolized antimicrobials: another look. Crit Care Med 1998;26:5–6.

31. Ramsey BW, Pepe MS, Quan JM, et al. Intermittent administration of inhaled tobramycin in patients with cystic fibrosis. N Engl J Med 1999; 340:23–26.

32. Soler N, Torres A, Santiago E, et al. Bronchial microbial patterns in severe exacerbations of chronic obstructive pulmonary disease (COPD) requiring mechanical ventilation. Am Rev Respir Crit Care Med 1998;157:1498–1505.

33. Eller J, Ede A, Schaberg T, et al. Infective exacerbations of chronic bronchitis-relation between bacteriologic etiology and lung function. Chest 1998;113:1542–1548.

34. Raimondi AC, Schottlender J, Lombardi D, et al. Treatment of acute severe asthma with inhaled albuterol delivered via jet nebulizer, metered dose inhaler with spacer, or dry powder. Chest 1997; 97(1):24–28.

35. Dhand R, Fink J. Dry powder inhalers. Respir Care 1999;44:940–951.

36. Pauwels R. Inhalation device, pulmonary deposition and clinical effect of inhaled therapy (review). J Aerosol Med 1997;10:S17–S21.

37. Lewis RA, Fleming JS. Fractional deposition from a jet nebulizer: how it differs from a metered dose inhaler. Br J Dis Chest 1985;79:361–367.

38. Newman DP, Pavia D, Moren F, et al. Deposition of pressurized aerosols in the human respiratory tract. Thorax 1981;36:52–55.

39. Lipworth BJ, Clark DJ. Lung delivery of salbutamol by breath activated pressurized aerosol and dry powder inhaler devices. Pulmon Pharmacol Ther 1997;10:211–214.

40. Newman SP. Aerosol generators and delivery systems. Respir Care 1991;36:939–951.

41. Hess DR. Aerosolized medication delivery. In: Branson RD, Hess DR, Chatburn RL, eds. Respiratory Care Equipment. Philadelphia: Lippincott, 1999:133–156.

42. Hess D, Fisher D, Williams P, et al. Medication nebulizer performance: effects of diluent volume, nebulizer flow and nebulizer brand. Chest 1996; 110:498–505.

43. Clay MM, Pavia D, Newman SP, et al. Assessment of jet nebulizers for lung aerosol therapy. Lancet 1983;2:592–594.

44. Loffert DT, Ikle D, Nelson HS. A comparison of commercial jet nebulizers. Chest 1994;106: 1788–1793.

45. Coates AL, MacNeish CF, Meisner BR. The choice of jet nebulizer, nebulizing flow, and addition of albuterol affects the output of tobramycin aerosols. Chest 1997;111:1206–1212.

46. Hess DR, Acosta FL, Ritz R, et al. Effect of helix on nebulizer function. Chest 1999;115:184–189.

47. Newman SP, Pellow PGD, Clarke SW. In vitro comparison of DeVilbiss jet and ultrasonic nebulizers. Chest 1987;92:991–994.

48. Phipps PR, Gonda I. Droplets produced by medical nebulizers: some factors affecting their size and solute concentration. Chest 1990;97:1327–1332.

49. Byron RR. Performance characteristics of pressurized metered dose inhalers in vitro. J Aerosol Med 1997;10:S3–S6.

50. Hess D, Daugherty A, Simmons M. The volume of gas emitted from five metered dose inhalers at three levels of fullness. Respir Care 1992;37: 444–447.

51. Berg E. In vitro properties of pressurized metered dose inhalers with and without spacer devices. J Aerosol Med 1995;8:S3–S11.

52. Kacmarek RM, Hess D. The interface between patient and aerosol generator. Respir Care 1991; 36:952–976.

53. Hess D. Aerosol therapy. Respir Clin North Am 1995;1:235–263.

54. Shultz RK. Drug delivery characteristics of metered dose inhalers. J Allergy Clin Immunol 1995; 96:284–287.

55. Everard ML, Devadason SG, Summers BG. Factors affecting total and "respirable" dose delivered by a salbutamol metered dose inhaler. Thorax 1995;50:746–749.

56. Guidry GG, Brown WD, Stogner SW. Incorrect use of metered dose inhalers by medical personnel. Chest 1992;101:31–33.

57. Barry PW, O'Callaghan C. The effect of delay multiple actuations and spacer static change on the in-vitro delivery of budesonide from the nebuhaler. Br J Clin Pharmacol 1995;40:76–78.
58. Newman DP, Weisz AWB, Talau N, et al. Improvement of drug delivery with a breath activated pressurized aerosol for patients with poor inhaler technique. Thorax 1991;46:712–716.
59. Ganderton D. The generation of respirable clouds from coarse powder aggregates. J Biopharm Sci 1992;3:101–105.
60. Dolovich M, Rheim R, Rashid F, et al. Measurement of the particle size and dosing characteristics of a radiolabelled albuterol-sulphate lactose blend used in the SPIROS dry powder inhaler. In: Dalby RN, Byron P, Farr S, eds. Respiratory Drug Delivery V. Buffalo Grove: Interpharm Press, 1996:332–345.
61. Dalby RN, Hickey AJ, Tiano SL. Medical devices for the delivery of therapeutic aerosols to the lungs. In: Hickey AJ, ed. Inhalation Aerosols: Physical and Biological Basis for Therapy: Lung Biology in Health and Disease. New York: Marcel Dekker, 1996;94:441–473.
62. Hansen OR, Pederson S. Optimal inhalation technique with terbutaline Turbuhaler. Eur Respir J 1989;2:637–639.
63. Pedersen S, Hansen OR, Fuglsang G. Influence of inspiratory flow rate upon the effect of a Turbuhaler. Arch Dis Child 1990;65:308–310.
64. Crompton GK. Delivery systems. In: Kay AB, ed. Allergy and Allergic Diseases. London: Blackwell Science, 1997:1440–1450.
65. Rajkumari NJ, Byron PR, Dalby RN. Testing of dry powder aerosol formulations in different environmental conditions. Int J Pharmacol 1995;113:123–130.
66. Pedersen S. Delivery systems in children. In: Barnes PJ, Grunstein MM, Leff AR, Woolcock AJ, eds. Asthma. Philadelphia: Lippincott-Raven, 1997:1915–1929.

9 Oxygen Therapy in Pulmonary Rehabilitation

Walter J. O'Donohue Jr.

⊳ Professional Skills

Upon completion of this chapter, the reader will:

- Understand the benefits of long-term oxygen therapy (LTOT) in pulmonary rehabilitation
- Recognize the cost and economic issues in supplying home oxygen therapy (HOT)
- Understand the new Medicare regulations and documentation necessary to prescribe HOT
- Recall requirements for appropriate use of home oxygen
- Recognize the options available for oxygen delivery, including new ambulatory systems

EFFICACY OF LTOT IN PULMONARY REHABILITATION

No therapy available today is more effective than continuous or near-continuous oxygen to increase survival and improve quality of life for patients with advanced chronic obstructive pulmonary disease (COPD) and hypoxemia. Multicenter clinical trials conducted in North America and the United Kingdom[1,2] have demonstrated the value of LTOT to prolong survival in patients with COPD. Furthermore, these studies found that near-continuous oxygen (18 h/d) was superior to oxygen provided only for 12 to 15 hours daily, including the nocturnal hours. In the North American Nocturnal Oxygen Therapy Trial (NOTT), neuropsychologic function was improved to a significantly greater degree in patients receiving near-continuous oxygen.[3]

Analysis of data from the National Institutes of Health multicenter Intermittent Positive-Pressure Breathing Study,[4] when correlated with the NOTT,[5,6] reveals that correction of hypoxemia in patients with COPD improves survival to levels expected for patients with similar degrees of obstructive lung disease without hypoxemia. Hypercapnia was present in about 50% of the NOTT study patients but did not seem to alter the outcome when hypoxemia was corrected. The factors that seem to have the greatest relevance to survival in COPD patients are (*a*) hypoxemia, (*b*) pulmonary hypertension,[7] and (*c*) the severity of the fixed obstructive dysfunction. Hypoxemia and pulmonary hypertension are physiologically related, and treatment with oxygen can correct hypoxemia and reduce, but not totally eliminate, pulmonary hypertension.[8-10] In addition to the increased survival and improved neuropsychologic function, oxygen can increase exercise tolerance and reduce dyspnea.[11-13] Some studies suggest that the mode of oxygen delivery (e.g., nasal cannula versus transtracheal catheter or high-flow versus low-flow) may alter exercise tolerance substantially.[14-16] Oxygen therapy also can reduce the hematocrit in patients with hypoxemia and erythrocytosis.[8,12] These are all important physiologic effects that are essential to optimize pulmonary rehabilitation.

When used in conjunction with a program for pulmonary rehabilitation, oxygen therapy allows patients with hypoxemia to exercise more safely, to increase exercise tolerance, and to experience a better quality of life. An exercise prescription can be developed, while monitoring cardiac and pulmonary function, with the oxygen flow adjusted to avoid arterial oxygen desaturation. Patients can then continue this program either at a rehabilitation center or at home, with periodic modifications in the prescription based on appropriate reassessment. Thus, many patients with chronic pulmonary disease not only have been able to live longer but also have enjoyed more active lives and, in some cases, have been able to maintain gainful employment.

ECONOMICS AND NEW REGULATORY ISSUES REGARDING HOT

Estimates of the magnitude of use and cost of HOT, based on Medicare data from 1993, indicate that 616,000 patients were receiving HOT at an annual cost of $1.4 billion.[17] The frequency of use of HOT in Medicare beneficiaries was reconfirmed by Silverman et al.[18] in a 1997 report. The cost of HOT in the United States exceeds the entire budget of the National Heart, Lung, and Blood Institute by approximately 40%. Each physician and respiratory care provider has a responsibility to be sure that oxygen is used appropriately and only when medically indicated. The Health Care Financing Administration (HCFA) has established precise guidelines for oxygen reimbursement based on the consideration that oxygen is "durable medical equipment" (DME). Medically, oxygen is considered to be a drug, but Medicare coverage does not include outpatient medications for any medical conditions. Fortunately, for patients with hypoxemia, the HCFA pays for home oxygen as DME; however, one of the prices we pay for this coverage is a complex certificate of medical necessity (CMN) form that must be completed by a physician or a member of the physician's staff and signed by the physician. It is considerably easier to prescribe dangerously addicting narcotics than it is to order HOT.

In 1988, Congress legislated a new system for reimbursement of DME known as the "6-Point Plan." This plan provided for prospective reimbursement of all DME, with oxygen and oxygen equipment constituting approximately 45% of the total cost. The 6-Point Plan for oxygen was based on the assumption that all oxygen delivery systems are clinically equal and cost neutral. The major safeguard for patients resulted from the physician being allowed to order the specific type of equipment that was judged to be medically necessary and appropriate.

The Balanced Budget Act of 1997 created major changes in oxygen reimbursement for Medicare patients beginning in 1998. Both Congress and the HCFA had assumed that Medicare was paying too much for oxygen therapy, particularly compared with Veterans Administration contracts, which often included only an oxygen concentrator and steel cylinders mounted on wheels for portability. As of January 1, 1998, a 25% across-the-board reduction occurred in reimbursement for home oxygen, with an additional 5% reduction scheduled for January 1, 1999. Neither Congress nor the HCFA acknowledged that they had any information on the effect of these cuts on patient access to appropriate equipment and therapy, but they were aware that access problems would be difficult to document and prove. A recent analysis of HOT for Medicare recipients performed by persons associated with the HCFA indicates that minority and rural patients were having difficulty with access even before the cuts in reimbursement.[18] Congress did direct the HCFA to undertake a study on access to oxygen service by Medicare patients, but it is doubtful that this study will ever be conducted.

The DME Regional Medical Directors have recently designed a new CMN form. This is Form HCFA-484.2, which was introduced just before the first cut in Medicare reimbursement for home oxygen (Fig. 9-1). This new CMN form no longer allows the physician to indicate the type of equipment to be placed in the home and is designed

U.S. DEPARTMENT OF HEALTH & HUMAN SERVICES
HEALTH CARE FINANCING ADMINISTRATION

FORM APPROVED
OMB NO. 0938-0534

CERTIFICATE OF MEDICAL NECESSITY

DMERC 484.2

OXYGEN

SECTION A   Certification Type/Date: INITIAL __/__/__   REVISED __/__/__   RECERTIFICATION __/__/__

PATIENT NAME, ADDRESS, TELEPHONE and HIC NUMBER	SUPPLIER NAME, ADDRESS, TELEPHONE and NSC NUMBER
(___)___-____ HICN _____	(___)___-____ NSC # _____

PLACE OF SERVICE _____	HCPCS CODE	PT DOB __/__/__; Sex ___ (M/F); HT.____(in.); WT.____(lbs.)
NAME and ADDRESS of FACILITY if applicable (See Reverse)	_____ _____ _____ _____	PHYSICIAN NAME, ADDRESS, TELEPHONE and UPIN NUMBER (___)___-____ UPIN # _____

SECTION B   Information in This Section May Not Be Completed by the Supplier of the Items/Supplies.

EST. LENGTH OF NEED (# OF MONTHS): _____ 1-99 (99=LIFETIME) | DIAGNOSIS CODES (ICD-9): _____ _____ _____ _____

ANSWERS	ANSWER QUESTIONS 1-10. (Circle Y for Yes, N for No, or D for Does Not Apply, unless otherwise noted.)
a) _____ mm Hg b) _____ % c) __/__/__	1. Enter the result of most recent test taken on or before the certification date listed in Section A. Enter (a) arterial blood gas PO$_2$ and/or (b) oxygen saturation test. Enter date of test (c).
Y N	2. Was the test in Question 1 performed EITHER with the patient in a chronic stable state as an outpatient OR within two days prior to discharge from an inpatient facility to home?
1 2 3	3. Circle the one number for the condition of the test in Question 1: (1) At Rest; (2) During Exercise; (3) During Sleep
XXXXXXXXXXXXXX XXXXXXXXXXXXXX XXXXXXXXXXXXXX	4. Physician/provider performing test in Question 1 (and, if applicable, Question 7). Print/type name and address below: NAME: ADDRESS:
Y N D	5. If you are ordering portable oxygen, is the patient mobile within the home? If you are not ordering portable oxygen, circle D.
_____ LPM	6. Enter the highest oxygen flow rate ordered for this patient in liters per minute. If less than 1 LPM, enter a "X".
a) _____ mm Hg b) _____ % c) __/__/__ .	7. If greater than 4 LPM is prescribed, enter results of most recent test taken on 4 LPM. This may be an (a) arterial blood gas PO$_2$ and/or (b) oxygen saturation test with patient in a chronic stable state. Enter date of test (c).

IF PO$_2$ = 56–59 OR OXYGEN SATURATION = 89%, AT LEAST ONE OF THE FOLLOWING CRITERIA MUST BE MET.

Y N D	8. Does the patient have dependent edema due to congestive heart failure?
Y N D	9. Does the patient have cor pulmonale or pulmonary hypertension documented by P pulmonale on an EKG or by an echocardiogram, gated blood pool scan or direct pulmonary artery pressure measurement?
Y N D	10. Does the patient have a hematocrit greater than 56%?

NAME OF PERSON ANSWERING SECTION B QUESTIONS, IF OTHER THAN PHYSICIAN (Please Print):
NAME: _____   TITLE: _____   EMPLOYER: _____

SECTION C   Narrative Description of Equipment and Cost

(1) Narrative description of all items, accessories and options ordered; (2) Supplier's charge and (3) Medicare Fee Schedule Allowance for each item, accessory and option. (See instructions on back.)

SECTION D   Physician Attestation and Signature/Date

I certify that I am the treating physician identified in Section A of this form. I have received Sections A, B and C of the Certificate of Medical Necessity (including charges for items ordered). Any statement on my letterhead attached hereto, has been reviewed and signed by me. I certify that the medical necessity information in Section B is true, accurate and complete, to the best of my knowledge, and I understand that any falsification, omission, or concealment of material fact in that section may subject me to civil or criminal liability.

PHYSICIAN'S SIGNATURE _____ DATE __/__/__ (SIGNATURE AND DATE STAMPS ARE NOT ACCEPTABLE)

FORM HCFA 484 (5/97)

Figure 9-1. CMN (Form HCFA 484.2) now required by the HCFA for reimbursement of HOT.

primarily for adjudication of Medicare claims and not as a prescription for therapy. With this change, the HCFA assumed that therapy would be initiated by a prescription from the physician to the oxygen supplier and that the CNM form would be mailed to the physician after therapy is begun. Although the necessity for a prescription for therapy is essential before the physician can sign the CMN, the HCFA is silent on how the prescription is to be transmitted to the oxygen supplier. A separate written prescription is implied and is a requirement for Joint Commmission on Accreditation of Healthcare Organizations (JCAHO) accreditation of the supplier. A prescription form now used by the author for prescribing HOT is presented as Figure 9-2. A summary of the major changes in the new CMN form (Form HCFA 484.2) is as follows:

A. In section A, the physician must provide his or her address, telephone number, and UPIN number.
B. In section B, the specific *ICD-9-CM* diagnostic code(s) must be provided, whereas previously a checklist of the most common diseases for which home oxygen is prescribed was included. Section B also includes a series of questions and answers to document the need for oxygen therapy and to justify the Medicare reimbursement. This includes the new requirements to (a) provide an arterial partial pressure of oxygen (PaO_2) or arterial oxygen percent saturation (SaO_2) measurement within 2 days before discharge from the hospital if HOT is prescribed at discharge and (*b*) provide documentation of the PaO_2 or SaO_2 with 4 L/min of oxygen if more than 4 L/min is prescribed for any period during the day or night.

Home Oxygen Prescription

NAME _____

ADDRESS _____ DATE _____

℞

1. **Oxygen flow:**
   ☐ Continuous: Liters/min _____. (FiO2 _____ for assisted ventilation) <u>and/or</u>
   ☐ Noncontinuous: (liters/min) walking _____, sleeping _____, exercise _____.

2. **Oxygen equipment (check one):**
   ☐ Stationary only (eg nocturnal or bedbound)
   For portable or ambulatory* systems, patient regularly goes beyond the limits of a stationary system with 50-ft tubing for times indicated below:
   ☐ Stationary and portable
   (less than 2 hr/day, minimum 2 hr/wk)
   ☐ Stationary and ambulatory*
   (more than 2 hr/day, minimum 6 hr/wk)
   ☐ Portable only ☐ ambulatory* only
   (eg walking or exercise only)

   * Ambulatory systems weigh less than 10 lbs, are designed to be carried and will last at least 4 hrs at a flow equivalent to 2L/min (eg liquid refillable units or light-weight cylinders and regulators, with or without oxygen conserving devices)

3. **Delivery System:**
   ☐ Nasal Cannula
   ☐ Transtracheal catheter
   ☐ Reservoir cannula
   ☐ Mask (eg CPAP or BiPAP)
   ☐ Other: _____

_____M.D.

Figure 9-2. Example of a written prescription form that provides specific directions to the home oxygen supplier for initiation of HOT.

C. Section C is new and contains space for the DME supplier to provide a narrative description of the oxygen delivery system being used, including the specific type of equipment, for example, compressed gas, liquid, or concentrator, and whether the delivery system is stationary or portable. The HCFA instructions to the physicians state, "Suppliers must use the space in Section C for a written confirmation of other details of the oxygen order, which, after review, the physician should confirm with a signature in Section D if he or she agrees. If the confirmation in Section C does not accurately represent the order, the CMN should be returned unsigned by the physician to the supplier for correction. The additional order information confirmed in Section D should include the means of oxygen delivery, for example, cannula, mask, etc., and the specifics of varying oxygen flow rates and/or noncontinuous use of oxygen as appropriate."

D. Section D requires the physician's personal signature and date, confirming that the information in the previous three sections is correct and that the prescription recorded by the supplier in Section C correctly "restates" the written or oral orders provided at the initiation of therapy.

Because the DME supplier must confirm in Section C of the new CMN form that the specific equipment *ordered* is being provided before the physician signs the form and for the provider to be reimbursed by the HCFA, the physician still has control over the therapy if he or she is willing and knowledgeable enough to exercise control and oversight of the treatment. The physician must supply a comprehensive written or oral prescription and insist that it be implemented before signing the CMN. Without a specific prescription for the oxygen delivery system that is most appropriate for the patient, the supplier is free to provide the least expensive equipment possible to help defray the recent reimbursement reductions. Physicians must be attentive to this aspect of prescribing HOT because suppliers have a great incentive to take control of therapy to reduce their costs, and the CMN form makes it even easier if the physician fails to provide a written oxygen prescription.

Because most patients with COPD and hypoxemia are able to live active and longer lives with oxygen therapy, liquid oxygen systems with ambulatory units that can be transfilled by the patient or lightweight aluminum cylinders coupled with oxygen-conserving devices are necessary to allow full activity and to facilitate pulmonary rehabilitation. High-pressure steel cylinders on wheels (strollers) are portable, but not ambulatory, and are suitable only for patients who occasionally leave the home or who take infrequent trips away from their stationary unit. The "standard of care" for most patients receiving HOT is ambulatory oxygen, except in the few who may be homebound. Recently, oxygen concentrators designed to refill ambulatory aluminum cylinders in the home have been introduced, and this technology has the potential to reduce the cost of HOT (Fig. 9-3). Currently, the major cost of therapy is not in the cost of equipment or oxygen itself but is in the requirements for resupply and home visits. Oxygen concentrators that can refill cylinders in the home require only occasional visits for maintenance of equipment.

INDICATIONS AND REQUIREMENTS FOR HOT

The current HCFA requirements for documentation of hypoxemia are adapted from the NOTT,[1] which established the efficacy for continuous LTOT. Continuous oxygen therapy is authorized if the partial pressure of oxygen (PaO_2) is equal to or less than 55 mm of Hg or the PaO_2 is between 56 and 59 mm of Hg and evidence of cor pulmonale, congestive heart failure, or erythrocytosis is present. The HCFA has also added an SaO_2 measurement of equal to or less than 88% to correspond to a PaO_2 of equal to or less than 55 mm Hg and an SaO_2 of 89% to be equivalent to a PaO_2 of 56 to 59 mm Hg. The measurement of SaO_2 is also easier to obtain during sleep or exercise if these are the only periods of

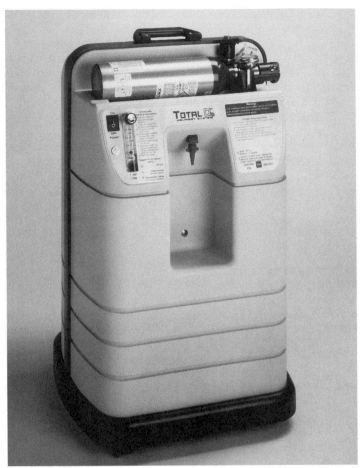

Figure 9-3. A new home oxygen concentrator that can provide continuous oxygen therapy while transfilling high-pressure aluminum cylinders for ambulation.

Box 9-1. Arterial Blood Gas or Arterial Oxyhemoglobin Saturation Indications for Home Oxygen Therapy

(A) Continuous oxygen therapy
    (1) $PaO_2 \leq 55$ mm Hg or $SaO_2 \leq 88\%$
    (2) $PaO_2 = 56$–59 mm Hg or $SaO_2 = 89\%$, with
        (a) Dependent edema owing to congestive heart failure, or
        (b) Cor pulmonale or pulmonary hypertension by electrocardiogram, gated
            blood pool scan, or pulmonary artery pressure measurement, or
        (c) Hematocrit greater than 56%
(B) Nocturnal oxygen only
    $PaO_2 \leq 55$ mmHg or $SaO_2 \leq 88\%$ during sleep or a drop in PaO_2 of more
        than 10 mm Hg or in SaO_2 of more than 5%, with signs or symptoms of
        hypoxemia (e.g., cognitive process, restlessness, or insomnia)
(C) Oxygen with exercise only
    $PaO_2 \leq 55$ mm Hg or $SaO_2 \leq 88\%$

PaO_2, arterial partial pressure of oxygen; SaO_2, arterial oxygen percent saturation.

Box 9-2. Medicare Requirements for Reimbursement of Home Oxygen Therapy

(A) Arterial blood gases or oxyhemoglobin saturation measurement performed by a Medicare-certified laboratory
(B) Clinical stability and optimum medical management before long-term oxygen therapy is prescribed
(C) Documentation of hypoxemia in hospitalized patients obtained within 2 d of discharge
(D) Provision of an oxygen prescription to the home oxygen supplier before initiation of therapy and completion of the CMN (Form HCFA 484.2)
(E) Retesting in 60–90 d if the blood gas is obtained on hospital discharge or in an unstable outpatient with a $PaO_2 > 55$ mm Hg or an $SaO_2 > 88\%$
(F) Measurement of PaO_2 or SaO_2 with the patient receiving 4 L/min oxygen if a flow rate of >4 L/min is prescribed
(G) Recertification, but not retesting, at the end of the first year
(H) Subsequent renewal only if the oxygen prescription changes
(I) Certification that the patient is mobile within the home if portable oxygen is ordered

CMN, certification of medical necessity; PaO_2, arterial partial pressure of oxygen; SaO_2, arterial oxygen percent saturation.

hypoxemia being encountered by the patient. In addition to these oxygen tension and saturation limits, the HCFA now recognizes that the patient should be clinically stable and receiving optimum therapy before LTOT is prescribed. The arterial blood gas or oxyhemoglobin saturation requirements for reimbursement of HOT are summarized in Box 9-1, and additional Medicare requirements for reimbursement are listed in Box 9-2.

APPROPRIATE OXYGEN THERAPY

In a five-state survey of patients using oxygen concentrators, the Office of the Inspector General[19] found that more than 30% of patients who were receiving oxygen concentrators because of abnormal blood gas measurements obtained during hospitalization were no longer using oxygen at all or to the extent being billed. The study also found that the physician often played a minor role in the entire process, commonly functioning only as the "signer of the CMN." This report of the Office of the Inspector General made both the HCFA and the medical community more aware that oxygen may be necessary for patients to be discharged from the hospital, but often it is not necessary for lifetime therapy. With increasing pressure for early hospital discharge brought about by the perspective payment system, many patients are still recovering from an acute respiratory illness when they leave the hospital and may need supplemental oxygen until full recovery has occurred. The Third National Oxygen Consensus Conference[20] recommended that when home oxygen is prescribed at the time of hospital discharge, arterial blood gasses should be repeated in 1 to 3 months when the patient is clinically stable and receiving optimum therapy. At this point, the decision for LTOT can be made, and if the patient qualifies for LTOT this is usually a lifetime commitment. Studies also indicate that oxygen can have a reparative effect on the lungs within 6 months that results in a reduction in alveolar-arterial oxygen gradient and an increase in the arterial PO_2 that is attributable to the beneficial effects of the oxygen therapy itself and not to changes in clinical stability.[21] On the basis of the best knowledge available today, when LTOT is prescribed for a clinically stable and appropriately managed patient who meets the current criteria for supplemental oxygen, it should not be discontinued later because the patient no longer meets *initial* blood gas requirements for therapy. Repeat arterial blood gas analysis should be used to follow the course of the disease and to guide overall management of the patient but not specifically to determine continuing need for oxygen therapy.

Although the HCFA allows SaO_2 measurements to be used to document the need for oxygen therapy, it is recommended that an arterial blood gas measurement be obtained to document the need for long-term (lifetime) continuous oxygen therapy.[22] SaO_2 measurements do not always correlate with the PaO_2 owing to multiple physiologic and technical factors that can affect the measurement. Measurement of SaO_2 is useful to document hypoxemia during sleep when evidence of clinical disease, such as cor pulmonale or erythrocytosis, is present in the absence of hypoxemia during the waking hours. In many patients other sleep disturbances may be present, such as obstructive or central sleep apnea, which may require treatment with modalities other than oxygen therapy. In some patients with chronic lung disease, the only abnormality associated with cor pulmonale may be nocturnal desaturation that is correctable by use of supplemental oxygen. Other patients with COPD and nocturnal desaturation may have no detectable disease attributable to tissue hypoxia or only a mild elevation in pulmonary vascular resistance without cor pulmonale, and no conclusive evidence exists of benefit from oxygen therapy in these individuals.[23]

Some patients with chronic lung disease may not have resting hypoxemia but may have desaturation during exercise. If dyspnea or exercise tolerance is improved with oxygen therapy, then oxygen should be prescribed during exercise and may be incorporated into a program for pulmonary rehabilitation. If desaturation occurs only with exercise, this should not be used as a means to justify continuous oxygen therapy. Often oxygen is prescribed indiscriminately for symptoms of dyspnea without documentation of benefit and without evidence of hypoxemia. Most often severe dyspnea is caused by mechanical dysfunction of the lungs and chest wall; if hypoxemia is not present, oxygen therapy is not justified unless it has been documented to increase exercise tolerance and is prescribed with specific activities of daily living or with a defined exercise program. A prescription for "oxygen as needed" (PRN) is never appropriate. In those patients who have qualified for LTOT, measurement of SaO_2 is useful to titrate the oxygen flow at rest, during various levels of exertion, and during sleep. In this context, SaO_2 measurements may be used to write a more complete oxygen prescription. It should also be noted that with many of the oxygen-conserving devices, the magnitude of oxygen conservation may be less with exercise or other activities of daily living, and an increase in flow rate is often necessary to prevent hypoxemia during these activities. In the NOTT,[1] oxygen flow was automatically increased by 1 L during both exercise and sleep. The usual goal of therapy is to maintain the PaO_2 at 60 to 65 mm Hg or the SaO_2 at $92 \pm 2\%$, especially when hypercapnia is present. The precise PaO_2 or SaO_2 that is best to improve quality of life or increase survival has not been well defined. In the NOTT,[1] the investigators attempted to maintain the PaO_2 between 60 and 80 mm Hg at all times. SaO_2 measurements are also useful to monitor acute changes in the respiratory status and may indicate that an arterial blood gas measurement is needed to completely assess the respiratory status of the patient.

HOME OXYGEN DELIVERY SYSTEMS

Compressed Gas Cylinders

Initially, all home oxygen was provided by use of compressed oxygen in large, steel cylinders that were regularly refilled by the home oxygen provider. Each cylinder contains enough oxygen to last 2 to 3 days at the usual flow rates, so several cylinders were usually placed in the patient's bedroom. The cylinders are large, bulky, and unattractive and because of their size and weight are not portable. Smaller E cylinders can be placed on wheels and have been used commonly for portability; however, these units weigh more than 20 lb and are difficult to manipulate on stairs and onto vehicles for public transportation. More recently, lightweight aluminum cylinders have been coupled with oxygen-conserving devices to provide ambulatory oxygen from units that can weigh as little as 4.5 lb, be carried in a fanny pack, and last up to 8 hours at flows equivalent to 2 L/min continuous oxygen. A family of these units, all weighing less than 10 lb when filled and lasting up to and beyond 24 hours at 2 L/min equivalent flow is demonstrated in Figure 9-4. As previously described, these units can now be transfilled in the home from specifically designed oxygen concentrators, avoiding the expense of home visits to refill or replace the cylinders.

Liquid Oxygen Systems

Liquid oxygen systems, which were first used by Dr. Thomas Petty and his associates in Denver, Colorado, had the important advantage of being the first oxygen delivery system to provide ambulatory oxygen therapy for extended periods of time.[24] Because liquid oxygen is cold, it is stored in insulated canisters at low pressure, and transfilling ambulatory units from large storage reservoirs in the home has been widely used for more than 3 decades. The reservoir units in the home may weigh from 60 to 120 lbs. The ambulatory units can weigh as little as 5.5 lb and, when combined with a built-in or external oxygen demand delivery device, can last up to 8 hours at a flow equivalent to 2 L/min. All liquid oxygen units vent gaseous oxygen when not in use and require regular refilling by the home oxygen supplier. Special equipment is required for transporting liquid oxygen and refilling home oxygen reservoirs, which, together with the frequent visits, make liquid oxygen the most expensive to supply. The Medicare reduction in reimbursement for home oxygen, along with the policy that all oxygen delivery systems are clinically equal (modality neutral), threatens the use of liquid oxygen in the future unless specifically ordered by the prescribing physician.

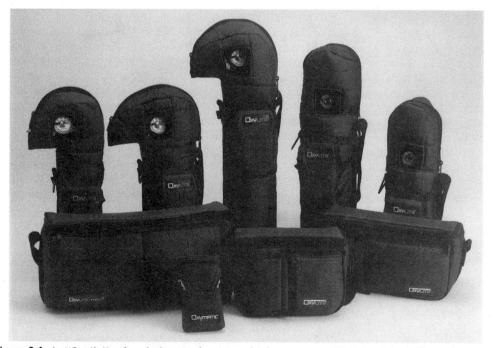

Figure 9-4. A "family" of ambulatory aluminum high-pressure cylinders with a demand oxygen delivery system, each weighing less than 10 lb and lasting from 4 1/2 to greater than 24 hours at 2 L/min equivalent flow.

Oxygen Concentrators

Oxygen concentrators use molecular sieves to separate nitrogen from oxygen in atmospheric gas. Modern oxygen concentrators for home use usually weigh 45 to 60 lb and can deliver up to 95% oxygen at flows of 4 to 6 L/min. The cost of purchasing and maintaining these units has made this the least expensive home oxygen supply system for DME providers. The cost of the newer units that can transfill aluminum cylinders in the home is greater, but less than the overall costs of delivery, supply, and maintenance of equipment necessary with liquid oxygen. The additional cost of electricity can be as great as $35 to $40 per month in some areas, and this cost is not reimbursed by any third-party payer.

Portable oxygen concentrators that can operate from both 12-volt DC current and standard house current (110-volt AC) are now available and weigh 32 lb or less. None of these units weigh less than 19 lb, and none are designed to be ambulatory. Continuous flow is limited to 2 L/min, but higher equivalent flow is available with oxygen-conserving devices internally or externally attached to the concentrator. The portable units are particularly useful with automobile travel because they can be plugged into the cigarette lighter when driving and into a standard electrical outlet in a motel or other dwelling.

Oxygen-Conserving Devices

Oxygen-conserving devices are of two types. They use either a reservoir for storage of 100% of oxygen that can be delivered early in inspiration or deliver a bolus or pulse of 100% oxygen during the first half of inspiration.[25] The reservoir oxygen conservers are marketed as either a nasal reservoir cannula or as a pendant reservoir cannula. The nasal reservoir uses a collapsible membrane with a 20-mL chamber that fills with oxygen during exhalation and empties early in inspiration. It is configured as a mustache that fits across the face under the nose. Because it is soft and increases the surface area of contact with the face, it is often more comfortable than a conventional nasal cannula but also more conspicuous. The pendant reservoir can be concealed under clothing and is less obtrusive when used in public. The actual reservoir with this device is the conducting tubing between the nasal cannula and the pendant; and the tubing tends to be somewhat larger in diameter, more rigid, and less comfortable when worn for prolonged periods of time. Both devices can provide oxygen conservation of up to 60% at rest.

The Demand Oxygen Delivery Systems (DODS) may vary substantially both in timing of oxygen delivery and in oxygen volume with each breath. They may be built into oxygen delivery systems or may be externally attached to any oxygen supply source. The DODS may be battery operated or pneumatically activated. The degree of oxygen conservation varies among the commercially available DODS, but it is usually greater than 50% at rest. As previously noted, with all oxygen-conserving devices, the degree of oxygen concentration may be less with exercise or when higher flows are necessary. The oxygen flow needed to correct hypoxemia both at rest and with usual activity should be determined for each patient. The oxygen flow also should be adjusted for exercise as part of a pulmonary rehabilitation program.

Transtracheal Oxygen

The use of a transtracheal oxygen catheter for LTOT has the advantage of both oxygen conservation and improved compliance with therapy. Oxygen conservation results from the use of the upper airway as an internal oxygen reservoir with overall oxygen conservation of about 55% at rest and 30% with exercise.[26] Increased compliance results from uninterrupted oxygen therapy 24 hours per day. Studies from several centers have shown that compared with oxygen by standard nasal cannula, exercise tolerance is increased, hematocrit is further reduced in patients with persistent erythrocytosis, and both pulmonary artery pressures and alveolar-arterial oxygen gradients are reduced.[15,21,27–30] Selinger and associates[31] found that in patients with COPD who were receiving oxygen therapy, removal of oxygen for only 3 hours per day resulted in increased pulmonary hypertension and impaired cardiac function. In the NOTT,[1] patients assigned to receive continuous oxygen therapy used oxygen only 18 hours each day and, therefore, continued to experience up to 6 hours of hypoxemia. Further discussion of oxygen delivery systems is found in Chapter 27.

CONCLUSION

LTOT can increase survival and improve quality of life in patients with COPD and hypoxemia and is a critical component of the rehabilitation program for any patient with hypoxemia owing to chronic lung disease. Indications and requirements for oxygen therapy have been defined by Medicare and are used by most third-party payers. New Medicare reimbursement policies for HOT that were implemented in 1998 and 1999 as part of the Balanced Budget Act of 1997 have substantially reduced reimbursement to oxygen suppliers (a 25% reduction in 1998 and an additional 5% in 1999). Recent changes in the CMN form have made it more difficult for the physician to transmit the details of the oxygen prescription to the oxygen supplier; thus, the oxygen supplier is provided the opportunity to reduce cost by providing less expensive equipment that may not fulfill the specific therapeutic requirements of the patient. This demands greater vigilance and knowledge by the physician. Ideally, a detailed written medical prescription for oxygen equipment and therapy should be provided to the oxygen supplier before initiation of therapy and issuance of the CMN. Advances in oxygen delivery systems allow greater freedom for patients, with lower maintenance costs. This now includes a new class of oxygen concentrators that can transfill aluminum cylinders in the home. Access to newer technology may be difficult, however, without physician involvement and knowledge of the oxygen system that is best for the comprehensive rehabilitation of each individual patient.

REFERENCES

1. Nocturnal Oxygen Therapy Trial Group. Continuous and nocturnal oxygen therapy in hypoxemic chronic obstructive lung disease: a clinical trial. Ann Intern Med 1980;93:391.
2. Report of the Medical Research Council Working Party: long-term domiciliary oxygen therapy in chronic cor pulmonale complicating chronic bronchitis and emphysema. Lancet 1981;1:681.
3. Heaton RK, Grant I, McSweeney AJ, et al. Psychologic effects of continuous and nocturnal oxygen therapy in hypoxemic chronic obstructive pulmonary disease. Arch Intern Med 1983;143:1941.
4. The Intermittent Positive-Pressure Breathing Trial Group. Intermittent positive-pressure breathing therapy of chronic obstructive lung disease: a clinical trial. Ann Intern Med 1983;99:612.
5. Anthonisen NR, Wright EC, Hodgkin JE, et al. Prognosis in chronic obstructive pulmonary disease. Am Rev Respir Dis 1986;133:14.
6. O'Donohue WJ Jr. The future of home oxygen therapy. Respir Care 1988;33:1125.
7. Neff TA, Petty TL. Long-term continuous oxygen therapy in chronic airway obstruction: mortality in relationship to cor pulmonale, hypoxia and hypercapnia. Ann Intern Med 1970;72:621.
8. Levine BE, Bigelow DB, Hamstra RD, et al. The role of long-term continuous oxygen administration in patients with chronic airway obstruction with hypoxemia. Ann Intern Med 1967;66:639.
9. Abraham AS, Cole RB, Bishop JM. Reversal of pulmonary hypertension by prolonged oxygen administration to patients with chronic bronchitis. Circ Res 1968;23:147.
10. Weitzemblum E, Sautegeau A, Ehrhart M, et al. Long-term oxygen therapy can reverse the progression of pulmonary hypertension in patients with chronic obstructive pulmonary disease. Am Rev Respir Dis 1985;131:493.
11. Cotes JE, Gilson JC. Effect of oxygen on exercise ability in chronic respiratory insufficiency: use of portable apparatus. Lancet 1956;1:872.
12. Petty TL, Finigan MM. Clinical evaluation of prolonged ambulatory oxygen therapy in chronic airway obstruction. Am J Med 1968;45:242.
13. Woodcock AA, Gross ER, Geddes DM. Oxygen relieves breathlessness in "pink puffers." Lancet 1981;1:907.
14. Wesmiller SW, Hoffman LA, Sciurba FC, et al. Exercise tolerance during nasal cannula and transtracheal oxygen delivery. Am Rev Respir Dis 1990;141:789.
15. Couser JL, Make BJ. Transtracheal oxygen decreases inspired minute ventilation. Am Rev Respir Dis 1989;139:627.

16. Dewan NA, Bell CW. Effect of high-flow and low-flow oxygen delivery via transtracheal catheter and nasal cannula on exercise tolerance and sensation of dyspnea. Chest 1991;100:52S.

17. O'Donohue WJ Jr, Plummer AL. Magnitude of usage and cost of home oxygen therapy in the United States. Chest 1995;107:301.

18. Silverman BG, Gross TP, Babish JD. Home oxygen therapy in Medicare beneficiaries, 1991 and 1992. Chest 1997;112:380.

19. US Department of Health and Human Services, Office of Inspector General, Office of Audit. National review of medical necessity for oxygen concentrators. 1990. Audit Control No. A-04-88-02058.

20. Conference report: new problems in supply, reimbursement and certification of medical necessity for long-term oxygen therapy. Am Rev Respir Dis 1990;142:721.

21. O'Donohue WJ Jr. Effect of oxygen therapy on increasing arterial oxygen tension in hypoxemic patients with stable chronic obstructive pulmonary disease while breathing ambient air. Chest 1991;100:968.

22. Conference report: problems in prescribing and supplying oxygen for Medicare patients. Am Rev Respir Dis 1986;134:340.

23. Fletcher EC, Luckett RA, Miller T, et al. Exercise hemodynamics and gas exchange in patients with chronic obstructive pulmonary disease, sleep desaturation, and a daytime PaO_2 above 60 mm Hg. Am Rev Respir Dis 1989;140:1237.

24. Petty TL. Historical perspective on long-term oxygen therapy. In: O'Donohue WJ Jr, ed. Long-term Oxygen Therapy. New York: Marcel Dekker, 1995:1.

25. O'Donohue WJ Jr. Oxygen conserving devices. Respir Care 1987;32:37.

26. Christopher KL, Spofford BT, Betrun MD, et al. A program for transtracheal oxygen delivery: assessment of safety and efficacy. Ann Intern Med 1987;107:802.

27. Benditt J, Pollock M, Roa J, et al. Transtracheal delivery of gas decreases the oxygen cost of breathing. Am Rev Respir Dis 1993;147:1207.

28. Bloom BS, Daniel JM, Wiseman M, et al. Transtracheal oxygen delivery in patients with chronic obstructive pulmonary disease. Respir Med 1989; 83:281.

29. Domingo C, Domingo E, Klamburg J, et al. Hemodynamic follow-up in COPD with 24 hour liquid oxygen therapy through transtracheal catheter. Chest 1991;100: 52S.

30. Hoffman LA, Wesmiller SW, Sciurba FC, et al. Nasal cannula and transtracheal oxygen delivery: a comparison of patient response after six months of each technique. Am Rev Respir Dis 1992; 145:827.

31. Selinger SR, Kennedy TP, Buescher P, et al. Effect of removing oxygen from patients with chronic obstructive pulmonary disease. Am Rev Respir Dis 1987;136:85.

10 Exercise in the Rehabilitation of Patients With Respiratory Disease

Bartolome R. Celli

Professional Skills

Upon completion of this the chapter, the reader will:

- Understand the effect and role of leg and arm training and give practical recommendations
- List important factors that contribute to decreased exercise in chronic obstructive pulmonary disease (COPD) patients
- Understand principles that apply to training patients with severe pulmonary problems

Patients with chronic respiratory diseases decrease their overall physical activity because any form of exercise will often result in debilitating dyspnea. The progressive deconditioning associated with inactivity initiates a vicious cycle in which dyspnea increases, at ever lower physical demands (Fig. 10-1). With time, the patients will also adopt a breathing pattern (shallow and rapid) that is detrimental to overall gas exchange, thus worsening their symptoms. In general, physical reconditioning is a broad therapeutic concept that has unfortunately been equated with simple lower extremity exercise training. This chapter reviews the current knowledge regarding exercise conditioning in much broader terms. The effect and role of leg and arm training will be critically analyzed, and practical recommendations will be given. Ventilatory muscle training will not be reviewed because it is addressed in a different chapter in this book.

The data that form the basis of our current knowledge about exercise conditioning have been obtained from patients with intrinsic lung disease, such as emphysema, bronchitis, bronchiectasis, cystic fibrosis, and acute respiratory failure. Little is known about reconditioning in patients with pure "pump failure," such as those with degenerative neuromuscular diseases. There is every reason to believe that in these patients, physical exercise may worsen rather than improve their overall function and sensation of well-being. Conversely, pure breathing retraining, such as slow deep breathing, could have a more universal application as long as extra loads are not placed on already weakened and dysfunctional respiratory muscles. As is reviewed in another chapter, patients with symptomatic pump failure may benefit more from ventilatory assistance and resting than from further training.

PHYSICAL RECONDITIONING

Exercise conditioning is the most important factor in the rehabilitation of patients with symptomatic respiratory disease. It is important to understand the principles and components of exercise training to adequately incorporate them in the treatment of these patients.

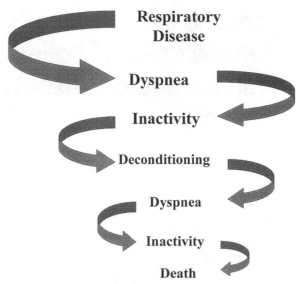

Figure 10-1. Respiratory disease is associated with progressive development of dyspnea at an even lower exercise level. This leads to progressive inactivity, which in turn induces further deconditioning and ever increasing dyspnea at lower exercise intensity. This "vicious cycle" can be reversed with exercise training.

General Principles

The short- and long-term effects of systematic exercise conditioning have been the subject of extensive investigation. In normal individuals, it is known that participation and completion of well-designed exercise training programs result in several objective changes:

1. Increase in maximal oxygen uptake, primarily owing to increases in blood volume, hemoglobin level, and heart stroke volume, with improvement in the peripheral use of oxygen.
2. Specific training increases muscular strength and endurance, primarily resulting from enlargement of muscle fibers, improved blood and energy supply, and change in the enzymes that help energy formation.
3. Improved muscle coordination.
4. Change in body composition with increased muscle mass and loss of adipose tissue.
5. Improved sensation of well-being.

In patients with obstruction to airflow, participation in a similar program will result in different outcomes depending on the severity of the obstruction. Patients with mild to moderate disease will, as a rule, manifest the same findings as healthy patients, whereas, as we shall discuss later, patients with the severe form will be able to increase exercise endurance and improve their sensation of well-being with little if any increase in the maximal oxygen uptake. Several recent studies have shown outcome improvement different from the specific effects of training on exercise performance in these patients, including improved muscle enzyme content, less dyspnea for similar work level, decreased lactic acid production at isowork, and improvement in activity of daily living and health-related quality of life. Once the benefits are achieved, information is available regarding the effect of maintenance programs on any of the outcomes, including exercise performance.

Patients with COPD manifest decreased exercise tolerance. The most important factors thought to contribute to this limitation are:

1. Alterations in pulmonary mechanics
2. Dysfunction of the respiratory muscles
3. Peripheral muscle dysfunction
4. Abnormal gas exchange
5. Alterations in cardiac performance
6. Malnutrition
7. Development of dyspnea

Other factors deserve to be mentioned but are less well characterized, including active smoking and polycythemia. Although the most severe patients cannot exercise to the levels where the training effect is thought to be optimal (above the anaerobic threshold), a large body of evidence supports exercise training as a beneficial therapeutic tool to help these patients achieve their full potential.

Physiologic Adaptation to Training

To train patients with severe pulmonary problems we must understand several principles that apply to exercise training:

1. Specificity of training
2. Intensity, frequency, and duration of the exercise load
3. Detraining effect

Specificity of Training
The training of muscles or muscle groups is beneficial only to the trained muscle. The response of the muscle depends on the stimulus.

Use of high-resistance, low-repetition stimulus (weight lifting) increases muscle strength, whereas low-resistance, high-repetition stimulus increases muscle endurance. Strength training is achieved by increasing myofibrils in certain muscle fibers, whereas endurance training increases the number of capillaries and enzymatic mitochondrial content in the trained muscles.

The training is specific to the trained muscle. Clausen et al. trained subjects with their arms or legs and observed that the decreased heart rate observed for arm muscle training could not be transferred to the leg group and vice versa.[1] Davis and Sargeant[2] showed that if training was completed for one leg, the beneficial effect could not be transferred to exercise involving the untrained leg. More recently, Belman and Kendregan[3] confirmed these findings in patients with COPD. They examined the effect of 6 weeks of training in eight patients who only trained their arms and seven patients who only trained their legs. They observed improved exercise only for the exercise for which the patients trained.

Intensity, Frequency, and Duration of the Exercise Load
These factors profoundly affect the degree of the training effect. Athletes will usually train at maximal or near-maximal levels to rapidly achieve the desired effects. Conversely, middle-aged nonathletes may require less intense exercise. Siegel et al.[4] showed that training sessions of 30 minutes close to three times a week for 15 weeks significantly improved maximal oxygen uptake if heart rate was raised above 80% of the predicted maximal rate. In patients with chronic lung disease, the issue of exercise intensity and duration has been studied by different authors, as we shall review later, but it seems that the larger the number of sessions and the more intense the sessions (as a function of maximal performance), the better the results.

In their work, Belman and Kendregan[3] exercised patients at 30% of maximal, and after 6 weeks of training four times weekly in which the load was increased as tolerated, they observed significant improvement in endurance time in 9 of the 15 patients. It is possible that the relatively low training level (30% of maximal) may help explain why six of their patients failed to increase the endurance time. In contrast, Niederman et al.[5] started the exercise at 50% of maximal cycle ergometer level and increased its intensity on a weekly basis and observed endurance improvement in most patients. Clark and coworkers[6] randomized 48 patients with severe COPD to training (n = 32) and control (n = 16). The training consisted of low-intensity aerobic exercise and isolated conditioning of peripheral muscles, including shoulder circling, abdominal exercise, wall press-up, quadriceps, and step-up exercise. The exercises were supervised in the hospital once weekly and were carried out daily at home for a total of 12 weeks. The trained group showed significant improvement in whole-body endurance, decreased ventilation for similar oxygen uptake, and decreased breathlessness.

Other authors have used higher starting exercise levels and have achieved higher endurance.[6-9] The best study in this regard is that by Casaburi et al.,[10] who studied 19 patients with COPD who could achieve anaerobic threshold (moderate COPD with a mean SD forced expiratory volume in 1 second [FEV_1] of 1.8 ± 0.53 L) before and after randomly assigned low-intensity (50% of maximal) or high-intensity (80% of maximal) exercise. The authors showed that the high-intensity training program was more effective than the low-intensity one. They also observed a drop in ventilatory requirement for exercise after training that was proportional to the drop in lactate at a given work rate. It therefore seems that training is achieved if the intensity of exercise is at least 50% of maximal and that it can be increased as tolerated. Conversely, any exercise is better than none, and indeed good results have been shown even for patients with minimal exercise performance when tested.[5,11]

The number of exercise sessions is also a matter of debate.[3,12] In general, as the number of sessions are increased, so is the change in observed endurance time. Because exercise cessation results in a loss of the training effect, the optimal plan should involve an intense training phase and a maintenance phase. The latter is difficult to implement and results in the frequently observed failure to maintain and preserve the beneficial effects achieved through the training. Unfortunately, only a limited number of studies have addressed this important issue. Foglio and coworkers[13] evaluated 35 asthma and 26 COPD patients before and immediately after discharge from an inpatient rehabilitation program and after 1 year of follow-up. Treatment improved muscle strength, exercise tolerance, dyspnea, and health-related quality of life. The improvement decreased with time but was maintained above baseline at 1-year follow-up. More studies are needed to verify this important finding.

Detraining Effect

This principle is based on observations that the effect achieved by training is lost after the exercise is stopped. Saltin et al.[14] showed that bed rest in normal subjects resulted in a significant decrease in maximal oxygen uptake within 21 days of resting. It took 10 to 50 days for the values to return to those seen before resting. Keens et al.[15] examined ventilatory muscle endurance after training in normal subjects who had undergone ventilatory muscle training. Within 1 month of having stopped training, the subjects had lost the training effect that they had achieved. Therefore, it seems important to continue to train, but the minimum practical and effective timing of maintenance training remains to be determined. Ries and coworkers[16] showed that after 12 weeks of intense exercise training, a once-a-month maintenance program maintained the benefit achieved for at least 1 year. A detailed review of the data from that study shows that continuous loss of the benefit occurred during that year. This suggests that a once-a-month session may not be enough and that a maintenance program that includes more sessions may be more effective.

Our exercise program is based on the data and concepts developed in the previous sections of this chapter. Patients are exercised at 70% of the maximal work achieved in a test day. This work is increased on a weekly basis as tolerated by the patient. We aim to complete 24 sessions, typically in an outpatient setting with sessions held three times weekly. The program may be completed quicker if the patient is in the hospital because

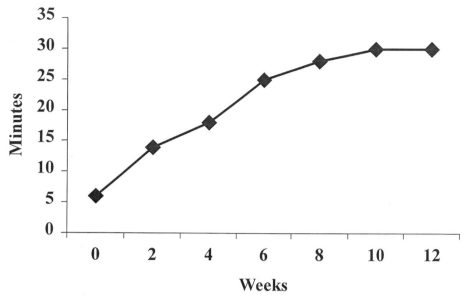

Figure 10-2. After initiation of a high-intensity training program, it takes 8 to 10 weeks for the patient to be able to maintain the targeted load for 25 to 30 minutes.

the sessions occur at least on a daily basis. Each session lasts 30 minutes if tolerated; otherwise, it is begun as guided by the patient's symptoms and no further load is provided until the patient can complete the 30 minutes of the session. Typically, it takes 6 to 8 weeks of high-intensity training to reach the targeted load (Fig. 10-2). A close communication exists between the person in charge of the training and the rehabilitation planning team. In those settings where metabolic measurements are not possible, the use of the perception of dyspnea using a Borg visual analog scale can substitute a target work rate. This has been shown in a series of studies of patients with COPD.[17,18] It is appealing to use dyspnea and not heart rate as the target to train patients with lung disease because breathlessness constitutes their most important complaint. The study by Mejia and coworkers[18] supports this concept and provides a useful, inexpensive, and rather accurate way to prescribe exercise in the simplest of settings.

LOWER EXTREMITY EXERCISE

Many uncontrolled studies have shown that the inclusion of leg exercise in the training of patients with lung disease is beneficial.[19-23] This has been confirmed in a series of controlled trials.

Cockcroft et al.[24] randomized 39 dyspneic patients younger than 70 years and not on oxygen to (*a*) a treatment group that spent 6 weeks in a rehabilitation center, where they underwent gradual endurance exercise training, and (*b*) a control group that received medical care but was given no special advice to exercise. The control group served as such for 4 months and was then admitted to the rehabilitation center for 6 weeks. Just like the treated patients, they were instructed to exercise at home afterward. Both groups were similar at baseline. Thirty-four patients completed the program. After rehabilitation, only 2 of the 16 control patients manifested improvement in dyspnea and cough, whereas 16 of the 18 patients included in the treatment group manifested improvement in these symptoms. More important, treated patients showed significant improvement in the 12-minute walk and in peak oxygen uptake (VO_2) compared with controls.

Sinclair and Ingram[25] randomized 33 patients with chronic bronchitis and dyspnea to two groups. The 17 patients in the treatment group exercised by climbing up and down on two 24-cm steps twice daily. Exercise time was increased to tolerance. Patients exercised at home and were evaluated by the treatment team weekly. The control group did not exercise, but all its members were reassessed after 6 months. The degree of airflow obstruction did not change in either group. Similarly, no improvement in strength of the quadriceps, minute ventilation, and heart rate occurred. In contrast, performance on the 12-minute walk test significantly increased in patients who were trained. These two studies are particularly important in that they were well designed and used randomization in the assignment of patients to the specific treatment groups.

More recently, O'Donnell et al.[26] compared breathlessness, 6-minute walking distance, and cycle ergometer work between two age-matched groups of patients with moderate COPD. The endurance exercise-trained group (n = 23) achieved significant reduction in dyspnea scores and increased the distance walked as well as the cycle ergometry work compared with the control group (n = 13). This trial is important in that it not only documented increased endurance but for the first time evaluated the patient's perception of dyspnea, which is the most problematic symptom and the one leading to physical limitation. Since those initial studies, several trials have documented the beneficial effect of lower extremity exercise.[16,27–31] Perhaps the most important one is the study by Ries et al.[16] In this study, 119 patents were randomized to an education support group (n = 62) or to a similar educational program with the addition of walking exercise three times weekly for 8 weeks (n = 57). At 2 months, and still seen at 4, 6, and 12 months, the patient who exercised manifested increased exercise endurance, less dyspnea with exercise, less dyspnea with activities of daily living, and a non–statistically significant increase in survival. This landmark study establishes the pivotal role of lower extremity exercise in the proven benefit of pulmonary rehabilitation. The results of all the studies are summarized in Table 10-1.

Numerous trials that have used patients as their own controls have shown similar results, with significant increased exercise endurance. The mechanism by which this improvement occurs remains a matter of debate. Some studies[7,23] have demonstrated a drop in heart rate at a similar work level, a hallmark of a training effect for the specific exercise. This is perhaps related to a decrease in exercise lactate level as suggested by Woolf and Suero.[32] More recent evidence in support of a training effect is provided by the study of Casaburi et al.[10] The patients showed a reduction in exercise lactic acidosis and ventilation after training. Furthermore, the reduction was proportional to the intensity of the training. A 12% decrease occurred in the lactic acidosis rise in patients trained with the low work rate (50% of maximum) and a 32% decrease occurred in the ones trained with the high work rate (80% of maximum). In both groups significant decreases occurred in heart rate after training. Other studies have failed to document either an increase in maximum oxygen uptake or a decrease in heart rate or lactate at a similar work level. The most important study in this group is that by Belman and Kendregan,[3] which failed to show a decrease in heart rate at the same work load as represented by the VO_2. These authors went further and analyzed muscle biopsy sample oxidative enzyme content before and after training. They observed no change in this parameter. Interestingly, 9 of the treated patients improved their exercise endurance. As stated previously, it is possible that this study used too low a training effort because training was started at 30% of the maximum achieved during their testing. That this may be so is supported by two studies from one group.[33,34] They first showed that muscle biopsy samples from the legs of patients with COPD had decreased content of oxidative enzymes in their mitochondria.[33] Subsequently, and extremely important for those who believe in the physiologic training, the mitochondrial enzymatic content significantly increased after exercise training.[34] In that same group of patients they also documented a delay of onset of the lactase threshold after training.

The evidence from all of these studies indicates that patients with COPD can be trained to a level that produces physiologic changes consistent with improved muscle

Table 10-1. Controlled Studies of Rehabilitation With Exercise in Patients With COPD

Study	No. of Patients	Duration	Course (wk)	Results
Cockcroft et al.[24]	18T	Daily	16	↑ 12 MW, ↑ VO$_2$
	16C	—	—	No change
Sinclair and Ingram[25]	17T	Daily	40	↑ FVC, ↑ 12MW
	16C	—	—	No change
O'Donnell et al.[26]	23T	Daily	8	↑ FVC, ↑ 12MW ↓ Dyspnea
	13C	—	—	No change
Reardon et al.[28]	10T	Twice weekly	6	↓ Dyspnea
	10C	—	—	No change
Ries et al.[58]	57T	Daily	8	↑ Exercise capacity ↓ Dyspnea ↑ Self-efficacy
	62C	Daily education	8	No change
Wykstra et al.[29]	28T	Daily at home	12	↑ Exercise capacity ↑ HRQoL
	15C	—	—	No change
Goldstein et al.[27]	45T	Daily	24	↑ 6MW VO$_2$ ↓ Dyspnea
	44C	None	24	No change
Strijboz et al.[30]	15 OP	Twice weekly	12	↑ 4MWD, ↑ work ↓ Dyspnea
	15 Home	Twice weekly	12	↑ 4MWD, ↑ work ↓ Dyspnea
	15 C	None	12	No change
Wedzicha et al.[31]	30 Ex, MRC/5	NA (home)	8	No change
	30 C, MRC/5	NA (home)	8	No change
	33 Ex, MRC/3-4	NA (hosp)	8	↑ WD, ↑ HRQoL
	33 C, MRC/3-4	NA (hosp)	8	No change

COPD, chronic obstructive pulmonary disease; T, treated; C, controls; 12MW, 12-min walk test; VO$_2$, peak oxygen uptake; FVC, forced vital capacity; HRQoL, health-related quality of life; 6MW, 6-min walk test; 4MWD, 4-min walk distance; OP, out-patient; Ex, exercise; MRC, Medical Research Council dyspnea scale; NA, not available; WD, walk distance.

performance. Figure 10-3 shows the average change of several important physiologic variables from some of these studies. It is interesting to note that the average improvement in outcomes, such as walking distance or exercise endurance, was similar whether high-intensity training,[10,34] lower-intensity training,[5] and even home training[30] was used.

Do All Patients Benefit?

Three studies addressed the issue of whether patients with the most severe COPD can undergo exercise training. This is an important question because many patients with the most severe COPD do not exercise to the intensity required to reach anaerobic threshold or to induce cardiovascular training. Niederman et al.[5] exercised 33 patients with different degrees of COPD (FEV$_1$ range, 0.33 to 3.82 L). After training, there was no correlation between the degree of airflow obstruction in these patients and their observed improvement. In other words, patients with very low FEV$_1$ were as likely to improve as were

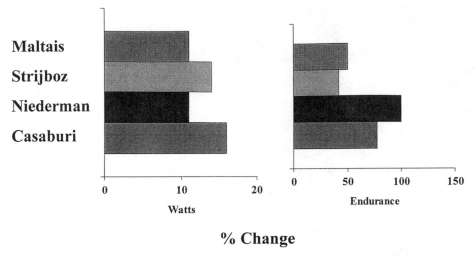

% Change

Figure 10-3. Improvement in work rate (watts) and exercise endurance time in selected series of exercise training in patients with COPD. Little differences in outcome occurred despite differences in the training programs.

patients with high FEV_1. Similarly, ZuWallack et al.[11] evaluated 50 patients with COPD (FEV_1 range, 0.38 to 3.24 L) before and after exercise training. They observed an inverse relationship between the baseline 12-minute walk distance and VO_2 and the observed improvement. They concluded that patients with poor performance on either the 12-minute walking distance or maximal exercise test are not necessarily poor candidates for an exercise program. Casaburi et al.[35] reported the effect of training 15 men and 10 women with severe COPD (FEV_1, 0.93 ± 0.27 L) with leg training at close to 80% of maximum. After training 3 times weekly for 6 weeks, a 77% improvement in the duration of a submaximal test, an improvement in oxygen kinetics, and a decrease in minute ventilation at the same work level were seen. Also, the respiratory rate decreased and tidal volume increased. From this data it seems prudent to conclude that most patients capable of undergoing leg exercise endurance training will benefit from a program that includes leg exercise. This overall principle is contradicted by the recent result of a randomized trial of pulmonary rehabilitation in patients with COPD who were stratified by the perception of dyspnea using the Medical Research Council (MRC) dyspnea scale. In that rather complex trial, patients with the most severe dyspnea (MRC = 5) failed to improve after exercise training, whereas patients with less dyspnea (MRC = 3/4) did show improvement in exercise performance. Of note, patients in the most severe group were treated at home, whereas those with less dyspnea were supervised at a rehabilitation institute, so it is possible that the exercise program was not the same for all groups. Nevertheless, this study is important in that it suggests that some patients may be too ill to benefit from exercise training. Certainly, more research is needed to clarify this important issue.

Type of Training

The type of exercise training to be prescribed and the testing modality are also subject to debate. Different studies have used different training techniques. Most studies include walking as both a measurement of exercise tolerance and of the training program, whereas others have relied on more precise methods, such as the cycle ergometer or treadmill.

The classic timed walk (6- or 12-minute walking distance), where the distance walked over 6 or 12 minutes is recorded, is good for patients with moderate to severe COPD but may not be taxing enough for patients with a lesser degree of airflow obstruction.[36]

We have found the 6-minute walking distance to be a reliable, inexpensive, and useful test. In at least two studies, the timed walked distance test has been shown to predict overall survival in patients with severe COPD.[37,38] Singh et al.[39] have reported a good correlation between the oxygen uptake measured with cycle ergometry and the "walking shuttle" test. This test progressively increases the demands on the patient being tested, thereby proving to be useful in patients with a lesser degree of airflow limitation.

We have evaluated stair climbing and shown that the VO_2 can be estimated from the number of steps climbed during a symptom-limited test.[40] Several studies have used treadmill testing and/or step testing even though the training has been done with the patient walking. Oxygen uptake is higher for stair climbing or treadmill testing than for the more commonly used leg ergometry, presumably because the former uses more body muscles than does leg cycling. Leg ergometry has become popular in its use as a testing device and has been the training apparatus for most recent studies. It is certainly smaller than the treadmill, and with relatively inexpensive units in the market, it is possible to place several together and to train groups of patients simultaneously.

Most of the studies quoted relied on either in-hospital or outpatient hospital training. Little information exists regarding implementation of such programs at home. In a unique report, O'Hara et al.[41] enrolled 14 patients with moderate COPD (FEV_1, 1.17 ± 0.76 L) in a home exercise program. The authors randomized the patients to daily walking while carrying a lightweight backpack (2.6 ± 0.5 kg) or the same backpacking regimen with additional weight lifting and strength limb exercises. These included wrist curls, arms curls, partial leg squats, calf raises, and supine dumbbell presses. The initial load was 4.3 ± 0.9 kg and was increased weekly by 1.2 ± 0.5 kg for 6 weeks to reach 10.4 ± 2.6 kg by the last week. The weigt lifters performed 10 repetitions 3 times, avoiding dyspnea, breathholding, and fatigue, for a total time of 30 minutes daily. Patients documented their exercises in a diary. Health care personnel visited the patients on a weekly basis. After training, all weight lifters had reduced their minute ventilation during bicycle ergometry compared with controls. Furthermore, the weight-trained patients showed a 16% increase in exercise endurance. This study suggests that exercise training can be achieved at home with relatively inexpensive programs, with the beneficial consequence of no hospital visits and in the comfort of a home. This initial report is supported by recent data that supervised exercise at home achieves the same outcomes as that obtained in the hospital.[29,30]

In our pulmonary rehabilitation program we complete testing using an electrically braked ergometer, while the training is done in a mechanically controlled ergometer, either as an outpatient or as an inpatient depending on the patients condition. Box 10-1 practically describes our training program. We believe that the training has to be tailored to each individual and to the available training equipment. The experience in less developed countries (as discussed elsewhere in this book) confirms that it is not necessary to have expensive equipment to successfully implement an exercise program for symptomatic patients with respiratory disease.

Although not all possible outcomes have been determined in every trial, it is possible

Box 10-1. Training Method for Leg Excrcise

1. Train at 60–80% of maximal work capacity[a]
2. Increase work every 5th session as tolerated
3. Monitor dyspnea and heart rate
4. Increase work after 20–30 min of submaximal targeted work is achieved
5. Aim for 24 sessions

[a]Work capacity as determined by an exercise test, not necessarily by evaluating heart rate. It is possible to substitute work capacity for dyspnea (see text for discussion).

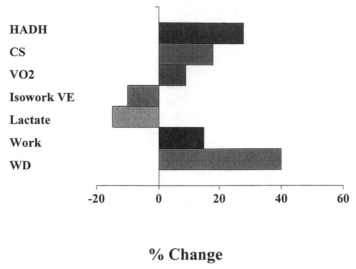

% Change

Figure 10-4. Lower extremity exercise training results in large increases in exercise endurances (*WD*) with lesser but significant increase in work rate and oxygen uptake (*VO*$_2$). Exercise training increases the mitochrondrial content of cytric synthase (*CS*) and 3-hydroxy-CoA-hydroxidase (*HADH*). After training, a decrease occurs in the generation of lactate and ventilation at any given work load (*isowork VE*). The data are the average of the results from references 5, 6, 10, 11, 16, 24, 25–31, and 34.

to obtain a picture of the most important benefits of lower extremity exercise. The average changes reported[5,6,10,11,16,24–34] until now are summarized in Figure 10-4. Most studies report a large improvement in walked distance or submaximal exercise endurance. This occurs with more modest, but still significant, increases in work rate or oxygen uptake. This is likely due to changes in the enzymatic content of muscle mitochondria such as cytric synthase and 3-hydroxy-acyl-CoA dehydrogenase. This change in enzyme content is associated with decreased lactate production and ventilatory requirement at similar work load. The overall consequence is a consistent improvement in exercise performance.

UPPER EXTREMITY EXERCISE

Most of our knowledge about exercise conditioning in patients undergoing rehabilitation is derived from programs emphasizing leg training. This is unfortunate because the performance of many everyday tasks requires not only the hands but also the concerted action of other muscle groups that partake in upper torso and arm positioning. Some muscles of the upper torso and shoulder girdle serve both respiratory and postural functions. Muscles such as the upper and lower trapezius, latissimus dorsi, serratus anterior, subclavius, and pectoralis minor and major possess a thoracic and an extrathoracic anchoring point. Depending on the anchoring point they may help position the arms or shoulder or, if given an extra thoracic fulcrum (such as fixing the arms in a supported position), they may exert a pulling force on the rib cage. We have shown that in patients with chronic airflow obstruction, as severity worsens, the diaphragm loses its force-generating capacity and the muscles of the rib cage become more important in the generation of inspiratory pressures.[42] When patients perform unsupported arm exercise, some of the shoulder girdle muscles have to decrease their participation in ventilation, and if the task involves complex purposeful arm movements, the pattern of ventilation may be affected.

Unsupported Arm Exercise

Tangri and Woolf[43] used a pneumobelt to study breathing patterns in seven patients with COPD while they performed simple activities of daily living such as tying their shoes and brushing their teeth. The patients developed an irregular and rapid pattern of breathing with the arm exercise. After the exercise, the patients breathed faster and deeper, which according to the authors was done to restore the blood gases to normal.

We have explored the ventilatory response to unsupported arm exercise and compared it with the response to leg exercise in patients with severe chronic lung disease.[44] Arm exercise resulted in dyssynchronous thoracoabdominal excursion that was not solely caused by diaphragmatic fatigue. The dyspnea that was reported by the patients was associated with a dyssynchronous breathing pattern. We concluded that unsupported arm exercise could shift work to the diaphragm and in some way lead to dyssynchrony. To test this hypothesis, we have used pleural pressure versus gastric pressure plots (with a gastric and endoesophageal balloon) and evaluated the changes as well as the ventilatory response to unsupported arm exercise and compared it with leg cycle ergometry in normal subjects and patients with airflow obstruction.[45,46] We documented increased diaphragmatic pressure excursion with arm exercise and alterations in the pattern of pressure generation with more contribution by the diaphragm and abdominal muscles of respiration and less contribution by the inspiratory muscles of the rib cage. These findings have been confirmed by others studying not only patients with COPD but also patients with cystic fibrosis.[47]

Our knowledge of ventilatory response to arm exercise was based on arm cycle ergometry. It is known that at a given work load in normal subjects, arm cranking is more demanding than leg cycling, as shown by higher VO_2, minute ventilation (V_E), heart rate, blood pressure, and lactate production.[48–51] At maximal effort, however, VO_2, V_E, cardiac output, and lactate levels are lower during arm than leg cycle ergometry.[48–52] Little is known about the metabolic and ventilatory cost of simple arm elevation. Some recent reports underscore the importance of arm position in ventilation. Banzett et al.[53] showed that arms bracing increases the capacity to sustain maximal ventilation compared with lifting the elbows from the braced position. Others have shown a decrease in the maximum attainable work load and increases in oxygen uptake and ventilation at any given work load when normal subjects exercised with their arms elevated.[54,55] We evaluated the metabolic and respiratory consequence of simple arm elevation in patients with COPD.[56] Elevation of the arms to 90° in front of them results in a significant increase in VO_2 and VCO_2. Concomitant increases occurred in heart rate and V_E. When ventilatory muscle recruitment patterns were evaluated with the use of continuous recording of gastric pressure and pleural pressure, the contribution to ventilation by the different muscle groups shifted, toward increased diaphragmatic and abdominal muscle use. The observations suggest that if we trained the arms to perform more work or if we decreased the ventilatory requirement for the same work, we should improve the patient's capacity to perform arm activity.

Effect of Arm and Leg Training

Several studies have used both arm and leg training and have shown that the addition of arm training results in improved performance and that the improved performance is for the most part task specific. In their study, Belman and Kendregan[3] showed a significant increase in arm exercise endurance after exercise training. Lake et al.,[57] randomized patients to arm exercise, leg exercise, and arm and leg exercise. There were increases for arm ergometry in the arm group and for leg ergometry in the leg group, and increased improvement in sensation of well-being when both exercises were combined. Ries et al.,[58] studied the effect of two forms of arm exercise, gravity resistance and modified proprioceptive neuromuscular facilitation, and compared them with no arm exercise in a group of 45 patients with COPD who were involved in a comprehensive, multidisciplinary pulmonary rehabilitation program. Although only 20 patients completed the program, they showed improved performance on tests that were specific for the training. The patients reported a decrease in fatigue in all tests performed. It is worth pointing out that in the study by Keens et al.[15] a group of patients with cystic fibrosis underwent upper extremity training consisting of swimming and canoeing for 1.5 hours daily. At the end of 6 weeks, upper extremity endurance increased but, most important, maximal sustainable ventilatory capacity had an increase similar to that obtained with ventilatory muscle training. This suggests that ventilatory muscles could be trained by using an arm exercise training program.

Because simple arm elevation results in a significant increase in V_E, VO_2, and VCO_2, we studied 14 patients with COPD before and after 8 weeks of 3 times weekly, 20-minute sessions of unsupported arm and leg exercise as part of a comprehensive rehabilitation program to test whether arm training decreases ventilatory requirement for arm activity.[59] A 35% decrease in the rise of VO_2 and VCO_2 was brought about by arm elevation (Fig. 10-5). This was associated with a significant decrease in V_E. Because the patients also trained their legs, we could not conclude that the improvement was caused by the arm exercise. To answer this question, we have recently completed a study of 25 patients with COPD who were randomized to either unsupported arm training (11 patients) or resistance breathing training (14 patients). After 24 sessions, arm endurance increased only for the unsupported arm training group and not for the resistance breathing training group. Interestingly, maximal inspiratory pressure increased significantly for both groups, indicating that by training the arms we could be inducing ventilatory muscle training for those muscles of the rib cage that hinge on the shoulder girdle.[60]

Practical Training of the Upper Extremity

Based on the information available, arm exercise has been recommended as an essential component of pulmonary rehabilitation programs.[61,62] As seen in Boxes 10-2 and 10-3 the methods for supported and unsupported arm vary in their implementation. Arm ergometry is performed for 20 minutes per session. We start at 60% of the maximal work achieved in the exercise test. The work is increased weekly as tolerated. Dyspnea and heart

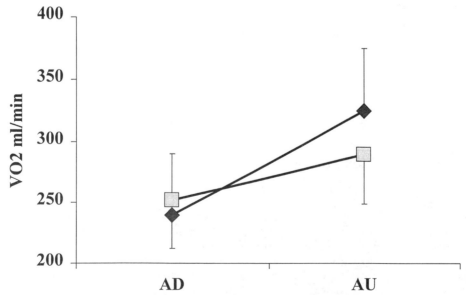

Figure 10-5. The oxygen uptake (VO_2) in 18 COPD patients with the arms down (AD) before rehabilitation (dark triangles). The VO_2 increases from baseline during arm elevation (AU). After arm training (light squares), the increase in VO_2 during AU is significantly lower than before.

Table 10-2. Controlled Studies of Arm Exercise in Patients With COPD

Study	No. of Patients	Duration	Course (wk)	Type	Results
Keens et al.[15]	7 Arms	1.5 h daily	4	Swimming/canoeing	↑VMT (56%)
	4 VMT	15 min daily	4	VMT	↑VME (52%)
	4 Controls	—	—	VMT	↑VME (22%)
Belman and Kendregan[3]	8 Arms	20 min 4× per wk	6	Arm Ergometry	↑ Arm cycle No ↑ PFT
	7 Legs	20 min 4× per wk	6	Cycle Ergometry	↑Leg cycle No ↑ PFT
Lake et al.[57]	6 Arms	1 h 3× per wk	8	Several types	No change PI_{max} VME
	6 Legs	1 h 3× per wk	8	Walking	No change PI_{max} VME
	7 Arms and legs	1 h 3× per wk	8	Combined	No change PI_{max} VME
Ries et al.[58]	8 Gravity resistance arms	15 min daily	6	Low resistance, high repetition	↑ Arm endurance ↓Dyspnea
	9 Neuromuscular facilitation	15 min daily	6	Weight lifts	↑ Arm endurance ↓Dyspnea
	11 Controls	—	6	Walk	No change
Epstein et al.[60]	13 Arms	30 min daily	8	UAE	↓VO_2 and V_E for arm elevation ↑PI_{max}
Martinez et al.[63]	10 VMT	30 min daily	8	VMT	↑PI_{max} and VME
	18 UAE	30 min 3× per wk	10	UAE	↑Work ↓ Isowork VO_2
	17 Ergometry	30 min 3× per wk	10	Arm ergometry	↑Work ↓ Isowork VO_2

COPD, chronic obstructive pulmonary disease; VMT, ventilatory muscle training; VME, ventilatory muscle endurance; PFT, pulmonary function tests; PI_{max}, maximal inspiratory pressure; UAE, unsupported arm exercise; VO_2, peak oxygen uptake; V_E, minute ventilation.

Box 10-2. Training Method for Supported
(Ergometry) Arm Exercise Training

1. Train at 60% of maximal work capacity[a]
2. Increase work every 5th session as tolerated
3. Monitor dyspnea and heart rate
4. Train for as long as tolerated up to 30 min

[a]Work capacity as determined by an exercise test, not
necessarily by evaluating heart rate (see text for discussion).

Box 10-3. Training Method for Unsupported Arm Training

1. Dowl (weight = 750 g)
2. Lift to shoulder level for 2 min; rate equal to breathing rate
3. Rest for 2 min
4. Repeat sequence as tolerated for up to 32 min
5. Monitor dyspnea and heart rate
6. Increase weight (250 g) every 5th session as tolerated

Table 10-3. Work of Breathing, Exercise Endurance,
and Maximal Transdiaphragmatic Pressure Before
and After Pulmonary Rehabilitation

Rehabilitation	Endurance Time (sec)	$\int$ Pesdt (cm $H_2O \cdot min^{-1}$)	Pdi$_{max}$ (cm H_2O)
Before	434	288	48
After	512[a]	219[a]	52

$\int$ Pesdt, work of breathing as estimated by the pressure time index calculated
from continuous recording of endoesophageal pressure; Pdi$_{max}$, maximal transdiaphragmatic pressure.
[a]$P < .05$.

Table 10-4. Evidence Benefits of Exercise Training in Patients With COPD

Type of Training	Outcome	Type of Evidence
Lower extremity	Improves exercise performance, dyspnea, and health-related quality of life	A
Upper extremity	Improves arm exercise endurance, decreases oxygen uptake during arm elevation	B

COPD, chronic obstructive pulmonary disease; A, evidence obtained from large controlled trials; B, evidence obtained from smaller controlled trials.

rate are monitored. Maximal work capacity is defined as the watts that the patient is capable of achieving. If the patient's limiting symptom is dyspnea at minimal work, we exercise him or her at 60% of the work that makes him stop. In the most severe patients, the heart rate is unreliable because they may be tachycardic even at rest and may not show any significant increase with exercise. In these patients, dyspnea may be a more reliable index to follow. In contrast, unsupported arm exercise training is achieved by having the patient lift a dowel (750 g in weight) to shoulder level at the same rhythm as the patient's breathing rate. The sequence is repeated for 2 minutes, with a 2-minute resting period. The exercises are repeated for 30 minutes. Dyspnea and heart rate are monitored. The load is increased by 250 g weekly as tolerated. We aim to complete 24 sessions.

Martinez et al.[63] compared unsupported arm training with arm ergometry training in a randomized clinical trial. Total endurance time improved significantly for both groups, but unsupported arm training decreased oxygen uptake at the same work load compared with arm cranking training. They concluded that arm exercise against gravity may be more effective in training patients for activities that resemble those of daily living.

An increasing body of evidence indicates that upper extremity exercise training results in improved performance for arm activities (Table 10-2). There also is a drop in the ventilatory requirements for similar upper extremity activities. All this should result in an improvement in the capacity of the patients to perform activities of daily living.

CONCLUSION

In summary, exercise training is the most important component in the rehabilitation of patients with obstructive airway disease. Table 10-3 shows the recommendation provided by the recent American College of Chest Physicians/American Academy of Cardiovascular and Pulmonary Rehabilitation evidence-based guidelines for pulmonary rehabilitation[61] and endorsed by the recent statement on pulmonary rehabilitation by the American Thoracic Society.[62] The benefits of lower and upper extremity exercise are multiple and seem to persist for at least 1 year after an 8- to 12-week program (Table 10-4). Because exercise can be performed by physically able patients regardless of age[64] or disease severity,[5,9] it should be the cornerstone of any program. Future research will clarify the issues of optimal duration and frequency of training so that the benefits last even longer.

REFERENCES

1. Clausen JP, Clausen K, Rasmussen B, et al. Central and peripheral circulatory changes after training of the arms or legs. Am J Physiol 1973; 225:675–682.
2. Davis CT, Sargeant AJ. Effects of training on the physiological responses to one and two legged work. J Appl Physiol 1975;38:377–381.
3. Belman MJ, Kendregan BA. Exercise training fails to increase skeletal muscle enzymes in patients with chronic obstructive pulmonary disease. Am Rev Respir Dis 1981;123:256–261.
4. Siegel W, Blonquist G, Mitchell JH. Effects of a quantitated physical training program on middle-aged sedentary man. Circulation 1970;41:19–29.
5. Niederman MS, Clemente PH, Fein A, et al. Benefits of a multidisciplinary pulmonary rehabilitation program: improvements are independent of lung function. Chest 1991;99:798–804.
6. Clark CJ, Cochrane L, Mackay E. Low intensity peripheral muscle conditioning improves exercise tolerance and breathlessness in COPD. Eur Respir J 1996;9:2590–2596.
7. Mohsenifar Z, Horak D, Brown H, et al. Sensitive indices of improvement in a pulmonary rehabilitation program. Chest 1983;83:189–192.
8. Holle RH, Williams DB, Vandree JC, et al. Increased muscle efficiency and sustained benefits in an outpatient community hospital-based pulmonary rehabilitation program. Chest 1988;94:1161–1168.
9. Zack M, Palange A. Oxygen supplemented exercise of ventilatory and nonventilatory muscles in pulmonary rehabilitation. Chest 1985;88:669–675.
10. Casaburi R, Patessio A, Ioli F, et al. Reductions in exercise lactic acidosis and ventilation as a result of exercise training in patients with obstructive lung disease. Am Rev Respir Dis 1991;143:9–18.
11. ZuWallack RL, Patel K, Reardon JZ, et al. Predictors of improvement in the 12-minute walking distance following a six-week outpatient pul-

monary rehabilitation program. Chest 1991;99: 805–808.

12. Make BJ, Buckolz P. Exercise training in COPD patients improves cardiac function. Am Rev Respir Dis 1991;143:80A.

13. Foglio K, Bianchi L, Brulette G, et al. Long-term effectiveness of pulmonary rehabilitation in patients with chronic airways obstruction. Eur Respir J 1999;13:125–132.

14. Saltin B, Blomquist G, Mitchell JH, et al. Response to exercise after bed rest and training. Circulation 1968;38:1–78.

15. Keens TG, Krastins IR, Wannamaker EM, et al. Ventilatory muscle endurance training in normal subjects and patients with cystic fibrosis. Am Rev Respir Dis 1977;116:853–860.

16. Ries AZ, Kaplan R, Linberg T, et al. Effects of pulmonary rehabilitation on physiologic and psychosocial outcomes in patients with chronic obstructive pulmonary disease. Ann Intern Med 1995;122:823–827.

17. Horowitz MB, Littenberg B, Mahler D. Dyspnea ratings for prescribing exercise intensity in patients with COPD. Chest 1997;109:1169–1175.

18. Mejia R, Ward J, Lentine T, et al. Target dyspnea ratings predict expected oxygen consumption as well as target heart rate values. Am J Respir Crit Care Med 1999;159:1485–1498.

19. Moser KM, Bokinsky GC, Savage RT, et al. Results of comprehensive rehabilitation programs. Arch Intern Med 1980;140:1596–1601.

20. Beaumont A, Cockcroft A, Guz A. A self-paced treadmill walking test for breathless patients. Thorax 1985;40:459–464.

21. Christie D. Physical training in chronic obstructive lung disease. BMJ 1968;2:150–151.

22. Hughes RL, Davidson R. Limitations of exercise reconditioning in COPD. Chest 1983;83:241–249.

23. Paez PN, Phillipson EA, Mosangkay M, et al. The physiologic basis of training patients with emphysema. Am Rev Respir Dis 1967;95:944–953.

24. Cockcroft AE, Saunders MJ, Berry G. Randomized controlled trial of rehabilitation in chronic respiratory disability. Thorax 1981;36:200–203.

25. Sinclair DJ, Ingram CG. Controlled trial of supervised exercise training in chronic bronchitis. BMJ 1980;1:519–521.

26. O'Donnell DE, Webb HA, McGuire MA. Older patients with COPD: benefits of exercise training. Geriatrics 1993;48:59–66.

27. Goldstein RS, Gork EH, Stubing D, et al. Randomized trial of respiratory rehabilitation. Lancet 1994;344:1394–1398.

28. Reardon J, Awad E, Normandin E, et al. The effect of comprehensive outpatient pulmonary rehabilitation on dyspnea. Chest 1994;105:1046–1048.

29. Wykstra PJ, Van Altens R, Kran J, et al. Quality of life in patients with chronic obstructive pulmonary disease improves after rehabilitation in house. Eur Respir J 1994;7:269–274.

30. Strijboz J, Postma D, Van Altena R, et al. A comparison between out-patient hospital-based pulmonary rehabilitation programs and a home-care pulmonary rehabilitation program in patients with COPD. Chest 1996;109:366–372.

31. Wedzicha J, Bestall J, Garrod R, et al. Randomized controlled trial of pulmonary rehabilitation in severe chronic obstructive pulmonary disease patients, stratified with the MRC dyspnea scale. Eur Respir J 1998;12:363–369.

32. Woolf CR, Suero JT. Alterations in lung mechanics and gas exchange following training in chronic obstructive lung disease. Chest 1969;55:37–44.

33. Maltais F, Simard A, Simard J, et al. Oxidative capacity of the skeletal muscle and lactic acid kinetics during exercise in normal subjects and in patients with COPD. Am J Respir Crit Care Med 1995;153:288–293.

34. Maltais F, Leblanc P, Simard C, et al. Skeletal muscle adaptation to endurance training in patients with chronic obstructive pulmonary disease. Am J Respir Crit Care Med 1996;154:442–447.

35. Casaburi R, Porszarz J, Burns M, et al. Physiologic benefits of exercise training in rehabilitation of patients with severe training in rehabilitation of patients with severe chronic obstructive pulmonary disease. Am J Respir Crit Care Med 1997; 155:1541–1551.

36. McGavin CR, Gupta SP, McHardy GJ. Twelve minute walking test for assessing disability in chronic bronchitis. BMJ 1976;1:822–823.

37. Gerardi D, Lovett L, Benoit-Connors J, et al. Variables related to increased mortality following outpatient pulmonary rehabilitation. Eur Respir J 1996;9:431–435.

38. Pinto-Plata V, Girish M. Taylor J, et al. Natural decline in the six minute walking distance (6MWD) in COPD. Am J Respir Crit Care Med 1998;157:20A.

39. Singh S, Morgan M, Hardman A, et al. Comparison of oxygen uptake during a conventional treadmill test and the shuttle walking test in chronic airflow limitation. Eur Respir J 1994;7:2016–2020.

40. Pollock M, Roa J, Benditt J, et al. Stair climbing (SC) predicts maximal oxygen uptake in patients with chronic airflow obstruction. Chest 1993; 104:1378–1383.

41. O'Hara WJ, Lasachuk BP, Matheson P, et al. Weight training and backpacking in chronic obstructive pulmonary disease. Respir Care 1984; 29:1202–1210.

42. Martinez FJ, Couser J, Celli BR. Factors influencing ventilatory muscle recruitment in patients with chronic airflow obstruction. Am Rev Respir Dis 1990;142:276–282.

43. Tangri S, Woolf CR. The breathing pattern in chronic obstructive lung disease, during the performance of some common daily activities. Chest 1973;63:126–127.

44. Celli BR, Rassulo J, Make B. Dyssynchronous breathing associated with arm but not leg exercise in patients with COPD. N Engl J Med 1968; 314:1485–1490.

45. Celli BR, Criner GJ, Rassulo J. Ventilatory muscle recruitment during unsupported arm exercise in normal subjects. J Appl Physiol 1988;64:1936–1941.

46. Criner GJ, Celli BR. Effect of unsupported arm

exercise on ventilatory muscle recruitment in patients with severe chronic airflow obstruction. Am Rev Respir Dis 1988;138:856–867.

47. Alison J, Regnis J, Donnelly P, et al. End expiratory lung volume during arm and leg exercise in normal subjects and patients with cystic fibrosis. Am J Respir Crit Care Med 1998;158:1450–1458.

48. Bobbert AC. Physiological comparison of three types of ergometry. J Appl Physiol 1960;15:1007–1014.

49. Steinberg J, Astrand PO, Ekblom B, et al. Hemodynamic response to work with different muscle groups, sitting and supine. J Appl Physiol 1967;22:61–70.

50. Davis JA, Vodak P, Wilmore JH, et al. Anaerobic threshold and maximal power for three modes of exercise. J Appl Physiol 1976;41:549–550.

51. Reybrouck T, Heigenhouser GF, Faulkner JA. Limitations to maximum oxygen uptake in arm, leg and combined arm-leg ergometry. J Appl Physiol 1975;38:774–779.

52. Martin TW, Zeballos RJ, Weisman IM. Gas exchange during maximal upper extremity exercise. Chest 1991;99:420–425.

53. Banzett R, Topulus G, Leith D, et al. Bracing arms increases the capacity for sustained hyperpnea. Am Rev Respir Dis 1988;138:106–109.

54. Dolmage TE, Maestro L, Avendano M, et al. The ventilatory response to arm elevation of patients with chronic obstructive pulmonary disease. Chest 1993;104:1097–1100.

55. Maestro L, Dolmage T, Avendano MA, et al. Influence of arm position in ventilation during incremental exercise in healthy individuals. Chest 1990;98(2):113(S).

56. Couser J, Martinez F, Celli B. Respiratory response to arm elevation in normal subjects. Chest 1992;101:336–340.

57. Lake FR, Hendersen K, Briffa T, et al. Upper limb and lower limb exercise training in patients with chronic airflow obstruction. Chest 1990;97:1077–1082.

58. Ries AL, Ellis B, Hawkins RW. Upper extremity exercise training in chronic obstructive pulmonary disease. Chest 1988;93:688–692.

59. Couser J, Martinez F, Celli B. Pulmonary rehabilitation that includes arm exercise reduces metabolic and ventilatory requirements for simple arm elevation. Chest 1993;103:37–38.

60. Epstein S, Celli B, Martinez F, et al. Arm training reduces the VO_2 and VE cost of unsupported arm exercise and elevation in chronic obstructive pulmonary disease. J Cardiopulmon Rehabil 1997;17:171–177.

61. Ries A, Carlin B, Carrieri-Colman V, et al. Pulmonary rehabilitation: joint ACCP/AACVPR evidence-based guidelines. Chest 1997;112:1363–1396.

62. Lareau S, ZuWallack R, Carlin B, et al. Pulmonary rehabilitation: American Thoracic Society. Am J Respir Crit Care Med 1999;159:1666–1682.

63. Martinez FJ, Vogel PD, DuPont DN, et al. Supported arm exercise vs. unsupported arm exercise in the rehabilitation of patients with chronic airflow obstruction. Chest 1993;103:1397–2002.

64. Couser J, Guthman R, Abdulgany M, et al. Pulmonary rehabilitation improves exercise capacity in older elderly patients with COPD. Chest 1995;107:730–734.

11 Ventilatory Muscle Training

Donald A. Mahler

Professional Skills

Upon completion of this chapter, the reader will:

- Understand the rationale for ventilatory muscle training (VMT)
- Describe the results of "appropriate" randomized, controlled studies of VMT in patients with chronic obstructive pulmonary disease (COPD)
- Prescribe specific goals or targets for the frequency, intensity, and duration of VMT

INTRODUCTION

In 1976, Leith and Bradley[1] demonstrated that ventilatory muscle strength and endurance could be specifically increased in normal individuals with appropriate VMT. They also proposed that VMT might be useful in three conditions: (*a*) for enhancement of sports performance; (*b*) for persons who must exercise with imposed ventilatory loads, such as respiratory equipment required by firefighters, miners, divers, etc.; and (*c*) for patients with respiratory disease in whom ventilatory loads are increased and/or ventilatory capacity is reduced.[1] Subsequent investigations of VMT have been performed in endurance athletes[2]; in patients with chronic respiratory disease (asthma, cystic fibrosis, and COPD),[3–5] chronic heart failure,[6] chronic cervical spinal cord injury,[7] and muscular dystrophy[8]; before cardiothoracic surgery[9]; and to assist weaning from mechanical ventilatory support.[10]

However, most published studies of VMT have focused on patients with COPD because of the high prevalence and morbidity (dyspnea and reduced functional status) of this condition. Selected studies have demonstrated that patients with COPD have inspiratory muscle weakness.[11,12] Furthermore, weakness of the respiratory muscles may contribute to dyspnea as well as reduced exercise performance.[13,14] Therefore, the *rationale* for VMT in individuals with respiratory disease is that increasing the strength and/or endurance of the respiratory muscles will reduce the severity of dyspnea and improve exercise capacity.

TYPES OF VMT

Skeletal muscles can be trained specifically for strength and endurance. In general, strength training requires high workloads with few repetitions, whereas endurance training incorporates low to moderate workloads with a high number of repetitions. For strength training of the respiratory muscles, a maximal inspiratory effort against an occluded airway can generate near-maximal inspiratory pressures. For endurance training of the respiratory muscles, maximal sustainable ventilation (usually 15 min) can be performed.[15] However, sustained hyperpnea causes hypocapnia, and carbon dioxide needs to be added to the inspired air to maintain *isocapnia* during hyperpnea. This training method requires monitoring of partial pressure of carbon dioxide as well as setting of a specific ventilatory target

165

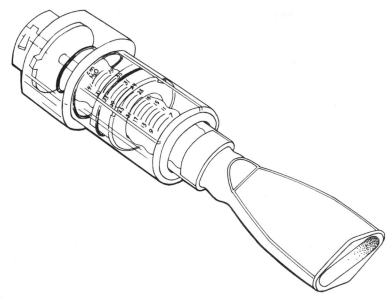

Figure 11-1. A schematic diagram of a targeted inspiratory muscle training device. By adjusting a spring coil, a specific pressure can be set so that the individual must generate a greater inspiratory pressure to open the valve and obtain air flow.

for each individual. Therefore, this approach requires that an experienced technician supervise and monitor an individual's training at a medical facility.

Most published studies of VMT in patients with respiratory disease have incorporated components of both strength and endurance training. For example, an inspiratory resistance system, such as the Threshold IMT (HealthScan; Cedar Grove, NJ) (see Fig. 11-1), can be used as a hand-held device by outpatients at a specific inspiratory pressure target for 15 to 30 minutes per day. Investigators have studied individuals with COPD because this patient population frequently seeks medical attention because of limitation in performing activities of daily living due to breathlessness.

For these reasons, this review will focus on the efficacy of inspiratory resistance training in patients with COPD.

CITED STUDIES

This review was based on information in the American College of Chest Physicians/American Association of Cardiovascular and Pulmonary Rehabilitation evidence-based guidelines published in 1997[5] as well as published studies of inspiratory resistance breathing in patients with COPD identified from a MEDLINE literature search. The following criteria were used to select "appropriate" studies:

- Randomized trial including treatment and control groups
- Use of a resistance or pressure device for VMT
- Use of an adequate training stimulus (i.e., overload principle of training)
- Inclusion of appropriate physiologic (inspiratory muscle strength, exercise capacity, etc.) and clinical (dyspnea ratings, health-related quality of life, etc.) outcomes

Seven randomized controlled trials of VMT were identified that met these criteria[16–22] (Table 11-1). In addition, five studies that examined VMT combined with general exercise training were also considered[23–27] (Table 11-2).

Table 11-1. Randomized Trials of Ventilatory Muscle Training

Study	Patients	Training Program	Outcomes
Pardy et al.[16]	9E	E: 15 min twice a day for 2 mo at an intensity "heralding fatigue"	E: ↑ 12MWD and exercise endurance
	8C	C: general exercise and weight lifting	C: no changes
	Age = 62 y	Duration: 8 wk	
Larson et al.[17]	10E	E: 15 min/d for week 1; 30 min/d thereafter at 30% PI_{max}	E: +9 cm H_2O PI_{max} (25%) ↑12MWD
	12C	C: same except at 15% PI_{max}	C: +5 cm H_2O PI_{max} (14%) No change in 12MWD
	Age = 64 y	Duration: 8 wk	
Harver et al.[18]	10E	E: 15 min twice a day with gradual ↑ in resistance	E: +15 cm H_2O PI_{max} (32%) +3.5 TDI
	9C	C: same except sham training with minimal resistance	C: +5 cm H_2O PI_{max} (12%) +0.3 TDI
	Age = 63 y	Duration 8 wk	
Guyatt et al.[19]	43E	E: 10 min five times a day with resistance ↑ as tolerated	E: +0.1 cm H_2O PI_{max} No change in 6MWD
	39C	C: same except sham training with minimal resistance	C: +0.9 cm H_2O PI_{max} No change in 6MWD
	Age = 66 y	Duration: 12 wk	
Lisboa et al.[20]	10E	E: 15 min twice a day at 30% PI_{max} with load increased as tolerated	E: +20 cm H_2O PI_{max} (31%) +3.8 TDI
	10C	C: same except sham training at 12% PI_{max}	C: +6 cm H_2O PI_{max} (11%) +0.6 TDI
	Age = 70 y	Duration: 5 wk	
Preusser et al.[21]	12E	E: 5 min/session at week 1 to 18 min/session at week 12, three times per week at 52% PI_{max}	E: +11 cm H_2O PI_{max} (35%) ↑12MWD
	10C	C: same except at 22% PI_{max}	C: +5 cm H_2O PI_{max} (12%) ↑12MWD
	Age = 65 y	Duration: 12 wk	
Lisboa et al.[22]	10E	E: 30 min/d at 30% PI_{max} for 6 d/wk	E: +23 cm H_2O PI_{max} (34%) +3.8 TDI; ↑6MWD
	10C	C: same except at 10% PI_{max}	C: +12 cm H_2O PI_{max} (19%) +1.7 TDI; no change in 6MWD
	Age = 62 y	Duration: 10 wk	

E, experimental group; C, control group; 12MWD, 12-minute walking distance; PI_{max}, maximal inspiratory pressure; TDI, Transition Dyspnea Index (measures change from the baseline state); 6MWD, 6-minute walking distance.

Table 11-2. Randomized Trials of Ventilatory Muscle Training *and* Exercise Training

Study	Patients	Training Program	Outcomes
Goldstein et al.[23]	6E	E: 15 min twice a day at a load that could be sustained for 10 min with a target of 20 min, 5 days per week	E: ↑ respiratory muscle endurance but no differences in 6MWD or treadmill endurance
	5C	C: same except sham training	
	Age = 66 y	Duration: 4 wk	
Dekhuijzen et al.[24]	20E	E: target flow with added resistance at 70% PI_{max} held for 3 sec for 15 min twice a day with load ↑ based on response	E: ↑ PI_{max} and ↑ 12MWD compared with exercise group
	20C	C: cycling and walking, but no VMT	
	Age = 59 y	Duration: 10 wk	
Weiner et al.[25]	12E	E: 15 min three times per week at 15% PI_{max} for 1 wk, then 60% PI_{max}	E: ↑ PI_{max} ↑ respiratory muscle endurance and ↑ cycle endurance compared with exercise only and control groups
	12C	C: cycle ergometry and sham VMT	
	12C	C: no VMT or exercise training	
	Age = 65 y	Duration: 6 mo	
Wanke et al.[26]	21E	E: 12 maximal static inspiratory efforts and 10 min at 70% PI_{max} daily	E: ↑ PI_{max} ↑ respiratory muscle endurance and ↑ VO_{2max} compared with exercise group
	21C	C: cycle ergometry 4 d/wk	
	Age = 56 y	Duration: 8 wk	
Berry et al.[27]	25E	E: 15 min twice a day at 15% (2 wk), 30% (2 wk), 60% (2 wk), and 80% (2 wk) of PI_{max} daily	E: ↑ 12MWD compared with control group, but no differences in VO_{2max}, PI_{max}, or treadmill time for the three groups
	9C	C: walking and upper extremity resistance training and sham VMT (15% PI_{max})	
	8C	C: flexibility training and sham VMT (15% PI_{max})	
	Age = 69 y	Duration: 12 wk	

E, experimental group; C, control group (exercise with or without sham ventilatory muscle training [VMT] or other control conditions); 6MWD, 6-minute walking distance; 12MWD, 12-minute walking distance; PI_{max}, maximal inspiratory pressure; VO_{2max}, maximal oxygen consumption.

TRAINING METHODS

The training characteristics of VMT programs have varied considerably:

- Frequency: 3 to 7 days per week
- Intensity: 10% (low) to 52% (high) of maximal inspiratory pressure (Pl_{max}). Although different inspiratory resistance devices have been used, the most commonly used training device in these studies was the Threshold IMT (Fig. 11-1).
- Duration: 5 to 12 weeks. Of the five studies in which VMT was combined with general exercise training (Table 11-2), the duration varied from a 4-week in-patient pulmonary rehabilitation program to a 6-month outpatient program.

OUTCOMES

Respiratory Muscle Function

Of the seven studies listed in Table 11-1, Pl_{max} was measured as an outcome variable in all except the one by Pardy et al.[16] However, in the study by Guyatt et al.,[19] neither the experimental nor the control group exhibited an improvement in respiratory muscle strength; this result indicates that the training load was inadequate. In the remaining five investigations significant increases in Pl_{max} occurred with VMT in the experimental group (Table 11-1). In fact, the studies were remarkably consistent in that Pl_{max} increased by 25%, 31%, 32%, 34%, and 35% in the training groups. To achieve this training response the workload was greater than 30% of the baseline Pl_{max}. The control group in these studies (sham or minimal-resistance "training") experienced increases of 11%, 12%, 12%, 14%, and 19% in Pl_{max}; these small increases are consistent with either learning from repeated testing or a minimal response to a low training load. In further support of the benefits of VMT, Villafranca et al.[28] reported that resistance training led to a significant increase in the maximal power output of the inspiratory muscles and that the resistive load was overcome with a shorter inspiratory time, with no change in tidal volume or total duration of the respiratory cycle.

Dyspnea

Only Harver et al.[18] and Lisboa et al.[20,22] measured breathlessness as an outcome as part of the VMT trials. Patients in the experimental group had significant improvements in the Transition Dyspnea Index of +3.5, +3.8, and +3.8 units (less breathlessness), whereas minimal changes (+0.3, +0.6, and +1.7 units) occurred in the control group of these three studies. Furthermore, the changes in Pl_{max} were correlated significantly with the *changes* in the Transition Dyspnea Index in the training group.[18,20]

Exercise Capacity

The changes in exercise performance were variable with VMT. Although Pardy et al.[16] and Larson et al.[17] demonstrated increases in the 12-minute walking distance after VMT, Guyatt et al.[19] and Preusser[21] showed no difference in the timed walking distance between the experimental and the control groups. However, in the experimental groups with improved Pl_{max}, walking distance also increased.

    In summary, the overall improvements in respiratory muscle function, dyspnea, and exercise capacity support the rationale for VMT.

STUDIES OF VMT COMBINED WITH EXERCISE TRAINING

Five studies examined the efficacy of VMT *combined* with general exercise training (Table 11-2).[23–27] In the study by Goldstein et al.,[23] VMT was part of a 4-week in-patient pulmonary rehabilitation program. The training group achieved an increase in inspiratory muscle endurance but no change in PI_{max} or exercise tolerance. This study was limited by the small sample size (6 patients in the training group and 5 in the control group). In studies from The Netherlands,[24] Israel,[25] and Austria,[26] investigators showed significant improvements in PI_{max} and exercise performance in the VMT plus exercise training group compared with the control group. However, neither dyspnea nor health status was measured in these studies. Berry et al.[27] showed that VMT combined with lower extremity exercise resulted in greater improvements in walking distance compared with a control group, but no differences in PI_{max} or exercise capacity were present compared with a group who only performed exercise training.

In general, these results show that the addition of VMT to standard exercise training can enhance exercise ability. It is possible, but unproved, that VMT plus lower extremity exercise training will also reduce dyspnea and improve health-related quality of life.

RECOMMENDATIONS

Who Is a Candidate for VMT?

Although this is a difficult question to answer, it seems reasonable to consider the following patient characteristics for an individual trial of VMT:

- Severe dyspnea
- Highly motivated
- Reduced respiratory muscle strength (PI_{max})
- Moderate to severe respiratory impairment, but not "end stage," with severe hyperinflation and flattened diaphragm

As an example, the ACCP/AACVPR Pulmonary Rehabilitation Guidelines Panel recommended that "VMT may be considered in individual patients with COPD who remain symptomatic despite optimal therapy."[5]

What Are the Exercise Prescription Guidelines for VMT?

The optimal VMT program has not yet been established.[29] However, studies of VMT (Table 11-1) that demonstrated clinical improvements included components of both strength and endurance training using inspiratory resistive loads. Based on these studies I recommend the following approach to VMT:

- Frequency: at least 5 days per week
- Intensity: greater than 30% PI_{max}
- Duration: 30 minutes per day (continuous or 15 minutes twice a day)
- Training device: a targeted inspiratory resistance system such as the Threshold IMT

The Threshold IMT can be adjusted to select an inspiratory pressure at a specific target (i.e., a percentage of the individual's PI_{max}). Typically, a breathing frequency of 12 to 15 breaths per minute is recommended. An alternative approach (i.e., strength training) is to instruct the individual to perform a certain number of sustained maximal inspiratory efforts (e.g., 20/d). Using this training technique, Redline et al.[30] reported that seven normal individuals increased their PI_{max} from 124 ± 10 to 187 ± 9 cm H_2O in 6 to 18 weeks.

What Outcomes Should Be Measured?

Specific physiologic and clinical outcomes should be measured at baseline and during and at completion of a trial of VMT. For example, inspiratory muscle strength (Pl_{max}) should be monitored because an increase in strength (if high pressures are generated during training) is expected if the training stimulus is adequate. An exercise performance test (e.g., submaximal exercise endurance) may be included as another physiologic measure. Important clinical outcomes such as ratings of dyspnea[31] and health-related quality of life[32] should be measured both to document and to quantify the anticipated benefits of VMT.

REFERENCES

1. Leith DE, Bradley M. Ventilatory muscle strength and endurance training. J Appl Physiol 1976; 41:508–516.
2. Boutellier U. Respiratory muscle fitness and exercise endurance in healthy humans. Med Sci Sports Exerc 1998;30:1169–1172.
3. Weiner P, Azgad Y, Ganam R, et al. Inspiratory muscle training in patients with bronchial asthma. Chest 1992;102:1357–1361.
4. Sawyer EH, Clanton TL. Improved pulmonary function and exercise tolerance with inspiratory muscle conditioning in children with cystic fibrosis. Chest 1993;104:1490–1497.
5. ACCP/AACVPR Pulmonary Rehabilitation Guidelines Panel. Pulmonary rehabilitation: joint ACCP/AACVPR evidence-based guidelines. Chest 1997;112:1363–1396.
6. Cahalin LP, Semigran MJ, Dec GW. Inspiratory muscle training in patients with chronic heart failure awaiting cardiac transplantation: results of a pilot clinical trial. Phys Ther 1997;77:830–838.
7. Rutchik A, Weissman AR, Almenoff PL, et al. Resistive inspiratory muscle training in subjects with chronic cervical spinal cord injury. Arch Phys Rehabil 1998;79:293–297.
8. Wanke T, Toifl K, Merkle M, et al. Inspiratory muscle training in patients with Duchenne muscular dystrophy. Chest 1994;105:475–482.
9. Nomori H, Kobayashi R, Fuyuno G, et al. Preoperative respiratory muscle training: assessment in thoracic surgery patients with special reference to postoperative pulmonary complications. Chest 1994;105:1782–1788.
10. Aldrich TK, Karpet JP, Uhrlass RM, et al. Weaning from mechanical ventilation: adjunctive use of inspiratory muscle resistive training. Crit Care Med 1989;17:143–147.
11. Begin P, Grassino A. Inspiratory muscle dysfunction and chronic hypercapnia in chronic obstructive pulmonary disease. Am Rev Respir Dis 1991;143:905–912.
12. Polkey MI, Kyroussis D, Hamnegard CH, et al. Diaphragm strength in chronic obstructive pulmonary disease. Am J Respir Crit Care Med 1996;154:1310–1317.
13. Killian KJ, Jones NL. Respiratory muscles and dyspnea. Clin Chest Med 1988;9:237–248.
14. O'Donnell DE. Exertional breathlessness in chronic respiratory disease. In: Mahler DA, ed.

Lung Biology in Health and Disease, Vol. III: Dyspnea. New York: Marcel Dekker, 1998: 97–148.
15. Levine S, Weiser P, Gillen J. Evaluation of a ventilatory muscle endurance training program in the rehabilitation of patients with chronic obstructive pulmonary disease. Am Rev Respir Dis 1986; 133:400–406.
16. Pardy RL, Rivington RN, Despas PJ, et al. Inspiratory muscle training compared with physiotherapy in patients with chronic airflow limitation. Am Rev Respir Dis 1981;123:421–425.
17. Larson JL, Kim MJ, Sharp JT, et al. Inspiratory muscle training with a pressure threshold breathing device in patients with chronic obstructive pulmonary disease. Am Rev Respir Dis 1988; 138:689–696.
18. Harver A, Mahler DA, Daubenspeck JA. Targeted inspiratory muscle training improves respiratory muscle function and reduces dyspnea in patients with chronic obstructive pulmonary disease. Ann Intern Med 1989;111:117–124.
19. Guyatt G, Keller J, Singer J, et al. Controlled trial of respiratory muscle training in chronic airflow limitation. Thorax 1992;47:598–602.
20. Lisboa C, Munoz V, Beroiza KT, et al. Inspiratory muscle training in chronic airflow limitation: comparison of two different training loads with a threshold device. Eur Respir J 1994;7:1266–1274.
21. Preusser BA, Winningham ML, Clanton TL. High- vs low-intensity inspiratory muscle interval training in patients with COPD. Chest 1994; 106:110–117.
22. Lisboa C, Villafranca C, Leiva A, et al. Inspiratory muscle training in chronic airflow limitation: effect on exercise performance. Eur Respir J 1997; 10:537–542.
23. Goldstein R, DeRosie J, Long S, et al. Applicability of a threshold loading device for inspiratory muscle testing and training in patients with COPD. Chest 1989;96:564–571.
24. Dekhuijzen PNR, Folgering HTM, van Herwaarden CLA. Target-flow inspiratory muscle training during pulmonary rehabilitation in patients with COPD. Chest 1991;99:128–133.
25. Weiner P, Azgad Y, Ganam R. Inspiratory muscle training combined with general exercise reconditioning in patients with COPD. Chest 1992; 102:1351–1356.
26. Wanke T, Formanek D, Lahrman H, et al. Effects of combined inspiratory and cycle ergometer

training on exercise performance in patients with COPD. Eur Respir J 1994;7:2205–2211.

27. Berry MJ, Adair NE, Sevensky KS, et al. Inspiratory muscle training and whole-body reconditioning in chronic obstructive pulmonary disease. Am J Respir Crit Care Med 1996;153:1812–1816.

28. Villafranca C, Borzone G, Leiva A, et al. Effect of inspiratory muscle training with an intermediate load on inspiratory power output in COPD. Eur Respir J 1998;11:28–33.

29. Belman MJ, Botnick WC, Nathan SD, et al. Ventilatory load characteristics during ventilatory muscle training. Am J Respir Crit Care Med 1994;149:925–929.

30. Redline S, Gottfried SB, Altose MD. Effects of changes in inspiratory muscle strength on the sensation of respiratory force. J Appl Physiol 1991;70:240–245.

31. Mahler DA, Guyatt GH, Jones PW. Clinical measurement of dyspnea. In: Mahler DA, ed. Lung Biology in Health and Disease, Vol. III: Dyspnea. New York: Marcel Dekker, 1998:149–198.

32. Maher DA, Jones PW. Measurement of dyspnea and quality of life in advanced lung disease. Clin Chest Med 1997;18:457–469.

12 Physical Therapy and Respiratory Care: Integration as a Team in Pulmonary Rehabilitation

Rebecca Crouch
Kevin Ryan

Professional Skills

Upon completion of this chapter, the reader will:

- Describe the role of physical therapists (PTs) and respiratory therapists (RTs) in pulmonary rehabilitation
- Describe the evaluation tools used for medical and surgical pulmonary rehabilitation patients
- Define the components of a comprehensive rehabilitation program for pulmonary rehabilitation candidates

INTERDISCIPLINARY APPROACH TO PULMONARY REHABILITATION

The history of PTs and RTs combining efforts to care for pulmonary patients is an interesting journey that closely parallels the beginnings of pulmonary rehabilitation itself. Miss Winifred Linton, an English nurse, initially treated traumatic respiratory complications during World War I. Following the war, she entered physical therapy training and began to teach localized breathing exercises to other PTs and surgeons at The Brompton Hospital. Her work continued through the 1940s and during the Second World War.[1]

A few PTs in the United States were instructed in chest physical therapy techniques and began to use and teach them during the polio epidemic of the 1940s. In the 1960s, the concept of inhalation therapy was developing with the use of artificial airways, positive-pressure ventilators, and supplemental oxygen.

Coinciding with these chest physical therapy and inhalation therapy techniques of the 1960s was the concept of pulmonary rehabilitation. Medical rehabilitation for neurologic and traumatic injuries had been recognized since 1923, when the American College of Radiology and Physiotherapy was founded. In 1937, the American Medical Association recognized the American Congress of Physical Therapy, which continued to foster the concept of rehabilitation. In the 1950s, Dr. Alvan Barach and his colleagues at the Goldwater Memorial Hospital in New York City were using supplemental oxygen, diaphragmatic breathing exercises, and progressive ambulation to treat the large population of patients with chronic lung disease.[2-4]

In the 1970s, RTs (no longer called "inhalation therapists") and PTs began to work together in a coordinated way to deliver pulmonary therapy in acute care settings.[1] The RT would initially treat the lung patient with intermittent positive-pressure breathing followed by the PT performing chest physical therapy, breathing exercises, range of motion (ROM), strengthening exercises, and progressive ambulation. The RT and PT would often work together, administering intermittent positive-pressure breathing in conjunction with breathing exercises, assisting with positioning during chest physical therapy (postural drainage and percussion), teaching the patient bed mobility and sitting for a more effective cough, assisting with sit to stand and transfers from bed to chair, and ultimately teaching progressive ambulation with supplemental oxygen and/or bagging for ventilator-dependent patients.

The advantage of an interdisciplinary team is that it allows each professional to assess, train, and treat the patient in their specialty discipline. RTs may lack the educational background and level of expertise in evaluation and muscle reeducation, chest mobilization, and therapeutic exercise to offer a comprehensive treatment program for the patient with lung disease.[1] Conversely, physical therapy curricula and clinical experiences may not include pulmonary pharmacology, detailed pulmonary evaluation skills (auscultation to assess breath sounds, cough, and sputum production), and diagnostic test interpretation (pulmonary function tests, arterial blood gases, chest radiology, and metabolic gas analysis). The respiratory and physical therapy discrepancies in educational backgrounds highlight mutual needs, areas for cooperation, and overlapping skills. The blending of talents from these two disciplines works extremely well to begin the process of treating, teaching, mobilizing, and rehabilitating the patient with lung disease in acute care and rehabilitation settings.

Team Communication

Although the purpose of this chapter is to outline the unique contributions PTs and RTs make to the pulmonary rehabilitation process, the work of other members of the pulmonary rehabilitation team cannot be ignored. The rehabilitation of pulmonary patients is a collaborative process that may use a variety of health care professionals.[5-8] The ultimate goal is to evaluate and treat individuals disabled by pulmonary disease. These individuals often have complex medical, psychosocial, and physical disabilities. The team goals are to aid the patient in achieving a higher functional level, an improved sense of well-being, and greater independence. These goals are especially challenging and require a group of health care professionals who possess special talents.

Communication and documentation are equally important in pulmonary rehabilitation. In a true "interdisciplinary" team approach, health care professionals from several specialties conduct separate assessments of the patient but through documentation and communication, converge to set goals, plan treatment, and evaluate progress.

The nucleus of the interdisciplinary team is the patient and his or her family.[4,7] The Joint Commission on Accreditation of Health Care Organizations and the Commission of Accreditation of Rehabilitation Facilities have placed the utmost of importance on identifying the goals of the patient as well as the team's short- and long-term goals.[8,9] Objective progress toward those goals must be demonstrated; therefore, team communication, coordination, and documentation are vital.

PATIENT EVALUATION

Diagnostic Tests

Pulmonary Function Tests

Pulmonary function tests provide the key information that defines the diagnostic classification and degree of impairment caused by diseases affecting the lung.[10] The failure of the respiratory system to effectively ventilate sufficient air to support gas exchange and ultimately the metabolic activity of the muscles results in the primary cause of functional limitations in patients with respiratory diseases. Measuring lung function with spirometry, lung volume, and diffusion studies is essential for a clear diagnostic assessment before starting pulmonary rehabilitation.[11] These studies provide the objective data that support the need for pulmonary rehabilitation training. They enable clinicians to define the degree of airway obstruction and to measure response to bronchodilators, amount of lung distention caused by hyperinflation, "lung stiffness" present in restrictive diseases, and gas exchange impairments. Pulmonary function test results provide clinicians with insights into the underlying cause and degree of lung tissue impairment that patients must work against to breathe. Understanding spirometry, lung volume, and diffusion test results is essential to see into the patient's disabling ineffectiveness to breathe at rest and during activity.

Spirometry

Spirometry is the most common and basic screening test for pulmonary disease. Spirometric studies of lung function collect air volume from a maximal inspiration to a complete exhalation (from "full to empty"). Spirometry measures the forced vital capacity (FVC), the forced expiratory volume in 1 second (FEV_1), and allows for calculation of the FEV_1/FVC ratio.[12] The FVC and FEV_1 decline with age and increase with height and are normally greater in men than in woman. Therefore, the percent predicted based on normal values for age, height, and gender provide the measured degree of severity and diagnostically classify patients of having obstructive and/or restrictive disease. For spirometry interpretation see Figure 12-1.

Lung Volumes

The studies of total lung capacity (TLC), residual volume (RV), and functional RV cannot be measured directly with a spirometer. Measured by either body plethysmography or helium dilution, these studies enable the clinician to evaluate the degree of hyperinflation caused by obstructive defects or the degree of "compressed" or stiff lung tissue present in restrictive defects.

The lower limit of the normal range for the TLC is about 80% of predicted—a decrease below this indicates a restrictive process. An increased TLC is classically defined as hyperinflation and is objectively evaluated by the presence of an RV:TLC ratio of greater than 140% of predicted. Air trapping is present when the RV is greater than 110% of predicted.[13]

Together with the chest radiograph, these studies can provide the visual picture and the measurable level of impairment that will help guide the therapist in evaluating the real limitations of chest wall excursion performed during breathing retraining exercises. Severely hyperinflated lungs may demonstrate little lateral or abdominal/diaphragmatic excursion owing to hyperextended chest wall muscles and flattened diaphragms. Instruction in breathing retraining techniques like pursed-lips breathing and gentle, rhythmic exhalation coordinated with activity can improve patients' breathing patterns and exercise tolerance in the presence of chronic lung disease. Restrictive lung tissue may create such a rigid chest wall that little movement is to be expected and the focus on more effective inspiratory efforts are required with therapist-assisted breathing retraining. Lung volume alterations in obstructive and restrictive patterns are illustrated in Figure 12-2.

Diffusion Capacity

The definitive test of the integrity of the alveolar capillary membrane is the measurement for diffusion of carbon monoxide into the blood. Diffusion is the movement of gases along a pressure gradient. Carbon monoxide is used because of its high affinity to hemoglobin and the usually small amounts present in the blood of normal healthy nonsmokers.

Diffusion capacity less than 80% of predicted is abnormal. The diffusion of carbon monoxide is low in emphysema, indicating destruction of alveolar septal walls and capillary beds, which reduces the surface area to effectively participate in gas exchange. In interstitial lung diseases, scarring and fibrotic changes thicken the alveolar wall, inhibiting diffusion of gases into the bloodstream. In pulmonary hypertension, the capillary wall is thickened, leading to deficiencies in gas exchange and resulting in decreased diffusion of carbon monoxide. The diffusion capacity may be normal or for unknown reasons increased in asthma.[10]

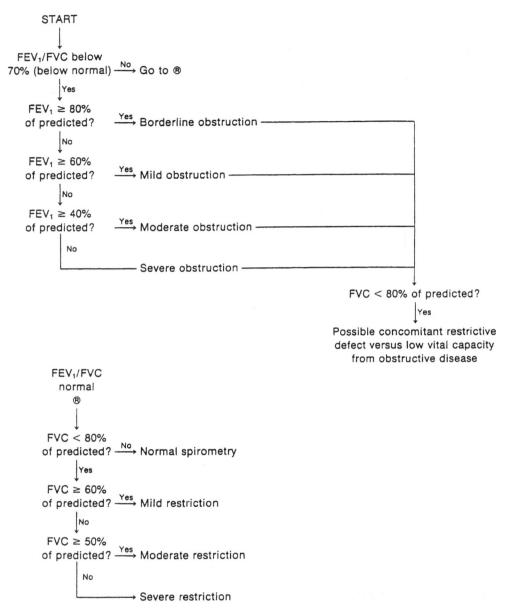

Figure 12-1. Spirometry interpretation. Always start by using the forced expiratory volume in 1 second/forced vital capacity (*FEV₁/FVC*) ratio to determine if obstruction exists. Grade the degree of obstruction using the percent of predicted FEV₁. If the FEV₁/FVC ratio and the FVC are above the lower limit of normal range, spirometry is normal. (Reprinted with permission from Burton GG, Hodgkin JE, Wald JJ, eds. Respiratory Care: a Guide to Clinical Practice. 4th ed. Philadelphia: Lippincott, 1997:230.)

Arterial Blood Gases

The essential diagnostic tool for the assessment of gas exchange to support life is the arterial blood gas. By extracting a blood sample from the artery, the arterial partial pressure of oxygen (PaO_2) and carbon dioxide ($PaCO_2$) are directly measured along with the blood pH. Normal levels of $PaCO_2$ are between 35 and 45 mm Hg. The pH of arterial blood is normally 7.35 to 7.45. Blood oxygen levels are age predicted and decline with age.

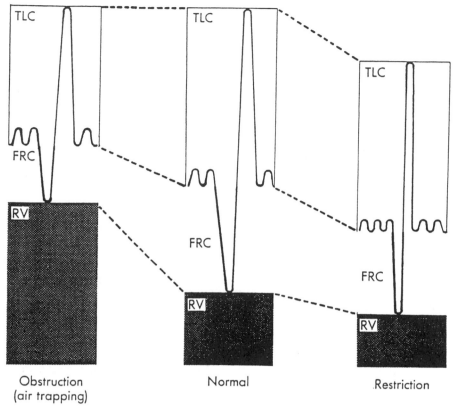

TLC

FRC

RV

TLC

FRC

RV

TLC

FRC

RV

Obstruction
(air trapping)

Normal

Restriction

Figure 12-2. Lung volume alterations in obstructive and restrictive patterns. A comparison of the changes in lung volume compartments in obstruction and restriction shows the following: in obstruction (with air trapping), the functional residual capacity (*FRC*) and residual volume (*RV*) are both increased at the expense of the vital capacity (VC), and hence total lung capacity (*TLC*) remains relatively unchanged; in restrictive patterns the FRC, RV, and VC are all decreased proportionately, resulting in a decrease in TLC. (Reprinted with permission from Roppel G. Manual of Pulmonary Function Testing. 4th ed. St. Louis: CV Mosby, 1986:9.)

Normal PaO_2 may be in the upper 90s at age 20 years and decrease to the mid 60s by age 90 years.[10]

Other values included in the blood gas report are calculated bicarbonate (HCO_3), normal range 22 to 26 meq, and arterial oxygen percent saturation (SaO_2). The SaO_2 can also be directly measured with co-oximetry and is directly proportional to partial pressure of oxygen (PO_2). The oxyhemoglobin dissociation curve in Figure 12-3 illustrates the relationship of PaO_2 to SaO_2. Changes in SaO_2 correlate closely with changes in PaO_2 on the upper, flat aspect of the curve. Drops in PO_2 below 60 result in exponential drops in oxygen saturation by pulse oximeter (SpO_2) and thereby eliminate any effective estimation of PaO_2 with oximetry trending at these low levels.[10]

Interpreting the arterial blood gas is essential in evaluating the pulmonary patient's degree of lung impairment effecting gas exchange and ultimately their acid base status. Arterial blood gas interpretation is necessary to identify acute changes that may need immediate treatment, such as hypercapnia, that may benefit from noninvasive ventilation or chronic changes that require ongoing management, such as hypoxemia requiring supplemental oxygen.

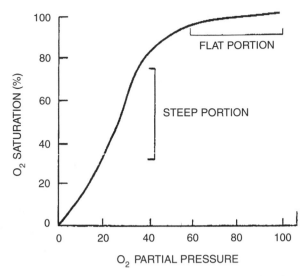

Figure 12-3. Oxyhemoglobin dissociation curve. O_2, oxygen. (Reprinted with permission from Brannon FJ, Foley MW, Starr JA, et al. Pulmonary assessment. In: Cardiopulmonary Rehabilitation: Basic Theory and Application. Philadelphia: FA Davis, 1993.)

Acidosis Versus Alkalosis

First, identify the pH as normal, acidotic (≤ 7.35), or alkolotic (≥ 7.45). Next, determine the cause of the low or high pH. Carbon dioxide will drive the pH down, resulting in respiratory acidosis. Hyperventilation and a low $PaCO_2$ will cause the pH to rise, resulting in respiratory alkalosis. HCO_3 secreted from the kidneys will drive the pH up when it is high (≥ 26 meq), resulting in metabolic alkalosis. Low blood HCO_3 (≤ 22 meq) causes the pH to drop, resulting in metabolic acidosis. A pH of less than 7.30 is a dangerous acidotic condition that usually indicates the need for aggressive acute care measures.

If the pH is normal and the $PaCO_2$ or HCO_3 levels are abnormal, compensation has occurred in blood acid base status. If the patient has chronic hypercarbia ($CO_2 \geq 45$) and the pH is normal, the HCO_3 will be high, creating a normal acid base status in the presence of respiratory failure. This is termed compensated respiratory acidosis. Respiratory muscle rest to provide for effective ventilatory muscle pump function is effective in the long-term management of chronic hypercapnic respiratory failure. Metabolic acidosis seen in diabetic ketoacidosis and chronic HCO_3 loss as a result of diarrhea may be compensated with increased respiratory drive and hyperventilation to lower PCO_2 and balance the pH. Correction of these metabolic deficiencies is essential to alleviating the excessive ventilatory efforts required to maintain normal acid base status.[14]

Hypoxemia

Low blood oxygen levels result in constriction of the pulmonary capillary bed, increased pulmonary artery pressures, right-sided heart failure, cardiac arrhythmia, and eventually death. Hypoxemia also results in impaired cognitive function owing to lack of sufficient oxygen to the brain. Correcting hypoxemia with supplemental oxygen is essential to avoid these untoward effects. PaO_2 less than 55 mm Hg or SaO_2 less than 88% is indication for supplemental oxygen by Medicare and most insurance carriers. Monitoring SpO_2 and trending with exercise, sleep, and rest compared with the measured SaO_2 from blood samples is effective in assessing the patient's needs for specific oxygen prescription flow rates during these activities. Estimating PaO_2 at altitude using nomograms for "educated guesses" or performing a high-altitude simulation test is beneficial in modifying the oxygen prescription for airline flight (estimated at 5000 to 8000 feet altitude) or when patients visit or vacation in mountain elevations.

Graded Exercise Test

One of the primary reasons pulmonary patients seek medical attention is because of shortness of breath with physical exertion.[15,16] This complaint offers a puzzling picture for the physician, who must determine if the cause of dyspnea is of cardiac or pulmonary origin. Although pulmonary function tests are helpful in the determination of airway flow dynamics and ventilatory capacities, they do not provide information about potential ventilatory limitations or cardiac abnormalities during physical exertion. The American College of Sports Medicine[15] cited the following indications to perform exercise testing with pulmonary patients:

- Cause of breathlessness remains unclear despite results from pulmonary function tests
- Patient's severity of breathlessness is disproportionate to objective data
- Both cardiac and respiratory diseases coexist
- Deconditioning, physiologic factors (e.g., anxiety), or obesity are suspected causes for exertional dyspnea
- To evaluate for exercise-induced oxygen desaturation
- Exercise prescription

The pulmonary exercise protocol may use either a cycle ergometer or a treadmill. The advantages and disadvantages of cycle ergometry versus treadmill for exercise testing are listed in Table 12-1. The exercise test protocol should be progressive, with equal stages of speed and grade. Small and short-duration exercise stages are preferable to larger and less frequent increases. Measurements of interest during the pulmonary exercise test include not only the workload (e.g., watts, METS, or kpm/min) but specific cardiovascular

Table 12-1. Advantages and Disadvantages of Bicycle Ergometry and Treadmill for Graded Exercise Testing

Bicycle Ergometry	Treadmill
Advantages	
Simple	Familiar
Inexpensive	Natural movement
Portable	Similar to exercise training
Ease of monitoring vital signs and EKG	Preferred method for obtaining max $\dot{V}O_2$
Eases work of breathing by stabilizing and elevating the chest when propping the arms on the handlebars	
Disadvantages	
Local muscle fatigue (quadriceps)	Expensive
Unaccustomed to riding	Noisy
Lower max $\dot{V}O_2$	Large
Speed dependent	Not easily portable
	Needs electrical source
	Difficult to obtain vital signs and EKG at high intensities

EKG, electrocardiogram; $\dot{V}O_2$, volume of oxygen consumed per minute.

and ventilatory parameters, rate of perceived exertion, and blood gases. Cardiovascular measurements should include the electrocardiogram, blood pressure, and heart rate. Ventilatory measurements are extremely useful in exercise testing of pulmonary patients. It is important to measure expired ventilation per minute, respiratory rate, tidal volume, volume of oxygen consumed per minute, and volume of carbon dioxide per minute. Subjective symptoms may be rated during the test by using a Borg or visual analog scale. The testing protocol should be low level and increase approximately 0.5 METs per stage.[17-19]

Determination of gas exchange can be pertinent information before beginning a pulmonary rehabilitation program. Although arterial blood gases (e.g., PaO_2 and $PaCO_2$) have been standardly measured in the past, noninvasive oximeters are available to detect oxygen desaturation within a ±3 to 5% confidence level. If carbon dioxide retention is suspected, the measurement of arterial blood gases with and without exertion is warranted to accurately make supplemental oxygen adjustments.[15-21]

6-Minute Walk Test

Many clinicians use the 6-minute walk test as a simple evaluation and outcome measurement tool. Specific equipment and instructions must be used when administering the test (Box 12-1). It is helpful to calculate the 6-minute walk speed when prescribing the walking speed for the exercise training sessions (i.e., free walking, treadmill) (Box 12-2).

Physical Therapy Evaluation

The physical therapy evaluation (Figure 12-4) begins with a thorough history that is essential to establishing rapport and to beginning to form a treatment plan for your patient. Comprehensive medical records are often unavailable before the initiation of the pulmonary rehabilitation program; therefore, a verbal account from the patient and/or family is helpful to the therapist. The pulmonary diagnosis and onset followed by a summary of other pertinent medical histories allows the therapist to establish a historical background for the rehabilitation patient's present respiratory and functional difficulties.

The smoking history is asked not only to assess the current smoking status but also to note the presence of smoking in the distant or near past. At this time, the exposure to passive smoking can be queried. The physical therapist should note medications and oxygen use and view the information more in terms of their musculoskeletal and functional ramifications as well as their clinical effects. If the pulmonary rehabilitation patient has been receiving prolonged systemic steroid therapy, he or she is at risk for the development of musculoskeletal complications (e.g., osteoporosis and proximal muscle weakness). The pulmonary rehabilitation history will allow the therapist to evaluate the types of exercises and equipment the patient may already be familiar with and to assess the patient's current exercise habits and capacities.

Assessing the pulmonary rehabilitation participant's psychosocial status and motivation will help the therapist adjust the educational training and treatment approach to a level that is most receptive to the patient. Understanding the family dynamics and enlisting the help and cooperation of family members may enhance the benefits of pulmonary rehabilitation and facilitate the formation of more realistic and achievable goals by the therapist, the patient, and the family. The therapist's goal should *always* be to facilitate the participant's individual level of success and a positive attitude about his or her accomplishments in pulmonary rehabilitation.[7]

The PT's pulmonary assessment should include an evaluation of the breathing pattern. Particular attention to the strength and coordination of the diaphragm muscle is a key component in the PT's evaluation. The use of accessory breathing muscles is prevalent among pulmonary rehabilitation patients and should be noted (Table 12-2). Patterns of holding the breath and pacing of breathing during movement are important to document. In addition, knowledge of and proficiency in using pursed-lips breathing are observed.[21-27]

Box 12-1. 6-Minute Walk Test Equipment and Procedure

Equipment required
  Measured walking distance in hallway or track—the recommended distance is
    100 feet uninterrupted before a turn is required
  Stopwatch
  Pulse oximeter
  Portable oxygen tank
  Nasal cannula, Venturi mask, or nonrebreather mask
  Blood pressure cuff and stethoscope
  Clipboard with a copy of the 10-point Borg scale on the back
  Assist devices—rolling walker, cart, or wheelchair for support if indicated to
    ensure safety
  Chairs positioned along the walkway for rests if needed
Procedure
  Document baseline data, including heart rate, blood pressure, SpO_2, and rate
    of perceived dyspnea (Borg scale)
  Patients should use all prescribed medications prior to performing the test; if
    supplemental oxygen is prescribed for exercise, the patient should begin the
    walk using the prescribed flow rate; the patient should carry or roll the
    portable oxygen tank to evaluate work under real life circumstances
  Assist devices such as rolling walkers, wheeled carts, or wheelchairs can be
    used as support devices; severely dyspneic patients or those who have
    orthopedic limitations or balance difficulties may require the assistance of
    this equipment
  A team member administering the test should instruct the person properly to
    ensure that a best effort is made during the test; written instructions should
    be given to the patient; it is also recommended that the instructions be
    read to the patient when they are ready to begin the walk
Patient instructions
  The 6-minute walk is a timed ambulation test to evaluate your functional
    capacity
  You are to walk back and forth from this point to a marked spot on the floor
    down the hall as many times as you can in 6 min
  You should cover as much ground as you can in 6 min; you should walk as
    fast as you can and as comfortably as you can
  You can rest any time, but the total time you have to cover this distance is 6
    min
  I will let you know when each minute has been completed
  You can speed up and slow down to keep whatever pace you feel is a
    comfortable pace for you to cover as much ground as you can in 6 min
  You should save your breath while walking, so do not carry on a conversation
    while performing the walk or during any rests you take
Documentation included in the test report
  Heart rate, SpO_2, rate of perceived dyspnea while walking; data are recorded
    at the end of each minute as appropriate
  Blood pressure at the completion of the walk before sitting down
  Number of rests and duration of each rest
  Oxygen flow rates used and the intervals at which oxygen flow was adjusted
  Lowest oxygen saturation and liter flow at which it occurred
  Oxygen flow or fraction of inspired oxygen required to keep $SpO_2 > 90\%$
  Assist device used
It is recommended to perform at least two walk tests to allow for a practice test
  and allow at least 10–15 minutes between each test; testing may also be
  performed on different days

Adapted with permission from AACVPR Guidelines for Pulmonary Rehabilitation Programs.
2nd ed. Champaign, IL: Human Kinetics, 1998:58.
SpO_2, oxygen saturation by pulse oximeter.

Box 12-2. Formulas for Calculating Functional Levels From the 6-Minute Walk Test

Average 6-min walk speed

Calculating the average walking speed from the 6-min walk can provide valuable information about gait and stride limitations when considering a target speed for the exercise program (i.e., free walking, treadmill). Using the average 6-min walk speed as a beginning target for exercise training may be a comfortable gait speed for the patient. Further increases in work when using the treadmill may be accomplished by adding elevation and/or speed during the exercise.

$$\text{Speed} = \frac{\text{Total Distance}}{\text{Time}} \times 0.01136$$

Distance is measured in feet
The constant 0.01136 is a conversion factor for turning "feet per minute" into "miles per hour": 60 min/h ÷ 5280 ft/mile = 0.01136
Example:

863 ft, 3 rests of 30 sec each $\dfrac{863}{6} = 143.833 \times 0.01136 = 1.63\,\text{mph}$
Total walking test time is 6:00

In addition to getting a baseline evaluation of a "comfortable speed" for walking on the treadmill, a more important purpose of the 6-minute walk test is its use as a functional evaluation that can be performed at the initiation of rehabilitation and before discharge as an objective outcome measure. Comparing total distance, heart rate, oxygen saturation, and rate of perceived dyspnea can provide a measure of the effectiveness of exercise training on the functional level of the patient.

MET level Calculation

One MET is the level of energy expenditure required at rest, and it has been standardized based on oxygen consumption as 3.5 mL/kg per minute

$$\text{METs} = \frac{(\text{mph})(26.83\,\text{m/min})(0.1\,\text{mL/kg/min}) + 3.5\,\text{mL/kg/min}}{3.5\,\text{mL/kg/min}}$$

Example:
Average 6-min walk speed = 1.63 mph

$$\text{METs} = \frac{(1.63\,\text{mph})(26.83\,\text{m/min})(0.1\,\text{mL/kg/min}) + (3.5\,\text{mL/kg/min})}{3.5\,\text{mL/kg/min}}$$

METs = 2.25
MET levels may be used to evaluate the functional expectations of performing various self-care activities in the home. Calculated MET levels provide target work levels of activity for exercise prescription on equipment other than the treadmill (such as bikes and rowers).

At the same time as the breathing pattern is being assessed, the PT may observe chest mobility. Over time, postural abnormalities are inevitable in chronic pulmonary disease patients. Lung hyperinflation leads to rib cage enlargement or "barrel chest" and diaphragmatic flattening. Joint mobility at the rib attachments to the sternum and vertebrae becomes limited, with a loss in overall rib cage mobility during respiration.

While the therapist is observing the breathing pattern and chest mobility, it is also appropriate to observe other abnormalities such as rib retractions, clubbing of the digits (Figure 12-5), and skin variations such as rashes or calluses over the elbows or feet.

Duke University Medical Center Pulmonary Rehabilitation
Physical Therapy Evaluation

Name:
History #:
MD:
Date:

Diagnosis: Age:

Onset:

Pertinent Medical History (PMH):

Pulmonary Rehabilitation History:

Mental Status:

Social/Family Status:

Medications:

Greatest Difficulties (Rank 3 most difficult):

Goals (Rank 3 most important):

Cough: Smoking History:

Oxygen: Pain:

Auscultation: Edema:

Breathing Pattern:

Range Of Motion (ROM):

Strength:

Posture/Skin/Other:

Foot Evaluation: Overpronator   Normal Pronator   Supinator   Heavy Runner
                 Other:

Assistive devices:

Gait:

PRECAUTIONS: Treatment/Plan:
_____Aspiration   _____Active cycle Breathing
_____Incision   _____PD and percussion
_____Osteoporosis   _____Flutter
_____Hypertension   _____3 Day Trial pulm hygiene
_____Hernia   _____Breathing retraining
_____Musculoskeletal   _____Cough retraining
_____Neurological   _____Postural exercises
_____Cardiac   _____Chair exercises
_____Diabetes   _____Rolling walker
_____Other: _____Ice
                                            _____Hot pack
Problems: _____TENS
1. Retained secretions   _____Individual nutrition consult
2. Ineffective breathing pattern/cough   _____Smoking cessation consult
3. Limited ROM   _____General conditioning
4. Postural deviations   _____Progressive ambulation
5. Decreased mobility   _____Strengthening/Stretching
6. Pain   _____Home exercise program
7. Oxygen desaturation
8. Decreased strength   Short-term Goals:
9. Altered nutritional status   1. _____
10. Smoking   2. _____
11. Altered mental status   3. _____
12. Decreased functional level   4. _____
    (ADLs, self-care)
                                            Long-term Goals:
Special Considerations: 1. _____
_____Use pillows/wedge for floor exercise 2. _____
_____Incisional precautions until _____   3. _____
_____No upper body flexion or rotation   4. _____
_____Give osteoporosis handouts
_____BP daily   Rehabilitation Potential:
_____Abdominal support   Poor   Fair   Good   Excellent
_____Monitor blood glucose
       _____pre _____post exercise

_____ P.T. Date: _____

Figure 12-4. Duke University Medical Center (*DUMC*) Pulmonary Rehabilitation Physical Therapy Evaluation form. *PD*, postural drainage; *TENS*, transcutaneous electrical nerve stimulation; *ADLs*, activities of daily living; *BP*, blood pressure. (Courtesy of the Pulmonary Rehabilitation Program, Duke University Medical Center, Durham, NC.)

Table 12-2. Muscles of Respiration

	Inspiration	Expiration
Normal	Diaphragm External intercostals	Passive process (relaxation of the diaphragm and external intercostals)

Accessory	Sternocleidomastoid
	Scalenes
	Serratus anterior
	Pectoralis major
	Pectoralis minor
	Trapezius (upper, middle, lower)
	Erector spinae
		Internal intercostals
		Abdominal muscles
		    Rectus abdominis
		    Obliquus externus abdominis
		    Transversus abdominis

Upper extremity and trunk observations are best performed with the patient's upper body clothing removed.

Prolonged steroid use may result in Cushing's syndrome (e.g., muscle atrophy, redistribution of fat from the extremities to the face and trunk), extensive bruising, and skin tears. Other side effects the therapist should be aware of with chronic steroid use include the development of osteoporosis, diabetes, behavioral changes, peptic ulcers, and glaucoma.[28]

Assessing the patient's cough history and mechanics as well as auscultating the chest may indicate the need for pulmonary hygiene. Others have reviewed the many qualities of cough and sputum production, as noted in Tables 3 and 4.

The musculoskeletal and functional assessment should begin with a gross manual muscle test of the upper and lower extremities and trunk. The ROM and flexibility evaluation must target key areas such as the shoulders, cervical spine, hamstrings, and

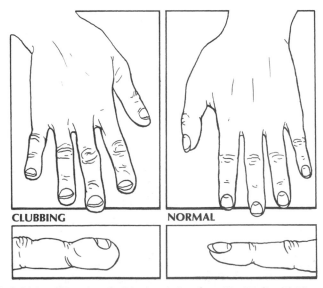

CLUBBING   NORMAL

Figure 12-5. Digital clubbing. (Reprinted with permission from DesJardins T, Tietsort JA. Assessment skills care to practitioner success. In: Burton GG, Hodgkin JE, Ward JJ, eds. Respiratory Care: A Guide to Clinical Practice. 4th ed. Philadelphia: JB Lippincott, 1997:168.)

Table 12-3. Guidelines for Evaluating Cough

Cough Characteristics	Possible Causes
Barking	Epiglottal disease, croup, influenza, laryngotracheal bronchitis
Brassy or hoarse	Laryngitis, laryngeal paralysis, laryngotracheal bronchitis, pressure on recurrent laryngeal nerve, mediastinal tumor, aortic aneurysm, left atrial enlargement
Inspiratory stridor	Tracheal or mainstem bronchial obstruction, croup, epiglottitis
Wheezy	Bronchospasm, asthma, cystic fibrosis, bronchitis
Dry	Viral infections, inhalation of irritant gases, interstitial lung diseases, tumor, pleural effusion, cardiac condition, nervous habit, radiation therapy, chemotherapy
Dry progressing to productive	Atypical and mycoplasmal pneumonia, Legionnaires' disease, pulmonary embolus and edema, lung abscess, asthma, silicosis, emphysema (late in disease), smoking, AIDS, acute bronchitis
Chronic productive	Bronchiectasis, chronic bronchitis, lung abscess, asthma, fungal infections, bacterial pneumonias, tuberculosis
Inadequate	Debility, weakness, oversedation, pain, poor motivation
Paroxysmal	Aspiration, asthma, left-sided heart failure, interstitial pulmonary fibrosis, viral pneumonia
Morning	Chronic bronchitis, smoking
Afternoon and evening	Exposure to irritants during the day
Associated with lying down or position change	Bronchiectasis, left-sided heart failure, chronic postnasal drip or sinusitis, gastroesophageal reflux with aspiration
Associated with eating or drinking	Neuromuscular disease of the upper airway, esophageal problems, aspiration
Violent cough and wheezing associated with eating	Aspiration of foreign body

Data from Fishman AP. Pulmonary Diseases and Disorders, Volume I. New York: McGraw-Hill, 1980; Humberstone N, Tecklin JS. Respiratory evaluation. In: Erwin S, Tecklin JS, eds. Cardiopulmonary Physical Therapy. 3rd ed. St. Louis: Mosby, 1995:338; and Krider SJ. Interviewing and the respiratory history. In: Wilkins RL, Sheldon RL, Krider SJ, eds. Clinical Assessment in Respiratory Care. St. Louis: Mosby, 1990:17.

gastrocnemius. The cervical spine and shoulders lose ROM as a result of poor posture and accessory muscle use. The lower extremity musculature typically loses ROM because of disuse.

Poor posture and pulmonary disease frequently develop simultaneously. The loss of chest wall mobility, assuming propping postures (e.g., professorial position) (Fig. 12-6), and the use of accessory breathing muscles in the cervical and shoulder girdle may lead to abnormal upper body postures. Scoliosis and kyphotic postures are associated with restrictive lung diseases.

All pulmonary rehabilitation patients should be questioned about pain. Fortunately, pulmonary diseases usually are not associated with pain; however, most patients will describe pain from other sources. The older age group diagnosed with chronic obstructive pulmonary disease often experiences pain from musculoskeletal causes (e.g., osteoarthritis of the cervical and lumbosacral spine, knees, hips, and shoulders). Those who have used

Table 12-4. Guidelines for Evaluating Sputum Samples

	Characteristics	Possible Causes
Source	Upper airway	
	Lower airway	
Quantity	Milliliters or cupsful per day	
Color	Red blood streaked or frankly bloody (hemoptysis)	**Pulmonary:** embolism with infarction, pneumonias, bronchiectasis, neoplasm, tuberculosis, abscess, trauma, arteriovenous malformation, aspiration of a foreign body, pulmonary hypertension
		Cardiac: mitral valve disease, pulmonary edema
		Systemic: coagulation disorders, Wegener's granulomatosis, Goodpasture's syndrome, sarcoidosis
		Other: emesis, oropharyngeal bleed rather than true hemoptysis
	Red currant jelly	Klebsiella pneumoniae
	Rust	Pneumococcal pneumonia
	Pink	Pulmonary edema, streptococcal pneumonia, staphylococcal pneumonia
	Frothy white	Asthma, pulmonary edema
	Black or flecked	Smoke or coal dust inhalation
	Apple green, thick	Haemophilus influenzal pneumonia
	Green or yellow, copious	Pus, bronchiectasis (separates into layers), infection, advanced chronic bronchitis, pseudomonas pneumonia
	Sand or small stone	Broncholithiasis, aspiration of foreign material
	Gray	Legionnaires' disease
Consistency	Thin, watery	
	Gritty	
	Layered	
	Frothy	
	Thick, mucoid	Bronchial asthma (small siliconelike casts), Legionnaires' disease, pulmonary tuberculosis, emphysema, neoplasms, early chronic bronchitis
	Mucopurulent (mucus and pus)	All of the above, infection, pneumonias, cystic fibrosis
	Purulent (pus)	
Odor	Foul	Lung abscess, bronchiectasis, anaerobic infections, aspiration

Data from Humberstone N, Tecklin JS. Respiratory evaluation. In: Erwin S, Tecklin JS, eds. Cardiopulmonary Physical Therapy. 3rd ed. St. Louis: Mosby, 1995:338; and Krider SJ. Interviewing and the respiratory history. In: Wilkins RL, Sheldon RL, Krider SJ, eds. Clinical Assessment in Respiratory Care. St. Louis: Mosby, 1990:19.

systemic corticosteroids for prolonged periods and in higher dosages may experience pain from vertebral compression fractures.

A key functional element for all pulmonary patients is the ability to walk. The PT assessment must identify any gait abnormalities and their origin (e.g., musculoskeletal, neurologic, or deconditioning). Several ambulatory assistive devices are now available to help pulmonary patients reinitiate ambulation or raise their ambulatory training to a higher functional level.

Reviewing the objective PT's evaluation will identify problems. Short- and long-term goals should be patient centered, realistic, and measurable. The treatment plan must be individualized and based on all objective test data and observations.

Respiratory Therapy Evaluation

Getting a medical history from the patient along with lists and use of medications is a valuable process and allows the clinician to gain important insights into the patient's knowledge of disease and how he or she manages and copes with it. Using questionnaires and interviewing patients about the information contained in their answers is an effective technique for getting the personal accounts necessary to get a view into patients' day-to-day routines as they manage their chronic lung condition. The initial evaluation is essential

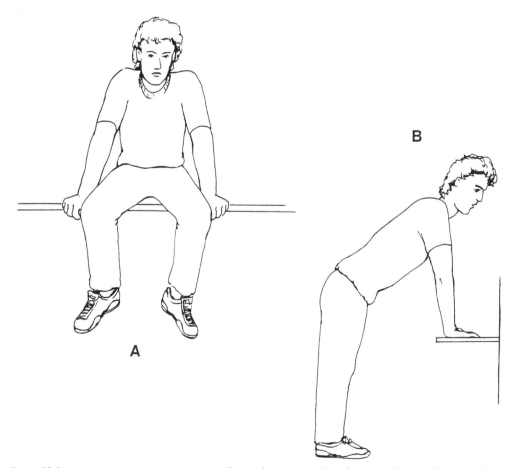

Figure 12-6. Postures that assist inspiratory efforts of patients with pulmonary disease. (Reprinted with permission from Brannon FJ, Foley MW, Starr JA, et al. Pulmonary assessment. In: Cardiopulmonary Rehabilitation: Basic Theory and Application. 2nd ed. Philadelphia: FA Davis, 1993.)

for developing an individualized treatment plan and establishing realistic goals that involve the patient as the most important member of the team.

Building rapport and trust during this time helps set the foundation for the relationship that must exist between the therapist and the patient. The statement "people want to know how much you care before they care how much you know" is more than just a cliché in this situation. It is important to consider the "real" expectations patients bring with them as they hope to be accepted not only into the program as a patient but as a person by the rehabilitation team members.[29] The assessment and interview time allows the rehabilitation staff to project a sense of true and honest regard for the patient's well-being.

Evaluation forms similar to that shown in Figure 12-7 are helpful in organizing this interview information to present findings that justify the skilled intervention of an RT for

---

Primary Diagnosis: _____

Chief Complaints: _____

Medical History:
_____ Cardiac Complications
_____ Hypertension
_____ Diabetes
_____ GI Problems
_____ Reflux/Hiatal Hernia
_____ Orthopedic Problems
_____ PND/Sinus Problems
_____ Vision/hearing
_____ Childhood Illnesses
_____ Other: _____

Past Surgical Hx: _____

Symptoms:
Y   N   Dyspnea
          Onset/Cause _____

Y   N   Cough Frequency _____
Y   N   Sputum
          Freq _____ Volume _____
          Viscosity _____ Color _____
Y   N   Wheezes
          Onset/Cause _____
Y   N   Fluid Retention/Edema
          Where _____ When _____

Y   N   Sleeping Problems # Hrs _____
Y   N   Extra Pillows   # _____

Dyspnea Index (Circle One)

Grade 1: SOB with heavy activity
         climbing stairs or walking up hills

Grade 2: SOB consistently with activity

Grade 3: Can walk at own slow pace but not at
         normal pace without SOB

Grade 4: SOB walking around the house
         dressing, grooming or talking

Allergies:
Food: _____

Medication: _____

Others: _____

Occupation: _____
Retirement/Disability: _____ (date)
Occupational Exposures:
_____ Farm/Ranch   _____ Pottery
_____ Welding   _____ Gases/Fumes
_____ Mines/Quarry   _____ Chemicals
_____ Sand Blasting   _____ Dust
_____ Foundry   _____ Asbestos

Respiratory Infections/Hospitalizations:
_____ Infections per year
          Antibiotic _____ Steroids: _____
_____ Hospitalizations per year
          When: _____
          Problem: _____

Aware of Signs/Symptoms of Infection: _____
Vaccines: Flu _____ Pneumovax _____ (year)

Smoking History:
Y   N   Quit Date: _____
          _____ Packs _____ Years
Y   N   Second Hand Smoke
          Family Member: _____

PHYSICAL EXAMINATION:
Breathing Pattern
Y   N   Pursed Lip Breathing
Y   N   Accessory Muscle use _____

Diaphragmatic/Abdominal Excursion
_____ Excellent _____ Good _____ Fair _____ Poor
Lateral Costal Excursion
_____ Excellent _____ Good _____ Fair _____ Poor

HR _____ B/P _____ SpO$_2$ (Rest) _____
RR _____ Edema _____ SpO$_2$ (PLB) _____
Breath Sounds _____

Figure 12-7. Respiratory Care Evaluation form from the St. Helena Hospital & Health Center Pulmonary Rehabilitation Program. *GI*, gastrointestinal; *PND*, post nasal drainage; *SOB*, shortness of breath; *Hx*, history; *HR*, heart rate; *B/P*, blood pressure; *SpO₂*, oxygen saturation by pulse oximeter; *RR*, respiratory rate; *PLB*, pursed-lips breathing. (Courtesy of the Pulmonary Rehabilitation Department at St. Helena Hospital, Deer Park, CA.)

<u>**Metered Dose Inhalers**</u>

MDI #1 _____

    Prescription: _____

MDI #2 _____

    Prescription: _____

MDI #3 _____

    Prescription: _____

MDI #4 _____

    Prescription: _____

Y   N   Needs Training

Y   N   Needs Spacer

<u>**Oral Medications**</u>

_____   _____

_____   _____

_____   _____

_____   _____

_____   _____

<u>**Stress Management:**</u>

Stressors: _____

          _____

Relaxation: _____

Leisure: _____

Exercise: _____

Aerosol Therapy:

Y   N   Hand-held Nebulizer

Medications: _____

Prescription: _____

Oxygen Therapy   Y   N

Prescription: ____ Rest ____ Sleep ____ Exercise

System: _____

Vendor: _____

<u>Non Invasive Ventilation:</u>   Y   N

System: _____ Vendor: _____

Prescription: _____

Nutrition:

Appetite: _____

Special Diet: _____

Weight Loss/Gain: _____

Salt use/restriction: _____

Vitamins/Supplements: _____

Fluid Intake:

Restrictions   Y   N

____Water   ____Juice   ____Soda

____Coffee   ____Tea   ____Alcohol

Total Fluids per day: _____

<u>**Assessment:**</u>

1. Understanding of Disease/Diagnosis Excellent Good Fair Poor Self Rated (0–10) _____
   One question he/she would like answered: _____
2. Personal goals: Short Term _____
                    Program Goals _____
                    Long Term _____

<u>**Plans:**</u>

1. _____

2. _____

3. _____

4. _____

5. _____

_____   _____

        Staff   Date

Figure 12-7 (*continued*)

pulmonary rehabilitation services and with sharing information with other team members. Asking simple, close-ended questions—such as *When did you first learn you had lung disease? Who told you? What were you told?*[30]—can give a wealth of insight into the diagnosis the patient has received and can provide specific information about his or her knowledge of the condition.

    Addressing the immediate needs of the patient regarding his or her diagnosis can be accomplished with another open-ended question—*If you could have one question answered right now about your lung disease, what would you like to know?* Asking a patient to rate his or her knowledge level on a scale from 0 to 10 is also helpful—*How would you rate your knowledge about your lung disease where 0 is "No Knowledge" and 10 is "I Know Everything About it"?* The answer may give you some insight into how much the person thinks he or she really knows about the lung condition and may want to learn.[31] Other open-ended questions—such as *What can you do to manage your lung disease, control your shortness of breath and make you feel better?*—provide a detailed view of what management skills patients use to minimize their symptoms. Often answers will involve the use of medications, oxygen, or rest techniques and allow the clinician the opportunity to assess the medical appropriateness of their use—whether they tend to be used as "rescue" techniques or "management tools" will be evident from a patient's answers. Supporting patients in the things that they are doing right and assisting them in developing more appropriate management skills are all evaluated in the initial assessment.

Addressing comorbid conditions that patients can recall and any detail they provide is important and can be backed up with hospital discharge summaries and physician office notes. The key issue here is not simply to replicate the medical records but to evaluate the patients' perspective, knowledge, and understanding of their overall condition. Keeping this perspective of the patients' answers in focus during the interview will help guide you in your role as health educator. By learning the manner how your patients (pupils) have interpreted the events over the course of their disease and understanding the perception they have about medical information they have heard or been taught will help you guide them to correct information and skills to help them in the long-term management of their disease.

Continued airway irritants that patients are exposed to are important to document to plan ways to limit additional lung irritation. History of airway exposure from occupational sources, allergy, flu, and pneumonia as well as smoking history provides an objective evaluation of the level of irritation that has led to current disease severity. Plans for eliminating current exposures include help in smoking cessation and strategies to eliminate second-hand smoke to limit further lung damage. Allergy to medications must be noted in the medical record for cases of emergency treatment and as a precautionary issue for recommending changes in prescriptions.

Symptom Assessment

Assessment of dyspnea, cough, sputum, wheezes, edema, fatigue, hemoptysis, postnasal drainage, heart burn, chest pain, swallowing problems, and nocturnal breathing difficulties can be accomplished with simple yes or no questions and asking for explanations of the onset, frequency, and impact these problems have on the patient's daily life. Classification of dyspnea is important documentation that provides quick, "at a glance" information to rate the degree of disability that the patient encounters on a routine basis.[32] Dependent edema with a history of heart disease is an important sign that may indicate the presence of pulmonary congestion and the need for diuretics.

Physical Examination

A physical examination evaluating the objective clinical data of heart rate, blood pressure, respiratory rate, breathing pattern, respiratory accessory muscle use, chest inspection, finger clubbing, edema, and breath sounds provides a baseline to compare with their status during subsequent visits. Evaluating the SaO_2 when at "normal" rest and with pursed-lips breathing is an excellent teaching opportunity on the benefit of this technique and also documents its effectiveness in the medical record.

Observation of the neck and shoulders for excessive accessory muscle use during quiet breathing will provide great insight into the severity of disease and the effect on ventilatory pump effort. Chest excursion, assessed with lateral costal and diaphragmatic/abdominal movement, will provide insights into the possible benefits of proprioceptive breathing retraining. The tactile cues used to elicit movement in the chest and abdominal wall when coordinated with breathing often provide patients with awareness to focus on lower thorax movement that they may lack as they rely on excessive accessory muscle use for the work of breathing. This hands-on technique will also provide the clinician with an assessment of the chest wall motion for symmetry.

Auscultation of the chest allows the quality of air movement within the lungs to be assessed. Listening with a stethoscope over the full area of the thorax overlying the lung tissue while the patient breathes in deeply with an open mouth will provide a full inspiratory and expiratory breath sound assessment. Wheezes indicating bronchoconstriction or airway collapse and crackles indicating excessive mucus, inflammation in the airways are the typical abnormal breath sounds that will be noted in auscultation. Crackles may also be present in fibrotic changes in lung tissue. Fluid in the lungs, as is common in congestive heart failure, will also be heard as high-pitched wheezes or high-pitched crackles. Normal, clear aeration in all lung fields will rarely be found in the patient being evaluated for pulmonary rehabilitation but may be the case with patients who suffer from chest wall deformities or primary pulmonary hypertension. Distant and decreased but clear breath sounds of the hyperinflated lung tissue of the emphysema patient is common.

Auscultation of wheezes and crackles when considered together with a history of symptoms that include a chronic cough with sputum production is a clear indication for an intensive bronchial hygiene regimen, which may include postural drainage therapy, directed cough, and positive airway pressure adjuncts. Excessive wheezing on inspiration and expiration may indicate an ineffective bronchodilator prescription.

Analysis of the patient's complete, prescribed drug regimen is best determined by the "grab bag" method. Be sure to ask patients to bring in all the medications they take (prescribed and over the counter) because this will allow for a comprehensive evaluation of the correct doses and frequency prescribed.[30] Asking the patient to describe the indication and use of each drug is effective for a baseline knowledge assessment regarding their medications. Using a placebo inhaler and asking them to demonstrate their technique will allow for assessment of the patient in the use of metered dose inhalers (MDIs). The method and coordination of the puff during a slow inhalation is necessary for effective use of the MDI. Be sure to ask patients to clarify their interpretation of "as needed," which is often part of the prescribed regimen for quick-acting or "rescue" bronchodilator MDIs.

The final aspect of the assessment will be to document the problems identified and a plan for interventions to address those problems. Getting the input from the patient regarding their needs at this point is essential in establishing a plan that can be accomplished and a therapeutic regimen that has meaning and value for the patient. The plan must address the issues surrounding the chief complaint that the patient arrived seeking help for. Patients usually have vague and ambiguous goals such as "I want to breathe better" and "I want to feel better so I can be healthier." The Personal Goals worksheet (Figure 12-8) can assist the patient in developing specific, measurable, and realistic goals that can be accomplished. This form can guide the patient in establishing short-term, intermediate (by program completion), and long-term goals.

Treatment plans usually involve most or, in some cases, all of the following measurable goals: correct use and adherence to the prescribed medication regimen; oxygen therapy equipment to best support the patient's lifestyle and activity; oxygen prescription with rest, sleep, and exercise; management of symptoms with breathing control; bronchial hygiene therapy; and infection control and reduction of exposure to lung irritants. All of these plans emphasize appropriate use of medical resources. A concept currently accepted as "collaborative self-management" places the responsibility on patients to take a more active role in their care. This concept emphasizes prevention by early intervention by patients through following a course of disease management skills directed by health care professionals.

These goals must be evaluated on an ongoing basis throughout the duration the patient is participating in the pulmonary rehabilitation program. Goals must be measurable and revised as the patient progresses toward achieving the demonstrated skills, which address these problems.

Physician's Evaluation

The therapist will find certain information helpful from the physician to plan an individualized pulmonary rehabilitation program. The medical history is invaluable in gathering information about the patient's pulmonary and nonpulmonary diagnoses. In addition to the medical history, a list of medications will allow the therapist to form ideas and questions

---

PERSONAL GOALS

The Rehabilitation Team has outlined specific goals for you during your Pulmonary Rehabilitation Program. However, we may not be aware of the personal goals you want to accomplish as a result of participating in the program. The following questions will guide you concerning your needs about living with Lung Disease.

1. What aspects of your Lung Disease do you know little about and wish that you knew more?

_____

_____

2. What activities do you enjoy but don't do much anymore because of Shortness of Breath?

_____

_____

3. What places do you enjoy going to but don't visit as much because of your breathing difficulties?

_____

_____

4. What things around the house would you like to do with more ease and less Shortness of Breath?

_____

_____

Based on the answers to the 4 questions above, what personal goals do you want to accomplish during:

A. The first few weeks of your Program?

My Immediate Goal is: _____

B. By the time you complete the Program?

My Short Term Goal is: _____

C. During the first 6 months after you complete the Program?

My Long Term Goal is: _____

_____   _____
Pulmonary Rehabilitation Candidate   Date

Although we cannot guarantee that you will reach these goals as a result of participating in our program, we do promise to help you work toward attaining them whenever possible.

Figure 12-8. Personal Goals worksheet. (Courtesy of the Pulmonary Rehabilitation Department at St. Helena Hospital, Deer Park, CA.)

to ask during the PT's and RT's evaluations. Having a complete and current medical history and a medication list from the physician can save a significant amount of time during the RT's and PT's interviews.

The physician's interpretation of diagnostic tests is beneficial in making plans regarding oxygen needs, medication training, and determination of the patient's status in the course of his or her disease (e.g., mild, moderate, or severe pulmonary disease). The physician may suggest additional diagnostic tests other than the standard tests that are done before beginning the rehabilitation program. Some diagnostics may clarify cardiaclike symptoms, whereas others may warrant adjustments in medication dosages.

The physician's recommended precautions are worthwhile to the therapist. No one wants to overlook a potentially harmful medication, concomitant disease, allergic reaction, or activity restriction and place the patient at risk for injury or exacerbation.

The physician's plan should consider all potential medication alterations, additional diagnostics, outside referrals, and medical options available to improve that patient's disease management. As a primary player on the rehabilitation team, the therapist looks to the physician for input based on his or her medical expertise and experience in the treatment of pulmonary patients at all levels of the disease process. With this information, the therapist can begin to form ideas and plans about the type of program that will be most appropriate for the participant.

EVALUATION PARAMETERS UNIQUE TO THE SURGICAL PULMONARY REHABILITATION PATIENT

Rehabilitating the pulmonary surgical patient can be challenging and exciting. Although many of the rehabilitation principles are the same for medical and surgical pulmonary rehabilitation patients, unique considerations exist for surgical rehabilitation.

Preoperative Goals

Fortunately, most pulmonary patients who require surgical intervention are not hospitalized before surgery. Consequently, this time is a window of opportunity to participate in pulmonary rehabilitation. The therapist must not expect significant central cardiopulmonary changes (i.e., heart and lung physiologic conditioning) in the patient's functional abilities; however, peripheral adaptations are common in this population.[33] Preoperative goals for the pulmonary rehabilitation participant include:

- Maximize function—this includes walking (with or without an assistive device) and the ability to move comfortably around their environment
- Reduce all musculoskeletal impairments to function—improve muscle strength, flexibility, and posture
- Improve the ability to perform the activities of daily living, such as bathing, shaving, dressing, cooking, cleaning, etc.
- Decrease sensitization to dyspnea—help the patient identify the causes of dyspnea and begin to exert greater self-control
- Improve breathing and cough techniques—teach breathing retraining, chest physical therapy, and cough techniques
- Improve activity endurance—increase the participant's ability for *sustained* activity while performing aerobic activities such as walking, bicycling, or arm ergometry
- Optimize medication use—review all medications and check for accurate usage
- Education—therapists have an opportunity to educate the patient and family about their pulmonary disease and review lifestyle changes that may occur after surgery
- Psychosocial support—pulmonary rehabilitation offers a support network for participants and family members who have similar diagnoses and are facing similar life events[34]

Incisions

Therapists must be familiar with the surgical procedures used in lung transplantation and/or lung volume reduction surgery (LVRS). Three types of incisions are commonly used for lung transplantation. For single lung transplantation, a unilateral thoracotomy is preferred. The incision is posterolateral, cutting between the fourth and fifth intercostal spaces. Occasionally, a portion of rib is resected to allow for better access to the lung.

The latissimus dorsi, lower trapezius, intercostals, rhomboids, and serratus anterior muscles are incised, allowing for greater access to remove and replace the lung.[21,35]

For double lung transplantation, the surgeon may use a clamshell incision. This is a horizontal incision above the level of the diaphragm. The pectoralis major and pectoralis minor muscles are incised. Occasionally, the surgeon may choose to use bilateral posterolateral thoracotomies for a double lung transplant. This procedure is usually by surgeon preference or occurs when the viability of both donor lungs is not known simultaneously.

Two types of incisions may be used for LVRS. The median sternotomy is a vertical incision along the sternal midline from the sternal notch distally below the xiphoid process. No muscles are incised and the sternum is closed with stainless steel staples or sutures. A thoracoscopic procedure may be used for LVRS or lung tumor resection. Two to three small incisions are made to allow for the insertion of a thoracoscope. Using the thoracoscope, the surgeon has the ability to visualize as well as resect lung tissue.[35]

Inpatient Postoperative Goals

Within 24 hours of surgery, the PTs and RTs begin acute postoperative treatment. The treatment plan and goals of this period are as follows:

- Aggressive pulmonary hygiene therapy—postural drainage therapy is necessary to mobilize secretions; it is important to consider that below the suture line, the lung is denervated and the patient may not be able to sense secretions that have moved cephaloid
- Review breathing and directed cough techniques—in this patient population, the therapist must think of breathing retraining in a different way; the therapist is actually retraining the diaphragm muscle, which now has a more normal environment in which to work; in the same sense, the rib cage and chest wall may now assume a more typical configuration; these changes, of course, do not happen quickly, but normal patterns of breathing and movement must be encouraged and taught at this early stage
- Maintain joint ROM and muscle strength—the patient will be reluctant to move voluntarily; the upper extremities and chest will be painful and stiff, but progressive ROM and movement must be encouraged
- Initiate self-care and activities of daily living—bed mobility, supine to sit, and sit to stand activities will allow the patient to begin bathing and dressing tasks
- Progressive ambulation and cardiopulmonary conditioning—ambulation within the room or in the hall with or without an assistive device is an essential element of early postoperative rehabilitation; in some cases, a treadmill or stationary bicycle may be moved into the patient's room to facilitate cardiopulmonary endurance training; cardiopulmonary parameters to monitor while conditioning the patient are SaO_2 and the use of supplemental oxygen, heart rate, blood pressure, respiratory rate, and the rate of perceived exertion

Exercise Limitations After Surgery

Following lung transplantation or LVRS, the patient should not lift more than 5 to 10 lb with the upper extremities for 6 to 8 weeks. Other upper body activities to avoid for the same period are trunk twisting, trunk bending, abdominal curl-ups, and arm ergometry. Swim strokes should be avoided for 3 months after surgery. The patient can usually resume driving after 6 weeks, or earlier with their physician's approval.

Outpatient Postoperative Goals

The pulmonary rehabilitation program must adopt a different set of objectives at this point in the rehabilitative process. Many patients describe this period as both exhilarating and frustrating. For the first time in a long while, they can breathe without a struggle.

Breathing is not the primary focus of every movement; however, their body cannot keep up with the level at which their lungs can perform, and nagging musculoskeletal aches and pains in the lower extremities may hamper them. Thus, the challenge for the pulmonary rehabilitation specialist is to gradually teach and guide the patient through an activity program that will achieve his or her highest functional level. The postoperative outpatient objectives are:

- To decrease incisional pain—moist heat, ice, or transcutaneous electrical nerve stimulation may be used for postoperative incisional pain control
- To increase strength and mobility—the level of postoperative strength depends on the preoperative strength and the length of hospitalization; mobility is highly influenced by pain and pain control
- To achieve good breathing and cough techniques—this is a continuation of the training that was initiated before surgery
- To improve stamina—the body must be trained to match the work that the lungs can now perform
- To adjust and titrate oxygen—some postoperative LVRS patients and occasionally lung transplant patients may continue to require oxygen; as the lungs and the body recuperate, the need for supplemental oxygen may be titrated down or possibly eliminated in certain patients; it is an unrealistic expectation to assume that all postsurgical pulmonary patients will no longer require supplemental oxygen either at rest or with exercise
- To assist with adjustments to a new and different lifestyle—it is important for the therapist to understand and help the patient adjust to potential changes in family dynamics, relationships with friends, and societal demands (e.g., return to work, a switch from disabled to "normal"); the patient should be encouraged to adopt a healthy lifestyle that includes a smoke-free environment, regular exercise, and compliance with medication and nutritional regimens[36]

Infection Control

With a postoperative lung transplant population in your rehabilitation program, special consideration must be given to infection control. Simple steps are usually most effective at keeping the spread of bacteria under control. Probably the most effective way to maintain good infection control is by regular hand washing by all of the patients and staff. Many excellent antibacterial soaps are available, and, when needed, the waterless antibacterial soaps are adequate until water is available. Maintaining a 3-foot distance from someone who has an upper respiratory tract infection is advised, especially when coughing is present.

Making clean linens accessible to all staff and participants is prudent. Equipment used by patients with known infections must be isolated and cleaned with an antibacterial solution before other participants use those same pieces of equipment. Examples of types of equipment that may be isolated include oximeters, dumbbells, cuff weights, therabands, timers, exercise mats, stationary bicycles, and others. Masks, gloves, and gowns are occasionally used depending on the circumstances.[37]

Organ Rejection Detection

Pulmonary rehabilitation program staff are excellent resources for recognizing early signs of organ rejection. All staff members must be knowledgeable about these warning signs and be able to distinguish between general complaints of fatigue, soreness, and actual troublesome indicators. A decrease in the FEV_1, shortness of breath, lower SaO_2 levels, and fever may be early signs of rejection that can be identified by the pulmonary rehabilitation staff.[37,38]

PLANNING AN INDIVIDUALIZED PULMONARY REHABILITATION PROGRAM

The team approach to pulmonary rehabilitation brings the expertise of many clinical disciplines to work toward the effective treatment of the whole patient. Understanding multiple needs of the patient justifies the skills of each discipline. As the patient progresses through the diagnostic testing, team evaluation, education training, and therapy sessions, their individual needs are identified and addressed. The patient will receive an accurate diagnosis from the physician. The most appropriate medications to treat their condition will be ordered. The patient should be prescribed the medical regimen that is best suited for his or her condition to address the primary respiratory diagnosis and any comorbid conditions. The patient will receive instruction in the proper use of all medications, including respiratory care interventions of aerosols, bronchial hygiene, and oxygenation to optimize respiratory function. Physical therapy assessments for addressing musculoskeletal and neuromuscular efficiency will be performed to develop exercises aimed at improving strength and endurance for enhancing physical function.[39] Occupational therapy involvement dovetails with physical therapy to identify the limited strength, breathing impairments, or anxiety/panic that impact the routine daily tasks for household and personal care needs. Nutritional services address the individual dietary and weight management issues that can have a significant effect on breathing. Counseling services are justified on an individual basis to deal with psychosocial issues involving the patient and family as well as to assist in long-term coping and end-of-life decisions. Often, home medical equipment and pharmacy personnel are consulted to assist in providing the best equipment or prescription recommendations for a particular patient's individual needs.

These services all provide patients with the well-rounded instruction and training for developing a balanced lifestyle that will help them optimize their lung health and enable them to manage the symptoms of their disease, participate in social activities, and cope with the day-to-day goal of living life to the fullest within the limitations of their condition. The form in Figure 12-9 provides the essential clinical information that can be distributed to each team member and discussed at the initial team meeting. Identification of target areas and goals for each of the areas may include statements similar to those found in Box 12-3.

Optimizing Medications

Optimal medical management for the effective treatment of the patient's lung disease and other comorbid conditions will ensure the best possible progress toward maximal improvements in functional capability. Providing the proper medication regimen available will minimize symptoms through stabilization of airways and maximize cardiopulmonary function to meet the metabolic demands of activity. Selection of an uncomplicated medication regimen with minimal dosing and side effects will promote adherence. Patients are often symptom motivated and will inappropriately use medications as the primary method of dyspnea management. Medications that reduce bronchospasm and airway inflammation as well as promote effective mobilization of secretions will enable the patient to optimize pulmonary function and reduce the debilitating symptoms of shortness of breath and cough.[11] Instruction in the proper use of medications along with proper instruction in breathing control and pacing will minimize overreliance on medications as rescue techniques and enhance their role as management tools for long-term disease control. Effective medical treatment of other conditions that contribute to breathing disorders such as congestive heart failure, gastroesophageal reflux, and postnasal drainage can help alleviate significant causes of respiratory symptoms and improve the patient's ability to function in daily life.

Suggestions for changes in the patient's medical regimen to the referring physician by the rehabilitation team is a common practice and can be made through the medical director or the rehabilitation coordinator. The intensive evaluation and identification of

PULMONARY REHABILITATION
Patient Profile

Name:	Address:	MRN:
Phone:		DOB:
Physician:	Phone:	Soc. Sec #

PAST MEDICAL HISTORY	

PAST SURGICAL HISTORY	

HISTORY PRESENT ILLNESS	

Medications			

Oxygen Prescription: Rest____lpm   Sleep____lpm   Activity_____lpm

Pulmonary Function Tests		
PRE	POST	% Change
FEV1	% Pred	% Pred	
FVC	% Pred	% Pred	
FEV1/ FVC%			
FEF25-75	% Pred	% Pred	
RV	% Pred		

Six Minute Walk Test		
Distance:	METS:	Lowest SpO2____ % on ____lpm O2
Speed:	# Rests:	Primary Limitation:

TEAM MEETING – Follow Up Issues	
PT	
OT	
RT	
Nutrition	
Psych	

Figure 12-9. Pulmonary Rehabilitation Patient Profile form. *MRN*, medical record number; *DOB*, date of birth; *Soc. Sec #*, social security number; *FEV₁*, forced expiratory volume in 1 second; *FVC*, forced vital capacity; *FEF*, forced expiratory flow; *RV*, residual volume; *METS*, metabolic equivalent values; *SpO₂*, oxygen saturation by pulse oximeter; *O₂*, oxygen; *PT*, physical therapist; *OT*, occupational therapist; *RT*, respiratory therapist; *Psych*, (Courtesy of the Pulmonary Rehabilitation Department at St. Helena Hospital, Deer Park, CA.)

Box 12-3. Pulmonary Rehabilitation Action Plan

Target area:	Improper metered dose inhaler use
Goal:	To use a metered dose inhaler properly
Plan:	Train patient in correct metered dose inhaler use and have patient practice correct technique with supervision; if difficulty continues, a spacer will be ordered
Target area:	Assessment of patient's need for oxygen therapy at rest, with exercise, and during sleep
Goal:	To meet the patient's oxygen needs before discharge
Plan:	Review ordered medical test, arterial blood gas, and exercise stress test to determine patient's oxygen needs for home
Target area:	Inadequate understanding of medications
Goal:	To understand medications prescribed
Plan:	Instruct patient on correct use of oral/inhaled medications prescribed, side effects, dosages, and contraindications
Target area:	Patient unsure of signs or symptoms appropriate to report to physician
Goal:	Patient will be able to differentiate between acute flare up of lung disease and ongoing difficulties of chronic lung disease
Plan:	Train patient in signs and symptoms of respiratory infection and how to report them to the physician in a timely manner
Target area:	Decreased knowledge of breathing control with activity
Goal:	To increase knowledge of the principles of breathing application with activity and patient ability to demonstrate application of these principles with activities of daily living
Plan:	Provide instruction and practice in coordinating breathing with activity
Target area:	Activity that causes the most dyspnea is _____
Goal:	To learn dyspnea management measures that will assist in _____
Plan:	Establish a daily exercise program to increase strength and endurance for _____
Target area:	Low exercise tolerance (6-min walk: _____ METs _____ ft distance)
Goal:	To raise exercise tolerance to _____ METs during 6-min walk
Plan:	Establish a safe exercise prescription for low exercise endurance and strength
Target area:	Poor understanding of effects of eating habits on breathing and pulmonary disease
Goal:	To provide information on the dietary needs of the pulmonary patient
Plan:	Instruct the patient on proper nutrition for the chronic obstructive pulmonary disease patient and to participate in the cooking class while in the program
Target area:	Social isolation, withdrawn behavior
Goal:	To be involved socially
Plan:	Explore support system and patient's feelings about self-image; discuss resources available in community and support groups

Adapted with permission from Morris K, Hodgkin JE. Pulmonary Rehabilitation Administration
and Patient Education Manual. Gaithersburg, MD: Aspen, 1996;2.3:7–17.

the patient's needs for day-to-day management of their lung disease enables the team to approach the treatment from a practical point of view that takes into consideration the patients desires for ease of the regimen with the least risk of side effects. Selection of the best drugs available to treat the primary pulmonary problem, other underlying causes of airway irritation, and other cardiopulmonary conditions is the primary goal of enhancing the patient's medical program. See Chapter 7, Pharmacologic Therapy, for detailed descriptions of medications.

Bronchodilators

Inhaled bronchodilators are the mainstay therapy in the management of chronic lung disease. Reduction of bronchoconstriction, by even a small amount, decreases airway resistance significantly and will allow patients to feel less breathless—enough to carry out their daily activities. Providing bronchodilators that maximize this effect will help patients optimize lung function and participate more fully in their activities for household and social roles.

β-Agonists relax bronchial smooth muscle and are also thought to increase cilliary action, thus aiding in mobilization of bronchial secretions. Since the development of this class of drugs in the 1950s, steady progress has resulted in more β_2 (lung)-specific drugs that also have progressively increased their duration of action. Older medications in this class, such as isoetherine (Bronchosol) and metaproterenol (Alupent), have significant side effects similar to epinephrine—increased heart rate, muscle tremors, and sense of anxiety. Their therapeutic effect also is relatively short and lasts for only 3 to 4 hours, resulting in the need for more frequent dosing. Newer medications such as albuterol (Proventil and Ventolin) and salmeterol (Serevent) have been reported to have minimal cardiac stimulation and other systemic sympathetic effects. They also have a much longer duration of action—albuterol up to 6 hours and salmeterol up to 12 hours.[11]

MDIs are a convenient route of administration that has been proven to be just as effective as using nebulized aerosols in the delivery of bronchodilators. They require coordination of the release of the medication from the canister together with a slow deep inhalation and 10-second breath hold. This technique promotes the best deposition of medication to the airways. Dry powder inhaler delivery systems are soon to become the norm. The propellants that activate MDIs have been shown as a chemical family to reduce the ozone layer in our atmosphere and are mandated by the government to be phased out. MDIs and the newer dry powder "puffers" are the delivery method of choice by most patients because of ease of use and convenience. Some patients, however, continue to prefer the nebulizer in promoting improved relief of symptoms. Often the nebulizer is prescribed on discharge from acute care stays, and these treatments can eventually be phased out and replaced with MDIs. Some patients enjoy the longer treatments with the nebulizer.[40] For most patients, the longer treatments, the need for frequent cleaning, sanitizing, and drying the equipment can be inconvenient and they will prefer the easier "quick puff" regimen of the MDI. Patient preference is a good guide to making the proper prescription recommendations.

The anticholinergic class of drugs decreases parasympathetic tone and keeps the airways from constricting. The effect of atropine on the airways has been realized since the early 1900s. An analog of atropine, iprotropium bromide (Atrovent), is available and acts as an airway stabilizer. Acting on a different pathway than the β-agonists, this drug is a compliment to the sympathomimetic medications in maintaining bronchodilation. The effect can last 4 to 6 hours, and dosing four times per day with 2 to 3 puffs is effective therapy.

Theophylline preparations have once again regained status as a mainstay in the management of chronic lung disease. With the previously held notion that a tight therapeutic range closely approaching toxicity (15–20 μg/mL) was required for effectiveness, these drugs fell out of popularity because of the frequent toxic side effect of gastrointestinal tract upset, tremors, anxiety, and loss of sleep reported by most patients. A caffeinelike compound, this drug has now been realized to have a greater benefit in stabilizing airway smooth muscle tone with a blood level less than previously believed to be required. Lower blood concentrations in the 5 to 10 μg/mL range have shown to be effective in promoting the beneficial effects of theophylline.[41]

Patients with frequent attacks of wheezing, chest tightness, and dry cough who show a significant response to bronchodilator by spirometry will usually benefit from a full regimen of medications aimed at relaxing bronchial smooth muscle spasm. Long-acting medications such as salmeterol, together with the anticholinergic effect of iprotropium, will maximize the prolonged relief patients appreciate and will enable them to maintain sufficient ventilation to remain as active as possible. Adding an oral theophylline product with twice- or once-per-day dosing can add additional benefits and provide a complete "bombardment" of the airways to maintain optimal patency. Prescribing a short-acting, quick-relief bronchodilator such as albuterol (if the main therapy is long-acting salmeterol) provides a rescue inhaler for attacks of wheezing, chest tightness, and shortness of breath not relieved with rest and breathing control.

Steroids

Relieving the chronic inflammatory response is now becoming understood as the essential precaution and treatment to minimize, reverse, or eliminate the risk of airway remodeling. Steroid medications address the issue of airway inflammation and may require frequent use to decrease the incidence of the effects of the chronic inflammatory response in the airway. Keeping these drugs to a minimum effective dose is important to control the potential problems of systemic side effects. Reducing oral steroids by prescribing higher doses of the more potent inhaled steroids now available is an important recommendation in the long-term management of hyperreactive airways disease. It is commonly accepted that oral steroids should be kept to less than 10 mg/d. This can be accomplished with the selection of the newer inhaled steroid preparations that have greater potency and effective dose per puff. Fluticasone (Flovent) has a decreasing dose availability. This drug dose can be tapered much the same way as oral prednisone is tapered to lower doses. Budesonide (Pulmicort) is delivered in a fine dry powder method and is potent enough to be used as 2 puffs twice per day. Potential side effects that patients often complain about with the use of inhaled steroids are hoarse throat and "raspy" voice. Steroid inhalers may take 3 to 4 weeks to effect inflammatory responses in the airways. The fact that patients will not experience rapid relief from symptoms and the uncomfortable fear of possible untoward side effects of steroids often causes patients to rely less and less on the use of these very effective medications. Educating patients about the long-term benefits of these inhaled drugs will improve adherence and minimize the need for systemic steroids to keep the airways stable.

Reviewing the medication list and grab bag of medications may in some cases reveal the use of older medications and even inhalers that expired months or even years earlier. Evaluating the patient's symptoms and reviewing pulmonary function tests for response to bronchodilators will guide the selection of the best medical management of airway disease that will include bronchodilator and possibly inhaled steroid therapy.

Oxygen

The complete oxygen prescription provides directives for use with rest, exercise, and sleep. Some patients who are hypoxemic (PaO_2 <55 mm Hg) at rest will require oxygen continuously. They may need adjustments to increase the liter flow for exercise and decrease the flow rate during sleep to maintain SpO_2 greater than 90%. Evaluating oxygenation needs with oximetry during sleep and exercise will enable the proper oxygen prescription to be generated. Getting the best home oxygen and portable system to meet the patient's needs can be a difficult endeavor in light of the current cutbacks in reimbursement for home oxygen by Medicare. Home medical equipment companies are in a modality neutral payment system and prefer to provide the least expensive system to the patient, thereby minimizing expenses in providing this service. Clinically, the best system for the patient will be one that maintains SaO_2 above 90% during all phases of daily life, allows mobility, and is the one the patient is able to operate best with the least amount of manual dexterity and fear.

Evaluating the patient's ability to ambulate with the type of portable system supplied to them is important. Some considerations include the weight of the tank, the ease and ability to maneuver carts, carrying shoulder bags, and transfilling the tanks. Choice of continuous flow or oxygen-conserving device is a required evaluation to best meet the patient's needs. Some conserving devices use a pulsed flow that senses the patient's inspiratory effort and delivers a bolus of oxygen with each breath. Others use a breath-to-breath or every-other-breath delivery based on the liter flow setting. All of the conserving systems eliminate flow of oxygen during the expiratory phase and thereby allow the system to conserve the volume of oxygen released during quiet breathing. This offers the potential to carry oxygen in a small-capacity reservoir and provide longer duration of use for each tank refill. During exercise or other activities requiring increased ventilatory needs, oxygen-conserving devices may not meet the demands for patients' oxygenation needs. Testing the system prescribed during ambulation and with exercise will likely require adjustments in the liter flow to maintain SpO_2 greater than 90%. This is an important assessment that must be done to document the system's ability to meet the patients needs.

Some patients may require mask oxygen during rehabilitation exercise sessions to maintain adequate oxygenation. Using the lowest fraction of inspired oxygen (F_IO_2) to maintain the SpO_2 greater than 90% is the best method of titrating oxygen to the patients needs. Patients with pulmonary fibrosis or primary pulmonary hypertension may even require a non-rebreather mask delivering up to 100% pure oxygen to overcome the gas exchange impairments in their lung.[42] As these patients become more conditioned, muscles become more metabolically efficient and oxygen demand decreases, and this will enable the patient to require less and less supplemental oxygen. Creative use of oxygen equipment may be needed to meet patients' inspiratory F_IO_2 needs. This can often be accomplished by using a Venturi mask at 50% together with a nasal cannula at 1 to 6 lpm. Eventually the F_IO_2 may be able to be decreased. First, decreasing the nasal cannula flow rate to 0 lpm over subsequent exercise sessions would be performed using oximetry monitoring as a guide. Then, decreasing the F_IO_2 on the Venturi mask to the lowest possible level while maintaining adequate oxygenation is the goal.

Designing the Exercise Program

Several physiological principles must be considered when designing the exercise training program.

- For a given workload, upper extremity work demands more energy than lower extremity work and is accompanied by a higher ventilatory demand[43]
- Upper body training is more likely to exacerbate breath holding, an asynchronous breathing pattern, and shortness of breath[44]
- Exercise benefits are muscle and task specific: strength and endurance gains cannot be expected in one muscle group (i.e., upper extremities) from training activities performed by a separate muscle group (i.e., lower extremities)[43,45]

These principles are the foundation for pulmonary rehabilitation exercise training and will ensure a sound and logical program of activity.

There are three basic components to exercise training with pulmonary rehabilitation patients: strength training, flexibility/stretching, and endurance training. Each of these components will be discussed separately.

Strength Training

Strength training programs for pulmonary rehabilitation programs are most effective when they are simple, practical, and widely applicable. Increasing strength and local muscle endurance improves the pulmonary patient's ability to perform functional activities, decreases local muscle fatigue, and enhances body image.[43,46–48] Each strength training regimen must be individually prescribed based on the initial physical therapy evaluation. Using the objective findings of diagnosis, medical history, muscle strength, and joint ROM, a safe and successful strength training program may be initiated with essentially all pulmonary rehabilitation participants. Generally, these programs are received enthusiastically by most individuals.

Many pulmonary patients describe disabling dyspnea with upper extremity activity. Consequently, self-care activities such as bathing, dressing, shaving, and hair grooming and household chores such as lifting pots and pans, lifting clothes from the washer and dryer, and preparing food become exhausting tasks that are dreaded. Several clinical studies have demonstrated that patients with pulmonary disease can train successfully with upper body resistive work, which promotes improved respiratory muscle function, less fatigue, and less dyspnea.[47-49]

Dumbbells, cuff weights, therabands, and weight machines may be used for strength training. The program for upper and lower extremities should begin with light weights and advance first by increasing repetitions. This method of progression facilitates the experience of almost immediate success. It also allows the muscles to adapt gradually to the additional demand while avoiding soreness and injury.

A strength program that begins with weights that feel "challenging but not easy or too difficult" is readily accepted by the patient. Repetitions begin with one set of 10 and progress to one set of 20 repetitions. Once the patient is able to perform 20 repetitions while using the guideline of being challenging on two separate days, the weight is increased by small increments (1 to 5 lb) and the repetitions are dropped back to one set of 10. The same progression pattern is used to gradually increase the repetitions and weight for all muscle groups. As an upper limit, the patient should not exceed their body weight on any strength training machine. If muscle or joint pain is experienced with strength training, the weight is initially dropped. Conservative treatment of the pain is initiated, which may include ice, moist heat, rest, splinting for joint support, elevation, or transcutaneous electrical nerve stimulation. If the pain continues, that particular strengthening exercise is discontinued until the pain and/or inflammation subsides.

Simple strengthening exercises using one's body weight may also be used effectively in a pulmonary rehabilitation program. Examples of these include stair climbing, toe raises, squats, and lunge steps. Exercises to challenge and improve balance and coordination may be used without additional equipment. Examples of balance exercises include standing hip rotation in clockwise and counterclockwise directions; standing unilateral hip hiking; standing unilateral toe pointing to the front, side, and back; and quadruped arm and leg extension.

Flexibility and Stretching

Most patients with chronic pulmonary disease have reduced joint and muscle flexibility primarily caused by inactivity and postural changes. Stretching exercises should be included in all pulmonary rehabilitation activity programs to increase joint ROM, improve muscle flexibility, discourage injuries, improve posture, and decrease stiffness.[50] Among the pulmonary rehabilitation population, specific areas of the body require attention. As a result of prolonged postural abnormalities, the cervical, thoracic, and lumbar spines; shoulders; and rib cage typically present with limited ROM. In the lower extremities, the hamstring and gastrocnemius muscles are often limited in ROM.

These muscles may be stretched in many different ways, but the most effective position for stretching these areas is supine. To assume the supine position, the therapist must instruct the patient in how to get up and down off of the floor, especially when stretching classes are taught in a group setting. Even though this activity may be difficult for the patient who is stiff and deconditioned, it is an extremely beneficial, functional, and important task to master. The only patients who should be excluded from learning this activity are those with severe osteoarthritis of the knees, or other musculoskeletal abnormalities that the PT has determined would absolutely prohibit this task. Osteoporosis, shortness of breath, or oxygen use are *not* contraindications for learning the standing to floor/supine activity.

Other simple pieces of equipment may be used for stretching. An "over the door" pulley system is frequently used for shoulder and rib cage stretching. Pulleys are particularly effective for postoperative chest incision stretching. Wand exercises using a dowel that is approximately 3 feet long may also be used for shoulder and rib cage mobility. An incline board easily accomplishes bilateral stretching of the gastrocnemius/soleus muscles and the Achilles tendons. The stretches should be held continuously for 20 to 30 seconds for three to five repetitions.

Endurance Training

Substantial evidence shows that lower extremity exercise training has both physiologic and psychologic benefit for pulmonary disease patients.[48] The exercise prescription for lower extremity endurance training may be based on the initial graded exercise test, using an initial intensity of 50% of the maximum workload for most rehabilitation participants. Examples of the equipment used for lower extremity endurance training include upright fixed handlebar stationary bicycles, recumbent bicycles, a recumbent stair stepper, and an upright reciprocal moving handlebar bicycle.

Upper extremity endurance training has been found to improve arm function in patients with pulmonary disease.[48] An upright reciprocal moving handlebar bicycle using the arms only, upper body ergometers, a recumbent stair stepper using the arms only, and continuous rhythmic arm movements with or without a wand are examples of upper extremity endurance exercise modalities. An initial workload of 25% of the maximum workload achieved on the exercise test is recommended for upper extremity endurance training.

Ambulation is a necessary mode of training for pulmonary patients because it is the basis of locomotion and is involved in many activities of daily living.[51] Modes of ambulation may include level-surface walking with or without an assistive device and treadmill ambulation. The importance of level surface walking must not be ignored in the pulmonary population. Ambulation training on level surfaces must include rolling or carrying one's own portable oxygen system if needed, propelling one's body over a surface, and supporting the body weight. Although the treadmill simulates these conditions, the total energy expenditure is measurably less. Consequently, it is important that all pulmonary rehabilitation programs include level-surface walking as part of the exercise protocol.

Pulmonary patients with mild or moderate disease may have the ability to expand their exercise regimen by using other types of equipment. Stair steppers, rowing machines, cross-country machines, and swimming offer a strenuous challenge to those patients who require a higher intensity of endurance training.

Paced Breathing With Exercise

With all forms of exercise, the pulmonary patient must be instructed in a paced breathing pattern. The patient should be instructed to inspire at rest and exhale during the more difficult phase of the exercise. The most effective breathing pattern encourages inhalation through the nose and exhalation through pursed lips. If the patient has difficulty and becomes anxious by an inability to accomplish this pattern of breathing, the therapist may instruct the patient to "simply pace the breathing with a comfortable pattern of inhalation and exhalation while performing exercise." All patients should be strongly encouraged *never to hold their breath* with activity. Breath holding is a common response of pulmonary patients to strenuous movement; however, this action only intensifies dyspnea, oxygen hunger, and physical distress.

Patient Training

They may forget what you said, but they will never forget how you made them feel.
Carl W. Buehner

Patient education takes patience. The process of learning can be a tedious work of helping a patient overcome the emotional barriers of fear of failure. Lecturing that simply presents information "at" program participants is not teaching. Education implies that a person is learning and is involved in the process of assimilating the information presented. In pulmonary rehabilitation, all members of the team must constantly maintain their role as health educators during therapy sessions as they interact with patients and family members. Whether in a formal lecture setting in a classroom or coaching a patient through a series of upper extremity exercises in the gym, team members should always be looking for the "teachable moment" when the pupil is ready to learn.[52] Guiding a patient successfully through the process of learning is an experience that neither the pupil nor the teacher forgets. Learning new information, clearing up misconceptions, and putting the new knowledge into practical actions results in a great sense of accomplishment for the teacher and the pupil. Assisting a patient to comprehend in simple terms a complex medical concept can be helpful in alleviating anxieties about the unknown. As one patient stated during his initial evaluation, "Knowledge is my antidote for fear" (Marty Sapp).

Many different situations can be created that will facilitate learning. Lively lectures on a specific health topic may be entertaining but have little impact on making a lasting impression that will be followed through into action. Giving patients and family members only a booklet or brochure about the management of their disease will be ineffective. Education is presenting information so that it can be retained. And it should also focus on *training* in skills that are essential to self-care and management of the disease. Box 12-4 provides common topics addressed in education and training sessions in Pulmonary Rehabilitation.[53]

Providing an interesting **"hook"** in the beginning of a presentation is essential in establishing the need for the information. Asking a thought-provoking question can often be the key to promoting the topic as something worthwhile for the patient to listen and learn, such as "*Why is it important to take all these different Metered Dose Inhalers? Did you know that it is helpful to take them in a specific order to get the most benefit from these medications?*

This type of question can lead to a lively discussion among program participants and lead directly to the formal lesson as found in the **"book,"** reference of an authoritative text (the program educational manual) that gives credibility to the presentation. The text can be used to help clarify or explain misconceptions that the participants have. This initial method of generating interest will get an individual or class in an attitude of readiness to **"look"** at the information and participate in the process of accepting new information and use information in developing a new skill to manage their lung disease.

Box 12-4. Common Topics Addressed in Educational Sessions

Anatomy and physiology of the lung
Pathophysiology of lung disease
Airway management
Breathing training strategies
Energy conservation and work simplification techniques
Medications
Self-management skills
Benefits of exercise and safety guidelines
Oxygen therapy
Environmental irritant avoidance
Respiratory and chest therapy techniques
Symptom management
Psychologic factors—coping, anxiety, panic control
Stress management
End-of-life planning
Smoking cessation
Travel/leisure/sexuality
Nutrition

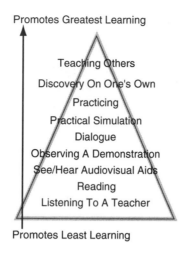

Figure 12-10. The learning pyramid.

Retention of information is the goal of any learning experience. To assess how well the information "took" it is important to ask questions at the conclusion of a lecture to evaluate the effectiveness of the presentation. A short "learning assessment" or test that is self-graded can be a helpful tool to evaluate how well the information presented has been assimilated and learned. Asking for a return demonstration in a one-on-one situation with guidance and cues will help the patient practice the new skill in an environment of encouragement that is nonthreatening.

The **"hook-book-look-took"** process of education is a method of guiding a patient through the often difficult progression of accommodating new information and understanding the essential information they need to develop the knowledge and practical skills of living life to the fullest within the limits of their disease.[54]

Improved retention and adherence to the established treatment plans is the goal of all educational and training methods used in pulmonary rehabilitation. Training to improve adherence can be accomplished through providing only the essential information for the patients and family members to understand the need for performing these skills. Getting feedback on barriers in their day-to-day life that may prevent them from performing the prescribed treatments is important. Counseling the patient and family to develop practical solutions to overcome these barriers will promote adherence to prescribed therapy.[55] The learning pyramid[56] in Figure 12-10 provides a list of activities from least to greatest retention. Asking group participants who have mastered a skill to share their expertise with a fellow member of the group will promote peer motivation and is a teaching method resulting in greatest learning and retention.

Setting Practical Goals and Facilitating Their Achievement

The SMART acronym is a good tool for developing individual patient goals. Goals that are specific, measurable, appropriate, realistic, and timely (SMART) will enable the team members to help patients accomplish effective progress in an efficient manner. Performance of a specific task or skill with decreasing need for tactile or verbal cues is a typical manner in which goals are stated and progress is measured. The skill should be one that is

St. Helena Hospital Pulmonary Rehabilitation
6 Week Program Schedule

	Week #1	MON	WED	FRI
1:00	Group Class	Program Orientation / Breaking the SOB Cycle	NO Group Class / Individual Appointments	How the Lungs Function / Breathing Retraining
2:00	Individual Education	Individual Appointments		Individual Appointments
2:30	Exercise	EXERCISE SESSION	EXERCISE SESSION	EXERCISE SESSION
4:00	Relaxation & Adjourn			

	Week #2	MON	WED	FRI
1:00	Group Class	Medications / Bronchial Hygiene	COPING / With Chronic Lung Disease	Nutrition for Breathing Easy
2:00	Individual Education	Individual Appointments		Individual Appointments
2:30	Exercise	EXERCISE SESSION	EXERCISE SESSION	EXERCISE SESSION
4:00	Relaxation & Adjourn			

	Week #3	MON	WED	FRI
1:00	Group Class	Activities of Daily Living	NO Group Class / Individual Appointments	A Balanced Life - ADLs / Occupational Therapy
2:00	Individual Education	Individual Appointments		Individual Appointments
2:30	Exercise	EXERCISE SESSION	EXERCISE SESSION	EXERCISE SESSION
4:00	Relaxation & Adjourn			

	Week #4	MON	WED	FRI
1:00	Group Class	12:00 Cooking Class / 1:00 Dietician Lecture	What are all these TESTS?	COPING / With Chronic Lung Disease
2:00	Individual Education	Individual Appointments	Individual Appointments	
2:30	Exercise	EXERCISE SESSION	EXERCISE SESSION	EXERCISE SESSION
4:00	Relaxation & Adjourn			

	Week #5	MON	WED	FRI
1:00	Group Class	Stress & Relaxation	COPING / With Chronic Lung Disease	Advanced Directives
2:00	Individual Education	Individual Appointments		
2:30	Exercise	EXERCISE SESSION	EXERCISE SESSION	EXERCISE SESSION
4:00	Relaxation & Adjourn			

	Week #6	MON	WED	FRI
1:00	Group Class	Medical Resources	NO Group Class / Individual Appointments	Home Recommendations / Benefits of Exercise
2:00	Individual Education	Individual Appointments		GRADUATION !
2:30	Exercise	EXERCISE SESSION	EXERCISE SESSION	EXERCISE SESSION
4:00	Relaxation & Adjourn			

Additional Tests			Individual Appointments		
Date	Time		Date	Time	

Figure 12-11. Six-Week Program Schedule for St. Helena Hospital Pulmonary Rehabilitation Department. *SOB*, shortness of breath; *ADLs*, activities of daily living. (Courtesy of the Pulmonary Rehabilitation Department at St. Helena Hospital, Deer Park, CA.)

reasonable and medically necessary and appropriate to the patient's condition. Taking into consideration the patient's level of function will help in developing goals that are attainable and realistic and can be achieved in a time span that is likely to demonstrate progress. The first 2 weeks of patient training in breathing control, use of medications, bronchial hygiene therapy, and exercise skills should demonstrate increasing independence with diminishing need for repeated individual instruction and cues. Nearly total independence in performing these and other techniques as previously listed should be accomplished by the time of discharge.

Many environmental considerations of the facility are essential to successful program participation. Handicapped parking and easy accessibility will ensure that patients will feel accommodated and will encourage attendance at each scheduled session. Ensuring patient comfort and convenience getting into the facility will decrease their frustration and anxiety about the walk to the center and their ability to participate in the therapy once they find their way. A detailed program schedule that lists days, dates, and times for group sessions for education and exercise as well individualized appointments for training will provide participants with a calendar of events showing when attendance is expected. Written instructions explaining exercises and appropriate clothing and footwear will keep the guesswork to a minimum for people who may have last exercised in high school gym class 45 years ago. (See the program schedule in Fig. 12-11.)

Group size is an important consideration in planning a program schedule. Group size may be mandated by third-party reimbursement or by diagnosis category. Too large a group will not allow the individual the attention required for training in the varied skills needed for managing chronic lung disease. A group large enough to promote camaraderie and peer motivation can be accomplished with 4 to 6 people. This group size may be effective for a single therapist and promotes efficiency of resources and allows for individual attention.

FACILITATING A LIFESTYLE CHANGE

Once the pulmonary patient has completed the basic pulmonary rehabilitation program, he or she should be encouraged to maintain and expand on the lifestyle changes that have been initiated. In a healthy population, the physical conditioning effects of an exercise program takes approximately 3 to 6 months. In a pulmonary population that is frequently deconditioned and older, conditioning adaptations may take twice as long.[51] With this fact in mind, the therapist must counsel the pulmonary participant to set gradual, realistic goals for rehabilitation.

It is important that the patient understand that noticeable changes in one's physical abilities and sense of dyspnea will come about in subtle ways after approximately 2 to 4 weeks of rehabilitation. When the therapist has carefully explained this phenomenon, most patients are able to sustain their motivation and effort during those first few grueling, exhausting weeks. The therapist should expect the patient to express feelings of doubt, discouragement, and even anger during this time when immediate gains are not obvious and the participant may be verbally and nonverbally expressing the question, "Is it worth all this effort?" In these situations, the therapist must be prepared to give realistic data and time lines concerning expectations and progress. Simultaneously, the therapist must offer optimistic and positive comments about their progress so far and anecdotes about other patients with similar diagnoses who have had successful outcomes. Ultimately, enlisting the assistance of other rehabilitation participants who have successfully completed the rehabilitation program and have moved beyond it to a true lifestyle change while managing their disease will have a profound impact on the novice rehabilitation participant.

DUKE UNIVERSITY MEDICAL CENTER
PULMONARY REHABILITATION
HOME EXERCISE PROGRAM

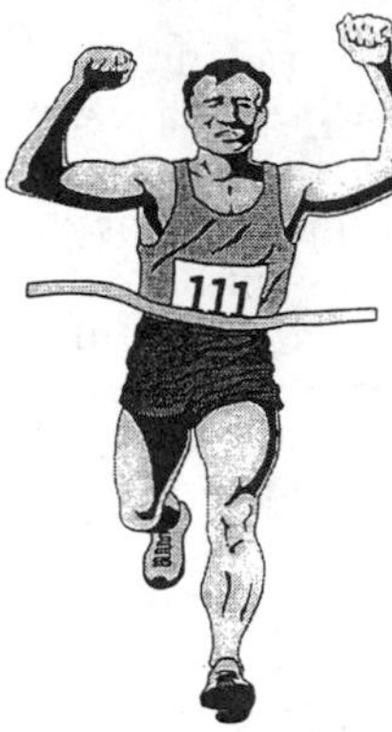

FOR: _____

DATE: _____

FLOOR EXERCISES: Do 4-5 times/week. Gradually increase repetitions to a maximum of 10 then increase weights.
Cuff Weights:_____
Dumbbells:_____
Therabands:_____

WALKING: Make walking a daily activity (5-7 times/week). Keep a record of time and distance for each walk. See the **attached** progressive walking schedule for the next 8 weeks. Use_____LPM oxygen.

STRENGTH TRAINING: If available, use cybex-type strength training equipment 2-3 times/week. Or you may use therabands and free weights to simulate the equipment. Remember to breathe properly---**DON'T HOLD YOUR BREATH!!!!!** Increase your repetitions to 20 then increase the weight.

UPPER BODY: Use an upper body ergometer if available to continue your exercise at a workload of_____.
Perform the exercise for 15 minutes 2-3 times/week. Use_____LPM oxygen.

BICYCLE: Set tension or level at_____. Pedal at 50-60 RPM. Perform a minimum of 15-20 minutes, 3-5 times/week. Your heart rate should be_____ to_____beats/minute. Use_____LPM oxygen.

BREATHING EXERCISES: Do diaphragmatic and pursed lip breathing twice daily for 2 minutes each session.

Figure 12-12. Duke University Medical Center Pulmonary Rehabilitation Home Exercise Program form. (Courtesy of the Pulmonary Rehabilitation Program, Duke University Medical Center, Durham, NC.)

Every participant who completes the basic pulmonary rehabilitation program should leave with an *individualized* home exercise program (see Fig. 12-12). Patients respond best to specific guidelines based on modes, frequency, and duration of exercise achieved in the last few days of the rehabilitation program. The therapist may add a schedule for gradual advancement of the exercises for those highly motivated participants or as a bridge of instruction until a solid maintenance regimen can be established.

Graduation from the basic pulmonary rehabilitation program should be recognized as a significant accomplishment by the staff. A graduation ceremony or party, diplomas, and written and/or verbal acknowledgment among peers are effective ways to celebrate the participant's completion of the program.

Near the conclusion of the program, the staff should provide information and resources regarding continuation of involvement. Maintenance or graduate pulmonary rehabilitation programs and other low-level or nonintimidating exercise programs may be suggested. Members of a maintenance exercise and follow-up program form a close support network for each other and encourage continued activity compliance by organizing telephone trees, holiday parties, travel opportunities, and scholarship fund-raising events. Local better breathers clubs are excellent avenues to "stay in touch" with others who have similar diagnoses. For the pulmonary transplant population, the opportunity exists to participate in athletic events such as the biannual Transplant Olympics sponsored by the National Kidney Foundation.

CONCLUSION

PTs and RTs have a long history of providing care to the pulmonary patient. Because of their educational backgrounds, each has unique approaches to treating these patients; combined, each therapist may complement the other to offer an unparalleled pulmonary rehabilitation program. The process of evaluating the physical and respiratory care needs of medical and surgical pulmonary patients are specific and are used to directly plan the appropriate treatment program in the rehabilitation setting. With thoughtful instruction, compassion, and skill, therapists may navigate the way for a successful lifestyle change among the pulmonary rehabilitation population.

REFERENCES

1. Frownfelter D. Introduction. In: Frownfelter D, ed. Chest Physical Therapy and Pulmonary Rehabilitation: An Interdisciplinary Approach. Chicago: Year Book, 1978:xvii–xx.
2. Barach A. The treatment of pulmonary emphysema in the elderly. J Am Geriatr Soc 1956; 4:884–887.
3. Fishman A. Forward. In: Fishman A, ed. Pulmonary Rehabilitation. New York: Marcel Dekker, 1996:xxv–xxvii.
4. Petty T. Pulmonary rehabilitation: a personal historical perspective. In: Casaburi R, Petty T, eds. Principles and Practice of Pulmonary Rehabilitation. Philadelphia: WB Saunders, 1993:1–8.
5. Ries A, Squier H. The team concept in pulmonary rehabilitation. In: Fishman A, ed. Pulmonary Rehabilitation. New York: Marcel Dekker, 1996: 55–65.
6. Southard D, Cahalin LP, Carlin BW, et al. Clinical competency guidelines for pulmonary rehabilitation professionals: American Association of Cardiovascular and Pulmonary Rehabilitation position statement. J Cardiopulm Rehabil 1995;15: 173–178.
7. Hilling L, Smith J. Pulmonary rehabilitation. In: Irwin S, Tecklin J, eds. Cardiopulmonary Physical Therapy. 3rd ed. St. Louis: Mosby, 1995: 445–470.
8. Program management. In: American Association of Cardiovascular and Pulmonary Rehabilitation: Guidelines for Pulmonary Rehabilitation Programs. 2nd ed. Champaign, IL: Human Kinetics, 1998:113–126.
9. Joint Commission on Accreditation of Healthcare Organizations. Hospital Accreditation Standards and Survey Process: The Advanced Course. 1st ed. Oakbrook Terrace, IL: Department of Education Programs, 1999.
10. Brannon FJ, Foley MW, Starr JA, et al. Pulmonary assessment. In: Cardiopulmonary Rehabilitation Basic Theory and Application. Philadelphia: FA Davis, 1996:253–277.
11. American Thoracic Society Standards for the Di-

agnosis and Care of Patients With Chronic Obstructive Pulmonary Disease (COPD) and Asthma. Am Rev Respir Crit Care Med 1995; 152:S77–S121.

12. Ruppel G. Manual of Pulmonary Function Testing. 4th ed. St. Louis: Mosby, 1986.

13. Enright PL, Hodgkin JE. Pulmonary function tests. In: Burton G, Hodkin JE, Ward JJ, eds. Respiratory Care: A Guide to Clinical Practice. 4th ed. Philadelphia: Lippincott, 1997:225–248.

14. Des Jardins T, Tietsort J. Assessment skills core to practitioner success. In: Burton G, Hodkin JE, Ward JJ, eds. Respiratory Care: A Guide to Clinical Practice. 4th ed. Philadelphia: Lippincott 1997:175–176.

15. Clinical exercise testing. In: American College of Sports Medicine's (ACSM) Guidelines for Exercise Testing and Prescription. 5th ed. Baltimore: Williams and Wilkins, 1995:86–109.

16. Frownfelter D. Exercise tolerance and training for patients with restrictive and obstructive lung disease. In: Hasson S, ed. Clinical Exercise Physiology. St. Louis: Mosby, 1994:85–100.

17. Exercise prescription for special populations. In: American College of Sports Medicine's (ACSM) Guidelines for Exercise Testing and Prescription. 4th ed. Philadelphia: Lea and Febiger, 1991: 161–186.

18. Weiser P, Mahler D, Ryan K, et al. Dyspnea: symptom assessment and management. In: Hodgkin J, Connors G, Bell C, eds. Pulmonary Rehabilitation: Guidelines to Success. 2nd ed. Philadelphia: JB Lippincott, 1993:478–511.

19. Exercise testing and training. In: American Association of Cardiovascular and Pulmonary Rehabilitation: Guidelines for Pulmonary Rehabilitation Programs. 1st ed. Champaign, IL: Human Kinetics, 1993:37–47.

20. Exercise assessment and training. In: American Association of Cardiovascular and Pulmonary Rehabilitation: Guidelines for Pulmonary Rehabilitation Programs. 2nd ed. Champaign, IL: Human Kinetics, 1998:51–69.

21. Watchie J. Cardiopulmonary Physical Therapy. Philadelphia: WB Saunders, 1995.

22. Brannon F, Foley M, Staff J, et al. Cardiopulmonary Rehabilitation: Basic Theory and Application. 2nd ed. Philadelphia: FA Davis, 1993.

23. Hammon L. Review of respiratory anatomy. In: Frownfelter D, ed. Chest Physical Therapy and Pulmonary Rehabilitation. Chicago: Year Book, 1978:3–39.

24. Wolfson M, Shaffer T. Respiratory muscle: physiology, evaluation, and treatment. In: Irwin S, Tecklin T, eds. Cardiopulmonary Physical Therapy. 3rd ed. St. Louis: Mosby, 1995:318–333.

25. Humberstone N. Respiratory assessment. In: Erwin S, Tecklin J, eds. Cardiopulmonary Physical Therapy. St. Louis: Mosby, 1985:208–229.

26. Crane L. Respiratory analysis. In: Scully R, Barnes M, eds. Physical Therapy. Philadelphia: JB Lippincott, 1989:548–586.

27. Hillegass E. Cardiopulmonary assessment. In: Hillegass E, Sadowsky H, eds. Essentials of Cardiopulmonary Physical Therapy. Philadelphia: WB Saunders, 1994:553–595.

28. Prancan A. Respiratory and cardiovascular drug actions. In: Frownfelter D, Dean E, eds. Principles and Practice of Cardiopulmonary Physical Therapy. 3rd ed. St. Louis: Mosby, 1996:775–787.

29. Gibbons M. RRT uses lumberjack background in rehab program. Adv Respir Care Pract 1991; 15:6, 7.

30. Ryan KP. Think rehab. Adv Manage Respir Care 1994;5:27–29.

31. Morris K, Hodgkin JE. Pulmonary Rehabilitation Administration and Patient Education Manual. Gaithersburg, MD: Aspen, 1996;23:7–17.

32. Mahler DA, Harver A. Clinical measurement of dyspnea. In: Mahler DA, ed. Dyspnea. Mount Kesco, NY: Futura, 1990:75–100.

33. Biggar D, Malen J, Trulock E, et al. Pulmonary rehabilitation before and after lung transplantation. In: Casaburi R, Petty T, eds. Principles and Practice of Pulmonary Rehabilitation. Philadelphia: WB Saunders, 1993:459–467.

34. Crouch R, Schein R. Integrating psychosocial services for lung volume reduction and lung transplantation patients into a pulmonary rehabilitation program. J Cardiopulm Rehabil 1997;17: 16–18.

35. Sadowsky H. Thoracic surgical procedures, monitoring, and support equipment. In: Hillegass E, Sadowsky H, eds. Essentials of Cardiopulmonary Physical Therapy. Philadelphia: WB Saunders, 1994:437–477.

36. Goldstein R, Hall M. Pulmonary rehabilitation before and after lung transplantation. In: Fishman A, ed. Pulmonary Rehabilitation. New York: Marcel Dekker, 1996:739–766.

37. Butler B. Physical therapy in heart and lung transplantation. In: Irwin S, Tecklin J, eds. Cardiopulmonary Physical Therapy. 3rd ed. St. Louis: Mosby, 1995:404–422.

38. Otulana B, Higenbottam T, Wallwork J. Causes of exercise limitation after heart-lung transplantation. J Heart Lung Transplant 1992;11:s244.

39. Hilling L, Smith J. Pulmonary Rehabilitation. In: Irwin S, Tecklin JS, eds. Cardiopulmonary Physical Therapy. St. Louis: Mosby, 1995:450–456.

40. Ward JJ, Hess D, Helmholz HF. Humidity and aerosol therapy. In: Burton G, Hodkin JE, Ward JJ, eds. Respiratory Care: A Guide to Clinical Practice. 4th ed. Philadelphia: Lippincott, 1997: 421–468.

41. Ziment I. Drugs used in respiratory care. In: Burton G, Hodkin JE, Ward JJ, eds. Respiratory Care: A Guide to Clinical Practice. 4th ed. Philadelphia: Lippincott, 1997:469–499.

42. Novitch R, Thomas H. Rehabilitation in chronic interstitial disease. In: Fishman, ed. Pulmonary Rehabilitation. New York: Marcel Dekker, 1996: 683–700.

43. American Thoracic Society. Comprehensive outpatient management of COPD. Am J Respir Crit Care Med 1995;152:584.

44. Celli B, Rassulo J, Make B. Dyssynchronous breathing during arm but not leg exercise in patients with chronic airflow obstruction. N Engl J Med 1986;314:1485–1489.

45. General principles of exercise prescription. In: American College of Sports Medicine (ACSM) Guidelines for Exercise Testing and Prescription. 5th ed. Baltimore: Williams and Wilkins, 1995: 153–176.

46. Strauss G, Osher A, Wang C, et al. Variable weight training in cystic fibrosis. Chest 1987;92(2): 273–276.

47. Ries A, Ellis B, Hawkins R. Upper extremity exercise training in chronic obstructive pulmonary disease. Chest 1988;93(4):688–692.

48. Ries A, Carlin BW, Carrieri-Kohlman V, et al. Pulmonary Rehabilitation. Joint ACCP/ AACVPR evidence-based guidelines. Chest 1997;112(5):1363–1396.

49. Lake F, Henderson K, Briffa T, et al. Upper-limb and lower-limb exercise training in patients with chronic airflow obstruction. Chest 1990;97(5): 1077–1082.

50. Barr R. Pulmonary rehabilitation. In: Hillegass E, Sadowsky H, eds. Essentials of Cardiopulmonary Physical Therapy. Philadelphia: WB Saunders, 1994:677–701.

51. Exercise prescription for pulmonary patients. In: American College of Sports Medicine (ACSM) Guidelines for Exercise Testing and Prescription. 5th ed. Baltimore: Williams and Wilkins, 1995: 194–205.

52. Ellers B. Innovations in patient-centered education. In: Gerteis M, Edgman-Levitan S, et al., eds. Through the Patient's Eyes: Understanding and Promoting Patient-Centered Care. San Francisco: Jossey-Bass Publishers, 1993:96–118.

53. American Thoracic Society. Pulmonary Rehabilitation—1999. Am J Respir Crit Care Med 1999;159:1666–1682.

54. Ryan KP. Patient education: special patients for special patients. Presented at the AACVPR Annual Meeting, Baltimore, MD, 1996.

55. Haynes RB, Wang E, Da Mota Gomes M. A critical review of interventions to improve compliance with prescribed medications. Patient Educ Counsel 1987;19:155–166.

56. Coyle J. Training That Works: Asthma Self Management Training Program. Washington, DC: Glaxo Welcome, The Business Communication Group of Washington, DC, 1994.

13 Occupational Therapy to Promote Function and Health-Related Quality of Life

Susan Coppola
Wendy Wood

⊘ Professional Skills

Upon completion of this chapter, the reader will:

- Understand the relationship of occupation and lifestyle redesign to health-related quality of life (HRQL) as the ultimate outcome of occupational therapy in pulmonary rehabilitation
- Understand how therapeutic occupations can enhance function relative to the World Health Organization's (WHO's) dimensions of participation, activity, and body functions and structure and service recipients' subjective views and experiences
- Relate the functional dimensions of participation, activity, and body functions and structure to the sequence and content of functional assessment and intervention in occupational therapy
- Explain evidence-based principles that should guide the selection of therapeutic occupation to be used in treatment and the construction of holistic and comprehensive total treatment programs
- Understand how to incorporate common therapeutic procedures and techniques in pulmonary rehabilitation within therapeutic occupations
- Understand how to run therapeutic groups focused on daily living skills and occupational projects

This chapter addresses pulmonary rehabilitation from the perspective of occupational therapy. It begins by discussing the field's core construct of *occupation* and then relating that construct to therapeutic programs of *lifestyle redesign*. To clarify the ultimate purpose of occupational therapy and also ensure a shared interdisciplinary language with respect to that purpose, the chapter proceeds by bridging the ideas of occupation and lifestyle redesign to commonly used terms within the rehabilitation field, specifically function as now defined by the WHO[1] and HRQL. The occupational therapy process of lifestyle redesign is next presented, including strategies for assessment and intervention pertaining to those areas of occupational functioning that people with pulmonary disorders deem vital to a high quality of life. Ultimately, the chapter has two purposes: (*a*) to offer clinical guidelines to occupational therapists in pulmonary rehabilitation that are optimally evidence based and theoretically sound, as gauged by contemporary standards of best possible practice in occupational therapy, and (*b*) to facilitate interdisciplinary understanding of the specific contributions of occupational therapy in pulmonary rehabilitation.

Throughout this chapter, it is understood that occupational therapists' involvement in pulmonary rehabilitation unfolds in many different treatment contexts across the continuum of care, from inpatient medical facilities and outpatient clinics to the institutional living environments, private homes, schools, work places, and communities of persons with pulmonary disorders. Accordingly, approaches to assessment and intervention described herein, as well as views of legitimate treatment goals, methods, and outcomes, are offered as vital guidelines to the practice of occupational therapy in pulmonary rehabilitation no matter where or when that practice occurs. At the same time, shifts in patients' functional capacities across the differing contexts of care often require that the focus of treatment shifts within the scope of these guidelines. It is recognized as well that the "natural" environments of home, school, community, and work place can be far more conducive to delivering robust programs of occupational therapy than medical facilities that offer only a limited range of treatment spaces. Across the continuum of care, therefore, occupational therapists are encouraged to implement these guidelines in ways that are resourceful, creative, flexible, and responsive to patients' current occupational needs.

OCCUPATION AND LIFESTYLE REDESIGN

The construct of occupation was central to the emergence of occupational therapy in the early 20th century and continues today to impart much influence on the field's evolution.[2] Although not prominently used by all health professionals, and used colloquially in the sense of paid work, "occupation" as used by occupational therapists refers to human activities that demark and define chunks of time in the stream of daily life, call forth the expression of dormant or undeveloped capacities, and relate directly to core motivations and identities. By so doing, occupations imbue people's everyday habits and routines—as well as their infrequent yet personally significant events, rituals, and celebrations—with shape, meaning, and purpose.

Put another way, one might say that occupation is as vital to people's lives as breathing is to their bodies. Like breathing, moreover, one's obligatory, productive, restful, leisurely, and celebratory occupations are often accomplished in relatively fluid, taken-for-granted fashions—at least, that is, until the onset of debilitating medical conditions. Thus, people seek the services of health professionals in pulmonary rehabilitation not only out of fundamental concerns about survival but also out of fundamental concerns that they might continue to have, or might once again have, lives worth living. If we listen, we hear their occupational identities: the meticulous homemaker, proficient gardener, avid reader, competent professional, devoted grandparent, expert golfer, and loyal church volunteer, all vital cues to successful programs of occupational therapy. Simultaneously, the meticulous homemaker may have become so physically deconditioned that making a bed requires that the balance of the day be spent recovering; the expert golfer may have given up hope of ever again playing nine holes; and the loyal church volunteer may have become homebound out of embarrassment in having to rely on portable oxygen in public. When valued undertakings such as these become compromised, or are cut altogether from the fabric of daily life, a spiraling cycle of losses in self-esteem, identity, hopefulness, functional capacity, and family and societal participation often ensues.

It is, accordingly, the work of occupational therapists in pulmonary rehabilitation to engage patients in collaborative processes of *lifestyle redesign* that place the precise occupations that both challenge and are deemed important by patients and their loved ones at the center of clinical intervention. Jackson et al.[3] defined lifestyle redesign as a therapeutic program of occupational therapy dedicated to empowering people to actively select and experience individualized patterns of occupations that are simultaneously health promoting and personally satisfying. As applied to pulmonary rehabilitation, effective programs of lifestyle redesign may be limited in focus and duration as well as broad. Yet, no matter where in this range a program falls, its effectiveness is gauged by the degree to which patients incorporate therapeutic experiences within those occupations that they want and need to do after discharge. Thus, the "proof" of occupational therapy is in how people learn to "do" life differently in their homes and communities and to the betterment of their health and satisfaction.

Relationship to HRQL and Function

Occupational therapy's emphasis on everyday occupations is congruent with contemporary emphasis on HRQL as a critical outcome of health care and rehabilitation in general[1,4–6] and of pulmonary rehabilitation in particular.[7–9] More specifically, being able to carry out *personally valued life activities* despite adverse health conditions is commonly viewed as one of several core elements of HRQL, a position that current research of both well and disabled persons strongly supports.[10–14] Furthermore, experiences of a good quality of life are increasingly acknowledged as being highly subjective and individualistic in nature.[15] Thus, as Browne et al.[15] noted with respect to quality of life, "It is of little use, for example, to observe that on average, the mobility of a sample of patients improved following an intervention, without knowing whether this domain is as important [to those patients] as other domains that may have disimproved." Hence, it is possible to impact "function" favorably while having no favorable impact on HRQL whatsoever, perhaps explaining why treatment areas traditionally favored by rehabilitation professionals, such as basic movement or self-care skills, have often not brought about better lives for those who have undergone extensive rehabilitation.[15–17] To understand how programs of lifestyle redesign strive to improve function in ways that also enhance HRQL, it is helpful to review the WHO's current views of function and disablement.

The WHO[1] recently revised its 1980 International Classification of Impairments, Disabilities, and Handicaps (ICIDH) to account more fully for environmental (social and physical) influences on ablement and also better represent the complex, varied, and dynamic nature of the disablement process. Although still being field tested, the WHO's new classification, International Classification of Functioning and Disability (ICIDH-2) (Fig. 13-1), has shifted away from terminology that emphasizes the negatives of incapacity and toward terminology that emphasizes meaningful activity and social participation.

Whereas the earlier ICIDH defined function as consisting of the three dimensions of impairment, disability, and handicap, ICIDH-2 now defines function in positive terms, describing the dimensions as body functions and structure, activity, and participation.[1]

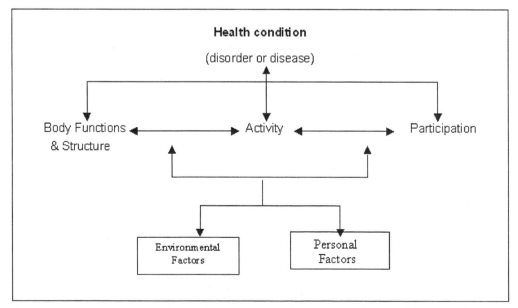

Figure 13-1. WHO International Classification of Impairments, Activities, and Participation. (Reprinted from International Classification of Functioning and Disability (ICIDH-2). Beta-2: draft for field trials: full version, July 1999. Available at: http://www.who.int/icidh/.)

ICIDH-2 addresses function at the level of the body, with problems at this level defined as *impairments*. Impairments are abnormalities in physiologic or psychologic functions or body structures. Also using more positive language, function at the level of the person is now described as *activity*, not disability. Activity refers to how people are able to perform activities of everyday life, from basic physical functions such as grasping, moving a leg, or hearing to complex physical and mental activities such as driving a car, playing a piano, or planning and cooking a meal. Problems of activity performance are called *activity limitations*. ICIDH-2 now addresses function at the level of society as *participation*, not handicap. Participation, the most elusive dimension of function, arises from a complex interplay of health conditions, body functions and structure, activities, and contextual factors that together influence the degree to which people participate in society to their own satisfaction. Participation restrictions arise when involvement in life situations is limited in manner or extent relative to the individual's desired level of participation.

As well as embracing terminology that speaks to human potential, ICIDH-2 emphasizes that simple, unidirectional, causal relationships do *not* exist between adverse health conditions and the three functional dimensions of body, activity, and participation. Instead, multiple pathways involving many mutually interacting variables, all of which are influenced by the contexts in which people "do" their lives, are viewed as potentially able to impact function profoundly. Emphasis on this complex nexus of factors and processes stems from a now large body of evidence showing that people with identical medical diagnoses, or similar health conditions, vary greatly in their actual functional capacities.

With respect to pulmonary rehabilitation, for example, although a diagnosis of emphysema may account for why a 60-year-old woman performs poorly on a pulmonary function test (functional dimension of body), neither her diagnosis nor her test performance is especially predictive of whether she carries out activities in her home (functional dimension of activity) or successfully works in a paid job (functional dimension of participation). Likewise, improving function with respect to her pulmonary impairments may very well *not* improve function with respect to her activities or social participation. That is, being able to perform daily activities at home may depend far more on learning how to integrate, within basic habits and routines, adaptations to single activities and also to ways of balancing the energy demands of multiple activities than on improved pulmonary function alone. In turn, improved function in home activities may bear no relationship to improved function at work if the woman's place of employment exposes her to poor air quality. Finally, even if this woman were unable to function independently in the home or at work after intensive rehabilitation, her HRQL may still have been greatly improved if therapy enabled her to participate once again in her most enjoyed activities as a grandmother and bridge club member (functional dimension of participation). As this example illustrates, processes of disablement are not only unique to individuals and the particulars of their life situations but defy reductions to simple causal relationships between illness, body functions and structure, activity performance, and participation.

Occupation, as used by occupational therapists in both language and as a therapeutic medium, bears a specific relationship to each of the ICIDH-2's three dimensions of function, with specific clinical implications for improving function in ways that promote HRQL. Just as the term "occupation" overlaps with colloquial use of the term "activity," so too does occupation encompass the more complex mental and physical activities within the activity dimension of ICIDH-2. For example, activities like cooking a meal or driving a car are regarded as occupations because they are purposeful, entail conscious perceptions of doing, tap many different skill areas simultaneously for their execution, and are also typically imbued with personal and sociocultural meanings. Conversely, basic functions that the ICIDH-2 also calls activities, such as grasping, moving a leg, remembering, and hearing, are viewed as discrete component functions embedded within the "doing" of occupations[18] but not as occupations per se. Keeping this distinction in mind, this chapter departs somewhat from ICIDH-2's terminology by using activity and occupation interchangeably to denote the complex "doing" experiences of people as whole beings. At the same time, as evidence reviewed later in this chapter suggests, occupation can influence basic physical functions and impairments favorably, such as when enriched rounds of daily activities promote both psychologic well-being and physical conditioning. Likewise, occupation is a key vehicle by which identity and social participation can be enhanced as when, say, playing the guitar is a source of personal pride and also the center of many songfests with family and friends.

Table 13-1 summarizes the previous discussion of occupation and its relationship to current WHO definitions, with relevant examples to pulmonary rehabilitation. As shown, occupation substantially overlaps with the functional dimension of participation and with complex mental and physical activities within the functional dimension of activity. Directional arrows are used to show that occupation can potentially influence function favorably with regard to (*a*) basic physical functions in the dimension of activity, (*b*) body functions and structure, and (*c*) participation.

THERAPEUTIC PROCESS OF LIFESTYLE REDESIGN

The therapeutic process of lifestyle redesign begins with a multidimensional functional assessment, proceeds to a series of interventions and ongoing evaluation of the effectiveness of those interventions, and concludes with evaluation of achieved outcomes pertaining to function and HRQL leading to discharge. This entire process unfolds within occupational therapy's established domain of expertise in *self-care activities* (e.g., bathing, toileting, bed mobility, emergency response), *work and productive activities* (e.g., child and elder care, housekeeping, shopping, transportation, cooking, management of money, household, or medication needs), *and play and leisure activities* (e.g., creative play, sports, recreational, and hobby interests).[19–22] To ensure that patients' particular occupational concerns are fully addressed, the occupational therapist acts throughout the therapeutic process as an expert educator, coach, ally, and advocate who empowers patients and their significant others as full cocollaborators in therapy.[23,24]

Multidimensional Functional Assessment

Effective and efficient intervention is more likely to ensue if the assessment has clearly delineated core problem areas and opportunities for improvement. Thus, this chapter emphasizes the assessment process as fundamental to best practice. A sample occupational therapy evaluation form serves as a summary and a guide to the reader on the sequence and content of this section on functional assessment (Fig. 13-2).

Before conducting actual assessments of a patient's functional status, the occupational therapist prepares by collecting background information from the medical record and through discussion with team members.[25] Information pertaining to medical diagnosis, medical history, medical precautions, documented impairments, and social and vocational history is especially important. *Medical diagnosis* is required for insurance reimbursement for occupational therapy, which serves as a clue to the types of impairments that the patient may experience. Onset of diagnoses indicates whether an acute problem or a chronic condition exists for which the patient may have already made many effective adaptations. *Medical history* includes secondary physical and psychologic diagnoses that may limit occupational performance, nutritional issues, and past and present use of medications and oxygen. *Medical precautions* indicate needed constraints in basic movements and activities. Data on *impairments* such as forced expiratory volume and endurance tests allow the occupational therapist to anticipate the patient's general level of physical capacity. When available, information pertaining to *social and vocational history* begins to paint a picture of the patient's culture, values, environment, and lifestyle. Education level will guide the selection of written instructional materials for use in therapy and also influence the extent to which a patient may or may not benefit from such materials.

Table 13-1. Relationship of Occupation to World Health Organization (WHO) International Classification of Impairment, Activity, and Participation (ICIDH-2)

Terminology	WHO Definitions	Occupation	Examples of Problems of Patients in Pulmonary Rehabilitation
Health condition	Disease or disorder of the body		COPD, asthma, ALS, major depression
Body functions and structure	Function at the level of the *body*; *impairment* is a loss or abnormality of bodily structures or function	Influence of function	Compromised pulmonary function, muscle weakness, anxiety, decreased range of motion, memory deficit
Activity	Function at the level of the *person*; activities may be limited in nature, duration, and quality; activities may range from basic movements to complex tasks	Occupation	Basic movements: difficulties lifting, breathing, or walking Complex activities: difficulties bathing, dressing, shopping, homemaking, or performing leisure interests and hobbies
Participation	Function at the level of *society*; refers to the outcome of complex relationships among health conditions, body functions and structure, and activities in context of persons' lived environments; context includes social, physical, and attitudinal features of environments that serve to facilitate or limit participation; participation can be restricted in nature, duration, and quality	Influence on function	Belief that assistive equipment is stigmatizing or symbolizes personal weakness; inaccessible physical environments in homes or places of work secondary to stairs, long distances, or challenging terrain; lack of knowledge of others about the effects of perfumes, humidity, or temperature on persons with pulmonary dysfunction

Data from International Classification of Functioning and Disability (ICIDH-2). Beta-2: draft for field trials: full version, July 1999. Available at: http://www.who.int/icidh/. COPD, chronic obstructive pulmonary disease; ALS, amyotrophic lateral sclerosis.

Name _____Medical Record #_____ Age_____ Date _____

Diagnosis_____ Onset _____ Precautions_____

Pertinent Medical History, Medications, Oxygen:

Social, Vocational, and Educational History:

PARTICIPATION

Extent of participation in:	Routines & Time Use Patterns:	Environmental Barriers/Resources:	Goals & belief in ability to change:
Activities of Daily Living			
Leisure & Social			
Work and Productive			

ACTIVITY PERFORMANCE

Problem activities:	Difficulty, Duration, Assistance, Outlook:	Strategies & breathing patterns:
1)	1)	
2)	2)	
3)	3)	
4)	4)	

BODY FUNCTIONS AND STRUCTURES, IMPAIRMENTS AND STRENGTHS AFFECTING ACTIVITY PERFORMANCE

Physical:	Cognitive:	Psychological:
Dyspnea:		
Activity Tolerance: MET level:		
Strength:		
Range of Motion:		
Other:		

Figure 13-2. Sample Occupational Therapy Assessment form. *MET*, table of metabolic equivalent values.

After pertinent background information has been obtained, direct assessment of the patient is undertaken with respect to ICIDH-2's functional dimensions of participation, activity, and body functions and structure. To understand sequencing of assessment across these dimensions, rationales underlying top-down approaches are next described. Table 13-2 shows how the ICIDH-2 classification system organizes functional assessment with respect to each dimension.

Top-Down Approach to Functional Assessment

State-of-the-art approaches to functional assessment in occupational therapy begin by ascertaining people's self-perceived capabilities, satisfactions, and dissatisfactions with regard to how well they are functioning within their family, school, work, or community lives.[26-28] This approach to functional assessment, in which the total contexts and meanings of occupational performance in everyday life constitute the starting point, is referred to as a "top-down approach."[28] In other words, the "top" of the assessment addresses the complex nexus of factors and dynamics that influence whether, how, and to what degree

Table 13-2. Occupational Therapy Multidimensional Functional Assessment Organized According to International Classification of Functioning and Disability (ICIDH-2) Dimensions of Function: Participation, Activity, and Body Functions and Structure

Dimensions of Function	Measurement of Dimension and Assessment Goals	Evaluation Methods and Tools
Participation	Determine impact of health conditions and of social and physical environment on everyday lifestyle, particularly social and productive activities Identify important activities for performance-based assessment	Interview Canadian Occupational Performance Measure School Function Assessment Functional Status Questionnaire Activity configuration Activity checklist Environmental assessment
Activity	Determine ability to perform specific activities relative to difficulty, assistance needed, duration limits, and outlook on activity Determine areas of strength that enable performance Determine which impairments should be evaluated in depth	Activity analysis Metabolic equivalent table Rate of perceived dyspnea Rate of perceived exertion Functional Independence Measure (FIM) Wee-FIM Assessment of Motor and Process Skills
Body functions and structure	Determine degree of severity, location, or duration of impairments that impede activities and social participation Determine whether the impairment can be remediated or whether it should be compensated for Determine areas of strength	Endurance: 6- or 12-minute walk test Strength: manual muscle test, grip strength Range of motion: goniometry Oxygen saturation: pulse oximetry Visual perception, cognitive performance, and motor control tools

Data from International Classification of Functioning and Disability (ICIDH-2). Beta-2: draft for field trials: full version, July 1999. Available at: http://www.who.int/icidh/.

a patient actually participates satisfactorily across all contexts of his or her life. Moving "downward" in functional complexity, the assessment next evaluates current performance abilities in occupations previously identified by the patient (or family) as especially important and also problematic. Finally, assessment proceeds further downward to the least complex elements of function, that is, a more detailed evaluation of distinct body functions and structure that directly impede activity performance. Thus, each phase of the top-down approach is designed to inform, delimit, and focus the next phase, thereby generating a fine-grained yet comprehensive picture of patients' occupational functioning.

Occupational therapy has moved toward top-down approaches to functional assessment during the past decade, and away from bottom-up approaches that start with and also emphasize evaluation of impairments, for several reasons. (*a*) By first ascertaining the perspectives of patients and their significant others, a foundation of mutual respect that empowers service recipients as full cocollaborators in therapy is immediately established.[29,30] In contrast, early emphasis on impairments places patients in passive and subservient roles relative to therapists. (*b*) Top-down approaches prevent subsequent imposition of treatment regimens by therapists that people are prone to dismiss as irrelevant to their postdischarge lives despite having willingly participated in those regimens when patients (see Trombly's[31] discussion of her father and works by DeJong,[17] Callahan,[32] Klein,[33] and Murphy[34]). (*c*) Patients often assume that what occupational therapists evaluate is what occupational therapists treat.[28] If occupational therapists focus initially on measuring impairments, then a false message is tacitly yet powerfully conveyed that treatment can and will "fix" those impairments. Conversely, although remediation of impairments such as muscle weakness or low endurance may be an element of treatment, patients need to understand that occupational therapy's greatest contribution to their postdischarge lives consists of helping them learn how to enact patterns of occupation in ways that promote their health and well-being. (*d*) Finally, the top-down approach is cost-effective and time-efficient as it guides the therapist to evaluate and treat only those occupational issues that, from patients' perspectives, adversely impact their quality of life.

First Phase: Dimension of Participation

The first phase of functional assessment targeting participation is accomplished primarily through interview of the patient and, ideally, important others (e.g., family, friends, caregivers, colleagues, and teachers) in the patient's life. If the patient has stopped a valued occupation, or reports impoverished rounds of occupations day in and day out, it is critical that the therapist uncover the real reasons why. Moreover, because processes of disablement cannot be reduced to simple causal relationships, a multiplicity of social, cognitive, emotional, physical, and contextual dynamics may be at play. For example, a person may stop doing volunteer work not because of any recent decline in physical capacity but out of embarrassment (an emotional issue) about chronic wheezing and coughing (a physical issue) in public (a social issue). In this phase of assessment, therefore, the occupational therapist explores the patient's involvement with meaningful occupations across multiple life contexts to reveal his or her personal characteristics, motivations, values, and beliefs about possibilities for healthful change. In addition, to whatever degree is possible, the occupational therapist evaluates the social and physical contexts of the patient's life.

Initial interview questions about participation and barriers to participation are geared to the patient's functional and educational level: How have pulmonary problems affected your ability to do the things you want to do? What are the most challenging things for you to do? What is the most important thing that you do or would like to do? What makes your spirit soar? What are you looking forward to? What would you be doing if you did not have pulmonary problems? How is your day and week typically organized? How do family, friends, and coworkers respond to your pulmonary problems? These questions illuminate who the patient is as a person and their lived experience of having a disability. In addition to informal interviews, several standardized tools have been published that address participation, initiating a top-down approach.

The Canadian Occupational Performance Measure (COPM)[35] is recommended as a standardized interview tool that can function as a valid outcome measure of occupational therapy with both adults and children. It begins by asking the patient to identify activities that he or she wants or needs to do. Using a scale from 1 to 10, the patient rates how well he or she is able to perform each activity and corresponding levels of satisfaction with performance. A list of five goal areas is generated from these responses to target subsequent interventions to the most critical areas of need identified by the patient. As long as the patient can communicate concerns and desires, or knowledgeable proxies are available to respond to the COPM's questions, it is an effective data-gathering tool with very debilitated patients and those with mild difficulties alike.

The School Function Assessment[36,37] is a standardized criterion-referenced tool that guides goal setting and treatment planning in the school environment. The School Function Assessment identifies both the strengths and the problems of a child with respect to his or her active participation in school activities within the classroom, science lab, playground, resource room, school bus, cafeteria, and restroom, among other contexts. In the interest of implementing pragmatic and sustainable solutions, the tool is designed to foster adult teamwork and interdisciplinary understanding of a child's unique constellation of abilities and difficulties across multiple performance contexts.

The Functional Status Questionnaire[38] is a standardized, self-administered screening tool that targets participation. The questions identify general physical, psychologic, and social role functions in the past month as well as satisfaction levels. In addition to being an appropriate tool to initiate a comprehensive top-down functional assessment, the Functional Status Questionnaire can be used to screen individuals to determine whether they might benefit from occupational therapy.

The activity configuration[39] is a nonstandardized written schedule of the patient's typical day or week. This tool uncovers temporal rhythms of the person's life, social contacts, and habits. In addition, the activity configuration can reveal adaptive strategies that the patient presently uses, ineffectively uses, or altogether fails to use with regard to managing the energy demands of everyday activities. Because energy level, dyspnea, and activity opportunities and demands can vary greatly from day to day, a weeklong activity configuration is useful for revealing whether or to what degree effective adaptive strategies are typically implemented.

Occupational therapists may also wish to use nonstandardized activity checklists that can ascertain patients' perspectives with regard to ability and interest in certain activities. A well-designed checklist can add efficiency to the interview by clarifying problem activities for the patient.[40] A checklist can also aid thoroughness by serving as an activity inventory for the therapist and patient to consider. If given in advance of interviewing, the occupational therapist should be aware that patients may have difficulty completing the checklist. Checklists can frustrate people with limited literacy, vision, writing, or information processing abilities. Checklists have also been found to frustrate patients with very mild or very severe limitations.[41]

Assessing Social and Physical Contexts of Participation
Assessment of the environment targets physical and social affordances and barriers that influence participation.[42] The extent to which the occupational therapist is able to evaluate a patient's actual life environments during initial assessment is greatly influenced by the therapist's work setting. Occupational therapists who see patients in medical facilities are most constrained in this regard, with access limited to important caregivers or family members who are present during assessment. Nevertheless, to ensure that all subsequent therapeutic recommendations are in fact workable in light of the core ethics, values, and emotions that motivate family members and caregivers,[43] the importance of incorporating such persons into this phase of assessment cannot be overstated. Dimensions of the social environment assessed include expectations that important others have regarding the patient's performance; their attitudes about the patient's capacities, weaknesses, and

potential, and their willingness to adapt, assist with, or back away from helping with occupations that are important to the patient.[44]

For example, it would ultimately be a waste of the patient's and the occupational therapist's time, and of health care dollars, to insist that a woman with COPM perform her self-care activities independently if (*a*) the woman prefers to be helped by her husband and (*b*) her husband regards such assistance as an expression of love and also deserved care for all the years in which she subjugated her needs to his. A far more fruitful course of action would instead be for the occupational therapist to ascertain during the first phase of functional assessment the patient's and her husband's perspectives on other areas of occupational functioning that each agree are troubling. Doing so might reveal, for instance, that increasing "homeboundness" and withdrawal from long-standing activities with family and friends are of concern to both husband and wife. Alternatively, the occupational therapist may come to "see" that although both are satisfied with their interdependence in her self-care, the husband still imposes considerable excess disability on his wife in all of her activities. In either of these scenarios, the occupational therapist would strive to find some acceptable "hooks" for intervention in which both husband and wife agree that she can far more actively take charge of her life and he can safely and guiltlessly be less consumed with her care. Such a "hook" may be greater independence in self-care, it may be resuming responsibility for feeding their dog and cat twice a day, it may be both or neither. Whatever the "hooks" are, however, they must reflect not a treatment regimen imposed by the therapist but healthful approaches to everyday occupations that have the greatest likelihood of being incorporated within the family's lifestyle after discharge. To this end, it is also critical that the occupational therapist educate husband and wife about the emotional and physical costs, including progressive debilitation, that helping where no help is needed imposes.

Occupational therapists who work in schools, places of work, private homes, or institutional living environments are in the advantageous position of immediately being able to assess how the physical contexts of daily life influence an individual's usual patterns of participation. Conversely, occupational therapists who work in medical facilities often must rely on a patient's or family members' descriptions, delaying evaluation until it becomes feasible to travel to relevant settings. Where such direct evaluations are not possible, photographs and drawings are used.

Regardless of whether an occupational therapist can assess the patient's everyday physical environments directly or must rely on secondary accounts, the occupational therapist needs to understand how various qualities of the physical environment influence a patient's abilities and motivations for activity. These qualities include *distances* that must be traveled to carry out activities in and outside of the home and *layout* of the living space, including *object availability; furnishings, obstructions,* and *lighting.* The investigation attends to issues of efficiency and safety, especially regarding falls, as well as to the patient's willingness to make home modifications. A recommended strategy for obtaining this information is to study typical pathways, including entryways and safe exits, and then examine each activity space used. The occupational therapist also explores how *air quality* (i.e., temperature, humidity, pollution, odors, and airborne compounds such as perfumes, cleaning agents, and coatings) influences participation in the different occupational contexts of home, school, work, and community. In so doing, the occupational therapist ascertains possibilities for modifying air quality.

Second Phase: Dimension of Activity

Whereas the first phase of assessment relies mainly on interview approaches to obtain information, the second phase of assessment relies mainly on *performance-based assessments* of function in single occupations and multiple occupations over time. Insisting that someone do a task that he or she rarely does compromises the clinical validity and utility of generated data while also risking alienating that person from occupational therapy—even when evaluative purposes are painstakingly explained.[33,34] Hence, to whatever degree is possible, patients are observed in those occupations they previously identified as high priorities for intervention. Occupational therapists working in medical facilities are once again most challenged in this regard and must strive to make available to patients possibilities for participating in a wide range of human occupations, or, alternatively, to simulate the demands of real life activities as closely as possible. Likewise, to whatever degree is pragmatically feasible, patients are to be encouraged to perform priority occupations at the same times and places, and in the same ways, as they usually do. Determining such things as whether someone stands or sits to groom, dresses in the bathroom or bedroom, uses a microwave or conventional oven, gardens in plots or in elevated planters, drives a car or uses public buses, or shops using a scooter or walker is critical. Because patients in medical facilities do activities in unfamiliar spaces with unfamiliar objects, their occupational therapists must also ascertain how observed performances depart (for better or worse) from those typically manifested in everyday environments.[19]

Another principle guiding selection of activities for performance-based assessment concerns the varying metabolic demands of different activities and, hence, the endurance of patients with respect to engaging in single activities as well as a round of multiple activities.[45–48] Occupational therapists can consult tables of metabolic equivalent values (METs) to help select activities of varying energy demands that fall within patients' priority lists of problematic occupations. METs are scaled from 1 to 10 based on the amount of oxygen consumed in the metabolic process to carry out a particular activity. One MET is the amount of energy used when a person is at rest. Thus, the endurance of a person who demonstrated hypoxemia and dyspnea when grooming (1.5 METs) would be much more compromised than that of a person who did not exhibit such symptoms until doing housework (3–4 METs) (Table 13-3). In addition to gauging tolerance for single activities, MET tables can help occupational therapists establish a baseline of endurance across multiple activities of varying energy demands. Ideally, during initial assessment or soon thereafter, patients enact some segment of their daily routines, encompassing activities at different MET levels (e.g., showering [4–5 METS], followed by grooming [1.5 METs], followed by dressing [3–4 METs]). Less ideally but still productive of much clinically useful information, patients perform activities out of their usual sequence during the assessment (e.g., ironing [2–3 METs], followed by bed making [3–4 METs], followed by sewing [1.5–2 METs]).

A final guiding principle for this phase of assessment concerns the occupational therapist's adoption of a conservative approach to intervening in the patient's performance. The patient is thus first given the opportunity to perform the activity as he or she normally would. While always ensuring safety, the occupational therapist intervenes only if and when problems arise and only then in incremental fashions corresponding to the nature of those problems, progressing from the least to the highest levels of verbal and physical assistance. This measured approach is particularly effective in revealing the patient's maximum functional capacity. As next described, the ways in which the patient responds to an activity's *physical, cognitive,* and *psychological demands* are also clearly revealed.[49] By analyzing such responses, the occupational therapist can further hone in on adaptive strategies that enable, and the nature of impairments that constrain, the patient's occupational performance.

Responses to Physical Demands

To gauge the patient's endurance and general activity tolerance, the occupational therapist keeps in mind the average MET values of activities published in tables, in addition to the specific strength and speed demands of those activities as actually enacted by patients during assessment.[50] For example, ironing with a heavy iron or quickly or while standing is more demanding of energy than is ironing with a light iron or slowly or while sitting. Also, use of the upper extremities is typically more taxing than the same amount of work done by the lower extremities.[51,52] In addition to these considerations, the occupational therapist watches for whether and how other common physical impairments in pulmonary

Table 13-3. Metabolic Equivalent (MET) Values for Some Occupational Performance Areas

MET Levels (Oxygen Consumed) [Level of Activity]	Self-care Activities	Work and Productive Activities	Play and Leisure Activities
1.5–2.0 METS (4–7 mL/kg/min) [Very light/minimal]	Eating Shaving, grooming Getting in and out of bed Standing	Desk work Typing Writing	Playing cards Sewing Knitting
2–3 METS (7–11 mL/kg/min) [Light]	Showering in warm water Level walking (3.25 km or 2 mph)	Ironing Light woodworking Riding lawn mower	Level bicycling (8 km or 5 mph) Billiards Bowling Golfing with power cart
3–4 METS (11–14 mL/kg/min) [Moderate]	Dressing, undressing Walking (5 km or 3 mph)	Cleaning windows Making beds Mopping floors Vacuuming Bricklaying Machine assembly	Bicycling (10 km or 6 mph) Fly-fishing (standing in waders) Horseshoe pitching
4–5 METS (14–18 mL/kg/min) [Heavy]	Showering in hot water Walking (5.5 km or 3.5 mph)	Scrubbing floors Hoeing Raking leaves Light carpentry	Bicycling (13 km or 8 mph) Table tennis Tennis (doubles)
5–6 METS (18–21 mL/kg/min) [Heavy]	Walking (6.5 km or 4 mph)	Digging in garden Shoveling light earth	Bicycling (16 km or 10 mph) Canoeing (6.5 km or 4 mph) Ice- or roller-skating (15 km or 9 mph)
6–7 METS (21–25 mL/kg/min) [Very heavy]	Walking (8 km or 5 mph)	Snow shoveling Splitting wood	Bicycling (17.5 km or 11 mph) Light downhill skiing Ski touring (4 km or 2.5 mph)

Reprinted with permission from Kohlmeyer K. Evaluation of sensory and neuromuscular performance components. In: Neistadt M, Crepeau E, eds. Willard and Spackman's Occupational Therapy. 9th ed. Philadelphia: Lippincott, 1998:255.

mL/kg/min, milliliters of oxygen consumed per kilogram body weight per minute; km, kilometer; mph, miles per hour.

disorders like dyspnea, fatigue, or limitations in upper extremity strength and range of motion affect performance.[25,53] If the patient experiences distress or if medical history or precautions indicate, the occupational therapist monitors the patient's heart rate, oxygen saturation rate, respiratory rate, or blood pressure before, during, and after the activity.[54] Table 13-4 offers general guidelines for monitoring vital signs in response to activity. Such monitoring gauges the severity of various physiological impairments *relative to actual occupational performance,* thereby providing contextually valid data that are extremely useful to patients and therapists alike.

For example, if the occupational therapist observes abnormal breathing patterns such as breath holding, forced exhalation, or gasping, then more measured assessment of how underlying physiologic impairments impact performance ought to be undertaken.[25] Pulse oximetry monitoring can be used to offer continuous information about oxygenation and heart rate during occupational performance for patients at risk for hypoxemia.[25] A portable pulse oximeter consists of a finger or ear clamp attached to a small monitor, which enables use of the device during most activities. Normal oxygen saturation values are 95 to 98%; a reading below 90% is a sign of hypoxemia. Oxygen saturation readings can offer early warnings that an activity should be modified or ceased. If decreasing the activity does not resolve the hypoxemia, oxygen can be increased through supplemental oxygen, use of breathing strategies, or shifts in body position such as propping on elbows. Of interest during assessment is how closely the patient's reported symptoms match changes in oxygenation and pulse, indicating the patient's ability to assess his or her status. If the symptoms and readings do not match, the patient may need pulse oximeter to ensure safety and may also benefit from biofeedback training.[25]

Table 13-4. Common Vital Signs Used to Monitor Physical Response to Activity[a]

Vital Signs	Evaluation	Normal Values	Abnormal
Pulse Heart rate (HR)	Index and first finger at radial or carotid artery; measured in beats per min: 15 sec × 4	Rate 60–100; avg. 75 Note: even rhythm and strength	Rate: >100—Tachycardia <60—Bradycardia
Respiratory rate (RR)	Observe rise/fall of abdomen/chest; listen; observe for distress and patterns (breath holding, irregular rate)	12–22 breaths per min (BPM)	Tachypnea Bradypnea (rare)
Blood pressure (BP)	Sphygmomanometer; seated, supine, and standing Measure: mm Hg	Systolic: 90–140 (avg. 120) Diastolic: 60–90 (avg. 80)	Hypertension Hypotension
Arterial blood gases (ABGs)	PaO_2—Partial pressure of oxygen in arterial blood	75–95 mm Hg on room air, age dependent	Hypoxemia
	SaO_2—Amount of oxygen bound to hemoglobin (oximeter)	>95%	Hypoxemia
	CaO_2—Total content of oxygen in arterial blood (A-line)	16–20 mL/dL blood	Decreased tissue oxygenation

[a]The physician sets guidelines for individual patients.

Table 13-5. Instructions for Evaluating Perceived Dyspnea and Perceived Exertion

1. Patient identifies an activity that is important and problematic and then performs that activity.
2. The patient is shown the following 10-point scales and asked to rate perceptions of dyspnea and exertion.
3. Descriptive terms in the scales serve as verbal anchors to assist the patient in rating.
4. To evaluate outcomes, retest using the same activity, rating scales, and instructions.
   Note: If assessing for change in activity performance, the patient uses newly acquired energy conservation and breathing strategies in the retest session. If assessing for impairment of endurance, the original activity is replicated.

Perceived Dyspnea Scale	Perceived Exertion Scale
Instructions: "How would you rate your shortness of breath during the activity? On a scale of 0 to 10, with 0 being no shortness of breath and 10 being shortness of breath so severe that you must stop and rest, what number best indicates your experience of shortness of breath?"	*Instructions:* "Rate how hard you were working (or the amount of physical effort) during the activity? On a scale of 0 to 10, with 0 being no effort and 10 being your maximum possible effort, what number best indicates your level of effort?"

My shortness of breath is:		My level of effort is:	
0	None	0	None
0.5	Very slight, just noticeable	0.5	Very slight
1		1	Slight
2	Mild	2	Mild
3	Moderate	3	Moderate
4	Somewhat heavy	4	Somewhat strong
5	Strong, heavy	5	Strong, heavy
6		6	
7	Severe	7	Very strong
8		8	
9		9	
10	Very, very severe; I must stop and rest	10	Very, very strong, almost the maximum possible

Adapted with permission from Borg G. Psychophysical bases of perceived exertion. Med Sci Sports Exerc 1982;14:377.

In addition to the previously mentioned objective measures, it is important that the occupational therapist determine the patient's subjective experience of the activity's difficulty. Borg[55] developed a scale with which patients can rate their perceived levels of dyspnea and exertion during an activity, using verbal anchors to assist in ratings (Table 13-5). An alternative subjective rating scale ranges from 6 to 20, with 6 being no effort and 20 being the maximum effort possible to complete the activity.[53] The 6 to 20 scale is useful for teaching patients to self-monitor heart rate for 6 seconds because of easier mathematical conversions. The counted number between 6 to 20 over a 6-second time interval is then multiplied by 10. A score of 6 has been found to often correlate with a heart rate of 60 beats per minute, and so on up the scale with 20 correlating with 200 beats per minute.

Responses to Psychologic Demands
Various psychologic dynamics in the patient's occupational experience are also carefully tuned into during performance-based assessment. A viscous cycle of dyspnea and anxiety can interfere with performance, leading a patient to avoid a particular activity after dis-

charge. Thus, it can be beneficial for this negative cycle to arise briefly during assessment to observe the patient's awareness and response. The patient is asked about feelings of satisfaction and dignity associated with performance. Motivation for treatment is likely to be enhanced if the patient is dissatisfied with performance or if receiving assistance is humiliating or unacceptable. If a large discrepancy exists between the performance as observed by the occupational therapist and the patient's subjective experience, the therapist is directed toward working with possible strategies to promote awareness and coping. At all times, frustration tolerance must be monitored so the occupational therapist can intervene to prevent new experiences of failure.

Responses to Cognitive Demands

Persons with pulmonary disorders may present with cognitive deficits owing to hypoxemia and given comorbidity with other conditions such as traumatic brain injury, stroke, late stage Parkinson's disease, alcoholism, schizophrenia, major depression, or dementia, among others. Although secondary diagnoses affecting cognition are often well documented, undocumented problems may still exist, such as when, for example, a patient incurred a mild brain injury during a recent fall or is in the earliest stages of dementia. The occupational therapist is thus always alert for cognitive deficits in context of occupational performance. To the extent possible given the cognitive demands of any one assessment activity, the occupational therapist observes the patient's attention span, immediate and short-term memory, organizational and sequencing skills, abilities to follow written or verbal instructions, decision-making capacities, and effectiveness in solving problems. As importantly, the occupational therapist watches for whether and how the patient employs adaptive strategies to accomplish the activity. Because such strategies suggest personal strengths with respect to cognitive processing, learning capabilities, and adaptability,[53] they can be expanded on in subsequent interventions. For example, it may become apparent while watching a patient dress that he takes frequent rest breaks, effectively uses a reacher, but demonstrates poor breathing techniques. In this case, the occupational therapist is cued to build on pacing strategies that are acceptable to the patient and to teach breathing strategies. Use of a reacher also suggests an openness to other assistive equipment in other occupations.

Standardized Performance-Based Assessments

Not all occupations that patients identify as high priorities can be assessed using standardized evaluation tools. For example, a city dweller's ability to use public transportation while reliant on portable oxygen may be the most daunting obstacle that person faces with regard to overcoming his or her spiraling social isolation, withdrawal from valued activities, and propensities to cancel outpatient appointments. Although perhaps not immediately able to be assessed, it is nonetheless critical that occupational therapists address capacities in those less routine activities that often prove to be the weakest link in a person's overall quality of life. The previously mentioned approach to performance-based assessment can be used to generate objective measures of functional capacity with regard to public transportation use, as well as any other occupational endeavor, be it horseback riding, mall walking, or gardening.

When, however, patients' occupational needs overlap with the content area of psychometrically sound, performance-based assessment tools, it is wise to use the established validity and reliability of such tools. Occupational therapists have access today to several good criterion-referenced tools that target the performance areas of self-care, work and productive activities (including driving), and play and leisure. Two well-established tools commonly used by occupational therapists that address basic self-care activities are the Functional Independence Measure (FIM)[56] and the Wee-FIM.[57] The FIM and Wee-FIM measure burden of care relative to assistance for adults and children, respectively. The FIM has been used to measure progress in persons with pulmonary disorders.[9] A recommended tool for instrumental activities of daily living such as homemaking activities is the Assessment of Motor and Process Skills (AMPS).[58] Because the AMPS allows patients to choose from among 56 possible evaluation activities and then perform chosen activities as typically undertaken, it powerfully instills a patient-centered approach to assessment and treatment. Also, through use of two subscales that analyze motor and cognitive processing in context of one activity, the AMPS allows occupational therapists to predict abilities in other activities of comparable difficulty. Because it is beyond the scope of this chapter to provide a more comprehensive overview of standardized assessments, readers are referred to contemporary textbooks in occupational therapy.[19–22,59]

Documenting Occupational Performance

Activity performance is described in terms of levels of *assistance, difficulty, duration,* and *outlook.* The patient's level of needed verbal and *physical assistance* with an occupation is the most common objective measure of functional capacity. When a standardized assessment has not been used, levels of assistance are typically described by the percentage of the activity the patient actually performed, as follows: independent, supervised or verbal cueing, minimum assistance (patient does approximately 75% of the activity), moderate assistance (patient does approximately 50% of the activity), maximum assistance (patient does approximately 25% of the activity), and dependent (patient does little or none of the activity). These levels of assistance are contained in the Medicare guidelines for occupational therapy.[60] *Difficulty* with an activity can be documented as changes in heart rate, respiration rate, breathing patterns, oxygen saturation levels, and blood pressure before, during, and after activities. Occupational therapists can track the patient's ability to continue with an activity, or *duration,* as another gauge of endurance and activity tolerance. Duration is measured by describing the length of time the patient is able to persist in an activity, as in a man tolerating washing his face while sitting on the edge of the hospital bed for one minute. Because the patient's position, materials used, pace, and environmental context will influence duration, these factors should be described as well. Again with regard to activity tolerance, the patient's perceived dyspnea, exertion, and experience of difficulty are important to document, as are psychologic responses, or *outlook.* Finally, to make all of these measures optimally meaningful with regard to endurance issues, metabolic demands of the activities used for assessment should be noted (Fig. 13-3).

Third Phase: Dimension of Body Functions and Structure

Evaluation of body functions and structure refers to various measurements of specific functions out of context of occupational performance. In a top-down approach, body functions and structure are evaluated in a conservative and streamlined fashion based on several principles: (*a*) Only body functions and structures that have already been directly observed to impede occupational performance are considered relevant for further evaluation. (*b*) Only impairments that require more finely grained measurements to guide intervention than that already obtained in context of activity performance are evaluated. Evaluating endurance using an ergometer may, after all, produce no new clinically useful data—and also less contextually valid data—than that already obtained in context of having the patient make a bed or breakfast. (*c*) Efficiency and comprehensiveness in evaluating body functions and structures is balanced across the interdisciplinary team. By not duplicating evaluations, the program becomes more cost-effective and patients are protected from undue frustrations in having to do the same tests over again. Thus, collaborations with the rehabilitation team to include psychologists and speech and language pathologists about cognitive, psychologic, and communication problems that arise during occupational performance are oftentimes vital. Moreover, when physical impairments can be capably evaluated by either occupational or physical therapists, occupational therapists may wish to "pass the baton" to their colleagues in physical therapy to free

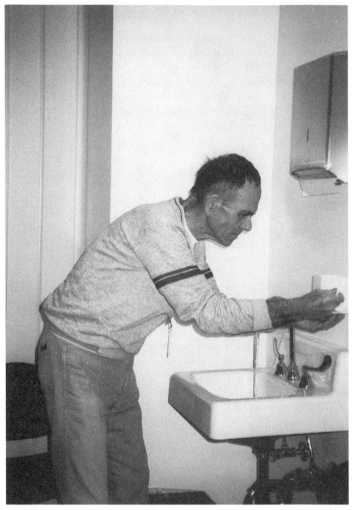

Figure 13-3. The occupational therapist observes performance of everyday activities. Assessment of impairments, such as shoulder range of motion, is done only when problems interfere with performance of important activities. (Courtesy of the Pulmonary Rehabilitation Program, Duke University Medical Center, Durham, NC.)

their own time for grappling with patients' various occupational challenges as thoroughly as possible. This is an especially critical issue in light of current cost-containment measures. Ultimately, a comprehensive program uses teamwork to integrate assessments by all involved professionals across multiple domains of function.[61] With these caveats in mind, occupational therapists may be called on to evaluate impairments in *upper body strength, range of motion, coordination, praxis,* and *sensation.* Occupational therapists may also evaluate swallowing difficulties, or *dysphagia,* that arise from muscle weakness or shortness of breath.[62]

Upper body and proximal muscle weaknesses, common limitations of the pulmonary patient, arise from multiple causes. Many patients have pulmonary problems associated with generalized weakness from neuromuscular diseases such as multiple sclerosis and amyotrophic lateral sclerosis. For patients with chronic pulmonary diseases, trunk, hip, and shoulder weakness can be caused by chronic steroid use.[63] Upper body weakness results from fatigue of the accessory muscles of respiration, propping on elbows to support the trunk, general debilitation, and posturing shoulders in adduction and elevation to expand the capacity of the lungs.[25,64] Further weakness results from disuse of the arms because of the greater energy expenditure required for upper body than lower body movement.

Measurement of strength is done using manual muscle testing. Instead of testing individual muscles, general movement strength is measured and rated on a scale from 0 to 5 from absent to normal. Movements that are often weak are shoulder flexion, external rotation, and abduction. The trunk should be supported when testing the upper extremity to isolate potential weakness areas. Trunk support can be provided by a chair with a back or by lying supine. Trunk strength is measured by first determining whether the patient can sit unsupported and whether that position can be maintained during perturbations in each direction—forward, backward, and to each side. Accessory muscles of respiration may be strong as a result of compensation for compromised lung capacity. Hand and finger strength is measured by dynamometer and pinch meter.

Range of motion limitations are often associated with weakness because they are caused by many of the same factors and are worsened by poor strength.[25] Decreased movement of the shoulders, neck, and trunk results from posturing of the shoulders in elevation and adduction to increase lung space. Posturing leads to a lack of arm swing during ambulation and neck stiffness that can, in turn, be particularly problematic for driving. Tight hip extensors limit the ability to reach the feet, which is worsened by fear or discomfort of flexing forward at the hips. Arthritis and osteoporosis often contribute to musculoskeletal problems of older adults with pulmonary dysfunction. The focus of occupational therapy is not to regain normal range of motion and strength but to improve or compensate for those limitations adequate to perform significant daily activities. Thus, a complete manual muscle test and goniometric evaluation is rarely needed. Gross functional range of motion can be efficiently tested by asking the patient to reach with both hands to toes, the small of the back, back of the head, and then raise arms overhead.

Finally, occupational therapists may engage patients in the 6- or 12-minute walk tests (see Chapter 12).[65] These tests offer objective baselines of endurance relative to estimated MET levels. As needed, upper extremity dowel exercises and upper body ergometers can also be used to reveal breathing strategies and delineate tolerance for upper body exercise.[7,25]

Outcomes of Multidimensional Functional Assessment

The first phase of assessment addressing ICIDH-2's functional dimension of participation brings immediate clarity to the occupational needs, problems, and issues of individual patients and their significant others. As concluded by Fisher,[66] this phase of assessment is thus "critical, and . . . must occur, even under the pressures of cost containment, reduced duration of care, [and] staff cuts, . . . [as it] results in overall outcomes being enhanced and overall costs reduced." The second phase of assessment addressing ICIDH-2's functional dimension of activity produces a wealth of clinically useful information pertaining to patients' functional capacities in valued occupations, including how impairments constrain performance and how areas of strengths might later be applied to resolve other problems. The third phase of assessment addressing ICIDH-2's functional dimension of body functions and structure refines understanding of specific deficit areas. Ultimately, this multidimensional assessment generates a clear picture of patients' current and desired participations across many life contexts, including problems and potentials in relevant activities. The outcome is a list of measurable and doable goals generated in collaboration with the patient, with specific intervention processes and time frames for accomplishing those goals. Table 13-6 offers examples of treatment goals and intervention for body functions and structures activities and participation. As next described, based on these goals, individualized programs are implemented to help people learn how to "do" valued occupations in ways that favorably influence and also optimally sustain their function and HRQL in postdischarge environments.

Table 13-6. Occupational Therapy Outcomes and Interventions Relative to ICIDH-2 Dimensions of Function

Descriptive Terms	Functional Outcomes: Sample Treatment Goals	Intervention Examples
Participation: Outcome is described in terms of engagement, participation, or occupation; occupational therapy intervention links to an outcome at the level of participation	*Patient will:* Return to half time work as a bank teller Participate in senior center activity programs three times per week Resume leisure participation of playing cards Participate in all aspects of public school program, including recess Engage in extended family gatherings Participate in church activities	Increase awareness of environmental barriers and individual's rights to an access under the Americans with Disabilities Act Modify physical environment; educate caregivers, family, employers, teachers, or other people who influence the patient's social and physical world
Activity: Ability to perform specific activities that are important to participation	*Patient will:* Use energy conservation strategies during homemaking activities to cook a family meal and then have the energy to sit with the family to eat Use assistive devices to bathe and dress self with minimum assistance Spontaneously use breathing techniques during yard work task to sustain the activity for 30 min with only mild shortness of breath	Education and training: Activity grading Breathing strategies Energy conservation techniques Assistive equipment Activity modification Environmental modification Assertiveness Relaxation
Body functions and structure: Impairments are addressed if they are remediable and if they enable the patient to perform an important activity	*Patient will:* Tolerate 10 min of upper extremity exercise on the ergometer set at zero resistance Increase strength in shoulder flexion and abduction to 4/5 ("good") Increase shoulder range of motion to 150° flexion and 70° external rotation	Graded tasks to increase endurance Upper extremity strengthening program Range of motion exercises

Data from International Classification of Functioning and Disability (ICIDH-2). Beta-2: draft for field trials: full version, July 1999. Available at: http://www.who.int/icidh/.

Intervention

In determining the best intervention for persons with pulmonary disorders, it is helpful first to consider a variety of evidence-based principles that can guide both the selection of specific activities for use as therapy as well as the construction of total treatment programs that, given available time and resources, are as comprehensive and holistic as possible. With this bigger picture in mind, occupational therapists can then attend to the more technical and procedural aspects of treatment in ways that are most likely to produce valuable outcomes pertaining to function and HRQL.

Evidence-Based Principles of Intervention

A growing body of evidence influencing occupational therapy today substantiates that therapeutic occupations are more efficacious in promoting function and HRQL than are clinically contrived tasks and exercises that lack the complexity of natural occupations. Research has shown, for instance, that interventions that subjugate the importance of the therapy task itself (e.g., dowel rod exercises or cone-stacking) to that which the task is supposed to teach or treat (e.g., pursed lips breathing and pulmonary dysfunction) typically fail to produce sufficient gains to meet the actual functional challenges of real life activities in real life contexts.[31,67,68] Likewise, considerable evidence has accumulated that traditional methods of prescribing exercise are ineffective in improving the cardiovascular fitness and overall activity levels of persons with sedentary lifestyles.[69] Looking at the same issues from the other side of what *works,* various studies have documented, in people with a wide range of disabling conditions, an array of healthful and adaptive benefits stemming from participation in therapeutic occupations, including, among others, skiing,[70] shopping at a mall,[13] working as a hospital volunteer,[71] playing electronic music,[72] eating at a restaurant,[73] arranging flowers,[12] or creating a make-believe subway station.[74] In addition, enriched patterns of everyday activities have been found to promote cardiovascular fitness,[71] reduce risk of falls,[75] slow the progression of impairments, improve psychologic well-being, and increase social participation.[10]

In light of such evidence, much consensus exists in occupational therapy today that top-down approaches are optimal not only to guide assessment but treatment as well.[76] By definition, top-down approaches to treatment are fully *occupation centered* and *patient centered*.[77] Occupation-centered approaches "cut to the chase"; that is, they do *not* assume that clinically contrived regimens that are not part of persons' usual lifestyles produce gains at the level of body functions and structures that, in turn, automatically translate into enhanced function in valued activities and social participation. Rather, based on current evidence, engagement in real life occupations is preserved as the most efficacious medium to treat deficit component areas of function, maximize strengths, and generalize abilities across multiple social and physical contexts. Moreover, several inherent qualities of everyday occupations are exploited as treatment mechanisms. Trombly[31] proposed that two such mechanisms are that therapeutic activities be simultaneously *purposeful* and *meaningful* from the patient's point of view. Pierce[78] further stipulated that activities be (*a*) *appealing* to the patient on face value alone (i.e., without the need for justification by the therapist to induce motivation); (*b*) *congruent* with the patient's goals; and (*c*) *intact* (i.e., be what people do for "real" and be undertaken in their lived environments).

By directly matching therapy activities to previously identified occupational needs and issues, occupational therapists can fully use the treatment mechanisms of purposefulness, meaningfulness, appeal, and goal congruence. The quality of intactness can also be readily used when working with patients in their homes, schools, work places, or communities. In addition, even if based in medical facilities, occupational therapists can take advantage of as many existing occupationally enriched spaces as patients can safely access, e.g., not just patients' rooms but rehabilitation kitchens and apartment areas, gift shops, public cafeterias, outside parks, and nearby restaurants, post offices, shops, public transportation stops, etc. Occupational therapists in medical facilities have also created occupationally enriched treatment spaces such as handyman work stations, occupation rooms, or home office areas. The quality of intactness also requires that patients' important others be substantively involved in treatment, just as they were in assessment. In addition to exploiting these treatment mechanisms, efficacious treatment programs couple didactic teaching with immediate experiential learning.

To incorporate all of these principles within a cohesive program of lifestyle redesign, occupational therapists often involve patients in daily living activities that are typically completed, start to finish, in one treatment session, e.g., basic self-care tasks, cooking a meal, writing a letter on a computer, or cleaning a room. In addition, occupational therapists can use individualized *occupational projects* that span multiple treatment sessions, involve outside "homework," require action in multiple physical and social contexts, and culminate in some kind of production, be it a physical object, social event, or both. The extent and number of occupational projects for any one patient can be geared to the number of available treatment sessions; occupational projects have been effectively used by the authors in as short a period as 1-week inpatient rehabilitation stays. Actual examples of projects undertaken by inpatients include planning and carrying out an outdoors family picnic; using the Internet to research an art history topic and then presenting a talk to the hospital staff; planning and carrying out a trip to the mall to buy glasses; and, for an intubated man with severe pulmonary dysfunction and physical disabilities, adapting the layout of his/her hospital room, procuring a tape-recorder and headphones, so he could listen to talking books and music without having to call for assistance (see examples by Jackson et al[3] and McLaughlin Gray[71]). Occupational projects are especially therapeutic because they build a momentum to therapy over sessions, imparting a narrative story line rife with risks, challenges, uncertain outcomes, and multiple possibilities of personal triumph: other inherent qualities of therapeutic occupation that are believed to have strong treatment effects.[74] Moreover, because such projects symbolize movement from disabled states to states of actively being in control and in charge of one's life, they can be catalytic in impact well beyond discharge. Finally, projects can help occupational therapists manage their time efficiently, as what to do does not have to be decided anew each treatment session and special events or trips can be planned in advance, especially with patient group occupational projects.

Incorporating Therapeutic Procedures and Techniques in Occupational Performance

Having ascertained the critical occupations and occupational projects that will constitute the core of patients' individualized treatment programs, occupational therapists then help patients learn how to incorporate relevant therapeutic strategies, techniques, and adaptations into their "doing" of activities. Especially relevant interventions for pulmonary rehabilitation include activity grading, breathing techniques, energy conservation, assertiveness and relaxation training, assistive device use, and modification of activities and the environment.

Activity Grading

Activity grading is a therapeutic strategy used by occupational therapists to promote progressively greater functioning that patients can also be taught to apply to their everyday lives. The purpose of activity grading is to provide a level of challenge that will help people progress in needed skill areas while not overwhelming them. To do so, selected therapeutic occupations are progressively modified, usually with regard to their levels of physical challenge pertaining to experienced difficulty, required physical assistance, or duration of time able to be tolerated. For example, a severely debilitated patient may begin light grooming such as face washing for 1 minute while in bed with the head of the bed elevated. Each day the patient may do this task for longer periods and in progressively more challenging positions, from seated in a chair with a back, to seated in a chair without a back, and, finally, to standing. In addition to grading the physical demands of an activity, occupational therapists can grade activities socially. That is, relative independence varies as a function of the social context in which an activity is undertaken. Generalizing highest levels of competence across differing expectations, needs, patience, and attitudes of different caregivers can be critical to maintaining functional gains long term. Hogan[54] offers an excellent description of activity grading for a ventilator-assisted man as he moved from an inpatient program to his home and community.

Breathing Techniques

The teaching of breathing techniques begins with awareness and ends when patients view the techniques as tools that they own and control. In other words, occupational therapists want to avoid the kind of situation as occurred to one of the authors when she asked participants in a group when they exhaled during an activity. Members of the group quietly looked at each other until one patient said, jokingly but earnestly, "Whenever the therapist tells us to!" Patients vary in their levels of awareness in respect to the influence of talking, concentrating, and body position on breathing patterns. During these activities, the occupational therapist asks the patient to observe and reflect on changes in breathing, to begin developing a sense of awareness and then control. Individualization in instruction coupled with immediate practice in selected therapeutic occupations is needed if healthful breathing techniques are to become habitual.

Pursed-lips breathing and *diaphragmatic breathing* are recommended breathing strategies for patients with lung disease. Pursed-lips breathing has been shown to improve gas exchange and respiratory muscle recruitment (Box 13-1).[79,80] Another possible benefit of pursed-lips breathing is that it helps keep airways open by maintaining positive airway pressure. Although many patients intuitively teach themselves this strategy, coaching by occupational therapists coupled with practice helps overcome tendencies to use inefficient breathing patterns such as breath holding during strenuous activities and, instead, to continue pursed-lips breathing before becoming short of breath. The practice of exhaling during the most strenuous part of an activity is taught as part of pursed-lips breathing training.

Research on diaphragmatic breathing has not produced evidence of its benefits on oxygen levels.[80] However, the clinical literature and anecdotal accounts suggest that diaphragmatic breathing does reduce dyspnea for some patients with lung disease.[80,81] The benefit of this technique seems to lie in the management of the stress and anxiety components of dyspnea; it may also influence perception of dyspnea.[80] Although further evidence is needed to explain and substantiate the effects of breathing training, many patients report that pursed lips and diaphragmatic breathing reduce dyspnea, improve relaxation, improve efficiency of breathing, and improve functional performance. In practice, occupational therapists systematically observe patient responses to breathing techniques to determine which patients benefit and document those results. Stress management and perception of control of breathing are legitimate benefits of breathing techniques that influence functional performance.

Energy Conservation

> *Common sense is genius dressed in working clothes.*
>
> Ralph Waldo Emerson

An extremely important dimension of occupational therapy has to do with helping patients learn how to balance satisfactory rounds of occupations over time. The activity configuration discussed previously in this chapter reveals both effective and problematic habits and routines. For example, compressing activities into the morning can lead to experiences of severe fatigue in the afternoon; similarly, overdoing one day can cause fatigue for several subsequent days. Some people learn how to adapt to such experiences by consciously

Box 13-1. Breathing Techniques and Training Process

Pursed-lips breathing
Used to reduce dyspnea during activities.
1. Initial instruction is in relaxed position, seated or supine
2. Patient closes mouth and slowly and deeply inhales through the nose
3. Exhalation is through firmly pursed lips, parted at the center, as in whistling
4. Prolong the exhalation phase to twice the length of the inspiration phase
5. Practice pursed lips breathing during an activity, which may be washing one's face for a very debilitated patient or vacuuming for another
6. Practice exhaling during the most strenuous part of a task, such as lifting an object or bending forward
7. Practice techniques in a variety of familiar activities as well as in moments of anxiety until they are automatic

Diaphragmatic breathing
Used to retrain muscles of breathing for improved efficiency and to promote relaxation.
1. Position in supine or seated
2. Place one hand on the abdomen just below the rib cage and the other hand on the chest
3. Patient observes the rise and fall of the abdominal wall during inspiration and expiration, respectively
4. Therapist explains the relationship between movement of the abdominal wall and the contraction (descending) of the diaphragm during inspiration and the patient's control of this action
5. Patient then practices consciously relaxing to expand the abdominal wall during inspiration; this can be done for up to an hour several times per day and whenever relaxation is needed
6. Diaphragmatic breathing may be done in conjunction with or before progressive muscle relaxation
7. Stronger pressure or a weight can be placed on the abdomen (ideally when supine) to improve strength
8. Diaphragmatic breathing can be done in conjunction with pursed-lips breathing

planning their time use over a week or month, regularly interspersing periods of activity with periods of rest, or conserving energy for the most valued activities. Others lack such proactive strategies, living a moment-by-moment existence with choice of activity subjugated to immediate opportunities and energy level. With this information as a baseline, the occupational therapist helps the patient devise an *occupational plan,* that is, activity schedules that ensure engagement in priority activities and minimize fatigue and frustration. Spontaneity, flexibility, and fun—all valued elements of a good day—are validated by being included in the development of such plans.[82] An effective tool to help patients devise and then implement their plans is that of an *occupational journal.* By keeping journals of usual routines and habits before trying to make substantive changes, patients grow more consciously aware of the effect that particular activities and their overall patterns of activity have on their physical conditioning and psychologic well-being.

As with breathing techniques, the teaching of energy conservation strategies begins with awareness and ends when patients view the strategies as tools that they own and control. Energy conservation strategies are common sense strategies that are not so common. Principles of efficiency enable patients to simplify their work and still accomplish what they set out to do. Box 13-2 contains a list of energy conservation principles geared to patients at high reading and motivation levels. Occupational therapy programs should have an array of written information, including simpler lists that focus on a few practical suggestions. Patients often benefit minimally from long lists of general principles, instead needing activity-specific recommendations such as "let your dishes air dry" or "place a chair in the bathroom for grooming." Therapeutic occupation provides a vehicle for practicing energy conservation principles, promoting learning and practical application. The occupational therapist can also model the use of language that is responsive to patients' expressions, concerns, and values yet evidences a stance of personal empowerment: "How can I outsmart this shortness of breath problem, and still go to the baseball game?" "I fatigue easily, so I will decide what is most important for me to do with that limited energy." "I am purchasing energy for the afternoon activity by resting this morning." "I am an efficiency expert." Once energy conservation strategies are part of a patient's routine activities, they are easily generalized to new activities. Ultimately, learning how to incorporate effective energy conservation strategies into everyday life relegates the presence of pulmonary impairments to a lower level of importance than that of human will and agency.

Occupational therapists should be aware that patients are sometimes confused when encouraged on the one hand to use activities and conditioning exercises to build and maintain their endurance and, on the other hand, to work smarter rather than harder using energy conservation strategies. As expressed by one patient, "Now who do we listen to, the physical therapist who tells us to exert ourselves or the occupational therapist who tells us to conserve our energy?" Patients must clearly understand not only the need for balance of exertion and rest, but when to emphasize one or the other. For patients who

Box 13-2. Energy Conservation Principles and Strategies

1. Limit the amount of work
   Prioritize activities
   Eliminate unnecessary tasks
   Delegate responsibilities
   Request assistance
2. Plan ahead and work according to the plan
   Allow sufficient time to complete activities
   Incorporate rest breaks into the plan
   Collect materials before you start
3. Organize your environment
   Place frequently used items in easy reach
   Organize the kitchen by function
   Eliminate clutter
4. Position yourself for comfort and efficiency
   Sit when possible
   Use proper body mechanics and posture
   Wear comfortable clothing and supportive footwear
5. Take control of your time
   Pace yourself to avoid rushing
   Spread activities over the day or week
   Plan rest breaks
   Rest before you are exhausted
6. Let tools do the work
   Use assistive devices such as reachers
   Use convenience items such as a microwave and an electric can opener
   Keep scissors and knives sharp
7. Tend to your mental hygiene
   Stay relaxed
   Use activities to take your mind off worries
   Get plenty of sleep
   Use relaxation techniques
   Have some fun in every day

do not maintain exercise programs following completion of a pulmonary rehabilitation program, it is especially important that they view an active lifestyle as sustaining of their functional capacities.

Relaxation and Assertiveness Training

Keys to enacting energy conservation principles are assertiveness and the ability to manage stress. Interpersonal relationships become complicated by disability and needs for assistance. Assertiveness training encompasses (a) validation of the patient's worth and right to express needs and opinions, (b) understanding the importance of honest and clear communication, and (c) skill training with the timing, words, and body language of assertive communication. Group settings offer role play opportunities, for example, telling someone their perfume is problematic. Ideally, practice of communication skills occurs with important others who are present for treatment.

Persons with lung disease often suffer from anxiety and may benefit from relaxation training.[62] Like assertiveness training, the occupational therapist first affirms the patient's right to relaxation and a sense of inner peace and points out the benefits of relaxation to performance and well-being. Techniques of relaxation include guided imagery, muscle relaxation, and breathing. Many disciplines teach relaxation and stress management. When the occupational therapist teaches or reinforces these techniques, the focus is on enabling the patient to engage in important daily life routines and occupations.

Assistive Devices

Assistive devices that enable physical performance can vary from simple long-handled shoe horns to complex computerized environmental control systems. Assistive devices such as calendar systems and computers can also augment cognitive performance. Bombarded with advertisements for energy-saving devices of varying quality, many patients have grown enamored of them, whereas others are put off. The occupational therapist's expertise in assistive devices can guide patients to make wise consumer decisions about which items will in fact be useful. The occupational therapist considers small differences in weight, size, grip, or the actual functioning of particular devices that can greatly alter their utility given a particular person's abilities and limitations. Also considered are subtle problems in motor planning, visual perception, learning ability, and frustration tolerance that can significantly influence a patient's capability with various devices. Symbolic meanings that assistive devices can hold are additionally important to regard. To one person, a reacher may be seen as a stigmatizing sign of personal weakness or incompetence; to another, it may symbolize mastery over disabilities. The occupational therapist further considers the patient's tolerance for using gadgets, for storing gadgets in their homes, and, of course, financial resources for purchasing gadgets. In summary, physical, psychologic, and cognitive capacities relative to personal preference and financial resources guide recommendations of assistive devices.

Activity and Environmental Modification

Table 13-7 offers a variety of specific suggestions to improve performance and safety for sample activities. Activity-specific recommendations incorporate energy conservation principles, environmental modification, assistive devices, and alternative techniques. Because patients vary in the amount of guidance needed to select and implement effective strategies, these suggestions should not be taken as a one-size-fits-all approach. For patients who need guidance, the occupational therapist collaborates with the patient and important other to target modifications that are both doable and personally acceptable, minimizing frustrating trial and error.

Therapeutic Groups

One distinct advantage of working in medical facilities is that of being able to offer therapeutic groups to patients with pulmonary disorders. Occupational therapists have used therapeutic groups as a cornerstone of treatment since the early 1900s.[83] Therapeutic groups are excellent vehicles for assessment and intervention, as well as for building support and sharing information among patients. Groups are often experienced as more fun and interesting for participants than are individual sessions.[25] When participants discuss problems of daily living with one another, they can receive empathy and praise for their clever adaptations from those with firsthand knowledge. Strategies suggested by peers and sanctioned by occupational therapists also seem more doable and legitimate. Moreover, groups are excellent vehicles for combining didactic information with immediate experiential learning (Fig. 13-4).

In creating therapeutic groups, it is important that occupational therapists distinguish between treating aggregates of people together in a group from groups that are truly therapeutic. Groups become therapeutic when the dynamics of the group process are advantageously exploited to promote learning and greater functional capacities. Therapist-led groups place patients in relatively passive and subservient roles, violate principles of adult learning, and are not therapeutic groups; therefore, they are not recommended for use. In contrast, in therapeutic groups, the occupational therapist plays a facilitative role, one that encourages interaction and exchange of information among group members. In so doing, the therapist validates the importance of continued involvement in peer networks for learning and support after discharge.

In constructing a group, it is useful to attend to issues of group membership. Although effective groups can vary in size from 3 to 12 members, 7 or 8 members offer an ideal balance of richness and manageability. Family members and important others should be encouraged to attend groups. Groups may consist of particular ages or stages of disease. Children with asthma, older adults, or individuals awaiting lung transplant may be able to relate better to others in similar circumstance. However, groups that effectively mix these populations can offer rich intergenerational support, hope, and wisdom.

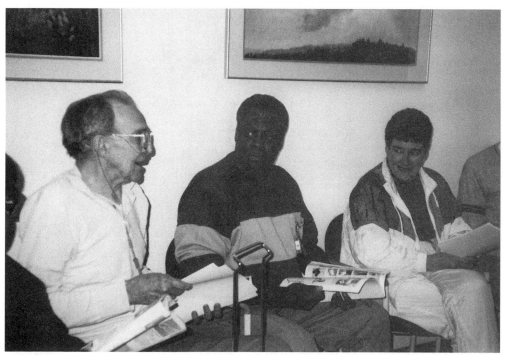

Figure 13-4. A daily living group involving patients and caregivers provides a context for support and mutual learning.

Table 13-7. Modifications for Specific Activities

Activity	Modifications	Prevention and Safety
Showering	Plan ahead by collecting all materials before starting; select a time when energy is high and ample time is available for the activity	Use chair, grab bars, and nonskid surface to prevent falls
	Minimize steam by using a well-ventilated room with an exhaust fan, avoiding very hot water, and turning on cold water first	Avoid getting into the tub unless someone is available to help with getting out
	Use assistive devices such as a shower chair, hand held shower head, long bath sponge, and soap on a rope; occupational therapists recommend specific types of shower chairs and grab bar locations for the individual	Emergency call system for problems
	Minimize effort for drying by use of a heat lamp, absorbent bathrobe, and slippers	
Dressing	Collect clothing in advance, possibly the evening before	Avoid rushing by allowing sufficient time to dress
	Sit to dress, in a chair with arms and a firm back	Put on all lower body clothing up to the knees, then stand up once to pull up over hips and fasten; if someone assists you to stand, this will save time
	Have any assistive devices used kept near the dressing location	
	Dress in segments, first upper body (rest), lower body (rest), then accessories	
	Set a comfortable room temperature; avoid chill by remaining covered, or replace one clothing item at a time	
	Use easy-to-manage clothing, e.g., slip-on or velcro shoes, loose socks, stretch or sweat pants, front button or loose pullover shirts and sweaters, loose-fitting dress, clip-on tie, a cape instead of a coat	
	Minimize fastener frustration: use velcro, elastic, zippers, large buttons	
	Use assistive devices: dressing stick, reacher, long-handled shoehorn, elastic shoelaces, sock aid	
Job	Modify work schedule, location, tasks, or equipment	Identify a job that offers flexibility of hours and allows for graded tasks
	Develop skills in areas for employment that require less physical activity	Find work that is satisfying and mentally challenging
	Increase value to employer and colleagues by identifying one's unique and creative contributions to the work setting	Develop collegial relationships that promote effective interdependence and helpfulness
	Utilize rights granted under the Americans with Disabilities Act (1990), which requires employers make reasonable accommodations for workers with identified disabilities	

Table 13-7 (*continued*)

Activity	Modifications	Prevention and Safety
Shopping	Prepare a shopping list arranged by the order in which items are found in the store	Stores are increasingly aware of the needs of older and disabled shoppers; get to know local retail personnel so that they will know your needs
	Use a shopping cart or motorized scooter	
	Shop frequently for fewer items or have assistance managing bags to the car and into the house	
	Have grocery bags packed with items to be refrigerated or frozen together so that they can be put away at home first, allowing a rest before the other bags need unpacking	Be aware of your rights under the Americans with Disabilities Act for access to public services
	Have bags packed light	
	Buy items in smaller containers and condensed forms such as frozen juice	
	Shop at times when the stores are not crowded and lines are short	
Golf	Plan optimal time of day based on energy level and congestion at the golf course	Have a call system if out alone
	Use assistive devices: gold cart, wheeled club carrier	
	Hire a caddy	
	Find a course with rest benches	
	Play every other hole or 9 holes	
	Have partner drive the ball and you putt	
Sexual intercourse	Identify times when rested, relaxed, and not hurried	Recognize that all individuals are sexual beings and accept one's desires for intimacy and sexual engagement
	Set temperature, ventilation, and humidity for comfort	
	Have an empty stomach	
	Use pillows for support	Seek information about any sexual restrictions that may apply to medical condition
	Position for minimal energy expenditure, such as side lying	
	Avoid positions that put pressure on chest or diaphragm	Open dialog between sexual partner about desires, physical limitations, and strategies for engaging in intercourse
	Maintain some awareness of breathing patterns so strategies can be used as needed, trying not to let that conscious attention to breathing detract from sexual engagement	Recognize that the respiratory rate may increase with sexual response

Two types of therapeutic groups used by the authors are recommended: (*a*) daily living groups that focus on problematic aspects of daily living, and (*b*) occupational project groups. In *daily living groups,* participants identify their most problematic aspects of daily living. Identified problems can be written on a board to help the group select priorities for discussion. Subsequent discussion addresses each problem activity, acknowledging psychosocial and physical issues and generating lists of solutions that participants have used. The occupational therapist facilitates this discussion by ensuring inclusion of all participants, endorsing key responses, and adding new information as appropriate. Following discussion, experiential learning on breathing strategies, relaxation, energy conservation, or adaptive equipment usage is undertaken. These mini-lessons can be led by the occupational therapist or a patient participant. Ideally, such learning is undertaken relative to the demands (actual or as closely simulated as possible) of problematic activities just discussed. Once problem areas have been addressed through informal sharing and experiential learning, the occupational therapist summarizes key principles generated by participants. Principles of energy conservation, such as planning ahead, using equipment, and sitting to work, often top the list. It is often useful at this point to provide a handout on these principles mentioning how many were generated by the group. The focus is shifted to how these principles can be generalized to new occupations and situations. Participants are given resources to obtain equipment, services, or support groups. In closing, participants are commended for their independent problem-solving and willingness to engage in the process of peer learning and support.

The aforementioned sequence is offered as a general guideline, as each therapeutic group is of course unique. A group may need to spend considerable time on a key issue, such as how to explain an invisible disability to others, the importance of having fun each day, or coping with anxiety. The occupational therapist must trust the group's ability to identify the most salient topics, facilitating a positive, problem-solving atmosphere. Participants may also vary a great deal in the amount of personal information they are comfortable sharing. Some may find the group a safer context for disclosing difficulties compared with individual sessions. Although it should not be assumed that verbal engagement is an indicator of learning, it is wise to follow up after the group with persons who seem particularly quiet, angry, or sad. Subsequent individual sessions can be arranged for patients whose questions and problems cannot be addressed sufficiently in the group format. Issues that arise in the group can be shared with the interdisciplinary team to learn how to best assist the patient.

Occupational project groups are organized, as the name suggests, around an occupational project of the group's choosing. An effective format is to have projects that are 1 week in duration. In these groups, participants decide on a fairly substantial project—usually involving travel outside of the health care facility—that will be planned, enacted, and then reviewed over the course of six consecutive group sessions. An important part of the projects is their inclusion of family and important others as well as access to the community. For example, completed weeklong occupational projects have included organizing a food drive for a local homeless shelter, putting on a magic show for family and hospital staff, organizing a potluck dinner for family and important others, shopping in malls, eating at restaurants, and visiting flea markets and museums. In a 6-day a week schedule, these projects were determined on a Monday, planned for Tuesday through Thursday, enacted on Friday, and reviewed on Saturday. Tasks related to the project address individual treatment goals and can be carried over into individual therapy sessions. For example, preparing a food item for the potluck meal becomes a vehicle for learning energy conservation and breathing strategies. Tasks can also consist of "practice homework" outside of therapy sessions, as when patients make phone calls to determine distance demands of the upcoming event or work on pursed lips breathing when posting flyers announcing the event. Typically, the event itself requires a longer session and, in the authors' experiences, is especially rich—for patients and therapists alike—when it involves multiple members of the interdisciplinary team.

Documentation of Intervention

Whether describing short- or long-term goals, narrative accounts of responses to intervention, or functional status at discharge, requires documentation of occupational therapy services at the level of occupational performance, and not impairments. Accordingly, relevant physiologic, musculoskeletal, or cognitive impairments as manifested in, say, dyspnea, heart rate, oxygen saturation levels, range of motion, or problem-solving skills are objectively described in context of occupational performance. As importantly, with regard to documenting functional status in the ICIDH-2[1] dimensions of activity and participation are (*a*) adaptive strategies or modified activity approaches that promote performance of valued activities, (*b*) environmental adaptations that reduce the physical demands of valued activities, (*c*) occupational plans that enable a richer round of personally satisfying activities, (*d*) social influences on occupational performance, and (*e*) subjective experiences of occupational performance.

SUMMARY

The purpose of occupational therapy in pulmonary rehabilitation is to help persons learn how to do the necessary and also spirit-enhancing occupations of their lives in ways that promote greater functional capacities and life satisfaction. Occupational therapists thus strive to improve function in ways that directly enhance HRQL. A multidimensional functional assessment determines status with regard to the dimensions of social participation, activity performance, and body functions and structure. To obtain outcomes of improved participation in meaningful life occupations, individualized programs of lifestyle redesign then target the particular occupational issues and concerns of individual patients and their important others. As the link between health and participation in meaningful occupations becomes clearer, occupational therapists will increase in availability and visibility on comprehensive pulmonary rehabilitation teams.[84]

REFERENCES

1. International Classification of Functioning and Disability (ICIDH-2). Beta-2: draft for field trials: full version, July 1999. Available at: http://www.who.int/icidh/.
2. Clark F, Wood W, Larson E. Occupational science: occupational therapy's legacy for the 21st century. In: Neistadt ME, Crepeau EB, eds. Willard and Spackman's Occupational Therapy. 9th ed. Philadelphia: Lippincott-Raven, 1998:13.
3. Jackson J, Carlson M, Mandel D, et al. Occupation in lifestyle redesign: the well elderly study occupational therapy program. Am J Occup Ther 1998;52:326.
4. Muldoon MF, Barger SD, Flory JD, et al. What are quality of life measurements measuring? BMJ 1998;316:542.
5. Robnett RH, Gliner JA. Qual-OT: a quality of life assessment tool. Occup Ther J Res 1995;15:198.
6. Jette A. Using health-related quality of life measures in physical therapy outcomes research. Phys Ther 1993;73:528.
7. Ries AL, Carlin BW, Carrieri-Kohlman V, et al. Pulmonary rehabilitation: joint ACCP/AACVPR evidence-based guidelines. J Cardiopulm Rehabil 1997;17:371–405.

8. Rodrigues JC, Ilowite JS. Pulmonary rehabilitation in the elderly patient. Clin Chest Med 1993; 14:429.
9. Rashbaum I, Whyte N. Occupational therapy in pulmonary rehabilitation: energy conservation and work simplification techniques. Phys Med Rehabil Clin N Am 1996;7:325.
10. Clark F, Azen S, Zemke R, et al. Occupational therapy for independent-living older adults: a randomized controlled study. JAMA 1997;278: 1321.
11. Yerxa E. Health and the human spirit for occupation. Am J Occup Ther 1998;52:412
12. Hasselkus E. Occupation and well-being in dementia: the experience of day care staff. Am J Occup Ther 1998;52:423.
13. Jackson J. The value of occupation as the core of treatment: Sandy's experience. Am J Occup Ther 1998;52:466.
14. Kane RA, Caplan AL, Urv-Wong EK, et al. Everyday matters in the lives of nursing home residents: wish for and perception of choice and control. J Am Geriatr Soc 1997;45:1093
15. Browne JP, Hannah MM, O'Boyle CA. Conceptual approaches to the assessment of quality of life. Psychol Health 1997;12:737.
16. Radomski MV. Nationally speaking: there is more

to life than putting on your pants. Am J Occup Ther 1995;49:487.

17. DeJong B. Independent living: from social movement to analytic paradigm. Arch Phys Med Rehabil 1979;60:435.

18. American Occupational Therapy Association (AOTA). Uniform terminology for occupational therapy. Am J Occup Ther 1994;48:1047.

19. Rogers JC, Holm MB. Evaluation of occupational performance areas. In: Neistadt ME, Crepeau EB, eds. Willard and Spackman's Occupational Therapy. 9th ed. Philadelphia: Lippincott, 1998:185.

20. Fenton S, Gagnon P. Evaluation of work and productive activities: work performance assessment measures. In: Neistadt ME, Crepeau EB, eds. Willard and Spackman's Occupational Therapy. 9th ed. Philadelphia: Lippincott, 1998:208.

21. Fenton S, Kraft W. Evaluation of work and productive activities: components of a therapeutic driving evaluation. In: Neistadt ME, Crepeau EB, eds. Willard and Spackman's Occupational Therapy. 9th ed. Philadelphia: Lippincott, 1998:213.

22. Knox S. Evaluation of play and leisure. In: Neistadt ME, Crepeau EB, eds. Willard and Spackman's Occupational Therapy. 9th ed. Philadelphia: Lippincott, 1998:215.

23. Law M. Client-Centered Occupational Therapy. Thorofare, NJ: Slack, 1998.

24. Egan M, Dubouloz CJ, von Zweck C, et al. The client-centred, evidence-based practice of occupational therapy. Can J Occup Ther 1998;65:136.

25. Scanlan M, Kishbaugh L, Horne D. Life management skill in pulmonary rehabilitation. In: Hodgkin JE, Connors JL, Bell CW, eds. Pulmonary Rehabilitation: Guidelines to Success. 2nd ed. Philadelphia: Lippincott, 1993:246.

26. Fisher AG, McGrath M. Nationally speaking: improving functional assessment in occupational therapy: recommendations and philosophy for change. Am J Occup Ther 1993;43:199.

27. Mathiowetz V. Role of physical performance component evaluations in occupational therapy functional assessment. Am J Occup Ther 1993;47:225.

28. Trombly CA. The issue is: anticipating the future: assessment of occupational function. Am J Occup Ther 1993;47:253.

29. Baum C. Client-centred practice in a changing health care system. In: Law M, ed. Client-Centred Occupational Therapy. Thorofare, NJ: Slack, 1998:29.

30. Fearing VG, Clark J, Stanton S. The client-centred occupational therapy process. In: Law M, ed. Client-Centred Occupational Therapy. Thorofare, NJ: Slack, 1998:67

31. Trombly CA. Occupation: purposefulness and meaningfulness as therapeutic mechanisms:1995 Eleanor Clarke Slagle lecture. Am J Occup Ther 1995;49:960.

32. Callahan J. Don't Worry: He Won't Get Far on Foot. New York: Vintage Books, 1989.

33. Klein BS. Slow dance: a story of stroke, love and disability. Knopf Canada, 1997.

34. Murphy RF. The Body Silent. New York: Henry Holt, 1987

35. Law M, Baptiste S, Carswell A, et al. Canadian Occupational Performance Measure Manual. 2nd ed. Toronto, Canada: CAOT Publications ACE, 1994.

36. Coster WJ, Deeny T, Haltiwanger J, et al. The School Function Assessment: Standardized Version. Boston: Boston University, 1998.

37. Coster W. Occupation-centered assessment of children. Am J Occup Ther 1998;52:337.

38. Jette AM, Davies AR, Cleary PD, et al. The Functional Status Questionnaire: reliability and validity when used in primary care. J Intern Med 1986;1:143.

39. Mosey AC. Activities Therapy. New York: Raven, 1973.

40. Phillips MA. A subjective ADL rating scale for the pulmonary patient. In: Occupational Therapy for the Energy Deficit Patient. New York: Haworth Press, 1986;1:79.

41. Pomerantz P, Flannery EL, Findling PK. Occupational therapy for chronic obstructive lung disease. Am J Occup Ther 1975;29:407.

42. Corcoran M, Gitlin L. The role of the physical environment in occupational performance. In: Occupational Therapy: Enabling Function and Well-being. Thorofare: NJ: Slack, 1997:336.

43. Hasselkus B. Ethical dilemmas in family caregiving for the elderly: implications for occupational therapy. Am J Occup Ther 1991;45:206.

44. McColl MA. Social support and occupational therapy. In: Occupational Therapy: Enabling Function and Well-being. Thorofare, NJ: Slack, 1997:410.

45. Kohlmeyer K. Evaluation of sensory and neuromuscular performance components. In: Neistadt ME, Crepeau EB, eds. Willard and Spackman's Occupational Therapy. 9th ed. Philadelphia: Lippincott, 1998:223.

46. Atchison B. Cardiopulmonary diseases. In: Trombly CA, ed. Occupational Therapy for Physical Dysfunction. 4th ed. Baltimore: Williams & Wilkins, 1995:875.

47. Brannon FJ, Foley MW, Starr JA, et al. Cardiopulmonary Rehabilitation: Basic Theory and Application. 2nd ed. Philadelphia: FA Davis, 1993.

48. Trombly CA. Cardiopulmonary rehabilitation. In: Trombly CA, ed. Occupational Therapy for Physical Dysfunction. 3rd ed. Baltimore: Williams & Wilkins, 1989.

49. Crepeau EB. Activity analysis: a way of thinking about occupational performance. In: Neistadt ME, Crepeau EB, eds. Willard and Spackman's Occupational Therapy. 9th ed. Philadelphia: Lippincott, 1998:135.

50. Minor MA. Promoting health and physical fitness. In: Christianson C, Baum C, eds. Occupational Therapy: Enabling Function and Well-being. Thorofare, NJ: Slack, 1997:256–287.

51. Berry MJ, Walschalger SA. Exercise training and chronic obstructive pulmonary disease: past and future research directions. J Cardiopulm Rehabil 1998;18:181.

52. Celli BR. The clinical use of upper extremity exercise. Clin Chest Med 1994;15:339.

53. Boissoneau CA. Breath of life: occupational therapy with ventilator assisted and pulmonary pa-

tients in a rehabilitation program. OT Practice 1997;July:28.

54. Hogan BM. Pulse oximetry for an adult with a pulmonary disorder. Am J Occup Ther 1994; 49:1062.

55. Borg GA. Psychophysical bases of perceived exertion. Med Sci Sports Exerc 1982;14:377.

56. Guide for the Uniform Data Set for Medical Rehabilitation (Adult FIM) Version 4.0. Buffalo, NY: State University of New York at Buffalo, 1993.

57. Msall ME, DiGaudio K, Duffy LC, et al. WeeFIM: normative sample of an instrument for tracking functional independence in children. Clin Pediatr 1994;44:431.

58. Fisher A. The assessment of instrumental activities of daily living motor skill: an application of the many-faceted Rasch analysis. Am J Occup Ther 1993;47:319.

59. Christiansen C, Baum C. Occupational performance assessment. In: Christiansen C, Baum C, eds. Enabling Function and Well-being. Thorofare, NJ: Slack, 1997:105.

60. Health Care Financing Administration. Medical review of part B intermediary outpatient occupational therapy (OT) bills. Washington, DC: US Government Printing Office, 1989. DHHS transmittal No. 1424.

61. Connors GL, Hilling LR, Morris KV. Assessment of the pulmonary candidate. In: Hodgkin JE, Connors JL, Bell CW, eds. Pulmonary Rehabilitation: Guidelines to Success. 2nd ed. Philadelphia: Lippincott, 1993:50.

62. Walsh LR. Occupational therapy as part of a pulmonary rehabilitation program. In: Occupational Therapy for the Energy Deficit Patient. New York: Haworth Press, 1986;1:65.

63. Bowyer SL, LaMothe ML, Hollister JR. Steroid myopathy: incidence and detection in a population with asthma. J Allergy Clin Immunol 1985; 76:234.

64. Strunk RE, Mascia AV, Lipkowitz MA, et al. Rehabilitation of a patient with asthma in the outpatient setting. J Allergy Clin Immunol 1991; 87:601.

65. McGavin CR, Gupta SP, McHardy GJR. Twelve-minute walking test for assessing disability in chronic bronchitis. BMJ 1976;1:822.

66. Fisher A. Uniting practice and theory in an occupational framework: 1998 Eleanor Clark Slagle lecture. Am J Occup Ther 1998;52:509.

67. Lin K, Wu C, Tickle-Degnan L, et al. Enhancing occupational performance through occupationally embedded exercise: a meta-analytic review. Occup Ther J Res 1997;17:25.

68. McClaughlin Grey J, Kennedy B, Zemke R. Dynamic systems theory: an overview. In: Zemke R,

Clark F, eds. Occupational Science: The Evolving Discipline. Philadelphia: FA Davis, 1996.

69. Dunn AL, Marcus BH, Kampert JB, et al. Comparison of lifestyle and structured interventions to increase physical activity and cardiorespiratory fitness. JAMA 1999;281:327.

70. Pasek P, Schkade S. Effects of a skiing experience on adolescents with limb deficiencies: an occupational adaptation perspective. Am J Occup Ther 1996;50:24.

71. McLaughlin Gray J. Putting occupation into practice: occupation as ends, occupation as means. Am J Occup Ther 1998;52:354.

72. Lee B, Nantais T. Use of electronic music as an occupational therapy modality in spinal cord rehabilitation: an occupational performance model. Am J Occup Ther 1996;50:362.

73. Clark F. Occupation embedded in real life: interweaving occupational science and occupational therapy: 1993 Eleanor Clarke Slagle lecture. Am J Occup Ther 1993;47:1067.

74. Mattingly C. The narrative nature of clinical reasoning. Am J Occup Ther 1991;45:998.

75. Law MR, Wald NJ, Meade TW. Strategies for prevention of osteoporosis and hip fracture. BMJ 1991;303:453–459.

76. Holm MB, Rogers JC, Stone RG. Person-task environment interventions: decision-making guide. In: Neistadt ME, Crepeau EB, eds. Willard and Spackman's Occupational Therapy. 9th ed. Philadelphia: Lippincott, 1998:471.

77. Wood W, guest ed. Special issue: occupation-centered practice and education. Am J Occup Ther 1998;52:313–496.

78. Pierce D. The issue is: what is the source of occupation's treatment power?. Am J Occup Ther 1998;52:490.

79. Breslin EH. The pattern of respiratory muscle recruitment during pursed-lips breathing in COPD. Chest 1992;101:75.

80. Breslin EH. Breathing retraining in chronic obstructive pulmonary disease. J Cardiopulm Rehabil 1995;15:25.

81. Berzins GF. An occupational therapy program for the chronic obstructive pulmonary disease patient. Am J Occup Ther 1970;24:81.

82. Ludwig FM. The unpackaging of routine in older women. Am J Occup Ther 1998;52:168.

83. Schwartzberg SL. Group process. In: Neistadt ME, Crepeau EB, eds. Willard and Spackman's Occupational Therapy. 9th ed. Philadelphia: Lippincott, 1998:120.

84. Glass TA, Mendes de Leon C, Marottoli RA, et al. Population based study of social and productive activities as predictors of survival among elderly Americans. BMJ 1999;319:478–483.

14 Nutritional Assessment and Support

A.M.W.J. Schols
E.F.M. Wouters

▷ Professional Skills

Upon completion of this chapter, the reader will:
- Know how to assess nutritional status in chronic obstructive pulmonary disease (COPD)
- Know the effects of nutritional depletion in COPD on functional performance, morbidity, and mortality
- Have insight into the causes of a negative energy balance in COPD
- Discuss the various strategies to improve nutritional status in COPD

INTRODUCTION

The association between weight loss and COPD has been recognized since the late 19th century. In the 1960s, several studies already reported that a low body weight and weight loss are negatively associated with survival in COPD.[1] Nevertheless, therapeutic management of weight loss and muscle wasting in patients with COPD has gained interest only recently because it was generally considered to be a terminal progression in the disease process and therefore inevitable and irreversible. Furthermore, weight loss has even been suggested as an adaptive mechanism to decrease oxygen consumption. Recent studies have challenged this attitude and showed that weight loss and a low body weight are associated with poor prognosis independent of, or at least not closely correlated with, the degree of lung function impairment.[2,3] Moreover, weight gain after nutritional support was associated with decreased mortality.[4]

The renewed interest in nutritional support as therapy in COPD runs parallel to changing concepts in the disease management not only predominantly aiming at the primary organ failure but also at the systemic consequences of the disease, including nutritional depletion.

RATIONALE FOR NUTRITIONAL SUPPORT

The most prominent symptoms of COPD are dyspnea and an impaired exercise capacity. During the past 10 years, research has shown that besides airflow obstruction and loss of alveolar structure, skeletal muscle weakness is an important determinant of these symptoms.[5] Recent studies have shown that peripheral skeletal muscle dysfunction is predominantly determined by skeletal muscle mass in COPD.[6,7]

Besides effects on peripheral skeletal muscle strength, several studies have also shown that body weight and particularly fat-free mass (FFM) as induced measures of muscle mass are significant determinants of exercise capacity and exercise response.[8-10] Patients with a depleted FFM were characterized by lower peak oxygen consumption and peak work rate and early onset of lactic acid compared with nondepleted patients. These findings suggest that the functional consequences of nutritional depletion not only relate to muscle wasting per se but also to alterations in muscle morphology and metabolism. Indeed, experimental studies and studies in other wasting conditions have shown that nutritional depletion causes generalized fiber atrophy but specifically decreases muscle fiber type II cross-sectional area.[11] Furthermore, altered levels of glycolytic and oxidative enzymes[11,12] and depletion of energy-rich substrates such as phosphocreatine and glycogen[13,14] have been described after nutritional depletion. It is furthermore clearly shown that nutritional depletion not only decreases peripheral muscle function but also affects respiratory muscle mass and strength.[15]

The functional consequences of being underweight and particularly of depletion of FFM are also reflected in a decreased health status as measured by the disease-specific St. Georges Respiratory Questionnaire.[16] Depletion of FFM is not only associated with weight loss but may also occur in normal-weight patients with a relatively increased fat mass.[17] Patients with depletion of FFM irrespective of body weight showed greater impairment in health status and quality of life compared with depleted patients with a relative preservation of FFM.[18]

Several studies using different COPD populations have now convincingly shown that a low body mass index (BMI) and weight loss are associated with an increased mortality risk.[2,4] Remarkably, overweight patients with moderate to severe COPD even have a lower mortality risk than normal-weight patients.[2,4] After adjustment for the effect of age, gender, lung function, smoking, and resting lung function, the increased mortality risk was found in patients with a BMI of less than 25 kg/m² (Fig. 14-1).[4] This could be related to the functional consequences of selective depletion of FFM in part of the patients but also to adverse effects of recent weight loss on other outcome measures. In this context it is interesting to note that recent weight loss is an important factor for outcome of acute

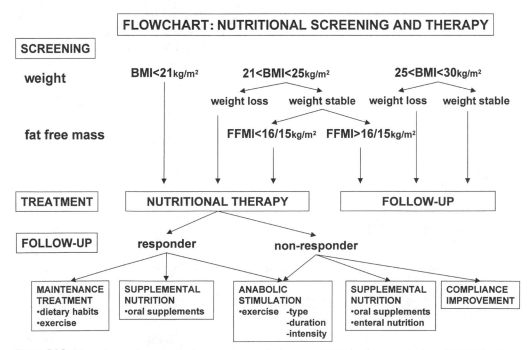

Figure 14-1. Flowchart of nutritional screening and therapy. *BMI,* body mass index; *FFMI,* fat-free mass index.

exacerbations as indicated by nonelective hospital readmission[19] and the need for and the outcome of mechanical ventilation.[20]

NUTRITIONAL ASSESSMENT

Based on the relationship between nutritional status and outcome, the following screening measures of nutritional status are recommended (Fig. 14-1).

Weight Indices

On the basis of the BMI, patients can be characterized as underweight, normal weight, and overweight. Underweight is normally defined as a BMI of less than 21 kg/m^2. In Caucasian people, this value is comparable to 90% of ideal body weight, based on the Metropolitan Life Insurance Tables. However, this value is rather arbitrary, and, according to recent recommendations, this cutoff point in elderly hospitalized patients should be extended to 24 kg/m^2.[21] Interestingly, this value strikingly corresponds to the increased mortality risk that was reported in patients with COPD and a BMI of less than 25 kg/m^2.

Weight Loss

Weight for height indices have limitations. Underweight patients are not necessarily in a poor nutritional status. This was illustrated by the fact that underweight patients with a relative preservation of FFM had a comparable muscle strength and exercise performance to normal-weight subjects with a normal FFM.[17] The adverse effects of involuntary weight loss, however, are well described, and progressive weight loss will ultimately lead to underweight and depletion of FFM. Therefore, recent involuntary weight loss should be considered in nutritional screening and follow-up. Commonly used criteria are weight loss of greater than 10% of usual body weight in the past 6 months or greater than 5% in the past month.

Body Composition

Weight is a rather global measure of nutritional depletion because it does not take body composition into consideration. Weight can be simply divided into fat mass and FFM. FFM consists of water (approximately 73%), protein, and minerals. Water is distributed intracellularly in the body cell mass and extracellularly. The largest single tissue of the body cell mass is muscle mass. In the absence of shifts between the water compartments, FFM is a useful measure of the body cell mass and thus of muscle mass. Depletion of FFM in COPD is defined as an FFM of less than 16 kg/m^2 in males and less than 15 kg/m^2 in females. This value is based on a linear gender-specific relationship between FFM and body weight (in the absence of obesity) using a cutoff point for BMI of 21 kg/m^2. Based on measurement of body weight and FFM, four groups of patients can be distinguished: (*a*) underweight and depletion of FFM, (*b*) underweight and relative preservation of FFM, (*c*) normal weight and depletion of FFM, and (*d*) normal weight and normal FFM.

Deuterium dilution and bioelectrical impedance analysis are relatively easy, noninvasive methods to assess FFM and have been used and validated extensively in COPD.[22,23] Dual-energy x-ray absorptiometry allows measurement of lean tissue mass, bone, and fat mass not only at the whole-body level but also at the various regions (trunk, arm, leg).[24] Biochemically, depletion of FFM is reflected in a decreased creatinine height index as calculated by the twenty-fourth urinary creatinine excretion of the patient divided by a reference value based on ideal body weight.[17]

In clinically stable patients with moderate to severe COPD, depletion of FFM has been reported in 20% of COPD outpatients[25] and in 35% of those eligible for pulmonary rehabilitation.[17] Limited data are available regarding the prevalence of nutritional depletion in representative groups of mild COPD as well as in patients with acute respiratory failure, although in the latter values up to 70% have been reported.[26] No clear relationship exists between measures of nutritional status and airflow obstruction, but weight loss and being underweight are associated with decreased diffusing capacity and are observed more frequently in emphysematous patients compared with those with chronic bronchitis.[6] The difference in body weight between the two COPD subtypes is merely a difference in fat mass. Depletion of FFM, despite a relative preservation of fat mass, also occurs in chronic bronchitis.[6]

CAUSES OF WEIGHT LOSS AND MUSCLE WASTING

To be able to judge the effectiveness of nutritional therapy as well as the optimal nutritional support strategy, insight is needed into the underlying mechanisms and contributing factors of overall weight loss and specific tissue wasting in COPD. Weight loss and in particular loss of fat mass occurs if energy expenditure exceeds dietary intake. More specifically, muscle wasting is a consequence of an inbalance between protein synthesis and protein breakdown. Alterations in both parts of the energy balance have been reported in COPD. Besides, increasing evidence points toward altered anabolic and catabolic mediators involved in the regulation of either protein synthesis or protein breakdown or both.

Energy Metabolism

Total daily energy expenditure (TDE) can be divided into different components. Basal metabolic rate is usually the largest component of TDE. Physical activity–induced thermogenesis can vary substantially between different individuals. Other components of TDE are diet-induced thermogenesis and components such as drug-induced thermogenesis and the thermoregular component. By gas exchange measurement of patients in awake, relaxed conditions after an overnight fast, it is now possible to conveniently measure so-called resting energy expenditure (REE). REE comprises the sleeping basal metabolic rate and the energy cost of arousal.

Based on the assumption that REE is the major component of TDE in sedentary persons, several studies have measured REE in COPD. After adjustment for the metabolically active FFM, REE was found to be elevated in COPD.[27] Although in healthy control subjects FFM could explain up to 84% of the individual variation in REE, this was only 43% in COPD patients.[28] Other factors, therefore, have been considered, such as work of breathing, hormone levels, drug therapy, and inflammation. A likely cause of the increased metabolic rate in COPD patients is increasing respiratory muscle work because the energy cost of increasing ventilation is higher in patients with advanced disease than in healthy controls of comparable age and gender. REE, however, correlates only weakly if all to individual or combinations of detailed lung function tests and blood gas values.[28] Thus, patients with the worst lung function, and in whom the work of breathing should be the highest, are not necessarily hypermetabolic. Nasal intermittent positive-pressure ventilation, which eliminates diaphragmatic and intercostal activity, did not reduce REE to normal in a group of hypermetabolic patients.[29] Furthermore, in COPD and in chest wall disease, airflow obstruction and oxygen cost of breathing were mutually related, but no correlation was found between oxygen cost of breathing and REE.[30]

Maintenance bronchodilating treatment for many patients consists of inhaled β-agonists. Two weeks of salbutamol increased REE by less than 8% in healthy males.[31] Acute inhalations of clinical doses of salbutamol, on the other hand, have been shown to increase REE in healthy subjects in a dose-dependent way up to 20%.[32] High doses of nebulized salbutamol are commonly administered during acute disease exacerbations. Nevertheless, no significant acute metabolic effects of this treatment were shown in elderly COPD patients compared with an age-matched control group.[33]

Another contributing factor of hypermetabolism may be related to inflammation. The polypeptide cytokine, tumor necrosis factor (TNF), is a proinflammatory mediator produced by different cell types. TNF inhibits lipoprotein lipase activity and is pyrogenic. It also triggers the release of other cytokines, which themselves mediate an increase in energy expenditure as well as mobilization of amino acids and muscle protein catabolism. Using different markers, several studies provided clear evidence for involvement of TNF-α–related systemic inflammation in the pathogenesis of tissue depletion. Elevated levels of TNF-α in (stimulated) plasma and of soluble TNF-receptors were found in patients with COPD,[34-36] particularly those with weight loss. Furthermore, several studies showed a relationship between TNF-α–related inflammation and resting metabolic rate.[37] Because diet-induced thermogenesis accounts only for 10% of total daily energy, expenditure will be small. Normal as well as increased diet-induced thermogenesis has been described in COPD patients.[38] Despite the methodologic difficulties in measuring TDE, recent studies focused attention on the activity-related energy expenditure in COPD patients. Using the doubly labeled water technique to measure TDE, it was demonstrated that COPD patients had a significantly higher TDE than did healthy subjects.[39] Remarkably, the nonresting component of TDE was significantly higher in the COPD patients than in the healthy subjects, resulting in a ratio between TDE and REE of 1.7 in COPD patients and 1.4 in healthy subjects. Otherwise, when TDE was measured in patients with COPD and in healthy persons in a respiration chamber, no differences in TDE were found between COPD patients and healthy persons, possibly by limitations of activities in the respiration chamber.[40] No difference in TDE between hypermetabolic and normometabolic COPD patients was found, and REE did not correlate significantly with TDE when FFM was taken into account.[41] The cause of an increased activity-related TDE is as yet unclear. It could be related to the observed decreased mechanical efficiency during leg exercise.[42] Part of this increased oxygen consumption during exercise can be explained by an inefficient ventilation in case of increased ventilatory demand, especially under conditions of dynamic hyperinflation. Furthermore, studies indicate a severely impaired oxidative phosphorylation during exercise in COPD, accompanied by an increased and highly anaerobic metabolism involving both the energy release from high-energy phosphate compounds as well as enhanced glucolysis.[43] Anaerobic metabolism is less efficient than aerobic metabolism.

Intermediary Metabolism

Besides an impaired oxidative phosphorylation during exercise, recent studies have shown alterations in resting cellular energy metabolism in peripheral muscle. A decrease in the activity of citrate synthase,[44] an increase in the glycolytic enzyme phosphofructokinase,[45] and (in hypoxemic patients) an increase in the activity and expression of cytochrome oxidase have been reported.[46] These enzymatic adaptations could indicate a shift toward a more glycolytic metabolism. At the substrate level, elevated muscular levels of lactic acid and pyruvate were shown to be associated in some circumstances with a decrease of muscle glycogen.[47] The functional consequences of these changes were reflected in alterations in adenosine nucleotide metabolism as reflected by a decreased plasma creatine/creatinine and detectable levels of inosine monophosphate, indicative of an imbalance between the use and resynthesis of adenosine triphosphate in resting muscle of patients with COPD.[48] It could be speculated that the observed changes in intracellular metabolites result in an increased overall energy metabolism. Limited data are available regarding possible alterations in substrate metabolism in COPD related to the overall and cellular energy metabolic state. On the muscular level, in addition to an altered energy state, alterations in the muscle amino acids profile have recently been described.[47,49] In contrast to the increased fat oxidation seen in other catabolic states, an increased use of carbohydrate was shown in depleted COPD patients compared with depleted patients without underlying lung disorders.[50] In severely hypoxemic COPD patients, an altered glucose metabolism was found that could not readily be explained by changes in glucoregulatory hormones or short-term alteration in oxygenation.[51] No evidence for insulin resistance is yet available.[52] Clearly, more data are needed, however, regarding substrate metabolism in well-defined subgroups of COPD based on the pattern and degree of tissue depletion, on the presence of tissue hypoxia, and perhaps also on the presence of systemic inflammation.

Dietary Intake

Hypermetabolism can explain why some COPD patients lose weight despite an apparent normal to even high dietary intake.[53] Nevertheless, it has been shown that dietary intake in weight-losing patients is lower than in weight-stable patients in absolute terms and in relation to measured REE.[54] This is remarkable because the normal adaptation to an increase in energy requirements in healthy men is an increase in dietary intake. The reasons for a relatively low dietary intake in COPD are not completely understood. It has been suggested that patients with COPD eat suboptimally because chewing and swallowing change their breathing pattern and decrease arterial oxygen saturation. Furthermore, gastric filling in these patients may reduce the functional residual capacity and lead to an increase in dyspnea. Intriguing is the role of leptin in energy homeostasis. This adipocyte-derived hormone represents the afferent hormonal signal to the brain in a feedback mechanism regulating fat mass. Besides, leptin has a regulating role in lipid metabolism and glucose homeostasis and increases thermogenesis. Furthermore, leptin has effects on T-cell–mediated immunity. Few data are reported on leptin metabolism in COPD. Circulating leptin correlates well with BMI and fat percentage as expected, but significantly lower values were observed compared with healthy subjects.[36] In experimental studies, administration of endotoxins or cytokines produced a prompt increase in serum leptin levels.[55] In COPD, one study also observed a relationship between leptin and soluble TNF-receptor 55, in particular in the emphysematous subtype. Leptin as well as soluble TNF-receptor 55 were in turn inversely related to dietary intake in absolute terms as well as adjusted for REE.[56] The exact regulation of leptin in COPD needs further explanation. Another factor of interest in evaluating dietary intake is the influence of psychologic dysfunctioning, such as anxiety, depression, and appetite. Although no systematic studies are available, limited physical abilities, financial constraints, and lack of supportive care should also be considered as factors that may interfere with dietary intake.

OUTCOME OF NUTRITIONAL INTERVENTION

Oral Nutritional Supplements

The first clinical trials to investigate the effectiveness of nutritional intervention consisted of nutritional supplementation by means of oral liquid supplements. All short-term studies (2–3 weeks)[57,58] showed a significant increase in body weight and respiratory muscle function. This short-term effectiveness is probably related partly to repletion of muscle water and potassium besides constitution of muscle protein nitrogen.[59] Only one study addressed the immune response to short-term nutritional intervention in nine patients with advance COPD.[60] Refeeding and weight gain were associated with a significant increase in absolute lymphocyte count and with an increase in reactivity to skin test antigens after 21 days of refeeding.

Significant improvements[61,62] in respiratory and peripheral skeletal muscle function but also in exercise capacity and health-related quality of life were observed in one inpatient and one outpatient study after 3 months of oral supplementation by about 1000 kcal daily. In other outpatient studies, however, despite a similar nutritional supplementation routine, the average weight gain was less than 1.5 kg in 8 weeks.[63-65] Besides noncompliance and biologic characteristics, the poor treatment response may be attributed at least partly to inadequate assessment of energy requirements and to the observation that the patients were taking supplements instead of their regular meals.

Despite the positive outcome of nutritional repletion in a controlled setting, the progressive character of weight loss in COPD demands appropriate feeding strategies to allow sustained outpatient nutritional intervention. To be able to provide a sufficient energy supply, the effect of an aggressive nutritional support regimen was studied in patients with severe COPD and weight loss not responding to oral supplementation.[66] During a prolonged interval of 4 months, nocturnal enteral nutrition support via percutaneous endoscopic gastrostomy tube was provided. The treated group had nightly enteral feeding adjusted to maintain a total daily caloric intake greater than two times the measured resting metabolic rate for sustained weight gain. Despite the magnitude of the intervention, a mean weight gain of only 3.3% (0.2 kg/week) was seen in the treated group. Weight gain seemed to be limited by the magnitude of the required caloric intake and by significant shifting of caloric intake between oral and enteral intake. Most of the increase in body weight was fat mass, and no significant improvement in physiologic function was observed. The limited therapeutic impact of isolated aggressive nutrition support could be related to the absence of a comprehensive rehabilitative strategy or to the fact that the selected patients were not only in a hypermetabolic state but also hypercatabolic.

Nutrition and Exercise

From a functional point of view it is obvious to combine nutritional support with exercise if possible. The effects of a daily nutritional supplement as an integrated part of a pulmonary rehabilitation program indeed resulted in significant weight gain (0.4 kg/week) despite a daily supplementation that was much less than in most previous outpatient studies.[67] The combined treatment of nutritional support and exercise not only increased body weight but also resulted in a significant improvement in FFM and respiratory muscle strength. The clinical relevance of treatment response was shown in a post hoc survival analysis of this study demonstrating that weight gain and increase in respiratory muscle strength were associated with significantly increased survival rates.[4] On Cox regression analysis weight gain during the rehabilitation period remained a significant predictor of mortality independent of baseline lung function and other risk factors, including age, sex, smoking, and resting arterial blood gases. In view of the ventilatory limitation and the experienced symptoms, exercise in most rehabilitation settings consists of general physical training, with emphasis on endurance exercise. Nutritional depletion, however, specifically impairs muscle strength. Studies in elderly subjects without pulmonary disease have shown that in particular strength training with nutritional support is superior to nutritional support alone in reaching an increase in FFM. No data are yet available regarding the effects of nutritional support and strength training in depleted patients with chronic respiratory disease.

TIMING AND NUTRITIONAL SUPPORT

Most studies have investigated the effects of nutritional supplementation in clinically stable patients. Anamnestic data, however, indicate that in some patients weight loss follows a stepwise pattern associated with acute (infectious) exacerbations. During an acute exacerbation, energy balance is often temporarily negative owing to a further increase in REE but particularly owing to a temporarily dramatic decrease in dietary intake.[68] Furthermore, these patients may have an increased risk for protein breakdown that may limit the effectiveness of nutritional supplementation.[69] Factors contributing to weight loss and muscle wasting during an acute exacerbation include an increase in symptoms, more pronounced systemic inflammation, alterations in leptin metabolism, and the use of high doses of glucocorticoids. One study showed a positive effect of nutritional support during hospitalization for an acute exacerbation, but clearly more research is needed to evaluate the relative effectiveness of nutritional support during or immediately after an acute exacerbation.[69]

MACRONUTRIENT COMPOSITION OF NUTRITIONAL SUPPLEMENT

Carbohydrate/Fat

Most intervention strategies are directed to balance energy expenditure by administration of nutritional supplements. Meal-related dyspnea and limited ventilatory reserves, however, may restrict the quantity and composition of nutritional support in patients with respiratory disease. Nutrient administration is associated with an obligate increase in ventilation and metabolic rate. The composition of the caloric intake can influence carbon dioxide production and therefore ventilatory demand. The respiratory quotient (or ratio carbon dioxide production/oxygen consumption) of glucose oxidation equals 1. The respiratory quotient of fat oxidation is 0.71, indicating a lower ventilatory load by reduced carbon dioxide production. Excessive carbon dioxide production by carbohydrate administration was observed in mechanically ventilated patients.[70,71] However, these effects only occurred in cases of caloric overload. Under these circumstances, triglyceride biosynthesis can be expected. Several studies in clinically stable COPD patients have studied the effects of a carbohydrate-rich drink on functional capacity in the immediate postprandial period. Using a high-caloric, carbohydrate-rich supplement (920 kcal, 53% carbohydrates), several studies reported significantly greater increases in minute ventilation, carbon dioxide elimination, oxygen consumption, respiratory quotient, arterial carbon dioxide tension, and fatigue score, together with a greater fall in the distance walked compared with a fat-rich drink.[72,73] After a more physiologic energy load (500 kcal), no difference in postprandial exercise capacity was shown between a high- versus a low-fat supplement.[74] Contraindications also exist for a high-fat supplement. A meal with a high fat content resulted in a significant delay in gastric emptying compared with feeding a meal with moderate fat.[74] Clinical ramifications exist to delayed gastric emptying, especially in patients with COPD. Because of the disease process itself, such patients already suffer from hyperinflation, a flattened diaphragm, and a reduction in abdominal volume, which results in feelings of bloating, abdominal discomfort, and early satiety. A significant delay in gastric emptying may lead to an extended time of abdominal distention, impacting on diaphragmatic mobility and thoracic expansion. High-fat diets may also cause bloating, loose stools, or diarrhea and may thus create tolerance problems. This finding is in line with a preferential use of carbohydrates in COPD patients during the acute phase of hospitalization for an exacerbation.[68] Furthermore, meal-related oxyhemoglobin desaturation may limit caloric intake and contribute to meal-related dyspnea in some patients, primarily in those who are hypoxemic at rest.[75] The degree of desaturation seemed to depend on meal type, being significantly higher after a fat-rich warm meal compared with a carbohydrate-right "cold" meal.[75]

Protein

The effects of wasting disease on protein metabolism is characterized by net protein catabolism owing to differences between protein synthesis and breakdown rates. This is seen in a negative nitrogen balance. The emphasis with respect to protein requirements in disease must be on optimal rather than minimal amounts of dietary proteins. Unfortunately, a clear clinical or physiologic end point for the determination of optimal protein requirements is not available. Only studies documenting the effects of dietary protein content on nitrogen balance or on protein kinetics have been published in various conditions. The available data suggest that in healthy subjects and in stable disease, protein synthesis is optimally stimulated during administration of 1.5 g protein/kg per day. Similarly, although the catabolic effects of acute disease cannot be manipulated merely by nutrition, net protein catabolic rates in these conditions are lowest by administration of 1.5 to 2.0 g protein/day.[76] Administration of proteins exceeding this quantity results only in increased protein catabolism.

Anabolic Agents

The difficulties encountered in nutritional support have led investigators to study alternative methods, in particular adjuvant treatment with recombinant human growth hormone (rhGH). Administration of this hormone induces lipolysis, protein anabolism, and muscle growth, either directly or through insulin-like growth factor-1. Thus, rhGH administration has been shown to improve nitrogen balance in various clinical conditions. Two uncontrolled studies reported the effects of rhGH in nutritionally depleted patients with COPD. Administration of rhGH for 8 days (0.03 mg/kg per day subcutaneously for 4 days, plus 0.06 mg/kg per day for another 4 days) failed to increase respiratory and peripheral skeletal muscle strength in COPD.[77] In contrast, an increase in inspiratory muscle strength was reported after 3 weeks of treatment (0.05 mg/kg per day subcutaneously).[78] Using a similar treatment regimen, however, but in a placebo-controlled fashion, the effects of administration of rhGH on body composition, resting metabolic rate, and functional capacity in underweight COPD patients in a stable clinical state were studied.[79] Although FFM increased significantly during the 3 weeks of treatment, no improvement was seen in muscle function, and exercise capacity even decreased in the treatment group. Furthermore, a significant increase in resting metabolic rate was observed. The effects of anabolic steroids have also been investigated in COPD. Nutritional repletion in combination with supportive treatment with the anabolic steroid nandrolone decanoate (males: 50 mg intramuscularly every 2 weeks; females: 25 mg intramuscularly every 2 weeks) during 8 weeks was studied in patients engaged in an inpatient pulmonary rehabilitation program.[67] Despite a similar weight gain to the group receiving nutritional support only, measurements of body composition indicated a favorable distribution of the body weight gain toward a larger increase in FFM in the group additionally treated with a short course of anabolic steroids and a larger improvement in respiratory muscle strength. Further studies are needed to investigate the extra effects of the supportive treatment procedures on exercise performance and quality of life.

Anticatabolic Agents

Even in a controlled setting such as an inpatient rehabilitation center, part of the patients do not respond to nutritional therapy. Besides noncompliance to therapy, an inadequate energy intake relative to energy requirements, and the inability of patients to ingest the extra calories, inadequate metabolic handling may contribute. The interaction between nutritional depletion and systemic inflammation has drawn attention to the potential beneficial effects of anticatabolic agents, in particular modulation of the inflammatory response. Several agents, such as n-3 fatty acids and nonsteroidal anti-inflammatory agents, have been investigated in other wasting conditions, such as human immunodeficiency virus, cancer, and sepsis. This may be an interesting therapeutic alternative for some patients with COPD because those exhibiting insignificant weight gain after nutritional support and anabolic stimulation (exercise, anabolic steroids) were characterized by an elevated systemic inflammatory response, as reflected by enhanced levels of soluble TNF-receptors, circulating leptin, and acute-phase proteins.[56,80]

PRACTICAL IMPLEMENTATION OF NUTRITIONAL SUPPORT

Based on the current insights into the relationship between nutritional depletion and outcome in COPD, a flowchart for nutritional screening and therapy is presented earlier in this chapter (Fig. 14-1). Simple screening can be performed based on repeated measurements of body weight. Patients are characterized by BMI (BMI = weight/height squared) and the presence or absence of involuntary weight loss. Nutritional supplementation is indicated for underweight patients (BMI < 21 kg/m²). Involuntary weight loss in patients with a BMI of less than 25 kg/m² should be monitored to assess whether it is progressive. If possible, measurement of FFM as an indirect measure of muscle mass may provide a more detailed screening of patients because this allows identification of normal-weight patients with a depleted FFM who, despite a normal body weight, should be considered for diet therapy.

Depending on the underlying cause of energy imbalance (decreased dietary intake or increased nutritional requirements), initial nutritional therapy may range from adaptations of the dietary behavior and food pattern followed by implementation of nutritional supplements. Nutritional support should be given as energy-dense supplements well divided during the day to avoid loss of appetite and adverse metabolic and ventilatory effects resulting from a high caloric load. When feasible, patients should be stimulated to follow an exercise program. For severely disabled cachectic patients who are unable to perform exercise training, even simple strength maneuvers combined with activities of daily living training and energy conservation techniques may be effective. Exercise not only improves the effectiveness of nutritional therapy but also stimulates appetite. After 4 to 8 weeks, therapy response can be determined. If weight gain and functional improvement are noted, the caregiver and the patient have to decide whether more improvement by a similar strategy is feasible or whether maintenance is the aim. It may then also be worthwhile to add or alter the exercise training program. If the desired response is not noted, it may be necessary to identify compliance issues. If compliance is not the problem, more calories may be needed by supplements or by enteral routes. Screening of nutritional status in relation to functional status can be done by the chest physician during hospitalization for an acute exacerbation or during outpatient follow-up. The chest physician can consult the dietitian for insight into the cause and treatment of impaired energy balance in weight-losing subjects and the physiotherapist for the type and intensity of an exercise program. The respiratory nurse or a nutrition therapist can play a valuable role in hospital and home care of patients with chronic lung disease during regular visits or telephone calls. They can monitor compliance and the weight course during diet therapy, give advice on meals and nutritional symptoms in the home setting to patient and family, and provide feedback to the other caregivers. Despite an optimal implementation of nutritional therapy as part of an integrated treatment approach to COPD, one should recognize that even then a subgroup of patients may not reach the intended effect because of underlying mechanisms of weight loss that are as yet unable to be reversed by merely caloric supplementation. Potential reversibility by means of specific nutrients (nutriceuticals) or pharmaceuticals will be a major focus of future research in this field.

REFERENCES

1. Vandenbergh E, Woestijne vdKP, Gyselen A. Weight changes in the terminal stages of chronic obstructive pulmonary disease. Am Rev Respir Dis 1967;95:556–566.
2. Wilson DO, Rogers RM, Wright EC, et al. Body weight in chronic obstructive pulmonary disease: the National Institutes of Health Intermittent Positive-Pressure Breathing Trial. Am Rev Respir Dis 1989;139:1435–1438.
3. Grey Donald K, Gibbons L, Shapiro SH, et al. Nutritional status and mortality in chronic obstructive pulmonary disease. Am J Respir Crit Care Med 1996;153:961–966.
4. Schols A, Slangen J, Volovics L, et al. Weight loss is a reversible factor in the prognosis of chronic obstructive pulmonary disease. Am J Respir Crit Care Med 1998;157(6):1791–1797.

5. ATS. Skeletal muscle dysfunction in chronic obstructive pulmonary disease: a statement on the American Thoracic Society and European Respiratory Society. Am J Respir Crit Care Med 1999; 159:S1–S40.

6. Engelen J, Schols A, Lamers R, et al. Different patterns of chronic tissue wasting among emphysema and chronic bronchitis patients. Clin Nutr 1999;18(5):275–280.

7. Bernard S, LeBlanc P, Whittom F, et al. Peripheral muscle weakness in patients with chronic obstructive pulmonary disease. Am J Respir Crit Care Med 1998;158:629–634.

8. Palange P, Forte S, Felli A, et al. Nutritional state and exercise tolerance in patients with COPD. Chest 1995;107:1206–1212.

9. Palange P, Forte S, Onorati P, et al. Effect of reduced body weight on muscle aerobic capacity in patients with COPD. Chest 1998;114:12–18.

10. Baarends EM, Schols AM, Mostert R, et al. Peak exercise response in relation to tissue depletion in patients with chronic obstructive pulmonary disease. Eur Respir J 1997;10:2807–2813.

11. Russell DM, Walker PM, Leiter LA, et al. Metabolic and structural changes in skeletal muscle during hypocaloric dieting. Am J Clin Nutr 1984;39:503–513.

12. Layman DK, Merdian Bender M, Hegarty PVJ, et al. Changes in aerobic and anaerobic metabolism in rat cardiac and skeletal muscles after total or partial dietary restrictions. J Nutr 1981;111: 994–1000.

13. Pichard C, Vaughan C, Struk R, et al. Effect of dietary manipulations (fasting, hypocaloric feeding, and subsequent refeeding on rat muscle energetics as assessed by nuclear magnetic resonance spectroscopy. J Clin Invest 1988;82:895–901.

14. Bissonnette DJ, Madapallimatiam A, Jeejeebhoy KN. Effect of hypoenergetic feeding and high-carbohydrate refeeding on muscle tetanic tension, relaxation rate, and fatigue in slow- and fast-twitch muscles in rats. Am J Clin Nutr 1997;66: 293–303.

15. Rochester DF, Braun NM. Determinants of maximal inspiratory pressure in chronic obstructive pulmonary disease. Am Rev Respir Dis 1985; 132:42–47.

16. Shoup R, Dalsky G, Warner S, et al. Body composition and health-related quality of life in patients with obstructive airway disease. Eur Respir J 1997;10:1576–1580.

17. Schols AMWJ, Soeters PB, Dingemans AMC, et al. Prevalence and characteristics of nutritional depletion in patients with stable COPD eligible for pulmonary rehabilitation. Am Rev Respir Dis 1993;147:1151–1156.

18. Goris A, Schols A, Weling-Scheepers C, et al. Tissue depletion in relation to physical function and quality of life in patients with severe COPD. Am J Respir Crit Care Med 1997;155(4):A498.

19. Pouw E, Ten Velde G, Croonen B, et al. Early nonelective readmission for chronic obstructive pulmonary disease is associated with weight loss. Clin Nutr 2000 (in press).

20. Vitacca M, Clini E, Porta R, et al. Acute exacerbations in patients with COPD: predictors of need

21. for mechanical ventilation. Eur Respir J 1996;9: 1487–1493.

21. Beck AM, Ovesen L. At which body mass index and degree of weight loss should hospitalized elderly patients be considered at nutritional risk? Clin Nutr 1998;17:195–198.

22. Schols A, Wouters EFM, Soeters PB, et al. Body composition by bioelectrical-impedance analysis compared with deuterium dilution and skinfold anthropometry in patients with chronic obstructive pulmonary disease. Am J Clin Nutr 1991; 53:421–424.

23. Baarends EM, Schols AMWJ, Van Marken Lichtenbeld WD, et al. Analysis of body water compartments in relation to tissue depletion in clinically stable patients with chronic obstructive disease. Am J Clin Nutr 1997;65:88–94.

24. Engelen MPKJ, Schols AMWJ, Heidendal GAK, et al. Dual-energy x-ray absorptiometry in the clinical evaluation of body composition and bone mineral density in patient with chronic obstructive pulmonary disease. Am J Clin Nutr 1998; 68(6):1298–1303.

25. Engelen MPKJ, Schols AMWJ, Baken WC, et al. Nutritional depletion in relation to respiratory and peripheral skeletal muscle function in out-patients with COPD. Eur Respir J 1994;7:1793–1797.

26. Fiaccadori E, Del Canale S, Coffrini E, et al. Hypercapnic-hypoxemic chronic obstructive pulmonary disease (COPD): influence of severity of COPD on nutritional status. Am J Clin Nutr 1988;48:680–685.

27. Fitting JW, Frascarolo P, Jequier E, et al. Resting energy expenditure in interstitial lung disease. Am Rev Respir Dis 1990;142:631–635.

28. Schols AM, Fredrix EW, Soeters PB, et al. Resting energy expenditure in patients with chronic obstructive pulmonary disease. Am J Clin Nutr 1991;554:983–987.

29. Hugli O, Schutz Y, Fitting JW. The cost of breathing in stable chronic obstructive pulmonary disease. Clin Sci Colch 1995;89:625–632.

30. Sridhar MK, Carter R, Lean MEJ, et al. Resting energy expenditure and nutritional state of patients with increased oxygen cost of breathing due to emphysema, scoliosis and thoracoplasty. Thorax 1994;49:781–785.

31. Wilson SR, Amoroso P, Moxham J, et al. Modification of the thermogenic effect of acutely inhaled salbutamol by chronic inhalation in normal subjects. Thorax 1993;48:886–889.

32. Amoroso P, Wilson SR, Moxham J, et al. Acute effects of inhaled salbutamol on the metabolic rate of normal subjects. Thorax 1993;48:882–885.

33. Creutzberg EC, Schols AM, Bothmer-Quaedvlieg FC, et al. Acute effect of nebulized salbutamol on resting energy expenditure in patients with chronic obstructive pulmonary disease and in healthy subjects. Respiration 1998;65:375–380.

34. De Godoy I, Donahoe M, Calhoun WJ, et al. Elevated TNF-alpha production by peripheral blood monocytes and weight-losing COPD patients. Am J Respir Crit Care Med 1996;153: 633–637.

35. Di Francia M, Barbier D, Mege JL, et al. Tumor necrosis factor-alpha levels and weight loss in

chronic obstructive pulmonary disease. Am J Respir Crit Care Med 1994;150:1453–1455.

36. Takabatake N, Nakamura H, Abe S, et al. Circulating leptin in patients with chronic obstructive pulmonary disease. Am J Respir Crit Care Med 1999;159(4):1215–1219.

37. Schols AMWJ, Buurman WA, Stall van der Brekel AJ, et al. Evidence for a relation between metabolic derangements and elevated inflammatory mediators in a subgroup of patients with chronic obstructive pulmonary disease. Thorax 1996; 51(8):819–824.

38. Hugli O, Frascarolo P, Schutz Y, et al. Total free living energy expenditure in patients with severe chronic obstructive pulmonary disease. Am Rev Respir Dis 1997;155:549–554.

39. Baarends EM, Schols AM, Pannemans DL, et al. Total free living energy expenditure in patients with severe chronic obstructive pulmonary disease. Am J Respir Crit Care Med 1997;155: 549–554.

40. Hugli O, Schutz Y, Fitting JW. The daily energy expenditure in stable chronic obstructive pulmonary disease. Am J Respir Crit Care Med 1996; 153:294–300.

41. Baarends EM, Schols AMWJ, Westerterb KR, et al. Total daily energy expenditure relative to resting energy expenditure in clinically stable patients with COPD. Thorax 1997;52:780–785.

42. Baarends, Schols A, Akkermans MA, et al. Decreased mechanical efficiency in clinically stable patients with COPD. Thorax 1997;52(11): 981–986.

43. Wuyam B, Payen JF, Levy P, et al. Metabolism and aerobic capacity of skeletal muscle in chronic respiratory failure related to chronic obstructive pulmonary disease [see comments]. Eur Respir J 1992;5:157–162.

44. Maltais F, Simard AA, Simard C, et al. Oxidative capacity of the skeletal muscle and lactic acid kinetics during exercise in normal subjects and in patients with COPD. Am J Respir Crit Care Med 1996;153:288–293.

45. Jakobsson P, Jorfeldt L, Henriksson J. Metabolic enzyme activity in the quadriceps femoris muscle in patients with severe chronic obstructive pulmonary disease. Am J Respir Crit Care 1995;151: 374–377.

46. Sauleda J, Garcia-Palmer F, Wiesner RJ, et al. Cytochrome oxidase activity and mitochondrial gene expression in skeletal muscle of patients with chronic obstructive pulmonary disease. Am J Respir Crit Care Med 1998;157:1413–1417.

47. Engelen M, Schols A, Does J, et al. Altered glutamate metabolism is associated with reduced muscle glutathione levels in patients with emphysema. Am J Respir Crit Care Med 2000;161(1):98–103.

48. Pouw EM, Schols AMWJ, Vusse vd GJ, et al. Elevated iosine monophosphate levels in resting muscle of patients with stable COPD. Am J Respir Crit Care Med 1998;157:453–457.

49. Pouw EM, Schols AM, Deutz NE, et al. Plasma and muscle amino acid levels in relation to resting energy expenditure and inflammation in stable chronic obstructive pulmonary disease. Am J Respir Crit Care Med 1998;158:797–801.

50. Goldstein SA, Thomashow BM, Kvetan V, et al. Nitrogen and energy relationships in malnourished patients with emphysema. Am Rev Respir Dis 1988;138:636–644.

51. Hjalmarsen A, Aasebo U, Kirkeland K, et al. Impaired glucose tolerance in patients with chronic hypoxic pulmonary disease. Diabetes Metab 1996;22:37–42.

52. Jakobsson P, Jorfeldt L, von Schenck H. Insulin resistance is not exhibited by advanced chronic obstructive pulmonary disease patients. Clin Physiol 1995;15:547–555.

53. Hunter AMB, Carey MA, Larsh HW. The nutritional status of patients with chronic obstructive pulmonary disease. Am Rev Respir Dis 1981; 124:376–381.

54. Schols AMWJ, Soeters PB, Mostert R, et al. Energy balance in chronic obstructive pulmonary disease. Am Rev Respir Dis 1991;143:1248–1252.

55. Grunfeld C, Zhao C, Fuller J, et al. Endotoxin and cytokines induce expression of leptin, the ob gene product, in hamsters. J Clin Invest 1996; 97:2152–2157.

56. Schols A, Creutzberg E, Buurman W, et al. Plasma leptin is related to pro-inflammatory status and dietary intake in patients with COPD. Am J Respir Crit Care Med 1999;160(4);1220–1226.

57. Wilson DO, Rogers RM, Sanders MH, et al. Nutritional intervention in malnourished patients with emphysema. Am Rev Respir Dis 1986;134: 672–677.

58. Whittaker JS, Ryan CF, Buckley PA, et al. The effects of refeeding on peripheral and respiratory muscle function in malnourished chronic pulmonary disease patients. Am Rev Respir Dis 1990; 142:283–288.

59. Russell DM, Prendergast PJ, Darby PL, et al. A comparison between muscle function and body composition in anorexia nervosa: the effect of refeeding. Am J Clin Nutr 1983;38:229–237.

60. Fuenzalada CE, Petty TL, Jones ML, et al. The immune response to short-term nutritional intervention in advanced chronic obstructive pulmonary disease. Am Rev Respir Dis 1990;142:49–56.

61. Rogers RM, Donahoe M, Constantino J. Physiologic effects of oral supplemental feeding in malnourished patients with chronic obstructive pulmonary diseases, a randomized control study. Am Rev Respir Dis 1992;146:1511–1517.

62. Efthimiou J, Fleming J, Gomes C, et al. The effect of supplementary oral nutrition in poorly nourished patients with chronic obstructive pulmonary disease. Am Rev Respir Dis 1988;137:1075–1082.

63. Otte KE, Ahlburg P, D'Amore F, et al. Nutritional repletion in malnourished patients with emphysema. JPEN J Parenter Enteral Nutr 1989;13: 152–156.

64. Knowles JB, Fairbarn MS, Wiggs BJ, et al. Dietary supplementation and respiratory muscle performance in patients with COPD. Chest 1988;93: 977–983.

65. Lewis MI, Belman MJ, Dorr Uyemura L. Nutritional supplementation in ambulatory patients

with chronic obstructive pulmonary disease. Am Rev Respir Dis 1987;135:1062–1067.

66. Donahoe M, Mancino J, Costatino J, et al. The effect of an aggressive support regimen on body composition in patients with severe COPD and weight loss. Am J Respir Crit Care Med 1994; 149 (abstract).

67. Schols AMWJ, Soeters PB, Mostert R, et al. Physiologic effects of nutritional support and anabolic steroids in patients with chronic obstructive pulmonary disease: a placebo-controlled randomized trial. Am J Respir Crit Care Med 1995;152:1268–1274.

68. Vermeeren MAP, Schols AMWJ, Quaedvlieg FCM, et al. The influence of an acute disease exacerbation on the metabolic profile of patients with chronic obstructive pulmonary disease. Clin Nutr 1994;13(Suppl 1):38–39.

69. Saudny Unterberger H, Martin JG, Gray Donald K. Impact of nutritional support on functional status during an acute exacerbation of chronic obstructive pulmonary disease. Am J Respir Crit Care Med 1997;156:794–799.

70. Talpers SS, Romberger DJ, Bunce SB, et al. Nutritionally associated increased carbon dioxide production: excess total calories vs high proportion of carbohydrate calories. Chest 1992;102:551–555.

71. Askanazi J, Elwyn DH, Silverberg PA, et al. Respiratory distress secondary to a high carbohydrate load: a case report. Surgery 1980;87:596–598.

72. Efthimiou J, Mounsey PJ, Benson DN, et al. Effect of carbohydrate rich versus fat rich loads on gas exchange and walking performance in patients with chronic obstructive lung disease. Thorax 1992;47:451–456.

73. Frankfort JD, Fischer CE, Stansbury DW, et al. Effects of high- and low-carbohydrate meals on maximum exercise performance in chronic airflow obstruction. Chest 1991;100:792–795.

74. Akrabawi SS, Mobarhan S, Ferguson PW. Gastric emptying (GE 1/2) and postprandial resting energy expenditure (REE), pulmonary function (PF) and respiratory quotient (RQ) of a high versus moderate fat enteral formula in chronic obstructive pulmonary disease (COPD) patients.

75. Schols AMWJ, Mostert R, Cobben N, et al. Transcutaneous oxygen saturation and carbon dioxide tension during meals in patients with chronic obstructive pulmonary disease. Chest 1991;100:1287–1292.

76. Hopkins B, Bristrian B, Blackburn G. Protein-calorie management in the hospitalized patient. In: Schneider H, ed. Nutritional Support in Clinical Practice. Philadelphia: Harper & Row, 1983.

77. Suchner U, Rothkopf MM, Stanislaus G, et al. Growth hormone and pulmonary disease: metabolic effects in patients receiving parenteral nutrition. Arch Intern Med 1990;150:1225–1230.

78. Pape GS, Friedman M, Underwood LE, et al. The effect of growth hormone on weight gain and pulmonary function in patients with chronic obstructive lung disease. Chest 1991;99:1495–1500.

79. Burdet L, de Muralt B, Schutz Y, et al. Thermogenic effect of bronchodilators in patients with chronic obstructive pulmonary disease. Thorax 1997;52:130–135.

80. Creutzberg E, Schols A, Weling-Scheepers C, et al. Characterization of non-response to high-caloric oral nutritional therapy in depleted patients with COPD. Am J Respir Crit Care Med 2000 (in press).

15 Tobacco Dependence: Pathophysiology and Treatment

David P.L. Sachs

◉ Professional Skills

Upon completion of this chapter, the reader will:

- Explain why tobacco dependence is a severe, life-threatening, chronic medical disease that requires long-term medical treatment and management, often for the life of the patient
- Describe the fundamental, genetically mediated, and not necessarily reversible alterations in brain neuronal structure and function caused by nicotine
- Describe the fundamental pharmacotherapeutic principles governing rational medical management of tobacco dependence
- List all classes of Food and Drug Administration (FDA)–approved medications for smoking cessation and provide examples
- Explain the difference between psychological dependence and nicotine addiction and why both must be treated during smoking cessation
- List the four Stages of Change that smokers go through to reach their goal of quitting smoking
- List the two key diagnostic questions that will help you determine whether a patient is ready to quit smoking
- Delineate a schedule of visits for the patient attempting to quit smoking

TOBACCO DEPENDENCE AS A CHRONIC DISEASE

Cigarette smoking is not a "habit," although many health care providers harbor this attitude, as do nearly all cigarette smokers. Unfortunately, the scientific facts do not support this point of view. Evidence shows that within 3 to 6 weeks of a child's beginning regular, daily cigarette smoking, even as few as one to two cigarettes per day, brain structure changes. The number of nicotine receptors within the cell membrane of brain neurons increases twofold to threefold. As David Kessler, MD, JD, former director of the FDA and currently dean of the School of Medicine, Yale University, determined in 1996, after the FDA's extensive review of the scientific evidence, "nicotine in tobacco smoke 'permanently alters the structure and function of the human body.'"[1] Approximately 1 year later, then-deputy director of the FDA, Curtis Wright, MD, PhD, summed up the FDA's scientific assessment of tobacco dependence: "Tobacco dependence is a . . .

[serious,] chronic, relapsing, life-threatening illness, that requires . . . long-term medical management" (pp. 221–223).[2]

This simple, yet profound, statement recast the conception of tobacco dependence from what it had been erroneously thought of—a short-term, self-limited disease, like pneumonia—to what it actually is—a chronic disease, like asthma, diabetes, or hypertension.

Cigarette smoking is the primary and cardinal symptom of the deadly disease of tobacco dependence. Before health care providers can effectively treat tobacco dependence and help their patients stop smoking, we need to review some of the exciting and groundbreaking research from the neurosciences, in particular, neurophysiology and neuropharmacology. In this chapter we first review the neurobiology of nicotine addiction. Then we review the medications currently available to treat tobacco dependence (both FDA approved and not FDA approved). This review also includes relevant clinical trial data, which will then lead to a practical, office practice paradigm.

NEUROBIOLOGY OF NICOTINE ADDICTION

Beneficial Effects of Nicotine

Nicotine affects how a person feels, thinks, and functions at a cellular level. Nicotine in tobacco smoke reaches the human brain a mere 7 seconds after the smoker inhales one puff. The nicotine is ultraconcentrated,[3] which is one of the reasons it can alter brain neuronal structure and function. It is 10 times more concentrated, puff-to-puff, in the systemic arterial circulation than it is in the mixed-venous circulation.

Nicotine in tobacco smoke increases the number of nicotine receptor sites in the brain by twofold to threefold (Fig. 15-1).[4–10] Moreover, this nicotine receptor proliferation is not necessarily reversible in humans.[11] Nicotine is one of the most potent central nervous system (CNS)–active drugs: milligram for milligram, it is 10 times more potent a euphoriant than heroin, cocaine, or *d*-amphetamine.[12]

The activation of nicotinic receptors throughout the brain increases brain production of numerous neurotransmitters, which, in turn, produce a wide range of effects (Fig. 15-2). Nicotinic receptors are particularly concentrated in several areas that are key to effective functioning, survival, and reproduction: the mesolimbic dopaminergic pathway, or "pleasure-reward pathway," and the locus ceruleus, a noradrenergic center in the brain. The locus ceruleus plays a critical role in cognitive processes and memory.

Dopaminergic Effects

The mesolimbic, dopaminergic pathway is normally activated in response to drinking, eating, and sexual/reproductive activity—activities essential for the survival of both the individual and the species. Dopamine is the neurotransmitter activated in this pathway.

When brain dopamine levels rise, the individual becomes cognitively aroused, feels more alert and vigorous, and perceives the sensation of pleasure.[13–20] In short, the person is energized and feels "really good." When brain dopamine levels fall, the opposite occurs. The individual feels moody, depressed, and dysphoric and experiences a loss of motivation (Table 15-1).

Acute nicotine administration produces increased CNS dopamine release, activating the mesolimbic dopaminergic system and *directly* causing the sensation of pleasure.[13–20] Consequently, the ultrahigh arterial nicotine levels that the cigarette delivers to the brain literally give the smoking patient fingertip control over mood, alertness, and vigor.

Noradrenergic Effects

Activation of the locus ceruleus causes norepinephrine levels to increase (see Table 15-1). The individual feels more alert and is cognitively aroused. Memory formation, storage,

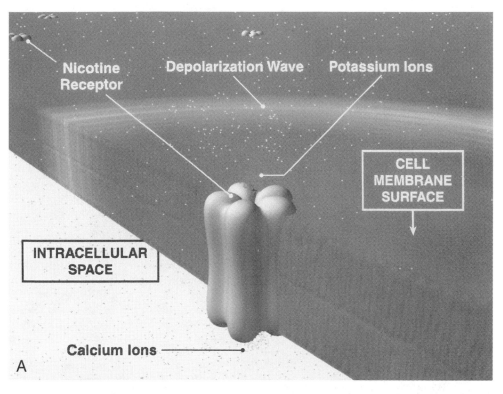

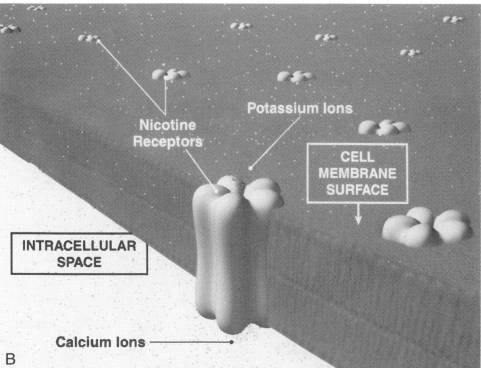

Figure 15-1. A. Cross section through the cell membrane of the postsynaptic surface of a dopaminergic neuron in the ventral tegmental area showing the "normal" density of nicotine receptors. **B.** Same as (A) except now showing the doubling to tripling of nicotine receptor density induced by tobacco smoke.

NEUROCHEMICAL EFFECTS OF NICOTINE

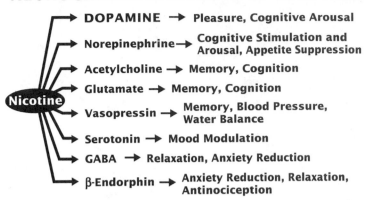

Figure 15-2. Nicotine induces the brain to increase its synthesis of a wide range of neurochemicals, with the results shown. (Adapted from Benowitz NL. Cigarette smoking and nicotine addiction. Med Clin North Am 1992;76:415–437; and Kellar KJ. Neuropharmacology and biology of neuronal nicotine receptors. In: Henningfield JE, Grunberg NE, eds. Addicted to Nicotine: A National Research Forum. Bethesda, MD: National Institute on Drug Abuse, National Institutes of Health, 1998:59–62.)

Table 15-1. Effects of Increased or Decreased CNS Dopamine and Norepinephrine Levels

Effects of Increased Levels	Effects of Decreased Levels
Dopamine	
Perception of pleasure and happiness	Feelings of depression
Increased energy and motivation	Dysphoria
Increased alertness	Loss of energy and motivation
Increased feeling of vigor	Decreased alertness
Increased cognitive arousal	Lethargy
Increased alertness	Decreased cognitive arousal
i.e., Person feels good	Decreased alertness
	i.e., Person feels depressed
Norepinephrine	
Increased alertness	Reduced alertness
Increased cognitive arousal	Decreased cognitive arousal
Enhanced memory formation, storage, retention, and recall	Impaired memory formation, storage, retention, and recall
Enhanced analytical skills	Impaired analytical skills
Enhanced arithmetic skills	Impaired arithmetic skills
Enhanced verbal skills	Impaired verbal skills
Appetite suppression	Increased appetite
i.e., Enhanced cognitive function	i.e., Reduced cognitive function

CNS, central nervous system.

retention, and recall are enhanced. Analytical, arithmetic, and verbal skills are also enhanced.[21–25]

As with the dopaminergic, pleasure-reward pathway, nicotine is a powerful activator of the locus ceruleus, causing norepinephrine release, leading to generalized brain activation and arousal; increased alertness, concentration, and intellectual skills; enhanced memory; and improved problem-solving behavior.[21,22,26,27] In addition, norepinephrine reduces appetite, contributing to smokers' lower weight compared with nonsmokers.[28] Thus, when a patient says that he or she thinks better when smoking, it is not merely "all in the head." It is a physiological, not a psychological, fact.

Nicotine Withdrawal

When smokers stop smoking "cold turkey," most experience one or more nicotine withdrawal symptoms (Table 15-2). These withdrawal symptoms are not "psychological"; they are physical and physiological. Their origin begins directly in altered CNS neurons. Nicotine withdrawal symptoms occur and are caused by nicotine's sudden removal from the increased number of nicotine receptor sites present in the smoker's brain.

The most common nicotine withdrawal symptoms are dysphoria and difficulty in thinking clearly. Symptom severity can range from being a minor nuisance to being truly disabling, totally disrupting all aspects of a person's life—family, marital, and occupational or professional. Although not all patients experience severe dysphoria, many comment

Table 15-2. Common Physiologically Induced
Nicotine Withdrawal Symptoms

Symptom	Frequency of Occurrence[127]
Anxiety[a]	87%
Irritability, frustration, or anger[a]	80%
Depression/depressed mood[a]	75%[b]/31%[c 138]
Difficulty concentrating[a]	73%
Increased appetite or weight gain[a]	73%
Restlessness[a]	71%
Craving for cigarettes[a]	62%
Nocturnal awakenings[a]	24%
Headache	N/A
Constipation	N/A

N/A, not available.
[a] Included as a nicotine withdrawal symptom in the current version of the American Psychiatric Association's *Diagnostic and Statistical Manual of Mental Disorders, Fourth Edition*, also known as *DSM-IV*,[29] or the predecessor version, *DSM-IIIR*.[128] Other symptoms, although not necessarily included in these manuals as nicotine withdrawal symptoms, are regarded by many experts in the field as nicotine withdrawal symptoms. All of these symptoms show a beneficial dose-response effect, being relieved by nicotine medications and/or bupropion.
[b] Frequency of occurrence when cigarette smokers with a history of depression stopped smoking cold turkey.
[c] Frequency of occurrence when cigarette smokers without a history of depression stopped smoking cold turkey.

that within 1 or 2 days of stopping smoking cold turkey they cannot think clearly and cannot do their job properly or adequately.

For example, one successful accountant of 20 years was dismayed that only 1 day after he had stopped smoking cold turkey he simply did not have the concentration skills to make sense out of basic financial spreadsheets. He described them as a "sea of numbers swimming before me." After 4 days of struggling unsuccessfully to practice accountancy, he smoked 1 cigarette and found that he could immediately think clearly again—his mind was functioning in its usual, keen fashion.

All of the CNS-induced symptoms caused by abrupt discontinuation of tobacco use (i.e., ultrahigh-dose nicotine intake) are promptly reversed, in dose-dependent fashion, by resumption of tobacco use[29] or administration of any nicotine pharmaceutical agent via any route, for example, intravenous, transdermal, or nasal spray.[30-32] Generally, nicotine withdrawal symptoms can be completely relieved within minutes after the patient smokes only one cigarette.

Genetics of Nicotine Addiction

CNS sensitivity and responsiveness to nicotine is genetically determined.[33-41] Without the proper genetic substrate, a smoker cannot become nicotine dependent. About 10% of cigarette smokers lack the requisite genes and have no physiological nicotine dependence. These individuals do not experience any of the nicotine withdrawal symptoms shown in Table 15-2. Rather, they can smoke 1 or 2 cigarettes every now and then, or even 10 or 30 cigarettes in a social setting one evening and then nothing for days, weeks, or longer, and not even think about cigarettes. These individuals are truly social smokers and do have complete, volitional control over when and under what circumstances they will smoke tobacco. Scientifically, they are called "chippers."[42-47] These people never seek assistance stopping smoking because they have no difficulty stopping smoking. Most patients at the lower end of the nicotine-dependency spectrum have only mild nicotine withdrawal symptoms. They too can readily stop smoking without any medical assistance. However, most tobacco users—about 75%—are sufficiently nicotine dependent so that their nicotine withdrawal symptoms are severe enough or last long enough that they will seek (or should seek) medical assistance.

Thus, with the appropriate genetic substrate, a tobacco user can become nicotine addicted (Fig. 15-3). About 90% of cigarette smokers are, in fact, physiologically nicotine addicted. As noted previously, they fall into a spectrum ranging from minimally nicotine addicted to severely nicotine addicted. As a general rule, the more severe an individual patient's nicotine addiction, the more severe will that patient's nicotine withdrawal symptoms be. Also, the more severe a patient's nicotine addiction, the more intensive will the medical treatment plan need to be.

For the approximately 90% of nicotine-addicted cigarette users, genetics accounts for about 53% of the phenotypic variance and environmental and social factors account for the other 47%.[48] For this 90%, stopping smoking is not a matter of "choice" or "free will." It is a medical and physiological problem that requires accurate diagnosis and appropriate medical treatment.

Development of Nicotine Addition

Figure 15-3 (left-hand portion) graphically shows the requirements for nicotine addiction. The individual, usually a child or early adolescent, must possess those genotypes that form the biological basis for nicotine addiction. Then, environmental and social factors must act on the child to induce genetic expression. Typically, these factors include peer pressure to smoke "because it's cool and all the movie stars do it"; rebelling against authority figures, either at home or at school; wanting to be more like adults they respect, for example, a parent or teacher who smokes; etc. Once the environmental and social factors

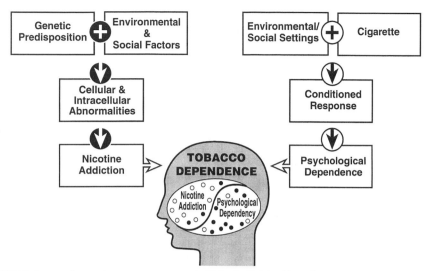

Figure 15-3. Tobacco dependence can occur only if the individual has the requisite genetic predisposition *and* is exposed to an environment that encourages experimenting with cigarettes. This combination (left-hand portion) then induces a wide range of brain neuronal cellular, intracellular, and cell-receptor changes that directly produce the physiological base for nicotine addiction. The right-hand portion of this illustration shows how an individual develops psychological dependence on tobacco products. To effectively treat tobacco dependence, *both* of these driving forces, nicotine addiction and psychological dependence, must be adequately treated.

lead the child to experiment with cigarettes, the ultrahigh doses of nicotine in tobacco smoke induce genetic expression in the genetically predisposed child to create the CNS cellular and intracellular abnormalities discussed previously that directly cause nicotine addiction. If the experimenting child does not have the genetic predisposition, then nicotine addiction cannot and will not occur. This child could well become psychologically dependent, only, on cigarettes but will have a vastly easier time stopping smoking later in life, if that individual desires to do so. It seems, though, that about 90% of human beings have the genes that will produce true physical addiction to nicotine, of greater or lesser severity.

Toxicology and Safety of Nicotine

Nicotine is neither a carcinogen nor a cocarcinogen.[49,50] Tobacco smoke contains at least 42 carcinogens and cocarcinogens, but nicotine is not one of them, despite thousands of basic science and clinical studies examining this point. Nicotine's toxicological profile is totally different from that of tobacco smoke. Tobacco smoke is highly carcinogenic, cardiotoxic,[51,52] and toxic to the pulmonary and vascular systems; in general,[49,50] nicotine alone, as would be used in nicotine medications, is not.[49-53]

MEDICATIONS TO TREAT TOBACCO DEPENDENCE

All FDA-approved medications for treating tobacco dependence increase immediate, end-of-treatment, and long-term (off-treatment) smoking cessation rates twofold to threefold.[49,54-73] In 1996, the Agency for Health Care Policy and Research Task Force recommended that essentially *all* patients who smoke, and want to try to quit, should be prescribed at least one medication.[70,74,75]

Pharmacologic Classes

Presently, four categories, or classes, of medications are available to treat tobacco dependence (Table 15-3). Effectiveness varies widely across medication class, and not all drugs that are effective are FDA approved for this indication.

Class 1: Nicotine Receptor Agonists

To date, the only nicotine receptor agonist medication available is nicotine itself. It is available in four different delivery formulations: patch, polacrilex ("gum"), inhaler, and nasal spray. A fifth, a lozenge, is due soon. Each delivers nicotine to the CNS via the systemic capillary bed, not the pulmonary capillary bed as with cigarettes, and are exceedingly slow at doing that compared with cigarette smoke inhaled into the lungs. Each system, however, has a different nicotine absorption profile. The patch is the slowest to reach the brain and the nasal spray is the fastest. Nonetheless, compared with the speed with which the cigarette delivers nicotine to the brain, even the nasal spray is glacially slow. Speed of nicotine delivery to the CNS might be thought of this way:

$$\text{Patch} <<< \text{Polacrilex} \approx \text{Inhaler} <<<<<< \text{Nasal Spray} <<<<<<...<<<<<<< \text{Cigarette}$$

In addition to the much slower speed of delivery, the nicotine dose delivered to the CNS by any of these medications is far below what the cigarette, puff to puff, delivers. Each tobacco smoke puff may deliver 10^{6-7} nicotine molecules to each synapse in an area of the CNS, whereas nicotine medications deliver many orders of magnitude less, probably in the range of 10^{2-3} nicotine molecules to each synapse.

Nicotine Patch

Clinical Trial Data Studies consistently show that short-term treatment with the nicotine patch (6-12 weeks of medication use only) typically doubles end-of-treatment smoking cessation rates, for example, approximately 60% versus 30% in the placebo-control group.[58,59] However, once medication use is stopped, because we are treating a chronic medical disease that is pathophysiologically like asthma, relapse usually increases substantially in active treatment groups. Even so, most studies that have presented data up to 9 months off medication still show a significant residual benefit to having received active nicotine patch during the short treatment period: for example, 25% versus 9%, a nearly threefold improvement in outcome.[59] The more office visit follow-up that occurs, the better controlled the tobacco dependence.[70,74,76]

Table 15-3. Fundamental Pharmacologic Classes of Medications for the Treatment of Tobacco Dependence

Class	Type	Example	FDA Approved	Class Effective
Class 1	Nicotine receptor agonist	Nicotine patch, nicotine nasal spray	Yes	Yes
Class 2	Nicotine receptor antagonist	Mecamylamine (Inversine)	No	Theoretically
Class 3	Nonnicotine receptor agents	Bupropion SR	Yes	Yes
Class 4	Combination medications	Bupropion SR + nicotine medication	Yes	Yes

FDA, Food and Drug Administration; SR, sustained release.

Dose-Response Effect Most large-scale (N>900 for each), traditional, dose-response nicotine patch trials have shown a clear-cut benefit to higher nicotine patch dosing when used as monotherapy, particularly during the weeks that medication was actually used.[58,72,77] One trial testing only two nicotine patch doses, and therefore not a true dose-response trial, failed to show any benefit of the higher patch dose.[78] The magnitude of the dose-response effect varied from study to study at the time medication use stopped, but the trends are all consistent.

Taking a closer look at the Transdermal Nicotine Study Group trial data is informative. As Figure 15-4*A* shows, the smoking cessation rate at the end of the 6-week treatment phase is a straight-line relationship with the dose of nicotine delivered. The curve is not plateauing between 14 mg of nicotine/24 hours and 21 mg of nicotine/24 hours. One could imagine that if the dose had been increased, then one of two hypothetical curves might have appeared: 21 mg of nicotine/24 hours is as good as it gets, so the efficacy curve plateaus with higher doses (Figure 15-4*B*, curve A), or the straight-line relation continues, with the end-of-treatment smoking cessation rates proportionately better with 42 mg of nicotine/24 hours compared with 21 mg of nicotine/24 hours (Fig. 15-4*B*, curve B). In fact, the data from Hughes et al.[77] would suggest that curve A is the correct one: 21 mg of nicotine/24 hours is as good as it gets.

It is important to note, however, that the standard dose-response paradigm, as used in these studies, is probably not the best design to use with nicotine because transdermal absorption varies nearly threefold across patients[79] and nicotine metabolism varies fourfold across patients.[80] Therefore, the resultant therapeutic serum nicotine level is unpredictable. To remedy this effect, two independent research teams have studied the serum nicotine level during treatment, *not* the dose of nicotine originally administered. Their findings suggest that individualizing and optimizing each patient's serum nicotine level during treatment significantly and substantially improves treatment results, including smoking cessation rates and also relief of nicotine withdrawal symptoms.[73,81]

Accomplishing this can require substantially higher nicotine patch doses, for certain patients than have been used heretofore.[58,72,77] In fact, although the average patch dose necessary to achieve a therapeutic nicotine level is three patches, the range, based on our clinical trial, is one to six patches. (The highest dose used in the Transdermal Nicotine Study Group trial[58] was one patch, in Hughes et al.[77] was two patches, and in Tonnesen et al.[72] was 1⅔ patches.) Our data show that the distribution curve of patch-dose × number of patients is normally distributed, so only about 1 to 5% of patients are at either patch-dose extreme, needing only one patch or as high as six patches (DPL Sachs, unpublished data, 1999).

The bottom line remains, however, that with standard nicotine patch dosing, transdermal nicotine doubles to triples end-of-medication-treatment and off-medication smoking cessation rates,[68] and the better the physician follow-up the better the smoking cessation rates.[74,76]

Nicotine Nasal Spray

The nicotine nasal spray (available by prescription only in the United States) seems, on the surface, to be equally effective as the nicotine patch.[62,63,82] However, it has a radically different pharmacokinetic profile, delivering nicotine to the CNS much faster than any other nicotine medication (but not nearly as fast as the cigarette). In fact, nicotine nasal spray may be preferentially beneficial for smokers with high nicotine dependency.[62] As discussed below, it also has particular benefit for all dependence levels of smokers when used in combination with the nicotine patch.[71]

Patients generally report marked relief of nicotine withdrawal symptoms, such as cigarette craving, irritability, or short temperedness, within 90 to 120 seconds of taking one dose (one spray in each nostril; 0.5 mg of nicotine/spray or 1 mg of nicotine/dose). Although this is far slower than the 7 seconds it takes a much higher nicotine dose to

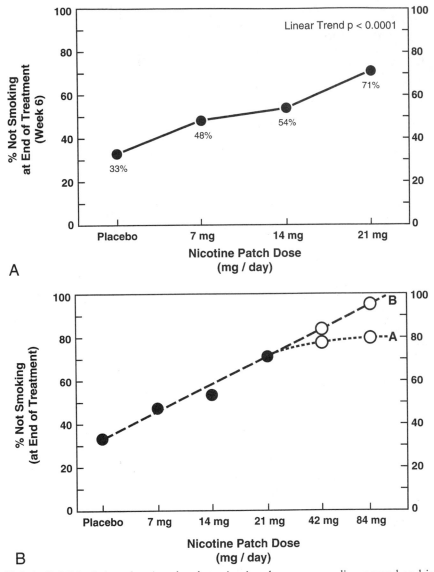

Figure 15-4. A. Published data showing the clear nicotine dose-response linear trend and improved smoking cessation rates at the end of a short (6-week) treatment period. **B.** Extrapolating the data from (A) to illustrate the theoretical limits if the nicotine patch dose had been increased in this study. Curve A shows what would have happened if 21 mg of nicotine delivered over 24 hours is "as good as it gets." That is, higher patch doses produce minimal further improvement in smoking cessation rates at the end of treatment. Curve B postulates a continuation of the straight-line linear trend until 100% not smoking is reached, at about 90 mg of nicotine per 24 hours. In fact, subsequent work would suggest that using the classic dose-response paradigm, the actual result is a little better than Curve A, but nowhere near curve B.[77] To get closer to curve B, the dose-response clinical trial design is inadequate. Rather, individualizing nicotine patch dose to optimize each patient's serum cotinine level, in relation to the serum cotinine level while the patient was smoking, is necessary. Then, but only then, can results closer to curve B be attained.[73] (Data from Sachs DPL. The use and efficacy of nicotine patches. Journal of Smoking Related Disorders 1994;5[suppl 1]:183–193.)

reach the brain after one puff on a tobacco cigarette, it is fast enough to make this medication particularly useful in "crisis" situations for the patient.

Nicotine Polacrilex

Nicotine polacrilex (Nicorette), commonly known by its inaccurate slang name, "nicotine gum," is also consistently effective in doubling to tripling the end-of-treatment smoking cessation rates.[68,83] Available in two dosage strengths, 2 and 4 mg, it requires a careful use technique. If it is chewed like regular chewing gum, it will not have any therapeutic effect. Also, during the first 1 to 2 months of treatment, patients must use a minimum of 9 pieces/day or they will not receive any therapeutic benefit.[55,56] The 4-mg strength is far more effective than the 2-mg strength for high–nicotine-dependent smokers,[54–56,84] with 6-week end-of-treatment smoking cessation rates as high as 85%, 29%, and 33% for 4, 2, and 0 mg of nicotine/piece, respectively ($P < .01$). The mean number of pieces of medication used daily for the entire 6-week treatment period was identical for the three treatment conditions: 10.3, 10.1, and 10.2, respectively.

Nicotine Inhaler (Oral)

The nicotine inhaler is the newest prescription medication to become available in the United States. It, too, is significantly more effective than placebo and shows end-of-treatment and 1-year smoking cessation survival curves similar to those found with the nicotine patch.[64–66] The nicotine inhaler is cleverly packaged and easy to use. Nicotine absorption does not occur in the tracheobronchial tree or the lung parenchyma, as initially thought, but strictly from the oral mucosa.[85,86] If used as a single medication, to achieve a therapeutic nicotine blood level patients need to use a minimum of 4 nicotine cartridges/day. Some may need to use as many as 20. In addition, patients need to take 100 to 200 puffs during the first 30 to 45 minutes after the cartridge is activated. One to two hours after being activated, most of the nicotine in the cartridge will have vaporized into the ambient air. The nicotine inhaler allows weaning from nicotine while maintaining partial reinforcement of the rituals associated with smoking, as well as some of the sensory aspects of smoking. The nicotine inhaler is the only medication presently available that gives even a modicum of "respiratory bite," or respiratory tract sensory stimulation, which is an independent reinforcer for cigarette smoking.[87]

Class 2: Nicotine Receptor Blockers

The only agent currently available is mecamylamine (Inversine), which has been used in various research studies over the years. Mecamylamine, however, has too many side effects (e.g., orthostatic hypotension, urinary retention in males with prostatic hypertrophy, and ileus) when used as a single agent to be practically useful. (However, see the "Class 4: Combination Medications" section.)

Class 3: Nonnicotine Receptor Agents

This class has many potential subclasses, including selective serotonin reuptake inhibitors (SSRIs), tricyclic antidepressants, and anxiolytics.[88,89] Only one subclass, dopaminergic/noradrenergic reuptake inhibitors (DNRIs),[90] contains a medication that is FDA approved for tobacco-dependence treatment: bupropion hydrochloride sustained release (SR) (Zyban).[67,91] A second subclass has compelling data to support clinical use of tricyclic antidepressants, specifically nortriptyline,[92] although FDA approval is doubtful, because no commercial interest stands to gain.

Selective Serotonin Reuptake Inhibitors (SSRIs)

One of the SSRIs, fluoxetine (Prozac), was subjected to at least two large, phase III multicenter trials under a formal Investigational New Drug (IND) application to the FDA for the tobacco-dependence treatment indication. Neither study showed a smoking cessation difference between any active dose and placebo. This IND application was withdrawn. No other SSRI has been systematically tested, and no clinical, anecdotal information indicates that any SSRI might be useful therapy in tobacco dependence.

Dopaminergic/Noradrenergic Reuptake Inhibitors (DNRIs)

In marked contrast to SSRIs, bupropion SR, a member of the DNRI subclass, has shown a consistent tobacco-dependence, therapeutic effect in all studies conducted to date.[67,91–95] Moreover, bupropion SR shows a clear dose-response treatment effect (see Table 15-4),[67] unequivocally proving a pharmacologic effect on underlying CNS neuronal cellular or subcellular pathophysiology. Bupropion's therapeutic effect not only extends to substantially and significantly improved smoking cessation rates[67,91] but also relief of nicotine withdrawal symptoms.[67,91] Of particular importance, bupropion also significantly reduces weight gain associated with stopping smoking by 50%.[67] This weight-suppressant effect of bupropion also demonstrated a significant dose-response relationship. Of particular value, this significant suppressant effect on weight gain persisted at least 1 year after bupropion therapy was stopped.[96]

The optimal duration of use for bupropion SR in the treatment of tobacco dependence is not known. The published studies were not designed to determine whether 6 (or 8) weeks was sufficient treatment duration. Because of the high relapse rate during the 45-week off-medication follow-up period,[67,91] some patients will definitely need a longer medication treatment phase.

Bupropion SR acts at a totally different site on central dopamine and noradrenergic neurons than does nicotine. Bupropion SR is a weak inhibitor of dopamine and norepinephrine reuptake. Consequently, a higher concentration of dopamine and norepinephrine molecules is maintained in their respective synaptic clefts.

Class 4: Combination Medications

Overview

Taking advantage of the different pharmacokinetic and pharmacodynamic properties of nicotine and nonnicotine medications to provide individualized, combination pharmacotherapy is the wave of the immediate future and produces the most effective results. Only a few of the possible combinations of already FDA-approved medications have undergone clinical trials. And no controlled clinical trials have been conducted to date using 3 or more different tobacco-dependency treatment medications, for example, bupropion SR + nicotine patch + nicotine nasal spray.

Table 15-4. Effect of Bupropion SR on Point Prevalence Smoking Cessation Rates (Objectively Validated)[67]

| Time After TQD | Patients Not Smoking, % | | | | |
	Placebo (n = 153)	Bupropion SR, 100 mg/d (n = 153)	Bupropion SR, 150 mg/d (n = 153)	Bupropion SR, 300 mg/d (n = 156)	Linear Trend P
Week 6[a]	19	29	39	44	<.001
Month 3	14	24	26	30	.003
Month 6	16	24	28	27	.03
Month 12	12	20	23	23	.02

SR, sustained release; TQD, Target Quit Date.
[a] Medication was stopped at week 6.

Only one combination treatment, bupropion SR + nicotine patch, is currently FDA approved for tobacco-dependence treatment. However, any combination of buproprion SR and another medication—two through five-at-a-time (e.g., bupropion SR plus the nicotine patch, polacrilex, nasal spray, and inhaler)—makes pharmacokinetic and pharmacodynamic sense and may be suitable for individual patients on a case-by-case basis. Many experts in the field are already using such combinations (LH Ferry, MD, MPH, personal communication, 1999; RD Hurt, MD, personal communication, 1999; DPL Sachs, MD, personal communication, 1999).

Buproprion SR + Nicotine Patch
The published data from the combination medication study (buproprion SR [Zyban] and nicotine patch [Habitrol]) reveal that at the end of the sixth week of treatment, just before initiating 2 weeks of nicotine patch tapering, the smoking cessation rate for bupropion SR (300-mg daily dose) and a placebo Habitrol-like patch alone was significantly higher than that for the nicotine patch alone (a Habitrol patch): 61% versus 44%.[91,97] The nicotine patch alone, however, was not significantly more effective than placebo: 44% versus 33% ($P =$ NS). The combination of bupropion SR + nicotine patch tended to produce higher smoking cessation rates than did bupropion SR alone and was significantly more effective than the nicotine patch alone: 66% versus 61% versus 44%, respectively. In a slightly different analysis, submitted to the FDA as part of the New Drug Application database, the bupropion SR + nicotine patch combination was significantly more effective at the end of the sixth week of treatment ($P =$ .04 or better for each pairwise comparison) than either active medication alone or placebo: 60% versus 51% versus 37% versus 24% (bupropion SR + nicotine patch vs. bupropion SR alone vs. nicotine patch alone vs. placebo, respectively).

The clinical experience of some expert clinicians in this field clearly shows that some patients definitely benefit from combination treatment with bupropion SR and nicotine patch (LH Ferry, MD, MPH, personal communication, 1999; RD Hurt, MD, personal communication, 1999; DPL Sachs, MD, personal communication, 1999). This makes physiological sense because each medication is acting at a different site on the dopamine and norepinephrine neuron. Also, the published clinical trial used only the standard nicotine patch dosage, which (see below) underdoses about 80% of users. Clinical experience indicates that an individualized nicotine patch dosage, in conjunction with bupropion SR, substantially increases smoking cessation rates and also withdrawal symptom relief (LH Ferry, MD, MPH, personal communication, 1999; RD Hurt, MD, personal communication, 1999; DPL Sachs, MD, personal communication, 1999).

An unexpected but encouraging finding from the published, combination medication study was the long-term smoking cessation benefit provided by bupropion SR + nicotine patch or bupropion SR only. Although relapse was considerable from the time medication use stopped, 8 weeks after the target quit date (TQD), to 1 year after the TQD, the treatment effect was still highly significant and clinically relevant. This occurred even though all patients had been off all tobacco-dependence medication for 43 weeks at the long-term, 1-year follow-up time point.

Mechanism of Action In the case of combination use of bupropion SR + a nicotine medication, we are accomplishing precisely the same type of pharmacologic/physiological objective that we have when we use two or more medications to optimally manage an asthmatic's bronchospastic airways (e.g., a β_2-inhaled bronchodilator, such as salmeterol [SereVent], combined with an inhaled corticosteroid, such as fluticasone [FloVent]). Namely, we are using two different biochemical pathways to achieve the same goal: in the case of asthma, increased airway diameter; in the case of tobacco dependence, using bupropion SR + a nicotine medication, enhanced activation of the dopaminergic and noradrenergic systems in the brain.

Nicotine Patch + Nicotine Nasal Spray

In another recent study, Bläondal et al.[71] showed that combination long-term use (up to 1 year) of two different nicotine medications, one with slow absorption and the other with rapid absorption, was both effective and safe. Nicotine nasal spray use alone for up to 1 year following a 3-month induction phase of nicotine nasal spray + standard-dose nicotine patch doubled the continuous smoking cessation rates compared with those who, in effect, received only 3 months of nicotine patch treatment alone (see Fig. 15-5). (This group used placebo nasal spray + standard-dose nicotine patch for the first 3 months, then placebo nasal spray for up to an additional 9 months.) At 3 months, 37% of nicotine nasal spray + nicotine patch–treated patients were continuous nonsmokers compared with 25% of placebo nasal spray + nicotine patch–treated patients ($P = .045$). At 1 year, 27% versus 11%, for patients continuing to use nicotine nasal spray versus placebo nasal spray, respectively ($P = .001$), after the first 3 months were continuous nonsmokers. Even after all medication use had been stopped for 5 years (6 years from the TQD), patients who had originally received both active medications 5 years earlier did better: 16% versus 9% (log rank $P = .004$).

Other insights that emerged from this large-scale trial ($N = 239$) include:

1. Adding nicotine nasal spray to nicotine patch therapy significantly and substantially improved the treatment results produced by nicotine patch alone.
2. Adding nicotine nasal spray to nicotine patch therapy reduced relapse during the first 3 weeks of combined treatment and also the first month of tapering.
3. Stopping nicotine nasal spray, even after treatment for as long as 1 year, was too soon for some patients.
4. Combining these two medications, even for those who were not successful in stopping smoking and *continued to smoke while using both active nicotine medications,* was safe and did not increase medical risk, cardiac or otherwise.
5. Some patients clearly needed and benefited from the relatively rapid delivery of nicotine to the CNS that the nicotine nasal spray provided, in addition to the steady-state nicotine level that standard-dose patch provided.
6. Some tobacco-dependent patients clearly benefit from longer than 3 months or 1 year of nicotine medication treatment (with either one or both medications). For some patients, medication treatment duration may need to last years to a lifetime to keep their tobacco dependency under adequate and sufficient control.

Nicotine Patch + Nicotine Polacrilex

Adding Nicotine Polacrilex to Nicotine Patch Similar to the above nicotine combination study, adding nicotine polacrilex (2-mg dose, only about 5-6 pieces/day) to standard, single nicotine patch treatment (12 weeks' duration followed by 12 weeks of tapering), doubled the odds ratio in 374 patients at the end of medication treatment + tapering: odds ratio = 2.04 (95% confidence interval = 1.14–3.57, $P = .018$).[98] This combination was both significantly more effective than nicotine patch alone and as safe as the placebo patch + placebo polacrilex.[98]

Adding Nicotine Patch to Nicotine Polacrilex Adding the nicotine patch (standard, single-patch dose) to ad lib use of 2-mg nicotine polacrilex (patients were instructed to use only ≥4 pieces/day) also significantly and safely increased end-of-treatment continuous smoking cessation rates (12 weeks after the TQD) for 300 patients: 39% versus 28% ($P = .038$).[99]

Nicotine Patch + Nicotine Inhaler (Oral)

Finally, a study recently presented at an international meeting, similar in design to those above, showed that combining nicotine inhaler with standard-dose nicotine patch was as safe as the placebo inhaler/placebo patch treatment condition and significantly more effective than either medication alone.[100]

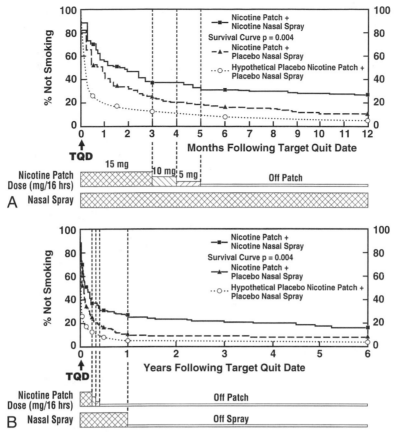

Figure 15-5. A. Life table analysis, a Kaplan-Meier plot, showing the continuous, objectively validated nonsmoking rate in patients treated with combination nicotine patch and nicotine nasal spray. The study was randomized and double blind. The 120 smokers randomized to receive nicotine patch (15 mg of nicotine per 16 hours) for 3 months + nicotine nasal spray had significantly higher smoking cessation rates than the 119 smokers randomized to receive the same nicotine patch treatment but with a placebo nasal spray (log-rank $P = .04$). This study did not have a placebo patch + placebo nasal spray condition. Because, as discussed in detail in the text, clinical trial data are so robust, showing that the nicotine patch alone doubles smoking cessation rates, to facilitate understanding of these data, a hypothetical curve has been added showing results that could reasonably have been expected had there been a placebo patch + placebo inhaler arm. Results, such as this hypothetical curve may be readily found in any number of published sources.[58,59] **B.** This same study followed patients double blindly for an additional 5 years after the assigned inhaler use was stopped. Note the relatively higher relapse rate when those using the active nicotine nasal spray had to stop use, suggesting what is supported by clinical experience: some patients need long-term medication treatment to remain tobacco free. (Data from Blondal T, Gudmundsson LJ, Olafsdottir I, Gustavsson G, Westin A. Nicotine nasal spray with nicotine patch for smoking cessation: randomised trial with six-year follow up. BMJ 1999;318:285–289.)

Summary of Combination Medication Studies
Any of the pairwise medication combinations tested in the studies briefly summarized above was always and consistently more effective than either medication alone or placebo during the period of active medication treatment. Moreover, the risk of cardiac or other clinically relevant medication side effect was no greater in combination medication–treated patients than in patients treated with either nicotine medication alone or dual placebos.

Clearly, all available clinical trial data show that at least two nicotine medications can be safely combined to substantially (usually by twofold) and significantly increase the treatment results that would be produced by either medication alone. Nicotine patch and bupropion SR can also be safely combined to likely boost treatment effectiveness. Clinical experience would suggest that more than two nicotine medications, in addition to bupropion SR, can be safely used to individualize and optimize the treatment and improve treatment results for specific patients (LH Ferry, MD, MPH, personal communication, 1999; RD Hurt, MD, personal communication, 1999; DPL Sachs, MD, personal communication, 1999).

The best results are seen when patients are actually using the medication(s). Relapse after medication use stops, 6, 12, 26, or 52 weeks after the TQD, depending on the study, generally increases sharply in all active medication-treated patients. All of the few studies, which have actually conducted formal hazard analysis to compute whether the risk, or hazard, of relapse increases above the ongoing relapse rate when active medication use stops, have shown a significant increase in that risk.[63,101] This effect appears true, in fact, whether looking at single- or double-medication trials involving nicotine medications only or nicotine + nonnicotine medications. This result should be no surprise because as with asthma medications, we have no specific evidence that any of the current generation of tobacco-dependence medications reverse the underlying neuropathologic effects in nicotine addiction. Thus, most patients undergoing medical treatment for tobacco dependence will permanently relapse, unless they are able to be managed as any other chronic disease patient: lapse, or even relapse, is to be expected; this can usually be treated if the patient wishes to be treated again and the physician has established a regular follow-up visit plan, as would be used for asthma, diabetes, or hypertension.

Safety of FDA-Approved Medications for Tobacco-Dependence Treatment

All currently available, FDA-approved, tobacco-dependence medications have a wide safety margin.

Nicotine Medications

In particular, all four of the currently marketed nicotine medications, regardless of the relative speed of nicotine delivery to the CNS, are extraordinarily safe medications,[49,50–52,102] even when used in individualized, higher-than-"standard" dosages[73,81,103,104] or when the patient is using multiple nicotine medications.[71,98–100] None cause or increase the risk of myocardial infarction, even when used with concomitant cigarette smoking.[51–53,98–100,104,105] None cause or increase the risk of neoplastic disorders,[49,50] stroke,[49,50,53] or peripheral vascular disease.[49–52] Short-[105] and long-term[53] use of nicotine medications in ex-smokers may even have a cardioprotective effect.

Bupropion SR

Bupropion SR is also exceptionally safe.[67,91,106] Only two side effects were directly caused by bupropion, 300 mg/d, and occurred with greater than 1% incidence: insomnia and xerostomia, or dry mouth. Insomnia occurred in 35%[67] to 42%,[91] and xerostomia occurred in 3%[91] to 11%.[67] Both side effects were generally mild at onset and decreased in intensity during the first few weeks of bupropion use.

Bupropion SR causes only one potentially serious side effect, seizure, with an occurrence rate of only 0.1%[107]—less than that of fluoxetine (Prozac). No seizures occurred in any of the nearly 2000 smokers who received an active dose of bupropion SR in the tobacco-dependence treatment trials. These five randomized, double-blind, placebo-controlled clinical trials excluded patients with:

- Seizure history
- History of severe head trauma

- History of brain tumor or stroke
- History of anorexia nervosa or bulimia
- Current alcohol abuse
- Use of a medication known to lower seizure threshold, for example, theophylline

Bupropion SR + Nicotine Patch (Habitrol)

This FDA-approved combination is also exceptionally safe. Only four side effects are directly caused by this combination and occur with greater than 1% incidence, with two of those, patch-site cutaneous reaction and dream abnormalities, specifically caused by the Habitrol patch. These two adverse events have not been reported to occur with this frequency with patches of different design, for example, the Nicotrol patch. As with the side effects with bupropion alone, side effects with the combination tended to be mild and well tolerated. The four side effects from bupropion SR and Habitrol and their frequency of occurrence are[91]:

- Insomnia—48%
- Patch site cutaneous erythema, edema, or pruritus—15%
- Dream abnormalities—14% (dream abnormalities for nicotine patch [Habitrol] alone—18%, also $P < .05$ compared with placebo)[91]
- Nausea—12%

The incidence of xerostomia with the combination was 9%, but that percentage was not significantly greater than that which occurred with placebo patch and placebo bupropion. A nonsignificant trend was seen for increased blood pressure, 6% versus 3%, $P = .24$, combination versus placebo.[91] No seizures occurred in the 244 smokers who received this combination therapy for 9 weeks, starting 1 week before the TQD.[91]

A PRACTICAL PARADIGM FOR SMOKING CESSATION

Randomized, double-blind, controlled clinical trials do not tell us how to optimally treat a specific patient sitting in our examination room. This is true for asthma medications, hypertension medications, or diabetic medications. It is also true for tobacco-dependence medications. Such randomized trials do tell us whether a given medication is effective. Depending on how such a trial is designed, it may also provide practical information that can assist us in treating a particular patient.

Office treatment for tobacco dependence is clinically most effective if the health care provider follows a plan similar to that recommended by the National Heart, Lung, and Blood Institute Expert Panel II for asthma diagnosis and management:

1. Assessment
2. Diagnosis, including contributing factors
3. Treatment
4. Follow-up
5. Patient and family education

Assessment

Although most smokers (about 70%) want to stop smoking, only a minority, about 15%, are ready to stop smoking at any given time. Of the remaining 85% of smokers, 15% are actually in the process of stopping smoking, and 70% of smokers are not actively thinking about stopping smoking (see Fig. 15-6). For the 70% of smokers not thinking about stopping smoking, the health care provider need not spend much time, but the time that

STAGES OF CHANGE IN SMOKING CESSATION
DEFINITIONS

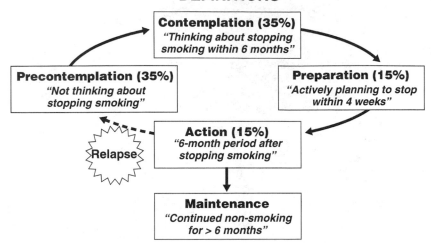

Figure 15-6. Although approximately 70% of cigarette smokers would like to stop smoking, at any given time only the 15% in the Preparation Phase are actually planning to stop. Another 15% have already stopped smoking (Action Phase), and a full 70% (Precontemplation + Contemplation Phases) are not at all ready to stop smoking. (Cancer 1996;67:805–807. Copyright © 1991 American Cancer Society. Reprinted by permission of Wiley-Liss, Inc., a subsidiary of John Wiley & Sons, Inc.)

is spent can be critically important. The patient should clearly and unambiguously hear from the health care provider that stopping smoking is the single most important thing the patient can do to improve health.

The health care provider can determine whether a specific patient is in the 15% ready and wanting to quit smoking by simply stating: "Stopping smoking is the single most important thing you can do to improve your health. Have you thought about stopping smoking?" About 15%—those who are in the *Action Phase*[108]—will say something like, "Not only have I thought about it, but I stopped smoking 5 days ago!" Another 15%, those in the *Preparation Phase,*[108] will say something like, "Yes, I have. Is there anything you can do to assist me? The last time I tried to quit, I had some real problems." About 35%, who are in the *Contemplation Phase,*[108] will indicate, on further questioning from you, that they are thinking about stopping smoking within the next 6 months, but are not ready to stop smoking now. The final 35% is in the *Precontemplation Phase.* As the name implies, they are not thinking about stopping smoking and they do not have plans to stop within the next 6 months. Interventions for tobacco-dependent patients in each of these four phases differ. In general, you match your intervention to the specific stage-of-change your patient is in: most intense for those in the Preparation or Action Phases and least intense (and geared toward helping the patient move toward the Preparation Phase) for those in the Contemplation or Precontemplation Phases. The following section focuses on interventions for patients in the Preparation and Action Phases.

Diagnosis (Including Contributing Factors) for the Patient in the Preparation Phase

Once you have assessed your patient and determined that that individual is in the Preparation Phase, you should reassure the patient that, indeed, you can do a great deal to assist in and simplify the smoking cessation process as well as minimize, if not eliminate, the pain caused by nicotine withdrawal symptoms.

What follows is the practical, pragmatic medical approach I use in my pulmonary medical clinic to diagnose and treat tobacco-dependent patients. Since adopting this clinical practice approach in 1995, we have been able to effectively treat about 70% of the patients we see for tobacco dependence. That is, 70% stop smoking and stay stopped. (Reasons for treatment failures are interesting and are presented later in this chapter.) Using this approach in a medical office setting requires somewhat more time and effort on the part of the physician and office staff than diagnosing and treating asthma, but less than diagnosing and treating a diabetic.

You will not find this approach or the algorithms I use in the conclusions of any randomized, double-blind clinical trial. Rather, this approach is rooted in the many randomized, double-blind (and open-label) clinical trials I have conducted during the last 25 years and my own clinical experience in the diagnosis and treatment of tobacco dependence during the last quarter century. Such an approach has the benefit of ultimate pragmatism. It also allows me to precisely individualize the treatment I prescribe for treating tobacco dependence in a specific patient. As a patient's needs change during treatment, I can modify the treatment to meet those needs.

Two Key Diagnostic Factors

Basic information about the questions you should ask an individual during the first diagnostic and treatment visit for tobacco dependence has already been provided in materials produced by the National Cancer Institute[109] and the American Academy of Family Physicians.[110] The answers to two key questions I now ask all my new tobacco-dependent patients will provide you with the most important information you will need to help your patients and effectively treat their tobacco dependence.

Why Do You Want to Stop Smoking?

For most tobacco-dependent patients in the Preparation Phase, health and medical concerns usually appear as one of the top three reasons that the patient has for wanting to stop smoking. Also, becoming increasingly important is the loss of self-control. Many patients do not like it that their cigarettes control them.

The fact is, if tobacco use did not incur such a high risk of morbidity and mortality, few smokers would really want to stop. Most cigarette smokers will tell you if you ask that their cigarette is their closest friend. As one individual I was treating phrased it: "My cigarette is my best and closest friend. It's always there for me. It picks me up when I'm down. It calms me when I'm tense. And I don't have to iron its shirts or make it lunch!"

In addition, at some point in the treatment process, the patient who has stopped smoking is wondering, at some level, "O.K., I've given up one of the most treasured aspects in my life. What am I getting in return?" Although such sentiments might seem bizarre to most health care providers, those readers who may be current or former smokers will doubtless recognize these thoughts. The information you learn from this first question, "Why do you want to stop smoking?" will often give you the information you will need weeks, months, or even years later when you sense your patient wondering, "So, what have I gained since I gave up smoking? What's the up side?" Drawing this question from your patient, whenever you sense it is arising, and being able to point them toward an answer can sometimes be crucial to maintaining continued treatment success.

What Concerns Do You Have About Stopping Smoking This Time?

Most tobacco-dependent patients have not thought about this question. Sometimes they do not even understand the question. Avoid the more typically used question to ascertain the "chief complaint," such as "How can I help you today?" to which patients will usually answer something like, "Well, I don't know . . ." with their voice trailing off. Changing the phrasing of the original question, for example, to "What fears do you have about stopping smoking this time?" will resonate better with some patients. With this question, you are helping the patient identify barriers that have blocked the path to stopping smoking in the past. Then you can help your patients make certain they do not experience the pain and suffering they experienced during a previous quit attempt from physiologically caused nicotine withdrawal symptoms. You may have to probe a bit to draw this kind of information out of your patient, but it is every bit as crucial as, for example, knowing the settings that will trigger an asthmatic attack in one of your asthmatic patients.

Specific Diagnostic Factors to Assess

Patients in the Preparation Phase should be evaluated for the presence or absence of the diagnostic factors in Box 15-1. Presence of any of these diagnostic factors, based on currently available studies, indicates the need for more intensive medical management, including the use of combination medications and also higher, individualized, nicotine patch dose.

In addition, women will have a much greater probability of successfully stopping smoking if they set their TQD during the first 15 days of their menstrual cycle (follicular phase).[111] Even for those women who do not have premenstrual syndrome, trying to stop smoking during the last half of their menstrual cycle, particularly the late luteal phase, is much more difficult.[111] The health care provider should therefore recommend to a female patient that she select a TQD that will fall during her follicular phase.

Treatment (including Pharmacotherapy)

Preparation Phase

As basic science knowledge—genetic, biochemical, physiological, pharmacologic, and behavioral—has evolved as new clinical insights have been published, and as new medications have become available, I have modified and refined my diagnostic and therapeutic approaches for tobacco dependence. All gets molded, refined, revised, and shaped in the crucible of clinical experience.

Fifteen years ago I used an approach analogous to hypertension treatment: start simple, adding interventions and medications until the blood pressure was brought under control. Despite establishing a "no-fault," no-guilt environment and carefully implementing a similar "stepped" approach for treating their tobacco dependence, patients would simply "disappear into the woodwork" if they did not succeed in stopping smoking with the first intervention. Controlled clinical research being conducted at about the same time at the Johns Hopkins Medical School found the same result (SJ Leischow, personal

---

Box 15-1. Prognostic Factors That Indicate the Need for Longer and More Intense Duration of Treatment, Use of Combination Medication Therapy, Use of Higher-Than-Standard Nicotine Patch Dose, or All of the Above

High nicotine dependence (Fagerström Test for Nicotine Dependence, ≥5 points)[54–56,59,62,115,129]
High serum cotinine level (serum cotinine, ≥250 ng/mL)[130,131]
Number of previous smoking cessation attempts ≥ 1[112,132]
Heavy cigarette smoker (≥20 cigarettes/day)[72,133,134]
Presence of nicotine withdrawal symptoms on previous quit attempt[114,115,116]
Began smoking cigarettes at a younger age (≤17 years old)[112,131]
Other smoker in household[112,132]
Patient is a woman and is:
    About to be treated with bupropion sustained release alone[132] or
    About to be treated with nicotine polacrilex alone[135,136]
History of depression or dysphoria[137,138]
History of alcohol or drug abuse[139]

communication, 1990): give the patient the best shot to successfully stop smoking the first time; you usually won't get a second chance. Our own subsequent research, as well as that of others, showed that smokers making their first smoking cessation attempt were twice as likely to succeed as those who had already tried one or more times to stop smoking.[112]

Therefore, my current approach in initially planning the treatment for a new patient in the (Preparation Phase) is to carefully think through how to best help the patient attack the two major forces driving tobacco dependence: nicotine addiction and psychological dependence (Fig. 15-3). If both etiologies are not adequately addressed, the patient will have no chance to successfully stop smoking.

Managing Psychological Dependence

Psychological Dependence Demystified. Psychological dependence refers to those settings and situations that serve as triggers for lighting up a cigarette. For most smokers, these triggers fall into four types: (*a*) neutral, habit-type settings, such as making a telephone call; (*b*) pleasurable situations, such as finishing a meal or having a cocktail; (*c*) distressing situations, such as an anxiety-provoking deadline; or (*d*) boring, monotonous situations, such as having to carry out an uninteresting, repetitive task.

The right-hand portion of Figure 15-3 shows schematically how psychological dependence develops. Both a trigger-type setting *and* a cigarette have to be present for a conditioned response to develop. Once a conditioned response has been established for a particular setting—smoking a cigarette while drinking a glass of wine, for example—then the smoker becomes dependent, psychologically dependent at this point, on having a cigarette while drinking a glass of wine. If the individual has never had access to a cigarette while drinking a glass of wine, that conditioned response, quite simply, cannot develop. Similarly, if the individual never experienced that setting, that is, drinking a glass of wine, even though cigarettes were readily available, then that conditioned response could never have developed, for example, drink wine → light up cigarette → enjoy both.

Once the conditioned response is formed, the smoker becomes psychologically dependent. The smoker wants a cigarette when having wine and will light up a cigarette, presuming one is available. (At this point we are ignoring the nicotine addiction side of the equation.) As discussed at the beginning of this chapter, about 10% of smokers are not physiologically addicted to nicotine at all. When an individual's smoking is solely driven by psychological dependence, then to smoke or not to smoke is, indeed, a matter of choice—most of the time. Such individuals are those who wake up one morning, look at the pack of cigarettes, wonder "why am I wasting my money on these?" throw them in the wastebasket, and never think about them again for the rest of their lives. These smokers are also the type who may smoke with friends while having a glass of wine —1 cigarette or 30—one evening, but not smoke any cigarettes the next evening when having a glass of wine.

Such persons may enjoy smoking but they can control when, with whom, and how much to smoke. They are *not* dependent on tobacco. For that to occur, for the smoker to also be tobacco dependent, then the individual *must* be physiologically addicted to nicotine. Tobacco dependence requires that the smoker be *both* addicted to nicotine and psychologically dependent on having cigarettes in certain types of situations. As also discussed earlier, about 90% of smokers develop true nicotine addiction. All such smokers also have plenty of situations that serve as cues for wanting a cigarette. So both requirements for tobacco dependence are fulfilled.

Treatment of Psychological Dependence. Treatment for psychological dependence is usually fairly straightforward, but a surprising proportion of patients try to ignore what they need to do. Table 15-5 reviews the basic steps for effectively treating psychological dependence. In most cases, any competent general health care provider can provide the guidance the patient needs for this part of the treatment. A psychiatrist, clinical psychologist, or clinical social worker is not usually necessary. There are exceptions, of course, as in any complex, organically based disease. Some patients should be referred to a specialist. For example, most patients who have an underlying depressive or anxiety disorder will benefit from concomitant care by a psychiatrist. Patients who have a major depressive disorder, dysthymia, panic attacks, or phobias would definitely benefit from concomitant psychiatric care. As a different example, tobacco-dependent patients who also have asthma or chronic obstructive lung disease should also receive concomitant care from a pulmonologist in addition to their primary care physician.

Developing the "Action Plan." You need to help patients develop their own unique "Action Plan" (see Tables 15-5 and 15-6) to handle external triggers for lighting up and smoking a cigarette. One way to assist your patients is by providing or recommending a well-prepared self-help book, audiotape, or videotape. A variety of excellent materials are available (see "Resources"). Any good self-help manual should contain material to help the patient perform each of the three steps listed in Table 15-6. Patients frequently will ask questions such as, "How do you think I should deal with the strong desire I have for a cigarette when I . . .?" However, patients are far more innovative and creative than we could ever be. They also know themselves best. They are in the best position to devise solutions to their specific triggers. Therefore, when patients ask me a question of this type, I encourage them to figure out their own solutions, using their self-help book as a resource, not a cookbook, to help guide them to developing effective coping strategies for each setting or situation that causes them to want a cigarette.

Offering yourself and staff as a sounding board for patient ideas is an effective tool to help patients develop the best solutions for their triggers. Let patients know that during the standard duration, follow-up office visits, the "door is always open" and they should feel free to ask any questions that have occurred to them since the last visit. Also, encourage them to talk about any problems that have occurred since the last visit and how they overcame them. Numerous controlled clinical trials have shown that regular, medical office,

Table 15-5. Steps the Patient Must Take in the Treatment of Psychological Dependence

Before Target Quit Date	After Target Quit Date
Develop the "Action Plan" (see Table 15-6)	Implement the Action Plan
	Modify the Action Plan, as needed, to improve its weak aspects
Determine whether you, the patient, want any outside support other than from your physician	Use outside sources of support, as desired
	Add new outside sources of support, as desired
If so, then determine potential outside sources of support, such as family, friends, minister or rabbi, support groups, etc.	
Know the basic nicotine withdrawal symptoms and recognize when you experience them (even while you are still smoking)	Advise treating health care provider of any nicotine withdrawal symptoms that are occurring, particularly those that are interfering, in any way, with the conduct of your (the patient's) life
Feel comfortable with medication(s) that will be used and, if using bupropion SR, identify any side effects that may occur	Report to the treating health care provider any benefits and also any side effects you think you are experiencing from the medication(s) you are using

Table 15-6. How the Patient Can Develop the "Action Plan"

What to Do	How to Do It
Identify and list each trigger setting (e.g., making a phone call, having a glass of wine, or going to a stressful meeting)	Literally, patients need to note what they are doing each time they want to have a cigarette and also light up a cigarette
Rate the strength of each trigger setting	Use a 0–4 scale: 0 = not a trigger and 4 = extremely strong trigger
Decide how to neutralize each trigger setting (AKA developing new "Coping Skills")	Patient needs to think through what has and has not worked in the past in those trigger settings with previous settings
	Patient needs to obtain new ideas from supportive friends and family members, whether ex-smokers, current smokers, or never smokers
	Patient needs to obtain new ideas from self-help materials: books, audiobooks, videobooks, and other resources

follow-up visits are essentially as effective as well-run, psychological, group counseling sessions.[76] Adding effective pharmacotherapy improves the treatment results even further. Next I describe how I integrate pharmacotherapy into the structure and treatment I provide for the psychological dependence aspects of tobacco dependence.

Managing Nicotine Addiction: Pharmacotherapy to Eliminate Nicotine Withdrawal
The greatest deficiency of most well-designed group counseling or behavior modification programs is their failure to adequately address the nicotine addiction side of the tobacco-dependency equation (Fig. 15-3). This is also the greatest deficiency of office practices.

Providing effective pharmacotherapy to treat the nicotine addiction side of the equation is at the same time simple and not so simple. The goal of effective pharmacotherapy is to completely suppress all of the physiologically caused nicotine withdrawal symptoms (See Table 15-2), from the morning of the TQD forward. Failure to do so results in the incredibly high relapse rates seen in the tobacco-dependence natural history studies: greater than 40% relapse within 7 days of a cold turkey quit attempt; greater than 50% relapse within 14 days of a cold turkey quit attempt.[113]

Monitoring nicotine withdrawal symptoms with patients is particularly critical in the first weeks after the TQD. Those scientific studies that have looked at the issues support clinical experience: the extent and the severity of nicotine withdrawal symptoms directly predict relapse during the first 2 to 6 weeks of treatment after the TQD.[114–116] The more withdrawal symptoms the patient experiences and the greater their severity, the more likely the patient will resume smoking to eliminate the nicotine withdrawal symptoms being experienced. The converse is also true: the fewer the nicotine withdrawal symptoms and the less their severity, the less likely will the patient be to slip, have occasional cigarettes, and then resume regular smoking. With more effective use of medications currently available to eliminate nicotine withdrawal symptoms, patients will experience less relapse. **Steps to Take Before the Target Quit Date to Maximize Smoking Cessation Success.** Before starting a patient on pharmacotherapy, the health care provider must take certain steps, as outlined in Box 15-2. Some of these steps can be accomplished during the initial tobacco-dependence evaluation; others, such as, "Make certain the patient has been developing an 'Action Plan,'" are best done at the visit shortly before the patient's TQD. **The Foundation.** Based on the clinical trial data summarized earlier in this chapter, coupled with my own clinical experience treating thousands of patients for tobacco dependence, since 1995 I have used bupropion and an adequate, individualized dose of transdermal nicotine as the patient's pharmacotherapeutic foundation. The FDA's approval, in 1997, of bupropion SR (Zyban) has simplified this approach. Box 15-3 summarizes the pharmacotherapeutic treatment recommendations, based on the approaches I use in my clinic every day.

Bupropion SR. The overwhelming majority of patients with tobacco dependence will benefit from treatment with bupropion SR. It should be started well before the patient's TQD. The FDA-approved prescribing information recommends 7 to 14 days. Some patients find that a longer bupropion lead-in period before the TQD is beneficial. Some patients (~25%) actually report not only a decreased desire to smoke but note that, without trying to reduce their cigarette consumption, they are smoking less. Some of these patients are eager to wait a little longer before actually quitting cigarette use, until they feel they are experiencing a maximum pre-TQD effect from bupropion. Other patients, once perceiving this benefit, want to stop smoking immediately. Conversely, some patients may experience one or more of the adverse events discussed earlier, most often mild insomnia or mild headache. I want to see these events controlled before the TQD because both are also physiologically caused nicotine withdrawal symptoms. For either reason, it is certainly appropriate to delay the TQD another week or 2. Treatment for these symptoms is different if they are caused by nicotine withdrawal or bupropion SR.

Box 15-2. What the Treating Physician Must Do While the Patient Is Still Smoking, Before Initiating Tobacco-Dependence Medications

Make certain the patient has been developing an "Action Plan" (see Table 15-6)
Have the patient set a "Target Quit Date" at least 2 weeks in the future
Make certain the patient understands that the treatment goal is not merely to stop smoking but also to be able to live life normally, feeling, thinking, and interacting with others in ways that are normal for that individual
Make certain the patient understands that you will individualize comprehensive medical treatment to maximize that individual's chances of stopping smoking and staying stopped (realizing that tobacco dependence is a chronic, relapsing disease)
Make certain the patient understands that you cannot predict how long that specific individual will need to be taking medication (including tapering), but it will be longer than he or she was likely thinking:
Average duration (for effective treatment): 6–9 months
Range: 6 weeks to years
25–35% of tobacco-dependent patients will need lifetime treatment, with at least one medication, to remain tobacco free
Make certain the patient understands that medication tapering will not begin until two criteria have been met:
The patient has been tobacco free for 30–60 consecutive days (clinical judgment call on your part) and
The patient feels comfortable beginning medication tapering
Make certain the patient understands that medication tapering is not a down escalator (see Box 15-6)
Make certain the patient understands that if he or she even thinks a nicotine withdrawal problem might be developing, the patient should promptly call you
Obtain Fagerström Test for Nicotine Dependence (see Box 15-1)
Obtain a blood specimen for serum cotinine analysis (see Boxes 15-1 and 15-3)

Box 15-3. Pragmatic Method to Initiate Tobacco-Dependence Medications

If using bupropion sustained release (recommended for most patients):
Start bupropion at least 1–2 weeks *before* the TQD
Initial dose: 150 mg every morning for 3–7 days or longer if necessary or desired
Then, increase to the therapeutic dose of 150 mg every 12 hours (300-mg total daily dose) at least 5–7 days before the TQD

If using the nicotine patch (recommended for most patients) determine initial dose:
Serum cotinine[a] ≥250 ng of cotinine/cc: start with two nicotine patches delivering a total of 30 mg of nicotine/16 hours (I advise that all nicotine patches be removed after approximately 16 hours of use, otherwise the patient will be at high risk for severe insomnia or bizarre dreams)
Serum cotinine <250 ng of cotinine/cc: start with one nicotine patch delivering a total of 15 mg of nicotine/16 hours[b]

Realize that the above, "simple" algorithm is going to underdose a large proportion of patients, so be prepared to increase the dose, even on the TQD

Instruct the patient to start using your prescribed nicotine patch dose beginning the morning of the TQD

See the patient back in your office 3–5 days after the TQD
Have the prescribed medication(s) produced the desired therapeutic effect?
Has the patient been able to completely (and relatively easily) stop smoking?
Are *all* nicotine withdrawal symptoms (see Table 15-2) negligible or nonexistent?
Is the patient experiencing any medication side effects?

Adjust medication dose(s), as required

Add booster medications—nicotine nasal spray, inhaler, and/or polacrilex (4-mg dose)—as necessary (see text)
Prescribe these as you would a metered dose inhaler for asthma:
You or your office staff must train the patient in the proper use technique *and*
Have the patient demonstrate the correct use technique before leaving your office

If the patient is doing well, without any problems, then have him or her return in about 3 weeks

If the patient is having difficult nicotine withdrawal symptoms, is smoking, or both, then have the patient come back in another 5–10 days, after dose adjustments (use clinical judgment to determine time interval between appointments); base visit frequency on how the patient is responding to revised treatment

[a] Cotinine can be assayed on serum by most commercial labs, such as BioScience, SmithKline, etc. Cost varies, ranging from $35–$75/assay.
[b] During the 16 hours that the patient is awake, you want nicotine delivery to be approximately 0.9 mg of nicotine per hour per patch. This is accomplished by all the largest-size nicotine patches (30 cm²) currently on the market, including Habitrol (Nicotinell in Europe), NicoDerm, Nicotrol (Nicorette in Europe), and ProStep.[69] Note that these are labeled on the package and the patch itself as delivering 21-mg nicotine/24 hours, 21-mg nicotine/24 hours, 15-mg nicotine/16 hours, and 22-mg nicotine/24 hours, respectively. They all, in fact, deliver 15 mg of nicotine during the first 16 hours of "wear" time. The major difference, in terms of nicotine delivery, occurs if the patch is worn for 24 hours. Then, each patch will deliver an additional 6, 6, 1, and 7 mg of nicotine, respectively, during the 8 hours the patient is asleep. The more nicotine delivered to the central nervous system during the 8-hour sleep cycle, the greater the incidence of sleep disturbances and bizarre dreams.
TQD, target quit date.

Because bupropion SR is so safe and shows a linear dose-response relationship, patients should take the maximal tolerable dosage (usually 300 mg/d, given in divided doses, about 12 hours apart) before the TQD, feel comfortable with that dosage, and not be experiencing any intolerable side effects.

Transdermal Nicotine (Nicotine Patch). I aim to individualize the nicotine patch dosage so that the venous cotinine level, during patch treatment after the TQD, is at least equal to what it was during baseline smoking. Our clinical experience has shown that doing so, alone, comes close to eliminating nicotine withdrawal symptoms. Then, in the first few days after the TQD, based on presence, absence, or severity of nicotine withdrawal symptoms, dosing adjustments can be fine-tuned. Also, agents such as nicotine nasal spray or nicotine polacrilex can be added to give patients both a sense of control and actual control over their nicotine intake, enabling small nicotine boluses at needed times, such as during a stressful meeting.

The nicotine patch dosage must be close to optimal from the TQD for two simple reasons:

1. If the dose is too high, patients will develop nausea or vomiting, which may lead them to stop patch treatment and resume smoking.
2. If the dose is too low, patients will be plagued with nicotine withdrawal symptoms of varying severity, which may prevent them from stopping smoking.

In an attempt to meet this goal, some researchers suggest using two standard 30-cm^2 nicotine patches (delivering 15 mg of nicotine per 16 hours or 21 mg of nicotine per 24 hours) as initial treatment if the patient smokes more than 20 cigarettes daily or one patch if the patient smokes fewer than 20 cigarettes daily.[103] In the first day or two after the TQD, the dosage can be increased or decreased as clinically indicated.

Using a nicotine patch dosing algorithm to compute the starting patch dosage may provide a more precise approach. Such an algorithm could use multiple cigarette smoking; baseline factors, such as venous cotinine level while smoking; age; sex; and body weight.[73] The benefit of this approach would be that the initial patch dosage would be close to optimal for each specific patient based on that patient's specific, easily determined, pretreatment factors. Our work to date indicates that three nicotine patches, delivering 45 mg of nicotine per 16 hours is the mean dosage necessary to achieve 100% venous cotinine replacement; however, the range varies from a low of 15 mg of nicotine per 16 hours (one "full-strength" patch) to 75 mg of nicotine per 16 hours (five patches).[73] This seems to be a normally distributed curve, so only a few patients need either one or five patches per day to achieve 100% replacement. Research also shows a highly significant linear correlation, $P < .01$, between percentage of nicotine replacement in venous blood by patch treatment and probability of stopping smoking. When the percentage of nicotine replacement is less than 50%, then the effectiveness of nicotine patch therapy is no better than that of placebo patch (DPL Sachs, Percent cotinine replacement by nicotine patch and probability of stopping smoking, unpublished data, 1995; RD Hurt, Percent cotinine replacement and probability of stopping smoking, unpublished data, 1995).[73]

The Critical First 7 Days After the Target Quit Date. If the starting medication dosages are close to optimal, the patient will simply not be bothered by nicotine withdrawal symptoms (see Table 15-2). Cravings for cigarettes will be easy to control. The patient will have a relatively easy and pain-free time not smoking. Remain alert, however, to underdosing. Careful questioning, which takes only a few minutes, will clearly establish whether the nicotine patch dosage should be increased.

Most of the time, patients feel and function much better than with any previous quit attempt. Consequently, if you do not show them a list of common nicotine withdrawal symptoms and explicitly ask whether any of these symptoms are worse than usual for them—"Are any of these symptoms more severe now than when you were smoking?"— you will miss diagnosing inadequate medication dosage or combination and thus miss the opportunity to optimize treatment. You will miss the opportunity to intervene in treatment at the single most critical time in therapy to help your patient continue not smoking. Remember that most patients in the early stages of treatment relapse because of uncontrolled nicotine withdrawal symptoms. (Later in treatment, after the third to twelfth month, unanticipated stress is the leading cause of relapse.)[117]

Some patients in the first week after the TQD (or the first few weeks, for that matter) have virtually no nicotine withdrawal symptoms, most of the time, but find that craving for cigarettes becomes uncontrollable when they are under severe stress, either at home or at work. At these times, they may slip and have several cigarettes (see Box 15-4). Slipping indicates medication underdosing and the need to increase the dosage of one or more medications and/or to add a relatively faster release form of nicotine medication: nicotine nasal spray (Nicotrol NS), nicotine polacrilex, 4-mg dose (Nicorette), or nicotine inhaler (Nicotrol Inhaler). Box 15-5 summarizes options to consider if the patient is having difficulty stopping smoking after the TQD or is experiencing disruptive nicotine withdrawal symptoms.

Important Add-On or Booster Medications. Nicotine nasal spray (Nicotrol NS), nicotine polacrilex, 4-mg dose (Nicorette), and nicotine inhaler (Nicotrol Inhaler) are all effective medications in the treatment of tobacco dependence. To be effective as primary monotherapy, however, and to achieve a therapeutic serum nicotine level, the nicotine nasal spray must be used 20 to 40 times per day, which is often impractical for many patients. Similarly, nicotine polacrilex needs to be used a minimum of nine times each day and preferably once per hour. The nicotine inhaler is even more demanding: four to six nicotine-containing cartridges, *minimum*, must be used per day (up to a maximum of 16 cartridges). Each cartridge must then be puffed on 100 to 200 times within about 20 minutes after the patient has activated the cartridge.

Although each of these medications can be used alone to treat tobacco dependence, as discussed earlier in this chapter, I have found that it makes the most sense, physiologically and practically, to use these medications as "booster" medications, on top of a foundation of an adequate nicotine patch dosage, as Box 15-4 shows with nicotine polacrilex.

Nicotine nasal spray, polacrilex, and inhaler are not FDA approved for use in combination, and they likely never will be for several reasons. First, such multicombination trials are difficult and costly. Second, different companies manufacture these products and have competing economic visions. Consequently, it is *not* likely that any of the pharmaceutical companies will conduct the relevant trials, let alone make the submission to the FDA that would then lead to FDA approval of that combination, whether involving two, three, four, or five medications. Therefore, *medical* practice will have to be guided by the clinical trials that do get conducted and published in the peer-reviewed, scientific literature, combined with an understanding of the basic pathophysiological features of tobacco dependence, the pharmacologic features of each medication available, and clinical judgment. Nonetheless, well-controlled, well-designed, randomized, double-blind trials, as discussed in depth earlier in this chapter, consistently show that combination use is more effective than use of either medication alone. One of the virtues of these medications is that from a pharmacokinetic standpoint it is virtually impossible for patients to overdose, particularly when used in addition to the nicotine patch. CNS-mediated nicotine regulation[118,119] prevents overdose.[120]

My clinical experience shows that each of these three relatively more immediate-release nicotine medications is important in the methods to help effectively treat the patient with tobacco dependence. Skillful prescription of one or more of these medications, in addition to the foundation of bupropion SR + individualized nicotine patch dose, can make all the difference between effective and ineffective treatment of tobacco dependence.

Box 15-4. Clinical Case #1: Effective Medical Management of Cigarette Slips Secondary to Acute Work-Related Stress During the First 6 Weeks of Tobacco-Dependence Treatment

The patient was a 54-year-old male Silicon Valley CEO presenting for tobacco-dependence treatment because his shortness of breath was interfering with all aspects of his life. He had only mild obstructive airway disease (mixed emphysematous and chronic bronchitic type) by pulmonary function testing but had hypoxemia, SpO$_2$ 91% on room air. He was smoking 1½ packs/day and was highly nicotine dependent, using the Fagerström Tolerance Questionnaire scale, with 8 points of a maximum of 11. He set his TQD for 9/13/93 using three standard-strength nicotine patches (delivering 45 mg of nicotine per 16 hours). The patient was delightfully surprised at how well he did initially. For the first 2 days he had no nicotine withdrawal symptoms of any kind, including craving for cigarettes. (He also had no signs or symptoms of nicotine toxicity.) As the first week wore on, however, he noticed that he was becoming progressively more irritable. Also, he was becoming plagued by intermittent, incredibly intense, and frequent cigarette urges.

Then late in the afternoon of his fourth day after stopping smoking, in response to severe stress at work, he had three cigarettes in rapid succession. He had no more cigarettes after that time, through the time he came to the clinic about 24 hours later. Because of those slips, however, as well as the increased cigarette craving and irritability, his nicotine patch dose was increased by 33% so that he was wearing four nicotine patches delivering 60 mg of nicotine per 16 hours. Moreover he was given a prescription for 4 mg of nicotine polacrilex as needed so that he felt that he could actively do something to immediately control intense cigarette urges.

Because of the medication changes and also because of the patient's smoking in response to an acute stress situation, the patient was seen 10 days later, on 9/27/93. He had used the four nicotine patches as prescribed and without difficulty. He was also using approximately four pieces of the 4-mg nicotine polacrilex daily. He had no medication side effects whatsoever. The patient reported that after his previous visit on 9/17/93, within 1 hour of putting on the fourth patch later that day he noted a marked decrease in irritability, anger, and cravings for cigarettes. During these preceding 10 days, however, he slipped on 4 separate days, having 1 cigarette on each of those days. Generally the trigger was work-related stress, but on one morning he rushed out of his house, forgetting to put on his four nicotine patches. He continued to have intermittent slips, nearly all secondary to sudden work-related stress for 6 weeks after his TQD. Finally, after he increased his daily usage of 4-mg nicotine polacrilex, while continuing to wear four nicotine patches/day, he was able to stop smoking completely on 10/27/93. Over the next 6 months, while not decreasing this nicotine patch dose, he slowly tapered off nicotine polacrilex. Then, during the next 4 months, he slowly tapered off his four nicotine patches. Throughout this time, he was seen about every 4 weeks. He knew to call immediately if he had any flare-ups in nicotine withdrawal symptoms, such as cigarette craving, irritability, or anger as this nicotine dose-reduction process was going on. (Of course, if he had a slip and smoked even part of a cigarette, that would be reason for a STAT phone call!)

Finally, 11 months after his quit date, he successfully tapered off all his nicotine medications. He had definitely needed the steady-state serum nicotine level that the four nicotine patches provided, but he also needed to be able to provide his central nervous system with periodic nicotine boosts, which the 4-mg dose of nicotine polacrilex provided. For approximately 2 months, from October to December 1993, his therapeutic nicotine dose, from both medications, was about 90 mg/d. This is what he needed to control his nicotine withdrawal symptoms to enable him to successfully stop smoking (dose to therapeutic effect). He had no nicotine toxicity symptoms or adverse events of any kind.

This gentleman continues to be 100% tobacco free now, more than 6 years later. And, of course, his pulmonary status improved dramatically, both clinically and physiologically. In fact his SpO$_2$ is now normal at 98% on room air, and he can run the length of San Francisco International Airport, carrying his laptop and garment bag, without any shortness of breath. (Of note, his symptoms and physiology improved substantially, even during the first 2 weeks after the TQD, despite the occasional cigarette slips, with dyspnea on exertion decreasing by 50% chronic productive cough completely resolving, and SpO$_2$ increasing from 91 to 95%.)

SpO$_2$, oxygen saturation by pulse oximeter; TQD, target quit date.

Box 15-5. Options If the Patient Is Having Difficulty Stopping Smoking
or With Nicotine Withdrawal Symptoms

Identify the problems specifically and precisely

Consider adding a more rapid-release nicotine medication—nicotine nasal spray, inhaler, or polacrilex (4-mg dose)—that the patient can use if episodic, severe cravings or intermittent stress seem to be part of the problem (see Box 5-4)

Consider increasing the nicotine patch dose if the patient has more persistent problems throughout the day[a] (see Box 5-4)

Reduce the nicotine patch dose if the patient develops nausea or vomiting and there is no other obvious explanation

Ask yourself if your patient might have an underlying depressive or anxiety disorder that the ultrahigh nicotine doses, puff-to-puff, from tobacco smoke were masking; if so, consider psychiatric consultation

Are there any other lifestyle, behavioral, personal, professional, or family issues that the patient needs to address? If so, then suggest that the patient re-review the Action Plan and the self-help material used; also, consider referral to a tobacco-dependence specialist, psychologist, or psychiatrist

[a] Some patients (~1–5%) will need to have their dose escalated as high as five patches (delivering 75 mg of nicotine over 16 hours) to be able to stop smoking and adequately suppress nicotine withdrawal symptoms so that they are functioning normally.

It is important to instruct patients in the use of each of these three nicotine medications before their TQD. The instructional protocol is virtually identical to that used when training an asthmatic to use a metered dose inhaler:

1. Health care provider *describes* correct use of the nicotine delivery medication
2. Health care provider *demonstrates* correct use technique
3. Health care provider has *patient describe* correct use technique
4. Health care provider *observes patient demonstrating* correct use technique

Patients frequently have distinct preferences for a particular device. Encourage them to learn to use all of them, before their TQD, so that after their TQD they can experiment with each to determine which device or devices provide the best relief of nicotine withdrawal symptoms. Patients should be instructed to use these medications on an as-needed basis. Typically, patients will use six to nine nasal spray doses or pieces of nicotine polacrilex per day or two to three nicotine inhaler cartridges per day.

Duration of Medication Use. No studies have been published to date that have been designed to determine the optimal duration of treatment. In fact, no studies have been conducted to determine whether such a thing as "an optimal treatment duration" even exists. (What is the optimal treatment duration for inhaled corticosteroids in Step 3 or 4 asthma? Two years? Five years? Lifetime? Does it even exist? No such studies have been carried out with asthma medications, either.)

In the tobacco-dependence literature, with only a few exceptions, medications have been provided for only a relatively short time: 6 to 12 weeks. The Agency for Health Care Policy and Research Guideline recommendations notwithstanding, the FDA's expert Drug Abuse Advisory Committee flatly stated in its summary discussion more than a year later, at the end of a 1-day special hearing including this issue, that no study design had been adequate to determine how long treatment should be carried out. They further stated, based on the growing body of knowledge relating to the fundamental neurophysiological changes that exist in the tobacco-dependent patient, that short-term treatment, for example, 6 to 12 weeks, is clearly inadequate. Much longer treatment is required; for life in many cases.[2] Both the FDA and the FDA Drug Abuse Advisory Committee explicitly stated that they wanted to see study designs to address these critical issues surrounding treatment duration.

In my experience, the duration of medication use for patients who are effectively treated is indeed wide. The average duration of use of one or more tobacco-dependence medications is about 9 months. A few may successfully taper off after 6 to 8 weeks; many will still be taking at least one medication, perhaps at lower dosages than at the start of treatment, 1, 2, 3, or even more years later. The yardstick my patients and I use is that no nicotine withdrawal symptoms should occur while slowly reducing the dosage of a medication (and medications should be tapered one at a time). Sometimes, when a patient is given a few days to stabilize at a lower dosage of a medication, nicotine withdrawal symptoms will resolve completely. If they do not, however, the dosage should be increased to the level at which the patient felt comfortable and had no withdrawal symptoms. A few weeks later, I will again try to reduce the medication, but more gradually than with the first attempt. Some patients find that they simply cannot accomplish dosage reduction without return of one or more nicotine withdrawal symptoms that are severe enough to begin interfering with their life. In such cases, the patient and I usually decide that the benefit of long-term, indefinite medication use, perhaps for life, far outweighs the medical risk of smoking relapse.

Practical Approach for Medication Tapering. Because controlled trial data are totally lacking, I have adopted an approach similar to that pulmonologists use in tapering asthmatic medications for tapering tobacco-dependence medications. This approach has worked well in practice and is summarized in Box 15-6. I advise patients at their first visit that they should not even contemplate tapering medications until they have met two criteria:

1. They have been completely tobacco free for 30 to 60 consecutive days.
2. They feel fully comfortable in starting to taper medications.

I also reiterate that tapering is not a down escalator, so to speak. The primary clinical management goal during medication tapering is the same as it was during treatment. Stopping smoking is not good enough. The patient should also be able to live life normally. The patient should feel normal; think normally; and interact with friends, family, and colleagues in the manner that is normal, typical, and usual for that individual. Only then will we taper one, and only one, medication at a time, starting with the most rapid-release nicotine medication the patient is taking, for example, nicotine nasal spray, nicotine polacrilex, or nicotine inhaler.

Box 15-6. Pragmatic Method for Tapering Tobacco-Dependence Medications

---

Medication tapering is not a down escalator
No "optimal" treatment length exists
Begin tapering only after the patient has been tobacco free for 30–60 consecutive
    days AND
The patient feels confident to start tapering
Taper one, and only one, medication at a time
Taper the most rapid-release nicotine medication first:
    Nicotine nasal spray, then
    Nicotine inhaler or nicotine polacrilex, then
    Nicotine patch
Taper or stop bupropion sustained release last
If nicotine withdrawal symptoms occur at any tapering step, revert to the previous
    dose, restabilize, then try a smaller dose reduction
Remember: About 25–35% of tobacco-dependent patients will require lifetime
    medication use (like most asthmatics) to remain tobacco free

---

For example, say the patient has been taking bupropion SR, 150 mg, every 12 hours, + nicotine patch (×3), delivering 45 mg of nicotine per 16 hours, + nicotine nasal spray, 7 to 8 doses per day (7-8 mg of nicotine/day from nasal spray), for the past 60 days, has been completely tobacco free since the TQD, and feels comfortable starting to taper. I would then advise the patient, over the next month, to continue using the same bupropion and nicotine patch dosages but to progressively reduce the number of nicotine nasal spray doses used per day. If nicotine withdrawal symptoms occur (see Table 15-2), then the patient needs to reduce more slowly. (Most patients have little difficulty tapering off nicotine nasal spray while they have an adequate, individualized nicotine patch dose + bupropion SR to continue providing a therapeutic foundation.) Keeping in mind the primary objective of continuing to keep nicotine withdrawal symptoms suppressed, tapering off regular, daily nicotine nasal spray use generally takes about 4 weeks, with an individual patient range of 2 to 6 weeks. I then advise the patient to keep the nasal spray readily available in pocket or purse as emergency therapy in case a severe nicotine withdrawal symptom suddenly erupts.

Once off regular, daily use of nicotine nasal spray, I then have the patient commence gradual reduction of the nicotine patch dosage, keeping the bupropion SR dosage unchanged. Most patients will readily tolerate a one-third dosage reduction, down to two patches delivering 30 mg of nicotine per 16 hours. Some, however, cannot and will report feeling strong cravings for cigarettes, becoming cranky, or developing any constellation of nicotine withdrawal symptoms. If so, the patient should increase back to three patches to restabilize. After 2 to 4 weeks back at the higher dose, the patient reduces the patch dose again, but this time by only one-third to one-half of one patch. (Both NicoDerm and Nicotrol are solid-state patches and may be easily and safely cut into any fractional dosage that the treating health care provider and patient desire. Because these patches are solid state, neither will "dump" nicotine, which could happen with either the Habitrol or ProStep patches, which are not solid-state patches.) Thus, for example, the patient would be receiving a total nicotine patch dose of 2½ patches delivering 37.5 mg of nicotine per 16 hours. The patient should stay at each patch dose reduction for a minimum of 2 weeks, and longer if necessary, before reducing the nicotine patch dose again. Thus, successful tapering off three nicotine patches will take a minimum of 6 weeks and can take many months—as long as a year. Some patients find, after they reduce the patch dosage to only one patch per day, that no matter how gradually they try to further reduce the patch dosage, intolerable nicotine withdrawal symptoms appear. The chief symptoms in my experience causing this problem have been difficulty concentrating, severe craving for cigarettes (in certain, usually highly specific, settings), and/or increased irritability. When this happens, I advise the patient that their brain cells are not yet capable of normal function without nicotine being present and that tapering should be postponed for a few months.

Approximately 25 to 35% of patients find that they cannot taper all medications without return of nicotine withdrawal symptoms that are disruptive to their lives. Because they generally know, from previous quit attempts, that these symptoms will completely resolve if they resume cigarette use, the decision becomes: (*a*) resume smoking or (*b*) continue use of one or more tobacco-dependence medications indefinitely. Most patients have no desire to resume smoking at this point because they have usually been in treatment for 6 to 18 months and have noted marked improvement in their health. Not surprisingly, they usually opt to continue one or more tobacco-dependence medications indefinitely.

Reasons for Treatment Failure
The reasons for treatment failure are fairly complex but usually center around one of the following basic issues: (*a*) the patient retains the belief that stopping smoking is merely a matter of willpower, (*b*) the patient cannot or will not accept that he or she is physically addicted to nicotine, and (*c*) the patient does not want to accept the fact that tobacco dependence is a chronic medical disease. Other reasons for treatment failure are outlined

in Box 15-7. Finally, of course, the initial diagnosis may be incorrect. Instead of being in the Preparation or Action Phases, the patient may be in, say, the Precontemplation Phase and nowhere near ready to stop smoking.

Action Phase

When you discover that one of your patients has recently stopped smoking (whether or not that individual used an over-the-counter nicotine medication), you should inquire whether your patient is living life normally. Specifically, determine if the patient is more anxious, restless, irritable, short-tempered, moody, sad, or depressed than usual. The patient should also be asked whether he or she is experiencing any difficulty thinking, at work or at home, or is having difficulty concentrating or focusing thought. In short, merely stopping smoking is not good enough. Your patient should not be suffering from nicotine withdrawal. If nicotine withdrawal is present, then the risk for relapse will be extremely high.

Most patients who stop smoking either cold turkey or by using standard-dose nicotine patch will experience nicotine withdrawal symptoms. They will not be aware, however, that the symptoms they are experiencing are directly caused by nicotine withdrawal, that they do not need to endure the pain and discomfort these symptoms cause, and that these symptoms are treatable. They will not be aware that untreated, these symptoms presage relapse.

Box 15-7. Reasons Tobacco-Dependence Treatment Is Not Effective

Patients refuse to accept that they are physically addicted to nicotine
Patients refuse to accept that stopping smoking is not merely a matter of willpower
Patient belief that all this work is not really necessary, "All I really have to do is try harder and exert more self-control"
Patient cannot accept the diagnosis of having a chronic medical disease
Patient wants a quick fix ("make it better, doctor; make it go away")
Patients do not like the thought of contemplating the possibility of long-term to lifetime use of one or more medications to keep tobacco dependence controlled and therefore enable them not to need to use tobacco products, such as cigarettes
Patient makes the decision, explicitly or tacitly, that, despite the medical consequences, they would rather be smoking cigarettes, i.e., "I'd rather live a shorter (medically disabled) life with cigarettes than a longer (healthier, less medically disabled) life without cigarettes"
Patient just gives up
Patient does not use medications as prescribed
Patient does not communicate occurrence of nicotine withdrawal symptoms to treating health care provider, leading to relapse
Patient does not communicate medication side effects to treating health care provider, leading patient to reduce or stop one or more medications, leading to intolerable (to the patient) nicotine withdrawal symptoms, in turn leading to relapse
Patient self-tapers one or more medications too rapidly, leading to onset of one or more nicotine withdrawal symptoms, such as craving for cigarettes, in turn leading to relapse
Patients have a cigarette slip, or partial relapse, leading to self-recrimination, self-flagellation, and/or guilt, preventing them from returning to the treating health care provider for treatment modification
Patient has or develops the attitude: failure begets failure
Patient has or develops an attitude in which failure becomes a self-fulfilling prophecy
Patient can no longer afford the cost of medications
Patient can no longer afford the cost of treatment

For example, a young software engineer had stopped smoking using one nicotine patch daily. She had not smoked anything since her TQD. When I saw her 1 week after her TQD I asked her if she could write computer code normally for her. She paused a moment, then said not only had she been unable to write a line of code since stopping smoking 1 week ago but she could not even conceptualize the algorithms. I asked her if this had ever happened before, to which she responded, "never." She also commented that this past week she had been extremely rude and short-tempered with the software team she supervised. This was not like her. I advised her to double her nicotine patch dose and return to see me in a week. When I saw her 1 week later, she reported that the day after I last saw her, on the increased patch dose, she could think again, she was working productively again, and she was her usual self in interactions with her colleagues.

Precontemplation and Contemplation Phases

The health care provider's goal here is to help move patients out of these phases into the Preparation Phase (Fig. 15-6). Medications, such as bupropion or nicotine patch, should not be prescribed for patients in these stages. Rather, they should be informed that when they decide they would like to stop, you are there to help them; to make the process easier, less of a struggle, and less painful; and, in short, to provide effective treatment. Two things that the health care provider can do for patients in these phases are as follows:

- Point out that scientific studies repeatedly show that *each* cigarette smoked knocks 6½ minutes off the individual smoker's life expectancy.[121,122] Thus, at the end of only 1 day, the two packs-per-day smoker will have reduced his or her life expectancy by more than 4 hours!
- Have brochures (see "Resources") available in the waiting and examination rooms, such as "Facts About Chronic Bronchitis" or "Facts About Second-Hand Smoke." Most patients in these phases will not ask for such information but will take it if it is made available to them. Such material can help keep lines of communication open and, over time, move patients to the Preparation Phase.

Follow-Up

The optimum follow-up schedule for treating a patient with tobacco dependence is similar to that used in the treatment of a patient with newly diagnosed asthma. The following is the schedule of visits I use for managing a tobacco-dependent patient:

- Visit #1: Before the Target Quit Date (TQD)

    Perform a standard medical history and physical examination
    Obtain blood for serum cotinine determination
    Measure Fagerström Test for Nicotine Dependence

- Visit #2: Before the TQD

    Review any diagnostic study results with the patient
    Make certain the patient understands the basic biologic features of nicotine addiction as well as the goals of treatment
    Outline the basic treatment plan
    Provide the patient with instructions and resources for developing an individualized Action Plan
    Have the patient set a tentative TQD
    Presuming I am going to prescribe bupropion SR, start the patient on a low dose—150 mg of bupropion SR every morning

Following visit 2, check with the patient by telephone after 3 to 7 days on low-dose bupropion to make certain the patient is not having any side effects; if any side effects are present, then institute appropriate treatment before increasing the dosage to 150 mg every 12 hours.

- Visit #3: Before the TQD (about 7 days after the patient has been advanced to 150 mg of bupropion SR twice daily, and also about 1-3 days before the TQD)

    Make certain that the higher dosage of bupropion SR is well tolerated
    Review the patient's Action Plan
    Review the previously selected TQD to determine if it still makes sense for the patient
    Prescribe individualized nicotine patch dose and inquire whether the patient would like to discuss the strengths and weaknesses of the relatively more rapid-release nicotine medications, that is, nasal spray, inhaler, or polacrilex

- Visit #4: 3 to 5 days After the TQD

    Determine presence or absence of disruptive nicotine withdrawal symptoms
    Optimize medication dosages to further suppress nicotine withdrawal symptoms and add additional medications, if necessary

Visit frequency thereafter depends on how the patient is doing medically and what you and the patient assess the patient's needs to be from a human contact perspective. In general, frequency is every 3 to 4 weeks until the start of medication tapering. If their treatment course has been rocky, these patients should be seen more often. If the patient decides to remain on the "maintenance" treatment medications and dosages for longer than 2 months, then I will plan to see the individual every 1 to 3 months until the patient feels ready to initiate medication tapering. Once medication tapering starts, I will see the patient every month or so until tapering is either completed or the patient has hit a plateau and cannot taper any further. If the patient requires long-term (>1 year) use of one or more tobacco-dependence medications, then I will generally see the patient every 6 to 12 months, or more often if needed. Always before, during, and after medication treatment I remind my patients to call or page if they have *any* questions, problems, or concerns, just as they would if they were being treated for asthma.

Follow-up office visits are critical to successful long-term medical management of any chronic disease. Tobacco dependence is no exception. Such follow-up in tobacco dependence is particularly important even after the patient discontinues all tobacco-dependence medications. Will patients keep these follow-up appointments? Some do; others do not, just as we see when treating other chronic medical diseases, once patients feel that their disease is stable.

What the Patient Must Hear From the Treating Clinician at the Start of Treatment

Because patient misunderstanding about tobacco dependence—the disease, its origins, and its treatment—is so rampant, your patients must hear several points from you before they actually commence treatment for their tobacco dependence. These critical points and concepts are summarized in Box 15-5.

A LOOK TO THE FUTURE

Twenty-five years ago cigarette smoking was thought to be a habit that could be "kicked" just like any other habit. All it took was willpower. Now we know that is not the case.

Twenty-five years ago we barely had the capability of measuring nicotine or cotinine levels in body fluids. Now we have the beginnings of a solid understanding of the neuronal genotypes that predispose to nicotine addiction, without which tobacco dependence cannot occur. We are also beginning to understand how nicotine affects—generally quite beneficially—the CNS at a cellular, subcellular, and molecular level. As this fundamental research continues in neurogenetics, neurophysiology, neuropathology, and neuropharmacology, our understanding of the real nature and natural history of tobacco dependence will continue to grow. As that happens, our treatment paradigms will continue to evolve. Such basic research will lead to the development of entirely new treatments and medications. For example, a completely new research area that seems to hold considerable therapeutic promise is nicotine immunology (Torgny H. Svensson, MD, PhD, personal communication, 1999).

It would seem, however, that the tremendous advances that will come in the next 10 years will be primarily through the academic and government sectors. Although the pharmaceutical industry grosses more than one-quarter of a billion dollars per year in the United States alone, it is currently investing little in research and development into advancing therapeutic approaches to nicotine addiction.

Fortunately, in 1999 the National Cancer Institute, in conjunction with the National Institute on Drug Abuse, embarked on an ambitious new tobacco control research program that is exceptionally well funded. Already these two National Institutes of Health institutes have established seven transdisciplinary research centers with leading investigators in the field. The academic disciplines involved range from molecular genetics to neurosciences to behavioral sciences to epidemiology, with the ultimate focus being to develop totally new and innovative strategies to prevent the onset of tobacco dependence in children and teenagers and to more effectively treat it in those who are or become tobacco dependent. The National Cancer Institute and the National Institute on Drug Abuse anticipate funding an additional five centers within the next 2 years. Thus, the United States will have a total of 12 basic and clinical science research and treatment centers by 2002. These centers will provide a solid funding, research, and training base that the tobacco-dependence field has sorely needed. An additional benefit of this initiative is that it will help to confer academic, scientific, and medical legitimacy and credibility to the tobacco-dependence field, which has certainly been wanting in most American medical schools.[123,124] Perhaps, then, as major new discoveries and insights emerge from these endeavors, our university and government scientists and clinicians will drag the pharmaceutical industry into the new millennium.

SUMMARY

Smoking cessation paradigms dating from the 1960s are based on the incorrect assumption that tobacco dependence is a short-term, nonchronic, self-limited matter of willpower, much less a disease, for which short-term treatment of a few days to 8 to 12 weeks should be sufficient. It can be effectively managed and treated, but only when recognized that tobacco dependence is a serious, life-threatening, chronic medical disease. Tobacco dependence is not a habit, and neither is its cardinal symptom, cigarette smoking. Tobacco dependence has distinct, defined, neurogenetic and neuropathological bases. Merely stopping smoking is an insufficient goal in tobacco-dependence treatment and sets the patient up for failure. What is required is rational pharmacotherapy based on the "treat-to-effect" or "dose-to-effect" model used to effectively treat many other complex chronic diseases, such as asthma, hypertension, or diabetes. This model includes providing adequate pharmacotherapy to suppress physiologically caused nicotine withdrawal symptoms, such as craving for cigarettes, increased anxiety, irritability, restlessness, dysphoria, depression, short-temperedness, increased appetite, or difficulty concentrating.

Treat-to-effect also means providing assistance, resources, and referral, if necessary, so that patients adequately attend to the psychological dependence side of tobacco dependence. Although medications suppress nicotine withdrawal symptoms, patients need to actively restructure their lives to undo the decades-long set of conditioned responses that causes them to want a cigarette in certain "trigger" settings, such as after a meal, when under stress, or when making a telephone call. For tobacco dependence to be effectively treated, nicotine addiction and psychological dependence must both be treated.

Throughout treatment and during medication tapering, the therapeutic goal must continue to be enabling the patient to lead as normal a life as possible, that is, nicotine withdrawal symptoms must be as completely suppressed as possible. If any start to occur, or recur, as medication(s) are tapered, one at a time, then the dosage needs to be increased to restabilize the patient then reduced more gradually.

None of the medications currently available for tobacco-dependence treatment are known to reverse the underlying neuronal pathology of tobacco dependence. Consequently, we have to anticipate that, as with asthma, some patients will need to take effective tobacco-dependence medications for many years to life if they are to be able to remain tobacco free.

Of all the clinical treatment trials conducted to date, *none* have been based on the fundamental neuropathologic factors that underpin tobacco dependence. Until studies are conducted that address these scientific insights, treatment must be empirically based, based on the scientific information we do have, and focused initially on complete suppression of all nicotine withdrawal symptoms. Then the patient will have the mental energy required to try to figure out how to live life without cigarettes.

ACKNOWLEDGMENTS

This chapter was funded entirely by the personal funds of the author, his family, and one of this book's editors. No pharmaceutical company underwrote this chapter, in whole, in part, or in any way. The opinions expressed herein are solely those of the author. They do not necessarily reflect the views of any of the many pharmaceutical companies whose products are discussed herein or of the US Food and Drug Administration (FDA). Many of the author's therapeutic recommendations go well beyond any FDA label. All such recommendations, however, are solidly based on currently available scientific information.

RESOURCES

Several self-help smoking cessation resources are available to health care providers and their patients:

- Dr. Art Ulene. How to Stop Smoking [Audiobook (audiotape)].Ulene A, Sachs DPL. New York: Random House, 1986. It may be ordered directly from Art Ulene, MD, Feeling Fine, 13160 Mindanao Way, Suite 270, Marina del Rey, CA 90292; 800-332-3373, Ext. 103, Attn: Jamie. The book part only of this audiobook is also available directly from the American Academy of Family Physicians (AAFP), 800-274-2237 or 816-333-9700. It is also available from the AAFP as part of the AAFP's Physician's Office *Stop Smoking Kit*. (Call the AAFP at 800-944-0000 and ask for Product #900. The complete kit costs $60 for AAFP members and $95 for non-AAFP members.)
- "Facts About Chronic Bronchitis" or "Facts About Second-Hand Smoke," brochures from the local chapter of the American Lung Association.

- The American Medical Association's videobook, *Stop [Smoking] For Good: A Video Housecall.*
- The National Cancer Institute has many useful resources and may be reached at 1-800-4-CANCER or http://nci.nih.gov.

REFERENCES

1. Food and Drug Administration. Regulations Restricting the Sale and Distribution of Cigarettes and Smokeless Tobacco to Protect Children and Adolescents: Final Rule. 21 CFR Part 801, et alia ed. Vol. 61. Washington, DC: US Department of Health and Human Services, 1996.
2. Food and Drug Administration. Open public hearing on improving the prescription labeling of smoking cessation products. In: CDER, ed. Drug Abuse Advisory Committee Meeting, With Representation From the Nonprescription Drugs Advisory Committee. Washington, DC: SAG Corp, 1997:251.
3. Henningfield JE, Stapleton JM, Benowitz NL, Grayson RF, London ED. Higher levels of nicotine in arterial than in venous blood after cigarette smoking. Drug Alcohol Depend 1993;33: 23–29.
4. Benwell ME, Balfour DJK, Anderson JM. Evidence that tobacco smoking increases the density of H3-nicotine binding sites in human brain. J Neurochem 1988;50:1243–1247.
5. Breese CR, Marks MJ, Logel J, et al. Effect of smoking history on H3-nicotine binding in human, post-mortem brain. J Pharmacol Exp Ther 1997;282:7–13.
6. Terry DC, Davila-Garcia MI, Stockmeier CA, Dilley GE, Shapiro LA, Kellar KJ. Binding to nicotinic receptors labeled by H3-epibatidine and H3-cytisine is increased in brains of smokers. Society for Neuroscience, 1996;22:1273.
7. Schwartz RD, Kellar KJ. Nicotinic cholinergic receptor binding sites in brain: in vivo regulation. Science 1983;220:214–216.
8. Schwartz RD, Kellar KJ. In vivo regulation of [3H]acetylcholine recognition sites in brain by nicotinic cholinergic drugs. J Neurochem 1985; 45:427–433.
9. Marks MJ, Burch JB, Collins AC. Effects of chronic nicotine infusion on tolerance development and nicotine receptors. J Pharmacol Exp Ther 1983;226:816–825.
10. Marks MJ, Stitzel JA, Collins AC. Time-course study of the effects of chronic nicotine infusion on drug response and brain receptors. J Pharmacol Exp Ther 1985;235:619–628.
11. Hughes JR. Tobacco withdrawal in self-quitters. J Consult Clin Psychol 1992;60:689–697.
12. Henningfield JE. Behavioral pharmacology of cigarette smoking. Adv Behav Pharmacol 1984; 4:131–210.
13. Nisell M, Nomikos GG, Svensson TH. Infusion of nicotine in the ventral tegmental area or the nucleus accumbens of the rat differentially affects

accumbal dopamine release. Pharmacol Toxicol 1994;75:348–352.
14. Nisell M, Nomikos GG, Svensson TH. Systemic nicotine-induced dopamine release in the rat nucleus accumbens is regulated by nicotinic receptors in the ventral tegmental area. Synapse 1994; 16:36–44.
15. Nisell M, Nomikos GG, Svensson TH. Nicotine dependence, midbrain dopamine systems and psychiatric disorders. Pharmacol Toxicol 1995; 76:157–162.
16. Tung C-S, Grenhoff J, Svensson TH. Nicotine counteracts midbrain dopamine cell dysfunction induced by prefrontal cortex inactivation. Acta Physiol Scand 1990;138:427–428.
17. Grenhoff J, Aston-Jones G, Svensson TH. Nicotinic effects on the firing pattern of midbrain dopamine neurons. Acta Physiol Scand 1986; 128:351–358.
18. Grenhoff J, Svensson TH. Selective stimulation of limbic dopamine activity by nicotine. Acta Physiol Scand 1988;133:595–596.
19. Svensson TH, Tung C-S. Local cooling of the prefrontal cortex induces pacemaker-like firing of dopamine neurons in rat ventral tegmental area in vivo. Acta Physiol Scand 1989;136: 135–136.
20. Marshall DL, Redfern PH, Wonnacott S. Presynaptic nicotinic modulation of dopamine release in the three ascending pathways studied by in vivo microdialysis: comparison of naive and chronic nicotine-treated rats. J Neurochem 1997;68:1511–1519.
21. Svensson TH, Engberg G. Effect of nicotine on single cell activity in the noradrenergic nucleus locus coeruleus. Acta Physiol Scand 1980; 479(Suppl):31–34.
22. Svensson TH, Grenhoff J, Engberg G. Effect of nicotine on dynamic function of brain catecholamine neurons. In: Foundation C, ed. The Biology of Nicotine Dependence: Ciba Foundation Symposium 152. New York: John Wiley and Sons, 1990:169–185.
23. Snyder FR, Henningfield JE. Effects of nicotine administration following 12h of tobacco deprivation: assessment on computerized performance tasks. Psychopharmacology 1989;97:17–22.
24. Snyder FR, Davis FC, Henningfield JE. The tobacco withdrawal syndrome: performance decrements assessed on a computerized test battery. Drug Alcohol Depend 1989;23:259–266.
25. Nemeth-Coslett R, Henningfield JE. Effects of nicotine chewing gum on cigarette smoking and subjective and physiologic effects. Clin Pharmacol Ther 1986;39:625–630.
26. Svensson TH. Peripheral, automatic regulation of locus coeruleus noradrenergic neurons

in brain: putative implications for psychiatry and psychopharmacology. Psychopharmacology 1987;92:1–7.

27. Grenhoff J, Svensson TH. Pharmacology of nicotine. Br J Addict 1989;84:477–492.

28. Klesges RC, Meyers AW, Klesges LM, LaVasque ME. Smoking, body weight, and their effects on smoking behavior: a comprehensive review of the literature. Psychol Bull 1989;106(2):204–230.

29. American Psychiatric Association. Nicotine-induced disorder. In: Diagnostic and Statistical Manual of Mental Disorders. 4th ed. Washington, DC: American Psychiatric Association, 1994:244–245.

30. Hughes JR, Hatsukami DK, Pickens RW, Krahn D, Malin S, Luknie A. Effect of nicotine on the tobacco withdrawal syndrome. Psychopharmacology 1984;83:82–87.

31. Nemeth-Coslett R, Henningfield JE, O'Keefe MK, Griffiths RR. Nicotine gum: dose-related effects on cigarette smoking and subjective ratings. Psychopharmacology 1987;92:424–430.

32. Sachs DPL, Benowitz NL. Are smokers trying to stop and smokers not trying to stop the same experimental model? In: Harris et al. ed. Proceedings of the Annual Meeting of the Committee on Problems of Drug Dependence; NIDA Research Monograph 95. Washington, DC: DHHS, PHS, NIDA, 1989:366–367. Publication ADM90-1663.

33. Kendler KS, Neale MC, MacLean CJ, Heath AC, Eaves LJ, Kessler RC. Smoking and major depression: a causal analysis. Arch Gen Psychiatry 1993;50:36–43.

34. Henningfield JE, Schuh LM, Jarvik MI. Pathophysiology of tobacco dependence. In: Bloom FE, Kupfer DJ, eds. Psychopharmacology: The Fourth Generation of Progress. New York: Raven Press, 1995;1:1715–1730.

35. Hughes JR. Genetics of smoking: a brief review. Behav Ther 1986;17:335–345.

36. Heath AC, Cates R, Martin NG, et al. Genetic contribution to risk of smoking initiation: comparisons across birth cohorts and across cultures. J Subst Abuse 1993;5:221–246.

37. Pomerleau OF. Individual differences in sensitivity to nicotine: implications for genetic research on nicotine dependence. Behav Genet 1995; 25:161–177.

38. Nakajima M, Yamamoto T, Nunoya K, et al. Role of human cytochrome P4502A6 in C-oxidation of nicotine. Drug Metab Dispos 1996; 24:1212–1217.

39. Morgan JI, Curran TE. Proto-oncogenes: beyond second messengers. In: Bloom FE, Kupfer DJ, eds. Psychopharmacology: The Fourth Generation of Progress. New York: Raven Press Ltd, 1995:631–642.

40. Chergui K, Nomikos GG, Math JM, Gonon F, Svensson TH. Burst stimulation of the medial forebrain bundle selectively increases FOS-like immunoreactivity in the limbic forebrain of the rat. Neuroscience 1996;72(1):141–156.

41. Svensson TH. Interview with Professor Torgny H. Svensson, MD, PhD, Regarding the Biology of Nicotine Addiction, Conducted by David P.L. Sachs, MD. Palo Alto, CA: Palo Alto Center for Pulmonary Disease Prevention, 1997.

42. Shiffman SM, Paty JA, Gnys M, Kassel JD, Elash C. Nicotine withdrawal in chippers and regular smokers: subjective and cognitive effects. Health Psychol 1995;14(4):301–309.

43. Shiffman SM. Tobacco "chippers": individual differences in tobacco dependence. Psychopharmacology 1989;97(4):539–547.

44. Shiffman SM, Fischer LB, Zettler-Segal M, Benowitz NL. Nicotine exposure among nondependent smokers. Arch Gen Psychiatry 1990; 47(4):333–336.

45. Shiffman SM, Zettler-Segal M, Kassel J, Paty J, Benowitz NL, O'Brien G. Nicotine elimination and tolerance in non-dependent cigarette smokers. Psychopharmacology 1992;109(4):449–456.

46. Shiffman SM, Kassel JD, Paty J, Gnys M, Zettler-Segal M. Smoking typology profiles of chippers and regular smokers. J Subst Abuse 1994;6(1): 21–35.

47. Brauer LH, Hatsukami D, Hanson K, Shiffman SM. Smoking topography in tobacco chippers and dependent smokers. Addict Behav 1996; 21(2):233–238.

48. Heath AC, Martin NG. Genetic models for the natural history of smoking: evidence for a genetic influence on smoking persistence. Addict Behav 1993;18:19–34.

49. Office on Smoking and Health, ed. The Health Consequences of Smoking: Nicotine Addiction: A Report of the Surgeon General. Washington, DC: US Department of Health and Human Services, 1988. DHHS Publication CDC 88-8406.

50. Benowitz NL, ed. Nicotine Safety and Toxicity. New York: Oxford University Press, 1998.

51. Benowitz NL, Gourlay SG. Cardiovascular toxicity of nicotine: implications for nicotine replacement. J Am Coll Cardiol 1997;29(7): 1422–1431.

52. Benowitz NL, Fitzgerald GA, Wilson M, Zhang Q. Nicotine effects on eicosanoid formation and hemostatic function: comparison of transdermal nicotine and cigarette smoking. J Am Coll Cardiol 1993;22(4):1159–1167.

53. Murray RP, Bailey WC, Daniels K, et al. Safety of nicotine polacrilex gum used by 3,094 participants in the Lung Health Study. Chest 1996; 109:438–445.

54. Tonnesen P, Fryd V, Hansen M, et al. Effect of nicotine chewing gum in combination with group counseling on the cessation of smoking. N Engl J Med 1988;318(1):15–18.

55. Sachs DPL. Effectiveness of the 4-mg dose of nicotine polacrilex for the initial treatment of high-dependent smokers. Arch Intern Med 1995;155:1973–1980.

56. Glover ED, Sachs DPL, Stitzer ML, et al. Smoking cessation in highly dependent smokers with 4-mg nicotine polacrilex. Am J Health Behav 1996;20(5):319–332.

57. Tonnesen P, Norregaard J, Simonsen K, Sawe U. A double-blind trial of a 16-hour transdermal nicotine patch in smoking cessation. N Engl J Med 1991;325(5):311–315.

58. Transdermal Nicotine Study Group. Transdermal nicotine for smoking cessation: six-month results from two multicenter controlled clinical trials. JAMA 1991;266:3133–3138.

59. Sachs DPL, Sawe U, Leischow SL. Effectiveness of a 16-hour transdermal nicotine patch in a medical practice setting, without intensive group counseling. Arch Intern Med 1993;153:1881–1890.

60. Hurt RD, Dale LC, Fredrickson PA, et al. Nicotine patch therapy for smoking cessation combined with physician advice and nurse follow-up: 1-year outcome and percentage nicotine replacement. JAMA 1994;271:595–600.

61. Fiore MC, Kenford SL, Jorenby DE, Wetter DW, Smith SS, Baker TB. Two studies of the clinical effectiveness of the nicotine patch with different counseling techniques. Chest 1994; 105:524–533.

62. Sutherland G, Stapleton JA, Russell MAH, et al. Randomised controlled trial of nasal nicotine spray in smoking cessation. Lancet 1992;340: 324–329.

63. Schneider NG, Olmstead R, Mody FV, et al. Efficacy of a nicotine nasal spray in smoking cessation: a placebo-controlled, double-blind trial. Addiction 1995;90:1671–1682.

64. Tonnesen P, Norregaard J, Mikkelsen K, Jorgensen S, Nilsson F. A double-blind trial of a nicotine inhaler for smoking cessation. JAMA 1993; 269(10):1268–1271.

65. Leischow SJ, Nilsson F, Franzon M, Hill A, Otte P, Merikle EP. Efficacy of the nicotine inhaler as an adjunct to smoking cessation. Am J Health Behav 1996;20(5):364–371.

66. Schneider NG, Olmstead R, Nilsson F, Mody FV, Franzon M, Doan K. Efficacy of a nicotine inhaler in smoking cessation: a double-blind, placebo-controlled trial. Addiction 1996;91(9): 1293–1306.

67. Hurt RD, Sachs DPL, Glover ED, et al. A comparison of sustained-release bupropion and placebo for smoking cessation. N Engl J Med 1997; 337(17):1195–1202.

68. Silagy C, Mant DC, Fowler G, Lodge M. Meta-analysis on efficacy of nicotine replacement therapies in smoking cessation. Lancet 1994;343: 139–142.

69. Fagerström KO, Sachs DPL. Medical management of tobacco dependence: a critical review of nicotine skin patches. Curr Pulmonol 1995; 16:223–238.

70. Fiore MC, Bailey WC, Cohen SJ, et al. Smoking Cessation. Rockville, MD: US Department of Health and Human Services, Public Health Service, Agency for Health Care Policy and Research, 1996. AHCPR Publication No. 96-0692, Clinical Practice Guideline No. 18.

71. Blondal T, Gudmundsson LJ, Olafsdottir I, Gustavsson G, Westin A. Nicotine nasal spray with nicotine patch for smoking cessation: randomised trial with six-year follow up. BMJ 1999;318:285–289.

72. Tonnesen P, Paoletti P, Gustavsson G, et al. Higher dosage nicotine patches increase one-year smoking cessation rates: results from the European CEASE trial. Eur Respir J 1999; 13(2):238–246.

73. Sachs DPL, Benowitz NL, Bostrom AG, Hansen MD. Percent serum replacement and success of nicotine patch therapy. Am J Respir Crit Care Med 1995;151:A688.

74. Fiore MC, for The Smoking Cessation Clinical Practice Guideline Panel and Staff. Smoking cessation clinical practice guideline. JAMA 1996; 275:1270–1280.

75. Fiore MC, Bailey WC, Cohen SJ, et al. Smoking Cessation: Information for Specialists: Clinical Practice Guideline. Rockville, MD: US Department of Health and Human Services, Public Health Service, Agency for Health Care Policy and Research, 1996. AHCPR Publication No. 96-0694, Quick Reference Guide for Smoking Cessation Specialists No 18.

76. Kottke TE, Battista RN, DeFriese GH, Brekke ML. Attributes of successful smoking cessation interventions in medical practice: a meta-analysis of 39 controlled trials. JAMA 1988;259:2883–2889.

77. Hughes JR, Lesmes GR, Hatsukami DK, et al. Are higher doses of nicotine replacement more effective for smoking cessation? Nic Tobacco Res 1999;1:169–174.

78. Jorenby DE, Smith SS, Fiore MC, et al. Varying nicotine patch dose and type of smoking cessation counseling. JAMA 1995;274(17):1347–1352.

79. Benowitz NL, Zevin S, Jacob P III. Sources of variability in nicotine and cotinine levels with use of nicotine nasal spray, transdermal nicotine, and cigarette smoking. Br J Clin Pharmacol 1997;43(3):259–267.

80. Benowitz NL, Jacob P III, Jones RT, Rosenberg J. Interindividual variability in the metabolism and cardiovascular effects of nicotine in man. J Pharmacol Exp Ther 1982;221:368–372.

81. Dale LC, Hurt RD, Offord KP, Lawson GM, Croghan IT, Schroeder DR. High-dose nicotine patch therapy: percentage of replacement and smoking cessation. JAMA 1995;274(17):1353–1358.

82. Hjalmarson A, Franzon M, Westin A, Wiklund O. Effect of nicotine nasal spray on smoking cessation. Arch Intern Med 1994;154:2567–2572.

83. Silagy C, Mant D, Fowler G, Lodge M. The effectiveness of nicotine replacement therapies in smoking cessation. Online J Curr Clin Trials 1994;3(113).

84. Herrera N, Franco R, Herrera L, Partidas A, Rolando R, Fagerström KO. Nicotine gum, 2 and 4 mg, for nicotine dependence: a double-blind placebo-controlled trial within a behavior modification support program. Chest 1995; 108(2):447–451.

85. Bergsträom M, Nordberg A, Lunell E, Antoni G, LangsträoB. Regional deposition of inhaled 11C-nicotine vapor in the human airway as visualized by positron emission tomography. Clin Pharmacol Ther 1995;57:309–317.

86. Lunell E, Bergsträom M, Nordberg A. Nicotine deposition and body distribution from a nico-

tine inhaler and a cigarette studied with positron emission tomography. Clin Pharmacol Ther 1996;59(5):593–594.

87. Rose JE, Zinser MC, Tashkin DP, Newcomb R, Ertle A. Subjective response to cigarette smoking following airway anesthetization. Addict Behav 1984;9:211–215.

88. Sachs DPL, Leischow SJ. Pharmacologic approaches to smoking cessation. Clin Chest Med 1991;12:769–791.

89. Sachs DPL, Fagersträom KO. Medical management of tobacco dependence: practical office considerations. Curr Pulmonol 1995;16:239–249.

90. Ascher JA, Cole JO, Colin JN, et al. Bupropion: a review of its mechanism of antidepressant activity. J Clin Psychiatry 1995;56(9):395–401.

91. Jorenby DE, Leischow SJ, Nides MA, et al. A controlled trial of sustained-release bupropion, a nicotine patch, or both for smoking cessation. N Engl J Med 1999;340:685–691.

92. Hall SM, Reus VI, Mūnoz RF, et al. Nortriptyline and cognitive-behavioral therapy in the treatment of cigarette smoking [see comments]. Arch Gen Psychiatry 1998;55(8):683–690.

93. Ferry LH, Robbins AS, Scariati PD, Masterson A, Abbey DE, Burchette RJ. Enhancement of smoking cessation using the antidepressant bupropion hydrochloride. Circulation 1992;86(4): 1-167.

94. Ferry LH, Burchette RJ. Efficacy of buproprion for smoking cessation in non-depressed smokers. J Addict Dis 1994;13(4):9A.

95. Ferry LH, Burchette RJ. Evaluation of bupropion versus placebo for treatment of nicotine dependence. Presented at the 147th Annual Meeting of the American Psychiatric Association, Philadelphia, 1994.

96. Hays JT, Hurt RD, Rigotti N, et al. A randomized controlled trial of sustained-release bupropion for pharmacologic relapse prevention following smoking cessation. JAMA (under review).

97. Food and Drug Administration Freedom of Information Office (FOI) (US Public Health Service). Open Public Hearing on Bupropion Sustained Release Tablets as an Aid to Smoking Cessation Treatment. December 12, 1996. Report No. NDA 20-711.

98. Kornitzer M, Boutsen M, Dramaix M, Thijs J, Gustavsson G. Combined use of nicotine patch and gum in smoking cessation: a placebo-controlled clinical trial. Prev Med 1995;24(1): 41–47.

99. Puska P, Korhonen HJ, Vartiainen E, Urjanheimo EL, Gustavsson G, Westin A. Combined use of nicotine patch and gum compared with gum alone in smoking cessation: a clinical trial in North Karelia. Tobacco Control 1995;4: 231–235.

100. Bohadana AB, Nilsson F, Martinet Y. Nicotine inhaler and nicotine patch: a combination therapy for smoking cessation. Nic Tobacco Res 1999;1:189.

101. Sachs DPL, Bostrom AG, Hansen MD. Relapse Hazard Functions During and After Nicotine Patch Smoking Cessation Treatment. Boston: Society of Behavioral Medicine, 1994.

102. Sachs DPL, Sawe U. Transdermal nicotine patch and absence of myocardial infarction risk. Paper presented at the American College of Chest Physicians 59th International Scientific Assembly, Cardiology Section. Orlando, FL, October 1993.

103. Fredrickson PA, Hurt RD, Lee GM, et al. High dose transdermal nicotine therapy for heavy smokers: safety, tolerability and measurement of nicotine and cotinine levels. Psychopharmacology 1995;122:215–222.

104. Zevin S, Jacob III P, Benowitz NL. Dose-related cardiovascular and endocrine effects of transdermal nicotine. Clin Pharmacol Ther 1998;64: 87–95.

105. Working Group for the Study of Transdermal Nicotine in Patients With Coronary Artery Disease. Nicotine replacement therapy for patients with coronary artery disease. Arch Intern Med 1994;154:989–995.

106. Food and Drug Administration, ed. Zyban: Prescribing Information. Washington, DC: US Department of Health and Human Services, 1997.

107. Johnston JA, Lineberry CG, Ascher JA, et al. A 102-center prospective study seizure in association with bupropion. J Clin Psychiatry 1991; 52:450–456.

108. Prochaska JO. Assessing how people change. Cancer 1991;67:805–807.

109. Glynn TJ, Manley M. How to Help Your Patients Stop Smoking: A National Cancer Institute Manual for Physicians. Washington, D.C. National Cancer Institute, 1990. Publication No. 90-3064.

110. American Academy of Family Physicians. Physician's Office Stop Smoking Program Kit. Kansas City: American Academy of Family Physicians, 1986. Product No. 900.

111. Allen SS, Hatsukami DK, Christianson D, Nelson D. Withdrawal and pre-menstrual symptomatology during the menstrual cycle in short-term smoking abstinence: effects of menstrual cycle on smoking abstinence. Nic Tobacco Res 1999; 1:129–142.

112. Sachs DPL, Bostrom AG, Hansen MD. Nicotine patch therapy: predictors of smoking cessation success. Am J Respir Crit Care Med 1994; 149(42):A326.

113. Garvey AJ, Bliss RE, Hitchcock JL, Heinold JW, Rosner B. Predictors of smoking relapse among self-quitters: a report from the normative aging study. Addict Behav 1992;17:367–377.

114. West RJ, Hajek P, Belcher M. Severity of withdrawal symptoms as a predictor of outcome of an attempt to quit smoking. Psychol Med 1989;19(4):981–985.

115. Norregaard J, Tonnesen P, Petersen L. Predictors and reasons for relapse in smoking cessation with nicotine and placebo patches. Prev Med 1993;22(2):261–271.

116. Killen JD, Fortmann SP. Craving is associated with smoking relapse: findings from three prospective studies. Exp Clin Psychopharmacol 1997;5(2):137–142.

117. Shiffman SM. Relapse following smoking cessation: a situational analysis. J Consult Clin Psychol 1982;50(1):71–86.
118. Sachs DPL. Pharmacologic, neuroendocrine, and biobehavioral basis for tobacco dependence. Curr Pulmonol 1987;8:371–405.
119. Sachs DPL. Advances in smoking cessation treatment. Curr Pulmonol 1991;12:139–198.
120. Foulds J, Stapleton J, Feyerabend C, Vesey C, Jarvis M, Russell MAH. Effect of transdermal nicotine patches on cigarette smoking: a double blind crossover study. Psychopharmacology 1992;106:421–427.
121. Rogot E. Smoking and life expectancy among U.S. veterans. Am J Public Health 1978;68(10): 1023–1025.
122. Schuman LM. The benefits of cessation of smoking. Chest 1971;59(4):421–427.
123. Ferry LH, Grissino LM, Runfola PS. Tobacco dependence curricula in US undergraduate medical education. JAMA 1999;282(9):825–829.
124. Ferry LH. Overcoming barriers to nicotine dependence treatment. Prim Care 1999;26(3): 707–746.
125. Benowitz NL. Cigarette smoking and nicotine addiction. Med Clin North Am 1992;76:415–437.
126. Kellar KJ. Neuropharmacology and biology of neuronal nicotine receptors. In: Henningfield JE, Grunberg NE, eds. Addicted to Nicotine: A National Research Forum. Bethesda, MD: National Institute on Drug Abuse, National Institutes of Health, 1998:59–62.
127. Hughes JR, Hatsukami DK. Signs and symptoms of tobacco withdrawal. Arch Gen Psychiatry 1986;43:289–294.
128. American Psychiatric Association. Nicotine-induced organic mental disorder. In: Diagnostic Statistical Manual of Mental Disorders. Third ed rev. Washington, DC: American Psychiatric Association, 1987:150–151.
129. Heatherton TF, Kozlowski LT, Frecker RC, Fagerstraom KO. The Fagerstraom test for nicotine dependence: a revision of the Fagerstraom Tolerance Questionnaire. Br J Addict 1991;86:1119–1127.
130. Paoletti P, Fornai E, Maggiorelli F, et al. Importance of baseline cotinine plasma values in smoking cessation: results from a double-blind study with nicotine patch. Eur Respir J 1996;9(4): 643–651.
131. Sachs DPL, Benowitz NL. Individualizing medical treatment for tobacco dependence [editorial; comment]. Eur Respir J 1996;9(4):629–631.
132. Dale LC, Glover ED, Sachs DPL, et al. Bupropion for smoking cessation: predictors of successful outcome. Chest (under review).
133. Killen JD, Fortmann SP, Telch MJ, Newman B. Are heavy smokers different from light smokers? a comparison after 48 hours without cigarettes. JAMA 1988;260(11):1581–1585.
134. Hajek P, Jackson P, Belcher M. Long-term use of nicotine chewing gum: occurrence, determinants, and effect on weight gain. JAMA 1988; 260(11):1593–1596.
135. Killen JD, Fortmann SP, Newman B, Varady A. Evaluation of a treatment approach combining nicotine gum with self-guided behavioral treatments for smoking relapse prevention. J Consult Clin Psychol 1990;58(1):85–92.
136. Sachs DPL, Leischow SJ. Differential gender treatment response: effectiveness of the 4 mg dose of nicotine polacrilex to treat low nicotine dependent male smokers but not women. In: Problems of Drug Dependence 1992: Proceedings of the 54th Annual Scientific Meeting, National Institute on Drug Abuse. Keystone, CO, 1992.
137. Glassman AH, Helzer JE, Covey LS, et al. Smoking, smoking cessation, and major depression. JAMA 1990;264:1546–1549.
138. Covey LS, Glassman AH, Steiner F. Depression and depressive symptoms in smoking cessation. Compr Psychiatry 1990;31(4):350–354.
139. Hughes JR. Treatment of smoking cessation in smokers with past alcohol/drug problems. J Subst Abuse Treat 1993;10:181–187.

16 Behavioral Medicine in Pulmonary Rehabilitation: Psychological, Cognitive, and Social Factors

Charles F. Emery
Kim R. Lebowitz

⟩ Professional Skills

Upon completion of this chapter, the reader will:

- Describe the psychologic sequelae of pulmonary disease and the treatment strategies for improving psychologic well-being
- Identify tools that assess levels of depression, anxiety, and psychologic adjustment
- Describe the cognitive deficits that may be associated with pulmonary disease
- Identify instruments used to assess cognitive functioning
- Describe the effects of pulmonary disease on social relationships and identify tools for assessing social support
- Understand the physical and role limitations experienced by the chronic obstructive pulmonary disease (COPD) patient and understand how psychologic and social factors can influence performance of daily activities
- Identify instruments that assess quality of life
- Describe psychologic factors associated with smoking cessation and understand ways to incorporate this knowledge into a treatment program
- Describe the relationship between nutrition and general well-being of pulmonary patients
- Identify the effects of exercise rehabilitation on the psychologic well-being, behavioral functioning, and cognitive functioning of pulmonary patients
- Understand the role of psychologic factors in medication compliance

Behavioral medicine is a multidisciplinary approach to understanding the mechanisms by which physical health is associated with health behavior (e.g., exercise, smoking, and diet) and psychologic well-being. The multidisciplinary approach in behavioral medicine facilitates examination of multiple influences of psychologic and social factors on physical functioning and the way in which these factors may interact to influence functioning

Table 16-1. Common Symptoms Observed in Behavioral Medicine Evaluation
of Patients in Pulmonary Rehabilitation

Emotional	Cognitive	Social	Behavioral
Depressed mood	Mild deficits	Reduced social activity	Impaired ADL
Anxiety	Impaired psycho- motor speed	Change in family roles	Smoking
Anger		Reduced independence	Malnourishment
Guilt	Impaired problem- solving		Decreased exercise capacity
Embarrassment	Impaired attention		Medication non- compliance
Avoid expressing strong emotions			

ADL, activities of daily living.

among patients with pulmonary disease. The purpose of this chapter is to discuss four primary areas of functioning (psychologic well-being, cognitive performance, social functioning, and behavioral adaptation) in patients with pulmonary disease. Common symptoms associated with each area of functioning are summarized in Table 16-1. In addition to describing symptoms in each of the four areas of functioning, this chapter will address the following issues: (*a*) available research literature supporting the relevance of each area of functioning for pulmonary disease and pulmonary rehabilitation, (*b*) relevant clinical data, (*c*) outcome assessment, and (*d*) treatment recommendations.

PSYCHOLOGIC FUNCTIONING

Psychiatric symptoms and diminished psychologic well-being frequently are observed among patients with pulmonary disease. Psychologic sequelae of pulmonary disease may influence functional status and physical well-being, independent of disease severity. Thus, assessment and treatment of psychologic factors are critical for effective treatment of the patient with pulmonary disease. For example, a recent study of 16 male veterans with COPD suggested that psychologic factors may be more relevant than medical factors. Survival among the veterans at 4-year follow-up was predicted by general psychologic distress but not by disease severity, comorbid illness, blood oxygenation, or previous medical treatment.[1] Common psychologic reactions among patients with pulmonary disease include anger, frustration, guilt, dependency, and embarrassment.[2,3] However, the most frequently observed psychologic symptoms among patients with pulmonary disease are symptoms of depression and anxiety.

Depression

Depression is perhaps the most commonly reported psychologic factor associated with COPD. Although the prevalence of depression in patients with COPD is not greater than that found in other chronically ill groups, studies have reported anywhere from 26% of patients being depressed to as many as 74% of COPD patients presenting with a "crippling degree of depression."[3-5] Depression in this population is typically characterized by hopelessness, a pessimistic outlook, reduced sleep, decreased appetite, increased lethargy, difficulties in concentration, and increased social withdrawal.[3]

Depression in COPD patients may significantly influence daily functioning. Studies consistently report that depressed mood predicts behavioral, social, and mental functioning; and greater depressive symptoms have been associated with higher levels of impairment in activities of daily living.[6-8] Although the correlation between depressed mood and disease severity is modest,[9] depression may have an influence on daily functioning that is independent of pulmonary functioning and disease severity. Because of the independent influence of depression on daily functioning, it has been suggested that treatments devised to increase physical health and quality of life should focus on reducing depressed mood.

Anxiety

Anxiety is another common psychologic consequence of COPD, having a disabling effect on as many as 96% of patients in one early study.[5] Symptoms of anxiety are manifested in various ways, including accelerated speech, exaggerated body movements, and physiologic signs of arousal such as tachycardia, sweating, and dyspnea.[10] Up to 37% of patients with COPD may experience one or more panic attacks, as defined by bouts of intense anxiety, physiologic arousal, temporary cognitive impairment, and a desire to flee the situation.[11] Those who experience panic report more catastrophic misinterpretations of their bodily symptoms but do not differ from patients without panic on measures of physical functioning, disease severity, shortness of breath, or psychologic distress. Thus, the experience of panic may reflect a cognitive interpretation of pulmonary symptoms rather than objective pulmonary status.[11]

Dyspnea itself, in conjunction with a fear of suffocation and death, is a source of significant anxiety in this population.[3] The emotional arousal of anxiety then increases ventilatory demands on the body, which may lead to hypoxia or hypercapnia. As shown in Figure 16-1, increased physiologic arousal, in turn, exacerbates anxiety symptoms, which then produce greater physiologic insufficiency, resulting in a circular pattern that is difficult to break.[3] Although anxiety symptoms are commonly reported in COPD patients, anxiety has not been found to predict quality of life or directly influence functional status in this population.[8,12] Thus, fluctuation of pulmonary symptoms associated with daily stressors does not seem to be influenced by anxiety symptoms per se.[13] However, the few published studies in this area are confounded by variability in the measurement of anxiety.

Personality

Several studies have evaluated personality functioning among patients with COPD, but no specific personality profile for COPD patients has been described. One recent study of 59 patients with COPD found that the prevalence of personality disorders (i.e., long-standing distress and difficulty with interpersonal relationships) was similar to that of a normal control group[14] and that no specific personality pathology could be associated with COPD. Strong emotional reactions such as anxiety, anger, and euphoria may exacerbate pulmonary symptoms by increasing energy expenditure, resulting in increased demands on ventilation and oxygenation. Emotions associated with decreases in arousal, such as feelings of depression and apathy, may decrease energy expenditure and result in decreased ventilatory demands and lower oxygen consumption. Because either hyperarousal or hypoarousal may lead to exacerbations in pulmonary symptoms, it has been

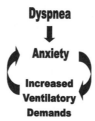

Figure 16-1. Hypothetical model of the dyspnea-anxiety relationship.

suggested that patients with COPD may avoid expressing strong emotions to prevent physiologic changes that affect pulmonary symptoms.[15] However, no data exist to suggest that COPD patients are more likely to avoid emotional expression than other groups with chronic illness. Thus, no reliable pattern of personality functioning or personality disorder among COPD patients has emerged.

Coping Skills and Self-Efficacy

Few studies have examined coping styles among patients with pulmonary disease, but the extant data suggest stability in coping over time. In a study of 40 patients with severe COPD, Parsons[16] found a tendency to use more problem-focused coping strategies (as opposed to emotion-focused strategies) and stability of perceived well-being during a 1-year interval. However, it was found that women in the study tended to use more emotion-focused coping than did men and that emotion-focused coping was associated with lower levels of perceived well-being. Similarly, more recent studies indicated that patients with COPD used rational coping strategies more than emotional coping or avoidance and that passive coping was associated with poorer social and role functioning.[17,18]

Self-efficacy can be defined as the expectation of one's own ability to complete a task, and it has been associated with health outcomes among COPD patients. Self-efficacy expectations for walking were found to be a significant predictor of survival among patients with COPD.[19] In addition, self-efficacy expectations are important for smoking cessation and exercise participation among patients with pulmonary disease.[20,21]

Assessment

Evaluation of psychologic functioning often includes both general assessment tools and specific indicators. Two common tools used for evaluating psychologic symptoms are the Brief Symptom Inventory[22] and the Profile of Mood States–Short Form.[23] The Brief Symptom Inventory is a 53-item multidimensional symptom inventory providing an overall index of symptoms as well as nine specific clinical subscales, including depression, anxiety, and hostility. The Profile of Mood States–Short Form is a 30-item list of adjective ratings providing an overall mood score as well as six mood subscores.

Symptom-specific indicators of psychologic distress include measures of depression and anxiety. Common measures of depression include the Beck Depression Inventory,[24] a widely used 21-item measure of depressive symptoms, and the Center for Epidemiological Studies–Depression Inventory,[25] a 20-item measure validated in samples of community-residing older adults. Anxiety measures include the Beck Anxiety Inventory,[26] a 21-item measure of symptoms of anxiety, and the State-Trait Anxiety Inventory,[27] a 40-item measure with 20 items assessing transient (state) anxiety and 20 items assessing long-standing (trait) symptoms of anxiety.

Treatment

Psychologic distress among patients with COPD may be treated by means of group counseling, psychotherapy, medication, exercise rehabilitation, or a combination of several of these modalities. Psychologic treatments targeting catastrophic misinterpretations of bodily symptoms are thought to decrease experiences of panic in COPD patients.[11] Although research in this area has not yet targeted symptoms of panic, one study suggests that cognitive restructuring may not significantly alter levels of overall anxiety or depression.[28] Relaxation training, however, in which the patient is taught strategies for relaxing muscle groups throughout the body, may improve symptoms of anxiety, dyspnea, and airway obstruction in COPD patients.[29]

One prototype for treatment of pulmonary patients is the cognitive-behavioral group format in which patients are taught relaxation skills combined with cognitive restructuring

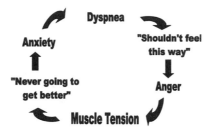

Figure 16-2. Model of interactive cycle of physical symptoms, cognitive distortions, and emotions used in behavioral medicine treatment of patients in pulmonary rehabilitation.

and identification of emotional changes. Cognitive restructuring includes identifying stress-producing thought patterns (e.g., "I should have quit smoking 10 years ago") and replacing them with more adaptive thoughts (e.g., "I wish I had quit smoking 10 years ago, but I wasn't ready at that time"). Patients are also encouraged to identify emotions (e.g., depression, anxiety, anger, or guilt) and stress-producing thoughts that are contributing to the emotional state. This approach, in either a group or individual format, provides patients with a model for approaching psychologic distress that can be used by the patient after pulmonary rehabilitation. An example of the stress-producing physical-cognitive-emotional cycle is shown in Figure 16-2.

Psychotropic medications are sometimes included in the treatment of psychologic distress among patients with pulmonary disease, and several studies have demonstrated benefits of psychotropic medication for reducing not only psychologic symptoms, such as depression and anxiety, but also physical symptoms (e.g., feelings of suffocation and dizziness).[30,31] Medications may be used in conjunction with individual or group counseling, and behavioral approaches are often important in facilitating the patient's efforts to follow the treatment regimen or, alternatively, to work toward reducing the need for medication.

COGNITIVE FUNCTIONING

Mild cognitive deficits have been observed among patients with COPD. However, the nature of the deficits and the extent to which they are related to hypoxemia are debated. Studies have described impaired neuropsychologic functioning among COPD patients in problem-solving, psychomotor speed, attention, and verbal memory.[32-35] However, verbal intelligence does not seem to be affected.[32] Recent studies confirm that cognitive performance of patients with COPD reflects isolated deficits and does not resemble cognitive performance among patients with dementia.[4,34] Greater hypoxia has been associated with more impairment in cognitive performance, but cognitive performance of severely hypoxic subjects remains better than performance of demented patients.

Data from the combined Nocturnal Oxygen Therapy Trial and the Intermittent Positive Pressure Breathing Trial have demonstrated a positive correlation between neuropsychologic impairment and hypoxemia. Control subjects performed better than mildly hypoxemic patients, who in turn performed better than patients who were moderately or severely hypoxemic. However, data from these studies and others have indicated that neuropsychologic functioning is not associated with standard pulmonary function variables (e.g., forced expiratory volume in 1 second) and is only moderately associated with hypoxemia.[36] Age and education accounted for the greatest amount of variance in neuropsychologic performance in the studies by Grant and colleagues.[32] Sleep disorders also are associated with hypoxemia and neuropsychologic dysfunction.[37] Rourke and Adams[38] thus suggest that sleep-disordered breathing and sleep apnea may represent additional risk factors for neuropsychologic impairment among patients with COPD.

Although past studies have evaluated self-perceptions of cognitive performance, studies have not evaluated the extent to which self-perceptions reflect objective cognitive performance. Mood or psychologic functioning may be a confounding variable in the self-assessment of cognitive functioning because previous studies have demonstrated an association of depression and anxiety with perceptions of poorer cognitive performance despite no impairment of objective indicators.

Assessment

Several neuropsychologic measures have been used in studies evaluating cognitive performance among patients with COPD. Instruments include comprehensive indicators of intellectual functioning as well as measures tapping specific domains. The most common assessment battery, which provides measures of overall intellectual ability as well as subscale scores in verbal and performance domains, is the recently revised Wechsler Adult Intelligence Scale–III.[39] Additional neuropsychologic measures commonly used in evaluation of COPD patients and patients with chronic illnesses include (*a*) the Trail Making Test, evaluating sequencing ability and visual motor tracking,[40] and (*b*) the Stroop Interference Test, designed to evaluate the patient's ability to shift perceptual set and meet changing demands of a task.[41]

Treatment

Intervention studies have demonstrated that treatment with supplemental oxygen may reverse some of the deficits in neuropsychologic functioning observed among patients with COPD.[42,43] However, improvements observed in neuropsychologic performance are relatively mild and would not be considered clinically significant.[43] In addition, blood oxygen levels must be diminished to an extreme extent for metabolic alterations to occur in energy-producing pathways in the brain. Instead, the role of oxygen in neurotransmitter regulation has been outlined as the most probable cause of neuropsychologic changes resulting from hypoxemia and from supplemental oxygen use.[38,44]

SOCIAL FUNCTIONING

The physical limitations of COPD may have far-reaching effects on family relations and lifestyle. Five areas cited by Clough and colleagues[45] include diminished wage-earning ability, changes in family roles, reduced independence, reduced social activities, and effects of oxygen use in the home. Sexual functioning may be impaired,[46] and spouses of COPD patients may be prone to both depression and anxiety.[47] Important gender and individual differences may affect attitudes of the patient with COPD. For example, women with COPD report lower marital satisfaction than men with COPD.[48] Furthermore, perceived social support contributes to enhanced well-being among patients with COPD[12] and may indirectly predict functional capacity.[6]

Assessment

Social support has been broadly conceptualized in two domains: structural support and functional support.[49] Structural support refers to the number of social relationships and the connections between individuals in the network. Functional support refers to the support role (e.g., companionship, instrumental or material assistance, or information providing) of the social relationships. Therefore, measures of structural support typically evaluate the number of individuals in the support network, whereas measures of functional support assess the needs fulfilled by individuals in the social network. Both forms of assessment are subjective, relying on respondent perceptions, but structural measures may facilitate a somewhat more objective analysis.

Social support is typically assessed via self-report measures, sometimes within a larger multidimensional assessment of functional status or quality of life. For example, the Sickness Impact Profile (SIP)[50] and the Medical Outcomes Study 36-Item Short Form Health Survey (SF-36)[51] both assess social functioning as one area of overall patient functioning. In addition, specific measures of social support are also available and used widely. The Interpersonal Support Evaluation List–Short Form is a 16-item measure of functional support assessing four different functions of the social support network: appraisal, self-esteem, belonging, and tangibility.[52] The Multidimensional Scale of Perceived Social Support is a 12-item measure of structural support that assesses potential sources of social support, including family, friends, and significant others.[53] Social support has also been assessed using study-specific questions designed by an investigator or staff member. Although such measures may provide useful data, they may have limited utility in other clinical or research settings. Findings regarding social support among patients with COPD are based on a variety of social support measures, including measures targeting both the structure and the function of the support network.

Treatment

Because of the importance of social support for the health and psychologic well-being of patients with pulmonary disease, pulmonary rehabilitation programs ideally would include spouses/caregivers in the educational components of the program. Inclusion of spouses/caregivers conveys to the patient the importance of the treatment (exercise) and contributes to the ability of the spouse/caregiver to facilitate exercise and proper medical care after the rehabilitation program has been completed. Psychologic counseling may include spouses/caregivers to provide a forum for discussion of distress resulting from changes in the patient and additional burdens of caregiving. For some patients, the spouse/caregiver may be providing more functional support than is required, which may undermine the patient's efforts at independent functioning. In such cases, the rehabilitation program may serve the important function of separating the patient from the spouse/caregiver for periods of time to allow the patient to engage in independent activities.

BEHAVIORAL FUNCTIONING

Activities of Daily Living

The lifestyle of individuals with COPD is often altered as a result of declining physical functioning associated with disease progression. Patients with COPD are typically confronted with difficulties in numerous areas of life functioning and may report significant impairments in bathing, grooming, dressing, eating, sleeping, and mobility.[9,54] In addition to difficulties in ambulation and home management, COPD also tends to hinder recreational activities and social interactions.[7,9,55]

Disease severity has long been thought to be the primary factor causing functional impairments in this population. Research conducted during the past several years, however, has indicated that disease severity may not directly affect functional performance.[7] Similarly, no direct relationship between pulmonary function and functional status has been observed, but pulmonary function may indirectly affect functional status via its effect on exercise capacity.[8] In general, however, pulmonary function seems to be no more important in predicting functional capacity than other more subjective factors, including indicators of psychologic well-being.[6–8,55]

Several psychologic factors and behavioral symptoms seem to affect patient functioning, both directly and indirectly. In a study of patients with COPD, Graydon and Ross[6] found that predictors of functional status varied according to whether patients used oxygen. Among non–oxygen-dependent subjects, negative mood, not pulmonary functioning, was found to be the strongest predictor of functional capacity; however, among oxygen-dependent subjects, impaired functioning was found to be directly influenced by self-report ratings of somatic symptoms and indirectly influenced by pulmonary functioning.[6] Recent literature suggests that depressed mood may be a better predictor of functional status than other mood states. In a sample of 104 COPD patients, depressed mood, exercise capacity, and dyspnea were the only factors that directly influenced functional status, whereas anxiety only had an indirect impact through the pathways of depressed mood and dyspnea.[8] Additional findings further suggest that depressed mood is a stronger predictor of functional capacity than are anxiety or optimism.[12] Self-esteem has also been found to play a role in patient functioning, with at least two studies reporting direct effects on functional status[12,56] and at least one study reporting indirect effects through the pathway of depressed mood.[8] Although psychologic factors may be less influential for patients receiving oxygen therapy, the literature consistently suggests that subjective factors, especially depressed mood, are important when considering a patient's functional impairments.

Perceived social support and satisfaction with social resources also seem to affect functional status, although data are inconsistent as to whether this influence is direct or indirect.[6,7,12,55] Some studies have found that social support directly influences functional status, whereas other studies indicate that the influence may be indirect, through the pathways of negative mood and somatic symptoms.[6,12] This discrepancy may be caused by variability in the measures used to assess social support across studies.

In summary, functional capacity is most likely influenced by a variety of factors, including pulmonary function, psychologic well-being, and social support, as shown in Figure 16-3. Several models have been tested, resulting in support for the notion that functional capacity is best predicted by a combination of factors rather than by any single factor in isolation.[8,12,55,56] Thus, numerous areas of functioning should be included in assessing functional capacity of patients and in developing an optimal treatment plan. Enhancement of patient functioning may best be addressed by targeting factors that directly influence functional capacity, such as depressed mood, self-esteem, exercise tolerance, dyspnea, or social satisfaction.

Assessment

Functional capacity can be assessed in several ways, most often using self-report instruments. One measure that has been used regularly with this population is the Sickness Impact Profile (SIP).[50] This 136-item questionnaire evaluates 12 areas of daily functioning (ambulation, mobility, body care and movement, social interaction, communication, alert-

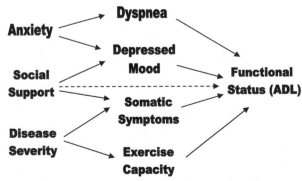

Figure 16-3. Model of psychologic, social, and physical variables with direct and indirect influence on functional status among patients with pulmonary disease.

ness behavior, emotional behavior, sleep and rest, eating, employment, home management, and recreation and pastimes), reflecting limitations in physical, psychologic, and social functioning. More recently, a short form of the SIP has been developed, the SIP-68, with 68 items covering six dimensions of functioning (somatic autonomy, mobility control, psychic autonomy and communication, social behavior, emotional stability, and mobility range).[57] Another measure that has come into widespread use in the past several years is the Medical Outcomes Study 36-Item Short Form Health Survey,[51] evaluating nine health-related dimensions: physical functioning, role functioning-physical, role functioning-emotional, social functioning, bodily pain, mental health, vitality, general health perceptions, and change in health. In addition to self-report instruments, functional capacity is also commonly assessed via a 6- or 12-minute walk test.

Treatment

Treatment strategies incorporate activity planning and pacing. Patients are encouraged to plan daily activities, to list them on a daily planner, and to mark off each activity as it is completed. Planning pleasurable activities is integral to this program to facilitate the patient's sense of control and to prevent depressive symptoms. Patients are encouraged to accept the pace at which they complete physical activities and are helped to identify new aspects of their daily activities to enjoy.

Smoking Cessation

Recent behavioral research suggests that comprehensive treatments targeting psychologic functioning may increase the efficacy of smoking cessation among individuals with COPD. Specifically, empiric evidence suggests that multicomponent smoking cessation treatment may be more effective than treatment in a single modality. In addition, psychologic variables seem to play a role in both the ability to quit smoking and the likelihood of relapse.

Several researchers have documented the beneficial effects of using a comprehensive treatment package for smoking cessation. Ockene and colleagues[58] randomly assigned 1200 healthy adult smokers to one of three conditions: (*a*) physician advice to stop smoking, (*b*) counseling in addition to advice, or (*c*) nicotine-containing gum in addition to counseling and advice. Rates of cessation were highest among subjects assigned to the most comprehensive treatment program. Additional studies have suggested that nicotine patches or nicotine nasal sprays may be ineffective unless combined with additional elements of a treatment plan, even with something as minimal as a self-help booklet.[59,60] According to Kottke et al.,[61] no single strategy is more effective than another. Instead, the most important factor in smoking cessation is consistent repetition of the stop smoking message. Thus, multimodal approaches and consistency of communications regarding smoking cessation seem to be critical to the success of smoking cessation interventions.

Psychologic factors, particularly self-efficacy and depressed mood, have been implicated in smoking cessation and relapse. In a study of smoking cessation among COPD patients with at least a 15-year smoking history, self-efficacy was the strongest predictor of cessation at 1 and 3 months after baseline assessment. In addition, patient behaviors, motivation, and outcome expectancies were predictors, but only when they were combined with self-efficacy expectations.[20] Thus, it seems that smoking cessation interventions would benefit by targeting self-efficacy expectations.

Negative mood also may be associated with smoking cessation and abstinence. Depressed smokers may have more difficulty quitting than nondepressed smokers and may be more likely to relapse several months later.[62] In a sample of patients with COPD, depressed mood was significantly associated with reduced ability to quit smoking.[63]

Treatment

Behavioral medicine treatment of smoking often includes relaxation training, group support, nicotine fading via brand switching, and training in relapse prevention. Patients are encouraged to modify the home/work environment to minimize smoking temptations and to enlist supportive allies in the home and work environments. Much of the initial work is devoted to establishing the patient's motivation and readiness for smoking cessation. Later sessions are devoted to preparing for becoming a nonsmoker and to developing strategies for coping with smoking relapses.

The amount of support that a smoker receives while trying to quit is thought to be an important factor in predicting success. Therefore, patients should be encouraged to seek the support of a spouse or friend.[64] Smoking cessation treatment groups may be beneficial in this regard. Cognitive coping strategies also may influence success at maintaining abstinence. In a sample of 91 healthy adult ex-smokers, successful abstinence at 3-month follow-up was associated with subjects' ability to use cognitive restructuring to modify an urge to smoke into an acknowledgment that smoking is not an optimal response. This cognitive process was associated with greater abstinence than was suppressing thoughts of smoking.[65]

Although much of the empiric evidence suggests the important role of psychologic factors in smoking cessation, few investigations have examined psychologic factors in the COPD population. The data to date, however, suggest that treatment programs for smoking cessation should emphasize psychologic factors such as mood, self-efficacy, social support, and cognitive restructuring. Further investigations are needed to evaluate the effectiveness of treatments aimed at modifying psychologic variables in patients with COPD.

Dietary Factors

Studies indicate that a significant number of patients with COPD are malnourished, as indicated by lower than normal body weight, triceps muscle skin fold, arm muscle circumference, and caloric intake. The most recent behavioral research has indicated that malnourishment may be associated with psychologic well-being and that dietary supplements may reverse the deterioration in psychologic and physical functioning associated with depleted nutrition.

Although few studies have investigated the degree to which nutrition is associated with psychologic and behavioral factors, Efthimiou and colleagues[66] found that perceptions of general well-being were significantly greater in 7 well-nourished COPD patients than in 14 malnourished patients. Although a similar degree of breathlessness and physical capacity was observed in the two groups, well-nourished patients demonstrated greater respiratory muscle strength and handgrip strength, as well as less muscle fatigue, which, in turn, may have contributed to greater feelings of well-being in the well-nourished group.[66]

Treatment

Dietary supplementation has been found to reverse some of the associated features of malnourishment, but the psychologic effects may not be evident with short-term use. Although an 8-week course of dietary supplements has been associated with weight gain and increased caloric intake,[67,68] a 3-month course of supplements contributed to general well-being in addition to increases in percentage of ideal body weight, caloric intake, respiratory muscle functioning, handgrip strength, and physical capacity (as measured by the 6-minute walk test), as well as decreases in levels of breathlessness.[66] Thus, psychologic and somatic symptoms may be improved via nutritional manipulations.

Behavioral approaches to weight management include activity planning, meal planning, and helping the patient develop realistic goals for body weight. For patients who experience anxiety associated with eating, relaxation training may be useful. Stimulus control approaches (e.g., eating only while seated, avoiding other activities while eating) are also important behavioral strategies for patients attempting weight loss.

Thus, evidence supports the idea that nutrition affects functioning of pulmonary patients. Future research is needed to clarify the relationship of psychologic well-being with nutritional intake in patients with pulmonary disease. No investigations to date have examined the effects of mood on nutritional and caloric intake, the effects of nutrition on cognitive functioning and mood, or psychologic factors that may predict nutritional status among pulmonary patients.

Exercise

Several studies evaluating psychologic outcomes of exercise rehabilitation have been conducted. Two observational studies (i.e., studies without control groups) found reductions in depression and anxiety associated with exercise, as well as increases in positive affect.[69,70] One of the studies found improved cognitive performance associated with exercise rehabilitation.[70] Two additional observational studies found reductions in affective distress associated with exercise.[71,72] However, randomized studies of exercise rehabilitation provide less evidence of effects on psychological or behavioral functioning. Two studies found no decrease in depression,[21,73] and a third study found no change in hostility, self-esteem, or social inadequacy.[74] One study did observe a significant increase in self-efficacy for walking,[21] and a recent randomized study reported reductions in symptoms of anxiety and depression among patients with COPD participating in a 10-week exercise rehabilitation program.[36] Exercise in the latter study was also associated with reductions in illness-related impairment (as measured by the SIP) and improved cognitive performance on a task evaluating frontal lobe functioning.

Treatment

Exercise seems to be an important component of treatment to facilitate psychologic gains. Indeed, the study by Emery et al.[36] found no changes in psychologic symptoms in a control group participating in education and social support without exercise, and similar negative results were observed in a 6-week nonexercise treatment of pulmonary patients.[75] Thus, these studies suggest that psychologic change in rehabilitation results from more than social support and knowledge. Increased physical fitness seems to be an operative component.

One of the significant contributions of the behavioral medicine literature has been in the area of compliance. Exercise compliance is at the heart of any rehabilitation program, and continued compliance (adherence) is essential for patients to maintain gains after the program. The relapse prevention strategy seems to be useful with this patient group in that it prepares patients to acknowledge and cope with the inevitable occasions when they are reluctant or unable to exercise. In addition, because negative mood states may be associated with reduced energy and interest in activities such as exercise, strategies for improving mood also, in turn, are likely to contribute to better exercise performance.

Medical Compliance

The medical regimen of individuals with COPD is often complex, with an average of 6.3 medications per patient.[76] Consequently, nonadherence is high, with about half of patients overutilizing or underutilizing their medications.[76,77] Unfortunately, little is known about factors associated with noncompliance in patients with COPD or about ways in which compliance can be increased in this population. One study of medication compliance in the COPD population found that forgetting to use medication and declining to use medication were the two most frequent reasons for noncompliance and that these reasons for noncompliance resulted from the patient feeling well enough without the medication.[76] Side effects, changes in daily routines, and running out of medication were also frequently reported as factors associated with noncompliance. In addition, impaired long-term memory has been associated with poor adherence among patients with COPD.[33]

Although no study to date has examined ways to increase medication compliance among patients with COPD, studies using nonpulmonary patients suggest that drug feedback approaches, in which patients are given feedback about blood serum levels, are the most effective method of increasing compliance. Reinforcing patients for medical compliance or symptom reduction may be somewhat effective, but little evidence supports the use of self-monitoring techniques.[78]

Treatment

Treatment of noncompliance must address the source of the problem (e.g., lack of patient understanding, appropriateness of the intervention, absence of support at home for medication compliance, or patient not trusting physician). Once the source of noncompliance has been established with the patient, then problem-solving can help the patient determine the extent to which medication compliance is feasible. Future investigations must address the role of behavioral and psychologic factors in medical compliance among COPD patients. Cognitive factors, mood, and social support should be examined further to determine their role in predicting or increasing medical compliance. Treatment efforts should then target modifiable factors associated with poor compliance.

SUMMARY

Behavioral medicine may incorporate evaluation and treatment of psychologic functioning, cognitive performance, social functioning, and behavioral performance among patients with pulmonary disease. A substantial database of research and clinical observation suggests the importance of each of these factors in the treatment of patients in pulmonary rehabilitation. In addition, increasing evidence supports the notion that behavioral and psychologic factors may interact to have a profound influence on health status. However, relatively few studies or reports document such interactions, highlighting the importance of this area for future work in the field of pulmonary rehabilitation.

REFERENCES

1. Ashutosh K, Haldipur C, Boucher ML. Clinical and personality profiles and survival in patients with COPD. Chest 1997;111:95.
2. Guyatt GH, Townsend M, Berman LB, et al. Quality of life in patients with chronic airflow limitation. Br J Dis Chest 1987;81:45.
3. Sandhu HS. Psychosocial issues in chronic obstructive pulmonary disease. Clin Chest Med 1986;7:629.
4. Isoaho R, Puolijoki H, Huhti E, et al. Chronic obstructive pulmonary disease and cognitive impairment in the elderly. Int Psychogeriatr 1996; 8:113.
5. Agle DP, Baum GL. Psychological aspects of chronic obstructive pulmonary disease. Med Clin North Am 1977;61:749.
6. Graydon JE, Ross E. Influence of symptoms, lung function, mood, and social support on level of functioning of patients with COPD. Res Nurs Health 1995;18:525.
7. Leidy NK. Functional performance in people with chronic obstructive pulmonary disease. Image J Nurs Sch 1995;27:23.
8. Weaver TE, Richmond TS, Narsavage GL. An explanatory model of functional status in chronic obstructive pulmonary disease. Nurs Res 1997; 46:26.
9. Engstrom C-P, Persson L-O, Larsson S, et al. Functional status and well being in chronic obstructive pulmonary disease with regard to clinical parameters and smoking: a descriptive and comparative study. Thorax 1996;51:825.
10. Dudley DL, Glaser EM, Jorgenson BN, et al. Psychosocial concomitants to rehabilitation in chronic obstructive pulmonary disease—part 2: psychosocial treatment. Chest 1980;77:544.
11. Porzelius J, Vest M, Nochomovitz M. Respiratory function, cognitions, and panic in chronic obstructive pulmonary patients. Behav Res Ther 1992;30:75.
12. Anderson KL. The effect of chronic obstructive pulmonary disease on quality of life. Res Nurs Health 1995;18:547.
13. Goreczny AJ, Brantley PJ, Buss RR, et al. Daily stress and anxiety and their relation to daily fluctuations of symptoms in asthma and chronic obstructive pulmonary disease (COPD) patients. J Psychopathol Behav Assess 1988;10:259.
14. Bauer H, Duijsens IJ. Personality disorders in pulmonary patients. Br J Med Psychol 1998;71: 165.
15. Dudley DL, Wermuth C, Hague W. Psychosocial aspects of care in the chronic obstructive pulmonary disease patient. Heart Lung 1973;2:289.
16. Parsons E. Coping and well-being strategies in individuals with COPD. Health Values 1990; 14:17.

17. Ketelaars C, Schlosser M, Mostert R, et al. Determinants of health-related quality of life in patients with chronic obstructive pulmonary disease. Thorax 1996;51:39.

18. Scharloo M, Kaptein A, Weinman J, et al. Illness perceptions, coping and functioning in patients with rheumatoid arthritis, chronic obstructive pulmonary disease and psoriasis. J Psychosom Res 1998;44:573.

19. Kaplan RM, Ries AL, Prewitt LM, et al. Self-efficacy expectations predict survival for patients with chronic obstructive pulmonary disease. Health Psychol 1994;13:366.

20. Devins GM, Edwards PJ. Self-efficacy and smoking reduction in chronic obstructive pulmonary disease. Behav Res Ther 1988;26:127.

21. Ries AL, Kaplan RM, Limberg TM, et al. Effects of pulmonary rehabilitation on physiologic and psychosocial outcomes in patients with chronic obstructive pulmonary disease. Ann Intern Med 1995;122:823.

22. Derogatis LR, Spencer PM. Brief Symptom Inventory: Administration, Scoring, and Procedures Manual–I. Baltimore: Clinical Psychometric Research, 1982.

23. McNair DM, Lorr M, Droppelman LF. Profile of Mood States. San Diego: Educational and Testing Service, 1981.

24. Beck AT. Depression Inventory. Philadelphia: Center for Cognitive Therapy, 1978.

25. Radloff LS. The CES-D Scale: a self-report depression scale for research in the general population. Appl Psychol Meas 1977;1:385.

26. Beck AT, Epstein N, Brown G, et al. An inventory for measuring clinical anxiety: psychometric properties. J Consult Clin Psychol 1988;56:893.

27. Spielberger CE, Gorsuch RL, Luschene RE. Manual for the State-Trait Anxiety Inventory. Palo Alto, CA: Consulting Psychologist Press, 1970.

28. Lisansky DP, Clough DH. A cognitive-behavioral self-help educational program for patients with COPD. Psychother Psychosom 1996;65:97.

29. Gift AG, Moore T, Soeken K. Relaxation to reduce dyspnea and anxiety in COPD patients. Nurs Res 1992;41:242.

30. Borson S, McDonald GJ, Gayle T, et al. Improvement in mood, physical symptoms, and function with nortriptyline for depression in patients with chronic obstructive pulmonary disease. Psychosomatics 1992;33:190.

31. Gordon GH, Michiels TM, Mahutte CK, et al. Effect of desipramine on control of ventilation and depression scores in patients with severe chronic obstructive pulmonary disease. Psychiatry Res 1985;15:25.

32. Grant I, Prigatano GP, Heaton RK, et al. Progressive neuropsychologic impairment and hypoxemia. Arch Gen Psychiatry 1987;44:999.

33. Incalzi RA, Gemma A, Marra C, et al. Verbal memory impairment in COPD: its mechanisms and clinical relevance. Chest 1997;112:1506.

34. Stuss DT, Peterkin I, Guzman DA, et al. Chronic obstructive pulmonary disease: effects of hypoxia on neurological and neuropsychological measures. J Clin Exp Neuropsychol 1997;19:515.

35. Vos PJE, Folgering HTM, van Herwaarden CLA. Visual attention in patients with chronic obstructive pulmonary disease. Biol Psychol 1995;41: 295.

36. Emery CF, Schein RL, Hauck ER, et al. Psychological and cognitive outcomes of a randomized trial of exercise among patients with chronic obstructive pulmonary disease. Health Psychol 1998;17:232.

37. Grant I, Heaton RK, McSweeny AJ, et al. Neuropsychologic findings in hypoxemic chronic obstructive pulmonary disease. Arch Intern Med 1982; 142:1470.

38. Rourke SB, Adams KM. The neuropsychological correlates of acute and chronic hypoxemia. In: Grant I, Adams KM, eds. Neuropsychological Assessment of Neuropsychiatric Disorders. 2nd ed. New York: Oxford, 1996:379–402.

39. Wechsler D. Wechsler Adult Intelligence Scale: Administration and Scoring Manual. 3rd ed. New York: The Psychological Corporation, 1997.

40. Reitan RM. Validity of the trail making test as an indicator of organic brain damage. Percept Mot Skills 1958;8:271.

41. Stroop JR. Studies of interference in serial verbal reactions. J Exp Psychol 1935;18:643.

42. Krop H, Block AJ, Cohen E. Neuropsychologic effects of continuous oxygen therapy in chronic obstructive pulmonary disease. Chest 1973;64: 317.

43. Heaton RK, Grant I, McSweeny AJ, et al. Psychologic effects of continuous and nocturnal oxygen therapy in hypoxemic chronic obstructive pulmonary disease. Arch Intern Med 1983;143: 1941.

44. Dustman RE, Emmerson RY, Ruhling RO, et al. Age and fitness effects on EEG, ERPs, visual sensitivity, and cognition. Neurobiol Aging 1990;11:193.

45. Clough P, Harnisch L, Cebulski P, et al. Method for individualizing patient care for obstructive pulmonary disease patients. Health Soc Work 1987;12:127.

46. Rabinowitz B, Florian V. Chronic obstructive pulmonary disease: psycho-social issues and treatment goals. Soc Work Health Care 1992;16:69.

47. Keele-Card G, Foxall MJ, Barron CR. Loneliness, depression, and social support of patients with COPD and their spouses. Public Health Nurs 1993;10:245.

48. Isoaho R, Keistinen T, Laippala P, et al. Chronic obstructive pulmonary disease and symptoms related to depression in elderly persons. Psychol Rep 1995;76:287.

49. Cohen S, Wills TA. Stress, social support, and the buffering hypothesis. Psychol Bull 1985;98:310.

50. Bergner M, Bobbitt RA, Carter WB, et al. The Sickness Impact Profile: development and final revision of a health status questionnaire. Med Care 1981;19:787.

51. Ware JE, Sherbourne CD. The MOS 36-Item Short Form Health Survey (SF-36), I: conceptual framework and item selection. Med Care 1992; 30:473.

52. Cohen S, Mermelstein RL, Kamarck T, et al. Measuring the functional components of social support. In: Sarason IG, Sarason B, eds. Social

Support: Theory, Research, and Applications. The Hague, Holland: Martines Niijhoff, 1985.

53. Zimet GD, Dahlem NW, Zimet SG, et al. The Multidimensional Scale of Perceived Social Support. J Pers Assess 1988;52:30.

54. Barstow RE. Coping with emphysema. Nurs Clin North Am 1974;9:137.

55. Leidy NK, Traver GA. Psychophysiologic factors contributing to functional performance in people with COPD: are there gender differences? Res Nurs Health 1995;18:535.

56. Weaver TE, Narsavage GL. Physiological and psychological variables related to functional status in chronic obstructive pulmonary disease. Nurs Res 1992;41:286.

57. De Bruin AF, Diederiks JPM, De Witte LP, et al. The development of a short generic version of the Sickness Impact Profile. J Clin Epidemiol 1994; 47:407.

58. Ockene JK, Kristeller J, Goldberg R, et al. Increasing the efficacy of physician-delivered smoking interventions: a randomized clinical trial. J Gen Intern Med 1991;6:1.

59. Fiore MC, Baker LJ, Deeren SM. Cigarette smoking: the leading preventable cause of pulmonary diseases. In: Bone RC, ed. Pulmonary and Critical Care Medicine. St. Louis: Mosby-Year Book, 1993;1–19.

60. Glover ED, Glover PN, Abrons HL, et al. Smoking cessation among COPD and chronic bronchitis patients using the nicotine nasal spray. Am J Health Behav 1997;21:310.

61. Kottke T, Battista RN, DeFriese GH, et al. Attributes of successful smoking cessation interventions in medical practice: a meta-analysis of 39 controlled trials. JAMA 1988;259:2883.

62. Hall SM, Munoz RF, Reus VI, et al. Nicotine, negative affect, and depression. J Consult Clin Psychol 1993;61:761.

63. Daughton DM, Fix AJ, Kass I, et al. Smoking cessation among patients with chronic obstructive pulmonary disease (COPD). Addict Behav 1980; 5:125.

64. Glynn TJ. Methods of smoking cessation: finally, some answers. JAMA 1990;263:2795.

65. Haaga DA, Allison ML. Thought suppression and smoking relapse: a secondary analysis of Haaga (1989). Br J Clin Psychol 1994;33:327.

66. Efthimiou J, Fleming J, Gomes C, et al. The effect of supplementary oral nutrition in poorly nourished patients with chronic obstructive pulmonary disease. Am Rev Respir Dis 1988;137:1075.

67. Lewis MI, Belman MJ, Dorr-Uyemura L. Nutritional supplementation in ambulatory patients with COPD. Am Rev Respir Dis 1987;135:1062.

68. Knowles JB, Fairbarn MS, Wiggs BJ, et al. Dietary supplementation and respiratory muscle performance in patients with COPD. Chest 1988; 93:977.

69. Agle DP, Baum GL, Chester EH, et al. Multidiscipline treatment of chronic pulmonary insufficiency, 1: psychologic aspects of rehabilitation. Psychosom Med 1973;35:41.

70. Emery CF, Leatherman NE, Burker EJ, et al. Psychological outcomes of a pulmonary rehabilitation program. Chest 1991;100:613.

71. Fishman DB, Petty TL. Physical, symptomatic and psychological improvement in patients receiving comprehensive care for chronic airway obstruction. J Chronic Dis 1971;24:775.

72. Ojanen M, Lahdensuo A, Laitinen J, et al. Psychosocial changes in patients participating in a chronic obstructive pulmonary disease rehabilitation program. Respiration 1993;60:96.

73. Gayle RC, Spitler DL, Karper WB, et al. Psychological changes in exercising COPD patients. Int J Rehabil Res 1988;11:335.

74. Deckhuijzen PN, Beek MM, Folgering HT, et al. Psychological changes during pulmonary rehabilitation and target-flow inspiratory muscle training in COPD patients with a ventilatory limitation during exercise. Int J Rehabil Res 1990;13:109.

75. Sassi-Dambron DE, Eakin EG, Ries AL, et al. Treatment of dyspnea in COPD: a controlled clinical trial of dyspnea management strategies. Chest 1995;107:724.

76. Dolce JJ, Crisp C, Manzella B, et al. Medication adherence patterns in chronic obstructive pulmonary disease. Chest 1991;99:837.

77. James PNE, Anderson JB, Prior JG, et al. Patterns of drug taking in patients with chronic airflow obstruction. Postgrad Med J 1985;61:7–10.

78. Epstein LH, Cluss PA. A behavioral medicine perspective on adherence to long-term medical regimens. J Consult Clin Psychol 1982;50:950.

17 Sexuality in the Pulmonary Patient

Paul A. Selecky

Professional Skills

Upon completion of the chapter, the reader will:

- Understand the integral role that sexuality plays in all human beings, both patients and caregivers
- Grasp the clinical responsibility of sexual health care
- Embrace the concept that sexuality lasts a lifetime
- Learn the role of a health care provider in sexual counseling
- Understand the potential positive and negative ways that sexuality can impact the caregiver–patient relationship

INTRODUCTION

The primary basis for pulmonary rehabilitation is to help the patient understand and cope with his or her lung disease and to attempt to help the patient achieve the goal of "optimizing physical and social performance and autonomy."[1] We therefore are interacting with the patient as a person, which includes his or her sexuality. Our patients are men and women of various ages who have differing sexual roles as husbands or wives or single adults who are involved in relationships in various ways. Caregivers also are sexual beings. Our sexuality impacts our interpersonal relationships, including the interactions with our patients.

It is evident, therefore, that because sexuality is a far-reaching subject, addressing sexuality clearly comes within the scope of our responsibilities as members of a pulmonary rehabilitation team. It is our job to help our patients cope with the impact of the disease process on their lives in all its intricacies, including their lives as sexual beings. We should help them better understand this impact as a part of the rehabilitative process.

SEX VERSUS SEXUALITY

A discussion of sex within the context of a pulmonary rehabilitation program often begins with the focus on the physical aspects of sex, namely, sexual intercourse and other physical expressions of sexual functioning. This is understandably an area of great interest, but it is important that we paint a broader picture for ourselves and our patients. The word *sex* triggers many different images in each individual, depending on his or her experience and expectations as well as on the contact in which the word is being used. *Sexuality* is a more complex term because it involves the total personality of an individual—how he or she thinks, how he or she acts and feels; in essence, who he or she is. It has been said that sex is something we do; sexuality is something we are.[2] Both are important and unique in each of us.

Table 17-1. Sex vs. Sexuality

Sex as Biology	Sexuality as Total Person
Facts	Attitudes
Male/female	Maleness/femaleness
Genitality	Personality
Physical pleasure	Intimacy
Doing	Being
Self-oriented	Relational

As described in Table 17-1, sex is a biologic term; sexuality addresses the total person. Our sex is our gender; it also establishes our role as male or female with a varying combination of masculine and feminine traits. Our sexuality colors our emotions, our understanding of ourselves, and our interactions with others. Together, sex and sexuality encompass the whole individual. Men and women respond differently to many situations in life because they are men or women. It is our responsibility as health care workers to better understand those differences if we are to be useful to our patients.

SEXUAL HEALTH CARE

The World Health Organization defines sexual health as "the integration of somatic, emotional, intellectual, and social aspects in ways that are positively enriching and will enhance personality, communication, and love."[3] Health care workers must attempt to achieve this objective through *sexual health care,* a concept that may seem a bit foreign to our roles as respiratory care professionals. It requires us to focus on the impact of chronic lung disease and its attendant symptoms on the sexual health of the patient. It is not sufficient for us to inquire about physical sexual dysfunction alone, such as impotence, decreased libido, or ejaculatory problems. We must gain an understanding of the impact of chronic lung disease on the sexuality of our patient as a total person.

The delivery of sexual health care is a responsibility of the entire pulmonary rehabilitation team, which should integrate discussions of sexuality into the entire rehabilitative process. This is in contrast to assigning the team coordinator the responsibility to elicit responses to specific questions about sexual functioning, and then to refer the patient as needed for specialty evaluation determined by any dysfunction that is uncovered. Schover and Jensen[4] describe this as a kind of "relay race" in which one health care worker passes the "baton" to the next. Instead, a more appropriate integrative approach should be applied that involves the entire rehabilitation team in a process that ideally includes the patient's sexual partner in the evaluation and treatment plan.

SEXUALITY LASTS A LIFETIME

The delivery of sexual health care is based on the thesis that sexuality lasts a lifetime, in contrast to the popular view expressed by the media that sexuality is relegated to the young. As Kaiser[5] has pointed out, "there is no age at which sexual activity, thoughts, or desire end." Sexual expression may change, but interest does not diminish. The significance of sexuality in later life is an extension of an individual's past life experiences, with the addition of (*a*) the normal expected aging process, (*b*) the availability of a sexual partner, and (*c*) one's general health. Alex Comfort, the noted gerontologist, and coauthor Lanyard Dial use a practical analogy, stating "most of our aged stop having sex for reasons similar to those why they stop riding a bicycle: general infirmity, fear that it would expose them to ridicule, and for most, lack of a bicycle."[6]

In simple analysis, a person who is sexually active during younger years is expected to become less active in later years, whereas the younger person who is sexually less active may likely become inactive. Comfort and Dial[6] point out that "as we age, the vast majority of us will notice little change in sexual function, except in the attitudes of other people. Sexuality will simply be transformed into a slightly different, probably quieter experience than it was in youth, but a no less sexual and no less worthwhile experience." Thienhaus[7] states that a reasonable attitude for caregivers to assume concerning sexual activity in later life is that "some do, some don't, and there's nothing wrong with either."

The patient with lung disease fits well into this concept of a lifetime of sexuality. He or she most often is an older individual who is facing the impact of aging on sexuality and sexual functioning, may be lacking a sexual partner, and is trying to cope with progressive breathing problems. It is important that the rehabilitation team be knowledgeable of these factors if it is to minister to the patient's concerns about sexuality.

Sexuality and the Aging Process

Aging is an ongoing process that affects all individuals and all bodily functions. Sexual health is not immune. Comfort and Dial[6] have pointed out, however, that "compared with the age changes in . . . the eyes' focusing ability or the lungs' vital capacity, sexual-organ changes are minimal." Nonetheless, despite the process of natural aging that one expects, changes in sexual functioning somehow seem to catch patients by surprise. This is more apparent in the aging male, largely because of the noticeable changes in his ability to achieve and maintain an erection. As a result, more studies and writings focus on the changes in the human sexual response during intercourse, as defined many years ago by Masters and Johnson.[8] Details regarding both sexes are listed in Box 17-1. For the male, orgasm and sexual intercourse are of shorter duration, have fewer secretions, and the force and volume of ejaculation is less. A variety of factors are responsible for the physical changes, including a decrease in testosterone, although the aging male quickly forgets or ignores the fact that the peak of testosterone occurs around age 20 years, with a steady decline thereafter.[9] Conversely, testosterone replacement therapy for normal elderly men will not restore libido to the level of younger men, and it will not aid the problem of impotence.[10]

The aging female continues to have the ability to have satisfying sexual relations despite a reduction in physiologic response as described in Box 17-1. In fact, surprisingly

Box 17-1. Impact of Aging on Sexual Response

Female
Decrease in vaginal length and width
Less vaginal elasticity
Longer to achieve vaginal lubrication
Less vaginal lubrication
Decrease in frequency of orgasms
Male
Longer to achieve erection
Less firm erection
Longer to ejaculate
Lower ejaculate volume
Longer recovery time

little change occurs in sexual activity across the average woman's life span, except for the impact of social factors and general health.[11] Menopause, which occurs in most women at about age 50 years, is associated with substantial reductions in hormonal levels, leading to a variety of physical changes in genital anatomy and functioning, which can lead to dyspareunia, the most common sexual complaint among older women seeking gynecologic consultation.[9] This is less pronounced in women who continue to be sexually active, giving a biologic credence to the adage "use it or lose it."[12] The dyspareunia is often linked to delayed and reduced vaginal lubrication, which can be aided by topical lubricants or local or systemic estrogen replacement therapy. The latter remains a controversial subject but is generally recommended for women who do not have an increased risk for breast or endometrial malignancy.

Hysterectomy does not impair sexual function, although it can have a negative psychologic effect on some women, who feel it has removed an essential part of their femininity.[13] Mastectomy can have even a greater impact on a woman's sense of her sexual attractiveness. Counseling by her physician and others can help the patient resolve these issues.

The expected physical changes associated with aging in both genders do not necessarily indicate that sexual desire and/or activity have ground to a halt, despite the myth and public perception that sexual functioning belongs to the younger set. Numerous studies have dispelled the myth of a declining sexual interest with advancing age.[5] Data from the National Survey of Families and Households revealed that 53% of married persons 60 years and older, and 24% of those 76 years and older, have reported having sexual intercourse four times within the last month.[14] The study further found that these practices often were tied to the individual's sense of self-worth and competence and to his or her partner's health status. A study of sexual interest and behavior in healthy 80- to 102-year-olds revealed that the frequency of masturbation and sexual intercourse did not change greatly after age 80 years.[15] Both sexes who remain sexually active are likely to be more physically fit and to feel younger and are more likely to achieve sexual satisfaction.[16] Sexual dysfunction is more likely to be related to comorbid illnesses and/or psychosocial factors rather than aging along.[17–20]

Ebersole and Hess[21] state that sexuality "is an affirmation that one's body functions well, maintains a strong sense of self-identity, and provides a means for self-assertion." It is a veritable measure of the quality of life.[6] Moreover, a study in the *British Medical Journal* revealed that mortality risk was 50% lower in men who had a high frequency of sexual intercourse and orgasm.[22] An accompanying editorial compared this to the findings that suggest that alcohol might make one live longer. It stated "what we thought was bad for you may actually be good for you, but it may not be good to tell you in case you do it too much, and it is certainly not good to tell you it is good for you if you do too much of it already—assuming we could agree what was too much in the first place."[23] The study suggested tongue-in-cheek that public health intervention programs be considered, comparing them to the efforts at improving health by encouraging fruit and vegetable consumption with the phrase "at least 5 a day."

Andrew Greeley,[24] renowned sociologist and author who studied the sexual practices of aging Catholics, concluded that "one suspects that the older lovers for whom passion and play have not stopped after a long life together of cherishing one another will have the last laugh. They are entitled to that laugh and they can afford to have it."

Availability of a Sexual Partner

One of the greatest barriers to sexual activity in later life is the lack of a healthy sexual partner. It has long been known that women's life expectancy is much greater than men's, causing most married women to face a long period of widowhood. Data from the 1997 report of the Bureau of the Census reveals that there are eight women for every five men 75 years and older.[25] It is estimated that after age 80 years, there are about four women for every man.[26] Despite their diminishing numbers, approximately two-thirds of men 75 years and older are married. Two-thirds of women in the same age group are widowed. As a result, simple arithmetic indicates that older unmarried men have a greater likelihood of finding a female partner.

On the other hand, fate has dealt a cruel blow to many older women. Although they live longer, they are more likely to spend their later years alone because of the loss of their spouse. Some women may be open to choosing a second partner, but often this is thwarted by the progressively diminishing number of available male partners their age, particularly those men who remain healthy and active. They could seek the company of younger men, but their families and society in general seem to frown on such unions, whereas an older man is often applauded for being able to successfully win the heart of a younger woman.

These statistics are confirmed by a household survey in Michigan of individuals 60 years and older. Approximately 74% of married men responded as being sexually active compared with 31% of unmarried men. In contrast, 56% of married women were sexually active, whereas only 5% of unmarried women gave the same response.[27] Interestingly, the daily consumption of coffee correlated with sexual activity in women and potency in men.

Both genders may have the additional obstacle of lacking adequate privacy, either because of their living situation, such as rooming in their adult children's home, or concern about "what the neighbors might say." Health care institutions and staff may be another source of problems. For example, nursing home personnel generally frown on if not prohibit conjugal visits between residents, even though Medicaid-supported institutions are required to allow requesting married couples to be housed together.[21] Understandable concern exists that elderly residents not be abused by other residents, but a more liberal attitude would allow greater freedom of sexual interaction between consenting residents. Richardson and Lazur[28] describe several interventions that could lower the barriers.

Sexuality and Chronic Illness

Sexual functioning can be affected by chronic illness in a variety of ways. Sometimes the effect is related to the specific disease, for example, impotence in diabetes, angina in coronary occlusive disease, or sometimes general frailty. Dyspnea is the major symptom of the patient with lung disease, but studies reveal that this does not seem to be a major obstacle to successful sexual intercourse, except perhaps for those with severe impairment who are dyspneic at rest.[29] Although the scientific data are somewhat contradictory, the impact of lung disease on sexual functioning is not to be measured by pulmonary function tests; rather, it is found in an understanding of the psychosocial impact of disease on the patient, as depicted in Box 17-2 (see Chapter 16).[30] Regardless of these factors, some patients have good coping skills and stand out as model patients because they are able to maintain an active lifestyle despite their chronic illness. This ability generally flows into their sexual functioning.

Box 17-2. Psychosocial Composite
of the Patient With Chronic
Lung Disease

Social, family, and sexual roles altered
Limited activities of daily living
Limited recreation
Preoccupied with body functions
Increased anxiety
Decreased self-esteem
Depressed
Overdependent

Wise[31] organizes the obstacles to sexual functioning into three categories. The lung disease patient has to struggle with *impersonal factors,* such as limited exercise tolerance, chronic cough, sputum production, and the potential side effects of medications. He or she also often struggles with *intrapersonal* obstacles such as decreased self-esteem and an altered view of his or her masculine or feminine role with the accompanying anxiety. These then lead to *interpersonal* obstacles with a spouse or intimate other, including the fear of sexual failure and ultimately a suppression of sexual desire. It is important to realize, however, that this is not a universal finding linked only to chronic illness. Many healthy couples also complain of sexual problems. Moreover, many patients do continue to live full and satisfying sexual lives.

WHAT CAN A HEALTH CARE PROVIDER DO?

Our primary role as health care professionals is to attend to our patient's needs. In the field of sexual health care, this must begin with a self-examination of our knowledge and attitudes about sexuality. Any deficits in sexual information can be corrected by further study of a variety of published resources, but the facts we know are not nearly as important to our patients as are our attitudes concerning sex and sexuality. Ideally, we want our attitude to be "sex positive" and accepting of others' points of view and lifestyles, and we want to avoid making value judgments. Our lack of sexual knowledge can be an obstacle in communicating with our patients, but this obstacle is worsened by their perceiving negative nonverbal messages or hearing negative attitudes expressed concerning their sexual interests and behavior. Our patients plead for our help as health care providers,[26] as is revealed in the list of suggestions in Box 17-3 from a survey on this issue of almost 1500 persons 50 years and older.[32]

Before introducing the subject of sexuality in a rehabilitation program, it is important that the rehabilitation team conduct an introspective evaluation of their sexual attitudes. This can be accomplished by conducting discussions of sexuality at team conferences. Team members might respond to probing questions such as "What are your attitudes about sexual activity in the elderly, masturbation, homosexuality, oral sex, and a wide variety of sexual subjects and practices?" and "How comfortable are you talking about sex?"[33] Oregon State University has developed a 30-minute board game to help caregivers examine their attitudes about aging and sexuality.[34]

Ideally, training in the diagnosis and treatment of sexual dysfunctions should be sought. Schover and Jensen[35] describe a model for a 1-day training session. At the very least, we need to be good listeners. We must respond to our patients' needs and concerns and not shut them out or turn them away.

Box 17-3. Older Adults' Suggestions for Health Care
Providers Regarding Discussion About Sex

Spend time with older adults
Use clear and easy-to-understand words
Help older adults feel comfortable talking about sex
Be open minded and talk openly
Listen closely
Treat older adults with a respectful and nonjudgmental
    attitude
Encourage discussion
Give advice or suggestions
Understand that sex is not just for the young

SEXUAL COUNSELING

Many health care workers feel unprepared to become involved in sexual counseling and feel more comfortable with discussion of almost every other subject in the field of pulmonary rehabilitation. Regardless of our hesitancy in discussing sexuality with our patients, we may have no choice other than to become involved when our patients ask questions. It is a subject for which the entire team should be prepared. The team should not relegate the responsibilities to just one member, such as the coordinator. Although the responsibility is often placed on the coordinator, the patient may feel more comfortable discussing questions concerning sexuality with some other members of the team. It is likely to be someone who appears to the patient to be most comfortable with the subject, someone who is approachable, or someone who appears able to discuss such intimate subjects in a relaxed and nonjudgmental manner. The coordinator may be the one to introduce the subject, but all members of the team should be open to continuing that discussion in their interactions with the patient.

Most questions can be addressed from the resource of our own life experiences without the need for specialized training. Francoeur[36] offers three cautions in this regard: (*a*) be aware of your limitations; (*b*) be sensitive to your position within the health care team so as not to interfere with the role of others, such as the primary care physician; and (*c*) avoid making a detailed recommendation to a patient that may go beyond the team's limitations.

A model for sexual counseling that many have found useful has been described by Annon[37] as the PLISSIT model, a four-step process progressing from simple to complex counseling. The caregiver proceeds through the four steps guided by the patient's needs and his or her own professional judgment and personal comfort. The steps are described in Box 17-4.

Permission Giving

The steps of this first level of counseling are listed in Box 17-5. They begin by merely introducing the subject to the pulmonary rehabilitation patient, and in doing so "give permission" to the patient to discuss his or her sexual concerns. It delivers a message from your team that says "It is OK to talk about sex here." This can be done by asking a few open-ended questions on the intake questionnaire and allowing time for the patient to elaborate on the responses during the intake interview. It is best to avoid questions that require a "yes" or "no" answer and instead to use proving and/or permission-giving questions, such as:

1. How has your breathing problem affected your view of yourself as a man or woman?
2. How does your breathing affect your sexual desire and activity?
3. You mentioned you were limited by your shortness of breath. How has it affected your sexual desire and functioning?
4. What do you find are the most troubling changes in your sexuality?
5. Many people have sexual concerns. What concerns you about your sexual functioning? What concerns your partner?

Box 17-4. PLISSIT Model for
Sexual Counseling

P = Permission giving
LI = Limited Information
SS = Specific Suggestions
IT = Intensive Therapy

Box 17-5. Giving Permission to be Sexual

Introduce the subjects of sex and sexuality
Communicate acceptance by your words and behavior
Use open-ended questions in the intake interview
Use terms comfortable to you and the patient
Be "sex positive"
Be a good listener
Encourage and support the patient
Do not stereotype the patient's behavior
Provide educational materials
Consider using a structured survey tool

Ebersole and Hess[21] provide more detailed questions in their text *Toward Healthy Aging* that can be asked if the patient expresses greater interest.

It is important that the interviewer asks questions in a relaxed and comfortable manner, and then waits for the patient to respond. We must be cautious of our body language that may be telling the patient that we really do not want to hear about his or her sexual problems because they embarrass us. The look on our faces is more important than the words we use. Structured survey tools are available to conduct a more formal inquiry.[38–40]

Ideally, such an interview should be conducted in privacy to maintain patient confidentiality. The interviewer should allow sufficient time for discussion, pointing out to the patient that additional opportunities will be available for addressing his or her concerns during the rehabilitation program. The patient's sexual partner should be involved in these discussions at some point, although initially it may be more comfortable for the patient to address the subject alone with the interviewer. Schover and Jensen[41] point out that *couple therapy* is more productive than addressing the patient alone. The interviewer often is able to assess the potential benefit of involving the patient's sexual partner in the discussion by assessing the role that the partner is already playing in the patient's illness. These authors point out that "general coping skills and sexual function are linked in the chronically ill" and advise the clinician that the best way to treat any sexual concerns is by fostering the strengths of the couple's relationship. They identify a strong relationship as one in which the couple has developed four important skills: (*a*) they are comfortable and flexible in allocating their individual roles, (*b*) they respect each other's boundaries and allow these boundaries to change over time, (*c*) they have achieved good communication, and (*d*) they have reached agreement on the rules of their relationship that govern its daily functioning. The same four skills apply to their sexual relationship as well.

The first step of *permission giving* may generate no response from the patient. It should be remembered that "some do, some don't, and there is nothing wrong with either."[7] Nonetheless, sexual concerns are common. Giving permission to discuss them is likely to bring results. A study in a general practice of adults of all ages, both sexes, different marital statuses, and different education levels revealed that more than 50% reported sexual problems or concerns, for example, frequency of intercourse, lack of sexual desire, marital or relationship problems, painful intercourse, and difficulties achieving an erection.[42] We should be prepared to address these concerns.

The solution to many patients' sexual concerns lies in education. Various institutions have produced printed materials that can be offered to patients or placed in the packet of education materials that they receive as part of the rehabilitation program.[43,44] Information for patients is also available on the Internet, for example, on the website of the National Institute on Aging at www.nih.gov/nia/.[45] Such educational efforts introduce the subject of sexuality but are of only limited usefulness unless the patient is given an opportunity to discuss individual concerns. Some programs introduce the topic of sexuality for discussion in patient support groups; this requires the presence of an experienced facilitator to make the discussion productive.

Limited Information

Introducing the topic of sexuality may open the door to further discussion. If such is the case, the clinician should be prepared to offer at least *limited information* of a general nature, such as listed in Box 17-6. The first step is to broaden the patient's focus from genital functioning to the impact of sexuality on their total being, explaining that sexuality also includes how a person thinks and feels, not just what he or she does. This is particularly important for the patient with lung disease who has often developed a negative self-image and who chooses to focus on his or her own frailties and limitations. This negative attitude often springs from society's image of the sexually active person as being young and attractive. Many patients unfortunately succumb to these myths, feeling that they are too old, too unattractive, or too sickly to have sexual feelings, let alone to consider being sexually active.

It is important that patients understand the impact of normal aging on sexual functioning, as described in Box 17-1. Although this knowledge does not resolve patients' concerns entirely, it often alleviates their fear that they are not normal. Patient education materials are available on this subject as well.[46]

Although there are no true aphrodisiacs, some medications can improve sexual desire and/or functioning by having a beneficial effect on an underlying medical disorder. Certain drugs used to treat Parkinson's disease, for example, have resulted in improved sexual functioning. Some antidepressants have improved libido in the absence of any antidepressant effect.[47]

More likely, medications can be the source or an aggravating factor for sexual dysfunction, particularly contributing to impotence in the male. Antihypertensive medications are commonly the culprit, but not all are known to cause this problem. Patients should be made aware of the potential for this side effect and advised to discuss it with their prescribing physician or a clinical pharmacist to see if an alternative medication can be substituted. Other medications may result in decreased libido in both sexes, as noted in Table 17-2.[48] Fortunately, few of the pulmonary medications suppress sexual functioning, and they in fact may enhance it by decreasing exertional dyspnea. On the other hand, decreased testosterone levels in men with chronic lung disease have been correlated with glucocorticoid therapy and with hypoxemia.[49]

Patients and their sexual partners may limit sexual activity because they fear that the physical exertion and associated increase in breathing may trigger an attack of coughing or dyspnea. They need to be reassured that although the breathing rate increases, the physical stress of sexual intercourse is limited and often lasts only a few minutes in most circumstances.[50] Individual styles of lovemaking, however, are varied.

Box 17-6. Provide Limited Information

Sexuality involves the total person
Aging has predictable effects on sexual function
Fears and myths about sex are to be dispelled
Physiologic stress of lovemaking is limited
Some medications can impair or aid sexual function
Sexual dysfunction can be treated
Discuss sexual concerns with your partner
Address and resolve impact of any comorbid conditions

Table 17-2. Some Medications That Can Affect Sexual Functioning

Erectile Dysfunction	Decreased Libido
Diuretics	Antihypertensive drugs
Antihypertensive drugs	Antihistamines
Anticholinergic drugs	Psychiatric drugs
Antihistamines	Sedatives
Antidepressants	Alcohol
Anorectic drugs	Anxiolytics
Alcohol	
Anxiolytics	

Specific Suggestions

As we move through this model of progressive counseling in sexual health, patients may ask for *specific suggestions* to address their problems or concerns. These also may be presented in a general way as one of the lectures given to patients in the pulmonary rehabilitation program or to patient support groups or at general patient education forums, such as the Better Breathers Clubs of the American Lung Association. A list of suggestions that focus on ways to enhance sexual performances is found in Box 17-7. Many of these suggestions are based on common sense but are worth reiterating for the patient and his or her sexual partner. Making these suggestions often reassures both partners and may encourage their discussing the subject further in private.

The rehabilitation team can advise patients to schedule lovemaking for the "best breathing" time. This usually is in the late morning or early afternoon after their daily morning bronchial hygiene has been completed and before late afternoon fatigue has begun to set in. In addition, older men often are better able to achieve an erection in the morning.[21] Advise patients to be creative and romantic in their sexual encounters, and urge them to avoid the "touchdown" mentality that often has been the driving force for many patients, that is, attempting to achieve orgasm or "score" on every sexual encounter. They need to be reminded of the sexual benefits of touch, for example, cuddling, caressing, and just spending some sexual time together.[21] They should be encouraged to explore a wide range of sexual behaviors "from smiling to orgasm."[51]

Specific variations on body position can be offered as an alternative to their usual habits of lovemaking.[52,53] For the male patient, the female-on-top position has been shown to have a lower metabolic expenditure.[50] Such a suggestion is less important if the change

Box 17-7. Specific Suggestions for Lovemaking

Be physically and emotionally rested
Ensure your privacy
Start and progress slowly
Choose the "best breathing" time
Avoid a "touchdown" mentality
Concentrate on mutual touch
Avoid after alcohol and heavy meals
Use oxygen and/or medications to your advantage
Choose less stressful positions
Be creative and romantic

Box 17-8. Intensive Therapy
for Sexual Problems

Training in communication
techniques
Marriage counseling
Urologic/gynecologic consultation
Psychologic counseling
Psychiatric counseling
Sex therapy

in position appears too unnatural to the couple. The male patient using the male-on-top position with someone other than his spouse expends the greatest amount of energy. For the male or female patient with coexisting symptomatic coronary occlusive disease, obtaining guidance from his or her physician on a safe level of physical activity would be an appropriate suggestion. Our role is simply to offer the suggestions in an attempt to give them permission to change their habits if they so desire and to point out the wide variety of ways in which couples conduct their lovemaking.

The team can remind patients to avoid lovemaking after a heavy meal or the use of alcohol because of the tendency to generate fatigue. Alcohol also can be a risk factor for male impotence, as Shakespeare pointed out in *Macbeth,* stating that "drink . . . provokes desire, but it takes away the performance." Cigarette smoking also is a risk factor for male impotence because the vasoconstrictive effects of nicotine alter the complex vascular mechanism associated with erection of the penis. More often than not, physicians have convinced their male patients to stop smoking because of its impact on their lung disease.

Intensive Therapy

If our suggestions have not resolved the patient's concerns up to this point, or if we detect problems that need specialty care, appropriate referrals should be made. Care options are described in Box 17-8. Referral requires our having knowledge of appropriate resources that are available in the community. Types of sexual dysfunction are listed in Box 17-9.

Erectile dysfunction, that is, impotence, can be a problem for the aging male. Estimates indicate that as many as 55% of men report problems with impotence by age 75 years.[9] It is not an all-or-nothing symptom. Impotence is defined as "the inability to attain and/or maintain penile erection sufficient for satisfactory sexual performance."[54] Regardless of the expected increase in incidence with age, impotence in elderly men should not be accepted as a normal course of events. Many patients can be successfully treated.

An erection is the result of a complex physiologic process that can go awry in a variety of ways.[21] This emphasizes the importance of appropriate diagnosis and treatment, which usually begins with the primary care physician. The patient can be referred for evaluation as needed to such specialists as an endocrinologist, urologist, vascular surgeon, or perhaps

Box 17-9. Sexual Dysfunctions

Erectile dysfunction/impotence
Premature ejaculation
Dyspareunia
Vaginismus
Inhibited sexual desire
Inhibited sexual arousal
Inhibited orgasm

sex therapist. The population being studied influences the results of studies that identify the various causes, but most indicate that most patients with impotence have an organic cause. Possible organic causes include medication effects, endocrine abnormalities, neurologic diseases, and vascular dysfunction. The effects of alcohol and nicotine have already been mentioned.

The complex nature of impotence requires the physician to perform a physical examination and compile a thorough history that includes a detailed discussion of the sexual dysfunction. This often is supplemented by appropriate laboratory studies as needed. A variety of treatment modalities are available, guided by evaluation. It includes such therapies as testosterone supplementation for the rare patient with hypogonadism, oral drug therapy, intracavernous injections of vasoactive medications, vacuum constriction devices, and penile prosthesis implantation.[55] Particular to our patients, a study of a small number of male patients with chronic obstructive pulmonary disease placed on long-term oxygen therapy to treat hypoxemia revealed an improvement in oxygenation followed by a reversal of sexual impotence in 42% after 1 month of oxygen use.[56] Regardless of the modality, sexual counseling is often an important part of each of these varied therapies.

Oral medications for the treatment of erectile dysfunction did not show reliable results until the introduction of sildenafil (Viagra®) in the United States dramatically revolutionized the awareness and treatment of this sexual dysfunction.[57] Originally introduced as a vasodilator for the treatment of coronary artery disease, sildenafil quickly gained greater use for the treatment of impotence. The new drug became the topic of discussion in newspapers, magazine, and talk shows. Its popularity soared, with pharmaceutical sales increasing dramatically in just the first few months of use.

Subsequent clinical experience has revealed that sildenafil improves erections in 63 to 82%, depending on the dose.[58] Its pharmacologic effect is to increase blood flow to the penis in response to sexual stimulation, not causing penile erections directly, and it has been shown to be effective in many causes of erectile dysfunction, including diabetes.[59] Its principal side effects relate to the vasodilatation and include headache, flushing, and small decreases in blood pressure. Although generally well tolerated by healthy individuals, serious cardiovascular events can occur in patients who are concurrently taking organic nitrates because the drug can cause potentially life-threatening hypotension. The deaths that have been reported to the Food and Drug Administration were related to probably cardiac events in patients who already were at risk because of their underlying cardiovascular disease. As a result, it has been difficult to discern whether the drug or the associated increase in physical sexual activity played the major role in these incidents.

The same caution applies to the use of sildenafil when used in postmenopausal women with sexual dysfunction.[60] The effect of the drug in this population in limited studies revealed that although overall sexual function did not improve significantly, vaginal lubrication and clitoral sensitivity changed. The role of this medication in this population thus remains to be determined. It is expected that other drugs of this nature will become available.

Review of Box 17-10 indicates that there are also many nonorganic causes of sexual problems that can occur at any age and that can be corrected or alleviated by ongoing counseling.[21] The patient and his or her sexual partner should focus on the problems they

Box 17-10. Nonorganic Causes
of Sexual Problems

Lack of a partner
Monotonous sexual interactions
Marital disharmony
Unreasonable sexual expectations
Fear of failure in sexual performance

are having in their sexual interactions, but these problems may be a symptom of a more general problem with their relationship.[61]

Couples need to be reminded that their lovemaking at night is an extension of their daytime interactions. They may be suffering from monotony and boredom in their daily life together, which can flow over into their love life. Both partners need to be reminded that each needs to continue to work on their relationship on an ongoing basis and to continue to romance each other. Patients with lung disease are often so involved in the management of their illness that they neglect their personal relationships. They may need to be reminded that they must work at being feminine or masculine and focus on expressing their sexuality in the way they dress, their general attitude, and how they interact with others. Most individuals enjoy being attractive and gaining the attention of others. We may need to remind patients how they pursued those goals in the past.

SEXUALITY AND THE CAREGIVER-PATIENT RELATIONSHIP

To a certain extent, our own sexuality has an effect on all the relationships we have with our patients. Sometimes this effect is brief and passing, such as when a caregiver administers a nebulizer treatment to a patient during a hospital stay. On the other hand, it can be ongoing over a period of time, such as in a pulmonary rehabilitation program or when delivering home care on a recurring basis to a patient. As discussed previously, we are sexual beings as males or females and thus cannot divorce sexuality from our interpersonal relationships. Male and female caregivers may act differently with male patients than with female patients. The difference in these interactions is not necessarily good or bad, but it is important that the caregiver be aware of how sexuality might have a negative impact on these relationships.

It is natural that a caregiver might be sexually attracted to a patient. Many people in the world are beautiful in mind, body, and soul, and it is understandable that we might be sexually attracted to them. These feelings are neither right nor wrong; they simply exist. However, we must recognize our sexual feelings and deal with them if they interfere with the professional nature of our relationship.

We are told to be loving and caring individuals, and at the same time we are expected to be scientifically objective. This combination can be difficult. We must compromise each of these goals in some way. If we are to be successful caregivers, we must be loving and caring, but we must also be aware of our own sexual feelings, needs, and desires to guard against their interfering with our roles as loving and caring health care professionals.

The relationship with our patients is unique. It has been described as a *fiduciary* relationship, that is, the patient has the trust and confidence that the caregiver will act in his or her best interest.[62] By its very nature, this relationship is asymmetric, with the patient being in a dependent and vulnerable role. The patient entrusts us with many personal and sometimes intimate aspects of his or her life, and we are obliged to preserve the patient's dignity and privacy. This ranges from how we address the patient to how we physically touch the patient and maintain an ongoing relationship.

As professionals, we have developed a sensitivity of calling the patient by his or her proper name and to avoid using familiar and potentially insulting labels. We have also learned about respecting the patient's "personal space" and about assessing when and how it is appropriate to touch the patient, either in the process of physical examination or in social touching. Touch can be an important part of healing, but limits and boundaries to touching exist and may vary from patient to patient.[21] It may seem appropriate at times to hold the hand of a depressed patient to offer comfort and support. Other patients may consider this gesture an intrusion. Our actions are generally guided by our own common sense and by the awareness of our own personal level of comfort. Regardless, the asymmetric and fiduciary nature of the relationship must be kept in mind, particularly when we may sense sexual feelings rising to the surface, either in ourselves or in our patients.

ETHICAL ISSUES IN SEXUAL HEALTH CARE

Acknowledging the impact of sexuality on our professional relationships brings the realization that sexual feelings sensed or expressed by either the caregiver or the patient can disrupt and alter the goals of the professional relationship. This leads to a variety of concerns regarding medical ethics. The caregiver may inadvertently or sometimes consciously become involved in circumstances with a patient that might be termed "boundary violations," which implies that the professional nature of the relationship has been breached. The "violations" by either the caregiver or the patient may at times be seemingly innocent and perhaps trivial—such as an inappropriate word or unwelcome familiarity—and simply be excused as a brief intrusion into the privacy of either the caregiver or the patient. On the other hand, more significant violations can occur, which, if not corrected, can lead to complete disruption of the relationship and sometimes become associated with charges of impropriety or ethical misconduct.

Most health care professionals have had little or no training on how to identify and avoid or correct sexually oriented disruptions in the professional relationship. Those in the field of psychiatry and related professions who become involved in long-term counseling have been the most vocal in addressing these issues. We can learn from their experiences as they apply to the field of pulmonary rehabilitation.

Seductive Behavior

The caregiver may sometimes find that a patient exhibits behavior that is sexually seductive, and he or she may be at a loss as to how to respond, except for the instinctual urge to turn and run. Such seductive behavior may be subtle and actually may be innocent, such as a wink of an eye, a touch, or other behavior by the patient that makes the caregiver feel uncomfortable. On the other hand, the behavior may be blatant, such as the male patient exposing his genitals to the female caregiver when she enters his hospital room or the female patient whose manner of dress becomes progressively seductive over time with a male caregiver. Regardless of the intent of the behavior, its sexual content is disruptive to the relationship and needs to be recognized and perhaps addressed.

At times, the caregiver may sense a sexual attraction to the patient, which by itself is neither right nor wrong but clearly must be recognized by the caregiver and suppressed. Sexual feelings are natural and spontaneous in each of us and should be recognized for what they are, that is, simply feelings. Acting on those feelings, on the other hand, is inappropriate and unethical. Seductive behavior by a patient to a vulnerable caregiver is understandably a formula for disaster for both individuals.

The caregiver should try to analyze and interpret the motivation for the patient's behavior. Is it expressing a truly sexual need or physical urge, or is the patient lonely and depressed and craving personal attention? Is the patient using this inappropriate behavior in an attempt to fulfill those needs? Perhaps the behavior is merely representative of the patient's personality, that is, he or she might be flirtatious or a sexual tease by nature. Conversely, the behavior may represent the patient's attempt to control the relationship by manipulating the caregiver's feelings. Under these circumstances, the caregiver should suppress the urge to "play along," however tantalizing it might appear. It is important to realize that the patient is responding to the relationship with the caregiver, not to the caregiver as an individual. It is at this point that the caregiver should identify what it is in his or her own behavior that may be generating sexual attraction by the patient.

If possible, the caregiver should try to preserve the relationship unless the behavior is totally disruptive. Suggestions for this are listed in Box 17-11.[62] It is important to reaffirm the professional nature of the relationship. Words or touches by the patient that

Box 17-11. Responses to a Seductive Patient

Do not play along
Identify patient's motive
Indicate your discomfort
Reaffirm the professional relationship
Preserve patient's self-esteem
Acknowledge patient's sexuality
Address patient's emotional needs
Transfer care to a different caregiver if necessary

are blatantly sexual must be addressed, and it must be pointed out to the patient that such liberties are not acceptable. The male patient who exposes his genitals during the female caregiver's visit to his hospital room should be told to cover up and that such actions are not welcomed and that they make the caregiver uncomfortable. More subtle behavior by the patient may be more difficult to address. The situation may be resolved simply by refocusing the relationship, pointing out to the patient that the behavior suggests that his or her feelings for the caregiver may be other than professional and thus are not appropriate.

It is important to preserve the patient's self-esteem by acknowledging and affirming his or her sexuality. The patient may feel sickly and unattractive and fear that the caregiver looks on him or her with pity or disgust. A negative response by the caregiver would then confirm the patient's low self-worth. The caregiver should try not to focus on the actual behavior but rather on the reason for the behavior. At times, unfortunately, the professional nature of the relationship is beyond repair, and this relationship must be severed. In such cases, the caregiver should transfer the patient to the care of another if possible. It is wise that the caregiver discuss this problem with the rehabilitation team or an appropriate supervisor.

Sexual Bias

Another sexual issue that may impact negatively on the caregiver–patient relationship is a preexisting sexual bias. As discussions concerning sexuality ensue in a pulmonary rehabilitation program, the caregiver may learn of sexual behavior or preferences of the patient that the caregiver finds personally unacceptable. Learning about a patient's homosexual preference, for example, may activate a sexual bias in the caregiver if he or she feels that homosexual behavior is morally wrong or somehow abnormal. As has been stated many times, feelings about sexuality are an integral part of our personality. The rightness or wrongness of a sexual bias is not the subject of this discussion. Rather, it is important that the caregiver recognize a personally sexual bias and take precautions that it does not interfere with the professional relationship.

This reemphasizes the importance of preparing for patient encounters by examining one's feelings and attitudes about sexuality and sexual behavior and by coming to grips with one's own sexual values and levels of comfort. It is not our place to make value judgments about sexual preferences or behavior of our patients, unless we feel that the behavior is harmful to the patient or to others. Although we may avoid making any comments to the patient, we must guard against sending nonverbal messages and disapproval, such as the look on our face or our body language or how we choose to continue the discussion. We may not agree with the patient's choices, but we must accept them and work to accept the patient unconditionally as a person.

Sexual Abuse

Our interactions with patients may reveal evidence or generate suspicion of sexual abuse of the patient. It most commonly involves individuals who depend on others for their care and support, such as children and the elderly. All health care professionals are legally required in most states to report suspected incidents of abuse and neglect, and legally immunity is provided for those making such reports. Victims of such abuse would seem to be unlikely participants in a pulmonary rehabilitation program, but this depends on the age and nature of the population that the program is serving.

The sexual abuse of children is a major problem in the United States, and we must be knowledgeable of the behavioral and physical signs that indicate that such abuse is taking place. This is particularly important in caregivers who serve children and young adults.[63] Although we often think of sexual abuse as occurring mainly in children, the caregiver must also consider whether elderly patients have been abused sexually.

Most commonly, the patient who has been abused will be an elderly woman who has lost her spouse and is physically or mentally dependent on another person for care. Often the abused person will be unwilling to talk about the abusive incidents because he or she is afraid that the abuser will find out and that the abuse will worsen. The caregiver is obliged to protect the patient from injury and thus should be familiar with the necessary steps to obtain protection or to seek appropriate professional resources.[64,65]

Sexual Interactions

It is difficult for a caregiver to know how to respond when the patient expresses attraction or "makes a pass" at him or her. The initial reaction may be one of flattery, the caregiver feeling pleased that the patient has found him or her to be attractive. However, it is important to focus on the nature of the relationship. The patient's response may seem genuine, but it is more commonly an expression of *transference*.[62] This is a behavioral phenomenon first identified by Freud, who noted that patients displace previous experiences, behavior, and emotions onto the caregiver. This can be a source of confusion for both the patient and the caregiver. Transference is not necessarily pathologic or sexual, but it can be either or both. Regardless of its nature, it must be recognized and understood by the caregiver and be addressed when their behavior oversteps the boundary limitations of the relationship.

It is understandable that patients may confuse their feelings toward the caregiver with feelings that may have been expressed to others in intimate relationships in their past. The patient may feel lonely and unloved and sense that the caregiver is beginning to fill those needs. After all, our professional behavior is to focus on the patient as a person, giving him or her our attention and addressing his or her needs and desires. Our actions tell the patient that we think he or she is a special person and worthy of our attention. The patient may feel the desire to respond to that attention, even though that desire is misguided.

Countertransference is a caregiver's return response to the patient. Again, such interaction is not necessarily bad and can sometimes act to cement the relationship, such as talking about things that both have in common, for example, a certain hobby, travel experiences, or interest in sports. Such discussions make the patient and caregiver feel more familiar and thus more comfortable with each other. Conversely, *sexual transference* and *countertransference* are generally disruptive. In these circumstances, the caregiver must be reminded of the asymmetric nature of the relationship and the fact that the patient is vulnerable and at risk for exploitation. Any encouragement that the caregiver gives to the patient's expression of sexual interest is a violation of the trust that the patient has placed in the relationship, with the patient suffering the consequences of the breach of that trust. Even if the patient continues to pursue the caregiver and seems to consent to an ongoing sexual relationship, many would argue that the initial fiduciary basis for the relationship prevents any true consent from occurring.[66] As a result, sexual interactions between caregiver and patient, particularly sexual intercourse, are unethical.[67]

SUMMARY

Sexuality is an integral part of the human experience and thus is an integral part of the rehabilitative process of an individual disabled by a chronic illness, often complicated by the natural aging process. We as health caregivers have a responsibility to understand this aspect of our patients' lives and to be prepared to minister to their needs. As our country ages, we must strive to meet this challenge and, as Comfort and Dial[6] state, strive "to make them welcome—now, because they include our parents, and in the future, because they will include ourselves."

Note: the section on Ethical Issues in Health Care in this chapter has been adapted from Selecky, PA. Sexuality and the patient with lung disease. In: Casaburi R, Petty TL, eds. Principles and Practice of Pulmonary Rehabilitation. Philadelphia: WB Saunders, 1993:387–390.

REFERENCES

1. American Thoracic Society. Pulmonary rehabilitation—1999. Am J Respir Crit Care Med 1999; 159(5 Pt 1):1666–1682.
2. Selecky PA. Sexuality and the patient with lung disease. In: Casaburi R, Petty TL, eds. Principles and Practice of Pulmonary Rehabilitation. Philadelphia: WB Saunders, 1993:382.
3. World Health Organization. Education and treatment in human sexuality: the training of health professionals. Geneva: World Health Organization, 1975. Technical Report Series 572.
4. Schover LR, Jensen SB. Sexuality and Chronic Illness: A Comprehensive Approach. New York: The Guilford Press, 1988:3.
5. Kaiser FE. Sexuality in the elderly. Urol Clin North Am 1996;23(1):99–109.
6. Comfort A, Dial LK. Sexuality and aging. Clin Geriatr Med 1991;7:1.
7. Thienhaus OJ. Practical overview of sexual function and advancing age. Geriatrics 1988;43(8): 63–67.
8. Masters WH, Johnson VE. Human Sexual Response. Boston: Little Brown, 1966.
9. Meston CM. Aging and sexuality. West J Med 1997;167(4):285–290.
10. Schow DA, Redmon B, Pryor JL. Male menopause: how to define it, how to treat it. Postgrad Med 1997;101(3):62–64, 67–68, 71–74.
11. Barber HR. Sexuality and the art of arousal in the geriatric woman. Clin Obstet Gynecol 1996; 39(4):970–973.
12. Gentili A, Mulligan T. Sexual dysfunction in older adults. Clin Geriatr Med 1998;14(2):383–393.
13. Goldstein MK, Teng NN. Gynecologic factors in sexual dysfunction of the older woman. Clin Geriatr Med 1991;7(1):41–61.
14. Marsiglio W, Donnelly D. Sexual relations in later life: a national study of married persons. J Gerontol 1991;46(6):S338–S344.
15. Bretschneider JG, McCoy NL. Sexual interest and behavior in healthy 80- to 102-year-olds. Arch Sex Behav 1988;17(2):109–129.
16. Bortz WM II, Wallace DH. Physical fitness, aging, and sexuality. West J Med 1999;170(3):167–169.
17. Mulligan T, Retchin SM, Chinchilli VM, et al. The role of aging and chronic disease in sexual dysfunction. J Am Geriatr Soc 1988;36(6): 520–524.
18. Mooradian AD. Geriatric sexuality and chronic diseases. Clin Geriatr Med 1991;7(1):113–131.
19. Zeiss RA, Delmonico RL, Zeiss AM, et al. Psychologic disorder and sexual dysfunction in elders. Clin Geriatr Med 1991;7(1):133–151.
20. Chiechi LM, Granieri M, Lobascio A, et al. Sexuality in the climacterium. Clin Exp Obstet Gynecol 1997;24(3):158–159.
21. Ebersole P, Hess P. Intimacy, sexuality, and aging. In: Ebersole P, Hess P, eds. Toward Healthy Aging. 5th ed. St. Louis: Mosby, 1998:583.
22. Davey Smith G, Frankel S, Yarnell J. Sex and death: are they related? findings from the Caerphilly Cohort Study. BMJ 1997;315(7123): 1641–1644.
23. Cleare AJ, Wessely SC. Just what the doctor ordered—more alcohol and sex. BMJ 1997; 315(7123):1637–1638.
24. Greeley A. Sex: The Catholic Experience. Allen, TX: Tabor, 1994:149.
25. US Bureau of the Census. Statistical Abstract of the United States: 1998. 118th ed. Washington, DC: US Bureau of the Census, 1998.
26. Holzapfel S. Aging and sexuality. Can Fam Physician 1994;40:748–750, 753–754, 757–758.
27. Diokno AC, Brown MB, Herzog AR. Sexual function in the elderly. Arch Intern Med 1990; 150(1):197–200.
28. Richardson JP, Lazur A. Sexuality in the nursing home patient. Am Fam Physician 1995;51(1): 121–124.
29. Fletcher EC, Martin RJ. Sexual dysfunction and

erectile impotence in chronic obstructive pulmonary disease. Chest 1982;81(4):413–421.

30. Emery CF. Psychosocial considerations among pulmonary patients. In: Hodgkin JE, Connors GL, Bell CW, eds. Pulmonary Rehabilitation: Guidelines to Success. 2nd ed. Philadelphia: JB Lippincott, 1993:279.

31. Wise TN. Sexual dysfunction in the medically ill. Psychosomatics 1983;24(9):787–801, 805.

32. Johnson B. Older adults' suggestions for health care providers regarding discussions of sex. Geriatr Nurs 1997;18(2):65–66.

33. Drench ME, Losee RH. Sexuality and sexual capacities of elderly people. Rehabil Nurs 1996; 21(3):118–123.

34. Oregon State University Extension Service. Sex and Aging: A Game of Awareness and Interaction (board game). Corvallis: Oregon State University, 1980.

35. Schover LR, Jensen SB. Sexuality and Chronic Illness: A Comprehensive Approach. New York: The Guilford Press, 1988:293.

36. Francoeur RT. Sexual components in respiratory care. Respir Management 1988;March-April:35.

37. Annon JS. Brief therapy. In: Annon JS, ed. The Behavioral Treatment of Sexual Problems. Honolulu: Enabling Systems, 1974;1.

38. Taylor JF, Rosen RC, Leiblum SR. Self-report assessment of female sexual function: psychometric evaluation of the Brief Index of Sexual Functioning for Women. Arch Sex Behav 1994;23(6): 627–643.

39. Clayton AH, McGarvey EL, Clavet GJ. The Changes in Sexual Functioning Questionnaire (CSFQ): development, reliability, and validity. Psychopharmacol Bull 1997;33(4):731–745.

40. Derogatis LR. The Derogatis Interview for Sexual Functioning (DISF/DISF-SR): an introductory report. J Sex Marital Ther 1997;23(4):291–304.

41. Schover LR, Jensen SB. Sexuality and Chronic Illness: A Comprehensive Approach. New York: The Guilford Press, 1988:14.

42. Ende J, Rockwell S, Glasgow M. The sexual history in general medicine practice. Arch Intern Med 1984;144(3):558–561.

43. Selecky PA. Sexuality and Chronic Breathing Problems (brochure). Santa Ana, CA: American Lung Association of Orange County, 1989.

44. Eckert RC, Bartsch K, Dowell D, et al. Being Close. Denver: National Jewish Hospital, 1984.

45. National Institute on Aging Information Center, PO Box 8057, Gaithersburg, MD 20898-8057, 1-800/222-2225.

46. Oregon State University. Sexuality in the Later Years (video). Corvallis: Oregon State University.

47. Yates A, Woman W. Aphrodisiacs: myth and reality. Med Aspects Hum Sexuality 1991;December:58.

48. Deamer RL, Thompson JF. The role of medications in geriatric sexual function. Clin Geriatr Med 1991;7(1):95–111.

49. Kamischke A, Kemper DE, Castel MA, et al. Testosterone levels in men with chronic obstructive pulmonary disease with or without glucocorticoid therapy. Eur Respir J 1998;11(1):41–45.

50. Cheitlin MD, Hutter AM Jr, Brindis RG, et al. Use of sildenafil (Viagra) in patients with cardiovascular disease: Technology and Practice Executive Committee. Circulation 1999;99(1):168–177.

51. Romano MD. Sexuality and the disabled female. Accent Living 1973;18:28.

52. Sipski ML. Sexuality and individuals with respiratory impairment. In: Bach JR, ed. Pulmonary Rehabilitation. Philadelphia: Hanley & Belfus, 1996:203.

53. Cole SS, Hossler CJ: Intimacy and chronic lung disease. In: Fishman AP, ed. Pulmonary Rehabilitation. New York: Marcel Dekker, 1996:251.

54. NIH Consensus Development Panel on Impotence. NIH consensus conference: impotence. JAMA 1993;270(1):83–90.

55. Montague DK, Barada JH, Belker AM, et al. Clinical guidelines panel on erectile dysfunction: summary report on the treatment of organic erectile dysfunction: the American Urological Association. J Urol 1996;156(6):2007–2011.

56. Aasebo U, Gyltnes A, Bremnes RM, et al. Reversal of sexual impotence in male patients with chronic obstructive pulmonary disease and hypoxemia with long-term oxygen therapy. J Steroid Biochem Mol Biol 1993;46(6):799–803.

57. Goldstein I, Lue TF, Padma-Nathan H, et al. Oral sildenafil in the treatment of erectile dysfunction. Sildenafil Study Group. N Engl J Med 1998; 338(20):1397–1404; published erratum appears in N Engl J Med 1998;339(1):59.

58. Sildenafil: an oral drug for impotence. Med Lett 1998;40:5–8.

59. Rendell MS, Rajfer J, Wicker PA, et al. Sildenafil for treatment of erectile dysfunction in men with diabetes: a randomized controlled trial: Sildenafil Diabetes Study Group. JAMA 1999;281(5): 421–426.

60. Kaplan SA, Reis RB, Kohn IJ, et al. Safety and efficacy of sildenafil in postmenopausal women with sexual dysfunction. Urology 1999;53(3): 481–486.

61. Plaud JJ, Dubbert PM, Holm J, et al. Erectile dysfunction in men with chronic medical illness. J Behav Ther Exp Psychiatry 1996;27(1): 11–19.

62. Selecky PA. Sexuality in respiratory care. In: Pierson DJ, Kacmarek R, eds. Foundations of Respiratory Care. New York: Churchill Livingstone, 1992:1237.

63. AMA issues diagnostic and treatment guidelines on child sexual abuse. Am Fam Physician 1993; 47(6):1519–1520.

64. Aravanis SC, Adelman RD, Breckman R, et al. Diagnostic and treatment guidelines on elder abuse and neglect. Arch Fam Med 1993;2(4): 371–388.

65. Council on Scientific Affairs. Elder abuse and neglect. JAMA 1987;257(7):966–971.

66. Kennedy E. Sexual Counseling: A Practical Guide for Those Who Help Others. New York: Continuum, 1989:63.

67. American Psychiatric Association. The Principles of Medical Ethics With Annotations Especially Applicable to Psychiatry. Washington, DC: American Psychiatric Association, 1998.

18 Preventive Aspects for the Patient with Chronic Lung Disease

Brian W. Carlin
Marie Lingat

◈ Professional Skills

Upon completion of this chapter, the reader will:

- Identify the various types of preventive measures available for the management of a patient with lung disease (e.g., primary, secondary, and tertiary measures)
- Identify measures used to detect abnormalities in lung function before the development of signs and symptoms associated with chronic obstructive pulmonary disease (COPD)
- Describe measures used to reduce the complications resulting from chronic lung disease (e.g., smoking cessation, pulmonary rehabilitation, supplemental oxygen use [Fig. 18-1], and vaccination)

COPD, including emphysema, chronic bronchitis, and asthma, is a considerable cause of morbidity and is currently the fourth leading cause of death in the United States. An estimated 14 million people have chronic bronchitis, 2 million have emphysema, and at least another 6 million have asthma. Of all the leading causes of death in the United States, COPD is the only one that has shown a relative increase during the past 20 years. Although the incidence of death owing to coronary heart disease has declined by 66% during that time, the incidence of death owing to COPD has increased by 47%.

Patients with very mild to moderate disease often have minimal, if any, symptoms and thus do not seek medical attention. It is only when symptoms develop that interfere with lifestyle that a patient seeks medical attention. An increase in morbidity and mortality thus can be expected. Strategies designed to diagnose the disease earlier in its course and to alter the progression of the disease are of vital importance when attempting to decrease morbidity and mortality.

Opportunities for the prevention of chronic lung disease (including obstructive, restrictive, and vascular lung diseases) exist. Health promotion requires the active participation of the patient in the treatment plan. Disease management requires the input of the patient along with many health care providers. This combination, can provide the person with chronic lung disease the ability to optimally function within the community.

Prevention strategies can occur at several levels (primary, secondary, and tertiary). Primary strategies focus on prevention of development of the disease, secondary strategies focus on early detection and prevention of symptomatic disease, and tertiary strategies focus on reduction of complications in patients who have symptomatic disease (Box 18-1). Comprehensive pulmonary rehabilitation often only includes tertiary prevention strategies; however, incorporation of primary and secondary prevention strategies into comprehensive pulmonary rehabilitation should be considered.

335

Box 18-1. Opportunities for Preventing Chronic Lung Disease

Primary strategies
  Smoking/nicotine abstinence, cessation
  Education (health)
  Components of comprehensive pulmonary rehabilitation
Secondary strategies
  Smoking cessation
  Spirometric measurement of expiratory flow rates in high-risk persons (e.g., smokers)
  Alpha-one-antitrypsin replacement therapy (for patients with the genetic deficiency
    syndrome)
  Components of comprehensive pulmonary rehabilitation
Tertiary strategies
  Smoking cessation
  Vaccination (pneumococcal, influenza)
  Pulmonary rehabilitation
  Oxygen supplementation (for patients with hypoxemia)
  Nutritional support (for malnourished patients)
  Antibiotic therapy for exacerbations
  Pulmonary hygiene

PRIMARY PREVENTION

The greatest risk factor for the development of chronic lung disease is cigarette smoking. Up to 90% of cases of COPD in the United States are caused by cigarette smoking.[1] Smoking rates are declining but because of the long latency period from the initiation of cigarette smoking to the development of chronic lung disease, the overall incidence of lung disease will continue to increase. If initiation of cigarette smoking could be prevented, the overall incidence of the development of chronic lung disease will be reduced eventually.

The greatest potential for such preventive efforts occurs by encouraging children and teenagers to abstain from smoking. Although most teenagers who begin to smoke stop by early adulthood, ongoing strategies to encourage abstinence must be promoted continually. Health care professionals are important role models in community antismoking campaigns. Educational efforts beginning with grade school children may be the most effective method to prevent the later development of chronic lung disease.

How important is it to encourage smoking cessation in patients who are older or who have already developed chronic lung disease? Although most of the smoking-related changes on lung function are irreversible and function may not improve significantly after cessation of cigarette smoking, the rate of decline of lung function will be reduced and may eventually approach the usual age-related rate of decline.[2] Smoking cessation even after the development of symptomatic disease is of great importance in the reduction of morbidity and mortality of patients with chronic lung disease.[3]

SECONDARY PREVENTION

Secondary prevention includes the early detection of disease and the prevention of symptomatic disease. Early detection of obstructive lung disease is problematic. Each person has a significant amount of "reserve" lung function, so it is not until relatively late in the disease course that a patient will exhibit symptoms. A person can lose up to half of his or her "lung function" (as measured by lung volumes and/or flow rates) with little or no effect on functional capacity or symptoms. Early detection of lung disease cannot be based solely on the patient's symptoms.

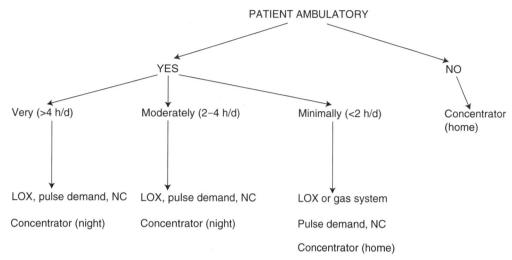

Figure 18-1. Oxygen delivery device selection. *LOX*, liquid oxygen system; *pulse demand*, pulse demand valve device; *NC*, nasal cannula.

Early detection efforts must be based on a simple reproducible means of assessing airway function. The clinical examination may be helpful in the evaluation of a patient suspected of having airway obstruction. Observation of a forceful exhalation time can be helpful in the clinical assessment. An exhalation time up to 3 seconds is normal, whereas an exhalation time of greater than 6 seconds suggests significant airflow obstruction. Should a prolonged expiratory time be noted clinically, spirometric confirmation should then be performed.

Simple spirometry offers the most advantageous way to assess airway function. Population screening through the measurement of flow rates might seem to be beneficial, but no data exist to support its use for this purpose. Spirometry is recommended as part of the routine management of patients at high risk for the development of lung disease (e.g., smokers). The National Lung Health Education Program recommends that anyone who currently smokes or is routinely exposed to environmental tobacco smoke or work place irritants and who has symptoms of chronic cough, wheezing, persistent mucus, or shortness of breath should have simple spirometry performed. Serial determination of the flow rates over time can then be used to determine if, in the individual patient, a greater than usual decline in flow rates is occurring.[4] Intervention (e.g., intensive smoking cessation for patients who continue to smoke) could then be afforded to such patients in an attempt to minimize ongoing decline of lung function and to improve functional status.

One of the problems with spirometry involves the quality of performance of this testing in primary care practices. As most patients with symptoms of cough, dyspnea, and sputum production will be initially evaluated by a primary care physician or primary caregiver, the importance of being able to perform spirometry accurately in the primary care setting is necessary.[5] In a recent study involving 30 primary care practices, acceptable results from spirometry were obtained in only a few patients evaluated (3.4% of patients in practices that received no training in the performance of spirometry and 13.5% of patients in practices that received minimal training).[6] These findings were observed despite the use of quality assurance devices that were built into the equipment being used for the testing. The availability and reliability for such screening thus needs to be more completely evaluated to ensure that accurate testing is performed.

Another tool that can be used to assess the effects of smoking or other lung disease on the individual's spirometry test results is the "lung age."[7] Lung age equations have been developed from reference linear regression equations and nomograms, thus allowing

Box 18-2. Equations for Estimation of Lung Age

Women
FEV$_1$ (L)
Lung age = 3.560H − 40.000(Obs FEV$_1$) − 77.280
FEF$_{25-75\%}$ (L/sec)
Lung age = 2.000H − 33.333(Obs FEF$_{25-75\%}$) + 18.367
Men
FEV$_1$ (L)
Lung age = 2.870H − 31.250(Obs FEV$_1$) − 39.375
FEF$_{25-75\%}$ (L/sec)
Lung age = 1.044H − 22.222(Obs FEF$_{25-75\%}$) + 55.844

FEV$_1$, forced expiratory volume in 1 second; L, liters; H, height (inches); Obs, observed; FEF$_{25-75\%}$, forced expiratory flow during the middle half of the forced vital capacity. Lung age is given in years.

lung age estimation in terms of ventilatory function (Box 18-2). Lung age can be compared with the person's chronologic lung age and can then be used during patient counseling (particularly with people who continue to smoke to help encourage discontinuation of smoking).

The early detection of lung function abnormalities could be used in the individual patient to encourage smoking cessation (if the patient remains a smoker), other risk reduction interventions (e.g., annual influenza vaccination), and entry into a comprehensive pulmonary rehabilitation program. Although definitive studies using such assessment and intervention techniques have yet to be performed, ultimately such an approach to the person at high risk for the development of chronic lung disease should result in a reduction of the associated morbidity and mortality.

TERTIARY PREVENTION

The focus of tertiary prevention is the reduction of complications resulting from a disease process. Smoking cessation, comprehensive pulmonary rehabilitation, supplemental oxygen administration (when significant hypoxemia is present), and immunization therapy are types of tertiary preventive measures available for patients with chronic lung disease.

Although many people who smoke try to quit each year, only about 6% are successful in the long term.[8] Many smokers have made a visit to their primary care physician within the past year, and a significant proportion say they would quit smoking had they been advised to do so by their physician. But many also say that they have not been advised by their physician to quit smoking. Physicians may not feel comfortable, however, in the process of assisting a patient to quit smoking.[9] Physician counseling, even if limited, can result in a doubling of the annual rate of smoking cessation. The "4 As" can be an effective means to inquire about the patient's smoking habits and can assist the patient with smoking cessation: *ask* (the patient about tobacco use at every office visit), *advise* (the patient of the dangers associated with smoking in a compassionate way), *assess* (the patient's readiness to quit smoking), and *assist* (the patient who is ready to quit).

Smoking cessation can result in a reduction of the decline in lung function in patients with established disease, as noted in the Lung Health Study. A significant reduction in the rate of decline of forced expiratory volume in 1 second (FEV$_1$) was noted in the cohort of patients who quit smoking and continued as nonsmokers during the 5 years of the trial.[2] This cohort underwent a comprehensive management program, including the use of nicotine replacement, psychosocial counseling, and frequent evaluation (with subsequent intervention) of the patient's adherence to the regimen.

The addiction associated with cigarette smoking arises from the nicotine delivered to the bloodstream. The physiologic withdrawal symptoms occurring with the decrease in the blood level of nicotine cause the patient to want to continue smoking. Several formulations of nicotine replacement therapy are currently available, including nicotine in patch, gum, or inhaler form. All modalities are effective for the delivery of nicotine to the bloodstream and have resulted in a doubling of the abstinence rates.[10] Physician counseling during this process is important to adjust the medication as necessary, to assess for side effects from the medication, and to offer ongoing support for the patient. Several office visits during the 2 months following initiation of the medication are advisable.

Several other aids are available to assist with smoking cessation. Sustained-release bupropion hydrochloride, an antidepressant, has recently been approved as such an aid.[11] Although its exact mechanism of action is unknown, its use has been shown to increase abstinence rates up to 23% at 1 year. Several other medications (caffeine, buspirone, and mecamylamine) have been used; however, little data are available regarding their overall effectiveness. Combination medication therapy has been shown to result in an increase in abstinence rates. Treatment with sustained-release bupropion hydrochloride alone or in combination with a nicotine patch resulted in significantly higher long-term rates of smoking cessation than did use of either the nicotine patch alone or placebo (35.5% rate in the group receiving bupropion hydrochloride and nicotine patch, 30.3% in the group receiving bupropion, 16.4% in the group receiving the nicotine patch, and 15.6% in the group receiving placebo). One concern of many patients is the potential weight gain associated with smoking cessation. In this study the weight gain noted with smoking cessation was only up to 2.1 kg.[12]

Many formal smoking cessation programs are available within the community. The most successful programs include those that are 2 weeks in duration with a minimum of four to seven sessions, those that offer a variety of interventions from a variety of professionals, and those that offer social support. Such programs may be found through the local lung association or local hospital.

The comprehensive management of smoking cessation (including education, psychologic counseling, medication administration, and social support) has been shown to result in 1-year abstinence rates of up to 44%. Smoking cessation is probably the most important factor responsible for a reduction in the number of complications in patients with symptomatic disease. A smoking cessation program can be a component of the pulmonary rehabilitation program itself or can be a part of another community-based program (e.g., in association with the local lung association or a hospital). Practice guidelines for smoking cessation have been developed (Box 18-3).[13]

Comprehensive pulmonary rehabilitation has been shown to effectively reduce dyspnea, improve exercise tolerance, improve health-related quality of life, and reduce hospitalizations necessary for COPD-related problems. Comprehensive pulmonary rehabilitation includes the assessment and evaluation of an individual patient, education regarding lung

Box 18-3. Smoking Cessation Practice Guidelines

Each person who smokes should be offered cessation treatment at every office visit
The clinician should ask and record the tobacco status of every patient
Counseling, even as brief as 3 minutes, is effective
The more intense the treatment the more effective it is in producing long-term abstinence from tobacco use
Nicotine replacement treatment (patches, gum, inhaler), clinician-delivered social support and teaching skills are effective components of smoking cessation treatment
The health care system should be modified to actively inquire about tobacco use or exposure at every visit

disease, psychosocial intervention, methods to minimize dyspnea, upper and lower extremity exercise in a monitored setting, measurement of various types of outcomes reflecting the patient and the program, and follow-up. Initially performed in an outpatient setting during an 8- to 12-week period, pulmonary rehabilitation offers another modality of therapy for patients with established, symptomatic lung disease. Evidence-based guidelines are available showing the essential components of a pulmonary rehabilitation program and the benefits noted following completion of comprehensive pulmonary rehabilitation for patients with COPD.[14] Recently, studies have shown benefit to the continuation/follow-up of pulmonary rehabilitation following the initial outpatient program. Unfortunately, many physicians are unaware of these potential benefits or have failed to accept pulmonary rehabilitation as an important and effective modality of therapy and thus have not offered comprehensive pulmonary rehabilitation to their patients with symptomatic lung disease.

Administration of supplemental oxygen to patients with COPD and resting hypoxemia has been shown to reduce morbidity and improve survival. Two landmark studies (the British Medical Research Council and the Nocturnal Oxygen Therapy Trial) performed in the early 1980s documented such benefits for patients who had a resting arterial partial pressure of oxygen of less than 55 torr.[15,16] Such benefits include not only a reduction in mortality but also a decrease in pulmonary artery pressure, an improvement in exercise tolerance, and an improvement in cognitive function. Patients who have COPD and arterial hypoxemia should thus be offered long-term oxygen therapy (Box 18-4). The beneficial effects of the administration of oxygen for patients who exhibit oxyhemoglobin desaturation only during exercise or during sleep are less well documented; however, most physicians would offer supplemental oxygen to those patients as well.

Supplemental oxygen can be administered in a variety of types (gas, concentrator, or liquid) and modalities (nasal cannula, conserving device, pulse demand device, or transtracheal). The most important aspect that needs to be considered when prescribing oxygen therapy is the ambulatory status of the individual patient. The system that allows for the maximum patient ambulation should be afforded to the patient who needs long-term oxygen therapy. Combinations of oxygen delivery modalities can be administered given the patient's clinical status (e.g., the use of an oxygen concentrator during sleep and a liquid system during ambulation for the patient who is ambulatory). A suggested approach to the choice of delivery method for patients who require supplemental oxygen can be seen in Figure 18-1.

Respiratory tract illness is a particularly worrisome complication for patients with chronic lung disease. Disruption of the epithelial surface of the airways promotes microbial colonization and, in some instances, invasive infection. Other abnormal host defenses present in a patient with COPD include loss of normal mucociliary function and production

Box 18-4. Indications for the Prescription of Long-Term Oxygen Therapy

Clinical stability of the patient
Demonstration of arterial hypoxemia or oxyhemoglobin desaturation
$PaO_2 < 55$ torr
or
PaO_2 56–59 torr and one of the following:
P pulmonale noted on electrocardiogram
Presence of edema
Cor pulmonale
This demonstration can be made with the patient during rest, exercise, or sleep conditions.

PaO_2, arterial partial pressure of oxygen.

of abnormal mucus and immunoglobulins. In addition, many factors (e.g., older age, structural abnormalities of the head and neck, or impaired level of consciousness) may promote the aspiration of oropharyngeal secretions in patients with respiratory disease. The effectiveness of cough is often impaired, leading to yet another pathway for the retention of potential microbial organisms within the tracheobronchial tree.

Acute exacerbations of chronic bronchitis and pneumonia account for more than 500,000 hospitalizations in the United States each year. The morbidity associated is significant, approximating 80,000 deaths per year. Up to half of all exacerbations of underlying COPD are related to viral illnesses, and a significant increase in hospitalization rates for patients with COPD is noted during months associated with outbreaks of influenza. The prevention of pneumonia in patients with chronic lung disease is an important part of the management of these patients.

Influenza viruses A and B, rhinovirus, respiratory syncytial virus, and adenovirus are a few of the viruses noted to be causative of exacerbations in underlying COPD. Viral infections usually occur during the winter months and may occur within the community or within the hospital setting. Prevention of influenza can be successfully accomplished with the use of a vaccine. The vaccine is commercially prepared from purified egg-grown viruses that are inactivated and is administered by an intramuscular injection. A trivalent, live, attenuated virus vaccine is also now available and is administered by an intranasal spray.[17] Antigens from the influenza A and influenza B viruses are contained within the vaccines, and protective antibodies can be expected to rise in the individual patient within several weeks of vaccination. The antibody response will depend on the individual's general health and immune status. Because the antibody response decreases with time and the influenza virus exhibits antigenic drift from one year to the next, annual vaccination is recommended.

Vaccination of patients at increased risk for infection is the single most important method to reduce the morbidity associated with influenza. The efficacy rate varies depending on the patient population being studied but ranges from 30 to 85%.[18,19] Despite these efficacy rates and the data showing a reduction in morbidity and mortality associated with vaccine administration, few people at risk for influenza infection are actually vaccinated each year.[20] The influenza vaccine is recommended for patients (adults and children) who have chronic lung and/or cardiac disease, are immunosuppressed, have diabetes, have renal disease, are older than 65 years, are residents of chronic care facilities (including personal care homes and nursing homes), or personnel in contact with high-risk patients (e.g., physicians, nurses, and hospital workers). It is important to encourage the vaccination of all members of the medical community who are in contact with high-risk patients. The vaccine should be administered in the fall on a yearly basis. Side effects are usually of minimal consequence (e.g., soreness around the injection site, fever, malaise, and myalgias). The only absolute contraindication to administration of the vaccine is an egg allergy.

Several antiviral medications (amantadine and rimantidine) have been shown to reduce the signs and symptoms associated with influenza A infection by up to 50%. Up to 90% effectiveness has been shown when using amantadine as a prophylactic agent. When used for the treatment of influenza, amantadine should be first given within 48 hours of the onset of clinical symptoms and should be continued for 48 hours following resolution of symptoms.[21] A daily dosage of either 100 or 200 mg is administered, but a maximum dosage of 100 mg should be used in patients older than 65 years. The major side effects from amantadine include drowsiness, insomnia, nervousness, and lightheadedness. These medications should not be considered as a substitute for administration of the vaccine, however.

Recently zanamavir (a viral neuraminadase inhibitor) has been approved for use in the treatment of influenza infection. It is delivered as a dry powder via oral inhalation. This medication has been shown to reduce the rate of viral shedding and the duration of clinical symptoms associated with influenza in healthy adults.[22,23] The use of zanamavir is discouraged, however, in patients with airway disease (e.g., asthma) because of its potential for airway irritation and potentiation of an exacerbation.

Pneumococcal vaccine is the other vaccination recommended for patients with chronic lung disease. The 23-valent vaccine contains serotypes that are responsible for more than 85% of invasive pneumococcal infections. Although some debate exists as to the efficacy of the vaccine and duration of protection in patients with COPD, efficacy for such patients approached 65% in one study.[24,25] The vaccine is recommended for use in persons older than 65 years.[26]

Revaccination with the pneumococcal vaccine is recommended after 6 years for patients with a high risk of fatal complications from pneumococcal infection (e.g., a patient with asplenia or chronic lung disease). Whether revaccination should be given routinely in other patient groups has not been answered to date. The side effects associated with revaccination are minimal, usually pain and induration at the injection site, but more serious local effects (e.g., skin necrosis) have been noted.[27]

The administration rates of both the influenza and pneumococcal vaccinations are low across the potential at-risk population for the development of either type of infection. Vaccination rates as low as 20% of the potential at-risk population have been reported. A well-designed vaccination administration protocol is necessary and should be available in physician offices and hospitals to ensure that patients and health care workers who might benefit from the vaccination actually receive it.

It is important that each patient be aware of the signs and symptoms associated with an infection (e.g., bronchitis and pneumonia). The development of an increase in shortness of breath, an increase in sputum production, or a change in the character of the sputum should prompt immediate attention and early consultation with the primary care physician. Other symptoms such as chest pain, fever, sore throat, and myalgias should also be of concern. In patients with at least two of the symptoms mentioned (increase in dyspnea, increase in sputum production, or sputum discoloration), antibiotic therapy has been shown to result in an improvement in the patient's clinical condition.[28,29] Existing guidelines for the treatment of patients with exacerbations of chronic bronchitis and community-acquired pneumonia can be helpful in the management of such patients.[30,31]

General measures regarding the health maintenance of patients with chronic lung disease should be discussed with each patient. The avoidance of groups of people who might potentially have influenza or other respiratory illnesses (e.g., shopping centers, health care facilities, and children) is an important component of these preventive efforts. Routine hand washing is important in the prevention of the transmission of infection, especially when one is caring for children. We commonly accept and return handshakes, and the transmission of infection is possible by this route as well. Although hand washing is not possible after each handshake, it could be performed frequently as able, thus ultimately decreasing the potential for the transmission of infection. Each of these measures can be discussed as part of the educational component associated with a pulmonary rehabilitation program.

One the most significant difficulties encountered in the management of a person with any type of chronic illness is the issue of adherence with the medical regimen. Even the most complete medical assessment and treatment plan can only be effective if the patient adheres with the recommendations made by the primary care provider. The primary care provider must be cognizant of the fact that most patients do not satisfactorily comply with the suggested medical regimen. To gain such adherence, the patient must become an active participant in the evaluation and treatment plan. Adherence to the medical regimen (both the daily regimen and the regimen associated with an acute illness, e.g., use of antibiotics for an acute exacerbation in a patient with underlying chronic lung disease), smoking cessation, and exercise program need to be assessed continually during the treatment program. Such adherence can be assessed during a comprehensive pulmonary rehabilitation program.

OTHER PREVENTIVE MEASURES

The American Cancer Society estimates that more than 170,000 Americans will be diagnosed with lung cancer during the upcoming year and that more Americans will die of lung cancer than of colon, breast, and prostate cancer combined.[32] The Lung Health Study showed that in middle-ages men and women with even mild degrees of airflow obstruction, deaths from lung cancer outnumbered deaths from COPD, coronary artery disease, or stroke.[2]

Treatment of early-stage lung cancer (stage 1) with surgical resection is effective, with a 5-year survival of about 70%. Unfortunately, by the time most lung cancers are detected, only 25% are resectable, and 5-year survival in this group is only 14%. Because of its significant association with the development of lung cancer, abstinence from cigarette smoking must be addressed in each smoker.[33] Prevention of the initiation of smoking or abstinence from smoking are of utmost importance in an attempt to reduce the overall morbidity and mortality caused by lung cancer.

Identification of lung cancer at earlier stages should also afford a reduced morbidity and mortality. Screening for lung cancer is feasible given a detectable presymptomatic phase of the disease (i.e., the development of increasing cellular atypia eventually progressing to invasive carcinoma) and an established means of intervention during this presymptomatic phase (i.e., surgical resection). Patients at high risk for the development of lung cancer include those with a family history of lung cancer, preexisting COPD, a history of previous smoking-associated cancer (of the lung or head and neck), occupational exposures (e.g., silica, heavy metals, radon, and asbestos), or preexisting pulmonary fibrosis.[34] The early identification of lung cancer in patients at high risk has been shown in several studies. In one study, 51 consecutive patients with either clinical symptoms of or occupational exposures to uranium or asbestos were identified by sputum cytology to have lung carcinoma. Forty-six of these patients had early-stage disease. Of 27 patients who were deemed to be surgical candidates, the 5-year actuarial survival, including deaths from all causes, was 55%.[35] In another study of 632 patients who had a greater than 40 pack-year smoking history and an FEV_1 of less than 70% predicted, screening sputum cytology revealed nine carcinomas (in situ or invasive).[36]

Sputum and bronchoalveolar lavage cytology studies have been the primary means to detect lung cancer. Radiographic and bronchoscopic techniques are also being used in the early identification of lung cancer. Computed tomography (CT) (particularly spiral CT) scanning offers a method for early detection. In a group of Japanese patients, the effectiveness of spiral CT in reporting the incidence of lung cancer was shown. In one group of male smokers older than 50 years, 14 of the 15 cancers detected by spiral CT were stage 1, and only 4 of these were visible by chest radiograph.[37] In a recent study, the use of CT scanning of the chest detected a significantly increased number of patients with lung cancer who would not have been otherwise diagnosed at that time because of their lack of symptoms.[38]

Autofluorescence bronchoscopy offers yet another technique for early detection. It has been shown to achieve an 89% improvement in the sensitivity for identification of moderate to severe endobronchial dysplasia.[39]

Newer biochemical and immunologic methods (e.g., the use of monoclonal antibodies for small cell and non–small cell carcinoma on sputum cytologic specimens) may allow lung cancer to be detected months to years earlier than would be possible with routine sputum cytology.[40] Eventually, hematologic gene markers for cancer will be used to detect lung cancer. Further investigations must be performed to determine the exact role for each of these techniques in the early detection of lung cancer.

Currently, an annual chest roentgenogram coupled to sputum cytology for people at high risk for lung cancer has been recommended.[41] Current studies are under way to more fully evaluate the value of obtaining yearly spiral CT and sputum cytology for patients in high-risk groups in regards to the early detection (and thus early treatment) of lung cancer.[42]

A potential approach to the prevention of lung disease and any associated complications involves the early identification of lung disease at a genetic level. Symptomatic lung disease develops in only 15 to 20% of whites who are heavy cigarette smokers, and airflow obstruction develops at earlier ages in some patients, thus suggesting that genetic factors may be playing a role.[43] Differences have been noted in the development of lung disease in different ethnic groups (e.g., the low prevalence of COPD noted in China).[44] The prevalence of airflow obstruction and pulmonary disease symptoms in Japanese-Americans who reside in Hawaii is significantly lower than in white Americans who reside there.[45] An increased prevalence of airflow obstruction within families not accounted for by smoking has also been suggested.[46] The Framingham Study provided the ability to analyze a subset of more than 5000 subjects from more than 1000 families, suggesting that after correction for smoking, polygenic gene effects and other environmental factors determine FEV_1.[47]

The importance of the various factors involved in the development of chronic lung disease (whether it be inflammatory cells, proteases and antiproteases, inflammatory mediators, or immunoglobulins) has yet to be fully defined from a genetic perspective. With identification of genes by the techniques of positional cloning, candidate genes, whole genome screens, or finding new genes, patients who are at risk for the development of lung disease may be detected early, and appropriate intervention at much earlier stages in the patient's life can be made.[48]

SUMMARY

The prevention of chronic lung disease can be afforded through a variety of strategies (Box 18-5). Primary strategies (e.g., health promotion), secondary strategies (e.g., spirometry in high-risk patients and smoking cessation, components of comprehensive pulmonary rehabilitation), and tertiary strategies (e.g., comprehensive pulmonary rehabilitation, administration of long-term oxygen therapy) can be used. A reduction in the morbidity and mortality associated with chronic lung disease can then successfully be afforded.[49]

Box 18-5. Prevention Measures to be Included as Part of a Pulmonary Rehabilitation Program

Smoking cessation, nicotine intervention
Controls of environment (crowds, humidity)
Proper hand-washing technique
Vaccination (influenza, pneumococcal)
Diet
Exercise
Mental wellness
Knowledge of course of lung disease
Knowledge of warning signs of an infection
Adherence to medication program, smoking cessation, and exercise program

REFERENCES

1. US Department of Health and Human Services. Chronic obstructive lung disease: the health consequences of smoking: a report of the Surgeon General. Washington, DC: US Office of the Assistant Secretary for Health, Office of Smoking and Health, 1984. DHHS Publication 84–2677.
2. Anthonisen NR, Connett JE, Kiley JP, et al. Effects of smoking intervention and the use of an inhaled anticholinergic bronchodilator on the rate of decline of FEV_1: the Lung Health Study. JAMA 1994;272:1497–1505.
3. Fletcher C, Peto R. The natural history of chronic airflow obstruction. BMJ 1977;1(6077):1645–1648.
4. The National Lung Health Education Program Executive Committee. Strategies in preserving lung health and preventing COPD and associated diseases: the National Lung Health Education Program (NLHEP). Chest 1998;113(suppl): 123S–155S.
5. Hankinson JL. Office spirometry: does poor quality render it impractical? Chest 1999;116:276–277.
6. Eaton T, Withy S, Garrett JE, et al. Spirometry in primary care practice. Chest 1999;116:416–423.
7. Morris JF, Temple W. Spirometric "lung age" estimates for motivating smoking cessation. Prev Med 1985;14:655–662.
8. Smoking cessation during previous year among adults—United States 1990 and 1991. MMWR Morb Mortal Wkly Rep 1993;42:504–507.
9. Russell MAH, Wilson C, Taylor C, et al. Effects of general practitioner's advice against smoking. BMJ 1989;2:231–235.
10. Henningfield JE. Nicotine medications for smoking cessation. N Engl J Med 1995;333(18):1196–1203.
11. Hurt RD, Sachs DPL, Glover ED, et al. A comparison of sustained release bupropion and placebo for smoking cessation. N Engl J Med 1997;337:1195–1202.
12. Jorenby DE, Leischow SJ, Nides MA, et al. A controlled trial of sustained release bupropion, a nicotine patch, or both for smoking cessation. N Engl J Med 1999,340.685–691.
13. Fiore MC, Bailey WC, Cohen SC, et al. Smoking cessation: clinical practice guideline No. 18. Rockville, MD: Agency for Health Care Policy and Research, 1996. AHCPR publication 90–0692.
14. American College of Chest Physicians/American Association of Cardiovascular and Pulmonary Rehabilitation. Pulmonary rehabilitation: evidence-based guidelines. Chest 1997;112(5):1363–1396.
15. Medical Research Council Working Party. Long-term domiciliary oxygen therapy in chronic hypoxic cor pulmonale complicating chronic bronchitis and emphysema. Lancet 1981;1:1681–1686.
16. Nocturnal Oxygen Therapy Trial Group. Continuous or nocturnal oxygen therapy in hypoxemic chronic obstructive lung disease: a clinical trial. Ann Intern Med 1980;93:391–398.
17. Nichol KL, Mendelmann PM, Mallon KP, et al. Effectiveness of live, attenuated intranasal influenza virus vaccine in healthy, working adults. JAMA 1999;282:137–144.
18. Govaert TME, Thijs CTMCN, Masurel N, et al. The efficacy of influenza vaccination in elderly individuals: a randomized double-blind placebo-controlled trial. JAMA 1994;272:1661–1665.
19. Gross PA, Hermogenes AW, Sacks HS, et al. The efficacy of influenza vaccine in elderly persons: a meta-analysis and review of the literature. Ann Intern Med 1995;123:518–527.
20. Mostow SR, Cate TR, Ruben FL. Prevention of influenza and pneumonia. Am Rev Respir Dis 1990;142:487–488.
21. Atkinson WL, Arden NH, Patriarca PA, et al. Amantadine prophylaxis during an institutional outbreak of type A influenza. Arch Intern Med 1986;146:1751–1756.
22. Monto AS, Fleming DM, Henry D, et al. Efficacy and safety of the neuraminidase inhibitor zanamivir in the treatment of influenza A and B virus infections. J Infect Dis 1999;180:254–261.
23. Monto AS, Robinson DP, Herlacher ML, et al. Zanamivir in the prevention of influenza among healthy adults. JAMA 1999;282:31–35.
24. Shapiro ED, Berg AT, Austrian R, et al. The protective efficacy of polyvalent pneumococcal polysaccharide vaccine. N Engl J Med 1991;325:1453–1460.
25. Butler JC, Breiman RF, Campbell JF, et al. Pneumococcal polysaccharide vaccine efficacy: an evaluation of current recommendations. JAMA 1993;270:1826–1831.
26. ACP Task Force on Adult Immunization and Infectious Diseases Society of America. Guide for Adult Immunization. Philadelphia: American College of Physicians, 1990.
27. Jackson LA, Benson P, Sneller VP, et al. Safety of revaccination with pneumococcal polysaccharide vaccine. JAMA 1999;281:243–248.
28. Anthonisen NR, Manfreda J, Warren CPW, et al. Antibiotic therapy in exacerbations of chronic obstructive pulmonary disease. Ann Intern Med 1987;106:196–204.
29. Saint S, Bent S, Vittinghoff E, et al. Antibiotics in chronic obstructive pulmonary disease exacerbations: a meta-analysis. JAMA 1995;273:957–960.
30. Balter MS, Hyland RH, Low D, et al. Recommendations on the management of chronic bronchitis: a practical guide for Canadian physicians. CMAJ 1994;151(Suppl):8S–23S.
31. Bartlett JG, Breiman RF, Mandell LA, et al. Community-acquired pneumonia in adults: guidelines for management. Clin Infect Dis 1998;26:811–838.
32. Landis SH, Murray T, Bolden S, et al. Cancer Statistics 1999. CA Cancer J Clin 1999;49:8–11.
33. Tockman MS, Anthonisen NR, Wright EC, et al. Airways obstruction and the risk for lung cancer. Ann Intern Med 1987;106:512.
34. Saraceno J, Spivack SD. Strategies for early detection of lung cancer. Clin Pulm Med 1999;6:66–72.

35. Bechtel JJ, Kelley WR, Petty TL, et al. Outcome of 51 patients with roentgenographically occult lung cancer detected by sputum cytology testing: a community hospital program. Arch Intern Med 1994;154:975–980.

36. Kennedy TC, Proudfoot SP, Franklin WA, et al. Cytopathological analysis of sputum in patients with airflow obstruction and significant smoking histories. Cancer Res 1996;56:4673–4678.

37. Kaneko M, Eguchi K, Ohmatsua H, et al. Peripheral lung cancer: screening and detection with low-dose spiral CT versus radiography. Radiology 1996;201:798–802.

38. Herschke CI, McCauley DI, Yankelevitz DF, et al. Early Lung Cancer Action Project: overall design and findings from baseline screening. Lancet 1999;354:99–105.

39. Lam S, Kennedy T, Under M, et al. Localization of bronchial intraepithelial neoplastic lesions by fluorescence bronchoscopy. Chest 1999;113: 696–702.

40. Tockman MS, Gupta PK, Myers JD, et al. Sensitive and specific monoclonal antibody recognition of human lung cancer antigen on preserved sputum cells: a new approach to early lung cancer detection. J Clin Oncol 1988;6:1685–1693.

41. Midthun DE, Jett JR. Early detection of lung cancer: today's approach. J Respir Dis 1998; 19:59–70.

42. Saraceno J, Spivack SD. Strategies for early detection of lung cancer. Clin Pulm Med 1999;66–72.

43. Burrows B, Knudson RJ, Cline MG, et al. Quantitative relationships between cigarette smoking and ventilatory function. Am Rev Respir Dis 1977; 115:195–205.

44. Buist AS, Vollmer WM, Wu Y, et al. Effects of cigarette smoking on lung function in four population samples in the People's Republic of China: the PRC-US Cardiovascular and Cardiopulmonary Research Group. Am J Respir Crit Care Med 1995;151:1393–1400.

45. Marcus EB, Buist AS, Curb AJ, et al. Correlates of FEV_1 and prevalence of pulmonary conditions in Japanese-American men. Am Rev Respir Dis 1988;138:1398–1404.

46. Higgins M, Keller J. Familial occurrence of chronic respiratory disease and familial resemblance in ventilatory capacity. J Chronic Dis 1975;28:239–251.

47. Givelber RJ, Couropmitree NN, Gottlieb DJ, et al. Segregation analysis of pulmonary function among families in the Framingham study. Am J Respir Crit Care Med 1998;157:1445–1451.

48. Barnes PJ. Molecular genetics of chronic obstructive pulmonary disease. Thorax 1999;54:245–252.

49. Connors GL, Hilling L. Prevention, not just treatment. Respir Care Clin N Am 1998;4:1–12.

SPECIAL CONSIDERATIONS IN PULMONARY REHABILITATION

19 Adherence in the Patient With Pulmonary Disease

Robert M. Kaplan
Andrew L. Ries

◉ Professional Skills

Upon completion of this chapter, the reader will:

- Recognize the extent of nonadherence among patients with chronic obstructive pulmonary disease (COPD)
- Be able to differentiate different adherence behaviors
- Summarize unique medicine adherence problems for patients with COPD
- Define overadherence and rational nonadherence
- Describe steps to improve adherence with exercise for patients with COPD
- Discuss behavioral interventions to improve adherence
- Recognize problems of relapse among smokers
- Identify internet resources to help patients stop smoking

Nearly all medical encounters end with advice and recommendations. Patients are advised to fill a prescription, take a medication, stay on a prescribed diet, or give up cigarettes. Often medical advice is given by managed care organizations or nonprofit agencies such as the American Lung Association. For example, the American Lung Association recommends that people with chronic bronchitis receive a vaccination against influenza and pneumococcal pneumonia. Nonadherence is the failure to follow such advice.

THE EXTENT OF THE PROBLEM

Much literature suggests that failure to comply with medical advice is a major problem that results in adverse consequences for consumers of health care.[1-3] Published figures suggest that nonadherence rates vary between 15 and 93%, depending on the patient population and the definition of adherence. Most studies suggest that at least a third of patients fail to adhere to treatment recommendations.[2] Nonadherence rates tend to be much higher among patients with chronic conditions.[4]

347

PHYSICIAN AWARENESS OF THE PROBLEM

Although evidence consistently demonstrates that patient nonadherence is common, many physicians do not seem to appreciate the problem. DiMatteo and DiNicola[5] reviewed a variety of studies on practitioner awareness. They found that physicians most often overestimated the extent to which their patients cooperated with recommendations. Caron and Roth[6] found that 22 of 27 medical residents overestimated the degree to which their patients complied with a prescribed liquid antacid prescription. The same investigators found that correlations between estimates made by senior faculty physicians and actual patient adherence were near zero. Several studies (i.e., Norell[7]) have suggested that physicians typically are inaccurate in their estimates of patient adherence and that they generally overestimate correspondence between their orders and patient behavior. These problems raise serious doubts about the validity of physicians' predictions of future patient adherence.

ADHERENCE IN COPD

Despite major advances in diagnosis and medical therapeutics, many patients do not receive optimal benefit from standard medical care. Although some aspects of COPD are treatable, the medical regimen is extremely complex. Medical management of COPD requires multiple medications. However, treatment may also include respiratory chest physiotherapy techniques, exercise, and advice to quit smoking. Most patients are confronted with complex combinations of antibiotics, bronchodilators, anti-inflammatory drugs, and, in some cases, supplemental oxygen. In the following sections, we consider adherence with different components of the regimen for patients with COPD.

ADHERENCE WITH PHARMACOLOGIC INTERVENTIONS

Using MEDLINE searches, we identified all papers on adherence with the COPD regimen back to 1980. In addition, we examined literature reviews published before 1980.[4,8] Recent studies are summarized in Table 19-1. Overall, the search revealed few studies that have directly addressed adherence, especially regarding traditional medical regimens. The studies considered different treatments in diverse samples and used various definitions of and measurements for adherence. Unfortunately, few conclusions, if any, can be drawn from the current literature.

Published studies have considered adherence with regard to a variety of different regimens. Adherence with oxygen therapy in Scotland was reported by Morrison et al.[9] Among patients with COPD prescribed 24-hour oxygen, only 14% were in full adherence. The average use was 14.9 hours per day, and 44% used their oxygen less than 15 hours per day. These patients also had poor adherence with other aspects of the regimen. Although all patients were requested to have acute arterial blood gas measurements within 12 months, only about half obtained the tests. In another study from the United Kingdom, it was shown that patients who are prescribed oxygen for less than 24 hours, in this case 15 hours per day, obtained high levels of adherence with the prescription.[10]

Long-term adherence with inhaled medications was evaluated in the Lung Health Study.[11] This was one of the first trials to evaluate inhaled bronchodilator medication used regularly over time. The Lung Health Study was a large clinical trial (N = 3923) of smoking intervention and bronchodilator therapy for the early stages of COPD. Early in the trial, self-report data suggested that nearly 70% of the patients adhered to the regimen. This rate dropped only slightly during the next 18 months. In addition to self-reports, the investigators weighed the canisters containing the medications. Self-reports confirmed

Table 19-1. Summary of Selected Recent Studies on Adherence

Citation	Regimen	Sample	Measure	Definition	Adherence
Costello et al., 1995[83]	Low-flow oxygen	99 hospitalized patients	Delivery of oxygen	Number of nasal cannulae displaced during night	49% dislodged the oxygen delivery device during the night; dislodging was more common for Venturi face masks than for nasal cannulae
Morrison et al., 1995[9]	Long-term oxygen therapy	519 COPD patients (Scotland); approximately equal numbers of males and females; mean age, 85 years	Hours of therapy per day	Use of oxygen >15 h/d	56% met definition of adherence; study had a high mortality rate
Nides et al., 1993[18]	Metered dose inhaler	231 participants in the Lung Health Study	Nebulizer chronolog that records the date and time of each medication dose	Matching of dose to prescription	Adherence was variable; typically, adherence was highest before a follow-up visit and declined after the visit
Wise et al., 1998[84]	Aerosolized inhalers (either placebo or active)	3923 male and female participants in the Lung Health Study	Self-reports and canister weights	Reduced weight of aerosol canister	81% by self report and 66% by canister weight
Rand et al., 1995[11]	Metered dose inhaler	3923 male and female participants in the Lung Health Study	Self-reports and canister weights	Reduced weight of aerosol canister	After 2 y, self-reported adherence was 70%, with 48% confirmed by canister weight
Solomon et al., 1998[14]	Pharmacist delivered care	98 COPD patients randomly assigned to care by clinical pharmacy residents or to usual care	Self-report and service use	Not defined	No differences in adherence; trend toward higher hospital use in controls
Kampelmacher et al., 1998[85]	Long-term oxygen therapy	528 on oxygen therapy visited at home (in the Netherlands)	Observations by medical students and self-reports	Match to protocol	Only one-third of patients were adequately informed about treatment; most patients were noncompliant
Corden and Rees, 1998[17]	Home nebulized therapy	82 COPD patients using nebulizers	Self-report and St. Georges Respiratory Questionnaire	Taking <70% of prescribed dose	Adherence was poor in 56% of cases; poor adherence correlated with low quality of life

COPD, chronic obstructive pulmonary disease.

by canister weights showed that 48% of the patients had good adherence at one year. Some nonadherence involved overuse of medication. Further analysis demonstrated that those who overuse medication are also likely to incorrectly report their true smoking status.

Personality measures tend not to be good predictors of adherence. A scale designed to assess medication adherence in COPD has been developed and reported by Powell,[12] but it is not clear that it will be of great clinical value because it does not predict adherence well. A variety of studies have investigated demographic characteristics associated with COPD self-care behaviors. For example, the Lung Health Study[11] suggested that adherence was associated with being married, older, and white and with having more severe disease. More adherent patients also had less shortness of breath and were hospitalized or confined to bed less often.[11] Studies of adherence with nebulizer therapy from the Intermittent Positive-Pressure Breathing Study showed that about half of the patients were adherent and half were nonadherent. Predictors of adherence included white race, married, abstinence from alcohol and cigarette use, and more severe shortness of breath. Furthermore, patients with more severe disease were also more likely to adhere to the therapy.[13] Few trials have evaluated interventions to improve adherence. Solomon et al.[14] failed to demonstrate that instructions by clinical pharmacy residents significantly improved adherence over usual care.

Some variables thought to predict adherence often fail to do so. For example, it is commonly assumed that heavy drinkers will be less likely to follow the regimen than those who drink less. In the Lung Health Study,[11] alcohol consumption was used as a predictor of the ability to quit smoking. The results revealed that heavy alcohol use (>25 drinks/ wk) was not a significant predictor of relapse in smoking cessation. However, binge drinking, defined as eight or more drinks per occasion once a month or more, was associated with greater relapse.[15]

Estimated or measured adherence values do not seem to converge on a specific rate or even a specific pattern. James et al.[16] reported that only half of their patients took their medicine regularly. Corden and colleagues[17] also found that about half of their patients (56%) failed to comply with home nebulizer therapy. The Intermittent Positive-Pressure Breathing clinical trial, which used objective assessments of actual time on intermittent positive-pressure breathing therapy, found only half of the patients using the nebulizer at least 25 minutes per day. Interventions by clinical pharmacists seem to have relatively small effects on adherence.[14] Adherence seems to be related to health-related quality of life. Patients with higher scores on the St. George's Respiratory Questionnaire have been shown to be more likely to comply with nebulizer therapy.[17]

Electronic medication monitors may be valuable methods for improving adherence among patients with COPD. One study evaluated 251 COPD patients participating in a multisite clinical trial of nebulizer therapy with inhalers. Patients were divided into intervention and control groups. Using an electronic medication monitor known as the nebulizer chronolog, the intervention group received feedback on the accuracy of their medication use. Patients receiving feedback were significantly more likely to adhere to the regimen and to use medications correctly than were those in the control group.[18]

The traditional view of adherence/nonadherence, in which the patient either strictly follows or fails to follow a treatment recommendation, may no longer be the optimal direction of adherence research. The degree of adherence required for the desired outcome, be it adherence to a prescribed regimen or maximizing quality or life, varies from treatment to treatment and should be considered. To date, few studies have systematically evaluated adherence with regard to the COPD regimen, and in these few cases, the focus has been on drug and oxygen therapy. Furthermore, only a few studies evaluating interventions to improve COPD patients' ability to manage their disease have been reported. Several commentaries have offered strategies for enhancing adherence; however, none have been systematically studied. Some individuals with asthma mistakenly stop using steroid inhalers, but continue bronchodilator inhalers, because they do not notice any acute effect from the steroid inhaler.

Overadherence

Most of the literature on adherence behaviors focuses on the extent to which patients underuse medications. A less common, but perhaps equally important, problem involves the overuse of medication. Overadherence is a more common problem when medications provide prompt symptomatic relief. In the study by Chryssidis et al.,[19] for example, the use of high doses of aerosol therapy often exceeded prescription rates. The mean percentage of prescribed dose actually used was 98.5% at 1 month follow-up and 110.8% at 2-month follow-up. Because each of these estimates were variable, it seems that some portion of the patients took considerably more medication than was prescribed.[19] It is not surprising that patients with COPD, a highly symptomatic disorder, would overuse a medication that provides rapid symptomatic relief.

Some of the evidence for patient overadherence comes from innovative studies on the assessment of adherence. For example, in one clinical trial on antihypertensive medications, patients were asked to bring their medications with them for follow-up visits. Adherence rates were remarkably high—sometimes approaching 100%. However, considerable variability existed among subjects, with those at higher adherence levels obtaining better clinical results. Using innovative methods that attach microprocessors to pill blister packs or to the caps of standard pill bottles,[20,21] it was possible to estimate not only how many of the pills were removed from the packages but also specifically when they were removed. Studies using these methods suggest that patients often have lapses in adherence in periods between visits or that medicine taking is erratic. Also, they may overuse medication or engage in "pill dumping" just before a clinic visit. These findings imply that medications may not be used as prescribed. Often, patients overuse medications before a clinic visit. Erratic medication use may substantially bias estimates of dose-response in clinical trials and provides an inaccurate measure of treatment side effects.[22,23]

Rational Nonadherence

Several competing theories exist about why patients fail to comply with medical regimens. Explanations for why patients fail to adhere might be divided into three categories: those that focus on the patient, those that focus on the patient's environment, and those that focus on the interaction between the patient and the provider. Patient-oriented explanations suggest that certain personalities fail to adhere to medical treatments or that patients intentionally reject therapy because of some flaw in their personality.[24] These explanations have failed to gain empiric support. Some evidence suggests that patients misunderstand instructions,[25,26] but relatively little evidence suggests that patients intentionally try to harm themselves by ignoring advice.

Environmental explanations suggest that elements in the patient's environment, such as family influences, reminders, or other environmental stimuli, influence adherence behavior.[27] Evidence for this view of adherence is suggested by studies demonstrating that reminders and simple environmental cues increase adherence.[28] These simple reminders might be notes attached to a refrigerator or electronic devices that beep when a dose of medication is indicated.

The third view of adherence emphasizes the role of the patient–provider relationship. Although the evidence cannot be reviewed in detail here, a substantial literature demonstrates that information exchanged between patients and providers is often poor.[29,30] This view of adherence suggests that the remedy to the problem is to improve communication between patients and their health care providers.

In considering the three views of noncompliant behavior, we find little evidence that patient personality variables explain much of the variability in nonadherence.[31] The environmental view is valuable in identifying simple manipulations that may enhance adherence behavior in some settings. However, the environmental view is not a comprehensive explanation that considers the patient's role in the choice to use or not use medications.

The patient–provider interaction view comes closest to dealing with the realities of the problem. Substantial evidence suggests that patients often do not comprehend instructions offered to them by their providers.[5] Conversely, providers often have an inadequate picture of the responses their patients have to treatment recommendations. In the following sections we explore this issue in more detail.

Liang[32] offered reasons why his chronically ill patients failed to take their medications. Common explanations were "I forgot," "too expensive," "felt dopey," "felt constipated," and "didn't work." Patients often have poor responses to medications, find that the medications are not providing the expected benefit, or cannot afford to purchase the medications. These patients are taking several factors into consideration in their decision to use or not use a product. Although the provider may condemn the patient as irrational, the patient may be making what he or she considers to be an informed choice. Kaplan and Simon[31] suggested that patients are more likely to comply with treatment when they perceive a net health benefit. Nonadherence occurs when the perceived negative consequences outweigh expected benefits. In this decision process, patients may discount future benefits because of current side effects. A corollary of the theory is that treatments that produce a short-term benefit may evoke better adherence than those that produce a delayed benefit. For example, treatments that provide immediate symptomatic relief, such as inhalers, may be associated with higher adherence than those such as antihypertensive therapies that exchange current inconvenience for future benefit.

One major reason for nonadherence is that patients experience treatment side effects, and, therefore, increased medicine use results in increased discomfort.[33] In one study, 36% of patients in a large tertiary care hospital had some iatrogenic disease.[34,35] Older individuals may experience a sevenfold increase in adverse reactions compared with those aged 20 to 29 years.[36] Evidence from the United Kingdom indicates that as many as 10% of admissions in geriatric units result from adverse reactions attributable to drug interactions.[37] Observed nonadherence might reflect patient feedback about bad experiences with the regimen. Although patients may be less direct about their decision not to adhere, observations of nonadherence may be a stimulus for discussion of treatment side effects.

Several authors have argued that nonadherence can be rational.[1] Patients may adhere to a regimen but fail to obtain the desired benefit. If the probability of an expected benefit is low and undesirable side effects are experienced, nonadherence may enhance health outcome. For example, a patient with streptococcal pharyngitis who discontinues taking an antibiotic on the eighth day of a 10-day course might be regarded as a noncomplier. However, if the patient decides that the inconvenience and side effects associated with the medication are a greater concern than the low probability of developing rheumatic fever, the decision may be regarded as rational. Nonadherence might also be regarded as rational when the patient achieves the desired result despite nonadherence. Indeed, studies in many areas do not show a systematic relationship between adherence and health outcome.[28] Many studies in the adherence literature fail to take health outcomes into consideration.

Practical Suggestions on Medication Adherence

Several practical suggestions emerge from the review of research on adherence to medical regimens. These suggestions parallel discussions on the locus of the problem. First, alterations in the patient's environment may increase adherence behavior. Simple techniques, such as using mailed reminders, placing reminder magnets on refrigerators, or telephone call reminders, have been successful in several studies. Some new products provide auditory cues as reminders. Patients might also purchase digital watches that beep according to their medical regimen schedule.

Behavioral contracts have also been used with some success. These contracts specify precise regimens and often require the patient to make some desired event or activity contingent on medicine use. For example, the contract might make some highly probable behavior, such as watching television, contingent on medicine use.

A second approach to increasing medicine-taking adherence requires enhanced physician–patient communication. A major focus of pulmonary rehabilitation programs is educating patients and family members about their disease and treatments and enhancing their ability to communicate with their physicians. Several studies have shown that patients often have misconceptions about their illness and about the expected effects of medications.[38] Furthermore, patients often experience side effects of medication. Rarely is this information fully communicated to the provider. Physicians should ask about all reactions to medication, barriers to taking medication in the patient's environment, and should clarify the patient's view of why the medications may or may not be effective.

Finally, evidence suggests that interventions designed to increase the patient's involvement might increase adherence and ultimately affect patient outcome. In one experiment, patients were coached on which questions to ask their provider before their encounter. In comparison with a group that received traditional patient education, those in the coached group had actually achieved better health outcomes. Analysis of audiotapes of these physician–patient interactions demonstrated that those in the experimental group were twice as effective as those in the control group in obtaining appropriate information from their physician.[39,40] The patient counseling sessions involved the use of a disease-specific algorithm and a set of diagnostic and therapeutic guidelines presented in the branching logic format. The purpose of the session was to identify important components of medical decisions and to increase patient involvement at each decision point. Other algorithms have now been developed for several chronic disease conditions.

ADHERENCE WITH EXERCISE

An important component of most pulmonary rehabilitation programs has been the establishment of a regular exercise regimen. Specific physical conditioning exercises, such as walking, can be undertaken by the patient to help maintain lung function and improve the remainder of the oxygen delivery system.[41] In several published studies, the improvements in patients with COPD after rehabilitation training have been striking.[42] Specifically, appropriate physical conditioning exercises can improve maximum oxygen consumption and endurance, reduce heart rate, improve ventilator efficiency, and increase tolerance for exercise.

Few studies have evaluated factors associated with long-term exercise maintenance among COPD patients. However, a rich literature in cardiac rehabilitation may provide useful suggestions. One literature review analyzed 24 studies that had reported 12 or more months of follow-up.[43] Long-term maintenance of exercise was associated with supervision of the exercise, availability of equipment, more frequent contact with program staff, the inclusion of a behavioral component, maintaining moderate as opposed to high-intensity activity, and specific interventions to maintain the behavior. Some success has been shown for difficult-to-reach patients. For example, Friedman and colleagues[44] offered a rehabilitation program to the medically indigent. By individualizing instructions and providing guidance for specific community activities such as mall walking, stair climbing, and use of neighborhood facilities, they were able to obtain a self-reported adherence rate of 90%.

Exercise as a Component of Rehabilitation

A few controlled trials documented the benefits of exercise programs for patients with COPD.[42] Cockcroft et al.[45] randomly assigned 39 patients to a 6-week exercise program or to a no treatment control group. Compared with the control group, patients in the exercise group experienced subjective benefits and increased the amount of distance they could walk in 12 minutes. However, follow-up was only 2 months. McGavin and coworkers[46] randomly allocated 24 COPD patients to a 3-month unsupervised stair climbing home exercise program or to a nonexercise control group. The 12 patients in the exercise group noted subjective improvements and an increased sense of well-being and decreased breathlessness. They also reported an objective increase in the 12-minute walk distance and maximal level of exercise on a cycle ergometer. These changes did not occur in the control group. However, follow-up was limited to 3 months. Ambrosino and coworkers[47] randomly assigned 23 patients to a 1-month medical and rehabilitative therapy group and 28 patients to medical therapy alone without exercise training. The experimental group improved in exercise tolerance and respiratory pattern, as evidenced by a decrease in respiratory rate and an increase in tidal volume. Again, these changes were not present in the control group.

One argument for the importance of exercise is that programs that do not have an exercise component are less effective. Sassi Dambron et al.[48] conducted a randomized clinical trial to evaluate a modified pulmonary rehabilitation program focused on coping strategies for shortness of breath, but without exercise training. Eighty-nine patients with COPD were randomly assigned to the 6-week treatment or to a 6-week general health education control group.

The treatment consisted of instruction and practice in techniques of progressive muscle relaxation, breathing retraining, pacing, self-talk, and panic control. Outcomes included the 6-minute walk test, quality of well-being, depression and anxiety scales, and six commonly used dyspnea shortness of breath measures. No significant differences occurred between the treatment and control groups at the end of treatment or at 6-month follow-up. The authors concluded that although dyspnea management strategies are an important component of COPD management, they should be taught in combination with other aspects of comprehensive pulmonary rehabilitation, namely, structured exercise training.

Another trial randomly assigned patients to one of three conditions: (*a*) waiting list control; (*b*) education and stress management; or (*c*) exercise, education, and stress management. Compared with the other two groups, those whose program included exercise experienced reduced anxiety and improvements in endurance and cognitive functioning.[49]

Behavioral Interventions

Behavioral interventions may be helpful in achieving long-term changes in exercise behavior. Kaptein[50] reviewed randomized behavioral intervention studies involving patients with COPD. He found 15 published studies, of which 13 suggested some benefit of intervention. The outcome measures used in these studies vary considerably. Common outcome measures assess quality of life, knowledge, exercise duration, and mood.

Atkins et al.[51] reported the results of an experimental trial designed to evaluate behavioral and cognitive–behavioral programs for increasing exercise among patients with COPD. The patients underwent exercise testing on a treadmill and were given an exercise prescription. Then they were randomly assigned to one of five experimental or control groups. The experimental groups were designed to increase participation in regular exercise. They included behavior modification, cognitive–behavior modification, and a cognitive modification condition.

The behavior modification treatment included goal setting, functional analysis of reinforcers mediating walking, a behavioral contract, contingency management, and two sessions of relaxation training. In the cognitive treatment, subjects experienced didactic interactions in which they learned to identify negative self-statements and to replace them with positive thoughts, to identify specific cues for promoting positive self-talk, and other similar strategies. The experimenter attempted to challenge irrational beliefs about walking whenever possible. The cognitive–behavioral group experienced many of the same positive self-talk exercises. However, they also received training in contingency management and two relaxation sessions. The attention control group received attention but did not have training specifically directed toward increasing adherence. During six sessions, they completed a variety of questionnaires including the Minnesota Multiphasic Personality Inventory (MMPI), a life stress questionnaire, and the Trail Making Test from the Halstead–Reitan Battery.[52] The results of these tests and their relationship to lung disease were discussed during the sessions. A more detailed description of the treatments is given in Atkins et al.[51] The first four sessions were held weekly during the month after the initial interview. Sessions were held biweekly the second month. Three months after the initial assessment, patients were reevaluated on all measures in the clinic. Outcome measures included a general quality of life index, pulmonary function tasks, exercise tolerance tasks, and measures of self-efficacy.

Analysis of the data suggested that those in the cognitive behavior modification group increased their walking more than those in the other experimental or control groups. All three treatment groups walked more than those in the two control groups.[51] These changes were reflected in changes in exercise tolerance measured 1 month after the treatment. However, no significant changes were present in spirometric parameters. In the course of 18 months, the experimental and control groups showed significant differences on a quality of life index.[53] These differences were used to calculate quality-adjusted life years and to demonstrate that the program was relatively cost-effective.[54]

Two recently published randomized trials reported shorter-term benefits favoring pulmonary rehabilitation over conventional treatment. Goldstein and coworkers[55] reported significant improvement in exercise tolerance, dyspnea, and quality of life after 6 months in 45 patients receiving 8 weeks of inpatient pulmonary rehabilitation followed by 16 weeks of supervised outpatient care compared with 44 patients who received conventional care from their own physicians. Wijkstra and coworkers[56] reported significant improvement in exercise tolerance and quality of life in 28 patients who were randomly allocated to a home pulmonary rehabilitation program for 12 weeks compared with 15 patients who received no rehabilitation.

Although comprehensive rehabilitation is believed to improve functional and psychosocial outcomes in patients with COPD, studies have not typically followed up patients for longer than 6 months. This has been problematic because the effects of behavioral intervention are often short lived. A treatment effect that lasts only 1 year, for example, may be of limited value because behavior modification does not cure the condition. Instead, there must be continuing behavior change.

In one of our studies, 119 patients with COPD were randomly assigned to either comprehensive pulmonary rehabilitation or an education control group. Pulmonary rehabilitation consisted of twelve 4-hour sessions distributed over an 8-week period.[57] The content of the sessions was education, physical and respiratory care, psychosocial support, and supervised exercise. The education control group attended four 2 hour sessions that were scheduled twice per month but did not include any individual instruction or exercise training. Topics included medical aspects of COPD; pharmacy use; breathing techniques; and a variety of interviews about smoking, life events, and social support. Lectures covered pulmonary medicine, pharmacology, respiratory therapy, and nutrition. Outcome measures included lung function, maximum and endurance exercise tolerance, symptoms of perceived breathlessness, perceived fatigue, self-efficacy for walking, the Center for Epidemiological Studies Depression Scale and the Quality of Well-Being Scale.

Compared with the educational group, the pulmonary rehabilitation group showed greater improvements on measures of exercise performance of both maximum level and endurance. In addition, the rehabilitation groups showed greater improvements for symptoms of breathlessness and self-efficacy. No differences were present between groups for measures of lung function, depression, or general quality of life. However, both groups experienced equivalent reductions in quality of life. For exercise variables, benefits tended to relapse toward baseline after 18 months of follow-up.

Several potential explanations exist for the failure to demonstrate long-term benefits from comprehensive pulmonary rehabilitation. One explanation is that behavioral interventions, without long-term follow-up or maintenance sessions, such as rehabilitation, are inadequate to produce long-term change. Long-term maintenance of behavior change has also been difficult to demonstrate in research on smoking cessation,[58] weight loss,[59] and exercise adherence.[60] The finding that patients experience behavior change during treatment that is not maintained after treatment is consistent across a variety of different behavioral interventions.[3] Discovering ways to maintain behavior change over extended periods of time remains a high priority for research.

Practical Suggestions on Exercise Promotion

In summary, patient adherence to exercise is perhaps the most difficult and least studied component of pulmonary rehabilitation. Exercise requires alteration in lifestyle, coping with uncomfortable sensations, and changes in daily schedules. To improve adherence with an exercise program, we recommend the following:

1. *Set realistic goals.* Patients who set goals too high become discouraged.
2. *Perform a functional analysis.* This involves identifying highly probable enjoyable behaviors such as watching television, reading a novel, or having a cup of coffee. These activities will differ from patient to patient. Once identified, the highly probable behaviors can be used as reinforcers for the exercise activity. The patient might be asked to sign a contract in which he or she agrees to make enjoyable activities contingent on completion of an exercise session.
3. *Use cognitive techniques.* Identify negative things a patient may say to himself or herself during an exercise session. Then teach the patient to use realistic, but positive, self-talk. For example, for a person who says to himself or herself "This is painful, I can't stand this," the positive coping self-statements of "Although this is painful, I know it will be good for me in the end" might be substituted. These statements must be rehearsed and practiced. Techniques for developing these statements have been described elsewhere.[51]

ADHERENCE IN SMOKING CESSATION PROGRAMS

Because of the well-documented association between smoking and COPD, successful smoking prevention programs are expected to reduce the incidence of these diseases. Smoking cessation programs are also valuable. Considerable interest has focused on the effects of smoking cessation for smokers with mild airway obstruction who may be at risk for COPD. In addition to the role of smoking as a cause of COPD, active cigarette smoking also affects the course of the illness. For example, cigarette smoking is associated with mucous hypersecretion, acute respiratory illnesses, altered airway reactivity, and increased risk of mortality from other causes, including coronary heart disease. Some of the relations between smoking and problems in the airways have been reviewed elsewhere.[61] A variety of studies have suggested that loss in lung function is associated with total duration of cigarette use.[62] Longitudinal studies indicate that pulmonary function is progressively lost with continued cigarette smoking. However, some evidence suggests that lung function is partially recoverable for those who cease cigarette smoking, particularly for those who do so early in life.[63]

Because of the potential benefits of smoking cessation, efforts to improve adherence to smoking cessation programs are of great importance. Evidence has accumulated suggesting that the physician may play a critical role in helping patients to stop smoking and to maintain this behavioral change.[64] Several experimental trials have trained physicians to provide a smoking cessation intervention. The components of the intervention include approaches for taking a smoking history, personalizing the health risks, setting a quit date, prescribing nicotine chewing gum, and counseling techniques for follow-up. In one study, Ockene and associates[65] assigned physicians to receive training in behaviorally oriented counseling techniques or to a control group in which patients were provided with only brief advice to stop smoking. Some of the interventions involved the use of nicotine gum, whereas others did not. The results suggested that the behavioral intervention, with or without the use of nicotine gum, resulted in greater reductions in cigarette use among patients. Furthermore, differences between these groups remained at 6-month follow-up.[65]

The Agency for Health Care Policy and Research (AHCPR) offered guidelines for smoking cessation in primary care medicine.[66] Despite the well-established health consequences of tobacco use, less than half of all physicians commonly advise their patients to give up cigarettes.[67] Among those who discuss smoking with their patients, few go much further. For example, only about one in four physicians make any effort beyond simply stating that the patient should quit smoking.[67] One of the biggest challenges in getting patients to quit smoking is the recognition that relapse is common. Most smokers who stop will begin using cigarettes again within 3 months. Among smokers who have abstained for 48 hours, nearly 20% relapse within the first week and an additional 13% relapse during the second week.[68] About 23% remain smoke free for 6 months. Relapse rates among those who participate in formal programs are somewhat better than they are for self-quitters.[69] Recent studies suggest that those smokers who slip are most likely to relapse. For example, a smoker who takes an occasional cigarette is significantly more likely to relapse than one who does not slip.[15,69–71]

Perhaps the best predictor of relapse is low personal expectations for remaining smoke free.[68,72] Using electronic daily diaries, Shiffman and colleagues[73,74] have determined factors that precipitate relapse. These studies suggest that lapses associated with self-reported stress or good mood were more likely to progress to relapses than those associated with eating or drinking.

Practical Suggestions on Smoking Interventions

Much literature on smoking cessation techniques has been developed and is best summarized in the AHCPR Guideline.[75] Overall, self-help groups tend not to achieve better outcomes than control groups.[76,77] We urge the use of self-help materials in combination with some counseling intervention. Telephone counseling seems to offer significant benefits. In addition, several toll-free 800 numbers are now available.[78] Evidence suggests that physicians and other health care providers can offer brief smoking cessation counseling[75] and that these simple interventions enhance abstinence rates at 6 and 12 months.[79,80] The addition of nicotine replacement therapy has also been shown to increase long-term maintenance. Pharmacotherapy may be more effective for men than for women, particularly when it is used in combination with smoking cessation counseling.[81]

In an analysis of the potential for smoking cessation programs, the AHCPR considered the impact of applying their Smoking Cessation Clinical Practice Guidelines for the U.S. population. The guidelines identify 15 different smoking cessation guidelines, ranging from minimal counseling to intensive counseling. Each intervention is considered with and without concomitant use of nicotine replacement in the form of gum or patches. The analysis assumed that the interventions would be available to 75% of adult smokers, which corresponds to the proportion that made a previous quit attempt. The model assumes that the program would yield 1.7 million new quitters, of whom 40% would have quit on their own and 60% may have been influenced in some way by the program to quit. Furthermore, the model assumed that 8.8% of smokers would quit with no intervention, 10.7% would quit with minimal counseling, 12.1% would quit with brief counseling, and 18.7% would quit with counseling lasting more than 10 minutes. Use of nicotine replace-

Table 19-2. Self-Help Smoking Cessation Programs Available to Physicians

Program	Available From	Website
Quit Smoking Action Plan	American Lung Association	www.lungusa.org
Adherence Tools for Professions	American Heart Association	www.americanheart.org
Quitting Smoking	American Cancer Society	www.cancer.org/tobacco/quitSmok.html

ment would boost these effects further. The program would cost an estimated $6.3 billion, or about $32 per smoker. Cost per quality-adjusted life year was estimated at $1915, placing it well below most programs that have been analyzed.[82]

A variety of excellent materials are available to help the patient through the cessation process. Some of these are described in Table 19-2. Some excellent self-help websites include http://www.lungusa.org/tobacco, http://www.nicotine-anonymous.org, http://www.quitnet.org, and http://clever.net/chrisco/nosmoke/cafe.html. To be most effective, these materials should be used in combination with some counseling intervention.

SUMMARY

The typical regimen for patients with COPD requires many different behaviors. These might include the use of several different medications, exercise, oxygen, respiratory and physiotherapy techniques, and other aspects of self-care. Adherence to this regimen can be challenging. In contrast to nearly every other medical condition, relatively few published studies evaluate the benefits of interventions to improve adherence among patients with COPD. Furthermore, we do not know the extent to which overuse of medication is associated with poor outcomes for patients with COPD. Behavioral intervention may enhance adherence with medicine taking, smoking cessation, and exercise. However, considerably more research is necessary to evaluate the long-term benefits of these interventions.

REFERENCES

1. Becker MH. Patient adherence to prescribed therapies. Med Care 1985;23(5):539–555.
2. Becker MH, Maiman LA. Strategies for enhancing patient compliance. J Community Health 1980; 6(2):113–135.
3. Shumaker SA, Schron EB, Ockene JK, et al., eds. The Handbook of Health Behavior Change. 2nd ed. New York: Springer Publishing, 1998.
4. Haynes RB, Taylor DW, Sackett DL. Compliance in Health Care. Baltimore: Johns Hopkins University Press, 1979.
5. DiMatteo MR, DiNicola DD. Achieving Patient Compliance: The Psychology of the Medical Practitioner's Role. New York: Pergamon Press, 1982.
6. Caron HS, Roth HP. Objective assessment of cooperation with an ulcer diet: relation to antacid intake and to assigned physician. Am J Med Sci 1971;261:61–66.
7. Norell SE. Accuracy of patient interviews and estimates by clinical staff in determining medication compliance. Soc Sci Med 1981;15(1):57–61.
8. Atkins CJ, Kaplan RM, Timms RM, et al. Behavioral exercise programs in the management of chronic obstructive pulmonary disease. J Consult Clin Psychol 1984;52(4):591–603.
9. Morrison D, Skwarski K, MacNee W. Review of the prescription of domiciliary long-term oxygen therapy in Scotland. Thorax 1995;50(10):1103–1105.
10. Restrick LJ, Paul EA, Braid GM, et al. Assessment and follow up of patients prescribed long-term oxygen treatment. Thorax 1993;48:708–713.
11. Rand CS, Nides M, Cowles MK, et al. Long-term metered-dose inhaler adherence in a clinical trial: the Lung Health Study Research Group. Am J Respir Crit Care Med 1995;152(2):580–588.

12. Powell SG. Medication compliance of patients with COPD. Home Healthc Nurse 1994;12(3): 44–50.

13. Turner J, Wright E, Mendella L, et al. Predictors of patient adherence to long-term home nebulizer therapy for COPD: the IPPB Study Group. Chest 1995;108(2):394–400.

14. Solomon DK, Portner TS, Bass GE, et al. Clinical and economic outcomes in the hypertension and COPD arms of a multicenter outcomes study. J Am Pharm Assoc (Wash) 1998;38(5):574–585.

15. Nides MA, Rakos RF, Gonzales D, et al. Predictors of initial smoking cessation and relapse through the first 2 years of the Lung Health Study. J Consult Clin Psychol 1995;63(1):60–69.

16. James PN, Anderson JB, Prior JG, et al. Patterns of drug taking in patients with chronic airflow obstruction. Postgrad Med J 1985;61(711): 7–10.

17. Corden Z, Rees PJ. The effect of oral corticosteroids on bronchodilator responses in COPD. Respir Med 1998;92(2):279–282.

18. Nides MA, Tashkin DP, Simmons MS, et al. Improving inhaler adherence in a clinical trial through the use of the nebulizer chronolog. Chest 1993;104(2):501–507.

19. Chryssidis E, Frewin DB, Frith PA, et al. Compliance with aerosol therapy in chronic obstructive lung disease. N Z Med J 1981;94(696):375–377.

20. Cramer JA, Mattson RH, Prevey ML, et al. How often is medication taken as prescribed? a novel assessment technique JAMA 1989;261(22): 3273–3277.

21. Cramer JA. Practical issues in medication compliance. Transplant Proc 1999;31(4A):7S–9S.

22. Rudd P, Ramesh J, Bryant-Kosling C, et al. Gaps in cardiovascular medication taking: the tip of the iceberg. J Gen Intern Med 1993;8(12):659–666.

23. Rudd P. Compliance with antihypertensive therapy: raising the bar of expectations. Am J Manag Care 1998;4(7):957–966.

24. Appelbaum SA. The refusal to take one's medicine. Bull Menninger Clin 1977;41(6):511–521.

25. Burke LE, Dunbar-Jacob JM, Hill MN. Compliance with cardiovascular disease prevention strategies: a review of the research. Ann Behav Med 1997;19(3):239–263.

26. Burke LE, Dunbar-Jacob J. Adherence to medication, diet, and activity recommendations: from assessment to maintenance. J Cardiovasc Nurs 1995;9(2):62–79.

27. Lorish CD, Richards B, Brown S. Missed medication doses in rheumatic arthritis patients: intentional and unintentional reasons. Arthritis Care Res 1989;2(1):3–9.

28. Agras WS. Understanding compliance with the medical regimen: the scope of the problem and a theoretical perspective. Arthritis Care Res 1989; 2(3):S2–S7.

29. Inui TS. Establishing the doctor-patient relationship: science, art, or competence? Schweiz Med Wochenschr 1998;128(7):225–230.

30. Roter DL, Stewart M, Putnam SM, et al. Communication patterns of primary care physicians. JAMA 1997;277(4):350–356.

31. Kaplan RM, Simon HJ. Compliance in medical care: reconsideration of self-predictions. Ann Behav Med 1990;12(2):66–71.

32. Liang MH. Compliance and quality of life: confessions of a difficult patient. Arthritis Care Res 1989;2(3):S71–S74.

33. Green LW, Mullen PD, Friedman RB. An epidemiological approach to targeting drug information. Patient Educ Couns 1986;8(3):255–268.

34. Steel K. Iatrogenic disease on a medical service. J Am Geriatr Soc 1984;32(6):445–449.

35. Steel K, Gertman PM, Crescenzi C, et al. Iatrogenic illness on a general medical service at a university hospital. N Engl J Med 1981;304(11): 638–642.

36. Williamson J, Chapin JM. Adverse reactions to prescribed drugs in the elderly: a multicare investigation. Aging 1980;9:73.

37. Hurwitz N. Predisposing factors in adverse reactions to drugs. BMJ 1969;1:536.

38. Leventhal H. The role of theory in the study of adherence to treatment and doctor-patient interactions. Med Care 1985;23(5):556–563.

39. Greenfield S, Kaplan S, Ware JE Jr. Expanding patient involvement in care: effects on patient outcomes. Ann Intern Med 1985;102(4):520–528.

40. Greenfield S, Kaplan SH, Ware JE Jr, et al. Patients' participation in medical care: effects on blood sugar control and quality of life in diabetes. J Gen Intern Med 1988;3(5):448–457.

41. Ries AL. The importance of exercise in pulmonary rehabilitation. Clin Chest Med 1994;15(2): 327–337.

42. Resnikoff PM, Ries AL. Maximizing functional capacity: pulmonary rehabilitation and adjunctive measures. Respir Care Clin N Am 1998;4(3): 475–492.

43. Simons-Morton DG, Calfas KJ, Oldenburg B, et al. Effects of interventions in health care settings on physical activity or cardiorespiratory fitness. Am J Prev Med 1998;15(4):413–430.

44. Friedman DB, Williams AN, Levine BD. Compliance and efficacy of cardiac rehabilitation and risk factor modification in the medically indigent. Am J Cardiol 1997;79(3):281–285.

45. Cockcroft AE, Saunders MJ, Berry G. Randomised controlled trial of rehabilitation in chronic respiratory disability. Thorax 1981;36(3):200–203.

46. McGavin CR, Gupta SP, Lloyd EL, et al. Physical rehabilitation for the chronic bronchitic: results of a controlled trial of exercises in the home. Thorax 1977;32(3):307–311.

47. Ambrosino N, Paggiaro PL, Macchi M, et al. A study of short-term effect of rehabilitative therapy in chronic obstructive pulmonary disease. Respiration 1981;41(1):40–44.

48. Sassi-Dambron DE, Eakin EG, Ries AL, et al. Treatment of dyspnea in COPD: a controlled clinical trial of dyspnea management strategies. Chest 1995;107(3):724–729.

49. Emery CF, Schein RL, Hauck ER, et al. Psychological and cognitive outcomes of a randomized trial of exercise among patients with chronic obstructive pulmonary disease. Health Psychol 1998;17(3):232–240.

50. Kaptein AA. Assessing quality of life in respiratory

disorders: chronic nonspecific lung disease. Monaldi Arch Chest Dis 1997;52(6):521–524.

51. Atkins CJ, Kaplan RM, Timms RM, et al. Behavioral exercise programs in the management of chronic obstructive pulmonary disease. J Consult Clin Psychol 1984;52(4):591–603.

52. Crowe SF. The differential contribution of mental tracking, cognitive flexibility, visual search, and motor speed to performance on parts A and B of the Trail Making Test. J Clin Psychol 1998; 54(5):585–591.

53. Kaplan RM, Ganiats TG, Sieber WJ, et al. The Quality of Well-Being Scale: critical similarities and differences with SF-36. Int J Qual Health Care 1998;10(6):509–520.

54. Toevs CD, Kaplan RM, Atkins CJ. The costs and effects of behavioral programs in chronic obstructive pulmonary disease. Med Care 1984;22(12): 1088–1100.

55. Goldstein RS, Gort EH, Guyatt GH, et al. Economic analysis of respiratory rehabilitation. Chest 1997;112(2):370–379.

56. Wijkstra PJ, van der Mark TW, Kraan J, et al. Long-term effects of home rehabilitation on physical performance in chronic obstructive pulmonary disease. Am J Respir Crit Care Med 1996;153(4 Pt 1):1234–1241.

57. Ries AL, Kaplan RM, Limberg TM, et al. Effects of pulmonary rehabilitation on physiologic and psychosocial outcomes in patients with chronic obstructive pulmonary disease. Ann Intern Med 1995;122(11):823–832.

58. Daughton DM, Fortmann SP, Glover ED, et al. The smoking cessation efficacy of varying doses of nicotine patch delivery systems 4 to 5 years post-quit day. Prev Med 1999;28(2):113–118.

59. Anderson DA, Wadden TA. Treating the obese patient: suggestions for primary care practice. Arch Fam Med 1999;8(2):156–167.

60. Sallis JF, Calfas KJ, Nichols JF, et al. Evaluation of a university course to promote physical activity: project GRAD. Res Q Exerc Sport 1999;70(1): 1–10.

61. Redline S, Tager IB, Speizer FE, et al. Longitudinal variability in airway responsiveness in a population-based sample of children and young adults: intrinsic and extrinsic contributing factors. Am Rev Respir Dis 1989;140(1):172–178.

62. Dockery DW, Speizer FE, Ferris BG Jr, et al. Cumulative and reversible effects of lifetime smoking on simple tests of lung function in adults. Am Rev Respir Dis 1988;137(2):286–292.

63. Camilli AE, Burrows B, Knudson RJ, et al. Longitudinal changes in forced expiratory volume in one second in adults: effects of smoking and smoking cessation. Am Rev Respir Dis 1987;135(4): 794–799.

64. Ockene JK, Zapka JG. Physician-based smoking intervention: a rededication to a five-step strategy to smoking research. Addict Behav 1997;22(6): 835–848.

65. Ockene JK, Kristeller J, Pbert L, et al. The physician-delivered smoking intervention project: can short-term interventions produce long-term effects for a general outpatient population? Health Psychol 1994;13(3):278–281.

66. Fiore MC. Overview of the Agency for Health Care Policy and Research Guideline. Tob Control 1998;7(Suppl):S14–S16.

67. Ockene JK, Aney J, Goldberg RJ, et al. A survey of Massachusetts physicians' smoking intervention practices. Am J Prev Med 1988;4(1):14–20.

68. Gulliver SB, Hughes JR, Solomon LJ, et al. An investigation of self-efficacy, partner support and daily stresses as predictors of relapse to smoking in self-quitters. Addiction 1995;90(6):767–772.

69. Brandon TH, Tiffany ST, Obremski KM, et al. Postcessation cigarette use: the process of relapse. Addict Behav 1990;15(2):105–114.

70. Baer JS, Kamarck T, Lichtenstein E, et al. Prediction of smoking relapse: analyses of temptations and transgressions after initial cessation. J Consult Clin Psychol 1989;57(5):623–627.

71. Norregaard J, Tonnesen P, Petersen L. Predictors and reasons for relapse in smoking cessation with nicotine and placebo patches. Prev Med 1993; 22(2):261–271.

72. Baer JS, Lichtenstein E. Classification and prediction of smoking relapse episodes: an exploration of individual differences. J Consult Clin Psychol 1988;56(1):104–110.

73. Shiffman S, Hickcox M, Paty JA, et al. Individual differences in the context of smoking lapse episodes. Addict Behav 1997;22(6):797–811.

74. O'Connell KA, Gerkovich MM, Cook MR, et al. Coping in real time: using Ecological Momentary Assessment techniques to assess coping with the urge to smoke. Res Nurs Health 1998;21(6): 487–497.

75. Fiore MC, Jorenby DE, Baker TB. Smoking cessation: principles and practice based upon the AHCPR Guideline, 1996. Ann Behav Med 1997; 19(3):213–219.

76. Gritz ER, Berman BA, Bastani R, et al. A randomized trial of a self-help smoking cessation intervention in a nonvolunteer female population: testing the limits of the public health model. Health Psychol 1992;11(5):280–289.

77. Curry SJ. Self-help interventions for smoking cessation. J Consult Clin Psychol 1993;61(5):790–803.

78. Zhu SH, Stretch V, Balabanis M, et al. Telephone counseling for smoking cessation: effects of single-session and multiple-session interventions. J Consult Clin Psychol 1996;64(1):202–211.

79. Morgan GD, Noll EL, Orleans CT, et al. Reaching midlife and older smokers: tailored interventions for routine medical care. Prev Med 1996;25(3): 346–354.

80. Tonnesen P, Mikkelsen K, Markholst C, et al. Nurse-conducted smoking cessation with minimal intervention in a lung clinic: a randomized controlled study. Eur Respir J 1996;9(11):2351–2355.

81. Perkins KA, Grobe JE, Caggiula A, et al. Acute reinforcing effects of low-dose nicotine nasal spray in humans. Pharmacol Biochem Behav 1997; 56(2):235–241.

82. Cromwell J, Bartosch WJ, Fiore MC, et al. Cost-effectiveness of the clinical practice recommendations in the AHCPR Guideline for smoking cessation. JAMA 1997;278(21):1759–1766.

83. Costello RW, Liston R, McNicholas WT. Compliance at night with low flow oxygen therapy: a comparison of nasal cannulae and venturi face masks. Thorax 1995;50(4):405–406.

84. Wise RA, Enright PL, Connett JE, et al. Effect of weight gain on pulmonary function after smoking cessation in the Lung Health Study. Am J Respir Crit Care Med 1998;157(3 Pt 1):866–872.

85. Kampelmacher MJ, Van Kestern RG, Alsbach GP, et al. Characteristics and complaints of patients prescribed long-term oxygen therapy in the Netherlands. Respir Med 1998;92(1):70–75.

20 Outcome Assessment

Richard ZuWallack

⟩ Professional Skills

Upon completion of this chapter, the reader will understand:

- The importance and rationale of outcome assessment in pulmonary rehabilitation
- The availability of outcome assessment in several areas, including exercise ability, dyspnea, health-related quality of life (HRQL), functional status, and nutritional status
- The advantages and disadvantages of different forms of exercise testing for chronic lung disease, such as incremental exercise testing, endurance testing at a constant workload, the timed walk test, and the incremental shuttle walking test
- The two major forms of dyspnea assessment in chronic lung disease: the rating of exertional dyspnea during exercise testing and questionnaire-measured dyspnea, usually in association with daily activities
- The concept and rationale of HRQL measurement in respiratory assessment and appreciate the differences between generic and respiratory-specific instruments
- The differences between functional status and quality of life instruments and the importance of evaluating the effect of severe lung disease on activities of daily living (ADLs)
- The importance of nutritional and body composition abnormalities in advanced chronic lung disease

THE RATIONALE FOR OUTCOME ASSESSMENT

The goals of pulmonary rehabilitation are to reduce symptoms, increase functional performance, and improve HRQL. Outcome assessment is used to quantify the improvement in these areas. This can be in the form of documenting individual patient gains resulting from the intervention or assessing the overall effectiveness of the program in one or more areas.[1] Although the pulmonary physiologic abnormalities associated with advanced chronic lung disease are usually irreversible, pulmonary rehabilitation often leads to measurable and clinically meaningful benefits[2] because a substantial portion of the morbidity from chronic respiratory disease is not directly related to the irreversible respiratory disease. For instance, although pulmonary rehabilitation does not increase the forced expiratory volume in 1 second (FEV_1) in chronic obstructive pulmonary disease (COPD), it improves peripheral muscle and cardiovascular conditioning, alleviates dyspnea through better pacing and breathing strategies, and reduces anxiety associated with dyspnea-producing activities. The role of outcome assessment in pulmonary rehabilitation is to capture these and other favorable changes.

Box 20-1 lists some of the rationale for outcome assessment in pulmonary rehabilitation. In view of its complexity, no single outcome assessment can capture the degree and breadth of improvement from the pulmonary rehabilitation intervention. Therefore, assessment in multiple areas is often advisable. Areas of outcome assessment are listed in Box 20-2.

For scientific studies of pulmonary rehabilitation outcome, randomization of patients to a treatment or control group is usually necessary. However, the inclusion of an untreated or partially treated control group is not feasible for typical clinically oriented pulmonary rehabilitation programs. For these, simple assessment of prerehabilitation to postrehabilitation changes in a few outcome areas without a control group is usually sufficient to document individual patient gains and the program's overall effectiveness. Even in randomized, controlled clinical trials, the patient obviously cannot be blinded to the pulmonary rehabilitation intervention. Therefore, effort-dependent outcome measures, such as the timed walk test, are potentially influenced by motivation or encouragement.[3] Other outcome areas, such as questionnaire-measured HRQL, are subjective and potentially affected by the patient's desire to please the rehabilitation staff.

The mere demonstration that a change resulting from pulmonary rehabilitation is statistically significant is not sufficient for clinical purposes—ideally, the favorable effect should also be demonstrated to be clinically relevant and meaningful.[4] Established or suggested clinically meaningful changes for the 6-minute walk test ($\sim$50 m)[5] and two HRQL measures, the Chronic Respiratory Disease Questionnaire (CRDQ)[6] (0.5 units per question) and the St. George's Respiratory Questionnaire (SGRQ)[7] (4 units), are available at this time.

Although outcome assessments before and shortly following rehabilitation treatment are easiest to perform, the documentation of long-term benefit is also important. It has become clear that some of the gains made from pulmonary rehabilitation wane over the

Box 20-1. The Rationale for Outcome Measurement in Pulmonary Rehabilitation

1. Outcomes such as decreased dyspnea and improved quality of life are of paramount importance to the patient yet correlate poorly with physiologic abnormalities. These outcomes are easily measured before and after rehabilitation.
2. Baseline impairment in symptoms, exercise performance, functional status, and quality of life vary widely among patients entering pulmonary rehabilitation. Knowledge of baseline status might allow the rehabilitation staff to focus intervention on those areas most affected.
3. Although the individual program's pulmonary rehabilitation intervention is usually roughly the same for each patient, the degree of improvement among patients often varies widely.
4. Patients allowed to see objective evidence of their improvement might be better motivated to continue with long-term rehabilitation efforts.
5. Feedback on outcomes can be useful for rehabilitation staff in maintaining morale and in adjusting rehabilitation therapy components to provide optimal results.
6. Prerehabilitation to postrehabilitation outcome assessment provides objective evidence for third-party payers on the effectiveness of the individual pulmonary rehabilitation program.
7. Clinical research on the effectiveness of pulmonary rehabilitation or its components requires accurate outcome measurement.

Adapted with permission from ZuWallack RL. Outcome assessment for pulmonary rehabilitation. Eur Respir Monogr 2000;13.

Box 20-2. Examples of Outcome Assessment in Pulmonary Rehabilitation

Laboratory tests of exercise performance
    Incremental exercise test to peak workload
    Steady-state endurance test
Field tests of exercise performance
    Self-paced: the 6-minute timed walk test
    Externally paced: the incremental and steady-state shuttle walking tests
Dyspnea
    Exertional dyspnea: the visual analog and Borg category scales
    Overall dyspnea: the Baseline and Transitional Dyspnea Indexes and the
       Medical Research Council dyspnea scale
Questionnaire measures of health-related quality of life
    Generic: the Medical Outcomes Study Short-Form 36
    Respiratory specific: the Chronic Respiratory Disease Questionnaire and the St.
       George's Respiratory Questionnaire
Questionnaire measures of functional status
    Generic: the Extended Activities of Daily Living scale
    Respiratory-specific: the Pulmonary Functional Status Scale and the Pulmonary
       Functional Status and Dyspnea Questionnaire
Nutritional status
Survival
Health care utilization

ensuing year.[8,9] Therefore, consideration should be given to assessment at intervals of months or years after completion of the formal program.

TESTS OF EXERCISE PERFORMANCE

Incremental Exercise Testing

Incremental exercise testing on a bicycle ergometer or treadmill to maximal tolerance or to a heart rate of about 85% of predicted provides an objective and reproducible measurement of exercise performance. Measurements of heart rate, respiratory rate, blood pressure, electrocardiographic tracings, and oxygen saturation are routinely monitored. With analysis of expired gases, the determination or calculation of minute ventilation, oxygen consumption, carbon dioxide production, anaerobic threshold, and respiratory dead space is possible. Additional information can be obtained by having the patient rate the level of exertional dyspnea or leg fatigue at intervals during the testing.

A listing of randomized, controlled trials of pulmonary rehabilitation or exercise training demonstrating the usefulness of incremental exercise testing is given in Table 20-1. In general, these studies have shown relatively small increases in peak oxygen consumption but more impressive increases in peak exercise workload after the period of exercise training. For example, in a study by Ries and colleagues[9] comparing comprehensive outpatient pulmonary rehabilitation to education alone, the rehabilitation group did not significantly increase their peak oxygen consumption at 2 months after therapy ($+0.11$ L/min, $P = .10$) but did increase their maximal treadmill workload by 1.5 metabolic equivalents—a 33% improvement over baseline. Similarly, a randomized, controlled study of 6 weeks' supervised exercise training in COPD[10] showed no significant change in peak oxygen consumption after exercise training (0.92 vs. 0.97 L/min) but did show a 33% increase in peak cycle work rate, from 36 to 48 watts. Finally, in an 18-month study comparing hospital-based outpatient pulmonary rehabilitation with a home-based setting, the hospital-based program resulted in a 20% increase in peak workload at 3 months, with

Table 20-1. Examples of Incremental Exercise Testing in Pulmonary Rehabilitation Outcome Assessment

Investigator	Intervention	Incremental Test	Results
Casaburi et al., 1991[12]	8 wk of inpatient rehabilitation; low (n = 8) vs. high (n = 11) work rate exercise training groups	Cycle ergometer	Both groups had a low lactate threshold; the higher work rate group had more training effect demonstrated by greater decreases in HR, lactate, VE, VCO_2, and VE/VO_2 at identical postexercise work rates
Reardon et al., 1994[32]	6 wk of comprehensive outpatient rehabilitation (n = 10) vs. untreated control group (n = 10)	Treadmill	No significant improvement occurred in maximal exercise performance after pulmonary rehabilitation; the treatment group, however, did have significant decreases in VAS-rated dyspnea measured during incremental testing
Ries et al., 1995[9]	8 wk of outpatient rehabilitation (n = 57) vs. education alone (n = 62)	Treadmill	The rehabilitation group had greater increases in maximal exercise work load and VO_2 and greater decreases in and perceived dyspnea and fatigue at maximal workload than did the education control group
O'Donnell et al., 1995[10]	Outpatient exercise training (n = 30) vs. an untreated, matched control group	Cycle ergometer	The treatment group showed preintervention to postintervention improvement in peak work rate and significant reductions in dyspnea and leg effort
Strijbos et al., 1996[11]	Hospital-based outpatient (n = 15) vs. home care–based outpatient rehabilitation (n = 15) vs. an untreated control group (n = 15)	Cycle ergometer	The hospital-based outpatient group showed a 19.8% increase in W_{max} at 3 mo, then a gradual decrease in this improvement over time; the home-based group showed a more gradual increase in W_{max} over time, with a 20.7% increase over baseline by 18 mo
Wijkstra et al., 1996[85]	12 wk of comprehensive home rehabilitation (n = 23) vs. no rehabilitation (n = 15)	Cycle ergometer	Thirty-nine of 43 patients had a ventilatory limitation to their exercise; the rehabilitation group had a greater increase in W_{max} and peak VO_2 and a greater decrease in dyspnea at W_{max} than the control group

HR, heart rate; VE, minute ventilation; VCO_2, peak carbon dioxide uptake; VO_2, peak oxygen uptake; VAS, visual analog scale.
From Wijkstra PJ, Van der Mark TW, Kraan J, et al. Effects of home rehabilitation on physical performance in patients with chronic obstructive pulmonary disease (COPD). Eur Respir J 1996;9:104–110.

a gradual decrease in effectiveness at 12 and 18 months. In contrast, the home-based program resulted in a gradual increase in maximal workload during this time period, peaking at 21% over baseline at 18 months.[11]

In addition to quantifying improvement in peak exercise performance, incremental exercise testing is useful in demonstrating changes in physiology resulting from exercise training. This is usually accomplished by measuring variables at *identical* workloads before and after therapy. This utility is demonstrated in a study by Casaburi and colleagues,[12] who compared high- and moderate-intensity stationary bicycle exercise training in individuals with moderately severe COPD. Eleven patients were randomized to the high-intensity exercise and nine to the moderate-intensity exercise protocol. Lactate production and resultant increased ventilatory demand was present in both groups at low exercise workloads. After the course of exercise training, only the group given high-intensity exercise training showed a true physiologic training effect, with decreases in blood lactate and minute ventilation at identical levels of exercise at follow-up testing (Fig. 20-1). In addition, their reduction in minute ventilation was proportional to their decrease in lactate production.

As the previously described study illustrates, incremental exercise testing can uncover the physiologic basis for favorable effects of exercise training in pulmonary rehabilitation. Despite this advantage, this type of exercise testing is limited by the expertise it requires, its expense, and some inconvenience to the patient.

Endurance Exercise Testing

Endurance testing on a stationary bicycle or treadmill usually involves exercising at a constant work rate for as long as tolerated. The work rate is usually set at a constant fraction of peak work rate (such as 85%) determined at a previous incremental exercise

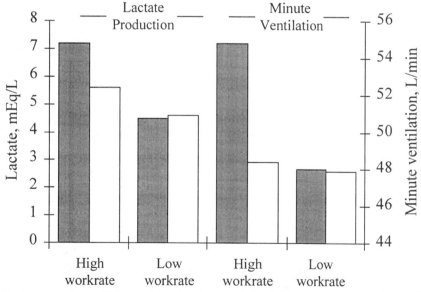

Figure 20-1. A comparison of high and low levels of exercise training on the physiologic adaptation to exercise. Eleven patients with COPD were given high-intensity exercise training and 9 were given low-intensity exercise training for 8 weeks. Baseline values are represented by the *shaded bars,* postexercise training values by the *white bars.* Posttraining responses were measured at the same work rate as in the pretraining study. The group given the high-intensity training had greater reductions in lactate and minute ventilation, indicating a greater physiologic training effect. (Adapted from Casaburi R, Patessio A, Loli F, et al. Reductions in exercise lactic acidosis and ventilation as a result of exercise training in patients with obstructive lung disease. Am Rev Respir Dis 1991;143:9–18.)

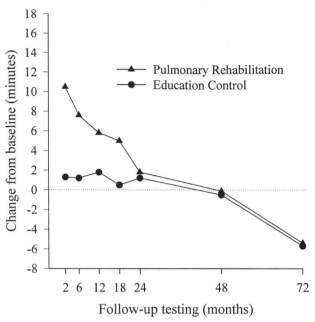

Figure 20-2. The effect of comprehensive pulmonary rehabilitation on treadmill exercise endurance time. (Adapted with permission from Ries AL, Kaplan RM, Limberg TM, et al. Effects of pulmonary rehabilitation on physiologic and psychosocial outcomes in patients with chronic obstructive pulmonary disease. Ann Intern Med 1995;122:823–832.)

test. The time the patient is able to tolerate this constant exercise is the outcome measure. Because the exercise work load is set by the investigator, self-pacing is not a potential confounding variable as with self-paced tests, such as the timed walk test. Exercise endurance measured in this fashion often shows considerable improvement after pulmonary rehabilitation,[9,13,14] probably reflecting the emphasis given to lower extremity exercise training.

The usefulness of endurance exercise testing is illustrated in the randomized, controlled study of pulmonary rehabilitation by Ries and associates.[9] One hundred nineteen patients with COPD were randomized to either comprehensive outpatient rehabilitation (n = 57) or education only (n = 62) groups. Treadmill exercise endurance testing was performed at approximately 95% of the patient's maximal exercise tolerance. The initial exercise endurance times in the rehabilitation and control groups (12.4 ± 8.4 and 11.8 ± 8.0 minutes, respectively) were similar. Figure 20-2 shows changes in this outcome measure over the study period. Treadmill endurance time was essentially unchanged in the control group, but did increase significantly in the rehabilitation group in the months immediately following pulmonary rehabilitation. For the latter group, the 10.5-minute increase in endurance time at 2 months represented an 85% increase over baseline. The favorable effects of rehabilitation remained statistically significant at 6 months and tended to be greater up to 18 months later. Following this, any beneficial effect was lost.

Walk Tests

The Timed Walk Test

The timed walk test has probably become the most widely used measure of exercise performance in pulmonary rehabilitation. For this test, the patient is given instructions to walk as far as possible in a corridor or large room during an allotted period of time, usually 6 or 12 minutes.[15,16] The distance covered is recorded as the outcome measure. The popularity of the timed walk test in pulmonary rehabilitation probably results from several features: (*a*) it is easy to administer, requires no special equipment, and is well tolerated by the patient; (*b*) the type and intensity of the exercise is relevant to many common daily activities; (*c*) it is very responsive to pulmonary rehabilitation intervention; and (*d*) reasonable estimates exist of what represents a clinically meaningful change in the walk distance.[5] The importance of the walk test is underscored by its incorporation as the major outcome variable in the National Emphysema Therapy Trial, a multicenter investigation to evaluate the effectiveness of lung volume reduction surgery for emphysema.[17]

Despite its advantages, the walk test is potentially biased by practice or learning effect and the positive effect of encouragement from rehabilitation personnel. For instance, in a study by Larson et al.[18] evaluating weekly 12-minute walk test performance in stable patients, a 7% increase in distance was present at the second walk, a 4% further increase was found at the third walk, and a 2% improvement at the fourth walk. Therefore, a minimum of two timed walks (with rests of approximately 15 minutes between them) is needed to reduce practice effect to a reasonably low level. Encouragement, supplied by the staff member administering the test, has been shown to increase the 6-minute walk distance by approximately 30 m[19]—a change not too different from that attributed to the rehabilitation intervention in some studies. For this reason, standardization of encouragement is also a necessary component of the timed walk test. A recommended protocol giving specific directions for 6-minute walk testing[20] is outlined in Box 20-3.

The timed walk test is usually very responsive to pulmonary rehabilitation intervention, probably reflecting the emphasis most programs give to lower extremity training. This is illustrated in Figure 20-3, which shows a meta-analysis of the effects of pulmonary

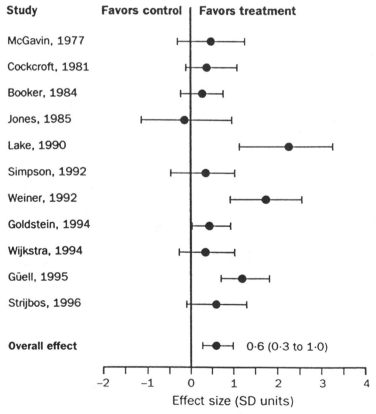

Figure 20-3. The effect of pulmonary rehabilitation on walking distance. (Reprinted with permission from Lacasse Y, Wong E, Guyatt GH, et al. Meta-analysis of respiratory rehabilitation in chronic obstructive pulmonary disease. Lancet 1996;348:117.)

Box 20-3. A Recommended Protocol for the Timed Walk Test

Equipment: Rolling distance marker and stopwatch; spirometer; pulse oximeter.

Exclusion criteria: Patients with musculoskeletal problems that significantly limit walking such as paralysis, pain, and psychiatric problems that would contribute to suboptimal walking performance; uncontrolled angina or hypertension, hypoxia, recent history of cardiac dysrhythmia or myocardial infarction; and other significant medical conditions that might be exacerbated by physical exertion.

Procedure:

1. Before the first walk, dyspnea (10-point Borg Scale), blood pressure, pulse, and respiratory rate are measured and recorded for all patients. In addition, any medications, such as an inhaled β-agonist or nitroglycerine, that might ordinarily be taken before activity should be self-administered. For COPD and asthma patients, postbronchodilator spirometry and baseline oximetry should be carried out 15 minutes after taking their β-agonist.

2. Walks will take place at approximately the same time of day, at least 2 hours after a meal.

3. Patients will be asked to walk from end to end of the walking track, covering as much ground as possible in 6 minutes.

4. The walks should be carried out in an area with minimal traffic that is at least 100 ft in length. Ambient temperature at that location should be recorded.

5. Two walks will be carried out with at least 15 minutes of rest between each walk. Consider carrying out the tests with more time between each walk or over two consecutive days for more disabled individuals.

6. The following instructions will be given to subjects:

   "The purpose of this test is to find out how far you can walk in 6 minutes. You will start from this point (indicate marker at one end of the course) and follow the hallway to the marker at the end, then turn around and walk back. When you arrive back at the starting point, you will go back and forth again. You will go back and forth as many times as you can in the 6-minute period. If you need to, you may stop and rest. Just remain where you are until you can go on again. However, the most important thing about the test is that you cover as much ground as you possibly can during the 6 minutes. I will tell you the time, and I will let you know when the 6 minutes are up. When I say 'stop,' please stand right where you are."

   Subjects are then asked to repeat the gist of the instructions to validate understanding.

7. During the first walk, pulse oximetry will be carried out during the test on everyone. Patients on supplemental oxygen will use their oxygen at the prescribed flow rate for exercise. Patients who desaturate to levels below 85% will be asked to stop walking and the walk test will be discontinued. Oxygen therapy may be considered, and if instituted, these patients may then be restudied.

8. During the walks, the following words of encouragement will be provided at 30-second intervals: "you're doing well," "keep up the good work," "good job," "you're doing fine."

9. With the exception of the first walk, during which pulse oximetry will be performed, staff will walk behind the patient so as not to influence his or her pace and will attempt to face the patient only when offering encouragement.

10. Patients are told when 2, 4, and 6 minutes (Stop) have elapsed.

11. The longest distance walked of the three trials will be noted, although all distances will be documented. Duration of time spent resting will also be recorded.

12. Immediately following completion of each walking test, patients will be asked to rate their level of breathing effort on the Borg scale and to indicate which symptom limited walking (shortness of breath, leg pain, etc.)

Reprinted with permission from Steele B. Timed walking tests of exercise capacity in chronic cardiopulmonary disease. J Cardiopulm Rehab 1996;16:25–33.

Table 20-2. A Comparison of the Timed Walk Test and Incremental Shuttle
Walking Test

Timed Walk Test	Incremental Shuttle Walking Test
Testing is done in the "field"	Testing is done in the "field"
Walking distance is the outcome measured	Walking distance is the outcome measured
More of a steady-state measure of exercise endurance	An incremental measure of exercise capacity
Self-pacing is potentially important in influencing performance	Speed is set externally, reducing or eliminating self-pacing effects

rehabilitation on walk test performance from 11 randomized, controlled clinical trials.
The favorable effect of treatment, which was +55.7 m, was not only statistically significant
but exceeds the estimated minimal clinically important difference for the 6-minute walk
distance of 54 m.[21]

The Shuttle Walking Test
The progressive 10-m shuttle walking test[22] is an externally paced measure of exercise
capacity for individuals with chronic lung disease. For this test the patient must walk up
and down a 10-m distance defined by marker cones 0.5 m from either end. Walking pace
is set by repetitive beeping signals from an audiocassette player. Instructions are given to
walk at a steady pace with a goal of reaching the opposite marker cone at the next beeping
signal. Initially, the time interval between the beeping signals is such that the patient must
walk at 0.5 m/sec to get to the opposite end in time. This speed is increased at 1-minute
intervals by shortening the time between beeping signals. The test end point is determined
when the patient becomes too breathless to keep up with the pace or is unable to complete
the shuttle in the time allowed. The total distance (number of completed shuttles times
10 m) is calculated as the outcome.

   Although the timed walk test and the shuttle walking tests are "field" measures of
distance walked, they differ in certain areas, as outlined in Table 20-2. Being incremental
in nature, the shuttle walking test is more a measure of exercise capacity. In contrast, the
timed walk test is probably more a measure of exercise endurance. In addition, unlike the
timed walk test, the shuttle test is not affected by self-pacing because pace is externally set.

   As might be expected, the shuttle walking distance correlates well with peak oxygen
consumption ($r = 0.88$) from incremental treadmill exercise.[23] Although to date it has
not been used extensively as an outcome measure for pulmonary rehabilitation, it seems
to be responsive to therapy. In a randomized, controlled trial of pulmonary rehabilitation
of COPD patients, those given hospital-based rehabilitation had an 88-m increase in
shuttle distance, representing a 46% increase over baseline.[24] If this impressive response
to therapy is replicated in subsequent rehabilitation studies, this test will probably grow
in popularity as an outcome measure.

DYSPNEA ASSESSMENT

Dyspnea, or breathlessness, is usually the principal symptom limiting exercise in patients
with advanced pulmonary disease and is probably the most important factor influencing
their HRQL.[25,26] In COPD patients, breathlessness is often most pronounced during tasks
requiring unsupported arm exercise, probably because this type of activity places both
ventilatory and nonventilatory burdens on the accessory respiratory muscles.[27] Although

dyspnea is correlated with respiratory physiologic abnormalities, such as airway obstruction or lung hyperinflation, it is also modulated by other factors, such as anxiety, depression, hysteria, social support, grief, fear, and past life experiences.[28] In addition, the effort component of dyspnea can be distinguished from its anxiety and distress components,[29] although the clinical importance of this distinction has yet to be determined.

In pulmonary rehabilitation outcome assessment, two forms of dyspnea measurement are generally used: (*a*) the level of exertional breathlessness during a specific task, such as exercise testing or a timed walk, and (*b*) overall breathlessness during daily activities.

Exertional Breathlessness

In moderately advanced respiratory disease, either dyspnea or leg discomfort (or both) usually limits exercise, whereas in severe disease dyspnea is usually the limiting symptom.[30] Exertional dyspnea can be measured with a 10- or 20-point category scale, such as the Borg scale,[31] or it can be rated using a visual analog scale. For the latter, the patient rates the intensity of dyspnea by pointing along a 100- or 200-mm vertical line. The vertical distance from the bottom of the line to this point is the level of dyspnea. The line is often anchored at either end with descriptors such as "greatest breathlessness" and "no breathlessness."

Pulmonary rehabilitation is an effective treatment for exertional dyspnea in patients with COPD. An example of its effectiveness is demonstrated in a study by Reardon and colleagues,[32] who randomized patients referred for pulmonary rehabilitation into either a treatment group (6 weeks of outpatient rehabilitation, n = 10) or a control group (6-week waiting period, n = 10). Incremental treadmill exercise testing was performed before and after the rehabilitation intervention or the waiting period. At 1-minute intervals during the testing, the patient rated his or her level of exertional dyspnea using a linear visual analog scale. Exertional dyspnea was unchanged in the control group but significantly reduced in the rehabilitation group. For the latter, the reduction in dyspnea was detectable early in the exercise and was maintained until peak workload was reached. The ratio of dyspnea to minute ventilation was also decreased in this study, suggesting that the improvement in dyspnea was not just owing to a decreased ventilatory demand resulting from exercise training. The changes in dyspnea at peak workload are depicted in Figure 20-4.

Another example of exertional dyspnea as an outcome measurement for pulmonary rehabilitation is given in a study by O'Donnell and colleagues,[10] who studied the impact of 6 weeks of exercise conditioning on dyspnea and leg fatigue of individuals with COPD. Results were compared with a control group that did not receive exercise training. Exercise was limited primarily by dyspnea and secondarily by leg fatigue, both before and after intervention. Despite an increase in exercise performance on cycle ergometer testing following the exercise training period, exertional dyspnea in the treatment group decreased, dropping from 5.3 to 3.8 ($P < .001$) on a 10-point Borg scale at peak exercise. The exercise training group also had a significant reduction in minute ventilation (due primarily to a decrease in respiratory frequency) at a standardized work rate. In multiple regression analysis, the reduction in dyspnea was predicted best by the reduction in ventilatory demand.

Breathlessness Associated With Activities

Overall dyspnea associated with daily activities is measured by questionnaire. Examples used as outcome measures for pulmonary rehabilitation include the Medical Research Council dyspnea scale; the Baseline Dyspnea Index and Transitional Dyspnea Index (BDI and TDI)[33,34]; the University of California, San Diego, Dyspnea Questionnaire[9]; and the dyspnea domain of the CRDQ.[35]

For the Medical Research Council dyspnea scale, the patient rates his or her level of dyspnea by choosing one of five responses that best describes the degree of overall

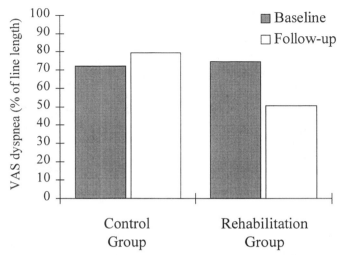

Figure 20-4. Changes in exertional dyspnea with pulmonary rehabilitation. Patients referred for out-patient pulmonary rehabilitation were randomized into a treatment group (n = 10) given 6 weeks of pulmonary rehabilitation or a control group (n = 10) who waited 6 weeks to begin rehabilitation. Dyspnea was measured using a visual analog scale (*VAS*) at regular intervals during incremental treadmill exercise. The bars represent VAS values at peak workload at baseline and after either the waiting period or the rehabilitation period. Maximal exercise capacity did not change significantly in either group. Pulmonary rehabilitation patients, however, had significant decreases in VAS-measured exertional dyspnea. (Data from Reardon J, Awad E, Normandin E, et al. The effect of comprehensive outpatient pulmonary rehabilitation on dyspnea. Chest 1994;105:1046–1052.)

breathlessness: (*a*) no breathlessness, (*b*) short of breath with strenuous exercise or when hurrying, (*c*) walk slower than people of the same age on the level or stop for a breath while walking at own pace on the level, (*d*) stop for a breath after 100 yd or after a few minutes on the level, and (*e*) too breathless to leave the house. As in most of these scales, the degree of breathlessness is rated by the degree of functional limitation it produces.

The BDI and TDI are interviewer-administered questionnaires that assess dyspnea through its effect on daily activities. The instrument takes about 3 to 4 minutes to complete.[36] The BDI has three scales: functional impairment, magnitude of task, and magnitude of effort. Each is scored on a 0 (severe) to 4 (no impairment) scale. The focal score, which sums the three, can therefore range from zero (most limitation from dyspnea) to 12 (no limitation from dyspnea). Changes in limitation in the areas of functional impairment, magnitude of task, and magnitude of effort are rated with the TDI. Each is scored on a −3 (major deterioration) to 0 (no change) to +3 (major improvement) scale. The focal TDI score, which sums the three, therefore, can range from −9 (greatest increase in limitation owing to dyspnea) to +9 (greatest reduction in limitation owing to dyspnea).

Some pulmonary rehabilitation studies using the BDI and TDI in outcome measurement are listed in Table 20-3. These studies indicate that the mean improvement in overall dyspnea during daily activities as reflected in the focal TDI score is between two and three units. In contrast, a recent clinical trial comparing the bronchodilators ipratropium and salmeterol in COPD demonstrated 1.18 and 1.07 units, respectively, in TDI dyspnea resulting from these drugs.[37]

The University of California, San Diego, Shortness of Breath Questionnaire is a 24-item instrument developed by the pulmonary rehabilitation program at that institution. It assesses dyspnea associated with 21 ADLs by having the patient rate each on a 6-point scale. The questionnaire also has three additional questions that assess limitations caused by shortness of breath, fear of overexertion, and fear of shortness of breath. The usefulness

Table 20-3. Examples of Randomized Controlled Studies of Pulmonary Rehabilitation With Dyspnea Measured by Questionnaire

Study	Treatment Intervention	Dyspnea Measure	Outcome
Reardon et al., 1994[32]	6 wk of OPR	BDI/TDI	TDI increased significantly in the treatment group (+2.3 units) compared with controls (0.2) ($P = .006$)
Goldstein et al., 1994[13]	8 wk of IPR and 16 wk of supervised outpatient training	BDI/TDI CRDQ dyspnea	TDI increased by 2.7 units ($P = .005$); CRDQ dyspnea increased by a clinically meaningful 3.0 units ($P = .006$)
Ries et al., 1995[9]	8 wk of OPR	UCSD Shortness of Breath Questionnaire	Improvement in questionnaire score by 7.0 units at 2-mo measurement following OPR ($P < .01$); beneficial effect gradually waned over ensuing months
O'Donnell et al., 1995[10]	6 wk of a multimodality exercise endurance program	BDI/TDI	TDI increased by 2.8 units ($P < .001$)
Cambach et al., 1997[86]	3 mo of home-based pulmonary rehabilitation	CRDQ dyspnea	Significant and clinically meaningful improvement in CRDQ dyspnea at 3 mo (+6 units) and 6 mo (+5 units) following pulmonary rehabilitation

OPR, Outpatient Pulmonary Rehabilitation; BDI, Baseline Dyspnea Index; TDI, Transitional Dyspnea Index; IPR, Inpatient Pulmonary Rehabilitation; CRDQ, Chronic Respiratory Disease Questionnaire; UCSD, University of California, San Diego.
From Cambach W, Chadwich-Straver RVM, Wagenaar RC, et al. The effects of a community-based pulmonary rehabilitation programme on exercise tolerance and quality of life: a randomized controlled trial. Eur Respir J 1997;10:104–113.

of this questionnaire as an outcome measure was demonstrated by the controlled trial of pulmonary rehabilitation by Ries et al.[9] Although the education-treated control group had no significant change in dyspnea by this measure, the rehabilitation group had a significant, 7.0-unit decrease in dyspnea by 2 months. This represents a 19.6% improvement over baseline.

The CRDQ is a 20-item instrument that measures HRQL for patients with COPD. This will be discussed in more detail later in this chapter. The dyspnea domain of this questionnaire consists of five questions that require the patient to rate five dyspnea-producing activities, each on a 1 to 7 scale. The activities must be dyspnea producing, performed regularly, and of importance to the patient. Thus, the dyspnea assessment is unique to the individual.

HEALTH-RELATED QUALITY OF LIFE (HRQL)

Quality of life is a somewhat nebulous concept that refers to the satisfaction or happiness with life that an individual has in domains that he or she considers important.[11,38,39] In this general sense, quality of life is affected by factors not necessarily related to health, such as job satisfaction, quality of housing, financial security, family and social interaction, and spiritual fulfillment.[40] HRQL focuses only on those areas of life satisfaction affected by alterations in health.[41] The HRQL measure must quantify the impact of the disease on important daily life activities and the sense of well-being.[42]

Because a cure for most chronic respiratory diseases such as COPD is not realistic and standard medical therapy is often only partially effective in relieving symptoms, improvement in HRQL has become an important outcome assessment in pulmonary rehabilitation. HRQL is, by nature, specific to the individual patient. Therefore, the questions are answered by the patient, never a spouse or a member of the pulmonary rehabilitation staff. Questionnaires can be generic and applicable to most disease states or respiratory specific, focusing on aspects of health influenced by lung disease. Areas of respiratory-specific HRQL measurement include respiratory symptoms (especially dyspnea or fatigue), social or role function, emotional function, ADLs, and the sense of mastery over disease.

The ideal HRQL questionnaire for pulmonary rehabilitation should be short and easy to understand and should be self-administered or easy for staff to administer. In addition, it should have both discriminative and evaluative properties. The former refers to its ability to distinguish individuals with better HRQL from those with worse HRQL, whereas the latter refers to its ability to detect small changes after therapy or over time.

In single studies, especially those evaluating patients with a relatively narrow spectrum of disease severity (such as in pulmonary rehabilitation), HRQL is poorly associated with pulmonary function abnormality, such as the FEV_1.[43] When results of multiple studies are used to capture the broad spectrum of airflow limitation, the correlation between respiratory function impairment and HRQL becomes more apparent.[44] However, for patients with advanced respiratory disease such as COPD, other measures of disease severity, especially the level of dyspnea and timed walk distance, are better predictors of HRQL than is the FEV_1.[25,43]

The following discussion touches on three HRQL questionnaires commonly used in pulmonary rehabilitation assessment: the respiratory-specific CRDQ and SGRQ and the generic Medical Outcomes Study Short-Form 36 (SF-36).

The CRDQ

The CRDQ[35] is perhaps the most widely used HRQL questionnaire in pulmonary rehabilitation assessment. This 20-item interviewer-administered questionnaire, which takes about 20 minutes to complete, has a total score and four domain scores: dyspnea, fatigue, emotion, and mastery—the sense of control over the disease. The dyspnea domain consists of five questions unique to the individual. For these, the patient must identify five activities from the preceding 2 weeks that were frequently done and were associated with breathlessness. A list of 26 activities is provided for suggestions. The dyspnea associated with each of the five chosen activities is then scored using a 7-point scale ranging from 1, extremely short of breath, to 7, not at all short of breath. The 15 questions used to assess the three remaining domains are also scored using a 7-point scoring system, with higher scores indicating less impairment in HRQL. A 0.5 unit per question change resulting from therapy is considered clinically meaningful.[45]

The tailoring of the dyspnea questions to the individual patient enhances the ability of the questionnaire to detect changes in HRQL, making this a desirable tool for outcome assessment in pulmonary rehabilitation. Its responsiveness is probably further enhanced by allowing patients to see their previous responses.[46] The five individual-specific questions rating dyspnea, however, diminish the discriminative abilities of this questionnaire. For example, one patient with mild respiratory disease might choose a dyspnea-producing activity such as jogging and another with severe disease might choose walking. Because the activities are so different, the dyspnea scores cannot be compared.

Controlled clinical trials of pulmonary rehabilitation using the CRDQ in outcome assessment are listed in Table 20-4.[24,47-50] An example of the utility of the CRDQ is the randomized, controlled trial of inpatient pulmonary rehabilitation for COPD by Goldstein and colleagues.[47] CRDQ domain score treatment effects are given in Figure 20-5. The postrehabilitation increases in all four domains were *statistically* greater than the corresponding changes for the untreated control group. However, using the 0.5 unit per question cutoff value for clinical significance,[6] only the dyspnea and mastery dimensions were *clinically* meaningful.

Table 20-4. Examples of Randomized, Controlled Studies of Pulmonary Rehabilitation Using the Chronic Respiratory Disease Questionnaire (CRDQ) to Measure HRQL

Study	Type of Rehabilitation	Change in CRDQ[a] in Treatment Group
Goldstein et al., 1994[13]	Inpatient pulmonary rehabilitation for 8 wk followed by supervised outpatient training for 16 wk	Improvements in dyspnea (0.6 units, $P = .006$), emotion (0.4 units, $P = .015$), and mastery (0.7 units, $P = .0002$) domains; the change in fatigue approached statistical significance (0.45, $P = .051$)[b]
Wijkstra et al., 1994[48]	Home-based comprehensive pulmonary rehabilitation for 12 wk	Improvements in dyspnea (0.9 units), emotion (0.6 units), fatigue (0.9 units), and mastery (0.6 units) domains (all, $P < .001$)
Cambach et al., 1997[49]	3 mo of home-based pulmonary rehabilitation	Improvements in dyspnea (1.2 units), fatigue (1.0 units), emotion (0.9 units), and mastery (0.75 units) domains at 3 mo[c]
Bendstrup et al., 1997[50]	Comprehensive outpatient pulmonary rehabilitation for 12 wk	Improvement in the total CRDQ score by 0.3 units at 6 wk, 0.4 units at 12 wk, and 0.6 units at 24 wk; the improvement in the 24-wk measurement was statistically significant
Wedzicha et al., 1998[24]	8 wk of comprehensive outpatient pulmonary rehabilitation; hospital based for those with moderate dyspnea, home based for those with severe dyspnea	For patients with moderate dyspnea given hospital-based intervention, the total CRDQ score increased by 0.7 units ($P < .0001$); for those given home pulmonary rehabilitation, total CRDQ score increased by 0.2 units, which was significantly greater than its baseline ($P < .05$), not different from the change in an education control group

HRQL, health-related quality of life; COPD, chronic obstructive pulmonary disease.
[a]CRDQ domain scores are expressed as mean change per question. Each question is scored on a 1–7 scale. A 0.5 unit change per question is considered clinically significant.
[b]Treatment effects (change in rehabilitation group CRDQ minus change in control group CRDQ).
[c]Asthma and COPD patients were studied. These results are from the subgroup (RC) with COPD.

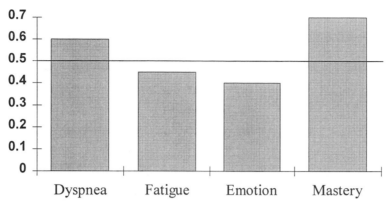

Figure 20-5. The effect of pulmonary rehabilitation on HRQL. The bars represent treatment effects: change in the CRDQ domain scores for rehabilitation patients minus corresponding changes in the domain scores for the untreated control group. Results are expressed in mean per-question changes. Each question can range from 1 (lowest score) to 7 (highest score). The *horizontal line* indicates a clinically meaningful change of 0.5 unit change per question. (Data from Goldstein RS, Gort EH, Stubbing D, et al. Randomized controlled trial of respiratory rehabilitation. Lancet 1994;344:1394–1397.)

The SGRQ

The SGRQ[7] is a 76-item respiratory-specific self-complete questionnaire requiring about 15 minutes to complete. Unlike the CRDQ, the instrument is proven valid for asthma as well as COPD patients. It measures HRQL in three domains: symptoms (distress owing to respiratory symptoms), activity (the effects owing to impairment of mobility or physical activity), and impacts (the psychosocial impact of the disease). A summary score can also be calculated. Another feature of the SGRQ is that the scoring of individual questions is weighted using empirically derived weights. Each of the three domains and the total score can range from 0 (no reduction in HRQL) to 100 (maximal reduction in HRQL). Questions specifically related to anxiety or depression were intentionally excluded from the SGRQ, so a separate questionnaire would have to be given to capture this outcome area.

Because HRQL is multidimensional, it is understandable that it is probably influenced by several aspects of the individual's morbidity. For example, a multiple regression analysis evaluating factors related to the SGRQ[51] identified dyspnea, depression, wheeze, and the 6-minute walk distance as predictors of the total SGRQ score. Interestingly, the FEV_1 was not significantly predictive in this model. These varied factors, however, explained less than 50% of the variance in HRQL. Dyspnea is a strong predictor of SGRQ measured HRQL,[25] as illustrated in Figure 20-6. Ketelaars and associates[43] evaluated the contributions of multiple factors to HRQL in 148 patients recruited for pulmonary rehabilitation. These factors included age, socioeconomic variables, respiratory disease severity, functional exercise capacity, and coping ability/strategy. Although no significant correlations were found between physiologic function and the SGRQ symptom score, a lower FEV_1, decreased maximum negative inspiratory pressure, and a decreased 12-minute walk distance all were associated with poorer SGRQ activity and impact domain scores. Interestingly, an avoidance coping strategy was related to less impairment in SGRQ activity and impact scores, suggesting that those individuals more likely to deny the significance of their disease are also more likely to report less impairment in HRQL.

A decrease in an SGRQ domain or total score by 4 or more units (i.e., 4% of its range) is considered a clinically meaningful improvement. The questionnaire has adequate reliability and validity and has been shown to be able to detect clinically meaningful

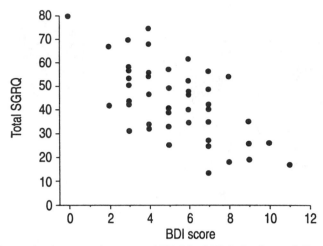

Figure 20-6. The relationship between dyspnea and HRQL. *SGRQ*, St. George's Respiratory Questionnaire; *BDI*, Baseline Dyspnea Index. (Reprinted with permission from Shoup R, Dalsky G, Warner S, et al. Body mass and quality of life in obstructive airway disease. Eur Respir J 1997;10:1578.)

changes in HRQL in COPD patients given the long-acting bronchodilator salmeterol (Fig. 20-7).[52] The SGRQ has also been able to detect the favorable change resulting from the use of nasal intermittent positive-pressure ventilation in hypoxemic, hypercapnic COPD.[53] The SGRQ has not been shown, however, to be particularly responsive to detecting favorable changes resulting from pulmonary rehabilitation. For instance, in a randomized, controlled study of pulmonary rehabilitation by Wedzicha and colleagues[24] that used both the CRDQ and the SGRQ as outcome measures, the investigators were able to show improvement in the treatment group in the CRDQ but not the SGRQ. The SGRQ, however, has been used successfully to discriminate between groups of patients with varying levels of disease severity. For example, in a study evaluating the effects of long-term oxygen therapy,[54] patients with hypoxemic COPD had much higher SGRQ scores (i.e., worse quality of life) than their nonhypoxemic counterparts.

The SF-36

The SF-36 is a 36-item self-complete questionnaire that measures general HRQL in eight areas.[55] Five of its scales (physical functioning, role-physical, bodily pain, social functioning, and role-emotional) define HRQL as the absence of limitation or disability. For these, a score of 100 indicates no limitations or disabilities. Three scales (general health, vitality, and mental health) are bipolar and measure negative and positive states. For these, a score of 50 indicates no limitations or disability and scores between 50 and 100 indicate positive health states. Two SF-36 summary scores, the physical component summary and the mental component summary, have been recently introduced.[56] These summary scores are standardized to have a mean of 50 and a standard deviation of 10 in normal populations. The SF-36 questionnaire takes just a few minutes to complete, but its scoring requires a considerable amount of hand calculation or computer assistance.

A general HRQL measure such as the SF-36 is less able to detect changes resulting from pulmonary rehabilitation intervention than respiratory-specific measures such as the CRDQ. However, its wider scope might allow for better detection of comorbidity, which is so common and important in individuals referred to pulmonary rehabilitation. To date, the ability of this instrument to detect changes resulting from pulmonary rehabilitation has not been clearly defined. Furthermore, the magnitude of change in the scales or component summary scores that is clinically meaningful for pulmonary rehabilitation

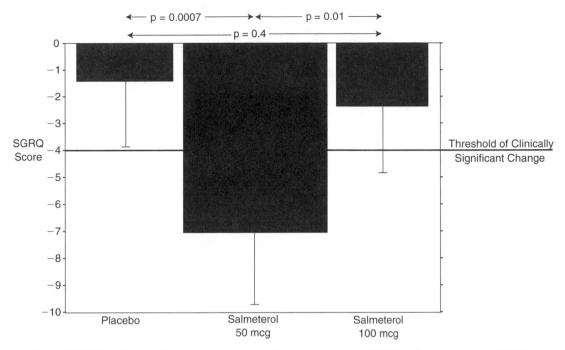

Figure 20-7. The effect of long-acting bronchodilator therapy on HRQL of patients with COPD. *SGRQ,* St. George's Respiratory Questionnaire. (Reprinted with permission from Jones PW, Bosh TK. In association with an international study group. Quality of life changes in COPD treated with salmeterol. Am J Respir Crit Care Med 1997;155:1286.)

patients is uncertain. Changes in the SF-36, however, have been shown to correlate with changes in patient-perceived health over time.[57] Several questionnaire scales, especially physical functioning, social functioning, role-physical, pain, vitality, and general health have been found to correlate well with measures of COPD disease severity.[58] In patients with COPD, dyspnea is, by far, the strongest predictor of SF-36 scores.[58]

QUESTIONNAIRE-MEASURED FUNCTIONAL STATUS

Functional status refers to the extent individuals perform their usual behaviors and activities without limitation from health problems.[59] For individuals with advanced lung disease, functional status relates predominantly to the individual's ability to perform ADLs.[60] ADLs serve to meet basic physical, psychologic, social, or spiritual needs; fulfill usual roles; and maintain health and well-being.[61] Functional status can be described as having four dimensions: capacity, performance, reserve, and capacity utilization (Fig. 20-8).[62] *Functional capacity* refers to the maximal potential to perform daily activities, analogous to the peak oxygen consumption in incremental exercise testing. *Functional performance* refers to the daily activities actually done, which for most individuals is considerably less than functional capacity. *Functional reserve* reflects the difference between performance and capacity, and *functional capacity utilization* indicates how close functional performance approaches functional capacity.

ADLs, which are physical components of functional performance, can be divided into basic and instrumental activities.[63] Basic ADLs include tasks concerned with daily self-care, such as feeding, dressing, personal hygiene, bowel function, and physical mobility. Many patients with chronic lung disease have dyspnea with these activities but remain able to perform them. Instrumental ADLs include higher-level tasks necessary to adapt

Table 1—*Relationships Among the Dimensions of Functional Status*

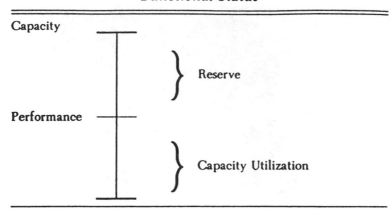

Figure 20-8. Functional status components. (Reprinted with permission from Leidy NK. Using functional status to assess treatment outcomes. Chest 1994;106:1645.)

independently to the environment,[64] such as cooking, shopping, home chores, walking outdoors, housework, doing laundry, driving a car, and gardening. Because they are more complex and require more energy expenditure than basic ADLs, they are more likely to be affected by respiratory disease. Limitation or elimination of instrumental ADLs, usually from associated dyspnea or fatigue, is a major component to the handicap from advanced chronic lung disease.

The concepts, functional status and HRQL, are not interchangeable. HRQL represents the gap between what is desired and what is achievable within the confines of the disease process.[65] In essence, it reflects in large part the impact of symptoms and limitation in ADL on the individual patient. Therefore, functional status is an important *component* of HRQL.

Patients with chronic respiratory disease that is severe enough to warrant referral for pulmonary rehabilitation often have significant impairments in ADLs. Although HRQL instruments have items pertaining to functional status, questionnaires that focus on ADLs explore this area of morbidity in more depth. The generic Extended Activities of Daily Living (EADL) scale[66] and two respiratory-specific questionnaires, the Pulmonary Functional Status Scale (PFSS)[67] and the Pulmonary Functional Status and Dyspnea Questionnaire (PFSDQ), which have been used in pulmonary rehabilitation assessment will be discussed.

The EADL Scale

This 22-item generic questionnaire[68] rates the performance (yes-no) in 22 extended (i.e., instrumental) ADLs in four domains: *mobility* (walking outside, climbing stairs, getting in and out of a car, walking over uneven ground, crossing the street, using public transport), *kitchen activities* (eating, making a hot drink, carrying hot drinks from room to room, washing, preparing a snack), *domestic tasks* (managing money, washing small clothing items, housework, shopping, full laundry), and *leisure activities* (reading newspaper or book, telephoning, writing letters, going out socially, gardening, driving a car).

The EADL scale was able to discriminate between 23 COPD patients who were oxygen dependent and 19 patients with slightly less severe airflow obstruction but no oxygen dependency.[69] In contrast, the HRQL measure, the SGRQ, was not significantly different in the two groups. EADL scores were related to the degree of airflow obstruction, HRQL, and mood state.

The PFSS

The PFSS is a 56-item, self-administered questionnaire that gives a total score and subscores of daily activities/social functioning, dyspnea, and psychological status. Completion time is about 15 minutes. The daily activities/social functioning subscore, which measures functional performance, has components of self-care, daily activities, household tasks, grocery shopping and meal preparation, transportation (mobility), and relationships. PFSS functional activities correlates strongly ($r = 0.76$) with the timed walk distance.[70] Although this questionnaire to date has not been used much as an evaluative instrument, two uncontrolled studies showed its ability to detect a positive response to rehabilitative intervention.[70,71] The responsiveness of the individual daily activities/social functioning component scores to inpatient pulmonary rehabilitation is depicted in Figure 20-9.

The PFSDQ[72]

The PFSDQ is a 164-item, self-administered questionnaire that requires about 15 to 20 minutes to complete. The limitation in performance and the level of dyspnea are rated

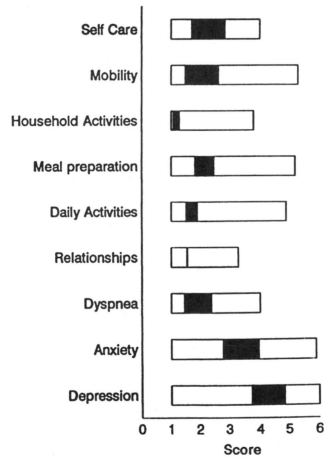

Figure 20-9. The effect of inpatient pulmonary rehabilitation on functional activities. The left and right margins of the *solid bars* indicate the pre- and post-inpatient pulmonary rehabilitation mean scores, respectively; the left and right margins of the *white bars* indicate minimum and maximum attainable scores, respectively. (Reprinted with permission from Votto J, Bowen J, Scalise P, et al. Short-stay comprehensive inpatient pulmonary rehabilitation for advanced chronic obstructive pulmonary disease. Arch Phys Med Rehabil 1996;77:1117.)

separately for each activity. The questionnaire has component scores of self-care, mobility, eating, home management, social activities, and recreational activities. Its activity total score correlates weakly with the percent-predicted FEV_1 and moderately with maximal oxygen consumption on exercise testing.[73] The PFSDQ can discriminate varying degrees of airway obstruction in COPD[74] and can detect change resulting from pharmacologic intervention.[75]

A much-shortened, modified version of the PFSDQ, the PFSDQ-M, was recently developed. Ten common activities are rated separately for activity (whether it is still done), associated dyspnea, and associated fatigue. These categories include brushing or combing hair, putting on a shirt, washing hair, showering, raising arms over head, preparing a snack, walking 3.5 m, walking on inclines, walking on bumpy terrain, and climbing three stairs.

Both the PFSDQ and the PFSDQ-M hold promise as measures of activity limitation and associated dyspnea for individuals with advanced lung disease. However, their ability to detect changes resulting from pulmonary rehabilitation has not been fully explored.

NUTRITIONAL STATUS

Abnormalities in nutritional status in individuals with chronic lung disease include increases or decreases in body weight and abnormalities in body composition. Body weight can be assessed as a percentage of ideal body weight or as the body mass index (expressed in kilograms per meters squared). In patients with COPD, decreased weight is associated with increased mortality independent of lung function.[76] Low body weight is also associated with decreased exercise performance on timed walk testing[77] and reduced muscle aerobic capacity during incremental stationary bicycle exercise.[78]

Body composition can be evaluated using anthropometry or bioelectrical impedance analysis, which estimate fat-free mass, or dual-energy x-ray absorptiometry, which estimates lean mass. Reductions in fat-free or lean body mass, which reflect the impact of advanced pulmonary disease on the peripheral musculature, may even be present in patients with normal weight.[79,25] Alterations in body composition are correlated with impaired performance on timed walk testing[79] and poorer HRQL independent of body weight.[25] An example of the effect of body weight and composition on HRQL is given in Figure 20-10.

In view of its prevalence and its relationship to the morbidity and mortality of patients with advanced chronic lung disease, the measurement of nutritional status should be considered as an outcome measure for pulmonary rehabilitation. However, to date, nutritional intervention has met with questionable success in COPD patients,[80] and recent studies have focused on hormonal supplementation to increase lean mass.[81] It remains unproved, however, whether nutritional or hormonal therapy will affect morbidity or mortality in COPD.

SURVIVAL

To date, only one randomized, controlled study of pulmonary rehabilitation has evaluated its effect on long-term survival. Ries and colleagues[9] randomly assigned patients with COPD to either an 8-week comprehensive outpatient pulmonary rehabilitation (57 patients) or a control group, where patients were given educational sessions (62 patients). Although 67% of the rehabilitation group versus 56% of the education control group were still alive at 6 years, this difference was not statistically significant ($P = .3$). The survival graph from this study is given in Figure 20-11.

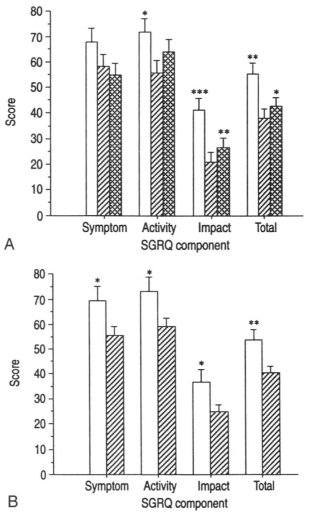

Figure 20-10. The relationship between body weight (**A**) and composition (**B**) and SGRQ-measured HRQL. *P < .05, **P < .01, and ***P < .001 versus patients with normal weight and normal composition. SGRQ, St. George's Respiratory Questionnaire (Modified with permission from Shoup R, Dalsky G, Warner S, et al. Body mass and quality of life in obstructive airway disease. Eur Respir J 1997;10:1579.)

HEALTH CARE UTILIZATION

Uncontrolled studies of health care utilization in pulmonary rehabilitation generally compare the number of hospital days or emergency department visits during a period of time before rehabilitation with a period of time after rehabilitation. These studies are subject to a regression to the mean bias because patients are often referred to pulmonary rehabilitation after a deterioration in condition that resulted in medical resource consumption. One relatively recent controlled study of outpatient pulmonary rehabilitation by Ries and colleagues[9] included an analysis of health care utilization, which consisted of self-reports of hospitalizations at each annual follow-up visit during a 6-year period. The mean number of hospital days in the year before randomization was not significantly different in the two groups: 6.4 days in the rehabilitation group and 3.6 days in the control group. At

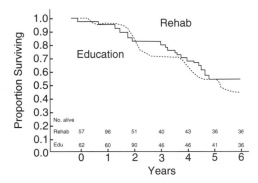

Figure 20-11. The effect of outpatient pulmonary rehabilitation on survival. (Reprinted with permission from Ries AL, Kaplan RM, Limberg TM, et al. Effects of pulmonary rehabilitation on physiologic and psychosocial outcomes in patients with chronic obstructive pulmonary disease. Ann Intern Med 1995;122:830.)

12 months, the mean number of days in the rehabilitation group decreased by 2.4 days, whereas it increased by 1.3 days in the control group. This difference, however, was not statistically significant ($P = .2$).

WHICH OUTCOME MEASURE(S) TO CHOOSE

Measurement of outcomes should be incorporated into every comprehensive pulmonary rehabilitation program. The extent of assessment will depend on the purpose of the

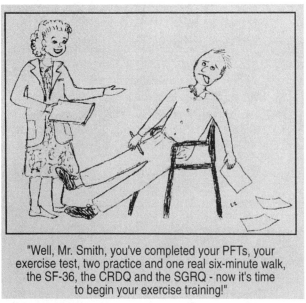

"Well, Mr. Smith, you've completed your PFTs, your exercise test, two practice and one real six-minute walk, the SF-36, the CRDQ and the SGRQ - now it's time to begin your exercise training!"

Figure 20-12. The potential effect of including too many outcome measures in pulmonary rehabilitation. *PFTs,* pulmonary function tests; *SF-36,* Medical Outcomes Study Short-Form 36; *CRDQ,* Chronic Respiratory Disease Questionnaire; *SGRQ,* St. George's Respiratory Questionnaire. (Reprinted with permission from ZuWallack R. Outcome assessment for pulmonary rehabilitation. Eur Respir Monogr, 2000.)

measurement, the goals of the program, and the level of clinician expertise in the evaluation of outcomes. Most clinical programs are not equipped to do a survival or cost-effectiveness analysis of their patients—that is best reserved for multicenter, controlled trials. For clinical purposes, assessment of exercise ability, dyspnea, and HRQL is reasonable and probably not too burdensome to the staff. The 6-minute walk test has proved to be an excellent field measure of functional exercise performance for pulmonary rehabilitation. The BDI and TDI, likewise, are valid and able to detect changes resulting from pulmonary rehabilitation. The CRDQ has the best track record as a responsive instrument for evaluating pulmonary rehabilitation. It does, however, require some expertise and time in administering it to the patient. The easier-to-administer SGRQ has good discriminant properties but has, to date, not shown improvement with pulmonary rehabilitation. Whichever measures are chosen, certainly the situation portrayed in Figure 20-12[82] is to be avoided.

REFERENCES

1. ATS statement on pulmonary rehabilitation. 1999, in press.
2. Pulmonary rehabilitation: joint ACCP/AACVPR evidence-based guidelines. J Cardiopulm Rehabil 1997;17:371–405.
3. Guyatt GH, Pugsley O, Sullivan MJ, et al. Effect of encouragement on walking test performance. Thorax 1984;39:818–822.
4. Juniper EF. Quality of life questionnaires: does statistically significant = clinically important? J Allergy Clin Immunol 1998;102:16–17.
5. Redelmeier DA, Bayoumi AM, Goldstein RS, et al. Interpreting small differences in functional status: the six minute walk test in chronic lung disease patients. Am J Respir Crit Care Med 1997;155:1278–1282.
6. Guyatt GH, Townsend M, Pugsley SO, et al. Bronchodilators in chronic air-flow limitation. Am Rev Respir Dis 1987;135:1069–1074.
7. Jones PW, Quirk FH, Baveystock CM, et al. A self-complete measure for chronic airflow limitation: the St. George's Respiratory Questionnaire. Am Rev Respir Dis 1992;145:1321–1327.
8. Vale F, Reardon JZ, ZuWallack RL. The long-term benefits of outpatient pulmonary rehabilitation on exercise endurance and quality of life. Chest 1993;103:42–45.
9. Ries AL, Kaplan RM, Limberg TM, et al. Effects of pulmonary rehabilitation on physiologic and psychosocial outcomes in patients with chronic obstructive pulmonary disease. Ann Intern Med 1995;122:823–832.
10. O'Donnell DE, McGuire M, Samis L, et al. The impact of exercise reconditioning on breathlessness in severe chronic airflow limitation. Am J Respir Crit Care Med 1995;152:2005–2013.
11. Strijbos JH, Postma DS, van Altena R, et al. A comparison between an outpatient hospital-based pulmonary rehabilitation program and a home-care pulmonary rehabilitation program in patients with COPD. Chest 1996;109:366–372.
12. Casaburi R, Patessio A, Loli F, et al. Reductions in exercise lactic acidosis and ventilation as a result of exercise training in patients with obstructive lung disease. Am Rev Respir Dis 1991;143:9–18.

13. Goldstein RS, Gort EH, Stubbing D, et al. Randomized controlled trial of respiratory rehabilitation. Lancet 1994;344:1394–1397.
14. Cambach W, Chadwick-Straver RVM, Wagenaar RC, et al. The effects of a community-based pulmonary rehabilitation programme on exercise tolerance and quality of life: a randomized controlled trial. Eur Respir 1997;10:104–113.
15. McGavin CR, Gupta SP, McHardy GJR. Twelve-minute walking test for assessing disability in chronic bronchitis. Br Med J 1976;1:822–823.
16. Mungall IPF, Hainsworth R. Assessment of respiratory function in patients with chronic obstructive airways disease. Thorax 1979;34:254–258.
17. http://www.nhlbi.nih.gov/nhlbi/lung/lvrspr.htm.
18. Larson JL, Covey MK, Vitalo CA, et al. Reliability and validity of the 12-minute distance walk in patients with chronic obstructive pulmonary disease. Nurs Res 1996;45:203–210.
19. Guyatt GH, Pugsley O, Sullivan MJ, et al. Effect of encouragement on walking test performance. Thorax 1984;39:818–822.
20. Steele B. Timed walking tests of exercise capacity in chronic cardiopulmonary disease. J Cardiopulm Rehab 1996;16:25–33.
21. Redelmeier DA, Bayoumi AM, Goldstein RS, et al. Interpreting small differences in functional status: the six minute walk test in chronic lung disease patients. Am J Respir Crit Care Med 1997;155:1278–1282.
22. Singh SJ, Morgan MDL, Scott S, et al. Development of a shuttle walking test of disability in patients with chronic airways obstruction. Thorax 1992;47:1019–1024.
23. Singh SJ, Morgan MDL, Hardman AE, et al. Comparison of oxygen uptake during a conventional treadmill test and the shuttle walking test in chronic airflow limitation. Eur Respir J 1994;7:2016–2020.
24. Wedzicha JA, Bestall JC, Garrod R, et al. Randomized controlled trial of pulmonary rehabilitation in severe chronic obstructive pulmonary disease patients, stratified with the MRC dyspnoea scale. Eur Respir J 1998;12:363–369.
25. Shoup R, Dalsky G, Warner S, et al. Body composition and health-related quality of life in patients with chronic obstructive airways disease. Eur Respir J 1997;10:1576–1580.

26. Siafakas NM, Schiza S, Xirouhaki N, et al. Is dyspnoea the main determinant of quality of life in the failing lung? A review. Eur Respir Rev 1997;7:53–56.

27. Celli B, Rassulo J, Make B. Dyssynchronous breathing during arm but not leg exercise in patients with chronic airflow obstruction. N Engl J Med 1986;314:1485–1490.

28. Sweer L, Zwillich CW. Dyspnea in the patient with chronic obstructive pulmonary disease: etiology and management. Clin Chest Med 1990; 11:417–439.

29. Carrieri-Kohlman V, Gormley JM, Douglas MK, et al. Differentiation between dyspnea and its affective components. West J Nurs Res 1996; 18:626–642.

30. Simoni P, Foglio K, Zanoni C, et al. Symptom limited exercise in COPD: do dyspnea and leg discomfort identify different groups of patients. Eur Respir J 1997;10:373s.

31. Borg GAV. Psychophysical bases of perceived exertion. Med Sci Sports Exerc 1982;14:377–381.

32. Reardon J, Awad E, Normandin E, et al. The effect of comprehensive outpatient pulmonary rehabilitation on dyspnea. Chest 1994;105:1046–1052.

33. Mahler DA, Weinberg DH, Wells CK, et al. The measurement of dyspnea: contents, interobserver agreement, and physiologic correlations of two new clinical indexes. Chest 1984;85:751–758.

34. Mahler DA, Wells CK. Evaluation of clinical methods for rating dyspnea. Chest 1988;93:580–586.

35. Guyatt GH, Berman LB, Townsend M, et al. A measure of quality of life for clinical trials in chronic lung disease. Thorax 1987;42:773–778.

36. Mahler DA, Tomlinson D, Olmstead EM, et al. Changes in dyspnea, health status, and lung function in chronic airway disease. Am J Respir Crit Care Med 1995;151:61–65.

37. Mahler D, ZuWallack R, Rickard K, et al. Effects of salmeterol and ipratropium on dyspnea as measured by the six minute walk and baseline dyspnea index/transitional dyspnea index (BDI/TDI). Am J Respir Crit Care Med 1997;155:A278.

38. Ferrans C, Powers M. Quality of life index: development of psychometric properties. Adv Nurs Sci 1990;8:15–24.

39. Quality of Life Database, 1998. In: American Thoracic Society Website. Available at: http://www.thoracic.org/qol/qoldata.html [August 18, 1998].

40. Gill TM, Feinstein AR. A critical appraisal of the quality of quality-of-life measurements. JAMA 1994;272:619–626.

41. Guyatt GH, Feeny DH, Patrick DL. Measuring health-related quality of life. Ann Intern Med 1993;118:622–629.

42. Jones PW. Issues concerning health-related quality of life in COPD. Chest 1995;107:187s–193s.

43. Ketelaars CAJ, Schlosser MAG, Mostert R, et al. Determinants of health-related quality of life in patients with chronic obstructive pulmonary disease. Thorax 1996;51:39–43.

44. Jones PW. Assessment of the impact of mild asthma in adults. Eur Respir Rev 1996;6:57–60.

45. Jaeschke R, Singer J, Guyatt GH. Measurement of health status: ascertaining the minimal clinically important difference. Control Clin Trials 1989; 10:407–415.

46. Guyatt GH, Berman LB, Townsend M, et al. Should study subjects see their previous responses? J Chronic Dis 1985;38:1003–1007.

47. Goldstein RS, Gort EH, Stubbing D, et al. Randomised controlled trial of respiratory rehabilitation. Lancet 1994;344:1394–1397.

48. Wijkstra PJ, Van Altena R, Krann J, et al. Quality of life in patients with chronic obstructive pulmonary disease improves after rehabilitation at home. Eur Respir J 1994;7:269–273.

49. Cambach W, Chadwick-Straver RVM, Wagenaar RC, et al. The effects of a community-based pulmonary rehabilitation programme on exercise tolerance and quality of life: a randomized controlled trial. Eur Respir J 1997;10:104–113.

50. Bendstrup KE, Ingemann Jensen J, Holm S, et al. Out-patient rehabilitation improves activities of daily living, quality of life and exercise tolerance in chronic obstructive pulmonary disease. Eur Respir J 1997;10:2801–2806.

51. Jones PW. Issues concerning health-related quality of life in COPD. Chest 1995;107:187s–192s.

52. Jones PW, Bosh TK. In association with an international study group. Quality of life changes in COPD treated with salmeterol. Am J Respir Crit Care Med 1997;155:1283–1289.

53. Meecham Jones DJ, Paul EA, Jones PW, et al. Nasal pressure support ventilation plus oxygen compared to oxygen therapy alone in hypercapneic COPD. Am J Respir Crit Care Med 1995; 152:538–544.

54. Okubadejo AA, Paul EA, Jones PW, et al. Does long-term oxygen therapy affect quality of life in patients with chronic obstructive pulmonary disease and severe hypoxaemia? Eur Respir J 1996; 9:2335–2339.

55. Ware JE. SF-36 health survey manual and interpretation guide. Boston, MA: The Health Institute, New England Medical Center.

56. Ware JE, Kosinski M, Keller SD. SF-36 Physical & Mental Health Summary Scales: A User's Manual. Boston: The Health Institute, New England Medical Center, 1994.

57. Harper R, Brazier JE, Waterhouse JC, et al. Comparison of outcome measures for patients with chronic obstructive pulmonary disease (COPD) in an outpatient setting. Thorax 1997;52:879–887.

58. Mahler DA, Mackowiak JI. Evaluation of the short-form 36-item questionnaire to measure health-related quality of life in patients with COPD. Chest 1995;107:1585–1589.

59. Ware JE. SF-36 Health Survey Manual and Interpretation Guide (Glossary:3). Boston: The Health Institute, New England Medical Center, 1993.

60. Lareau SC, Breslin EH, Meek PM. Functional status instruments: outcome measure in the evaluation of patients with chronic obstructive pulmonary disease. Heart Lung 1996;25:212–224.

61. Leidy NK. Functional status and the forward progress of merry-go-rounds: toward a coherent analytical framework. Nurs Res 1994;43:196–202.

62. Leidy NK. Using functional status to assess treatment outcomes. Chest 1994;106:1645–1646.

63. Guccione AA. Functional assessment. In: Physical Medicine and Rehabilitation: Assessment and Treatment. Philadelphia: 1994:193–208.

64. Spector WD, Katz S, Murphy JB, et al. The hierarchical relationship between activities of daily living and instrumental activities of daily living. J Chronic Dis 1987;40:481–489.

65. Jones PW. Issues concerning health-related quality of life in COPD. Chest 1995;107:187s–193s.

66. Lincoln NB, Gladman JRF. The extended activities of daily living scale: a further validation. Disabil Rehabil 1992;14:41–43.

67. Weaver TE, Narsavage GL. Physiological and psychological variables related to functional status in chronic obstructive pulmonary disease. Nurs Res 1992;41:286–291.

68. Lincoln NB, Gladman JRF. The extended activities of living scale: a further validation. Disabil Rehabil 1992;14:41–43.

69. Okubadejo AA, O'Shea L, Jones PW, et al. Home assessment of activities of daily living in patients with severe chronic obstructive pulmonary disease on long-term oxygen therapy. Eur Respir J 1997;10:1572–1575.

70. Haggerty MC, Stockdale-Wolley R, ZuWallack R. Functional status in pulmonary rehabilitation participants. J Cardiopulm Rehabil. 1999;19:35–42.

71. Votto J, Bowen J, Scalise P, et al. Short-stay comprehensive inpatient pulmonary rehabilitation for advanced chronic obstructive pulmonary disease. Arch Phys Med Rehabil 1996;77:1115–1118.

72. Lareau S, Carrieri-Kohlman V, Janson-Bjerklie Roos P. Development and testing of the pulmonary functional status and dyspnea questionnaire (PFSDQ). Heart Lung 1994;23:242–250.

73. Lareau SC, Breslin EH, Meek PM. Functional status instruments: outcome measure in the evaluation of patients with chronic obstructive pulmonary disease. Heart Lung 1996;25:212–224.

74. Lareau SC, Breslin EH, Anholm JD, et al. Reduction in arm activities in patients with severe obstructive pulmonary disease. Am Rev Respir Dis 1990;145:A476.

75. Borson S, McDonald GJ, Gayle T, et al. Improvement in mood, physical symptoms, and function with nortriptylline for depression in patients with chronic obstructive pulmonary disease. Psychosomatics 1992;33:190–201.

76. Gray-Donald K, Gibbons L, Shapiro SH, et al. Nutritional status and mortality in chronic obstructive pulmonary disease. Am J Respir Crit Care Med 1996;153:961–966.

77. Schols AMWJ, Mostert R, Soeters PB, et al. Body composition and exercise performance in patients with chronic obstructive pulmonary disease. Thorax 1991;46:695–699.

78. Palange P, Forte S, Onorati P, et al. Effect of reduced body weight on muscle aerobic capacity in patients with COPD. Chest 1998;114:12–18.

79. Schols AMWJ, Soeters PB, Dingemans AMC, et al. Prevalence and characteristics of nutritional depletion in patients with stable COPD eligible for pulmonary rehabilitation. Am Rev Respir Dis 1993;147:1151–1156.

80. Fitting JW. Nutritional support in chronic obstructive lung disease. Thorax 1992;47:141–143.

81. Casaburi R, Carithers E, Tosolini J, et al. Randomized controlled trial of growth hormone in severe COPD patients undergoing endurance training. Am J Respir Crit Care Med 1997;155:A498.

82. ZuWallack RL. Selection criteria and outcome assessment in pulmonary rehabilitation. Monaldi Arch Chest Dis 1998;53:429–437.

21 Home Mechanical Ventilation in the USA

Douglas C. Johnson

⧪ Professional Skills

Upon completion of this chapter, the reader will:

- Identify which patients might benefit from home mechanical ventilation (HMV)
- Describe the different modes of HMV, including both invasive and noninvasive
- Understand issues related to the costs of HMV
- Know issues related to training and nonventilator aspects of HMV

DEFINITION / HISTORY

HMV is a method of treating chronic respiratory failure in the home rather than in the hospital or another institution. Home ventilation first began in the United States in the late 1940s when some postpolio patients returned home using body ventilators (iron lungs). In the 1950s, intermittent positive-pressure ventilation (IPPV) via a mouthpiece was used in some centers for daytime support. In the 1960s and 1970s, chronic mechanical ventilation was usually performed through tracheostomy and IPPV. In recent years, ventilatory support without tracheostomy via noninvasive methods has become increasingly common.

GOALS

Advances in respiratory care have made it possible to prolong the life and improve the quality of life of many patients with chronic respiratory failure. Home care management of ventilator-assisted individuals has been promoted by concerns for improved quality of life and reduced costs. Important objectives of HMV[1] include (*a*) improvement in quality of life, (*b*) improvement in survival, (*c*) reduced hospitalization, and (*d*) reductions in cost. Common outcome indicators include improvement in arterial blood gases, hospitalizations, incidence of pneumonia, survival, exercise tolerance, and measures of quality of life.

EPIDEMIOLOGY

Although some countries have nationwide databases of patients receiving HMV,[2] no such database exists for the United States. A comprehensive evaluation of the numbers of patients undergoing HMV in the United States has not been successful, with a lack of an effective approach to track the use and practices of home ventilator use.[3]

Some state and regional studies of HMV use in the United States show a significant increase in the number of patients receiving long-term ventilator support in institutional settings and in the home.[4,5] Make and Gilmartin[6] estimated that about 7,000 persons were receiving HMV and about 11,400 long-term ventilator patients were being cared for in hospitals in the United States in 1986. According to a Gallup survey,[7] about 11,419 patients were chronically ventilated nationwide in 1990 in acute care hospitals, with chronic ventilation defined as requiring mechanical ventilation for 6 hours per day or longer for 30 days or longer. About 25% of these patients were discharged to HMV and 20% to alternate sites such as nursing homes, with most continuing to receive care in the acute care hospital. In 1990, Goldberg and Frownfelter[8] identified 453 long-term (>3 weeks) ventilator-assisted individuals in Illinois (a rate of 3.6/100,000). At this rate, about 11,000 patients would be receiving long-term ventilation in the United States.

METHODS OF HOME VENTILATION

HMV can be categorized in several different ways. Ventilation can be continuous or intermittent, with intermittent use usually at night only or at night with occasional daytime use. HMV can be invasive (administered by tracheostomy) or noninvasive. Noninvasive ventilation can be administered via negative-pressure or positive-pressure devices.

In a survey of HMV in neuromuscular patients (684 patients, 13,751 patient years), Bach et al.[9] found a variety of methods used. Daytime ventilation included mouthpiece IPPV, nasal IPPV, intermittent abdominal pressure ventilators, negative-pressure body ventilators, and tracheostomy IPPV. Nocturnal ventilation devices included negative-pressure body ventilators, nasal IPPV, mouthpiece IPPV, IPPV via strapless oral–nasal interfaces, and tracheostomy IPPV. Many patients switched from one mode of support to another during the course of their illness.

Although some patients require continuous mechanical ventilation, in many patients with chronic respiratory failure 4 to 6 hours of therapy per night improves daytime gas exchange and symptoms of dyspnea. Several theories have been proposed to explain why intermittent ventilation is effective.[10,11] One possible mechanism is that intermittent rest of chronically fatigued muscles improves respiratory muscle function. Diaphragmatic electromyographic activity and respiratory muscle work are reduced during ventilation.[12,13] Another possible mechanism is improvement in lung compliance in patients with neuromuscular or chest wall disease,[14] possibly by reexpansion of areas of microatelectasis. A third possible mechanism is that by preventing nocturnal hypoventilation, mechanical ventilation prevents the blunting of central ventilatory drive that occurs with hypercapnia.[15]

SELECTION OF PATIENTS FOR CHRONIC MECHANICAL VENTILATION

The selection of patients who require chronic mechanical ventilation ($\geq$6 h/d for $\geq$ 30 d) is sometimes clear-cut but often requires considerable judgment. The decision to initiate mechanical ventilation requires knowledge of the disease process, rate of progression, and risk of complication. Several studies have shown that mechanical ventilation is beneficial for patients with neuromuscular and chest wall diseases without acute respiratory failure. Bach et al.,[9] in a retrospective study, found that the incidence of hospitalizations and pneumonia was much lower in patients with neuromuscular diseases treated with HMV than in those managed with oxygen therapy alone.

Categories of diseases managed with chronic mechanical ventilation (Box 21-1) include those with abnormal ventilator control, chest wall disorders, neuromuscular disorders, primary pulmonary disorders, and other.

Box 21-1. Conditions That May Require Long-Term
           Mechanical Ventilation

Abnormal ventilatory control
    Central hypoventilation
    Poststroke
Chest wall disorders
    Kyphoscoliosis
    Postsurgical (thoracoplasty)
Neuromuscular disorders
    Amyotrophic lateral sclerosis
    Congenital myopathies
    Diaphragm paralysis (Guillain-Barré, postsurgical)
    Muscular dystrophy
    Poliomyelitis
    Spinal cord (injury, syringomyelia)
Primary pulmonary disorders
    Bronchiectasis
    Bronchopulmonary dysplasia
    Chronic aspiration
    Chronic obstructive pulmonary disease (emphysema)
    Cystic fibrosis
    Postsurgical
Other (nocturnal ventilation only)
    Congestive heart failure and sleep disturbance
    Obstructive sleep apnea

SELECTION OF PATIENTS FOR HMV

Patients requiring long-term mechanical ventilation are treated in many different settings, including respiratory care units in acute care hospitals, weaning units in non–acute care hospitals, general medical floors, specialized nursing homes, and the home.

Once it is determined that a patient will require chronic ventilatory support, an assessment should be made as to the best form of ventilatory support and whether the patient is appropriate for HMV. The intermediate ventilator care unit has played a role in several institutions in improving care, reducing costs, and preparing patients for HMV.[16–18]

HMV can be considered for most patients who are medically stable and have a supportive family situation. HMV has been found to work well for patients ranging in age from young children to the elderly.[19] Most ventilator-assisted children do well at home, including those with congenital central hypoventilation syndrome.[20,21] Care of the child with long-term ventilation in the home seems as safe as in the hospital.[22] Issues relevant to ventilation in children have been reviewed,[23–28] including those related to tracheostomy tubes in the young child.

INSTITUTING HMV

Once a patient has been identified as a candidate for HMV, several issues must be addressed, including patient training, family training, insurance approval, and arranging equipment and services. For the patient who requires only noninvasive ventilatory support at night, it is usually easy to arrange for the device and to train the patient and family. This contrasts with the patient requiring continuous home ventilation via tracheostomy, which entails more extensive patient and family training, many home services, and often difficulty with insurance approval.

OBSTACLES TO DISCHARGE FROM AN ACUTE CARE HOSPITAL

The U.S. health care system is largely free market, with involvement of state (Medicare and Medicaid), private, and charitable bodies. Home respiratory care providers are generally private, with reimbursement from the state, health maintenance organizations, or insurance. Large differences can exist in how different insurance providers deal with HMV.

DeWitt et al.[29] studied factors that contributed to delay in hospital discharge in 54 ventilator-assisted children discharged to HMV; 94% received positive-pressure ventilation (PPV) via tracheostomy and 6% received negative-pressure ventilation (NPV). These children often remained hospitalized for several months for nonmedical reasons, with time from medical stability to discharge of 118 ± 144 days. It took third-party payers more than 3 months (99 ± 141 days) to approve home care funding. Once funding was approved, it took 48 ± 87 more days to be discharged. The time for approval was about four times greater with public (184 ± 177 days) than private (52 ± 43 days) funding. Parent training took 52 ± 65 days, with some of this time owing to delays in insurance. Eighty percent of patients used in-home nursing care for 8 to 24 hours per day. The availability of home respiratory care vendors or visiting nurses did not affect the delays for any patients.

MANAGEMENT GUIDELINES

The American College of Chest Physicians[1] and the European Respiratory Society Rehabilitation and Chronic Care Scientific Group[30] have created guidelines for physicians about HMV. The American Thoracic Society[31] has developed guidelines for HMV of children. Committees of the American Society for Testing and Materials[32] developed voluntary consensus standards, and the Joint Commission for Accreditation of Health Care Organizations[33] established quality management accreditation for home care organizations providing support services related to medical technology. The Consensus Conference on Problems in Home Mechanical Ventilation[34] identified many areas of concern regarding HMV. These reports emphasize the need for proper patient selection, education of patients and family, and equipment and for providing adequate professional, daily care, and emergency services. Successful deployment of HMV requires a home care service with physician supervision. It also requires a supporting family or other care provider, adequate training of the patient and family, psychosocial support, and adequate financial support.

INVASIVE OR NONINVASIVE VENTILATION

An important decision to make is whether a patient needs a tracheostomy. Noninvasive ventilation, or ventilatory support without an endotracheal airway, can be given either by devices that apply intermittent negative extra-thoracic pressure or by using a nasal or face mask to deliver PPV.

Invasive ventilation, or ventilation via endotracheal airway, is often used for patients who are ventilator dependent for most of the time or who have significant swallowing disturbances. Tracheostomy offers dependable access to ventilation and allows for suction of secretions or aspirated material. Ventilation via a tracheostomy provides easy access for suctioning and secretion clearance, and with a cuffed tube it provides a means to prevent gross aspiration and to deliver higher pressures and volumes. Invasive ventilation has the advantages compared with NPV of having fewer restraints on posture, avoiding upper airway obstruction, and providing an increased tidal volume. However, the many disadvantages of invasive ventilation, including more frequent pulmonary infections and limitation of speech, make noninvasive ventilation preferable in patients who can be adequately ventilated with noninvasive means. A heated humidifier is usually required when the oropharynx is bypassed.

It is important to consider whether a given patient can be transitioned from tracheostomy to noninvasive ventilation. Many patients do well with noninvasive ventilation, even 24 hours per day. Although tracheostomy has traditionally been recommended for individuals who are ventilator dependent for more than 12 to 15 hours per day, considerable success has been achieved in avoiding the need for tracheostomy and in switching patients with neuromuscular and chest wall disorders from tracheostomy to noninvasive IPPV.[35,36] Although difficulty with retained secretions is cited as a reason for tracheostomy as opposed to noninvasive ventilation, use of manually or mechanically assisted coughing techniques can often provide adequate secretion clearance and allow noninvasive ventilatory support.[37]

NONINVASIVE VENTILATION

The advantages to using noninvasive ventilation are numerous.[38] Noninvasive approaches allow for normal swallowing, feeding, and speech. Cough and physiologic air warming and humidification are preserved. Noninvasive ventilation can often eliminate the need for intubation or tracheostomy, preventing such problems as injury to the vocal cords or trachea and nosocomial lower respiratory infections. Noninvasive ventilation can facilitate discharge to the home or the community.

Noninvasive PPV is commonly used at night for management of patients with chronic respiratory failure,[11] and it has proved useful in the long-term management of patients with neuromuscular disease.[39–42] Noninvasive PPV during sleep has also been shown to significantly improve daytime arterial blood gases, lung volumes, and respiratory muscle strength[43] and reduce hospitalizations[42] in patients with respiratory insufficiency caused by severe kyphoscoliosis. Noninvasive PPV improves nighttime oxygen desaturation and hypoventilation in patients with chest wall diseases without daytime respiratory failure.[44] The use of PPV and other options for ventilatory support in neuromuscular diseases has been reviewed.[45]

Noninvasive ventilation can be used as maintenance therapy in patients with intrinsic lung disease and marked hypercapnia, for example, partial pressure of carbon dioxide greater than 60 mm Hg.[46] Short-term use of a few hours per day improves respiratory pattern and blood gases in stable chronic obstructive pulmonary disease (COPD) patients with chronic hypercapnia.[47] Longer-term use of nasal PPV has been shown to benefit some hypercapnic COPD patients. A prospective randomized study found improvements in quality of life measures, sleep, arterial partial pressure of oxygen (PaO_2), and arterial partial pressure of carbon dioxide ($PaCO_2$) with 3 months of PPV.[48] However, many patients with severe chronic COPD do not tolerate long-term bilevel positive airway pressure (biPAP).[49]

NEGATIVE-PRESSURE VENTILATION

Negative pressure ventilators support ventilation by exposing the chest wall to subatmospheric pressure during inspiration, with expiration occurring as the pressure around the chest wall increases to atmospheric. The use of NPV has been reviewed.[50–52]

Body ventilators apply negative pressure to the entire body below the neck. The Emerson iron lung was widely used in the 1950s during the polio epidemic. Fiberglass descendents of the iron lung weigh less than 100 lb. Less bulky and more portable devices have been designed that primarily apply negative pressure to the thorax and abdomen. These include rigid, nonflexible cuirass shell devices and the ponchowrap, which uses a plastic grid covering the thorax that is covered with a windproof fabric sealed at the neck, waist, and arms.[53]

Uncontrolled studies uniformly show the benefit of intermittent NPV in patients with chronic respiratory failure caused by chest wall, neuromuscular, or central hypoventilation diseases.[54–57] However, for stable severe COPD patients, a large, double-blind, prospective study found no benefit of 12 weeks of NPV.[58]

Negative-pressure assisted ventilation has the advantage of not covering the face, but has not received widespread application because of poor patient acceptance, inadequate effectiveness in many patients, the awkward size of the devices, and the development of upper airway obstruction in some patients. However, patients with neuromuscular disease, chest wall deformity, central hypoventilation, or diaphragm paralysis often benefit from negative-pressure assisted ventilation.

NONINVASIVE PPV

Since the late 1980s, noninvasive PPV delivered by nasal or face mask has gained increasingly widespread acceptance for the treatment of ventilatory failure. This is largely because of the development of improved masks and improved ventilator technology. Many types and sizes of masks are available,[59] including face masks that cover the nose and mouth, nasal masks, "nasal pillows" that fit into the nostrils, and cushion devices that fit across the nostrils. An occasional patient requires a chin strap to prevent air leakage from the mouth.

VENTILATORS

Recent advances in technology have improved the types of ventilators used for both invasive and noninvasive ventilation in the home. Portable volume ventilators are much smaller and lighter than conventional hospital-based ventilators. Internal and external batteries allow ventilators to operate for 24 hours, enabling the patient to be more mobile. Portable ventilators typically provide high- and low-pressure alarms and extended battery power supplies.[60] Although home pressure support devices differ in terms of rebreathing and expiratory resistance, no significant differences in $PaCO_2$, tidal volume, or respiratory rate were found comparing an intensive care unit ventilator with a home ventilator.[61]

Positive-Pressure Ventilators

Noninvasive PPV can be given by a volume ventilator, a pressure-controlled ventilator, a bi-level positive airway pressure (PAP) ventilator, or a continuous positive airway pressure (CPAP) device. Small portable ventilators are available when nocturnal or intermittent home use is desired.[59] Relatively inexpensive, simple-to-operate portable ventilators capable of producing different inspiratory and expiratory pressures, that is, bi-level PAP, are produced by several manufacturers. These machines can maintain the pressure while providing adequate flow to meet patient need. For patients with apneas, a ventilator mode that provides a backup pressure-cycled rate is essential.

Volume Ventilators

Volume-cycled noninvasive ventilation, in which the ventilator delivers a set volume for each breath, is frequently used in management of chronic respiratory failure for HMV.[62–64] It can be used via tracheostomy, via nasal or face mask, or for day use via mouthpiece.

Some patients have poor tolerance of this therapy,[65,66] probably related to elevated inspiratory pressures related to increased airway resistance, which are uncomfortable to the patient or that cause leaks.[67]

Pressure Ventilators

Pressure-limited ventilation, in which the ventilator delivers a set pressure for each breath, can also be used via tracheostomy, nasal or face mask, or mouthpiece. This mode of ventilation, given with bi-level PAP, is frequently used for noninvasive ventilation.[38]

Bi-level PAP ventilators provide continuous high-flow positive airway pressure that cycles between a high-positive pressure and a lower-positive pressure. For spontaneous mode, bi-level PAP responds to patient flow rates to cycle between higher pressure (inhalation) and lower pressure (exhalation). It reliably senses a patient's breathing efforts, even with air leaks in the patient's circuit. When inspiration is detected, the higher pressure is delivered for a fixed time or until the flow rate falls below a threshold level.

With bi-level PAP, supplemental oxygen is diluted by a high flow of air through the system. Patients thus may require a higher liter flow of oxygen when they are receiving bi-level PAP than when using nasal cannula. A common inspiratory and expiratory line can lead to rebreathing of exhaled gas and persistent hypercapnea.[61] Rebreathing has been shown to occur with low expiratory pressure settings and the standard exhalation device during bi-level PAP.[46,68] Use of an alternative exhalation device or expiratory pressures of at least 4 cm H_2O reduces carbon dioxide rebreathing. Patients are usually started at low pressures and increased as tolerated to their final settings (usually 8 to 14 cm inspiratory pressure, 4 to 5 cm expiratory pressure).

For the standard volume ventilator, the peak inspiratory flow rate and trigger sensitivity should be set to minimize patients' effort. Ventilator circuit resistance should be kept low with the use of sufficiently large tracheostomy tube size and pass-over rather than cascade humidification systems. A low intermittent mandatory ventilation rate can contribute significantly to work of breathing.[69] So the rate should be high enough to provide most of the patient's ventilation.

So far, the Food and Drug Administration has not approved portable bi-level PAP ventilators for use with tracheostomy patients. This is primarily because of concerns about adequate alarms for totally ventilator-dependent patients. Standard ventilators can provide pressure-support or pressure-control ventilation via tracheostomy, but their size and cost make them unreasonable for home use.

LIMITATIONS OF NONINVASIVE PPV

When PPV is applied, patients should be monitored and attention should be given to comfort, level of dyspnea, respiratory rate, and oxygen saturation. Patients should be watched for signs of ventilator–patient asynchrony, nasal mask intolerance, significant air leaks, gastric distention, drying of the eyes, and facial skin breakdown, especially at the bridge of the nose. Some patients have claustrophobia with nasal or face masks.[70] Gastric distention is uncommon in the short term with pressure support levels less than 25 cm H_2O[12] but common with long-term noninvasive PPV.[71] Eye irritation or conjunctivitis has been reported in 16% of patients.[66] Facial skin necrosis has been reported in 2%[72] to 18%[73] of patients.

Intrinsic positive end-expiratory pressure is often present in patients with COPD and can lead to much respiratory effort to trigger the ventilator.[74] This can be alleviated by the addition of external positive end-expiratory pressure.[75]

Proper fit of a nasal mask is essential to provide an adequate seal and prevent nasal trauma or eye irritation. Humidification (dry or heated) may improve comfort and possibly reduce rhinitis. When a leak-tolerant noninvasive PPV system is used, it is not necessary to apply the interface so securely that it is airtight. The device can usually be loosened enough to be comfortable. Selecting masks that fit with low pressure to the skin, using nasal pillows, or alternating between different types of masks can reduce skin breakdown.

TRACHEOSTOMY TUBE SELECTION

The choice of tracheostomy tube is important for patients undergoing invasive ventilation. Types of tracheostomy tubes include cuffed or noncuffed; single cannula or double cannula, and fenestrated or nonfenestrated. The size of the cuff varies significantly between different manufacturers.

A cuffed tube is typically used with PPV. This allows a means to prevent air from leaking through the mouth and to prevent gross aspiration. However, some patients with relatively normal lungs (neuromuscular disease or cervical spine injury) can receive sufficient ventilatory support using uncuffed tubes. If an uncuffed tube is used, pressure-controlled ventilation has advantages over volume-controlled ventilation in some patients. A single-cannula tube has the advantage of having a larger inner airway for the outer size of the tube, whereas a double cannula tube is easier to clean secretions from in the tube. Fenestrated tubes have a hole or holes in the tube that, if lined up properly in the patient's airway, provide increased area to breathe through the mouth (e.g., with a speaking valve). However, if the fenestration abuts the tracheal wall it can induce granulation tissue, and a larger-sized outer diameter tube is required (compared with a single-cannula tube), which decreases the area to breathe through the mouth.

SECRETION CLEARANCE

A significant issue with HMV is adequate secretion clearance. Patients with difficulty clearing their own secretions often benefit from a mechanical insufflation-exsufflation (MIE) device. Candidates for nontracheostomy ventilator support need reliable, effective assisted coughing or MIE during respiratory tract infections. Tracheostomized patients can also benefit from MIE but frequently require suctioning as well. No standardized approach to regulations regarding tracheal suctioning exists. Typically the patient and family are trained, but some states restrict suctioning to nurses or respiratory therapists, which can significantly increase the costs of caring for patients on HMV. Bach et al.'s[76] extensive experience with HMV patients has been without incident regarding suctioning in tracheostomized patients without daily licensed nursing care.

EQUIPMENT

In the United States, every physician may prescribe home oxygen or HMV. Equipment is generally provided by commercial companies. Equipment needs vary depending on the type of ventilator support and the ability of the patient to breathe on his or her own, without the ventilator. Ventilator-dependent patients with tracheostomy have a wide variety of equipment needs (Box 21-2). Fully ventilator-dependent patients should have a backup power supply, a backup ventilator, and a manual resuscitator.

Box 21-2. Equipment for Those With Tracheostomy Receiving Home Ventilation

Suction—electric and portable
Charger for portable suction
Ventilator (e.g., positive-pressure ventilator with pressure alarms and batteries
    [2 ventilators if respiratory autonomy <4 h])
Self-inflating resuscitating bag
Suction catheters
Tracheostomy tube and tape
Syringe and needles
Sterile and clean gloves
Swedish nozzle or heat and moisture exchangers
Mechanical insufflator-exsufflator
Sterile normal saline (to loosen secretions)
Sterile dressing packs and tracheostomy gauze
Oxygen
Humidifier
Battery for ventilator, battery charger

PSYCHOLOGIC ASPECTS IN HMV

Patients receiving HMV can have a good quality of life.[77] Pehrsson et al.[78] found good psychosocial function in patients receiving HMV. However, long-term ventilator support often limits activities of daily living, restricts patient mobility, and interferes with the patient's ability to communicate verbally and eat. These can promote anxiety and a sense of isolation, with fears of death and abandonment.[79] In a survey of HMV,[5] 87% of patients felt there was a positive effect on lifestyle: life sustaining, facilitating mobility, and improved physical symptoms. Difficulties were more common early on, with 53% of patients having initial difficulties coping with the ventilator and 11% at the time of survey.[5]

IMPROVING COMMUNICATION IN THE VENTILATED PATIENT

Numerous devices allow tracheostomized patients to communicate verbally. Some devices can be used on full ventilator support (electrolarynx, talking trach, and buccal resonator) or during periods of spontaneous breathing via devices that provide airflow through the vocal cords (speaking valve with cuff deflated, with appropriately sized tube). Deflating the cuff and placing a speaking valve on the tracheostomy tube provides a means of talking during periods of spontaneous breathing. Some fully ventilator-dependent patients tolerate short periods with the cuff deflated and an "in-line" speaking valve.

Although fenestrated tracheostomy tubes have been advocated to permit speech, our experience is that speaking valves can be successfully used in most patients with appropriately sized single-cannula tubes. In addition, granulation tissue can grow into the fenestration. For patients with normal respiratory muscle strength, any of the speaking valves are well tolerated. However, for those with significant respiratory muscle weakness, a speaking valve with low inspiratory resistance, such as the Montgomery or Shiley valve, is preferable. We routinely measure airway pressures proximal to the speaking valve when assessing patients for use of the speaking valve. If the expiratory pressure is low (<6 cm H_2O with deep breathing), the speaking valve can be used with the current tracheostomy tube. If the expiratory pressure is high (>10 cm H_2O with deep breathing), a smaller outer

Box 21-3. Ventilator Training Checklist

The caregiver should be able to

- Demonstrate how to assemble and disassemble ventilator circuits
- Demonstrate how to operate ventilator controls and maintain settings
- Demonstrate how to change the ventilator setting
- Describe the ventilator alarm functions
- Demonstrate how to determine and correct the source of an alarm
- Demonstrate how to clean and maintain equipment
- Demonstrate how to set up and administer breathing treatments
- Describe how to perform emergency procedures in case of ventilator alarm failure, tracheostomy tube displacement, or mechanical airway blockage
- Demonstrate how to plug the tracheostomy tube and use supplemental oxygen for appropriate patients

diameter tube should be placed and the pressures reassessed. To provide a good seal with low cuff pressure with a small outer diameter tube, large-volume cuffs are needed.

TRAINING

Many families cope well with HMV,[80] but comprehensive training for the patient and family is essential. For noninvasive ventilation only at night, respiratory therapists can usually train the patient with the device in the home. For totally ventilator-dependent patients and those with tracheostomies, training is much more involved. Gracey[81] reviews many of the issues of home education and provides a comprehensive checklist for transition to HMV. Patients, family members, and home caregivers need to know about the ventilator, how to connect and disconnect the patient, tracheostomy tube and site care, and administering medications. Ventilator training issues are numerous (Box 21-3). Training should include the ability to handle emergency situations, including the ability to use a manual resuscitator, to connect the patient to a backup ventilator, and to clear secretions from patients (suction via tracheostomy tube and/or MIE via tube or face mask).

HOME CARE

Home supervision of patients is usually performed by medical and/or nursing personnel, who have many responsibilities.[82,83] Patients receiving full-time HMV have extensive needs for personal care tasks, with caregivers reporting an average of 8.4 hours per day caring for their family member receiving full-time HMV.[84] The range of care varies from less than 1 to 24 hours per day, with frequent use of home health care nurses or health care aides. More than 50% of caregivers care for equipment and prepare meals; more than 40% administer medications, bathe the patient, and take the patient outdoors; and more than 30% perform dressing, suctioning, and shopping for the patient.[83] Technical emergency service should be available 24 hours per day.

DISEASES APPROPRIATE FOR HMV

Neuromuscular Diseases

Bach et al.[9] conducted a survey that included 672 ventilator-dependent patients with neuromuscular diseases. A variety of methods were used for daytime ventilation, including mouthpiece IPPV, nasal IPPV, intermittent abdominal pressure ventilator, negative pressure body ventilators, and tracheostomy IPPV. For nocturnal ventilation, devices included negative pressure body ventilators, nasal IPPV, mouthpiece IPPV, IPPV via strapless oral–nasal interfaces, and tracheostomy IPPV.

Patients with gastric tubes had higher rates of pneumonia than those without gastric tubes. Among those without gastric tubes, pneumonia and hospitalizations were more common among those with tracheostomy IPPV than those who used noninvasive devices. The rates of hospitalizations and pneumonia were significantly reduced by undergoing tracheostomy for suctioning only in postpolio patients. Pneumonia and hospitalizations were more common among neuromuscular patients treated with body ventilators than with noninvasive IPPV users. The incidence of hospitalization and pneumonia increased significantly when the patients were prescribed supplemental oxygen alone and decreased significantly when they were treated by IPPV (noninvasive or tracheostomy). Once nocturnal ventilation was provided, their incidence of respiratory problems decreased. Noninvasive IPPV users did better than body ventilator users. The full-time noninvasive IPPV users had the lowest rates of pneumonia and hospitalizations—lower than with negative pressure body ventilators, and lower than with tracheostomy. Tracheostomy patients had .53/year re-admission and .36/year pneumonia rates. Cough assistance is essential for the success of noninvasive ventilation in this group.[85,86]

Hypoventilation and hypoxia at night is common when vital capacity is below 55% of predicted in postpolio patients.[87] Nocturnal assisted ventilation significantly improves $PaCO_2$ in these patients,[88] with most managed with noninvasive ventilation.

Moss et al.[89] found that fewer than 10% of amyotrophic lateral sclerosis (ALS) patients chose home ventilation, with only about 5% receiving chronic ventilation. Only a minority of ALS patients receiving home ventilation decided in advance to receive mechanical ventilation, with most initiating it in an emergency setting. In another study of 50 ALS patients receiving chronic mechanical ventilation, Moss et al.[90] found significantly lower costs and improved quality of life among those receiving HMV compared with institutional mechanical ventilation. These studies emphasize the importance of disclosing to patients and their families the benefits and burdens of HMV and the importance of advanced directives in these patients, as many go on to develop a locked-in syndrome.

Cervical Spine Injury

Patients with cervical spine injuries above C4 will be unable to breathe on their own. Many patients with cervical spine injuries to C4, C5, or C6 who are initially ventilator dependent become independent after a few to several months. For those patients who remain ventilator dependent, diaphragm pacing should be considered.

Thoracic Cage Abnormalities

Idiopathic kyphoscoliosis is the most common thoracic cage condition requiring ventilatory support. Others include congenital spinal developmental abnormalities, spinal tuberculosis, spinal cord injury, ankylosing spondylitis, and pectus excavatum. The use of long-term noninvasive ventilation in these patients has been reviewed.[91] Nocturnal hypoventilation often precedes daytime hypoventilation in these patients. NPV is often ineffective in chest wall diseases because of the distorted chest wall and possible induction of upper airway obstruction.

Noninvasive PPV is usually effective in patients with thoracic cage abnormalities,[91–93] but some require tracheostomy. Zaccaria et al.[94] studied 17 patients with kyphoscoliosis and respiratory failure, with all patients doing well with PPV. Six patients were managed by tracheostomy and IPPV and 11 patients were managed with nasal IPPV with volume-cycled pressure ventilator. $PaCO_2$ improved from 66 to 44 mm Hg after 1 month and 1 year.

Chronic Obstructive Pulmonary Disease

Although HMV clearly benefits patients with respiratory failure and neuromuscular or thoracic cage abnormalities, its use in patients with COPD is less clear. Patients with end-stage pulmonary disease often require higher pressures, tidal volumes, and rates for effective ventilation, which makes ventilation more difficult, particularly if given noninvasively. NPV has been shown to be of no benefit to patients with severe COPD in a large, double-blind study.[58]

PPV can effectively ventilate patients with COPD with respiratory failure, and good results have been obtained using noninvasive PPV for management of acute respiratory failure in COPD patients.[72] Invasive ventilation can support patients with COPD chronically, but studies using noninvasive IPPV for COPD have been variable.

Leger et al.[92] found improvements in $PaCO_2$ during spontaneous ventilation of 50 COPD patients in the first and second years of treatment with noninvasive PPV, without a change in PaO_2. Elliott et al.[95] studied 12 hypercapnic COPD patients treated by night HMV for 6 months. Eight patients completed the protocol. They also found a reduced $PaCO_2$, with unchanged PaO_2. Perrin et al.[96] studied 14 hypercapnic COPD patients and found that HMV with noninvasive IPPV in combination with oxygen therapy improved both PaO_2 and $PaCO_2$. Measures of quality of life also showed improvements in physical mobility, emotional reactions, and energy. Jones et al.[97] found reduced hospitalizations in 11 patients with severe hypercapnic COPD treated with noninvasive IPPV, with improved blood gases despite progression of airway obstruction.

Clini et al.[98] studied 34 patients with severe COPD (on long-term oxygen therapy [LTOT] and $PaCO_2$ >50 mm Hg) and treated (not randomized) either with biPAP and LTOT or LTOT alone. Neither group showed improved $PaCO_2$. Rates of hospitalization were lower among those with home programs (either LTOT or HMV and LTOT) than among historical controls.

Long-term mechanical ventilation via tracheostomy can be effective for patients with severe COPD. Muir[99] studied 259 patients with severe COPD and HMV who were tracheostomized for at least a year and followed up for up to 10 years: 67% had at least one episode of acute respiratory failure before tracheostomy, which was performed acutely in 89% of patients; 82% returned home after being discharged from the hospital; and 16% went to long-stay units. Of those in long-stay units, only 22% were kept because of medical causes, with the remainder kept mostly because of unfavorable home or sociofamilial conditions.

Bronchiectasis

Gacouin et al.[100] (France) studied 16 patients with bronchiectasis and chronic respiratory failure, providing noninvasive IPPV at night with volumetric ventilators in control mode, with oxygen as needed. $PaCO_2$ did not change significantly in up to 24 months, but the authors feel that the lack of worsening supports the belief that CPAP was helpful. CPAP was well tolerated, with all patients wanting to continue treatment after 1 year.

Cystic Fibrosis

A small study by Piper et al.[101] supports using noninvasive IPPV to treat patients with respiratory failure caused by end-stage cystic fibrosis. Each of their four patients tolerated nocturnal nasal IPPV well, improved blood gases and respiratory muscle strength, and had subjective improvements in sleep and daily level of activity.

Obstructive Sleep Apnea

For obstructive sleep apnea (OSA), nasal CPAP is the treatment of choice because it helps maintain patency of the airway, preventing obstruction. Some OSA patients who require but do not tolerate high CPAPs do well with biPAP. The inspiratory pressure is set high enough for full airway patency, and the expiratory pressure is set high enough for partial patency so the device can sense inspiration. Tracheostomy is seldom required for treatment of OSA, with dental appliances an option for patients who cannot tolerate nasal CPAP or biPAP.

Congestive Heart Failure

Some recent studies suggest that CPAP therapy may become an important modality in the treatment of patients with severe congestive heart failure (CHF). Nearly half of patients with stable and optimally treated CHF have significant sleep disturbances.[102] Nocturnal CPAP in patients with chronic CHF and sleep-related breathing disturbances improves apneas, nocturnal oxygenation, symptoms of heart failure, and left ventricular ejection fraction.[103–105] CPAP also decreases sympathetic nervous activity among these patients.[106] The role of CPAP in chronic CHF patients without significant sleep-related breathing disturbances is not yet known.

SAFETY

HMV has been shown to be safe. Srinivasan et al.[107] studied reports of home ventilator failure in 150 ventilator-assisted patients, finding 189 reports. Defective equipment or mechanical failure was found in 39% (73 reports), or one failure for every 1.25 years of continuous use. Other problems included improper care, damage, or tampering with the ventilator by caregivers (13%); equipment improperly used (30%); and equipment functional but the patient's condition changed, mimicking ventilator failure (3%). No problems were found in 16%. Ninety-three percent of the ventilator-associated problems could be solved at home, with hospitalization needed in 2 patients—related to changes in the patient's clinical condition. Failures were much more common among those receiving continuous ventilation (66% of episodes) than among those receiving nocturnal ventilation. Seventy-four percent of the time a backup ventilator was available at home. No adverse outcomes, deaths, or serious injuries were associated with home ventilator failure in this study.

COSTS

As opposed to in Europe, where National Health Services are responsible for the costs of HMV,[108] coverage in the United States is by a variety of private and public funding groups. The cost of HMV varies dramatically depending on the underlying condition of the patient and the need for home care nursing and personal care attendants. For patients receiving nocturnal noninvasive ventilation who can fully care for themselves, little cost is incurred beyond the rental or purchase of the ventilator. For patients who are fully ventilator dependent, the cost is much higher.

Various studies have found the yearly cost of HMV in the 1990s in the United States of $91,700,[109] $130,000,[110] and $153,000,[89] with the latter in a group of ALS patients. Other indirect costs are primarily of the opportunity cost (lost wages) of home caregivers.[111]

Studies have consistently found significant cost savings and improved quality of life with HMV compared with mechanical ventilation in an acute or chronic care facility. Fields et al.[112] estimate savings of about $80,000 per year per patient with tracheostomy managed at home, largely because of reduced costs for nursing care. A study of 50 ALS patients in 1996 found the yearly cost of home ventilation ($136,560) much less than for those in an institution ($366,852).[90]

Bach et al.[76] found considerable cost savings by transitioning patients from tracheostomy to noninvasive methods of ventilator support, then discharge to the home. All patients required 24-hour support and had been in respiratory units for an average of 9 years. The average cost at home was $235 per day, with the highest portion for attendant care, whereas the rehabilitation units received about $700 per day, thus yielding savings of $162,000 per year for each patient.

Some states restrict suctioning to nurses or respiratory therapists, which can markedly increase the costs of caring for patients receiving HMV. This restriction is not supported by evidence, with Bach et al.[76] finding no incidents regarding suctioning without daily licensed nursing care in a large group of tracheostomized HMV patients.

FUTURE OF HMV

HMV provides significant improvements in quality of life and health care costs compared with institutional mechanical ventilation. We have learned much about how to provide effective management of patients with chronic respiratory failure, including patient selection, ventilator issues, training of the patient and caregivers, transition from invasive to noninvasive ventilation, and transition from institution to home. Noninvasive PPV has become the preferable means of HMV for many patients. The major challenge for the upcoming years will be to disseminate and implement what we have learned. With the United States lacking any central mechanisms to manage chronic ventilator-dependent patients, these patients can be approached in a variety of ways. Respiratory centers can function as areas of expertise to facilitate discharge of individuals to the community, as well as to train health care professionals. The future of HMV in the United States will depend on the level of support provided by the wide variety of health care providers for ventilator management in general and for home ventilator care in particular.

REFERENCES

1. O'Donohue WJ, Giovannoni AM, Goldberg AL, et al. Long-term mechanical ventilation: guidelines for management in the home and at alternative community sites. 1986;90:1S–37S.
2. Chailleux E, Fauroux B, Binet F, et al. Predictors of survival in patients receiving domiciliary oxygen therapy or mechanical ventilation: a 10-year analysis of ANTADIR Observatory. Chest 1996;109:741–749.
3. Goldberg AL. Technology assessment and support of life-sustaining devices in home care: the home care physician perspective. Chest 1994; 105:1448–1453.
4. Adams AB, Whitman J, Marcy T. Surveys of long-term ventilatory support in Minnesota: 1986 and 1992. Chest 1993;103:1463–1469.
5. Goldstein RS, Psek JA, Gort EH. Home mechanical ventilation: demographics and user perspectives. Chest 1995;108:1581–1586.
6. Make BJ, Gilmartin ME. Rehabilitation and home care for ventilator-assisted individuals. Clin Chest Med 1986;7:679–691.
7. A Study of Chronic Ventilator Patients in the Hospital: A Patient Profile and Analysis Conducted by the Gallup Organization for the American Association for Respiratory Care. Dallas: American Association for Respiratory Care, 1991.

8. Goldberg AL, Frownfelter D. The Ventilator-Assisted Individuals Study. Chest 1990;98: 428–433.
9. Bach JR, Rajaraman R, Ballanger F, et al. Neuromuscular ventilatory insufficiency: effect of home mechanical ventilator use v oxygen therapy on pneumonia and hospitalization rates. Am J Phys Med Rehabil 1998;77:8–19.
10. Hill NS. Noninvasive ventilation: does it work, for whom, and how? Am Rev Respir Dis 1993;147:1050–1055.
11. Claman DM, Piper A, Sanders NM, et al. Nocturnal noninvasive positive pressure ventilatory assistance. Chest 1996;110:1581–1588.
12. Brochard L, Isabey D, Piquet J, et al. Reversal of acute exacerbations of chronic obstructive lung disease by inspiratory assistance with a face mask. N Engl J Med 1990;323:1523–1530.
13. Renston JP, DiMarco AF, Supinski GS. Respiratory muscle rest using nasal BIPAP ventilation in patients with stable severe COPD. Chest 1994;105:1053–1060.
14. Bergofsky EH. Respiratory failure in disorders of the thoracic cage. Am Rev Respir Dis 1979;119:643–669.
15. Hill NS, Eveloff SE, Carlisle CC, et al. Efficacy of nocturnal nasal ventilation in patients with restrictive thoracic disease. Am Rev Respir Dis 1992;145:365–371.
16. Scheinhom DJ, Artinian BM, Catlin JL. Wean-

ing from prolonged mechanical ventilation: the experience at a regional weaning center. Chest 1994;105:534–539.

17. Bagley PH, Cooney E. A community-based regional ventilator weaning unit: development and outcomes. Chest 1997;111:1024–1029.

18. Scheinhom DJ, Chao DC, Stearn-Hassenpfiug M, et al. Post-ICU mechanical ventilation: treatment of 1,123 patients at a regional weaning center. Chest 1997;111:1654–1659.

19. Janssens JP, Cicofti E, Fifting JW, et al. Noninvasive home ventilation in patients over 75 years of age: tolerance, compliance, and impact on quality of life. Respir Med 1998;92:1311–1320.

20. Oren J, Kelly D, Shannon D. Long-term follow-up of children with congenital central hypoventilation syndrome. Pediatrics 1987;80:375–380.

21. Marcus C, Jansen M, Poulsen M, et al. Medical and psychosocial outcome of children with congenital hypoventilation syndrome. J Pediatr 1991;119:888–895.

22. Wheeler WB, Maguire EL, Kurachek SC, et al. Chronic respiratory failure of infancy and childhood: clinical outcomes based on underlying etiology. Pediatr Pulmonol 1994;17:1–5.

23. Keens TG, Jansen MT, DeWitt PK, et al. Home care for children with chronic respiratory failure. Semin Respir Med 1990;11:269–281.

24. Nelson VS, Carroll JC, Hurvitz EA, et al. Home mechanical ventilation of children. Dev Med Child Neurol 1996;38:704–715.

25. Voter KZ, Chalanick K. Home oxygen and ventilation therapies in pediatric patients. Curr Opin Pediatr 1996;8:221–225.

26. Pilmer S. Prolonged mechanical ventilation in children. Pediatr Clin North Am 1994;41:473–512.

27. Robart P, Make B, Tureson DW, et al. AARC clinical practice guideline: long-term invasive mechanical ventilation in the home. Respir Care 1995;40:1313–1320.

28. Shneerson JM. Home mechanical ventilation in children: techniques, outcomes and ethics. Monaldi Arch Chest Dis 1996;51:426–430.

29. DeWitt PK, Jansen MT, Ward SL, et al. Obstacles to discharge of ventilator-assisted children from the hospital to home. Chest 1993;103:1560–1565.

30. Donner CF, Howard P, Robert D. Patient selection and techniques for home mechanical ventilation: European Respiratory Society Rehabilitation and Chronic Care Scientific Group. Monaldi Arch Chest Dis 1993;48:40–47.

31. American Thoracic Society. Home mechanical ventilation of pediatric patients. Am Rev Respir Dis 1990;141:259.

32. American Society for Testing and Materials. Committees F29.09.03 (Home Care Ventilators) and F31.01.02 (Home Respiratory Care). Philadelphia: American Society for Testing and Materials.

33. Joint Commission for Accreditation of Health Care Organizations. Accreditation Manual for Home Care. Oakbrook Terrace, Ill: Joint Commission for Accreditation of Health Care Organizations, 1993.

34. Plummer AL, O'Donohue WJ, Petty TL. Consensus conference on problems in home mechanical ventilation. Am Rev Respir Dis 1989;140:555–560.

35. Bach JR, Saporito LR. Indications and criteria for decannulation and transition from invasive to noninvasive long-term ventilatory support. Respir Care 1994;39:515–531.

36. Udwadia ZF, Santis GK, Steven NM, et al. Nasal ventilation to facilitate weaning in patients with chronic respiratory insufficiency. Thorax 1992;47:715–718.

37. Bach JR. Indications for tracheostomy and decannulation of tracheostomized ventilator users. Monaldi Arch Chest Dis 1995;50:223–227.

38. Hillberg RE, Johnson DC. Noninvasive ventilation. N Engl J Med 1997;337:1746–1752.

39. Bach JR, Alba AS. Management of chronic alveolar hypoventilation by nasal ventilation. Chest 1990;97:52–57.

40. Pinto AC, Evangelista T, Carvalho M, et al. Respiratory assistance with a non-invasive ventilator (Bipap) in N4ND/ALS patients: survival rates in a controlled trial. J Neurol Sci 1995;129 (Suppl):19–26.

41. Soudon P. Tracheal versus noninvasive mechanical ventilation in neuromuscular patients: experience and evaluation. Monaldi Arch Chest Dis 1995;50:228–231.

42. Leger P, Bedicam JM, Comette A, et al. Nasal intermittent positive pressure ventilation. Chest 1994;105:100–105.

43. Ellis ER, Grunstein RR, Chan S, et al. Noninvasive ventilatory support during sleep improves respiratory failure in kyphoscoliosis. Chest 1988;94:811–815.

44. Masa JF, Celli BR, Riesco JA, et al. Noninvasive positive pressure ventilation and not oxygen may prevent overt ventilatory failure in patients with chest wall diseases. Chest 1997;112:207–213.

45. Unterborn JN, Hill NS. Options for mechanical ventilation in neuromuscular diseases. Clin Chest Med 1994;15:765–781.

46. Ferguson GT, Gilmartin M. CO_2 rebreathing during BIPAP ventilatory assistance. Am J Respir Crit Care Med 1995;151:1126–1135.

47. Ambrosino N, Nava S, Bertone P, et al. Physiologic evaluation of pressure support ventilation by nasal mask in patients with stable COPD. Chest 1992;101:385–391.

48. Jones DFM, Paul EA, Jones PW, et al. Nasal pressure support ventilation plus oxygen compared with oxygen therapy alone in hypercapnic COPD. Am J Respir Crit Care Med 1995;152:538–544.

49. Strumpf DA, Milhnan RP, Carlisle CC, et al. Nocturnal positive-pressure ventilation via nasal mask in patients with severe chronic obstructive pulmonary disease. Am Rev Respir Dis 1991;144:1234–1239.

50. Hill N. Clinical applications of body ventilators. Chest 1986;90:897–905.

51. Ambrosino N, Rampulla C. Negative pressure

ventilation in COPD patients. Eur Respir Rev 1992;2:353–356.

52. Corrado A, Gorini M, Villella G, et al. Negative pressure ventilation in the treatment of acute respiratory failure: an old noninvasive technique reconsidered. Eur Respir J 1996;9:1531–1544.

53. Nava S, Ambrosino N, Zoechi L, et al. Diaphragmatic rest during negative pressure ventilation by pneumowrap: assessment in normal and COPD patients. Chest 1990;98:857–865.

54. Curran FJ. Night ventilation by body respirators for patients in chronic respiratory failure due to late stage Duchenne muscular dystrophy. Arch Phys Med Rehabil 1981;62:270–274.

55. Garay SM, Turino GM, Goldring RM. Sustained reversal of chronic hypercapnia in patients with alveolar hypoventilation syndromes: long-term maintenance with noninvasive mechanical ventilation. Am J Med 1981;70:269–274.

56. Goldstein RS, Molotiu N, Skrastins R, et al. Reversal of sleep-induced hypoventilation by nocturnal negative pressure ventilation in patients with restrictive ventilatory impairment. Am Rev Respir Dis 1987;135:1049–1055.

57. Jackson M, Kinnear W, King M, et al. The effects of five years of nocturnal cuirass-assisted ventilation in chest wall disease. Eur Respir J 1993; 6:630–635.

58. Shapiro SH, Ernst P, Gray-Donald K, et al. Effect of negative pressure ventilation in severe chronic obstructive pulmonary disease. Lancet 1992; 340:1425–1429.

59. Meduri GU, Turner RE, Abou-Shala N, et al. Noninvasive positive-pressure ventilation via face mask: first-line intervention in patients with acute hypercapnic and hypoxemic respiratory failure. Chest 1996;109:179–193.

60. Health devices: portable volume ventilators. ECRI 1992;21:255–291.

61. Lofaso F, Brochard L, Hang T, et al. Home versus intensive care pressure support devices: experimental and clinical comparison. Am J Respir Crit Care Med 1996;153:1591–1599.

62. Bach JR, Alba A, Mosher R, et al. Intermittent positive pressure ventilation via nasal access in the management of respiratory insufficiency. Chest 1987;94:168–170.

63. Leger P, Jemequin J, Gerard S, et al. Home positive pressure ventilation via nasal mask for patients with neuromusculoskeletal disorders. Eur Respir J 1989;2:640S–645S.

64. Gay PC, Patel AM, Viggiano RW, et al. Nocturnal nasal ventilation for treatment of patients with hypercapnic respiratory failure. Mayo Clin Proc 1991;66:695–703.

65. Marino W. Intermittent volume cycled mechanical ventilation via nasal mask in patients with respiratory failure due to COPD. Chest 1991; 99:681–684.

66. Foglio C, Vitacca M, Quadri A, et al. Acute exacerbations in severe COPD patients: treatment using positive pressure ventilation by nasal mask. Chest 1992:101:1533–1538.

67. Hoo GWS, Santiago S, Williams AJ. Nasal mechanical ventilation for hypercapnic respiratory failure in chronic obstructive pulmonary disease: determinants of success and failure. Crit Care Med 1994;22:1253–1261.

68. Lofaso F, Brochard L, Touchard D, et al. Evaluation of carbon dioxide rebreathing during pressure support ventilation with airway management system (BiPAP) devices. Chest 1995; 108:772–778.

69. Marini JJ, Smith TC, Lamb VJ. External work output and force generation during synchronized intermittent mechanical ventilation. Am Rev Respir Dis 1988;138:1169–1179.

70. Criner GJ, Tzouanakis A, Kreimer DT. Overview of improving tolerance of long-term mechanical ventilation. Crit Care Clin 1994;10:845–866.

71. Leger P. Noninvasive positive pressure ventilation at home. Respir Care 1994;39:501–510.

72. Brochard L, Mancebo J, Wysocki M, et al. Noninvasive ventilation for acute exacerbations of chronic obstructive pulmonary disease. N Engl J Med 1995;333:817–822.

73. Kramer N, Meyer TJ, Meharg J, et al. Randomized prospective trial of noninvasive positive pressure ventilation in acute respiratory failure. Am J Respir Crit Care Med 1995;151:1799–1806.

74. Elliott MW, Mulvey DA, Moxham J, et al. Inspiratory muscle effort during nasal intermittent positive pressure ventilation in patients with chronic obstructive airways disease. Anaesthesia 1993;48:8–13.

75. Appendini L, Patessio A, Zanaboni S, et al. Physiologic effects of positive end-expiratory pressure and mask pressure support during exacerbations of chronic obstructive pulmonary disease. Am J Respir Crit Care Med 1994;149:1069–1076.

76. Bach JR, Intintola P, Alba AS, et al. The ventilator-assisted individual: cost analysis of institutionalization vs rehabilitation and in-home management. Chest 1992;101:26–30.

77. Janssens JP, Penalosa B, Degive C, et al. Quality of life of patients under home mechanical ventilation for restrictive lung diseases: a comparative evaluation with COPD patients. Monaldi Arch Chest Dis 1996;51:178–184.

78. Pehrsson K, Olofson J, Larsson S, et al. Quality of life of patients treated by home mechanical ventilation due to restrictive ventilatory disorders. Respir Med 1994;88:21–26.

79. LaFond L, Homer J. Psychosocial issues related to long-term ventilatory support. Probl Respir Care 1988;1:241–256.

80. Smith CE, Mayer LS, Parkhurst C, et al. Adaptation in families with a member requiring mechanical ventilation at home. Heart Lung 1991;20:349–356.

81. Gracey DR. Options for long-term ventilatory support. Clin Chest Med 1997;18:563–576.

82. Thomas VM, Ellison K, Howell EV, et al. Caring for the person receiving ventilatory support at home: care givers' needs and involvement. Heart Lung 1992;21:180–186.

83. Findeis A, Larson JL, Gallo A, et al. Caring for individuals using home ventilators: an appraisal by family caregivers. Rehabil Nurs 1994;19: 6–11.

84. Sevick MA, Sereika S, Matthews JT, et al. Home-

based ventilator-dependent patients: measurement of the emotional aspects of home caregiving. Heart Lung 1994;23:269–278.

85. Bach JR. Mechanical insufflation-exsufflation: comparison of peak expiratory flows with manually assisted and unassisted coughing techniques. Chest 1993;104:1553–1562.

86. Bach JR. Update and perspectives on noninvasive respiratory muscle aids: part 2—the expiratory muscle aids. Chest 1994;105:1538–1544.

87. Bach JR, Alba A. Pulmonary dysfunction and sleep-disordered breathing as postpolio sequelae: evaluation and management. Orthopedics 1991;14:1329–1337.

88. Midgren B. Lung function and clinical outcome in postpolio patients: a prospective cohort study during 11 years. Eur Respir J 1997;10:146–149.

89. Moss AH, Casey P, Stocking CB, et al. Home ventilation for amyotrophic lateral sclerosis patients: outcomes, costs, and patient, family, and physician attitudes. Neurology 1993;43:438–443.

90. Moss AH, Oppenheimer EA, Casey P, et al. Patients with amyotrophic lateral sclerosis receiving long-term mechanical ventilation: advance care planning and outcomes. Chest 1996;110:249–255.

91. Leger P. Long-term noninvasive ventilation for patients with thoracic cage abnormalities. Respir Care Clin N Am 1996;2:241–252.

92. Leger P, Bedicarn JM, Comette A, et al. Nasal intermittent positive pressure ventilation: long-term follow-up in patients with severe chronic respiratory insufficiency. Chest 1994;105:100–105.

93. Simonds AK. Nasal intermittent positive pressure ventilation in neuromuscular and chest wall disease. Monaldi Arch Chest Dis 1993;48:165–168.

94. Zaccaria S, Zaccaria E, Zanaboni S, et al. Home mechanical ventilation in kyphoscoliosis. Monaldi Arch Chest Dis 1993;48:161–164.

95. Elliott MW, Simonds AK, Carroll MP, et al. Domiciliary nocturnal nasal intermittent positive pressure ventilation in hypercapnic respiratory failure due to chronic obstructive lung disease: effects on sleep and quality of life. Thorax 1992;47:342–348.

96. Perrin C, El FY, Vandenbos F, et al. Domiciliary nasal intermittent positive pressure ventilation in severe COPD: effects on lung function and quality of life. Eur Respir J 1997;10:2835–2839.

97. Jones SE, Packham S, Hebden M, et al. Domiciliary nocturnal intermittent positive pressure ventilation in patients with respiratory failure due to severe COPD: long-term follow up and effect on survival. Thorax 1998;53:495–498.

98. Clini E, Vitacca M, Foglio K, et al. Long-term home care programmes may reduce hospital admissions in COPD with chronic hypercapnia. Eur Respir J 1996;9:1605–1610.

99. Muir JF, Girault C, Cardinaud JP, et al. Survival and long-term follow-up of tracheostomized patients with COPD treated by home mechanical ventilation: a multicenter French study in 259 patients. Chest 1994;106:201–209.

100. Gacouin A, Desrues B, Lena H, et al. Long-term nasal intermittent positive pressure ventilation (NIPPV) in sixteen consecutive patients with bronchiectasis: a retrospective study. Eur Respir J 1996;9:1246–1250.

101. Piper AJ, Parker S, Torzillo PJ, et al. Nocturnal nasal IPPV stabilizes patients with cystic fibrosis and hypercapnic respiratory failure. Chest 1992;102:846–850.

102. Javaheri S, Parker TJ, Wexler L, et al. Occult sleep-disordered breathing in stable congestive heart failure. Ann Intern Med 1995;122:487–492.

103. Takasaki Y, Orr D, Rutherford R, et al. Effect of nasal continuous positive airway pressure on sleep apnea in congestive heart failure. Am Rev Respir Dis 1989;140:1578–1584.

104. Lapinsky SE, Mount DB, Mackey D, et al. Management of acute respiratory failure due to pulmonary edema with nasal positive pressure support. Chest 1994;105:229–231.

105. Naughton NT, Liu PP, Bernard DC, et al. Treatment of congestive heart failure and Cheyne-Stokes respiration during sleep by continuous positive airway pressure. Am J Respir Crit Care Med 1995;151:92–97.

106. Naughton MT, Bernard DC, Liu PP, et al. Effects of nasal CPAP on sympathetic activity in patients with heart failure and central sleep apnea. Am J Respir Crit Care Med 1995;152:473–479.

107. Srinivasan S, Doty SM, White TR, et al. Frequency, causes, and outcome of home ventilator failure. Chest 1998;114:1363–1367.

108. Fauroux B, Howard P, Muir JF. Home treatment for chronic respiratory insufficiency: the situation in Europe in 1992: the European Working Group on Home Treatment for Chronic Respiratory Insufficiency. Eur Respir J 1994;7:1721–1726.

109. Sevick MA, Kamlet MS, Hoffman LA, et al. Economic cost of home-based care for ventilator-assisted individuals: a preliminary report. Chest 1996;109:1597–1606.

110. Oppenheimer EA, Baldwin-Myers A, Tanquary P. Ventilator use by patients with amyotrophic lateral sclerosis. Denver, CO: International Conference on Pulmonary Rehabilitation and Home Ventilation, 1991.

111. Sevick MA, Bradham DD. Economic value of caregiver effort in maintaining long-term ventilator-assisted individuals at home. Heart Lung 1997;26:14–157.

112. Fields AI, Rosenblatt A, Pollack MM, et al. Home care cost-effectiveness for respiratory technology–dependent children. Am J Dis Child 1991;145:729–733.

22 Home Mechanical Ventilation in Europe

Jean-François Muir

⟳ Professional Skills

Upon completion of this chapter, the reader will:

- Identify the main centers in charge of home mechanical ventilation (HMV) in Europe
- Appreciate the real incidence of use of volumetric versus barometric respirators
- Have an estimation of the importance of HMV among the different European countries
- Compare the different insurance systems and conception of social security organization in Europe

Long-term HMV with intermittent positive-pressure breathing was introduced in clinical practice after the iron lung era at the end of the 1950s. This marked a period of rapid progress in ventilator technology, prompted by the worldwide polio epidemic of that time. This coincided with other important developments in the area of respiratory care such as endotracheal mechanical ventilation and tracheostomy. The application of all of these concepts improved survival after acute respiratory failure, which in turn led to a growing number of patients with chronic respiratory failure (CRF) who were candidates for home discharge but had no system in place to implement it.[1] The possibility to ventilate patients at home was further advanced by the development of long-term oxygen therapy (LTOT) in the late 1970s. The infrastructure required to efficiently provide oxygen at home served as a basis for the rapid introduction of HMV.

The first attempt to ventilate patients through the nares was reported by Rideau in patients with Duchenne de Boulogne myopathy in the middle 1980s. This was followed by the expanding use of noninvasive mechanical ventilation in patients with acute respiratory failure or CRF also at the end of the 1980s. The experience since then has mushroomed so that HMV is now widely used in Europe mainly in restrictive patients of various origin but also in patients with severe hypercapnic and unstable chronic obstructive pulmonary disease.[2,3] The French organization the Association Nationale pour le Traitement A Domicile de l'insuffisance Respiratoire Chronique (ANTADIR) reported a prevalence of 10/100,000 inhabitants[4] in 1991, which rose to 14/100,000 4 years later.

In 1992, an informal group from within the European Respiratory Society (Rehabilitation and Chronic Care) and the International Union Against Tuberculosis and Lung Disease gathered together specialists in chronic respiratory care from 13 countries. They attempted to evaluate the general organization of home care of CRF by means of a questionnaire. This included information on home treatment: LTOT, HMV, and nasal continuous positive airway pressure. It also attempted to characterize the prescribers, prescription trends, and practical organization of home care (supply of material, supervision of patients, and equipment). The format was similar to that used by ANTADIR in France.[5] The results of a similar but shorter version describing only the prevalence of HMV is shown in Table 22-1. Some registers similar to that of ANTADIR have

Table 22-1. The Current Status in Europe

Country/ Update/ Population	NO Pts Under MV			Nasal & Facial, %	% INPV	Est. NO Children <16 Yrs	Respirators %		Etiology of CRF			% CWD. & Tuberc. Seq.	Others Restrictive Pts.
	Est. Number	Prevalence (/100000)	% Trach.				Volume Cycled	Pressure Cycled	Obstructive %	Restrictive % (Total)	% NMD		
Belgium/ 1998 10.2 million	250	2.5	33	67	0	50	50	50	10 (only with tracheostomy)	90	30	40	20
Denmark/ Oct. 1999 5 million	475	9.5	30	70	0	50	30	70	5–10	90–95			
Finland/ 1997 5.1 million	201	4	22	78	0	10	70	30	10	90	49	16	
France/ 1998 59 million	10000	16.9	23	76	<1	568	60	40	29	52	49	43	8
Germany/ 1998 82 million	3500	4.26	9	90	<1	est. <3%	57	43	36	22	21	58	OHS:13
Iceland/ 1999 270,000	53	19.62	0	100	0	2	4	96	14 (overlap S.)	86	28	24	48
Italy/ 1998 57 million	9144	16.04	19	80.1	0.9	est. 3.4%	2639	3706	—	—	—	—	—
Spain/ 1998 40 million	1127	2.81	10	90	0	<2%	60	40	20	80	15	38	—
Sweden/ 1998 8.9 million	700	7.86	20	80	0	40	65	35	7	83	50	50	0
Switzerland/ 1998 7.1 million	474	6.67	—	—	—	—	—	—	—	—	—	—	—
UK/ 1998 59 million	4000	6.77	2.5	95	2.5	150	30	70	25	75	60	40	

been developed in some European countries since 1992. They provide interesting analyses on survival but are essentially devoted to LTOT, with limited information regarding HMV.[6,7]

QUANTITATIVE IMPORTANCE OF HMV IN EUROPE

The best available data on HMV comes from France. Since 1981, the associative system ANTADIR has managed 32 national regions, covering approximately 70% of patients receiving home treatment for CRF. Since 1984, a sample of about 80% of ANTADIR's patients has been surveyed to provide a precise annual report about patient status and their equipment.[4] A major outcome has been survival analysis, which has been published separately.[6]

The information is not as solid in other countries because of differences in organization and structure. Partial information (usually age and sex of the recipient) can be obtained from analysis of Health Service data in Belgium. The organization of the country into different districts, as in Denmark, Italy, or Germany, or community care areas, as in

Table 22-1. (*continued*)

Others Etiologies	Existence of a National Register	Prescriber of HMV?			Health Organization			Comments
		Pulmonologist	Anesthesiologist	Other	Public?	Private?	Other?	
	Yes (national health services)	Yes	—	—	Yes	Yes		Costs supported by NHS
	In constitution 2 centers: East (45% of the territory) and West (55%)	0	0	Intensivists (trained as anesthesiol.)	100% financed by the local county			Equipment and attendants regionally organized
	No	Responsible for obstructive and restrictive pts	If the treatment is started in the ICU and for trach. Pts	Specialists of the dis. Responsible for the CRF/team decision.	Near 100% #1/3 have a "resp. paralysis status"	1 private clinic (1/3 paid by public funds)		Old status of "respiratory paralysis pt status" where the hospital has to provide all the home care
19	Yes: ANTADIR	80%	5%	15%	Yes: Federation of 27 regional associations (#50000 pts)	Private resp. care network (#20000 pts)		100% reimbursement of expenses by public health funds
8	No	>90%			Public insur. pays for HMV	No specificity		Reimbursement if symptoms of CRF and daytime hypercapnia
0	Yes	Pulmonologists only	No	No	100%	0	0	—
—	No	Yes	Yes		Public insur. pays for HMV	No specificity		Medical certificate required
—	No	Yes	—	—	Yes	—	—	—
0	Yes	75% one centre	16% mainly in		100%	0	0	—
—	—	—	—	—	—	—	—	—
0	In pediatric pts only	#100%	No	Pediatricians	Equipment by NHS Carers by local authority	Only overseas pts not entitled to NHS	No	—

HMV, home mechanical ventilation; NHS, National Health Service; CRF, chronic respiratory failure.

Ireland, complicates the collection of national information.[8] Complete information can be obtained for home treatment via a reimbursement system in Spain.[5] In Great Britain, a national register of HMV is available for children but not for adults.[9]

The Swedish Society of Chest Medicine has started a national register of patients receiving HMV, collecting data both retrospectively and prospectively since January 1, 1996.[10] The introduction of the register was facilitated by the fact that the Swedish Society has run the national oxygen register successfully for almost 10 years.[7] The definitions of the variables collected in the Swedish register were elaborated on in close Swedish–Danish cooperation. Both countries have publicly financed health care systems and a similar cultural and socioeconomic structure. In Sweden (population 8.9 million), 541 patients (262 males) were reported to use HMV on January 1, 1996. This corresponds to a prevalence of 6.1/100,000 inhabitants. A total of 45 clinics reported patients to the Swedish register, with the 10 largest clinics accounting for more than two-thirds of the patients. The prevalence in the 26 health care regions varied between 1.2 and 20 per 100,000 inhabitants. Chest physicians cared for 70% of the patients, whereas 20% were cared for by anesthesiologists (mainly from one center). If we review the data provided by the Swedish register and the less complete data presented in Table 22-1, the median prevalence of HMV in Europe is close to 10/100,000 habitants.

EQUIPMENT PROVIDED

Currently, both adults and children receive HMV for chronic lung disease, neuromuscular disease, chest wall deformities, and central hypoventilation. Interestingly, the type of equipment used to provide ventilation varies from one region to another, although a progressive shift has occurred from volume-cycled to pressure-cycled ventilators. England uses more pressure-cycled than volumetric ventilators, plus a significant number of negative-pressure ventilators. Negative-pressure ventilation for neuromuscular disease is no longer used in Sweden but is still seen in Italy. Only 35 patients (0.5% of the patients under the auspices of ANTADIR receiving HMV) are thought to receive this treatment in France. In Sweden, volume-controlled ventilators were used by 75% of the patients, 25% having supplemental oxygen. Here again, the fraction of patients under pressure-controlled ventilators is rapidly increasing. The progressive integration of the different European societies will likely decrease these differences.

REGULATION OF PRESCRIPTION

In Europe, home HMV is prescribed by pulmonary specialists (Table 22-1), with national guidelines advising the correct prescription in some countries. In Germany, public health insurance services monitor the correct prescription. Prescription rules also exist in France, Germany, Spain, Belgium,[11] and Switzerland.[12] The latter is the only country with an element of tight control of prescription practices. Review of its experience on adherence to guidelines and patient's compliance has been published.[13] In Sweden,[10] Norway, and Italy, specialists have created recommendations in the absence of national guidelines.

ORGANIZATION OF EQUIPMENT AND HOME SUPERVISION

The actual equipment is supplied by commercial companies, hospitals, or national organizations and health services, both nationalized and private (Table 22-1). A combination of different suppliers exists in Belgium, Great Britain, France, and Switzerland. In Norway, the National Health Service exclusively buys the equipment for HMV and provides it, through local hospitals, to the patient for as long as necessary. Generally in Scandinavian countries, the development of HMV has been impaired by its costs, which sometimes have to be supported by the local hospital (as in Finland). The net effect is a difference in the use of pressure-cycled respirators (which are less costly) as the preferred form of HMV in the different European countries, especially for neuromuscular CRF.[14] Some of the large differences in the number of patients receiving HMV in different countries may be explained by different national systems of health care provision rather than by actual differences in the prevalence of the underlying diseases.[10]

Home supervision of patients is usually performed by medical and/or nursing personnel and occasionally by technical staff. Once more, the quality of service seems to be highly variable. Technical support for the equipment is usually provided by the commercial companies. The overall HMV is usually supervised by clinicians in the Netherlands, Ireland, Great Britain, and Switzerland. In Italy, parallel systems are used, with systematic home supervision provided by rehabilitation centers, home care services, and voluntary associations.

COMMUNITY SERVICES AND HOME CARE

Many patients receiving nocturnal ventilation do not need additional services. Conversely, patients who live alone, or those who have major disabilities (posttraumatic injuries, neuromuscular involvement of nonrespiratory areas), may need assistance for daily activities, such as cooking, body care, and bathing. In Europe, volunteers from churches or charity organizations frequently provide these services. In some instances, the service can be provided by the social assistance and reimbursed by the local health authority. Other more continuous services, such as "meals on wheels," transportation, and homemaking, are only seldom available. If the patient becomes too dependent on external help, the setting is changed to a sheltered facility. A home care program including these "social" needs is obviously desirable, but funding and organization limitations are usually major obstacles.

COSTS

In nearly all countries, the National Health Service is responsible for the costs of HMV (Table 22-1). Exceptions are Scandinavian countries, where the local county provides concentrators, ventilators, continuous positive airway pressure, and mobile oxygen. In Switzerland, all therapeutic costs are supported by medical insurance companies in collaboration with the specialized Association for Tuberculosis and Pulmonary Diseases. In Italy, patients have public reimbursement of their expenses. In Belgium, the national social security allows mutual medical insurance companies to pay for home treatment for CRF prescribed by approved hospital departments.[11] In all countries, cost includes home installation and supervision of equipment. Given the differences by which health care is paid for from country to country, it is not surprising that the situation in Europe is so diverse[15] (Table 22-1). In most European countries, a national policy regarding prescription modalities, reimbursement, assistance, and medical supervision does not exist, even though the National Health Service or other insurance companies usually reimburse the costs of LTOT and the ventilator. Only France, through ANTADIR, has developed an organization that includes a register of patients and equipment use as well as home care supervision.[4,5,15] A uniform European standard is lacking, and the uniformization of systems is consequently a challenging task.[15]

CONCLUSION AND PERSPECTIVES

This chapter provides information about HMV in European countries. For some countries, the information is as yet incomplete and characterized only by a paucity of outcome data. The cost of chronic care, including HMV, is important for most National Health Services. Cost-benefit analyses of treatment must eventually be possible. Currently, the major differences between countries depend on the existence or not of a national register. In addition, the differences are magnified by the form by which home treatment is prescribed, the monitorization of those rules, and the financial incentive that ultimately influences the equipment used at home. The differences are also explained by the historical origin of home care in each country, the different impact of commercial companies, and the supervision of insurance companies on doctor's prescriptions. The differences in reimbursement systems and in organization of home care explain the differences in costs. The multiplicity of systems throughout Europe demonstrates that no ideal mechanism has yet been found.

Several countries are capable of collecting data regarding HMV through their registers, and all should do so. Most countries know precisely or approximately how many patients are treated through data collection undertaken by national thoracic societies. In the meantime, therapeutic guidelines addressing noninvasive mechanical ventilation are being rewritten. In COPD, like LTOT, the objective of HMV is to increase survival and improve quality of life. Unfortunately, since the two large trials that showed the beneficial effect of oxygen therapy for COPD hypoxemic patients,[16,17] limited data concerning HMV have been published. The guidelines include criteria for patient selection, evaluation, and monitoring.

From the available data, we conclude that the prevalence of HMV will probably continue to rise in most countries, secondary to the extension of indications (chronic obstructive pulmonary disease, bronchiectasis, neuromuscular diseases) and to the increment of noninvasive use of pressure support ventilators. Systematic collection of the data related to this type of chronic care should provide us with a clearer scope of the problem and its consequences in the years to come.

ACKNOWLEDGMENTS

The following authors contributed to the generation of the data presented in this chapter: J.C. Chevrolet, MD, Département de Médecine Soins Intensifs Hôpital Cantonal CH 1211 Genève 14 Suisse; A. Corrado, MD, Terapia intensiva polmonare Azienda Ospedaliera-Careggi Firenze, Italy 50134; C. Donner, MD, Fondazione Salvatore Mauderi, Veruno 28010 Italy; J. Escarrabil, MD, Hospital de Bellvitge 08907 L'Hospitalet Spain; B. Fauroux, MD, Hopital Trousseau 75012 Paris, France; T. Gislason, MD, Vifilsstadir, 210 Gardabar, Iceland; J. Grebstadt, MD, University of Bergen, Norway; P. Hämäläinen, MD, University of Tampere Finland; B. Midgren, MD, Division of Lung Medicine, University Hospital 22185 LUND, Sweden; O. Norregaard, MD, Respiratory Center West, Aahrus, Denmark; D. Rodenstein, MD, Service de Pneumologie, Centre Universitaire St. Luc, Brussels 1180, Belgium; R. Sergysels, MD, Service de Pneumologie, Centre Universitaire St. Pierre Brussels 1180, Belgium; B. Schönhofer, MD, Krankenhaus Kloster Grafshatz Schmallenberg 57392 Germany; A. Simonds, MD, Royal Brompton & Harefield NHS Trust London, UK.

The authors want to thank Pr. K. Strom (Sweden) and Mr. Foret (ANTADIR) for their help.

REFERENCES

1. Donner CF, Howard P, Robert D. Patient selection and techniques for home mechanical ventilation. Monaldi Arch Chest Dis 1993;48:40–47.

2. Muir JF. Intermittent positive pressure ventilation in COPD. Eur Respir Rev 1992;10:335–345.

3. Adams AB, Whitman J, Marcy T. Surveys of long-term ventilatory support in Minnesota: 1986 and 1992. Chest 1993;103:1463–1469.

4. Muir JF, Voisin C, Ludot A. Organization of home respiratory care: the experience in France with ANTADIR. Monaldi Arch Chest Dis 1993; 48:462–467.

5. Fauroux B, Howard P, Muir JF. Home treatment for chronic respiratory insufficiency: the situation in Europe in 1992. Eur Respir J 1994;7:1721–1726.

6. Chailleux E, Faroux B, Binet F, et al. Predictors of survival in patients receiving domiciliary oxygen therapy or mechanical ventilation: a 10-year analysis of ANTADIR observations. Chest 1996;109: 741–749.

7. Ström K. Experience with an oxygen registry in Sweden. In: O'Donohue WJ, ed. Long-term Oxygen Therapy: Scientific Basis and Clinical Application. New York: Marcel Dekker, 1995: 331–346.

8. Healy E, Kelly P, Clancy L. Long-term home oxygen: current practice in Ireland. Ir Med J 1993;86:62–63.

9. Howard P. Home mechanical ventilation and respiratory care in the United Kingdom. Eur Respir Rev 1992;2:416–417.

10. Bengt MI, Olofson J, Harlid R, et al. Home mechanical ventilation in Sweden, with reference to Danish experiences. Accepted for publication in Respir Med.

11. Institut National Assurance-Maladie-Invalidité

(INAMI). Convention entre le Comité de Gestion du Service des Soins de Santé de l'INAMI et les Services hospitaliers. In: Assistance ventilatoire mécanique au long cours à domicile. Brussels, Belgium: INAMI ed., 1992:1–5.

12. Association Suisse contre la Tuberculose et les Maladies Pulmonaires. Lignes directrices pour la ventilation mécanique à domicile. Bull Office Santé Publ. 1991;1:5–10.

13. Chevrolet ICI, Fitting JW, Domenighetti G, et al. Ventilation mécanique à domicile en Suisse en 1990. Schweiz Med Wochenschr 1991;121: 368–377.

14. Bach JR. Ventilator use by muscular dystrophy association patients. Arch Phys Med Rehabil 1992;73:179–183.

15. Donner CF, Zaccaria S, Braghiroli A, et al. Organization of home care in patients receiving nocturnal ventilatory support. Eur Respir Monogr 1998;3:380–399.

16. Medical Research Council Working Party. Long-term domiciliary oxygen therapy in chronic hypoxic cor pulmonale complicating chronic bronchitis and emphysema. Lancet 1981;1:681–686.

17. Nocturnal Oxygen Therapy Trial Group. Continuous or nocturnal oxygen therapy in hypoxaemic chronic obstructive airways disease: a clinical trial. Ann Intern Med 1980;93:391–398.

23 Surgical Therapy for COPD

Fernando J. Martinez

ⓓ Professional Skills

Upon completion of this chapter, the reader will:

- Understand the history of surgical therapy for emphysema
- Be able to contrast standard bullectomy with lung volume reduction surgery (LVRS)
- Understand the clinical, physiologic, and radiographic indications for standard bullectomy
- Understand the clinical, physiologic, and radiographic indications for LVRS
- Understand the clinical, physiologic, and radiographic indications for lung transplantation
- Appreciate the current status of long-term results from standard bullectomy, LVRS, and lung transplantation

Chronic obstructive pulmonary disease (COPD) is a category of heterogeneous diseases with a varying pathophysiologic basis[1] but that manifest varying degrees of chronic airflow obstruction and hyperinflation. The incidence in the United States is estimated to be at least 14 million, and the prevalence is rising.[2-4] At least 2 million individuals suffer from predominantly emphysema, which is characterized by anatomic air space enlargement.[5] The economic burden of these disorders is huge and increases with more severe disease.[6] Furthermore, a marked impairment of quality of life is noted in these patients as the disease progresses.[7]

During the past 50 years many advances have been made in the management of COPD. The American Thoracic Society has recently published a detailed, evidence-based analysis of medical management that provides a stepped-care algorithm of bronchodilators and suggests a possible role for anti-inflammatory agents.[8] Furthermore, a recent comprehensive review of pulmonary rehabilitation has confirmed objective and subjective improvements with varying rehabilitation formats in patients with COPD.[9] Despite these advances, many patients continue to experience incapacitating breathlessness and exercise limitation. During the past 90 years this has led to numerous surgical approaches to ameliorate symptoms in these patients.

HISTORY OF SURGICAL THERAPY FOR EMPHYSEMA

Elegant discussions of the surgical history of emphysema management have been provided by Gaensler et al.[10] and more recently by Deslauriers.[11] The surgical attempts reflect the state of knowledge for their era. Early authors emphasized surgical attempts to improve thoracic mobility, including costochondrectomy and transverse sternotomy.[10,11] Results were unpredictable, however. As it became clearer that thoracic distention was the result and not the cause of emphysema, surgeons began to advocate techniques to decrease the size of the thoracic cage, including thoracoplasty and phrenicectomy.[10,11] Similarly, attempts were made to improve diaphragmatic architecture and function by inducing a pneumoperitoneum or by the use of abdominal belts. Although transient relief was noted, practical considerations limited widespread use of these techniques.[10,11]

Efforts to treat the airway component of chronic airflow obstruction included denervation procedures based on the assumption of an imbalance in the autonomic nervous system.[11] Some individuals addressed the problem of expiratory, tracheobronchial collapse by supporting the membranous trachea using various prosthetic devices.[10,11] Because of significant morbidity and unpredictable results, widespread enthusiasm never developed.

In an attempt to reduce hyperinflation, Brantigan and colleagues approached patients with emphysema in a unique fashion. They hypothesized that by surgically removing lung volume one could restore radial traction on the terminal bronchioles.[10–12] This was postulated to improve expiratory airflow obstruction and improve diaphragmatic position and function.[13,14] Although symptomatic improvement was reported in most patients, the operative mortality was significant (6/33, 18%).[13] As such, widespread application of this novel technique never materialized.

During the subsequent 40 years various groups applied similar principles in small case series.[15–18] In 1991 Wakabayashi and colleagues[19] reported preliminary results using laser shrinkage of target areas of emphysema via unilateral thoracoscopy. Although follow-up data were incomplete, moderate physiologic improvement was suggested.[19] The current era of LVRS was ushered in by Cooper and colleagues,[20] who reported dramatic improvement with a similar technique to Brantigan's although applied bilaterally via median sternotomy (MS).[20] Multiple subsequent investigators reported more limited improvements, as enumerated recently by Utz and colleagues[21] and Benditt and Albert.[22] Despite these results, the available literature has been limited by inconsistent follow-up, varying surgical techniques and patient selection criteria, and lack of control groups. As a result, many important questions remain.

Lung transplantation dates to the early 1960s, with a total of 36 transplants performed between 1963 and 1974, of which 14 were performed for patients with emphysema.[23] Unfortunately, uniformly poor results were noted, with only three patients living longer than 1 month and the longest living only 10 months. The major causes of death among patients who underwent transplantation with COPD were respiratory failure due to rejection, infection, or bronchial disruption.[24,25] The first successful lung transplantation occurred as part of a heart–lung block for pulmonary vascular disease in 1981,[26] in part owing to advances in immunosuppressive medications (particularly cyclosporine) and surgical techniques. In 1983 single lung transplantation (SLT) was successfully performed in patients with idiopathic pulmonary fibrosis (IPF), and it was reported in 1986. Because of differences in lung compliance, this form of therapy was believed to be inappropriate for patients with COPD. In fact, early reports of SLT in patients with COPD had suggested this. Stevens and colleagues[27] reported two patients who underwent left SLT for α_1-deficiency–related emphysema. Serial ventilation and perfusion to the lungs were measured in these patients (who survived 10 and 26 d). A gradual increase in perfusion to the transplanted lung accompanied by an increase in ventilation to the native lung was documented. The authors hypothesized that the highly compliant, native, emphysematous lung was contributing to the ventilation–perfusion mismatch. In an accompanying editorial, Bates[28] suggested double lung transplantation (DLT) as a potential surgical modality to avoid such mismatch.

Patterson and colleagues[29,30] reported successful DLT in patients with COPD. Subsequently, Hutchin and colleagues and Veith et al.[31] noted that significant ventilation–perfusion imbalance and/or impairment in the transplanted lung occurred predominantly during rejection, infection, or implantation injury. Mal et al.[32] reported successful SLT in two patients with severe COPD. Since that time, SLT has become the predominant surgical therapy for advanced COPD, with 74% of patients undergoing transplantation in 1997 for COPD receiving a single lung.[23]

WHICH SURGICAL TECHNIQUE SHOULD BE USED?

An exhaustive description of the surgical techniques is outside the scope of this chapter. Interested readers are referred to the published literature.[33,34] Points of importance to the practicing internist will be briefly discussed, contrasting the most frequently used techniques (bullectomy, LVRS, and lung transplantation). For the following discussion, LVRS will refer to surgical volume reduction in the absence of large bullae.

Bullectomy

Multiple techniques have been used to resect localized bullae, including standard lateral thoracotomy,[10] bilateral resection by median sternotomy (MS),[35] and video-assisted thoracic surgery (VATS) with stapling[33] or endoloop ligation.[36] Unfortunately, comparative studies are not available. As such, the surgical approach depends on the nature of the bullous disease (bilateral vs. unilateral), the severity of respiratory insufficiency, and the experience of the surgeon.[33]

Lung Volume Reduction Surgery

The surgical approach to LVRS has been similarly varied and includes MS,[34] standard thoracotomy, and VATS.[37] Some authors have promoted laser ablation,[38] although recent comparative trials have raised significant questions about this technique. McKenna and colleagues[39] described results of a prospective, randomized trial of laser versus stapled, unilateral LVRS. The mean postoperative improvement in forced expiratory volume in 1 second (FEV_1) and elimination of oxygen dependency were greater in the stapled group, whereas the incidence of delayed pneumothorax was higher in the laser-treated group. No cut plication has been advocated as an alternative with potentially less morbidity.[40]

Comparative studies are few but have confirmed greater improvement with bilateral procedures.[41,42] An advantage of MS over VATS has not been clearly established. Some authors suggest that this depends on surgeon preference and experience.[43] Kotloff and colleagues[44] retrospectively compared MS and VATS performed by different surgeons at the same medical center.[44] Similar improvement was noted in physiologic outcome, although no difference was seen in duration of air leak or length of stay. The overall incidence of respiratory failure and the total in hospital mortality was higher in the MS group. In a sequential, nonrandomized study, Wisser et al.[45] examined MS versus bilateral VATS procedures. No difference was seen in functional or physiologic results. In addition, postoperative morbidity and mortality were similar between the two groups. A definitive recommendation will require prospective, controlled data collection.

Lung Transplantation

The current surgical approaches and principles of postoperative management are outside the scope of this chapter. Interested readers may refer to recent, excellent reviews of the topic.[23,46,47] Briefly, SLT is generally performed via a posterolateral thoracotomy, with cardiopulmonary bypass rarely required in patients with severe COPD.[46] Although difficult to predict, patients with more severe pulmonary hypertension are more likely to require bypass.[46,48] Because of early problems with the healing of the tracheal anastomosis, DLT has evolved during the past decade with the introduction of the bilateral sequential operation.[49] This procedure, which is performed through a transverse thoracosternotomy with lungs implanted separately and sequentially, has become the standard approach.[46]

Much controversy continues to revolve around the optimal transplant procedure in patients with COPD. In some patients, DLT seems to be a better approach. This includes patients with septic disease (significant bronchiectasis, e.g.) or those with large bullae[46] and, potentially, those with elevated pulmonary artery pressure.[23] The last indication is suggested by the data of the University of Minnesota group, which has recently compared outcome in 93 consecutive patients.[48] In patients treated with SLT, a significantly lower 3-year survival was seen in those with an elevated pulmonary artery systolic pressure (>40 mm Hg; n = 16) (34 vs. 77%). No such difference was seen in patients undergoing DLT. Multiple authors have retrospectively compared results of SLT versus DLT when these indications are not present. Patterson et al.[50] compared 11 patients undergoing DLT with 7 treated with SLT. The operative course was similar between the two groups, although patients undergoing DLT suffered a greater incidence of airway complications. Similar data were presented by Low and colleagues,[51] who compared 16 patients undergoing DLT and 16 undergoing SLT. Although the immediate postoperative course was similar between the two groups, the 1-year survival was higher for those undergoing SLT (93 vs. 71%). Similarly, another group has reported improved 1-year survival in patients undergoing SLT versus DLT (77 vs. 35%).[52] Similar mortality data have been reported by Cooper et al.,[53] although only a fraction of the patients reported were transplanted for COPD. Al-Kattan and colleagues[54] compared 21 patients with emphysema treated with heart–lung transplantation (HLT) with 68 treated with SLT. A similar actuarial 5-year survival was reported for both groups (67% for SLT vs. 60% for HLT).

In contrast, Sundaresan et al.[55] reported a similar perioperative course in patients undergoing SLT versus DLT, although a trend toward better 5-year survival was seen in those treated with bilateral transplantation. These data are a bit difficult to interpret because the group undergoing SLT was older (55 vs. 49 years). Similarly, Bavaria et al.[56] retrospectively compared 47 patients undergoing SLT with 29 undergoing DLT for COPD. Perioperative course was more complicated in the SLT group, with a longer length of intubation (8.13 vs. 2.43 days) and a higher incidence of primary graft dysfunction (19.2 vs. 3.45%). These translated into a markedly higher 60-day mortality in the SLT group (21.3 vs. 3.45%). These data are difficult to interpret because the SLT group was significantly older (55.3 vs. 48.8 years) and had worse pulmonary function at baseline (forced vital capacity, 1.76 vs. 2.18). Most recently, the group at the University of Minnesota compared the results of 87 patients treated with SLT with 16 undergoing DLT for COPD.[57] A trend toward improved 5-year survival was demonstrated for the DLT group. All of these data are limited by the lack of prospective data collection and randomization to ensure comparable treatment groups. As such, clear recommendations require further data collection.

WHAT ARE THE RESULTS OF SURGERY?

Short-Term Results

Bullectomy

Bullectomy seems to be of short-term benefit in highly selected patients.[58–64] Snider[65] recently provided an elegant review of case series published since 1950. None of the 22 studies included a control group, and most were retrospective in nature. As such, firm conclusions were difficult to reach. In general, improvement in hypoxemia and hypercapnia were most frequently reported with greater heterogeneity in the improvement in airflow. When measured, total lung capacity (TLC), residual volume (RV), and trapped gas (measured as the difference between plethysmographic and dilutional lung volumes) generally decreased. Cor pulmonale reversed if hypoxemia and hypercapnia were present in highly selected patients. Most authors described improvement in dyspnea, with several groups reporting quantitative improvement in breathlessness. Little data were provided regarding improvements in health-related quality of life (HRQL), medication or oxygen requirements, or effects on subsequent hospitalizations.

Lung Volume Reduction Surgery

Since the early report of Cooper and colleagues,[20] numerous reports of LVRS have appeared in the literature. Summaries of these studies have been well described by Utz et al.,[21] Benditt and Albert,[22] and Sciurba.[66] It is evident that major problems are noted consistently, including (*a*) variable surgical techniques and selection criteria, (*b*) short and often incomplete postoperative follow-up, (*c*) retrospective data collection in most series, and (*d*) the absence of a control group in all published reports.

Clinical Results

A wide range of 30-day mortality, the classic surgical benchmark of operative mortality, has been reported after LVRS, ranging from 0 to 15%. The differences in morbidity and mortality may relate to varying definitions of surgical mortality, different inclusion and exclusion criteria, different surgical techniques and experience, and varying postoperative management.[21,67] The Health Care Finance Administration decided to deny coverage for LVRS in late 1995 on the basis of two independent assessments of available data.[68] A subsequent report to Congress included a supplemental analysis of Medicare claims identified by *International Classification of Diseases, Ninth Edition,* code for LVRS procedures performed from October 1995 to January 1996.[69] This database included 722 patients. The 3-month mortality was 14.4% and the 6-month mortality was 16.9%. In addition, a marked rise was noted in the number of acute care hospital days (11.8 days/patient in the year before surgery to 18.7 days/patient in the year after LVRS, exclusive of the surgical hospitalization). Furthermore, long-term care facility days, rehabilitation hospital days, and skilled nursing facility days rose in the year after surgery.[69] Although these data are flawed by the lack of standardized recording of the surgical procedure performed or patient characteristics, they suggest potentially significant short-term morbidity and mortality. More rigorous, prospective, controlled data are being collected to better define the risks of the procedure, particularly in an older, Medicare-insured population.

Pulmonary Function

The original report by Cooper et al.[20] reported an 82% improvement in FEV_1 (mean follow-up, 6.4 mo). Subsequent studies by this group and those of subsequent series by others confirmed significant mean improvements in spirometry, although to a lesser extent than initially reported.[21,22,66] Most published studies emphasized spirometric data, with mean improvements in FEV_1 ranging from 13 to 96%. Unfortunately, many authors failed to specify whether reported values are those obtained before or after the administration of bronchodilators, which makes interpretation of the results difficult. Nevertheless, given a preoperative FEV_1 that ranges from 15 to 33% predicted, the improvements seem to be significant.

In addition, close review of published data suggests that, in general, bilateral procedures are associated with greater short-term improvement. Of studies in which a unilateral procedure was used exclusively, the mean improvement in FEV_1 was 29%; in studies exclusively using a bilateral procedure, the mean improvement was 46%. Direct comparisons of unilateral versus bilateral reduction are scarce.[41,42,70] McKenna and colleagues[41] reported results in 166 consecutive patients undergoing volume reduction via thoracoscopic stapling (unilateral in 87 patients and bilateral in 79 patients). Those undergoing unilateral procedures experienced a 31% improvement in FEV_1 compared with 57% increases in those undergoing bilateral volume reduction 6 months after surgery. Mortality at 1 year was lower in the bilateral group compared with the unilaterally treated group (5 vs. 17%). Argenziano et al.[42] described results in 64 patients undergoing bilateral stapling procedures and 28 undergoing unilateral procedures. The indications for unilateral procedures included patients with asymmetric disease, previous thoracic surgery, or the presence of concomitant tumors. Improvement in FEV_1 was greater in the bilaterally treated group (70 vs. 28%). Finally, Eugene and colleagues[70] reported results of unilateral reduction in 34 patients compared with bilateral procedures in 10 patients. The surgical procedures included a mixture of stapling and laser procedures. The improvement in FEV_1 was much higher in those treated bilaterally (82%) compared with those treated unilaterally (45%). Although no well-performed, randomized trials have been published, greater improvement in spirometry is apparent in patients undergoing bilateral LVRS.

Similarly, limited data have been published regarding various surgical techniques. In general, laser procedures seem to result in worse outcomes than do stapling techniques. McKenna et al.[39] have reported the only prospective, randomized trial contrasting stapled versus laser lung reduction. These authors described results in 33 patients undergoing unilateral VATS with Nd:YAG laser reduction compared with 39 patients undergoing bilateral VATS with stapled resection. Those undergoing stapled resections experienced a greater short-term improvement in FEV_1 than those undergoing laser reduction (32.9 vs. 13.4%). In addition, Keenan and colleagues[71] noted much higher morbidity in a limited number of patients undergoing unilateral laser reduction (n = 10) compared with a group undergoing predominantly stapled resections (n = 57). Pulmonary function test results between the two groups were not reported, however. As such, the limited data suggest that current laser technology has a limited role in LVRS.

Several groups have compared short-term physiologic outcomes of bilateral surgery performed via VATS or MS. Kotloff and colleagues[44] reported a retrospective series from the same institution. Fifty-nine patients underwent bilateral LVRS via MS and 40 underwent bilateral reduction via VATS. No difference was noted in short-term spirometric outcomes, although total in hospital mortality was significantly higher in the MS group (13.8 vs. 2.5%). Wisser and colleagues[45] compared 15 patients undergoing bilateral LVRS via MS with 15 undergoing bilateral thoracoscopic LVRS. They noted little difference in all outcomes, including spirometry, between the two surgical groups. Hazelrigg et al.[72] published similar retrospective results. Interestingly, Ko and Waters[73] noted a much higher total mortality (25%) in 19 patients undergoing bilateral LVRS via MS compared with 23 patients treated thoracoscopically (8%). Furthermore, the improvement in FEV_1 was higher in the VATS group (62 vs. 28%). Unfortunately, none of these studies were randomized, which limits the conclusions that can be reached. Further prospective, randomized data collection is required to better define this important surgical question.

Importantly, most pulmonary function data reported represents the mean improvement in FEV_1. The variance around the mean is described in remarkably few studies.[44,74,75] Figure 23-1 illustrates the distribution of change in FEV_1 in the retrospective comparison of bilateral LVRS via MS and VATS reported by Kotloff et al.[44]; approximately one-third of patients in both groups experienced a less than 20% short-term rise in FEV_1. Other investigators have published qualitatively similar data.[71,75-77] As such, most investigators demonstrate a mean improvement in FEV_1, although a wide range of response is evident, with 20 to 50% of patients demonstrating little short-term spirometric improvement after LVRS.[67] Highlighting the limitation of FEV_1 as the sole measure of improvement, many patients who experience limited spirometric improvement demonstrate significant lessening of breathlessness.[76]

Although less frequently reported, lung volumes have generally decreased during short-term follow-up; the range of decrease in TLC varies from 2 to 23%, whereas the RV has dropped from 3 to 39%. Although rarely reported, the changes in diffusion capacity of carbon dioxide (DLCO) have been modest. Little data are available to judge the effects of surgical techniques on lung volume and DLCO changes. Changes in resting arterial blood gases have been heterogeneous, ranging from significant improvements in arterial partial pressure of oxygen (PaO_2) and decreases in arterial partial pressure of carbon dioxide ($PaCO_2$) to little change.[22,66,78] Albert and colleagues[79] have presented the most detailed data, which highlight significant improvement in arterial blood gases in some patients with worsening in others. For the group as a whole, minimal changes were noted. Furthermore, no correlation was seen between arterial blood gas changes and the change in spirometry, lung volumes, or DLCO. The authors believed that the effect of LVRS on

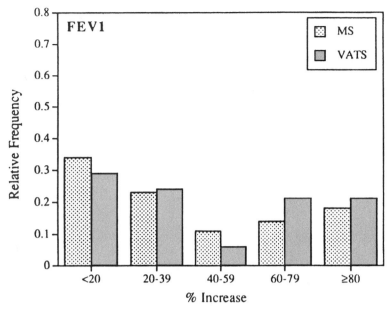

Figure 23-1. Distribution of percentage increases in forced expiratory volume in 1 second (*FEV₁*) after bilateral LVRS via median sternotomy (*MS*) and video-assisted thoracic surgery (*VATS*). (Reprinted with permission from Kotloff R, Tino G, Bavaria J, et al. Bilateral lung volume reduction surgery for advanced emphysema: a comparison of median sternotomy and thoracoscopic approaches. Chest 1996;110:1399–1406.)

blood gases resulted primarily from alterations in ventilation–perfusion heterogeneity and not mean alveolar ventilation.[79]

Exercise Capacity

Most investigators have used simple measures of exercise capacity, such as timed measures of walk distance. Consistent improvements in walk distance have been reported, ranging from 7 to 103%. Unfortunately, most investigators provide limited descriptions of the methods used. Six-minute walk distance, the most common test used, is highly dependent on testing format and patient encouragement.[80] In addition, pulmonary rehabilitation has been shown to improve walk distance.[80] Given the limited methodologic descriptions provided by most investigators, it is difficult to reach definite conclusions regarding the magnitude of improvement or the causal relation to LVRS versus the effects of continued, aggressive rehabilitation.

Recently, several groups have reported results of cardiopulmonary exercise testing suggesting consistent, short-term increases in maximal workload, peak oxygen uptake (VO_2), and minute ventilation (VE). Keller and colleagues[74] performed maximal cardiopulmonary exercise testing in 25 patients before and after unilateral LVRS, confirming increases in work load, VO_2, and VE. The latter was achieved through increased tidal volume, with little change in respiratory rate. Mean inspiratory and expiratory flows increased significantly in all patients, whereas PaO_2 improved in 20.[74] Benditt et al.[81] extended these findings in a study of patients performing maximal cardiopulmonary exercise testing before and after bilateral LVRS. They confirmed improved aerobic capacity but noted decreased heart rate at similar work loads. Ventilatory limitation was seen in most patients as they developed acute respiratory acidosis during maximal exercise before and after LVRS.

Martinez and colleagues[76] noted similar results at isowork but improved dyspnea. This correlated best with decreased dynamic hyperinflation.[76] In addition, Tschernko et al.[82] noted a significant decrease in the work of breathing during exercise after LVRS.

Ferguson et al.[83] confirmed improvement during maximal cardiopulmonary exercise testing but extended the findings by confirming improved tidal volume at submaximal work loads during steady-state testing. Furthermore, they noted improved physiologic dead space with decreased $PaCO_2$ during exercise, whereas the improvement in exercise capacity correlated with the improvement in FEV_1 and the maximal inspiratory mouth pressure. Most recently, the short-term effects of LVRS on the pulmonary vascular response to exercise have been described by two groups.[84,85] Neither group noted significant changes in pulmonary hemodynamics at rest or during exercise. In contrast, Weg and colleagues[86] recently reported an elevation of resting pulmonary artery pressures in nine patients 3 months after bilateral LVRS.

Medication and Oxygen Requirements

Several groups have described improvements in oxygen (O_2) requirement after surgery.[21] Keenan and colleagues[71] reported an elimination of O_2 requirement in 17% of patients and a decrease in O_2 requirement in 25% of patients 3 months after unilateral LVRS. Naunheim et al.[87] reported that 48% of patients had discontinued O_2 3 months after unilateral LVRS. Others have reported similar data after unilateral LVRS.[41,70,88–90] Cooper and colleagues[91] reported that of the 52% of patients using O_2 continuously before surgery, only 16% were using O_2 continuously 6 months after bilateral LVRS. In addition, of the 92% who were using O_2 with exertion before surgery, only 44% were doing so after surgery. Similar data have been reported by other investigators.[45,72,73,90,92–94] In the only randomized trial to examine bilateral versus unilateral LVRS, McKenna and colleagues[41] noted that 6 months after unilateral LVRS, 18 (36%) of 50 patients requiring O_2 before surgery did not require it after surgery. In the bilaterally treated group, 30 (68%) of 44 patients requiring O_2 before surgery required it after surgery. The difference between the two groups was significant ($P < .01$). Unfortunately, most studies have reported short-term data with little description of oxygen titration techniques. Furthermore, in many cases, follow-up is incomplete, which could inflate the percentage of patients liberated from O_2.

Several groups have reported significant steroid liberation rates after LVRS.[20,70,72,87,88,90,91,95,96] Cooper and colleagues[91] examined prednisone requirement in 56 of 76 patients eligible for 1-year follow-up after bilateral LVRS. Before surgery, 53% of patients required chronic steroid use; the percentage decreased to 17% six months and 19% one year after surgery. McKenna et al.[41] reported a resolution of steroid requirement in 54% of patients 6 months after unilateral LVRS and in 85% of patients after bilateral LVRS. The difference between the groups was significant ($P < .02$). Unfortunately, most studies provide little detail regarding steroid reduction protocols, thereby limiting the ability to adequately interpret these data. Further data must be prospectively collected before firm conclusions can be reached regarding the effect of LVRS on subsequent medication use.

Dyspnea and HRQL

Severe emphysema markedly impairs quality of life.[7] Most investigators have reported improvements in dyspnea after LVRS, although only a few have used validated instruments to quantify the degree of improvement. Most have used the Medical Research Council (MRC) dyspnea scoring system[97] to grade dyspnea; most investigations have demonstrated significant short-term improvements, with a range of 2.9 to 4.1 before surgery to 0.8 to 1.8 after surgery.[20,39,41,42,70,91,98–102] Other groups have used the Transitional Dyspnea Index of Mahler and colleagues.[103] The range of improvement has varied widely from Transitional

Dyspnea Index scores of 0.92 to 7.8, suggesting little to dramatic decreases in dyspnea.[20,71,74,76,87,89,91,94,96,104] Data comparing varying surgical techniques are scant, however. Argenziano et al.[42] noted little change in dyspnea improvement as measured using the MRC scale after unilateral or bilateral LVRS. McKenna and colleagues[41] reported a greater percentage of patients with higher-grade dyspnea (3–4 on the MRC scale) after surgery in patients treated with unilateral (44%) compared with bilateral (12%) LVRS. In contrast, Wisser et al.[45] noted no difference in dyspnea improvement whether patients underwent LVRS via bilateral VATS or MS. Importantly, few groups have examined the independent effect of aggressive pulmonary rehabilitation compared with LVRS. Cooper et al. noted little change from baseline dyspnea (MRC grade 2.9) to immediately after pulmonary rehabilitation (2.8), with a significant decrease after bilateral LVRS via MS (1.2) suggesting an independent effect of surgery.[91] As with spirometric data, most data have been reported as mean improvements. Few investigators have provided the range of improvement. Keller and colleagues[74] provided short-term Transitional Dyspnea Index scores in 25 patients after unilateral LVRS. Twenty-two patients demonstrated a change of +3 or more, suggesting moderate improvement.

The most detailed analysis of dyspnea after LVRS has been reported by Brenner et al.,[99] who recorded the MRC score before and after thoracoscopic LVRS in 145 patients. The distribution of improvement in breathlessness is illustrated in Figure 23-2. The baseline FEV_1 weakly correlated with baseline dyspnea, and the change in FEV_1 correlated poorly with the change in dyspnea ($r = 0.3$). A better correlation was noted between lesser improvement in dyspnea after LVRS and higher preoperative hyperexpansion. Nevertheless, a significant number of patients with severe hyperinflation (RV/TLC >0.7) noted improved breathlessness after surgery (8 of 36 patients). In addition, although 28% of patients had minimal or no improvement in FEV_1 after surgery, 10 of these 37 patients noted an improvement by 2 or more dyspnea scores. This discrepancy in improved breathlessness and improvement in FEV_1 has been described by others. Martinez and colleagues[76] noted improved breathlessness in 17 patients after bilateral LVRS via MS, although six patients experienced a less than 20% improvement in FEV_1 after surgery. A significant correlation was noted between decreased breathlessness during exercise and improvement in dynamic hyperinflation.

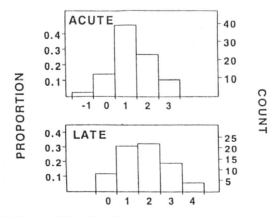

IMPROVEMENT IN DYSPNEA SCORE

Figure 23-2. Distribution of improvement in dyspnea score early and late after bilateral LVRS. The baseline dyspnea scores averaged 3.0 ± 0.7. (Reprinted with permission from Brenner M, McKenna R, Gelb A, et al. Dyspnea response following bilateral thoracoscopic staple lung volume reduction surgery. Chest 1997;112:916–923.)

The quantification of HRQL provides important additional information to gauge the impact of COPD.[105] This information is incremental to the quantification of breathlessness[106] and seems to loosely correlate with increasingly severe disease.[107] In fact, because HRQL measures how a person enjoys life it may be the most important of all functional measurements. Unfortunately, only a few investigators have reported formal measurement of HRQL. Furthermore, although optimal information is obtained with the use of both a generic instrument and a disease-specific instrument,[108] no group has reported these data before and after LVRS. The group at Washington University[20,91] has reported short-term improvements using the Medical Outcomes Study Short-Form 36 (SF-36) and the Nottingham Health Profile, generic instruments that have been validated in patients with COPD.[105,106,109] The improvement after LVRS was noted in measures of vitality, social functioning, physical functioning, and general health and in an increased ability to perform various roles. Hazelrigg et al.[89] noted improved HRQL measured with the SF-36 in 80% of patients after LVRS. They expanded these findings by noting a similar short-term improvement after bilateral LVRS via VATS or MS.[72] Ferguson and colleagues[83] reported improvement in HRQL as measured by the SF-36 after bilateral LVRS; the improvement in social functioning correlated well with the improvement in FEV_1, whereas the improvement in exercise capacity correlated directly with the improvement in physical functioning and inversely with dyspnea. The most detailed analysis to date has been published by Moy and colleagues,[110] who measured HRQL with the SF-36 before and after comprehensive pulmonary rehabilitation and again after bilateral LVRS via VATS in 19 patients. No significant change was noted in any of the domains after pulmonary rehabilitation, although significant improvement was noted in vitality after LVRS. Compared with baseline scoring, the combination of rehabilitation and bilateral LVRS resulted in significant improvement in four of the eight domains (physical functioning, role limitations owing to physical problems, social functioning, and vitality). Pulmonary rehabilitation accounted for most of the improvement in role limitations and LVRS accounted for most of the improvement in physical functioning, vitality, and social functioning. Cordova et al. used the Sickness Impact Profile[111] before and after LVRS, confirming significant improvements in overall, physical, and social scores 3, 6, and 12 months after surgery.[112] In a subsequent analysis, the same group confirmed a similar degree of improvement in HRQL in patients with hypercapnia compared with those who were normocapnic before surgery.[113]

Quantification of HRQL by disease-specific instruments is more limited in the literature. Bagley and colleagues[90] described changes measured with the Chronic Respiratory Questionnaire, the first disease-specific questionnaire developed for use in patients with COPD.[114] During short-term follow-up, improvements were noted in the four domains of dyspnea, fatigue, emotional function, and mastery. Most recently, Norman et al.[115] reported results using the St. George's Respiratory Questionnaire. Large improvements were noted in scores within all sections, with a mean reduction in the total score of 31 points 3 months after bilateral LVRS via MS.

Transplantation

Postoperative complications are frequent in patients undergoing SLT or DLT. These are described in detail by others[23,46,47] and include primary graft failure, airway complications, acute rejection, and infection. The latter includes community acquired bacterial pathogens from the donor or nosocomial bacterial pathogens early in the postoperative period.

Pulmonary Function

The published literature has consistently demonstrated spirometric improvement after both SLT and DLT. In general, the improvement is lesser for SLT, with peak FEV_1 ranging from 45 to 60% predicted.[50,51,53,55,56,116–122] These results are exemplified by the data presented by Levine et al.,[116] who described functional results in 28 patients undergoing 29 SLT procedures. A rise occurred in FEV_1 from a baseline of 16% predicted to 57% predicted 3 months and 60% predicted 6 months after SLT. These data are typical for

COPD patients undergoing SLT and are consistent with a mixed obstructive and restrictive picture. Several groups have examined the factors determining postoperative spirometry after SLT. Brunsting et al.[122] examined 14 patients and suggested that recipient chest wall factors determined postoperative pulmonary function in these patients. The importance of recipient factors was confirmed by Cheriyan and colleagues,[123] who concluded that pulmonary function after SLT reflected restriction of the transplanted lung and obstruction in the native lung with a decreased transpulmonary pressure. In an elegant study of 14 COPD patients studied after SLT, Estenne et al.[124] confirmed hyperinflation of the native lung in all patients with a lower, yet stable, TLC in the allograft. Interestingly, the graft exhibited a normal functional residual capacity, suggesting that the expansion of the rib cage allows preservation of the functional residual capacity in the transplanted lung. The discrepancy in function between the native lung and the allograft may produce an interesting spirometric abnormality.[125] This biphasic pattern has been shown to reflect the differing time constants of the normal transplanted lung and the emphysematous lung.[126] Importantly, when this abnormality develops after initial stabilization of lung function, a bronchial stenosis should be considered.[125]

In contrast, patients undergoing DLT experience a significantly higher FEV_1, with most series reporting values near normal. This is highlighted by the report by Gaissert et al.,[120] who described functional results in 33 patients undergoing bilateral LVRS (mean age, 57 years), 39 undergoing SLT for COPD (mean age, 55 years), and 27 undergoing DLT for COPD (mean age, 49 years). Figure 23-3 illustrates the short-term change in FEV_1 as a percent of predicted values. Clearly, a greater improvement is seen after DLT compared with SLT and LVRS. These data are qualitatively similar to those presented by other groups.[50,51,53]

The variability of spirometric indices has been examined by Martinez et al.[127] in 351 sequential spirometry measurements in 65 healthy recipients (18 HLT, 24 DLT, 23 SLT, 20 with emphysema) after the 80th postoperative day. The month-to-month variability

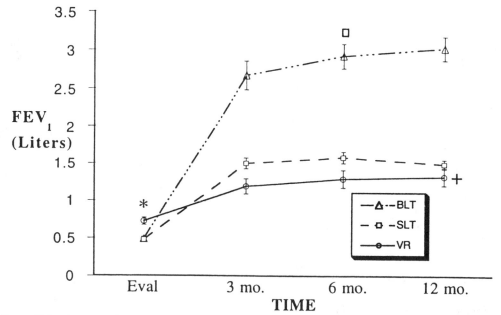

Figure 23-3. Change in forced expiratory volume in 1 second (*FEV₁*) before and after bilateral LVRS (*VR*), single lung transplantation (*SLT*), and bilateral lung transplantation (*BLT*) for COPD. (Reprinted with permission from Gaissert H, Trulock I, Cooper J, et al. Comparison of early functional results after volume reduction or lung transplantation for chronic obstructive pulmonary disease. J Thorac Cardiovasc Surg 1996;111:296–307.)

in forced vital capacity and FEV_1 was similar to that in healthy subjects and was, in part, dependent on time after transplantation. The significant value for change in FEV_1 was 18% in HLT recipients 1 year or less after transplantation, 9% in HLT recipients more than 1 year after transplantation, and 13% for SLT recipients throughout follow-up. Becker and colleagues[128] reported that the sensitivity and specificity of spirometry for suggesting acute changes in graft function was highest for FEV_1 in SLT recipients with COPD.

Exercise Capacity

Numerous groups have demonstrated improvement in 6-minute walk distance after both SLT and DLT. Kaiser et al.[117] described a rise in distance walk during the first 24 weeks after SLT in 11 patients with emphysema. Similar data were reported by Mal and colleagues.[118] Early comparisons between functional results in patients undergoing DLT suggested a greater improvement in walking distance than in emphysema patients undergoing SLT. Patterson et al.[50] confirmed a greater rise in DLT recipients (573.0 m) than in SLT recipients (528.0 m) 3 months after transplantation. Similar results were reported by this group in another report[55] and by another group of investigators.[56] In contrast, Low et al.[51] described a similar 6-minute walk distance in patients undergoing SLT and DLT for COPD. In the study by Gaissert and colleagues[120] described previously, little difference in 6-minute walk distance was seen up to 1 year after SLT or DLT for emphysema.[120] Interestingly, 6 months after LVRS the 6-minute walk distance was greater than for patients undergoing DLT. It is evident that most patients who survive the initial postoperative period experience an initial improvement in walk distance during short-term follow-up.

As with LVRS, several groups have described exercise capacity with formal measurement of cardiopulmonary response during maximal exercise. Interestingly, all investigators have demonstrated significant aerobic limitation after SLT or DLT with little evidence for ventilatory limitation. The earliest report of cardiopulmonary exercise testing after lung transplantation was that of Miyoshi et al.,[129] who described maximal exercise results in six patients with IPF studied a mean of 18 months (range, 6–43 months) after SLT and six patients treated with DLT (four with emphysema) a studied mean of 10 months earlier. Both groups demonstrated a significant aerobic limitation, with a maximum achieved VO_2 of 44.2% predicted in SLT and 48.5% predicted in DLT recipients. Neither group demonstrated ventilatory limitation as defined by maximal VE divided by maximum voluntary ventilation. These results were extended by Gibbons and colleagues,[130] who studied six patients treated with SLT for COPD with six treated with SLT for IPF. The results were remarkably similar between these two groups and those of previous investigators. Peak oxygen saturation was slightly lower in the IPF group (90.2%) than in the COPD group (95.2%), whereas the respiratory rate was higher (40.4 bpm in IPF vs. 26.5 bpm in COPD). Short-term data reported by other investigators have been consistent with these findings.[131,132] Orens et al.[133] extended these findings by contrasting maximal exercise response 3, 6, and 9 to 12 months after SLT for IPF, SLT for COPD, SLT for pulmonary vascular disease, and DLT. The maximal achieved VO_2 was remarkably similar in all patient groups and rose 3 to 6 months after transplantation but tended to fall by 12 months. Schwaiblmair and colleagues[134] studied a large number of patients with varying underlying disease (IPF, 32%; emphysema, 28%; and cystic fibrosis, 23%, were most common) before and after SLT (n = 46), DLT (n = 32), and HLT (n = 25). At a mean of 55 days after transplantation, all three groups reached a similar maximal achieved VO_2 (43.9% predicted in SLT, 40.2% predicted in DLT, and 38.4% predicted in HLT). Furthermore, the authors demonstrated a similar, severe aerobic limitation in all groups before transplantation, which improved significantly after surgery. Importantly, no evidence of ventilatory limitation was noted after transplantation, with a significant decrease in physiologic dead space and alveolar minus arterial gradient at peak exercise. This is in contrast to the data of Martinez and colleagues,[135] who demonstrated tidal flow loop encroachment in patients after SLT but not DLT. Interestingly, the maximal VO_2 was similar in both groups, although peak exercise breathlessness was lower in DLT recipients.

Evans et al.[136] have confirmed abnormality in quadriceps muscle pH and phosphorylation potential (using ^{31}P-magnetic resonance spectroscopy) during exercise in lung transplant recipients. This abnormality in peripheral muscle oxygen utilization during exercise is supported by the biopsy data of Wang and colleagues,[137] who demonstrated a lower mitochondrial adenosine triphosphate production rate, mitochondrial enzymes, and a higher reliance on anaerobic metabolism in seven stable recipients. These data may help explain the aerobic limitation consistently noted after transplantation.

Stiebellehner et al.[138] have recently demonstrated this aerobic limitation to be partly reversible. These authors studied nine lung transplant recipients (7 DLT, 2 SLT) a mean of 12 months after transplantation. Maximal exercise testing was performed at baseline, after 11 weeks of normal activity, and after a 6-week program of aerobic endurance training. As expected, a significant aerobic limitation was seen at baseline. This changed little after normal activity but improved after endurance training (see Fig. 23-4). In addition, at identical submaximal levels of exercise, a significant decrease in VE and

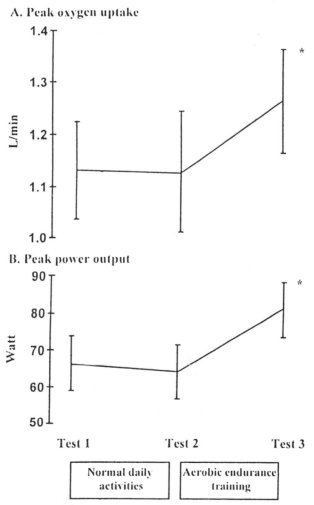

Figure 23-4. Peak oxygen uptake (**A**) and peak power output (**B**) at baseline (Test 1), after a period of normal activity (Test 2), and after a comprehensive exercise program (Test 3) in nine patients after lung transplantation. (Adapted with permission from Stiebellehner L, Quittan M, End A, et al. Aerobic endurance training program improves exercise performance in lung transplant recipients. Chest 1998;113:906–912.)

heart rate was seen after training. These data suggest that the aerobic limit seen after transplantation can be reversed, at least in part, with pulmonary rehabilitation.

Quality of Life

Limited data are available detailing changes in HRQL after lung transplantation. Gross et al.[139] administered lung transplant candidates and recipients the Medical Outcomes Study Health Survey, the Index of Well-Being, the Karnofsky Performance Status Index, and questions assessing work history. Lung transplant candidates, most of whom had obstructive disease, demonstrated significant impairment in HRQL. In those with sequential measurement, significant improvement was noted in multiple parameters 6 to 12 months after transplantation. In a longitudinal study, TenVergert and colleagues[140] prospectively evaluated 24 patients (13 with emphysema) before transplantation and at defined times after surgery. Before transplantation, major restrictions were noted, as measured by the Nottingham Health Profile. One month after transplantation, improvement was noted in several measures. In addition, further improvement was noted during the first four postoperative months such that Nottingham Health Profile scores were comparable to those of the general population. Cohen et al.[141] expanded on these findings by noting that pretransplant anxiety and psychopathology predicted posttransplant adjustment, with greater anxiety predicting worse posttransplant quality of life. Interestingly, despite these improvements, return to employment is seen in only a few transplant recipients during the first year after surgery.[142]

Long-term Results

Bullectomy

Many groups have described several years of follow-up after bullectomy. Fitzgerald et al.[59] described results in 84 patients who underwent 95 surgical procedures in more than 20 years; mean follow-up was 7.3 years. Long-term follow-up was available in 47 patients. Inconsistent maintenance of improvement was noted in 16 patients, with unilateral bullae occupying more than 70% of the hemithorax, although some patients demonstrated improvement for 3 to 5 years. Figure 23-5 illustrates the data of Pearson and Ogilvie,[143]

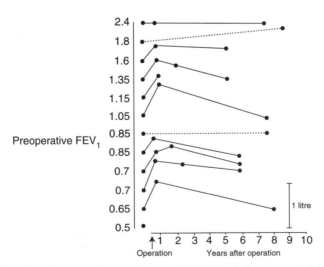

Figure 23-5. Serial forced expiratory volume in 1 second (*FEV₁*) measurements in 12 patients undergoing bullectomy (bilateral in 1, unilateral in 11) and followed up for a mean of 7.3 years. The size of bulla ranged from 20 to 80% of a hemithorax, with a median of 50%. (Reprinted with permission from Pearson M, Ogilvie C. Surgical treatment of emphysematous bullae: late outcome. Thorax 1983;38:134–137.)

who followed up 11 patients for a mean of 7.3 years. Short-term improvement was noted in all, but a gradual decrement in physiologic improvement was noted in most patients. Although not quantitated, the authors reported that dyspnea returned, with four of nine patients back to their preoperative level at last follow-up. A review of published data by Snider[65] suggests that one-third to one-half of patients maintain benefits for about 5 years. Importantly, most authors have reported poorest long-term outcome in those individuals with a greater degree of emphysema in the remaining lung and greater underlying chronic bronchitis.[59–61,64]

Lung Volume Reduction Surgery

Clinical Results
Data on long-term morbidity and mortality are limited. The reported mortality during long-term follow-up varies from 0 to 27%. The data presented by the Health Care Finance Administration to Congress in 1998 reported a 23% twelve-month mortality and a 28% eighteen-month mortality.[69] Brenner et al.[144] reported a prospective study of 256 consecutive patients with severe emphysema (mean FEV_1, ~25% predicted) who underwent bilateral LVRS via VATS or MS. Using standard survival analysis techniques, 1-year survival was 85% and 2-year survival averaged 81%. Interestingly, patients with the greatest short-term improvement in FEV_1 after surgery had the best long-term survival, as did those who were younger (<70 years), had a baseline FEV_1 greater than 0.5 L, and had a PaO_2 greater than 54 mm Hg. Unfortunately, comparison of these mortality figures to the expected mortality rate in a similar patient population is difficult, as reviewed by Fessler and Wise.[67] Most published data regarding survival in COPD have been collected in large epidemiologic studies that include individuals with pathophysiologically different causes, including emphysema, chronic bronchitis, bronchiectasis, and reactive airways disease. In fact, some investigators have clearly demonstrated an improved prognosis in patients with predominantly "asthmatic bronchitis" compared with those primarily with emphysema.[145] The Nocturnal Oxygen Therapy Trial Group[146] examined 203 patients with chronic airway obstruction, a mean FEV_1 of approximately 30% predicted, hypoxemia, and no other comorbid factors expected to influence survival. A total of 64 patients (31.5%) died during mean follow-up of 19 months, yielding 1-year mortality of 11.9% in the group treated with continuous O_2 therapy. In the Intermittent Positive-Pressure Breathing Trial, 985 nonhypoxemic patients with a postbronchodilator FEV_1 of approximately 41% were followed up for a mean of 34.7 months.[147] Patient age and postbronchodilator FEV_1 were the best predictors of mortality. In patients older than 65 years with an FEV_1 between 30 and 39% predicted, annual mortality was approximately 12%. This increased to almost 20% if the FEV_1 was below 30% predicted. Unfortunately, only the study by Burrows and colleagues[145] specifically examined prognosis in patients with emphysema. Meyers et al.[148] retrospectively compared a group of 22 patients denied surgery purely because of the withdrawal of Medicare funding with a group of 65 Medicare patients who underwent bilateral LVRS. No difference was seen in baseline age, clinical status, or pulmonary function. During 3 years of follow-up, 17% of patients undergoing bilateral LVRS had died compared with 36% of patients in the denied group. The difference in survival was not statistically different, however. Interestingly, only minor deterioration was seen in the spirometry of the denied group, whereas the LVRS group experienced an approximately 60% increase in FEV_1 24 months after surgery.

Pulmonary Function
Little long-term follow-up (>12 months) has been published after LVRS. The results in 13 patients treated with varying surgical techniques (unilateral in 11) were reported by Roue and colleagues.[149] An improvement in symptoms was noted in 12 of 13 patients 6 months after surgery; FEV_1 improved in the same 12 patients. Although data collection was incomplete, four of six patients maintained a greater than 20% improvement in FEV_1

at 2 years, but neither of the two evaluable patients maintained improvement at 4 years. The Washington University group reported the results of spirometry in their original 20 patients 24 months after bilateral LVRS.[91] FEV_1 had risen from 27% of predicted at baseline to 45% of predicted 1 year and 42% of predicted 2 years after surgery. This same group has presented 3-year follow-up data on this same cohort of patients.[150] Although data collection was incomplete, a trend toward declining pulmonary function was confirmed for the group as a whole by the second and third year. Nevertheless, the mean FEV_1 at 3 years remained elevated compared with baseline values (0.83 ±0.26 vs. 1.04 ±0.54 L).

Similarly, a significant improvement in pulmonary function in 10 patients undergoing bilateral thoracoscopic stapling was reported by Gelb and colleagues.[151] FEV_1 increased from 0.71 to 1.15 L 6 months after surgery but decreased to 0.95 L 1 year after surgery.[151] In a slightly different group of patients, the same investigators noted a further slight drop in FEV_1 24 months after surgery.[152] Cassina and colleagues[100] reported 2-year data in a group of 12 patients with α_1-antitrypsin–related emphysema who underwent bilateral LVRS via thoracotomies and a group of 18 patients with non–α_1-antitrypsin–related emphysema undergoing LVRS via MS. A decrement in pulmonary function was seen in both groups, although at a much faster rate in the α_1-antitrypsin–deficient patients. Investigators at Temple University reported follow-up to 18 months after bilateral stapling via MS.[112] The improvement in FEV_1 seemed to be maintained in the six patients with 18-month data (baseline mean FEV_1, 0.69 L compared with 0.91 L at 18 months), although significant variability was noted.

Brenner et al.[153] published the rate of FEV_1 change more than 6 months after LVRS in a retrospective analysis of 376 patients undergoing LVRS at the same institution. Patients underwent unilateral laser resection via thoracoscopy (n = 46), unilateral stapling via thoracoscopy (n = 111), bilateral thoracoscopic stapling (n = 184), and bilateral stapling via MS (n = 14), with the remainder undergoing a combination of unilateral thoracoscopic stapling and laser resection. Although follow-up was variable and a significant amount of data were missing, Figure 23-6 illustrates the time course of improvement in FEV_1. The peak improvement in FEV_1 was noted 3 to 6 months after surgery, with a

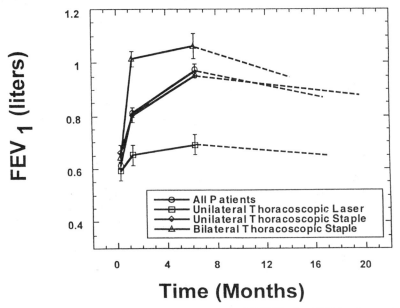

Figure 23-6. Change in forced expiratory volume in 1 second (FEV_1) after LVRS using various surgical techniques. (Reprinted with permission from Brenner M, McKenna R Jr, Gelb A, et al. Rate of FEV_1 change following lung volume reduction surgery. Chest 1998;113:652–659.)

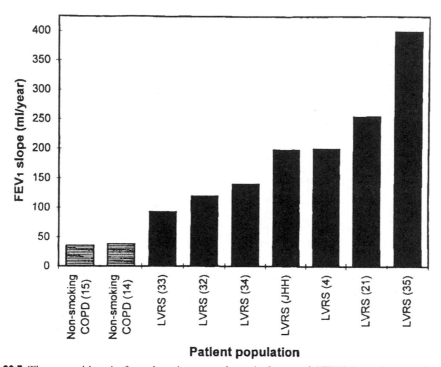

Figure 23-7. The annual loss in forced expiratory volume in 1 second (*FEV₁*) in patients with chronic obstructive pulmonary disease (*COPD*) or following lung volume reduction surgery (*LVRS*). *JHH,* Johns Hopkins Hospital. (Reprinted with permission from Fessler H, Wise R. Lung volume reduction surgery: is less really more? Am J Respir Crit Care Med 1999;159:1031–1035.)

greater improvement seen with bilateral procedures. A higher rate of drop in FEV_1 (0.255 ± 0.057 L/y) was seen in patients experiencing the greatest initial improvement (during the first 6 months after surgery, which were those treated with bilateral stapling). The least drop in FEV_1 was noted in patients with the least initial improvement (those treated unilaterally). The annualized rate of decline in FEV_1 after LVRS has been addressed by Fessler and Wise,[67] who compared this to that expected in previously reported groups of patients with COPD (see Fig. 23-7). These authors highlight the difficulty in identifying a cohort of well-described COPD patients to serve as appropriate control subjects for this analysis.[67] The need for a randomized trial of LVRS is strongly supported by these data.

Fewer data are available defining the time course of response in lung volumes and DLCO. Cooper and colleagues[91] have reported 24-month follow-up data suggesting that the initial decrease in RV and TLC seems to be maintained. Similarly, Cordova et al.[112] reported decreases in RV and TLC 6 and 12 months after bilateral LVRS that were maintained in the six patients with data collected 18 months after surgery. In contrast, Gelb et al.[152] noted a maintenance of the initial decrease in RV and TLC up to 12 months after surgery but a mild increase in both parameters 18 to 24 months after surgery. In addition, Cassina and colleagues[100] described a trough in RV and TLC 3 to 6 months after surgery but a rise by 12 months and a further rise 24 months after surgery. Because hyperinflation is of paramount importance in the genesis of breathlessness in patients with COPD,[76,154] further long-term data are required to define the potential clinical significance of these rising lung volumes.

Exercise Capacity
Limited data are available regarding long-term maintenance of improvements in exercise capacity. Cooper et al.[91] reported maintenance of the improvement in 6-minute walk

distance 24 months after surgery despite decrements in spirometry described earlier. Similarly, Cordova et al.[112] noted a higher 6-minute walk distance in six patients 18 months after surgery compared with preoperative values. In contrast, Cassina and colleagues[100] suggest a gradual, albeit mild, decline in 6-minute walk distance 24 months after LVRS. These data are difficult to interpret because little description is provided regarding continued participation in pulmonary rehabilitation after surgery, which could alter exercise capacity.

Cordova et al.[112] described improvements in VO_2 and VE over baseline in the 10 patients studied 12 months after surgery, whereas Gelb and colleagues[152] described a decrease in maximal VO_2 and VE 12 to 24 months after surgery in seven patients (although the 24-month values remained above the preoperative values). Unfortunately, these data are limited by small numbers and varying or undescribed postoperative rehabilitation schedules.

Medication and Oxygen Requirements

The Washington University group has described O_2 requirements in their original cohort of 20 patients.[91] Twenty-six percent had continuous O_2 requirements at baseline compared with no patients 12 and 24 months after bilateral LVRS. Interestingly, 84% of patients at baseline required O_2 with exertion, which decreased to 5% twelve months after surgery but rose to 32% two years after surgery. These data are limited by the lack of detailed descriptions of the O_2 titration protocols used by the investigators. Similar difficulties are encountered when examining postoperative steroid requirements. Cooper and colleagues[91] noted that 42% of their original cohort were steroid dependent at baseline, whereas only 6% were so 12 months after surgery and 11% were so 24 months after bilateral LVRS.

Improvement in Dyspnea and HRQL

A limited number of investigators have described the long-term change in dyspnea after LVRS. Roue et al.[149] quantified dyspnea using the Fletcher Scale,[155] noting an improved dyspnea in 12 of 13 patients 6 months after LVRS, with 11 of 13 maintaining improvement 12 months, 7 of 13 (54%) 18 months, 4 of 13 (31%) 24 months, and 4 of 13 (31%) 36 months after surgery. None of 3 eligible patients maintained an improvement in dyspnea 48 months after surgery. Brenner et al.[153] noted a similar distribution of improved dyspnea during long-term (>6 months after bilateral LVRS) as during short-term follow-up. Gelb et al.[152] noted a similar improvement in dyspnea (≥ 1 grade) in 12 patients 1 year after LVRS and in 10 of 12 two years after surgery. In contrast, Cassina and colleagues[100] noted an initial improvement in MRC dyspnea grade 3 months (grade 1.6) and 6 months (grade 1.5) after bilateral LVRS in non–α_1-antitrypsin–related emphysema. This improvement waned 12 months (grade 1.7) and 24 months (grade 2.2) after surgery.[100] The worsening dyspnea was more pronounced in patients with lower lobe, α_1-antitrypsin–related emphysema. Data regarding long-term improvement in HRQL are limited, with only Cordova and colleagues[112] reporting maintenance of an initial improvement in Sickness Impact Profile in five of six patients with 18-month follow-up.

Lung Transplantation

Clinical Results

Long-term results of lung transplantation are limited by significant complications that impair survival. Data from the Registry of the International Society for Heart and Lung Transplantation suggests an approximately 80% one-year, 70% two-year, and 60% three-year survival for emphysema patients.[156] This contrasts favorably with the survival for patients transplanted for IPF and primary pulmonary hypertension (see Fig. 23-8). Five-year mortality after transplantation seems positively related to increasing recipient age and the need for repeated transplantation but is less in patients with underlying emphysema.[142] The most frequent causes of late death include obliterative bronchiolitis (OB), infection,

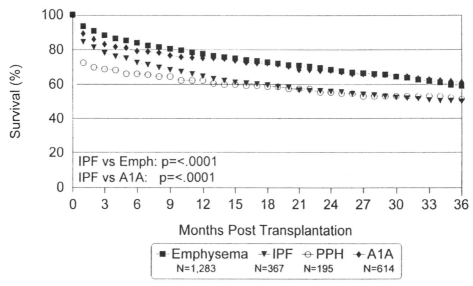

Figure 23-8. Survival up to 36 months after transplantation for emphysema (*Emph*), idiopathic pulmonary fibrosis (*IPF*), primary pulmonary hypertension (*PPH*), and $\alpha\alpha_1$-antitrypsin–related emphysema (*AIA*). (Reprinted with permission from Hosenpud J, Bennett L, Keck B, et al. The registry of the International Society for Heart and Lung Transplantation: fourteenth official report—1997. J Heart Lung Transplant 1997;16:691–722.)

and malignancy.[142] Interestingly, this same group recently presented a time-dependent, nonproportional analysis to assess the risk of mortality after transplantation relative to patients on the transplant waiting list.[157] Importantly, a survival benefit was not seen with end-stage emphysema by 2 years of follow-up.

Pulmonary Function
As with bullectomy and LVRS, long-term results of pulmonary function are scarce. In general, early reports noted that some patients demonstrated stability in FEV_1 improvement and others experienced a decline in pulmonary function after several months.[118] Levine et al.[116] noted FEV_1 rising from 16% of predicted before SLT to 57% of predicted 3 months, 60% of predicted 6 months, 54% of predicted 12 months, and 52% of predicted 24 months after transplantation. These differences did not achieve statistical significance, however. These authors believed that the longer-term decrease related to the development of OB in some of the patients after 6 months of follow-up. The importance of OB was highlighted by Bjortuft et al.,[158] who contrasted pulmonary function in stable recipients of SLT for COPD with that in recipients who developed histologic OB or obliterative bronchiolitis syndrome (BOS). Figure 23-9 illustrates the time course of FEV_1 in patients with COPD undergoing SLT. Stability is noted in patients without OB in contrast to the decrement noted in the other group. Several groups have suggested that this decrease in pulmonary function is particularly likely in SLT recipients. Sundaresan et al.[55] noted that SLT recipients experienced a gradual fall in FEV_1 after the first year following transplantation. In contrast, a lesser drop was seen in DLT recipients. Importantly, BOS (see below) was more prevalent in SLT recipients (51 vs. 33%, $P = .079$). Similarly, Al-Kattan et al.[54] noted a peak FEV_1 13 months after SLT for COPD followed by a progressive decline. This decline was not seen after HLT for COPD. The clinical importance of OB is highlighted by a drop in pulmonary function and the increased mortality associated with OB.[159] In fact, Becker et al.[128] noted that decrement in spirometric values was greatest for OB compared with acute rejection or infection in patients treated with SLT. Given the difficulty in

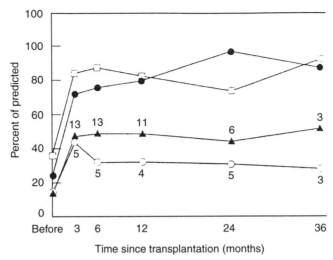

Figure 23-9. Change in DLCO corrected for alveolar volume up to 36 months after transplantation in patients with (*open square*) and without (*closed circle*) BOS. Change in FEV₁ up to 36 months after transplantation in patients with (*open circle*) and without (*closed triangle*) BOS. (Reprinted with permission from Bjortuft O, Geiran O, Field J, et al. Single lung transplantation for chronic obstructive pulmonary disease: pulmonary function and impact of bronchiolitis syndrome. Respir Med 1996;90:553–559.)

histologic confirmation of OB, BOS has been defined as a persistent, greater than 20% drop in FEV₁ from the posttransplant baseline value in the absence of other acute conditions (airway complications, infection, congestive heart failure, reversible airway reactivity, and systemic disease).[160] Furthermore, BOS can be staged according to the drop in FEV₁ from the peak posttransplant value. Interestingly, a drop in midflow rates (forced expired flows between 25% and 75% of the forced vital capacity) may be an earlier predictor of OB than changes in FEV₁.[161] In any case, the frequent development of OB more remote after transplantation can have a negative effect on long-term pulmonary function.

Exercise Capacity
Reports of long-term data after lung transplantation are few. Sundaresan et al.[55] noted persistent improvement in 6-minute walk distance after both SLT and DLT for COPD up to 4 years after transplantation. A greater degree of improvement was seen in DLT compared with SLT up to 3 years after transplantation but not 4 years after surgery. The same group, in an earlier publication, had noted improved walk distance 1 and 2 years after SLT for various disease states.[53] Interestingly, patients with COPD experienced a mild drop in 6-minute walk distance between these two times (473 m at 1 year vs. 435 m at 2 years). Similar data have been presented by Bavaria and colleagues[56] up to 24 months after transplantation. Maximal achieved VO₂ changed little in SLT or DLT recipients from 3 months to 1 to 2 years after transplantation in the report by Williams et al.[131] The most detailed report of long-term cardiopulmonary exercise response after SLT for COPD was presented by Levine and colleagues.[116] These investigators reported remarkably little change in maximal achieved VO₂ 3 (43% predicted), 6 (43% predicted), 12 (48% predicted), and 24 months (55% predicted) after transplantation. Similar results were noted in the ventilatory response to exercise at these follow-up times. Although limited data were presented, Al-Kattan et al.[54] reported a maximal achieved VO₂ of 58% predicted 5 years after HLT for COPD compared with 42% predicted for SLT. As such, a significant limitation to exercise remains for patients after lung transplantation, although the effect of long-term aerobic training has not been described in this patient population.

Quality of Life
Gross et al.[139] noted a similar result on the Medical Outcomes Study Health Survey in 17 recipients tested 19 to 36 months and 16 recipients tested more than 36 months after transplantation compared with responses 11 months after surgery. Importantly, recipients with BOS showed decrements in HRQL, particularly in physical and social functioning and bodily pain. Similar results were demonstrated by TenVergert and colleagues,[140] who administered the Nottingham Health Profile to 24 patients up to a median of 19 months after transplantation. These investigators and others have reported that approximately 20 to 40% of recipients are employed, at least part-time, long term after transplantation.[140,142,162]

WHICH PATIENTS SHOULD AND WHICH SHOULD NOT BE CONSIDERED FOR SURGERY?

Bullectomy

Based on the presumption that improvement depends on relief of compressed normal lung, most investigators have attempted to identify optimal surgical candidates on the basis of pulmonary function and radiographic features (Tables 23-1 and 23-2).

Clinical Features
In general, better candidates for bullectomy have persistent exertional limitation despite optimal medical therapy and pulmonary rehabilitation. In fact, a recent report has confirmed that preoperative pulmonary rehabilitation resulted in a lower incidence of postoperative pulmonary complications after upper abdominal surgery.[163] These data should apply to thoracic procedures. A worse surgical result has been associated with older age in some series. Laros et al.[60] noted a mean age of 56 years in patients who died of respiratory insufficiency after bullectomy compared with those who exhibited favorable long-term responses (mean age, <50 years). Similar results were published by Fitzgerald and colleagues.[59] In addition, several groups have reported higher morbidity and worse long-term results in the presence of superimposed chronic bronchitis.[59,60,64] Although imperfect, a history of chronic sputum production and recurrent respiratory infections may provide a suggestion of such primarily airway disease.[1]

Physiologic
In general, most authors have reported ideal patients to have a "restrictive" picture by spirometry with simultaneous elevation of functional residual capacity and TLC.[164] In addition, severe obstruction, particularly when associated with smaller bullae, has been associated with poor long-term results.[164] In a prospective study, Nakahara and colleagues[165] noted the best improvement in those with an FEV_1 greater than 40% predicted. Significant bronchoreversibility, as a surrogate of airway disease, has been proposed as an additional, relative contraindication (see Table 23-2).[10,164] Lung volume measurement has been studied to a lesser extent, although elevation of trapped gas has been seen in groups demonstrating better responses to classic bullectomy.[59,164] The DLCO has been used to identify greater underlying emphysema,[165,166] with two groups suggesting a better response in those patients with higher DLCO and lack of exertional desaturation.[58,165] Absolute thresholds for individual decision making are not available, however.

Imaging
Most of the literature has focused on radiographic imaging to identify the nonfunctioning lung to be resected and to assess the remaining lung for evidence of compression and preserved function. Multiple authors have noted poorer results in patients with bullae occupying less than one-third of the hemithorax.[61,167] This seems particularly true for

Table 23-1. Potential Indications for Classic Bullectomy, LVRS in the Absence of Giant Bullae, and Lung Transplantation in Patients With Advanced COPD

Parameter	Bullectomy[a]	LVRS Without Giant Bullae[b]	Lung Transplantation[c]
Clinical	Young age (<50 y)	Age <75 y	Age <65 y
	Rapid progressive dyspnea despite maximal medical therapy	Disability despite maximal medical treatment, including pulmonary rehabilitation	Chronic symptomatic disease despite maximal medical and surgical therapy
	Ex-smoker	Ex-smoker (>6 mo)	Ex-smoker (>6 mo)
Physiologic	Normal or slightly decreased FVC	FEV_1 after bronchodilator <40% predicted	FEV_1 after bronchodilator ≤25% predicted
	FEV_1 >40% predicted		
	Little bronchoreversibility		

	"High" trapped lung volume	Hyperinflation
		  TLC >120% predicted
		  RV >250%
		  Increased RV:TLC	

	Normal or near-normal DLCO	DLCO <50% predicted	$PaCO_2$ ≥55 mm Hg
	Normal PaO_2 and $PaCO_2$		
Imaging	CXR—bulla >1/3 hemithorax	CXR—hyperinflation	
	CT—large and localized bulla with vascular crowding and normal pulmonary parenchyma around bulla	CT—marked emphysema with heterogeneity	
	Angiography—vascular crowding with preserved distal vascular branching		
	Isotope scan—well-localized matching defect with normal uptake and washout for underlying lung	Isotope scan—target areas for resection	

[a]Martinez F. Diagnosing chronic obstructive pulmonary disease. Postgrad Med 1998;103:112–125; Feileib M, Rosenberg H, Collins J, et al. Trends in COPD morbidity and mortality in the United States. Am Rev Respir Dis 1989;140(Suppl):S9–S18; Higgins M, Thom T. Incidence, prevalence, and mortality; intra- and intercountry differences. Lung Biol Health Dis 1989;43:23–43; Petty T. A new national strategy for COPD. J Respir Dis 1997;18:365–369; and Casio M, Majo J. Overview of the pathology of emphysema in humans. Chest Surg Clin N Am 1995;5:603–634.

[b]Grasso M, Weller W, Shaffer T, et al. Capitation, managed care, and chronic obstructive pulmonary disease. Am J Respir Crit Care Med 1998;158:133–138; Corris P. Quality of life and predictions of survival in patients with advanced emphysema. Chest Surg Clin N Am 1995;5:659–671; American Thoracic Society. Standards for the diagnosis and care of patients with chronic obstructive pulmonary disease. Am J Respir Crit Care Med 1995;152:S77–S120.

[c]ACCP/AACVPR Pulmonary Rehabilitation Guidelines Panel. Pulmonary rehabilitation: joint ACCP/AACVPR evidence-based guidelines. Chest 1997;112:1363–1396; Gaensler E, Cugell D, Knudson R, et al. Surgical management of emphysema. Clin Chest Med 1983;4:443–463; and Deslauriers J. History of surgery for emphysema. Semin Thorac Cardiovasc Surg 1996;8:43–51.

LVRS, lung volume reduction surgery; COPD, chronic obstructive pulmonary disease; FVC, forced vital capacity; FEV_1, forced expiratory volume in 1 second; TLC, total lung capacity; RV, residual volume; DLCO, diffusion capacity of carbon dioxide; $PaCO_2$, arterial partial pressure of carbon dioxide; PaO_2, arterial partial pressure of oxygen; CXR, chest radiograph; CT, computed tomography.

Table 23-2. Potential Contraindications for Classic Bullectomy, LVRS in the Absence of Giant Bullae, and Lung Transplantation

Parameter	Bullectomy[a]	LVRS Without Giant Bullae[b]	Lung Transplantation[c]
Clinical	Age >50 y	Age >75–80 y	Age >65 y
	Cormorbid illness	Comorbid illness with 5-y mortality >50%	Nonpulmonary organ dysfunction (renal, hepatic, neurologic)
	Cardiac disease	Severe coronary artery disease	
	Pulmonary hypertension >10% weight loss	Pulmonary hypertension (PAsyst >45, PA mean >35 mm Hg)	Untreatable cornary artery disease or left ventricular dysfunction
	Frequent respiratory infections	Surgical constraints: previous thoracic, procedure, pleuradesis, chest wall deformity	
	Chronic bronchitis		
Physiologic	FEV$_1$ <35% predicted	FEV$_1$ >50% predicted	
	"Low" trapped gas volume	RV <150% predicted	
		TLC <100% predicted	
	Decreased DLCO	DLCO <10% predicted	
		PaCO$_2$ >60 mm Hg	
		6-min walk <400 ft. after rehabilitation	
		Increased inspiratory resistance	
Imaging	CXR—vanishing lung syndrome	CXR—no hyperinflation	
	Poorly defined bullae		
	CT—multiple ill-defined bullae underlying lung	CT—minimal emphysema; homogenous, severe emphysema	
	Angiography—vague bullae; disrupted vasculature elsewhere		
	Isotope scan—absence of target zones, poor washout in remaining lung	Isotope scan—absence of target zones	

[a]Martinez F. Diagnosing chronic obstructive pulmonary disease. Postgrad Med 1998;103:112–125; Feileib M, Rosenberg H, Collins J, et al. Trends in COPD morbidity and mortality in the United States. Am Rev Respir Dis 1989;140(Suppl):S9–S18; Higgins M, Thom T. Incidence, prevalence, and mortality; intra- and intercountry differences. Lung Biol Health Dis 1989;43:23–43; Petty T. A new national strategy for COPD. J Respir Dis 1997;18:365–369; and Casio M, Majo J. Overview of the pathology of emphysema in humans. Chest Surg Clin N Am 1995;5:603–634.

[b]Grasso M, Weller W, Shaffer T, et al. Capitation, managed care, and chronic obstructive pulmonary disease. Am J Respir Crit Care Med 1998;158:133–138; Corris P. Quality of life and predictions of survival in patients with advanced emphysema. Chest Surg Clin N Am 1995;5:659–671; American Thoracic Society. Standards for the diagnosis and care of patients with chronic obstructive pulmonary disease. Am J Respir Crit Care Med 1995;152:S77–S120.

[c]ACCP/AACVPR Pulmonary Rehabilitation Guidelines Panel. Pulmonary rehabilitation: joint ACCP/AACVPR evidence-based guidelines. Chest 1997;112:1363–1396; Gaensler E, Cugell D, Knudson R, et al. Surgical management of emphysema. Clin Chest Med 1983;4:443–463; and Deslauriers J. History of surgery for emphysema. Semin Thorac Cardiovasc Surg 1996;8:43–51.

LVRS, lung volume reduction surgery; PAsyst, systolic pulmonary artery pressure; PA mean, mean pulmonary artery pressures; FEV$_1$, forced expiratory volume in 1 second; RV, residual volume; TLC, total lung capacity; DLCO, diffusion capacity of carbon dioxide; PaCO$_2$, arterial partial pressure of carbon dioxide; CXR, chest radiograph; CT, computed tomography.

the long-term maintenance of functional improvement. Additional radiographic studies advocated by some have included inspiratory/expiratory chest radiographs. One group has emphasized that expiratory opacification of surrounding tissue is useful in identifying an individual with a better response to bullectomy.[59,164] Angiography was a popular method used to identify crowded vasculature in compressed lung,[164] although in the past 15 years computed tomography (CT) has demonstrated clear advantages. CT allows a clear assessment of the volume of air in bullae, the presence of compressed lung, and a view of the structure of the remaining lung tissue.[61,164,168,169] Some investigators have used radionuclide scans to assess the relative function of bullous and nonbullous areas. Nakahara et al.[165] used an index of dynamic ventilation to predict postsurgical function, although most have obtained qualitative data from isotope scans. These may be particularly useful in assessing lung zones that appear normal or minimally involved on CT or chest radiograph.[170]

Lung Volume Reduction Surgery

Because the main benefit from LVRS is believed to relate to the surgical relief of hyperinflation by removal of nonfunctioning lung, some authors have attempted to identify patients with lungs resembling a two-compartment model.[171] One compartment comprises emphysematous lung, which is volume occupying but nonfunctional and surgically accessible[171]; the other would comprise emphysematous lung with a relative preservation of function.[171] Potential criteria to identify such patients are enumerated in Table 23-1, although none of these criteria have been prospectively and rigorously validated, and they remain controversial.

Clinical Features

As with bullectomy, the clinical evaluation of the patient considered for LVRS should aim to identify patients with parenchymal destruction typical of emphysema. The presence of frequent respiratory infections and chronic, copious sputum production may be useful in identifying patients with primarily airway disease.[172] Furthermore, the history and physical examination should attempt to identify features that could predict a higher mortality or a high likelihood of poor functional result. Although controversial, advanced age has been suggested as a predictor of increased mortality.[41,75,89,171,173] In contrast, other investigations have not confirmed a higher risk in patients older than 75 years.[174]

Significant comorbidity, which will independently limit survival, has been considered a contraindication (see Table 23-2), including advanced cancer or multiorgan disease. The presence of significant coronary artery disease is frequently seen in this patient population,[175] although it may not be an absolute contraindication to surgery. Preliminary data from our institution[176] and others[177] suggest successful combined LVRS and cardiac surgery in patients with significant valvular or coronary disease and severe emphysema. Similarly, pulmonary hypertension has been reported to be a relative contraindication[171] as some authors have noted an elevation of resting pulmonary artery pressures in nine patients 3 months after bilateral LVRS.[86] In contrast, other groups have documented only modest effect on the pulmonary vascular response to exercise.[84,85] Because prohibitive pulmonary hypertension is infrequent in this patient population[178] and the effect of milder pulmonary vascular abnormality has not been prospectively studied,[21] further data are required to define absolute thresholds for exclusion of surgery. The presence of α_1-antitrypsin deficiency has been recently reported to be associated with less favorable outcome. Cassina and colleagues[100] compared 12 patients with α_1-antitrypsin deficiency with 18 patients with typical smoker's emphysema. Although short-term clinical and physiologic responses were similar, the long-term response (12–24 months) was clearly poorer in α_1-antitrypsin deficiency, as described above.[100] Whether this represents the presence of lower lobe emphysema or deficiency in α_1-antitrypsin remains unclear.

Clinical severity of disease has not proven to be an absolute contraindication. Two groups have reported acceptable results in patients undergoing LVRS despite requiring mechanical ventilation because of acute respiratory failure.[90,179] Patients who were prednisone dependent (>10 mg/d; mean dose, 24 mg/d) or had failed pulmonary rehabilitation (most secondary to frailty) did not experience a poorer outcome in the study by Argenziano et al.[96] The importance of preoperative pulmonary rehabilitation remains unclear. A review of 41 published series between 1994 and 1999 in which the use of pulmonary rehabilitation was described yields 21 studies in which preoperative rehabilitation was used and 20 in which it was not used. Comparison of these 2 study types demonstrates remarkable similarity in operative mortality (mean, 3.6 vs. 2.9%), total mortality (8.0 vs. 7.5%), length of stay (15.5 vs. 16.5 days), and improvement in FEV_1 (48.7 vs. 45.3%). Although these data are difficult to interpret because of widely varying surgical techniques and experience, a major difference is not apparent. Nevertheless, because of the significant morbidity and mortality of LVRS, a preoperative course of rehabilitation seems warranted. Because surgical volume reduction is a palliative procedure, the significant improvement noted in symptoms after rehabilitation may suffice for selected patients. In these patients, the chance of surgical complications could thus be avoided.

Physiologic

Most investigators have used pulmonary function testing to aid in identifying optimal candidates for surgery. In contrast to classical bullectomy, most authors agree that a postbronchodilator FEV_1 greater than 40 to 45% predicted does not justify the risks of LVRS (see Table 23-2). It is difficult to define a lower limit of FEV_1 that identifies individuals at prohibitive risk because some groups have demonstrated acceptable short-term results and morbidity in patients with severely decreased FEV_1. For example, Argenziano et al.[96] noted acceptable spirometric and functional improvements in patients with an FEV_1 less than 500 mL (mean, 368 mL), which is similar to data from other investigators.[70,174] If the mechanism of improvement in spirometry relates to improvement in elastic recoil,[180] patients with airflow obstruction from structural emphysema should benefit most from LVRS. Although a marked bronchodilator response has been touted by some as a spirometric method of identifying primarily airway disease, this has not been rigorously tested. In fact, data would support a significant bronchodilator response in a significant proportion of patients with emphysema.[181] Izquierdo-Alonso et al.[182] confirmed greater bronchoreversibility in patients with a normal DLCO compared with those with a low DLCO, suggesting a different pathophysiologic lesion. To better identify individuals with airway disease, Ingenito and colleagues[77] measured inspiratory resistance in patients undergoing thoracoscopic LVRS. In a multivariate analysis, only those patients with low inspiratory resistance demonstrated short-term improvements in FEV_1. In fact, a linear correlation could be demonstrated between resistance and the change in FEV_1 during short term follow-up, suggesting that LVRS should not be offered to patients when the pathophysiologic basis of obstruction is primarily airway in nature. Importantly, in individual patients, this clinical separation may be difficult.

LVRS has been suggested by some investigators to result in improved pulmonary function in patients with a significant elevation of TLC.[171] Others have argued that the RV and RV:TLC ratio may be better theoretical predictors of response.[183] Indeed, preliminary data have suggested that an elevated RV:TLC ratio may be the best physiologic parameter to identify patients demonstrating improved quality of life,[184] pulmonary function,[185,186] and exercise capacity after bilateral LVRS. Thurnheer et al.[102] have recently confirmed the importance of physiologic hyperinflation at baseline in predicting improvement in forced vital capacity after bilateral LVRS. Given the importance of hyperinflation in the genesis of dyspnea in patients with COPD, these findings would be expected.[154]

A very low DLCO has been suggested to be associated with increased risk after LVRS.[71,89,187] In fact, Keenan et al.[71] noted a bad outcome (death or length of stay ≥30 days) in patients with a DLCO of 25% predicted or less, particularly if associated with hypercapnia ($PaCO_2$, >50 mm Hg). Hazelrigg et al.[89] noted a lower DLCO (26.5% predicted vs. 38.1% predicted) in patients dying after LVRS. Other investigators have not confirmed these findings, however.[174]

Some have suggested poor outcome in patients with significant abnormalities of arterial oxygenation.[39] Interestingly, a subsequent analysis by the same group noted no worsening of outcomes in patients with a PaO_2 of less than 50 mm Hg.[174] Several groups have suggested impaired outcome and higher mortality in patients with hypercapnia.[71,83,89,188] As mentioned earlier, Keenan et al. noted a poor outcome in those patients with a $PaCO_2$ greater than 50 mm Hg (6 of 10 experienced death or prolonged length of stay compared with 5 of 28 normocapnic patients).[71] This was particularly likely if both an elevated $PaCO_2$ and low DLCO were present (5 of 6 patients experiencing a bad outcome). Similarly, Hazelrigg et al.[89] noted a higher $PaCO_2$ in patients dying after LVRS (mean, 48 mm Hg) compared with those surviving (mean, 42.5 mm Hg). Szekely and colleagues[188] compared a group of patients experiencing a bad outcome after LVRS (>3 weeks length of stay or death within 6 months) with a group experiencing an acceptable outcome. If either a $PaCO_2$ greater than 45 mm Hg or a 6-minute walk distance less than 200 m was present before surgery a bad outcome was more likely (6 of 16 patients died vs. 0 of 25 deaths). On the other hand, Argenziano et al.[96] noted an acceptable surgical outcome in a small group of patients (n = 9) with a $PaCO_2$ greater than 55 mm Hg (mean, 67 mm Hg). O'Brien and colleagues[113] compared results after bilateral LVRS in patients with a $PaCO_2$ greater than 45 mm Hg (n = 15; mean, 58 mm Hg) in contrast to normocapnic patients (n = 31; mean, 41 mm Hg), noting no difference in clinical or physiologic outcomes during short- or longer-term follow-up. The same group has subsequently demonstrated a significant correlation between a decrease in postoperative $PaCO_2$ and changes in FEV_1, DLCO, RV:TLC, and maximal inspiratory mouth pressures.[78] Importantly, patients with the highest preoperative $PaCO_2$ demonstrated the greatest decrease after LVRS. Similarly, little difference in surgical morbidity, mortality, and postoperative functional improvement was noted between hypercapnic (≥45 mm Hg) and normocapnic patients by another group of investigators.[189] Clearly, more prospectively collected data are required to define physiologic predictors of response to LVRS.

Preoperative exercise capacity has been examined as a predictor of outcome in a limited number of investigations. Hazelrigg et al.[89] demonstrated a lower 6-minute walk distance in patients dying after thoracoscopic laser LVRS (356 vs. 714 feet). Szekely and colleagues[188] noted a greater likelihood of poor outcome after bilateral LVRS if the initial 6-minute walk distance was less than 200 m, particularly if associated with an elevated $PaCO_2$. Interestingly, maximal VO_2 has demonstrated only a loose correlation with the change in aerobic capacity after LVRS[101] and has not proven to be a reliable predictor of mortality, although the number of patients studied is extremely limited. Data suggest that maximal VO_2 may predict complications after thoracotomy for the resection of suspected lung cancers.[190] As such, additional investigation is required to establish the role of cardiopulmonary exercise testing in predicting morbidity and mortality after LVRS.

Imaging

Thoracic imaging has assumed a primary role in the evaluation of patients for LVRS. In contrast to bullectomy, where CT is used to identify compressed lung and localized bullous change, in LVRS CT is used to identify the presence of moderate to severe emphysema with heterogeneity. Most authorities consider topographic heterogeneity a prerequisite for optimal response from LVRS.[21] Brenner et al.[187] noted greater spirometric improvement in patients with upper lobe–predominant emphysema. Similar results were reported by McKenna and colleagues[41] in patients undergoing unilateral LVRS. In a more detailed analysis, this group examined results in 138 patients surviving bilateral LVRS.[174] One hundred six patients (77%) had upper lobe–predominant emphysema, 10 (7%) had lower lobe–predominant emphysema, and 22 (16%) had diffusely homogenous emphysema. The greatest improvement in FEV_1 was noted in patients with upper lobe emphysema (73%), although patients with homogenous emphysema experienced a 38% improvement.

More detailed, CT-specific data have been provided by the group at Washington University in St. Louis. Slone and colleagues[191] used a qualitative scoring system to quantify the percentage of upper lobe–predominant emphysema, lung compression, and the percentage of normal or mildly emphysematous lung. In the 47 surviving patients (of 50 patients total), greater postoperative improvement was noted in those with a global pattern of upper lobe–predominant emphysema and in patients with more heterogeneous emphysema, more compressed lung, and a larger percentage of normal and mildly emphysematous lung. In fact, the combination of upper lobe severity and the percentage of mildly emphysematous or normal lung were the best predictors of improved FEV_1 ($r^2 = 0.49$). This group has confirmed qualitatively similar results using a quantitative high-resolution CT measure of emphysema heterogeneity.[192] A quantitative, computerized scoring system based on helical CT has been shown to provide an accurate index of emphysema heterogeneity by our group.[193] A high index, suggesting upper lobe–predominant emphysema, was the single best predictor of short- and long-term physiologic and functional outcomes after bilateral LVRS in one preliminary report.[185] The data from these groups are limited by the strong preexisting bias toward patients with heterogeneous emphysema, however.

Using a qualitative emphysema scoring system, Weder and associates[194] confirmed the value of emphysema heterogeneity but also noted improvement in patients with homogenous disease. Figure 23-10 illustrates the 34% improvement in FEV_1 noted in patients with homogenous emphysema compared with a 44% improvement in those with intermediately heterogenous emphysema and an 81% improvement in those with markedly heterogenous emphysema. A similar improvement in dyspnea was noted in all three groups. These findings are qualitatively similar to those reported by Wisser and colleagues.[195] These data support the theoretical model described by Fessler and Permutt[183] that suggests that disease heterogeneity may be a less important factor in spirometric improvement after LVRS. Clearly, controversy persists and confirms the need for additional, prospective data collection.

Isotope studies have been used to identify areas of decreased perfusion, which represent potential surgical "target zones."[43] In fact, some have suggested that evidence of functional

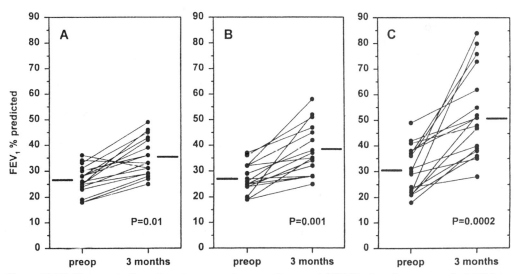

Figure 23-10. Change in forced expiratory volume in 1 second (*FEV₁*) after thoracoscopic LVRS in patients with predominantly homogenous emphysema (**A**), intermediately heterogeneous emphysema (**B**), and markedly heterogeneous emphysema (**C**). *Preop,* preoperative. The *P* values correspond to comparisons of postoperative with preoperative values. (Reprinted with permission from Weder W, Thurnheer R, Stammberger U, et al. Radiologic emphysema morphology is associated with outcome after surgical lung volume reduction. Ann Thorac Surg 1997;64:313–320.)

heterogeneity can be assessed using this technique.[196,197] Wang et al.[196] reported the results of qualitative scoring of perfusion in 103 patients undergoing bilateral LVRS. In the 96 survivors, short-term improvement in FEV_1 correlated best with the extent of upper lobe predominance of decreased perfusion, although the correlation was weak ($r = 0.38$). Recently, Thurnheer et al.[102] compared qualitative assessment of emphysema heterogeneity on high-resolution CT with qualitative assessment of impaired perfusion on lung scanning. Patients with homogenous perfusion experienced less short-term improvement in FEV_1 (23%) compared with those demonstrating intermediately heterogeneous perfusion (38%) and markedly heterogenous perfusion (57%). Importantly, in multivariate analysis, preoperative hyperinflation and emphysema heterogeneity on high-resolution CT proved to be more powerful predictors of improvement after bilateral LVRS. We have demonstrated that a quantitative index of perfusion heterogeneity correlated moderately with the change in FEV_1 3 ($r = 0.36$, $P = .04$), 6 ($r = 0.36$, $P = .05$), and 12 months ($r = 0.42$, $P = .03$) after bilateral LVRS.[197] A potential role for scintigraphy in identifying surgical target zones for resection in patients with more homogenous emphysema on high-resolution CT could not be excluded.

Lung Transplantation

Given the significant morbidity and mortality associated with lung transplantation, careful patient selection is crucial to an optimal outcome. In addition, to improve longevity and quality of life, optimal timing of referral and listing is paramount. A summary of potential selection criteria is contrasted with bullectomy and LVRS in Tables 23-1 and 23-2.

Clinical Features
The initial evaluation of patients considered for transplantation should include an assessment of the risks associated with age because older patients clearly have a significantly worse survival rate.[142] The Joint Statement of the American Society for Transplant Physicians, the American Thoracic Society, the European Respiratory Society, and the International Society for Heart and Lung Transplantation suggests that potential age limits included approximately 55 years for HLT, 65 years for SLT, and 60 years for DLT.[198] Although definitive data are few, several clinical characteristics are believed by most authorities to represent absolute contraindications. These include other major extrathoracic organ dysfunction (e.g., hepatic or renal insufficiency, untreatable coronary artery disease or left ventricular dysfunction, progressive neuromuscular disease), human immunodeficiency infection, active malignancy within the past 2 years (except basal or squamous cell carcinoma of the skin), hepatitis B surface antigen positivity, and hepatitis C infection with biopsy-proven histologic evidence of liver disease.[23,198,199] Relative contraindications include extracapsular renal cell tumor, breast cancer (stage 2 or higher), colon cancer (staged higher than Dukes A), and melanoma (level III or higher) within the past 5 years.[198] Additional relative contraindications include poorly treated or untreated symptomatic osteoporosis,[200] severe musculoskeletal disease involving the thorax, chronic steroid dose greater than 20 mg/day,[201] an ideal body weight of less than 70% or greater than 130%,[202] active substance addiction during the previous 6 months (including tobacco), psychosocial problems that are likely to impact negatively on outcome, need for invasive mechanical ventilation, and colonization with fungi or atypical mycobacteria.[198] Quiescent systemic illness is not believed to be a contraindication, although target organ involvement other than the lungs should be carefully excluded.[203]

Physiologic
Given the risks of lung transplantation, accurate assessment of disease prognosis is required for optimal timing of listing. Physiologic testing has been the most frequently used modality to assess prognosis in patients with COPD. Travers and colleagues[204] noted that after controlling for age, FEV_1 after bronchodilator administration was the best predictor of mortality in this patient population. In fact, patients younger than 65 years with an FEV_1

of 20 to 29% predicted had a cumulative survival of 0.65 at 2 years and 0.30 at 5 years. Furthermore, patients with signs and symptoms of cor pulmonale had a worse survival rate. As noted earlier, 1-year mortality in the Nocturnal Oxygen Therapy Trial was 11.9% in the group treated with continuous O_2. In the Intermittent Positive-Pressure Breathing Trial,[147] patient age and postbronchodilator FEV_1 were the best predictors of mortality. In a smaller study of 84 COPD patients requiring long-term O_2 therapy, cumulative survival was 71% at 3 years and 48% at 5 years.[205] Interestingly, 5-year survival was much lower (36.3%) in patients with a mean pulmonary artery pressure greater than 25 mm Hg compared with those with a pulmonary artery pressure of 25 mm Hg or less (62.2%). Similar data have been published in patients with α_1-antitrypsin–related emphysema. In the Danish registry, 2-year mortality was 50% for patients with an FEV_1 of less than 15% predicted and 35% for those with an FEV_1 between 15 and 20% predicted.[206] Expressed in a different fashion, the same group demonstrated median survival of 10.5 years for patients with an initial FEV_1 of less than 25% predicted and 14.2 years for those with an FEV_1 between 25 and 49% predicted.[207] Similarly, in a group of 158 patients with α_1-antitrypsin–related emphysema, 3-year mortality was 40% for those with an initial FEV_1 of less than 30% predicted and 59% at 5 years.[208] Three-year mortality was only 7% and 5-year mortality was only 19% in patients with an initial FEV_1 between 30 and 65% predicted. The data reported from the North American Alpha-1-Antitrypsin Deficiency Registry Study Group are similar, with 5-year mortality of 30.3% in patients with an FEV_1 of 35% predicted or less compared with 12.0% for an FEV_1 of 35 to 49% predicted and 4.3% for those with an FEV_1 of 50% predicted or higher.[209] Interestingly, this study group also suggested that augmentation therapy with α_1-antitrypsin was associated with a lower mortality rate. The importance of the postbronchodilator FEV_1 is highlighted in the current recommendation that an emphysema patient be considered an appropriate candidate for transplantation when the FEV_1 is below 25% predicted and/or the $PaCO_2$ is equal to or greater than 55 mm Hg.[198] Similarly, the presence of pulmonary hypertension with progressive deterioration should be considered an additional feature suggesting that transplantation should be considered an appropriate surgical intervention.

Imaging

Imaging techniques have a less defined role in the preoperative evaluation for lung transplantation than has been suggested for bullectomy or LVRS. It would seem intuitive that the presence of emphysema would be associated with a worse prognosis than chronic airflow obstruction primarily related to an airway process. For example, Gelb et al.[210] have reported detailed physiologic parameters in 10 patients with severe chronic airflow obstruction (mean FEV_1, 32% predicted) but little emphysema on high-resolution CT. All of these patients had significant hyperinflation, decreased DLCO, and abnormal pressure–volume curves. In the three patients who died, CT and anatomic scores for emphysema were closely correlated. In addition, the membranous-bronchiole and respiratory-bronchiole scores were markedly abnormal, suggesting that the major abnormality was severe, intrinsic "small airways disease." Whether these patients have a similar long-term mortality as patients with similar airflow obstruction but anatomic emphysema is unclear. The earlier work of the University of Arizona College of Medicine would support this hypothesis. These investigators examined the survival rate and rate of decline in FEV_1 during 10 years of follow-up in white, non-Mexican Americans with chronic airflow obstruction.[211] In this prospective study, patients with clinical features most consistent with chronic asthmatic bronchitis (a primarily airway process) were contrasted with patients believed to have nonatopic, smoking-related obstructive disease (more consistent with emphysema). The authors found the rate of decline in FEV_1 to be greater and survival to be decreased in patients with nonasthmatic airflow obstruction. Interestingly, Hughes et al.[212] noted that an upper lobe–predominant pattern of emphysema on chest radiography was associated with more exertional dyspnea and a greater decline in pulmonary function than in patients with lower lobe–predominant or diffuse emphysema. Further data are required to define the role of imaging in providing prognostic information in patients evaluated for lung transplantation.

CT has been demonstrated to alter the surgical approach to lung transplantation in selected patients. Kazerooni and colleagues[213] retrospectively examined the results of preoperative chest radiography and CT in 190 transplant candidates. CT prompted a change in the determination of which lung was more severely diseased for 27 of 169 patients. Of the 45 patients who subsequently underwent transplantation, CT prompted a change in the determination of which side to perform SLT in 4. This same group has identified pulmonary nodules, suspicious for malignancy, in 8 of 190 patients evaluated for lung transplantation.[214] Because an active malignancy precludes transplantation, such a finding would clearly alter the candidacy of a patient for lung transplantation. Finally, the presence of unsuspected bronchiectasis could alter the decision to perform DLT in contrast to SLT.

CONCLUSIONS

During the past decades extensive literature has been published regarding surgical therapies for advanced COPD. The most widely accepted have been directed at surgical relief of hyperinflation, bullectomy, and LVRS. During the past 10 years, lung transplantation has become a viable option for selected patients. Bullectomy is an established surgical technique for a limited number of patients, whereas LVRS could be an option for a significantly larger number of patients. The initial enthusiasm for this procedure has been tempered by major questions regarding the optimal surgical approach, safety, firm selection criteria, and confirmation of long-term benefits.[215] The long-term follow-up reported in patients undergoing classical bullectomy should serve to caution against unbridled enthusiasm for the indiscriminate application of LVRS. Patients with the poorest long-term outcome despite favorable short-term improvements after bullectomy have consistently been those with the lowest pulmonary function and significant emphysema in the remaining lung. These patients appear remarkably similar to those currently being evaluated for LVRS. As such, the National Heart, Lung, and Blood Institute partnered with the Health Care Finance Administration to establish a multicenter, prospective, randomized study of intensive medical management including pulmonary rehabilitation versus the same plus bilateral LVRS (via MS or VATS), the National Emphysema Treatment Trial, or NETT. The primary objectives are to determine whether LVRS improves survival and exercise capacity. The secondary objectives will examine effects on pulmonary function and HRQL, compare surgical techniques, examine selection criteria for optimal response, identify criteria to determine those who are at prohibitive surgical risk, and examine long-term cost effectiveness. It is hoped that data collected from this multicenter collaboration will place the role of LVRS in a clear perspective for the physician caring for patients with advanced COPD. Given the risks and expense of transplantation, additional data will be required to contrast mortality and improvement in HRQL between LVRS and lung transplantation. It may be that volume reduction will serve as a "bridge" to transplantation in a select few individuals.[120,216,217] With time and additional study, the optimal surgical approach to patients with advanced COPD should be better defined.

REFERENCES

1. Martinez F. Diagnosing chronic obstructive pulmonary disease. Postgrad Med 1998;103:112–125.
2. Feileib M, Rosenberg H, Collins J, et al. Trends in COPD morbidity and mortality in the United States. Am Rev Respir Dis 1989;140(Suppl): S9–S18.
3. Higgins M, Thom T. Incidence, prevalence, and mortality: intra- and intercountry differences. Lung Biol Health Dis 1989;43:23–43.
4. Petty T. A new national strategy for COPD. J Respir Dis 1997;18:365–369.
5. Casio M, Majo J. Overview of the pathology of

emphysema in humans. Chest Surg Clin N Am 1995;5:603–634.

6. Grasso M, Weller W, Shaffer T, et al. Capitation, managed care, and chronic obstructive pulmonary disease. Am J Respir Crit Care Med 1998;158:133–138.

7. Corris P. Quality of life and predictions of survival in patients with advanced emphysema. Chest Surg Clin N Am 1995;5:659–671.

8. American Thoracic Society. Standards for the diagnosis and care of patients with chronic obstructive pulmonary disease. Am J Respir Crit Care Med 1995;152:S77–S120.

9. ACCP/AACVPR Pulmonary Rehabilitation Guidelines Panel. Pulmonary rehabilitation: joint ACCP/AACVPR evidence-based guidelines. Chest 1997;112:1363–1396.

10. Gaensler E, Cugell D, Knudson R, et al. Surgical management of emphysema. Clin Chest Med 1983;4:443–463.

11. Deslauriers J. History of surgery for emphysema. Semin Thorac Cardiovasc Surg 1996;8:43–51.

12. Naef A. History of emphysema surgery. Ann Thorac Surg 1997;64:1506–1508.

13. Brantigan O, Kress M, Mueller E. A surgical approach to pulmonary emphysema. Am Rev Respir Dis 1959;39:194–202.

14. Brantigan O, Mueller E. Surgical treatment of pulmonary emphysema. Am Surg 1957;23:789–804.

15. Delarue N, Woolf C, Sanders D, et al. Surgical treatment for pulmonary emphysema. Can J Surg 1977;20:222–231.

16. Even P, Sors H, Safran D, et al. Hemodynamique des bulles d'emphyseme un nouveau syndrome: la tamponade cardiaque emphysemateuse. Rev Fr Mal Respir 1980;8:117–120.

17. Dahan M, Salerin F, Berjaud J, et al. Interet de l'exploration hemodynamique dans les indications chirurgicales des emphysemes. Ann Chir 1989;43:669–672.

18. Crosa-Dorado V, Pomi J, Perez-Penco E, et al. Treatment of dyspnea in emphysema: pulmonary remodeling: hemo- and pneumostatic suturing of the emphysematous lung. Res Surg 1992; 4:152–155.

19. Wakabayashi A, Brenner M, Kayaleh R, et al. Thoracoscopic carbon dioxide laser treatment of bullous emphysema. Lancet 1991;337:881–883.

20. Cooper J, Trulock E, Triantafillou A, et al. Bilateral pneumectomy (volume reduction) for chronic obstructive pulmonary disease. J Thorac Cardiovasc Surg 1995;109:106–116.

21. Utz J, Hubmayr R, Deschamps C. Lung volume reduction surgery for emphysema: out on a limb without a NETT. Mayo Clin Proc 1998;73:552–566.

22. Benditt J, Albert R. Surgical options for patients with advanced emphysema. Clin Chest Med 1997;18:577–593.

23. Dunitz J, Hertz M. Surgical therapy for COPD: lung transplantation. Semin Respir Crit Care Med 1999;20:365–373.

24. Wildevuur C, Benfield J. A review of 23 human lung transplantation by 20 surgeons. Ann Thorac Surg 1970;9:489–515.

25. Veith F, Koerner S. Problems in the management of lung transplant recipients. Vas Surg 1974; 8:273–282.

26. Reitz B, Wallwork J, Hunt S, et al. Heart-lung transplantation: successful therapy for patients with pulmonary vascular disease. N Engl J Med 1982;314:1140–1145.

27. Stevens P, Johnson P, Bell R, et al. Regional ventilation and perfusion after lung transplantation in patients with emphysema. N Engl J Med 1970;282:245–249.

28. Bates D. The other lung. N Engl J Med 1970; 282:277–279.

29. Patterson G, Cooper J, Goldman B, et al. Technique of successful clinical double lung transplantation. Ann Thorac Surg 1988;45:626–633.

30. Cooper J, Patterson G, Grossman R, et al. Double-lung transplant for advanced chronic obstructive lung disease. Am Rev Respir Dis 1989; 139:303–307.

31. Veith F, Koerner S, Siegelman S, et al. Single lung transplantation in experimental and human emphysema. Ann Surg 1973;178:463–476.

32. Mal H, Andreassian B, Pamela F, et al. Unilateral lung transplantation in end-stage pulmonary emphysema. Am Rev Respir Dis 1989;140:787–802.

33. Dartevelle P, Macchiarini P, Chapelier A. Operative technique of bullectomy. Chest Surg Clin N Am 1995;5:735–749.

34. Cooper J, Patterson G. Lung volume reduction surgery for severe emphysema. Semin Thorac Cardiovasc Surg 1996;8:52–60.

35. Iwa T, Watanabe Y, Fukatani G. Simultaneous bilateral operations for bullous emphysema by median sternotomy. J Thorac Cardiovasc Surg 1981;81:732–737.

36. Liu H, Chang C, Lin P, et al. An alternative technique in the management of bullous emphysema: thoracoscopic endoloop ligation of bullae. Chest 1997;111:489–493.

37. Brenner M, Yusen R, McKenna R Jr, et al. Lung volume reduction surgery for emphysema. Chest 1996;110:205–218.

38. Wakabayashi A. Thoracoscopic laser pneumoplasty in the treatment of diffuse bullous emphysema. Ann Thorac Surg 1995;60:936–942.

39. McKenna R, Brenner M, Gelb A, et al. A randomized, prospective trial of stapled lung reduction versus laser bullectomy for diffuse emphysema. J Thorac Cardiovasc Surg 1996;111:317–322.

40. Swanson S, Mentzer S, DeCamp M, et al. Nocut thoracoscopic lung plication: a new technique for lung volume reduction surgery. J Am Coll Surg 1997;185:25–32.

41. McKenna Jr R, Brenner M, Fischel R, et al. Should lung volume reduction for emphysema be unilateral or bilateral. J Thorac Cardiovasc Surg 1996;112:1331–1338.

42. Argenziano M, Thorashow B, Jellen P, et al. Functional comparison of unilateral versus bilateral lung volume reduction surgery. Ann Thorac Surg 1997;64:321–327.

43. Naunheim K, Ferguson M. The current status of lung volume reduction operations for emphysema. Ann Thorac Surg 1996;62:601–612.

44. Kotloff R, Tino G, Bavaria J, et al. Bilateral lung volume reduction surgery for advanced emphysema: a comparison of median sternotomy and thoracoscopic approaches. Chest 1996;110: 1399–1406.

45. Wisser W, Tschernko E, Senbaklavaci O, et al. Functional improvement after volume reduction: sternotomy versus videoendoscopic approach. Ann Thorac Surg 1997;63:822–828.

46. Trulock E. Lung transplantation. Am J Respir Crit Care Med 1997;155:789–818.

47. Arcasoy S, Kotloff R. Lung transplantation. N Engl J Med 1999;340:1081–1091.

48. DeHoyos A, Demajo W, Snell G, et al. Preoperative prediction for the use of cardiopulmonary bypass in lung transplantation. J Thorac Cardiovasc Surg 1993;106:787–796.

49. Pasque M, Cooper J, Kaiser L, et al. Improved technique for bilateral lung transplantation: rationale and initial clinical experience. Ann Thorac Surg 1990;49:785–791.

50. Patterson G, Maurer J, Willitams T, et al. Comparison of outcomes of double and single lung transplantation for obstructive lung disease. J Thorac Cardiovasc Surg 1991;101:623–632.

51. Low D, Trulock E, Kaiser L, et al. Morbidity, mortality, and early results of single versus bilateral lung transplantation for emphysema. J Thorac Cardiovasc Surg 1992;103:1119–1126.

52. Bando K, Paradis I, Keenan R, et al. Comparison of outcomes after single and bilateral lung transplantation for obstructive lung disease. J Heart Lung Transplant 1995;14:692–698.

53. Cooper J, Patterson G, Trulock E, et al. Results of single and bilateral lung transplantation in 131 consecutive recipients. J Thorac Cardiovasc Surg 1994;107:460–471.

54. Al-Kattan K, Tadjkarimi S, Cox A, et al. Evaluation of the long-term results of single versus heart-lung transplantation for emphysema. J Heart Lung Transplant 1995;14:824–831.

55. Sundaresan R, Shiraishi Y, Trulock E, et al. Single or bilateral lung transplantation for emphysema? J Thorac Cardiovasc Surg 1996;112:1485–1495.

56. Bavaria J, Kotloff R, Palevsky H, et al. Bilateral versus single lung transplantation for chronic obstructive pulmonary disease. J Thorac Cardiovasc Surg 1997;113:520–528.

57. King M, Savik K, Park S, et al. Similar outcomes after bilateral single lung transplantation for chronic obstructive pulmonary disease. J Heart Lung Transplant 1998;17:59.

58. Hugh-Jones P, Whimster W. The etiology and management of disabling emphysema. Am Rev Respir Dis 1978;117:343–378.

59. Fitzgerald M, Keelan P, Angell D. Long-term results of surgery for bullous emphysema. Surgery 1974;68:566–582.

60. Laros C, Gellisen H, Bergstein P, et al. Bullectomy for giant bullae in emphysema. J Thorac Cardiovasc Surg 1986;91:63–70.

61. Nickoladze G. Functional results of surgery for bullous emphysema. Chest 1992;101:119–122.

62. Potgieter P, Benatar S, Hewitson R, et al. Surgical treatment of bullous lung disease. Thorax 1981;36:885–890.

63. Sung D, Payne W, Black L. Surgical management of giant bullae associated with obstructive airway disease. Surg Clin North Am 1973;53:913–920.

64. Petro W, Hubner C, Greschuchna D, et al. Bullectomy. Thorac Cardiovasc Surg 1983;31: 342–345.

65. Snider G. Reduction pneumoplasty for giant bullous emphysema: implications for surgical treatment of nonbullous emphysema. Chest 1996; 109:540–548.

66. Sciurba F. Early and long-term functional outcomes following lung volume reduction surgery. Clin Chest Med 1997;18:259–276.

67. Fessler H, Wise R. Lung volume reduction surgery: is less really more? Am J Respir Crit Care Med 1999;159:1031–1035.

68. Holohan T, Handelsman H. Lung-Volume Reduction Surgery for End-stage Chronic Obstructive Pulmonary Disease. Rockville, MD: Agency for Health Care Policy Research, 1996.

69. Shalala D. Report to Congress: Lung Volume Reduction Surgery and Medicare Coverage Policy: Implications of Recently Published Evidence. Washington, DC: Department of Health and Human Services, 1998.

70. Eugene J, Dajee A, Kayaleh R, et al. Reduction pneumoplasty for patients with a forced expired volume in 1 second of 500 milliliters or less. Ann Thorac Surg 1997;63:186–192.

71. Keenan R, Landrenau R, Sciurba F, et al. Unilateral thoracoscopic surgical approach for diffuse emphysema. J Thorac Cardiovasc Surg 1996; 111:308–316.

72. Hazelrigg S, Boley T, Magee M, et al. Comparison of staged thoracoscopy and median sternotomy for lung volume reduction surgery. Ann Thorac Surg 1998;66:1134–1139.

73. Ko C, Waters P. Lung volume reduction surgery: a cost and outcomes comparison of sternotomy versus thoracoscopy. Am Surg 1998;64:1009–1013.

74. Keller C, Ruppel G, Hibbett A, et al. Thoracoscopic lung volume reduction surgery reduces dyspnea and improves exercise capacity in patients with emphysema. Am J Respir Crit Care Med 1997;156:60–67.

75. Yusen R, Trulock E, Pohl M, et al. Results of lung volume reduction surgery in patients with emphysema. Semin Thorac Cardiovasc Surg 1996;8:99–109.

76. Martinez F, de Oca M, Whyte R, et al. Lung-volume reduction improves dyspnea, dynamic hyperinflation, and respiratory muscle function. Am J Respir Crit Care Med 1997;155:1984–1990.

77. Ingenito E, Evans R, Loring S, et al. Relation between preoperative inspiratory lung resistance and the outcome of lung-volume-reduction surgery for emphysema. N Engl J Med 1998; 338:1181–1185.

78. Shade D Jr, Cordova F, Lando Y, et al. Relation-

ship between resting hypercapnia and physiologic parameters before and after lung volume reduction surgery in severe chronic obstructive pulmonary disease. Am J Respir Crit Care Med 1999;159:1405–1411.

79. Albert R, Benditt J, Hildebrandt J, et al. Lung volume reduction surgery has variable effects on blood gases in patients with emphysema. Am J Respir Crit Care Med 1998;158:71–76.

80. Sciurba F, Slivka W. Six-minute walk testing. Semin Respir Crit Care Med 1998;19:383–392.

81. Benditt J, Lewis S, Wood D, et al. Lung volume reduction surgery improves maximal O_2 consumption, maximal minute ventilation, O_2 pulse and dead space-to-tidal volume ration during leg cycle ergomerty. Am J Respir Crit Care Med 1997;156:561–566.

82. Tschernko E, Gruber E, Jaksch P, et al. Ventilatory mechanics and gas exchange during exercise before and after lung volume reduction surgery. Am J Respir Crit Care Med 1998;158:1424–1431.

83. Ferguson G, Femandez E, Zamora M, et al. Improved exercise performance following lung volume reduction surgery for emphysema. Am J Respir Crit Care Med 1998;157:1195–1203.

84. Kubo K, Koizumi T, Fujimoto K, et al. Effects of lung volume reduction surgery on exercise pulmonary hemodynamics in severe emphysema. Chest 1998;114:1575–1582.

85. Oswald-Mammosser M, Kessler R, Massard G, et al. Effect of lung volume reduction surgery on gas exchange and pulmonary hemodynamics at rest and during exercise. Am J Respir Crit Care Med 1999;158:1020–1025.

86. Weg I, Rossoff L, McKeon K, et al. Development of pulmonary hypertension after lung volume reduction surgery. Am J Respir Crit Care Med 1999;159:552–556.

87. Naunheim K, Keller C, Krucylak P, et al. Unilateral video-assisted thoracic surgical lung reduction. Ann Thorac Surg 1996;61:1092–1098.

88. Eugene J, Ott R, Gogia H, et al. Video-thoracic surgery for treatment of end-stage bullous emphysema and chronic obstructive pulmonary disease. Am Surg 1995;61:934–936.

89. Hazelrigg S, Boley T, Henkle J, et al. Thoracoscopic laser bullectomy: a prospective study with three-month results. J Thorac Cardiovasc Surg 1996;112:319–327.

90. Bagley P, Davis S, O'Shea M, et al. Lung volume reduction surgery at a community hospital: program development and outcomes. Chest 1997; 111:1552–1559.

91. Cooper J, Patterson G, Sundaresan R, et al. Results of 150 consecutive bilateral lung volume reduction procedures in patients with severe emphysema. J Thorac Cardiovasc Surg 1996;112:1319–1330.

92. Daniel T, Chan B, Bhaskar V, et al. Lung volume reduction surgery: case selection, operative technique, and clinical results. Ann Surg 1996;223:526–533.

93. Gaissert H, Trulock I, Cooper J, et al. Comparison of early functional results after volume reduction or lung transplantation for chronic obstructive pulmonary disease. J Thorac Cardiovasc Surg 1996;111:296–307.

94. Bousamra M II, Haasler G, Lipchik R, et al. Functional and oximetric assessment of patients after lung reduction surgery. J Thorac Cardiovasc Surg 1997;113:675–682.

95. Miller J, Lee R, Mansour K. Lung volume reduction surgery: lessons learned. Ann Thorac Surg 1996;61:1464–1469.

96. Argenziano M, Moazami N, Thomashow B, et al. Extended indications for lung volume reduction surgery in advanced emphysema. Ann Thorac Surg 1996;62:1588–1597.

97. American Thoracic Society Task Group on Screening for Respiratory Disease in Occupational Settings. Official Statement of the American Thoracic Society. Am Rev Respir Dis 1982; 126:952–956.

98. Bingisser R, Zollinger A, Hauser M, et al. Bilateral volume reduction surgery for diffuse pulmonary emphysema by video-assisted thoracoscopy. J Thorac Cardiovasc Surg 1996;112:875–882.

99. Brenner M, McKenna R, Gelb A, et al. Dyspnea response following bilateral thoracoscopic staple lung volume reduction surgery. Chest 1997; 112:916–923.

100. Cassina P, Teschler H, Konietzko N, et al. Two-year results after lung volume reduction surgery in α_1-antitrypsin deficiency versus smoker's emphysema. Eur Respir J 1998;12:1028–1032.

101. Stammberger U, Bloch K, Thurnheer R, et al. Exercise performance and gas exchange after bilateral video-assisted thoracoscopic lung volume reduction for severe emphysema. Eur Respir J 1998;12:785–792.

102. Thurnheer R, Engel H, Weder W, et al. Role of lung perfusion scintigraphy in relation to chest computed tomography and pulmonary function in the evaluation of candidates for lung volume reduction surgery. Am J Respir Crit Care Med 1999;159:301–310.

103. Mahler D, Weinberg D, Wells C, et al. The measurement of dyspnea: contents, interobserver agreement, and physiologic correlates of two new clinical indices. Chest 1984;85:751–758.

104. Sciurba F, Rogers R, Keenan R, et al. Improvement in pulmonary function and elastic recoil after lung-reduction surgery for diffuse emphysema. N Engl J Med 1996;334:1095–1099.

105. Nishimura K, Tsukino M, Hajiro T. Health-related quality of life in patients with chronic obstructive pulmonary disease. Curr Opin Pulm Med 1998;4:107–115.

106. Mahler D, Mackowiak J. Evaluation of the short-form 36-item questionnaire to measure health-related quality of life in patients with COPD. Chest 1995;107:1585–1589.

107. Ferrer M, Alonso J, Morera J, et al. Chronic obstructive pulmonary disease stage and health-related quality of life. Ann Intern Med 1997; 127:1072–1079.

108. Harper R, Brazier J, Waterhouse J, et al. Comparison of outcome measures for patients with chronic obstructive pulmonary disease (COPD) in an outpatient setting. Thorax 1997;52:879–887.

109. Prieto L, Alonso J, Ferrer M, et al. Are results of the SF-36 Health Survey and the Nottingham Health Profile similar? a comparison in COPD patients. J Clin Epidemiol 1997;50:463–473.

110. Moy M, Ingenito E, Menlzer S, et al. Quality of life domains of physical activity remain improved at greater than 9 months following lung volume reduction surgery (LVRS). Am J Respir Crit Care Med 1998;157(Suppl):A496.

111. Bergner M, Bobbitt R, Carter W, et al. The Sickness Impact Profile: development and final revision of a health status measure. Med Care 1981;19:787–805.

112. Cordova F, O'Brien G, Furukawa S, et al. Stability of improvement in exercise performance and quality of life following bilateral lung volume reduction surgery in severe COPD. Chest 1997;112:907–915.

113. O'Brien G, Furukawa S, Kuzma A, et al. Improvements in lung function, exercise, and quality of life in hypercapnic COPD patients after lung volume reduction surgery. Chest 1999; 115:75–84.

114. Guyatt G, Berman L, Townsend M, et al. A measure of quality of life for clinical trials in chronic lung disease. Thorax 1987;42:773–778.

115. Norman M, Hillerdal G, Orre L, et al. Improved lung function and quality of life following increased elastic recoil after lung volume reduction surgery in emphysema. Respir Med 1998;92: 653–658.

116. Levine S, Anzueto A, Peters J, et al. Medium term functional results of single-lung transplantation for endstage obstructive lung disease. Am J Respir Crit Care Med 1994;150:398–402.

117. Kaiser L, Cooper J, Trulock E, et al. The evolution of single lung transplantation for emphysema. J Thorac Cardiovasc Surg 1991;102: 333–341.

118. Mal H, Sleiman C, Jebrak G, et al. Functional results of single-lung transplantation for chronic obstructive lung disease. Am J Respir Crit Care Med 1994;149:1476–1481.

119. Briffa N, Dennis C, Higenbottam T, et al. Single lung transplantation for end stage emphysema. Thorax 1995;50:562–564.

120. Gaissert H, Trulock E, Cooper J, et al. Comparison of early functional results after volume reduction or lung transplantation for chronic obstructive pulmonary disease. J Thorac Cardiovasc Surg 1996;111:296–307.

121. Bjortuft O, Geiran O, Fjeld J, et al. Single lung transplantation for chronic obstructive pulmonary disease: pulmonary function and impact of bronchiolitis obliterans syndrome. Resp Med 1996;90:553–559.

122. Brunsting L, Lupinetti F, Cascade P, et al. Pulmonary function in single lung transplantation for chronic obstructive pulmonary disease. J Thorac Cardiovasc Surg 1994;107:1337–1345.

123. Cheriyan A, Garrity E, Pifarre R, et al. Reduced transplant lung volumes after single lung transplantation for chronic obstructive pulmonary disease. Am J Respir Crit Care Med 1995; 151:851–853.

124. Estenne M, Cassart M, Poncelet P, et al. Volume of graft and native lung after single-lung transplantation for emphysema. Am J Respir Crit Care Med 1999;159:641–645.

125. Neagos G, Martinez F, Deeb G, et al. Diagnosis of unilateral mainstem bronchial obstruction following single-lung transplantation with routine spirometry. Chest 1993;103:1255–1258.

126. Herlihy J, Venegas J, Systrom D, et al. Expiratory flow pattern following single-lung transplantation in emphysema. Am J Respir Crit Care Med 1994;150:1684–1689.

127. Martinez J, Paradis I, Dauber J, et al. Spirometry values in stable lung transplant recipients. Am J Respir Crit Care Med 1997;155:285–290.

128. Becker F, Martinez F, Brunsting L, et al. Limitations of spirometry in detecting rejection after single-lung transplantation. Am J Respir Crit Care Med 1994;150:159–166.

129. Miyoshi S, Trulock E, Schaefers H, et al. Cardiopulmonary exercise testing after single and double lung transplantation. Chest 1990;97:1130–1136.

130. Gibbons W, Levine S, Bryan C, et al. Cardiopulmonary exercise responses after single lung transplantation for severe obstructive lung disease. Chest 1991;100:106–111.

131. Williams T, Patterson G, McClean P, et al. Maximal exercise testing in single and double lung transplant recipients. Am Rev Respir Dis 1992; 145:101–105.

132. Levy R, Ernst P, Levine S, et al. Exercise performance after lung transplantation. J Heart Lung Transplant 1993;12:27–33.

133. Orens J, Becker F, Lynch J III, et al. Cardiopulmonary exercise testing following allogeneic lung transplantation for different underlying disease states. Chest 1995;107:144–149.

134. Schwaiblmair M, Reichenspurner H, Muller C, et al. Cardiopulmonary exercise testing before and after lung and heart-lung transplantation. Am J Respir Crit Care Med 1999;159:1277–1283.

135. Martinez F, Orens J, Whyte R, et al. Lung mechanics and dyspnea after lung transplantation for chronic airflow obstruction. Am J Respir Crit Care Med 1996;153:1536–1543.

136. Evans A, Al-Himyary A, Hrovat M, et al. Abnormal skeletal muscle oxidative capacity after lung transplantation by 31P MRS. Am J Respir Crit Care Med 1997;155:615–621.

137. Wang X, Williams T, McKenna M, et al. Skeletal muscle oxidative capacity, fiber type, and metabolites after lung transplantation. Am J Respir Crit Care Med 1999;160:57–63.

138. Stiebellehner L, Quittan M, End A, et al. Aerobic endurance training program improves exercise performance in lung transplant recipients. Chest 1998;113:906–912.

139. Gross C, Savik K, Bolman R III, et al. Long-term health status and quality of life outcomes of lung transplant recipients. Chest 1995;108: 1587–1593.

140. TenVergert E, Essink-Bot M, Geertsma A, et al. The effect of lung transplantation on health-related quality of life: a longitudinal study. Chest 1998;113:358–364.

141. Cohen L, Littlefield C, Kelly P, et al. Predictors of quality of life and adjustment after lung transplantation. Chest 1998;113:633–644.

142. Hosenpud J, Bennett L, Keck B, et al. The Registry of the International Society for Heart and Lung Transplantation: sixteenth official report—1999. J Heart Lung Transplant 1999;18: 611–626.

143. Pearson M, Ogilvie C. Surgical treatment of emphysematous bullae: late outcome. Thorax 1983;38:134–137.

144. Brenner M, McKenna R Jr, Chen J, et al. Survival following bilateral staple lung volume reduction surgery for emphysema. Chest 1999;115:390–396.

145. Burrows B, Bloom J, Traver G, et al. The course and prognosis of different forms of chronic airways obstruction in a sample from the general population. N Engl J Med 1987;317:1309–1314.

146. Nocturnal Oxygen Therapy Trial Group. Continuous or nocturnal oxygen therapy in hypoxemic chronic obstructive lung disease: a clinical trial. Ann Intern Med 1980;93:391–398.

147. Anthonisen N, Wright E, Hodgkin J, et al. Prognosis in chronic obstructive pulmonary disease. Am Rev Respir Dis 1986;133:14–20.

148. Meyers B, Yusen R, Lefrak S, et al. Outcome of Medicare patients with emphysema selected for, but denied, a lung volume reduction operation. Ann Thorac Surg 1998;66:331–336.

149. Roue C, Mal H, Sleiman C, et al. Lung volume reduction in patients with severe diffuse emphysema: a retrospective study. Chest 1996;110: 28–34.

150. Yusen R, Pohl M, Richardson V, et al. 3-year results after lung volume reduction surgery. Am J Respir Crit Care Med 1998;157(Suppl):A335.

151. Gelb A, Brenner M, McKenna R Jr, et al. Lung function 12 months following emphysema resection. Chest 1996;110:1407–1415.

152. Gelb A, Brenner M, McKenna R Jr, et al. Serial lung function and elastic recoil 2 years after lung volume reduction surgery for emphysema. Chest 1998;113:1497–1506.

153. Brenner M, McKenna R Jr, Gelb A, et al. Rate of FEV_1 change following lung volume reduction surgery. Chest 1998;113:652–659.

154. O'Donnell D. Dyspnea in advanced chronic obstructive pulmonary disease. J Heart Lung Transplant 1998;17:544–554.

155. Fletcher C. The clinical diagnosis of pulmonary emphysema: an experimental study. Proc R Soc Med 1952;45:577–584.

156. Hosenpud J, Bennett L, Keck B, et al. The registry of the International Society for Heart and Lung Transplantation: fourteenth official report—1997. J Heart Lung Transplant 1997; 16:691–722.

157. Hosenpud J, Bennett L, Keck B, et al. Effect of diagnosis on survival benefit after lung transplantation for end-stage lung disease. Lancet 1998;351:24–27.

158. Bjortuft O, Geiran O, Fjeld J, et al. Single lung transplantation for chronic obstructive pulmonary disease: pulmonary function and impact of

bronchiolitis syndrome. Respir Med 1996;90: 553–559.

159. Heng D, Sharples L, McNeil K, et al. Bronchiolitis obliterans syndrome: incidence, natural history, prognosis, and risk factors. J Heart Lung Transplant 1998;17:1255–1263.

160. Cooper J, Billingham M, Egan T, et al. A working formulation for the standardization of nomenclature and for clinical staging of chronic dysfunction in lung allografts. J Heart Lung Transplant 1993;12:713–716.

161. Patterson G, Wilson S, Whang J, et al. Physiologic definitions of obliterative bronchiolitis in heart-lung and double-lung transplantation: a comparison of the forced expiratory flow between 25% and 75% of the forced vital capacity and forced expiratory volume in one second. J Heart Lung Transplant 1996;15:175–181.

162. Paris W, Diercks M, Bright J, et al. Return to work after lung transplantation. J Heart Lung Transplant 1998;17:430–436.

163. Chumillas S, Ponce J, Delgado F, et al. Prevention of postoperative pulmonary complications through respiratory rehabilitation: a controlled clinical study. Arch Phys Med Rehabil 1998; 79:5–9.

164. Gaensler E, Jederlinic P, FitzGerald M. Patient work-up for bullectomy. J Thorac Imaging 1986;1:75–93.

165. Nakahara K, Nakaoka K, Ohno K, et al. Functional indications for bullectomy of giant bulla. Ann Thorac Surg 1983;35:480–487.

166. Pride N, Barter C, Hugh-Jones P. The ventilation of bullae and the effect of their removal on thoracic gas volumes and tests of over-all pulmonary function. Am Rev Respir Dis 1973; 107:83–98.

167. Kinnear W, Tatterfield A. Emphysematous bullae: surgery is best for large bullae and moderately impaired lung function. BMJ 1990;300: 208–209.

168. Carr D, Pride N. Computed tomography in preoperative assessment of bullous emphysema. Clin Radiol 1984;35:43–45.

169. Morgan M, Denison D, Strickland B. Value of computed tomography for selecting patients with bullous lung disease for surgery. Thorax 1986;41:855–862.

170. Mehran R, Deslauriers J. Indications for surgery and patient work-up for bullectomy. Chest Surg Clin N Am 1995;5:717–734.

171. Lefrak S, Yusen R, Trulock E, et al. Recent advances in surgery for emphysema. Annu Rev Med 1997;48:387–398.

172. Martinez F. Diagnosing chronic obstructive pulmonary disease. Postgrad Med 1998;103:112–125.

173. Brenner M, McKenna R Jr, Gelb A, et al. Objective predictors of response for staple versus emphysematous lung reduction. Am J Respir Crit Care Med 1997;155:1295–1301.

174. McKenna R Jr, Brenner M, Fischel R, et al. Patient selection criteria for lung volume reduction surgery. J Thorac Cardiovasc Surg 1997;114: 957–967.

175. Thurnher R, Muntwyler J, Stammberger U, et al.

Coronary artery disease in patients undergoing lung volume reduction surgery for emphysema. Chest 1997;112:122–128.

176. Whyte R, Bria W, Martinez F, et al. Combined lung volume reduction surgery and mitral valve reconstruction. Ann Thorac Surg 1998;66: 1414–1416.

177. Schmid R, Stammberger U, Hillinger S, et al. Lung volume reduction surgery combined with cardiac interventions. Eur J Cardiothorac Surg 1999;15:585–591.

178. Bach D, Curtis J, Christensen P, et al. Preoperative echocardiographic evaluation of patients referred for lung volume reduction surgery. Chest 1998;114:972–980.

179. Criner G, O'Brien G, Furukawa S, et al. Lung volume reduction surgery in ventilated-dependent COPD patients. Chest 1996;110:877–884.

180. Gelb A, Zamel N, McKenna R Jr, et al. Mechanism of short-term improvement in lung function after emphysema resection. Am J Respir Crit Care Med 1996;154:945–951.

181. Anthonisen N, Wright E, Group IT. Response to inhaled bronchodilators in COPD. Chest 1987;91:36S–39S.

182. Izquierdo-Alonso J, Sanchez-Hernandez I, Fernandez F, et al. Utility of transfer factor to detect different bronchodilator responses in patients with chronic obstructive pulmonary disease. Respiration 1998;65:282–288.

183. Fessler H, Permutt S. Lung volume reduction surgery and airflow limitation. Am J Respir Crit Care Med 1998;157:715–722.

184. Butler C, Benditt J, Lewis S, et al. Improvement in quality of life following lung volume reduction surgery correlates with changes in lung volume and exercise function but not with air flow limitation or dyspnea. Am J Respir Crit Care Med 1997;155(Suppl):A795.

185. Zisman D, Curtis J, Kazerooni E, et al. Emphysema heterogeneity and hyperinflation predict improvement after bilateral lung volume reduction surgery. Am J Respir Crit Care Med 1998;157(Suppl):A497.

186. Kurosawa H, Hida W, Kikuchi Y, et al. Hyperinflation estimated by residual volume can predict benefit of lung volume reduction surgery in patients with emphysema. Am J Respir Crit Care Med 1997;155(Suppl):A 605.

187. Brenner M, Kayaleh R, Milne E, et al. Thoracoscopic laser ablation of pulmonary bullae: radiographic selection and treatment response. J Thorac Cardiovasc Surg 1994;107:883–890.

188. Szekely L, Oelberg D, Wright C, et al. Preoperative predictors of operative morbidity and mortality in COPD patients undergoing bilateral lung volume reduction surgery. Chest 1997; 111:550–558.

189. Wisser W, Klepetko W, Senbaklavaci O, et al. Chronic hypercapnia should not exclude patients from lung volume reduction surgery. Eur J Cardiothorac Surg 1998;14:107–112.

190. Martinez F, Paine R. Medical evaluation of the patient with potentially resectable lung cancer. In: Pass H, Mitchell J, Johnson D, et al., eds.

Lung Cancer: Principles and Practice. Philadelphia: Lippincott-Raven, 1996:511–534.

191. Slone R, Pilgram T, Gierada D, et al. Lung volume reduction surgery: comparison of preoperative radiologic features and clinical outcome. Radiology 1997;204:685–693.

192. Gierada D, Slone R, Bae K, et al. Pulmonary emphysema: comparison of preoperative quantitative CT and physiologic index values with clinical outcome after lung-volume reduction surgery. Radiology 1997;205:235–242.

193. Kazerooni E, Whyte R, Flint A, et al. Imaging of emphysema and lung volume reduction surgery. RadioGraphics 1997;17:1023–1036.

194. Weder W, Thurnheer R, Stammberger U, et al. Radiologic emphysema morphology is associated with outcome after surgical lung volume reduction. Ann Thorac Surg 1997;64:313–320.

195. Wisser W, Klepetko W, Kontrus M, et al. Morphologic grading of the emphysematous lung and its relation to improvement after lung volume reduction surgery. Ann Thorac Surg 1998;65:793–799.

196. Wang S, Fischer K, Slone R, et al. Perfusion scintigraphy in the evaluation for lung volume reduction surgery: correlation with clinical outcome. Radiology 1997;205:243–248.

197. Jamadar D, Kazerooni E, Martinez F, et al. Semiquantitative ventilation/perfusion scintigraphy and single photon emission computed tomography for evaluation of lung volume reduction surgery candidates: description and prediction of clinical outcome. Eur J Nucl Med 1999; 26:734–742.

198. Maurer J, Frost A, Glaville A, et al. International guidelines for the selection of lung transplant candidates. Am J Respir Crit Care Med 1998; 158:335–339.

199. Lynch J III, Martinez F. Lung transplantation: who's a candidate? J Respir Dis 1996;17:393–412.

200. Di Boscio V, Sarli M. Lung transplantation and osteoporosis: a review. Clin Pulm Med 1999; 6:110–117.

201. Shafers H, Wagner T, Demertzis S, et al. Preoperative corticosteroids: a contraindication to lung transplantation? Chest 1992;102:1522–1525.

202. Grady K, Costanzo M, Fisher S, et al. Preoperative obesity is associated with decreased survival after heart transplantation. J Heart Lung Transplant 1996;15:863–871.

203. Levine S, Anzueto A, Peters J, et al. Single lung transplantation in patients with systemic disease. Chest 1994;105:837–841.

204. Travers G, Cline M, Burrows B. Predictors of mortality in chronic obstructive pulmonary disease. Am Rev Respir Dis 1979;119:895–902.

205. Oswald-Mammosser M, Weitzenblum E, Quoiz E, et al. Prognostic factors in COPD patients receiving long-term oxygen therapy. Chest 1995;107:1193–1198.

206. Seersholm N, Dirksen A, Kok-Jensen A. Airway obstruction and two year survival in patients with severe $\alpha\alpha_1$-antitrypsin deficiency. Eur Respir J 1994;7:1985–1987.

207. Seersholm N, Kok-Jensen A. Survival in relation to lung function and smoking cessation in patients with severe hereditary α_1-antitrypsin deficiency. Am J Respir Crit Care Med 1995;151: 369–373.

208. Wu M, Eriksson E. Lung function, smoking and survival in severe $\alpha\alpha_1$-antitrypsin deficiency PiZZ. J Clin Epidemiol 1988;41:1157–1165.

209. TA-ADRS Group. Survival and FEV_1 decline in individuals with severe deficiency of α_1-antitrypsin. Am J Respir Crit Care Med 1998;158: 49–59.

210. Gelb A, Zamel N, Hogg J, et al. Pseudophysiologic emphysema resulting from severe small-airways disease. Am J Respir Crit Care Med 1998;158:815–819.

211. Burrows B, Boom J, Traver G, et al. The course and prognosis of different forms of chronic airways obstruction in a sample from the general population. N Engl J Med 1987;317:1209–1214.

212. Hughes J, Hutchinson D, Bellamy D, et al. Annual decline of lung function in pulmonary emphysema: influence of radiological distribution. Thorax 1982;37:32–37.

213. Kazerooni E, Chow L, Whyte R, et al. Preoperative examination of lung transplant candidates: value of chest CT compared with chest radiography. Am J Roentgenol 1995;165:1343–1348.

214. Kazerooni E, Hartker F III, Whyte R, et al. Transthoracic needle aspiration in patients with severe emphysema: a study of lung transplant candidates. Chest 1996;109:616–619.

215. Fein A. Lung volume reduction surgery: answering the crucial questions. Chest 1998;113: 277S–282S.

216. Zenati M, Keenan R, Courcoulas A, et al. Lung volume reduction or lung transplantation for end-stage pulmonary emphysema? Eur J Cardiothorac Surg 1998;14:27–32.

217. Bavaria J, Pocettino A, Kotloff R, et al. Effect of volume reduction on lung transplant timing and selection for chronic obstructive pulmonary disease. J Thorac Cardiovasc Surg 1998;115: 9–18.

24 Ethical Issues in Patients With Advanced Lung Disease

John E. Heffner

> ## ◎ Professional Skills
>
> *Upon completion of this chapter, the reader will:*
>   - Understand the difficulties that exist with predicting which patients with advanced lung disease will benefit from intubation and mechanical ventilation for respiratory failure
>   - Recognize the role of advance care planning to assist patients in making their end-of-life decisions
>   - Identify the shortcomings of present efforts to promote the adoption of advance directives
>   - Denote the interests of patients with severe lung disease for advance care planning
>   - Select patients for advance care education
>   - Provide patients with chronic lung disease a framework for discussing advance directives with their families and physicians

INTRODUCTION

Patients with advanced lung disease frequently present difficult ethical dilemmas during the course of their care. Regardless of the nature of the underlying pulmonary condition, most patients with chronic respiratory disorders experience a slowly progressive course punctuated by episodes of acute worsening of their lung function. Each episode of pulmonary decompensation poses questions regarding the appropriateness of life-sustaining interventions, such as intubation and mechanical ventilation. For some patients, life-supportive care may promote survival and allow recovery to a baseline level of function. For others, intubation and mechanical ventilation may leave patients with a restricted level of activity or simply prolong the dying process when respiratory failure occurs at the terminal stage of disease. In an effort to assist patients with their decision regarding the acceptability of life-sustaining care, clinicians are often called on to estimate both the likelihood of survival for their patients and the anticipated quality of their postrecovery lives.

Unfortunately, clinicians have a limited ability to predict the outcome of acute respiratory failure for individual patients with chronic lung disease.[1] Multiple studies indicate that patients with chronic obstructive lung disease (COPD) admitted for an acute exacerbation of airway disease have an overall survival to hospital discharge that ranges from 66 to 94%.[2-11] Survival to hospital discharge of patients with COPD who require assisted ventilation is lower, ranging from 60 to 74%.[12-18]

Although overall survival is good, no clinical factors, including the severity of blood gas abnormalities or the presence of comorbid factors, identify the subset of patients who

453

will fail to survive.[1] Moreover, no studies have identified predictors that reliably identify patients who will survive hospitalization with a decreased functional level and diminished quality of life. Even fewer data exist to describe the probability of survival or postrecovery function of patients who present with respiratory failure caused by advanced lung diseases other than COPD.

In the absence of accurate prognosticating tools, the care of patients with advanced lung disease presents ethical dilemmas and challenging patient care considerations. The ethical dilemmas often focus on decisions regarding the withholding or withdrawal of life-supportive care, such as cardiopulmonary resuscitation, artificial airways, and mechanical ventilators. The patient care considerations encompass palliative care measures and social support for patients who are experiencing severe discomfort at the terminal stages of their disease. Considering that COPD is the fourth leading cause of death,[19] it is remarkable that few empiric studies have examined clinical approaches to these ethical dilemmas and unique management needs presented by patients with chronic lung disease at the end of life. This chapter reviews important ethical considerations in the care of these patients and provides recommendations for using opportunities provided by pulmonary rehabilitation to help patients as they prepare for and pass through the terminal stages of their disease.

RATIONALE FOR ADVANCE CARE PLANNING

Considerable ethical, social, and legal support exists for allowing patients to refuse medical care even when such refusal would result in their death.[20,21] In most jurisdictions, living wills and durable powers of attorney for health care are recognized instruments for conveying patients' health care wishes when they become incapacitated. These documents address the observation that most patients with advanced lung disease wish to direct their own end-of-life decisions even after they lose decision-making capacity. A questionnaire study of patients enrolled in pulmonary rehabilitation indicates that more than 80% of patients prefer to direct decisions regarding intubation and mechanical ventilation by either communicating with their physicians directly, through a written advance directive, or through their appointed surrogate decision makers.[22]

Patients' interests to direct their end-of-life decisions mandates that caregivers assist patients with advanced lung disease in making end-of-life decisions that reflect their unique clinical circumstances, life values, and goals. Unfortunately, most studies indicate that less than 15% of elderly patients under the long-term care of physicians and patients with chronic health conditions of a general nature have had discussions with their physicians about end-of-life care.[22-27] Similarly, only 19% of patients with advanced lung disease have complete discussions with their physicians about the appropriateness of life support in various clinical circumstances, and 15% have participated in discussions regarding the nature of life-supportive care.[22] Although most patients with chronic lung disease have formulated opinions regarding the acceptability of intubation and mechanical ventilation, less than 15% of these patients feel confident that their physicians understand their wishes.[22]

The importance of this patient–physician dialog is underscored by the observation that patients need medical information from their caregivers to formulate their advance care decisions. Patients often have an inflated estimation of the value of life-sustaining care.[28] When geriatric patients are presented with realistic estimations of the likelihood of survival after cardiopulmonary resuscitation, they often alter their willingness to undergo life-sustaining care.[29,30] Patients with chronic lung disease similarly demonstrate a lower interest in accepting intubation and mechanical ventilation as the probability of survival decreases and when baseline or postrecovery respiratory function diminishes.[22]

Patients with advanced lung disease, therefore, have a greater opportunity to make end-of-life decisions that result in the outcomes they desire if they gain an accurate knowledge of the nature of life-sustaining interventions and their probabilities of success in different clinical circumstances. Because this information needs to be tailored to the unique health circumstances of each patient, physicians and other caregivers with an awareness of the patient's condition are in the best position to inform their patients regarding these issues. Helping patients prepare for decisions that may entail the withholding or withdrawing of life-sustaining care should emulate the approach care providers use to inform patients about the nature of surgical procedures before requesting consent for an operative procedure.

BARRIERS TO ADVANCE CARE PLANNING

It remains uncertain as to why few patients with chronic health conditions have an opportunity to discuss end-of-life issues with their physicians. Physicians seem to wait for patients to request information on advance directives because they interpret such initiatives as evidence that patients are emotionally ready to discuss these topics.[24] Most patients do not demonstrate initiative and instead wait for their physicians to introduce advance care planning.[22] The resulting communication "standoff" leaves patients uninformed regarding the value of life-supportive care in their unique circumstances.

The barriers to communication are not entirely defined. Multiple studies indicate that most patients are receptive to advance care planning discussion.[22–27] In groups of patients with advanced lung disease, information is desired on advance directive by 89% and explicit explanations of the nature and value of life-supportive care by 69%.[22] It seems that most patients do not present barriers to greater communications about end-of-life care.

It has been suggested that several barriers exist for physicians to initiate these discussions, including time constraints,[31] physicians perceptions that they already understand their patients' end-of-life preferences,[32–34] and discomfort with discussing end-of-life issues.[35] Recent studies indicate that pulmonary physicians who feel personal discomfort discussing end-of-life decisions are more likely to postpone these discussions with their patients with COPD.[35]

POTENTIAL ROLE FOR PULMONARY REHABILITATION IN INITIATING ADVANCE CARE PLANNING

Programs directed toward physicians to promote more patient–physician discussions on advance care planning have produced mixed results. The SUPPORT investigators observed negligible effects of an inpatient program to notify physicians of patients who would benefit from end-of-life discussions.[34] In contrast, a comprehensive effort to change the culture within a medical center regarding the importance of advance directives promoted a greater patient–physician dialog.[36] This study, however, was limited to inpatient care and did not examine the effect of physician education on patient–physician discussions on advance care planning in the ambulatory setting. Other studies in general patient populations indicate that policy interventions, computer prompts to electronic medical records, and physician education have only marginal success in promoting these discussions and the proportion of patients with completed advance directives.[25,37–53]

Promoting discussions on advance planning in the ambulatory setting is important because most patients with advanced lung disease indicate a preference for such discussions to occur during periods of stable health.[22] Only 19% of patients with chronic lung disease would choose to defer advance care planning to an acute hospitalization, when the need for life-supportive care seems imminent.[22]

Unfortunately, observational studies indicate that most advance planning occurs during critical illnesses when patients have already lost their decision-making capacity.[35,54,55]

Only 20% of patients who have a do-not-resuscitate order placed in their medical record have had an opportunity to participate in the decision-making process.[56]

The reluctance of physicians to initiate end-of-life discussions has produced interest in promoting advance care planning by encouraging patients with chronic lung disease to initiate these discussions with their physicians. Physician behavioral studies indicate that patient expectations and requests for specific components of care are potent influences for altering physician practice patterns.[57] Enrollment in pulmonary rehabilitation seems to be an opportunity to inform patients regarding the importance of advance care planning and of discussing end-of-life issues with their physicians. Success of such a program would depend on patients' willingness to participate in advance care planning educational programs within pulmonary rehabilitation and their opinions regarding the suitability of receiving this information from nonphysician educators.

To address these issues, a recent study examined the attitudes of patients with advanced lung disease enrolled in pulmonary rehabilitation programs.[22] The authors found that patients identified pulmonary rehabilitation educators and lawyers in addition to physicians as the most sources of information on advance directives (Table 24-1). Pulmonary rehabilitation educators and physicians were identified as the preferred sources of information on life-supportive care. This receptiveness to information from a variety of sources provides an opportunity to develop curricula within pulmonary rehabilitation that prepare patients to initiate discussions with their physicians and approach advance care planning in an informed manner.

The effectiveness of advance care planning curricula in pulmonary rehabilitation, however, has received little investigational attention. One study examined a brief educational intervention about advance directives directed toward patients with chronic lung disease enrolled in pulmonary rehabilitation.[58] The study determined that education increased the proportion of patients who had completed written advance directives from

Table 24-1. Subject Preferences[a] for Sources of Information on Advance Directives and the Life Support Interventions of Intubation and Mechanical Ventilation

	Preference Rating	
Source	**Advance Directives**	**Life Support**
Pulmonary rehabilitation	1.75 ± 0.74^b	1.63 ± 0.67^e
Lawyer	1.77 ± 0.91^c	2.48 ± 0.92
Physician	1.80 ± 0.77^c	1.34 ± 0.50^f
Family	2.02 ± 1.01^d	1.74 ± 0.84^e
Reading	2.10 ± 0.74^d	NA
Community class	2.31 ± 0.81	2.38 ± 0.81^d
Clergy	2.58 ± 0.85	2.70 ± 0.80

Reprinted with permission from Heffner JE, Fahy B, Hilling L, et al. Attitudes regarding advance directives among patients in pulmonary rehabilitation. Am J Respir Crit Care Med 1996;154:1735.

NA, not assessed.

[a] Preference ratings calculated from the mean $\pm$ SD of a four-level Likert scale, with "1" corresponding to highly preferred and "4" corresponding to very undesirable.

[b] $P < .05$ compared with clergy, community class, or reading.

[c] $P < .05$ compared with clergy and community class.

[d] $P < .05$ compared with clergy.

[e] $P < .05$ compared with clergy, lawyer, or community class.

[f] $P < .05$ compared with clergy, lawyer, community class, or family.

34 to 86% but had a smaller effect on increasing the number of patients who had discussed these issues with their physicians (22–58%). Moreover, only 44% of patients had confidence at the end of the study that their end-of-life wishes were understood by their physicians. These results support the utility of end-of-life education within pulmonary rehabilitation, especially considering that the educational intervention was brief and did not provide follow-up monitoring of patients for completion of advance planning. The advantages of different approaches to advance care planning education within pulmonary rehabilitation warrant further evaluation.

Although pulmonary rehabilitation seems to be a potentially valuable site for advance planning information for patients with advanced lung disease, most programs do not offer end-of-life educational opportunities. In a recent survey study, fewer than 10% of pulmonary rehabilitation programs in the United States provide information on end-of-life issues.[59] More than 70% of nonphysician directors of rehabilitation programs, however, state a willingness to include such education into their curricula.[59] Some program directors responding to this survey, however, stated a reluctance to present sessions on advance care planning, voicing a concern that education on end-of-life issues might be unsettling or depressing to their patients.

The psychologic impact of advance care planning has been examined in several studies. These studies indicate that discussions on end-of-life issues do not cause the patient depression or provoke excessive anxiety or a sense of hopelessness.[55,56,60–62] Geriatric patients participating in end-of-life discussions with their physicians have demonstrated a decrease in measured anxiety and depression scores.[62] Elderly patients and patients with chronic health conditions identify loss of control over their lives and fears of becoming a burden to their families as their greatest concerns. Advance care planning may decrease anxiety and depression by providing patients with approaches to retaining control over their health care and avoiding prolonged illnesses before their deaths.[63]

The psychologic impact of advance care planning for patients with advanced lung disease has not been extensively investigated. Existing data, however, indicate that more than 88% of patients with advanced lung disease enrolled in pulmonary rehabilitation state an interest in learning more about advance care planning.[22] Nearly all (>99%) of these patients indicate that end-of-life discussions would not provoke unacceptable levels of concern or anxiety.[22]

ADVANCE PLANNING CURRICULA WITHIN PULMONARY REHABILITATION

The foregoing discussion indicates that patients wish to learn more about advance care planning so as to participate effectively in their end-of-life decisions. Presently, however, patients do not often participate in discussions on advance care planning with their physicians and have limited resources to learn about end-of-life issues tailored to their unique respiratory conditions. Limited data indicate that curricula on advance care planning within pulmonary rehabilitation would assist patients in making valid end-of-life decisions.

Unfortunately, formal curricula for educating patients on advance care planning have not been developed and validated to date. If such a curriculum were to be designed, it would need to contain elements that would assist rehabilitation directors to select patients for advance care planning and provide information that would allow patients to participate in a meaningful way in their end-of-life decisions.

Selecting Patients for Advance Care Planning

Although most patients want their caregivers to initiate discussions regarding end-of-life care, it should be noted that a small proportion do not.[22] In a survey of patients with advanced lung disease, 4% of patients indicated that they would prefer their caregivers to make all of their end-of-life decisions without being included in the decision-making process.[22] Similarly, although most patients do not think that end-of-life discussions would promote undo anxiety, 1% indicate that such discussion would be too anxiety provoking to pursue.[22] Also, some members of certain ethnic groups are reluctant to engage in discussions about end-of-life issues. Mexican-American, Korean-American, and Navajos are less receptive to making their own life support decisions.[64,65] Receptiveness to participating in advance planning increases as members of ethnic groups begin to assimilate into the dominant culture.[65] An educational program within pulmonary rehabilitation on advance care planning, therefore, would need to respect the reluctance of some patients to participate.

One acceptable approach for selecting patients for discussing end-of-life care entails presenting patients with an invitation to participate in educational sessions without exposing them to the contents of the program. End-of-life topics can be introduced while discussing other components of health care planning, such as vaccinations, health screening, and disease prevention activities. An appropriate invitation would come in the form of a statement of rationale and a question: "Patients with chronic lung conditions can develop respiratory complications that might require life-supportive care, such as mechanical ventilation. It is important for your physician to understand your attitudes and beliefs about life-prolonging care in different circumstances. Would you be willing to participate in an educational program intended to assist you with making decisions about your care if you developed a severe illness?"

Patients who voice a reluctance to participate may respond more favorably as they learn more about the nature of their lung conditions in pulmonary rehabilitation and the possibility for progressive deterioration. Periodic invitations to participate as patients demonstrate increasing trust and comfort within the rehabilitation program may allow patients to become more receptive to advance care planning. Also, some patients with anxiety about discussing life-sustaining treatment still want to have these discussions take place after receiving reading material on advance planning and additional opportunities and encouragement.[22,66]

Helping Patients Make Valid End-of-Life Decisions

An important component of advance care planning involves the completion of a written document that is intended to direct patients' care when they have lost their decision-making capacity or can no longer communicate their wishes. A living will provides caregivers a statement regarding a patient's wishes for life-supportive care in various clinical circumstances, often limited in some jurisdictions to the existence of a terminal disease. A durable power of attorney for health care provides an opportunity to appoint a health care proxy who can represent the patient's wishes through surrogate decision making.

Unfortunately, written advance directives have been only marginally successful in allowing patients to direct their end-of-life care.[67] As previously stated, only a small proportion of patients with general categories of disorders[23-26] and patients with advanced lung disease have completed these documents.[22] Also, physicians often are unaware of the existence of formal advance directives and do not adhere to the written directives when critical illnesses arise.[34,68,69] Moreover, patients with written advance directives frequently fail to understand the contents and implications of their complete documents,[70] and surrogate decision makers usually have a poor understanding of patients' end-of-life wishes.[71] These shortcomings have created concern that written advance directives have little utility for supporting patient autonomy at the end of life.[72,73]

Recent data indicate that emotional and societal barriers exist to valid advance care planning. Depression,[74,75] socioeconomic conditions,[76] the effects of disease on family units,[77] ethnic barriers,[77,78] disease discrimination,[78] and patient misunderstanding of the purpose of advance planning can influence the wishes of patients for end-of-life care as they complete their advance directives. Adequate caregiver training regarding the elements that influence patient decisions may safeguard patients from making decisions that do not reflect their personal wishes and goals. Caregivers can also direct patients to appropriate resources if depression or socioeconomic factors seem to influence patients' decisions away from their best interests.

Although advance directives have been promoted as instruments that direct patients' end-of-life care, most patients intend that their surrogates and physicians overrule their advance directives in some clinical situations as circumstances dictate.[79,80] Advance directives, therefore, should be considered for many patients to represent general statements regarding treatment preferences. Patients need to be asked how specifically their advance directives should be respected. Without an ongoing dialog, physicians generally demonstrate a poor understanding of their patients' preferences for overruling advance directives, which is associated with more interventional end-of-life care.[81]

Despite these efforts to assist patients to formulate valid written advance directives, it seems that written instruments will always fall short in providing accurate and comprehensive descriptions of patients' wishes in all conceivable clinical circumstances. Recent discussions on end-of-life planning have recommended a conceptual shift in our thinking about advance care planning.[82] This shift directs us to understand how patients rather than caregivers perceive advance care planning and to participate in an expanding definition of advance care planning.

AN EXPANDED DEFINITION OF ADVANCE CARE PLANNING

Caregivers tend to perceive written advance directives as operational tools that direct the selection of life-sustaining interventions when patients can no longer participate in health care decision making. From patients' perspectives, advance directives are only one of the many resources available to patients for achieving their end-of-life goals. These goals extend beyond the usual choices between specific life-supportive interventions presented to patients during episodes of respiratory failure. Patients' more comprehensive goals at the end of life center on preparing for death, achieving a sense of control over their lives, and fortifying personal relationships with friends and families.[82]

The goals of advance care planning from patients' perspectives, therefore, are more psychosocial and less operational or oriented toward accepting or rejecting specific interventions. The goals of advance care planning may consequently shift from patient–physician communication focused on the withholding or withdrawing of various life-sustaining interventions toward communication between family members. This communication within a patient's family has a purpose of strengthening family relationships and offering mutual support as patients anticipate the end of their lives.

Educators in pulmonary rehabilitation who care for patients with advanced lung disease nearing the end of life can facilitate this strengthening of family relationships. Appropriate efforts would involve families in advance care planning and promote a dialog between patients and their families regarding the prognosis of the patient's lung disease and the decisions regarding care that they will eventually face. Educators can identify patient and family needs for resources to enrich these discussions and provide specific respiratory-related information tailored to a specific patient's unique health circumstances and stage of disease. Educators can also make themselves available to respond to patients' questions and concerns. During enrollment in pulmonary rehabilitation, educators can monitor their patients' advance care planning and obtain copies of written directives to be certain that they accurately reflect their patients' stated preferences, life values, and goals.[82]

In this model, an ongoing dialog about end-of-life decisions—rather than a written advance directive itself—becomes the purpose of advance care planning. This purpose fulfills patients' needs to prepare for death, enhance family relationships, and receive the end-of-life care that best conforms to their wishes and preferences. Enrollment in pulmonary rehabilitation may provide the suitable environment to assist patients with initiating and maintaining this family-oriented dialog.

SUPPORTING PATIENTS' END-OF-LIFE NEEDS BEYOND ADVANCE DIRECTIVES

Many patients with advanced lung disease enrolled in pulmonary rehabilitation will experience progression of their respiratory condition. Eventually, coping mechanisms that previously alleviated the discomforts of chronic dyspnea will fail and patients will experience ongoing respiratory distress. If such patients elect to forego life-supportive care with ventilatory support, they require reassurance that effective palliative measures will limit suffering as they approach the end of life and that they will not be abandoned by their care providers.[83] Most pulmonary rehabilitation programs educate patients regarding the progressive nature of their disease.[59] Yet most programs have not included education on the availability and effectiveness of palliative care and community resources for managing the difficulties that progressive respiratory diseases present at the end of life. This omission may be unfortunate because patients with lung disease commonly harbor an unspoken fear of experiencing the pain of suffocating as they die. This fear seems reasonable considering that severe dyspnea is a common experience of patients dying from any cause.[84] Also, almost all of the patients with COPD monitored in the SUPPORT study experienced dyspnea during the last few days of their life.[85] Patients with advanced lung disease have an all too familiar understanding of the discomforts produced by unremitting dyspnea.

Unremitting dyspnea during terminal care requires directed efforts to improve patient comfort. Supplemental oxygen has been shown to offer marginal benefit in studies wherein patients with cancer were randomized to receive supplemental oxygen versus compressed air.[86] A cold stream of air across a patient's face generated by an electric fan has been shown to diminish dyspnea in some settings.[87,88]

Patients who elect not to undergo intubation during a terminal episode of respiratory failure often experience marked increases in work of breathing. A few studies have demonstrated that noninvasive positive-pressure ventilation can decrease dyspnea while still allowing patients to communicate with their families during periods of removal of face masks.[89] Noninvasive positive-pressure ventilation can be applied at home as a palliative measure for dying patients with advanced lung disease.

Most patients dying with advanced lung disease will require pharmacologic interventions for palliative care. Opioids offer the most effective relief for severe dyspnea at the end of life. These agents alter patients' perceptions of breathlessness and decrease the ventilatory response to hypercapnia and hypoxia. Although these agents can worsen gas exchange and accelerate death by depressing respiratory drive, their use for dying patients is justified through the principle of double effect. This principle deems interventions with potential for harm as being acceptable if the caregiver's intent in treating patients was to relieve pain and suffering and not to hasten death. Terminal sedation is appropriate to treat a dying patient's pain and dyspnea, recognizing that the patient may lose consciousness and experience an accelerated demise as an unintended side effect.[90]

Most patients with terminal dyspnea fail to experience an adequate response to oral opioids,[91] which produce considerable adverse side effects.[92] Limited experience exists with the use of nebulized opioids, which may diminish dyspnea without depressing ventilatory drive,[93,94] although one study indicates that respiratory depression can occur.[95] Most patients needing terminal dyspnea control require parenteral morphine. In this setting, patients should be reassured that morphine doses will be adjusted in anticipation of dyspnea rather than after intolerable dyspnea has already occurred.

Benzodiazepine drugs can supplement morphine during palliative care by relieving anxiety.[84] These agents are usually avoided until the last days of life because they cloud consciousness. Chlorpromazine has been shown to relieve dyspnea that was unresponsive

Box 24-1. Parameters for Identifying Patients Who Qualify for Hospice Services

> I. Severity of chronic lung disease documented by
>   A. Disabling dyspnea at rest; poorly or unresponsive to bronchodilators, resulting in decreased functional activity, e.g., bed-to-chair existence, often exacerbated by other debilitating symptoms such as fatigue and cough
> FEV_1 after bronchodilator, >30% predicted, is helpful supplemental objective evidence but should not be required if not already available
>   B. Progressive pulmonary disease
>   1. Increasing visits to the emergency department or hospitalizations for pulmonary infections and/or respiratory failure
>   2. Decrease in FEV_1 on serial testing of >40 mL/y is helpful supplemental objective evidence but should not be required if not already available
> II. Presence of cor pulmonale or right heart failure
>   A. These should be caused by advanced pulmonary disease, not primary or secondary to left heart disease or valvulopathy
>   B. Cor pulmonale may be documented by
>   1. Echocardiography
>   2. Electrocardiogram
>   3. Chest radiograph
>   4. Physical signs of right heart failure
> III. Hypoxemia at rest on supplemental oxygen
>   A. PO_2 ≤55 mm Hg on supplemental oxygen
>   B. Oxygen saturation ≤88% on supplemental oxygen
> IV. Hypercapnia
>   A. PCO_2 ≥50 mm Hg
> V. Unintentional progressive weight loss of >10% of body weight over the preceding 6 mo
> VI. Resting tachycardia >100/min in a patient with known severe chronic obstructive pulmonary disease

Data from Stuart B, Alexander C, Arenella C, et al. Medical Guidelines for Determining Prognosis in Selected Non-cancer Diseases. Arlington, VA: The National Hospice Organization, 1996.
FEV_1, forced expiratory volume in 1 second; PO_2, partial pressure of oxygen; PCO_2, partial pressure of carbon dioxide.

to opioids and benzodiazepine drugs.[96] Intractable cough at the end of life can be managed with opioid agents or nebulized anesthetic drugs.[97] Anticholinergic agents can alleviate the terminal airway secretions that may gag patients or distress families who are observing a prolonged "death rattle."

Community resources have not matured for patients with advanced lung disease as they have for patients with terminal malignancies. Alternatives to hospitalization for terminal patients with advanced lung disease, however, do exist. The National Hospice Organization recently revised their guidelines for selecting patients with noncancer diseases for access to hospice services.[98] These guidelines discuss the difficulties in accurately predicting the prognosis of patients with advanced COPD but recognize the appropriateness of providing hospice services for subsets of these patients (Box 24-1).[98] Educational programs within pulmonary rehabilitation can serve as contact resources to advise patients and their families regarding these community resources.

CONCLUSION

End-of-life care of patients with advanced lung disease can be enhanced with the adoption of well-conceived advance directives that reflect patients' end-of-life preferences. Advance directives by themselves, however, cannot communicate by themselves a full spectrum of patient preferences in all conceivable health care circumstances. They should serve as a component of an ongoing dialog between patients, families, and care providers that promotes an understanding of the patient's life values and goals. With this understanding, patients have the greatest opportunity to approach the end of their life with confidence that their wishes will be honored, their dying experience will strengthen their family relationships, and they will gain support from the family relationships that advance care planning engendered. Education on life-supportive interventions and end-of-life issues within pulmonary rehabilitation can foster this expanded role of advance care planning for patients with advanced lung disease.

REFERENCES

1. Heffner JE. Chronic obstructive pulmonary disease: ethical considerations of care. Clin Pulm Med 1996;3:1–8.
2. Asmundssen T, Kilburn KH. Survival of acute respiratory failure: a study of 239 episodes. Ann Intern Med 1969;70.
3. Vanderbergh E, van de Woestijne KP, Gyselin A. Conservative treatment of acute respiratory failure in patients with chronic obstructive lung disease. Am Rev Respir Dis 1968;98:60–69.
4. Sluiter HJ, Blokzyl EJ, van Dijl W, et al. Conservative and respirator treatment of acute respiratory insufficiency in patients with chronic obstructive lung disease: a reappraisal. Am Rev Respir Dis 1972;105:932–942.
5. Moser KM, Shibel EM, Beamon AJ. Acute respiratory failure in obstructive lung disease. Med Clin North Am 1973;57:781–792.
6. Kettel LH. The management of respiratory failure in chronic obstructive lung disease. Med Clin North Am 1973;57:781–792.
7. Burk RH, George RB. Acute respiratory failure in chronic obstructive pulmonary disease: immediate and long-term prognosis. Arch Intern Med 1973;132:865–868.
8. Seriff NS, Khan F, Lazo BJ. Acute respiratory failure: current concepts of pathophysiology and management. Med Clin North Am 1973;57:1539–1550.
9. Warren PM, Flenly DC, Millar JS, et al. Respiratory failure revisited: acute exacerbations of chronic bronchitis between 1961–68 and 1970–76. Lancet 1980;1:467–470.
10. Bone RC, Pierce AK, Johnson RL. Controlled oxygen administration in acute respiratory failure in chronic obstructive pulmonary disease: a reappraisal. Am Rev Respir Dis 1978;65:896–902.
11. Martin RT, Lewis SW, Albert RK. The prognosis of patients with chronic obstructive pulmonary disease after hospitalization for acute respiratory failure. Chest 1982;82:310–314.
12. Portier F, Defouilloy C, Muir JF. Determinants of immediate survival among chronic respiratory insufficiency patients admitted to an intensive care unit for acute respiratory failure. Chest 1992;101:204–210.
13. Rieves RD, Bass D, Carter RR, et al. Severe COPD and acute respiratory failure: correlates for survival at the time of tracheal intubation. Chest 1993;104:854–860.
14. Menzies R, Gibbons W, Goldberg P. Determinants of weaning and survival among patients with COPD who require mechanical ventilation for acute respiratory failure. Chest 1989;95:398–405.
15. Bradley RD, Spencer GT, Semple SJG. Tracheostomy and artificial ventilation in the treatment of acute exacerbations of chronic lung disease: a study in twenty-nine patients. Lancet 1964;1:854–859.
16. Jessen O. Tracheostomy and artificial ventilation in chronic lung disease. Lancet 1967;2:9–12.
17. Sukumalchantra Y, Dinakara P, Williams MH. Prognosis of patients with chronic obstructive pulmonary disease after hospitalization for acute ventilatory failure: a three-year follow-up study. Am Rev Respir Dis 1966;93:215–222.
18. Gillespie DJ, Marsh MM, Divertie MB, et al. Clinical outcome of respiratory failure in patients requiring prolonged (>24 hours) mechanical ventilation. Chest 1986;90:364–369.
19. Petty TL. Definitions, causes, course, and prognosis of chronic obstructive pulmonary disease. Respir Care Clin N Am 1998;4:345–358.
20. President's Commission for the Study of Ethical Problems in Medicine and Biomedical and Behavioral Research. Deciding to forego life-sustaining treatment: a report on the ethical and legal issues in treatment decisions. Washington, DC: US Government Printing Office, 1983.
21. Lanken PN, Ahlheit BD, Crawford S, et al. Withholding and withdrawing life-sustaining therapy. Am Rev Respir Dis 1991;144:726–731.
22. Heffner JE, Fahy B, Hilling L, et al. Attitudes regarding advance directives among patients in pulmonary rehabilitation. Am J Respir Crit Care Med 1996;154:1735–1740.
23. Emanuel LL, Barry MJ, Stoekle JD, et al. Advance directives for medical care: a case for greater use. N Engl J Med 1991;324:889–895.
24. La Puma J, Orentlicher D, Moss R. Advance directives on admission: clinical implications and analysis of the Patient Self-determination Act of 1990. JAMA 1991;266:402–405.
25. Rubin SM, Strull WM, Fialkow MF, et al. Increasing the completion of the durable power of attorney for health care: a randomized, controlled trial. JAMA 1994;271:209–212.
26. Virmani J, Schneiderman LJ, Kaplan RM. Relationship of advance directives to physician-patient

communication. Arch Intern Med 1994;142: 909–913.

27. Lo B, McLeod GA, Saika G. Patient attitudes to discussing life-sustaining treatment. Am J Med 1986;146:1613–1615.

28. Miller DL, Jahnigen DW, Gorbien MJ, et al. Cardiopulmonary resuscitation: how useful? attitudes and knowledge of an elderly population. Arch Intern Med 1992;152:578–582.

29. Murphy DJ, Burrows D, Santilli S, et al. The influence of the probability of survival on patients' preferences regarding cardiopulmonary resuscitation. N Engl J Med 1994;330:545–549.

30. Frankl D, Oye RK, Bellamy PE. Attitudes of hospitalized patients toward life support: a survey of 200 hospitalized medical patients. Am J Med 1989;86:645–648.

31. Wolf SM, Boyle P, Callahan D, et al. Sources of concern about the Patient Self-determination Act. N Engl J Med 1991;325:1666–1671.

32. Lo B. "Do not resuscitate" decisions: a prospective study at three teaching hospitals. Arch Intern Med 1985;145:1115.

33. Uhlmann RF, Pearlman RA, Cain KC. Physicians' and spouses' prediction of elderly patients' resuscitation preferences. J Gerontol 1988;43:115–121.

34. Connors AF Jr, Dawson NV, Desbiens NA, et al. A controlled trial to improve care for seriously ill hospitalized patients: the study to understand prognoses and preferences for outcomes and risks of treatments (SUPPORT). JAMA 1995;274: 1591–1598.

35. Sullivan KE, Hébert PC, Logan J, et al. What do physicians tell patients with end-stage COPD about intubation and mechanical ventilation? Chest 1996;109:258–264.

36. Reilly BM, Wagner M, Magnussen R, et al. Promoting inpatient directives about life-sustaining treatments in a community hospital: results of a 3-year time-series intervention trial. Arch Intern Med 1995;155:2317–2323.

37. Hanson LC, Tulsky JA, Danis M. Can clinical interventions change care at the end of life? Ann Intern Med 1997;126:381–388.

38. Cohen-Mansfield J, Droge JA, Billig N. The utilization of the durable power of attorney for health care among hospitalized elderly patients. J Am Geriatr Soc 1991;39:1174–1178.

39. Cohen-Mansfield J, Rabinovich BA, Lipson S, et al. The decision to execute a durable power of attorney for health care and preferences regarding the utilization of life-sustaining treatments in nursing home residents. Arch Intern Med 1991; 151:289–294.

40. Hare J, Nelson C. Will outpatients complete living wills? a comparison of two interventions. J Gen Intern Med 1991;6:41–46.

41. Sachs G, Stocking C, Miles S. Empowerment of the older patient? a randomized controlled trial to increase discussion and use of advance directives. J Am Geriatr Soc 1992;40:269–273.

42. High D. Advance directives and the elderly: a study of interventional strategies to increase their use. Gerontologist 1993;33:342–349.

43. Holley JL, Nespor S, Rault R. The effects of providing chronic hemodialysis patients written material on advance directives. Am J Kidney Dis 1993;22:413–418.

44. Luptak MK, Boult C. A method for increasing elders use of advance directives. Gerontologist 1994;34:409–412.

45. Markson LJ, Fanale J, Steel K, et al. Implementing advance directives in the primary care setting. Arch Intern Med 1994;154:2321–2327.

46. Cuglian AM, Miller T, Sobal J. Factors promoting completion of advance directives in the hospital. Arch Intern Med 1995;155:1893–1898.

47. Silverman HJ, Tuma P, Schaeffer MH, et al. Implementation of the patient self-determination act in a hospital setting. Arch Intern Med 1995; 155:502–510.

48. Duffield P, Podzamsky JE. The completion of advance directives in primary care. J Fam Pract 1996;42:378–384.

49. Meier DE, Fuss BR, O'Rourke D, et al. Marked improvement in recognition and completion of health care proxies: a randomized controlled trial of counseling by hospital patient representatives. Arch Intern Med 1996;156:1227–1232.

50. Meier DE, Gold G, Mertz K, et al. Enhancement of proxy appointment for older persons: physician counseling in the ambulatory setting. J Am Geriatr Soc 1996;44:37–43.

51. Sulmasy DP, Song KY, Marx ES, et al. Strategies to promote the use of advance directives in a residency outpatient practice. J Gen Intern Med 1996;11:657–663.

52. Landry FJ, Kroenke K, Lucas C, et al. Increasing the use of advance directives in medical outpatients. J Gen Intern Med 1997;12:412–415.

53. Richter KP, Langel S, Fawcett SB, et al. Promoting the use of advance directives: an empirical study. Arch Fam Med 1995;64:609–615.

54. Quill TE, Bennett NM. The effects of a hospital policy and state legislation on resuscitation orders for geriatric patients. Arch Intern Med 1992; 15:569–572.

55. Bedell SE, Belbanco TL. Choices about cardiopulmonary resuscitation in the hospital: when do physicians talk with patients? N Engl J Med 1984; 310:1089–1093.

56. Stolman CJ, Gregory JJ, Dunn D, et al. Evaluation of the do not resuscitate orders at a community hospital. Arch Intern Med 1989;149:1851–1856.

57. Maly RC, Abrahamse AF, Hirsch SH, et al. What influences physician practice behavior? an interview study of physicians who received consultative geriatric assessment recommendations. Arch Fam Med 1996;5:448–454.

58. Heffner JE, Fahy B, Hilling L, et al. Outcomes of advance directive education of pulmonary rehabilitation patients. Am J Respir Crit Care Med 1997;155:1055–1059.

59. Heffner JE, Fahy B, Barbieri C. Advance direction education during pulmonary rehabilitation. Chest 1996;109:373–379.

60. Reilly BM, Magnussen CR, Ross J, et al. Can we talk? inpatient discussions about advance directives in a community hospital. Arch Intern Med 1994;154:2299–2308.

61. Pfeifer MP, Sidorov JE, Smith AC, et al. Discussion of end of life medical care by primary care

physicians and patients: a multicenter study using qualitative interviews. J Gen Intern Med 1994; 9:82–88.

62. Kellogg FR, Crain M, Corwin J, et al. Life-sustaining interventions in frail elderly persons: talking about choices. Arch Intern Med 1992;152: 2317–2320.

63. Reid DW, Ziegler M. Validity and stability of a new desired control measure pertaining to psychological adjustment of the elderly. J Gerontol 1980;35:395–402.

64. Carrese JA, Rhodes LA. Western bioethics on the Navajo reservation. JAMA 1995;274:826–829.

65. Blackhall LJ, Murphy ST, Frank G, et al. Ethnicity and attitudes toward patients' autonomy. JAMA 1995;274:820–825.

66. Steinbrook R, Lo B, Moulton J, et al. Preferences of homosexual men with AIDS for life-sustaining treatment. N Engl J Med 1986;314:457–460.

67. Miles SH, Koepp R, Weber EP. Advance end-of-life treatment planning: a research review [review]. Arch Intern Med 1996;156:1062–1068.

68. Teno J, Lynn J, Wenger N, et al. Advance directives for seriously ill hospitalized patients: effectiveness with the Patient Self-determination Act and the SUPPORT intervention. J Am Geriatr Soc 1997;45:500–507.

69. Phillips RS, Wenger NS, Teno J, et al. Choices of seriously ill patients about cardiopulmonary resuscitation: correlates and outcomes. Am J Med 1996;100:128–137.

70. Jacobson JA, White BE, Battin MP, et al. Patients' understanding and use of advance directives. West J Med 1994;160:232–236.

71. Hare J, Pratt C, Nelson C. Agreement between patients and their self-selected surrogates on difficult medical decisions. Arch Intern Med 1992; 152:1049–1054.

72. Tonelli MR. Pulling the plug on living wills: a critical analysis of advance directives. Chest 1996; 110:816–822.

73. Heffner JE. End-of-life ethical decisions. Semin Respir Crit Care Med 1998;19:271–282.

74. Tsevat J, Cook EF, Green ML, et al. Health values of the seriously ill. Ann Intern Med 1994;122: 514–520.

75. Rosenberg M, Wang C, Hoffman-Wilde S, et al. Results of cardiopulmonary resuscitation: failure to predict survival in two community hospitals. Arch Intern Med 1993;153:1370–1375.

76. Schonwetter RS, Walker RM, Kramer DR, et al. Socioeconomic status and resuscitation preferences in the elderly. J Appl Gerontol 1994;13: 157–171.

77. Covinsky KE, Landefeld CS, Teno J, et al. Is economic hardship on the families of the seriously ill associated with patient and surrogate care preferences? Arch Intern Med 1996;156:1737–1741.

78. Curtis JR, Patrick DL. Barrier to communication about end-of-life care in AIDS patients. J Gen Intern Med 1997;12:736–741.

79. Seghal A, Galbraith A, Chesney M, et al. How strictly do dialysis patients want their advance directives followed? JAMA 1992;267:59–63.

80. Mazur DJ, Hickman DH. Patients' preferences for risk disclosure and role in decision making for invasive medical procedures. J Gen Intern Med 1997;12:114–117.

81. Teno JM, Hakim RB, Knaus WA, et al. Preferences for cardiopulmonary resuscitation: physician-patient agreement and hospital resource use. J Gen Intern Med 1995;10:179–186.

82. Martin DK, Thiel EC, Singer PA. A new model of advance care planning. Arch Intern Med 1999; 159:86–92.

83. Youngner SJ, Lewandowsky W, McClish DK, et al. "Do not resuscitate" orders: incidence and implications in a medical intensive care unit. JAMA 1985;253:54–57.

84. Rousseau P. Nonpain symptom management in terminal care. Clin Geriatr Med 1996;12:313–327.

85. Lynn J, Teno JM, Phillips RS, et al. Perceptions by family members of the dying experience of older and seriously ill patients. Ann Intern Med 1997;126:97–106.

86. Booth S, Kelly M, Cox N, et al. Does oxygen help dyspnea in patients with cancer? Am J Respir Crit Care Med 1996;153:1515–1518.

87. Friedman S. Facial cooling and perception of dyspnea [letter]. Lancet 1987;2:1215.

88. Schwartzstein R, Lahive K, Pope A, et al. Cold facial stimulation reduces breathlessness induced in normal subjects. Am Rev Respir Dis 1987; 136:58–61.

89. Meduri GU, Fox RC, Abou-Shala N, et al. Noninvasive mechanical ventilation via face mask in patients with acute respiratory failure who refused endotracheal intubation. Crit Care Med 1994; 22:1584–1590.

90. Sulmassy DP, Pellegrino ED. The rule of double effect: clearing up the double talk. Arch Intern Med 1999;159:545–550.

91. Woodcock AA, Gross ER, Gellert A, et al. Effects of dihydrocodeine, alcohol, and caffeine on breathlessness and exercise tolerance in patients with chronic obstructive lung disease and normal blood gases. N Engl J Med 1981;305:1611–1616.

92. Boyd KJ, Kelly M. Oral morphine as symptomatic treatment of dyspnea in patients with advanced cancer. Palliat Med 1997;11:277–281.

93. Farncombe M, Chater S, Gillin A. The use of nebulized opioid for breathlessness: a chart review. Palliat Med 1994;8:306–312.

94. Zeppetella G. Nebulized morphine in the palliation of dyspnea. Palliat Med 1997;11:267–275.

95. Jedeikin R, Lang E. Acute respiratory depression as a complication of nebulised morphine. Can J Anaesth 1998;45:60–62.

96. McIver B, Walsh D, Nelson K. The use of chlorpromazine for symptom control in dying cancer patients. J Pain Symptom Manage 1994;9:341–345.

97. Hsu DH. Dyspnea in dying patients. Can Fam Physician 1993;39:1635–1638.

98. Stuart B, Alexander C, Arenella C, et al. Medical Guidelines for Determining Prognosis in Selected Non-cancer Diseases. Arlington, VA: The National Hospice Organization, 1996.

25 Social and Recreational Support of the Pulmonary Patient

Mary R. Burns

▷ Professional Skills

Upon completion of this chapter, the reader will:

- Understand how to establish a Better Breathers' Club (BBC)
- Know how to encourage patient participation
- Be able to plan patient social activities
- Know how to increase physical involvement
- Be able to plan a rally or other large event

INTRODUCTION

Pulmonary rehabilitation (PR) is now accepted as the standard of care for most patients with respiratory disability.[1-4] Many studies have shown important benefits, including increased exercise tolerance, decreased number of symptoms, and improved quality of life, after PR.[3-5] Unfortunately, of the few studies looking at long-range benefits of this improvement, most show that 1 year after PR many of these benefits begin to diminish.[5]

What can we do to prevent this? A growing body of data seems to indicate that social support may ameliorate the slide back into inactivity, isolation, and depression so commonly seen in respiratory patients before PR.[6]

Therefore, offering a social and recreational support system becomes an integral part of the continuum of care for the long-range well-being of respiratory patients.[7]

ESTABLISHMENT OF A PATIENT SUPPORT GROUP

Once the need for a social and recreational support system for the respiratory patient population is agreed on, holding a monthly group meeting is usually the first step in implementing this support system. It is helpful to enlist the aid of the hospital respiratory committee, a supportive physician,[8] or a PR department manager to obtain the necessary cooperation of hospital administration usually needed to establish this group. The American Lung Association may also have suggestions for establishing a support group, often called a Better Breathers' Club (BBC).

Location

The next challenge is to find a suitable room or auditorium in which to hold BBC meetings. If the hospital does not have space, other areas to investigate are the local American Lung Association, YMCA or YWCA, church halls, and community centers. For the small group just getting started, a physician may offer his office waiting room. However, this will be only a temporary solution because the goal should be to eventually have a much larger group than can fit into the limited space of an office.

It is important to make sure that the meeting area is easy to reach, bearing in mind the physical limitations of this population. Parking access is important but difficult to obtain in some large facilities. Solutions include blocking off close parking spots for BBC members on the day of the meeting, valet parking, parking lot shuttle service, or arranging for volunteer assistance with wheelchairs for the most impaired patients. Hospital vans for transportation, or door-to-door dial-a-ride service, are offered for the disabled in some communities. The hospital social services department or the City Hall of your city might have other suggestions for assisting with transportation to the meetings.

Time of Meetings

The day of the week and time of day on which to meet are the next two items for consideration. Most BBC's meet once a month, although a few meet weekly. Depending on the weather, some BBC's may wish to skip a few meetings during the summer or worst months of winter. Once the program becomes established, however, you may find that your group does not wish any break in the schedule. For the most part, it is better to avoid Monday and Friday for meetings. Monday is sometimes a universal holiday and meetings on either of these two days may interfere with long weekends for staff, speakers, and attendees.

Respiratory patients often have trouble getting started in the morning and are reluctant to drive at night; therefore, midday meetings work best. Making a lecture part of the meeting provides a focal point. Scheduling the lecture to conclude before 2 PM makes it feasible for a busy physician to speak to the group and yet get back to the office in time for afternoon appointments. It is important to allow time before and after the lecture for socializing. If the meeting is held in a hospital, perhaps a buffet luncheon can be arranged. Bringing a box lunch, or sandwiches from home, is another option. Many groups serve beverages only, with members bringing snacks. Meals can then be reserved for special occasions once or twice a year.

The First Meeting

Plan the first BBC meeting far enough in advance to arrange for adequate publicity. If a PR program is already in operation, graduates, of course, are the first to be sent a printed invitation. Active members can be asked to assist with planning and hosting the event. Make sure the announcement makes it clear that a spouse or friend is equally welcome. The hospital newsletter, local newspaper, and local chapter of the American Lung Association may assist with publicizing the event. Often, local radio and TV stations have free public service announcements that can be used. Flyers can also be posted in offices of physicians. It is usually wise to enlist the help of the hospital public relations department for assistance, permission, and additional ideas. This is a good time to establish cordial relations with a department that can be of great assistance in the future.

Make this first meeting as special as circumstances allow. A few balloons, colorful napkins, and a little extra effort on refreshments go a long way. Have several chairs at the entrance, along with a table equipped with pens, name tags, and markers. Use PR graduates, or a nucleus of individuals interested in a support group, from the start. Two can sit at the sign-in table to ensure that everyone entering signs a sheet with their name, address, and telephone number before filling in a name tag to wear. Others can act as official hosts and hostesses to warmly welcome guests and help them find a seat. Make sure volunteers have a name tag or an official badge.

Introduce new guests to the person they are seated next to, even if it is necessary to read their name tag to do so. Do *everything* possible to provide a warm, welcoming atmosphere for this and all future meetings.

If a PR staff already exists, as many as possible should be present for this first meeting, wearing name tags that are easy to read. The staff also should mingle and welcome guests.

When the meeting starts, welcome the group and introduce all staff members who are present. If the group is small, each guest can also introduce himself or herself. Now is the time to discuss hopes and plans for the future. Ask for audience input. Suggest that a group of interested people meet to discuss further ideas. Set a date for the meeting at this time while interest is high. If a few in the group have shown great interest in forming a support group, they can specifically be asked to participate and help. They may become future leaders. If the group is totally new, this may have to be postponed for a few more meetings. Respiratory patients often need a great deal of encouragement before beginning to actively participate, so don't be discouraged by initial reticence.

The first speaker, of course, should be someone who will give an interesting talk that will stimulate the interest and enthusiasm of the group. A topic that includes the word "new" usually will guarantee a large audience. Asthma, medications, and discussions on how to handle stress are also high on the interest list of respiratory patients.

Have an audiocassette recorder or videotape camera ready to record the guest speaker. Consider asking a patient to be responsible for tending to the recording process. This can be the first item in the group library. The tapes can be used for future attendees who have missed a meeting, for those who are homebound, or for those who wish to hear the topic again. It also is useful for reviewing the lecture to summarize it for a patient newsletter. Be sure to have a camera and take a few pictures to document this special occasion. At least one of the patients is sure to have an interest in photography and may be willing to help in this area.

Guest speakers donating their time appreciate a thank you. Ask one or two patients to write short notes of appreciation.

Although a monthly patient meeting is an important part of the continuum of care for a PR program, it can also be of value if the PR program has not yet been established. The patient with respiratory disease is usually hungry for knowledge, help, and empathy from others with a similar disability. Although a BBC cannot take the place of PR, it does help to fulfill a need until the PR program can be established. At that time it will also become a referral source as well as being of key importance in maintaining social and recreational support while updating knowledge.

The Telephone Committee

At the first BBC meeting, or even before, solicit several patients to do the telephoning for the group. Even the most physically limited are able to assist in this way. It is a good way to establish group cohesiveness, which is so important, and to start involvement of even the homebound patient in the group process.

If the group is small, two or three callers are adequate. Involve as many as possible. If the group is large, appoint a chairperson to whom all other callers report. Have each caller be responsible for no more than 10 names, if possible.

Calls can be made several days before each monthly luncheon, or before other activities, to encourage people to come as well as to get an attendance count. Most people like being called and knowing that someone cares. Friendships develop, and some people on the calling list may like to be called more often, especially if they become homebound.

Callers should notify the chairperson of the telephone committee about attendance, illness in a family, or any special information that would be helpful to the PR staff. After all the information for the month is collected, the chairperson telephones a member of the staff to report. This means that only one telephone call each month to the staff will keep them informed about the entire patient population. This committee is of *major* importance. It helps the busy staff keep in close contact with support group members with a minimum expenditure of time.

Patient Board of Directors

A patient Board of Directors (BOD) designed to oversee BBC operations can be established in several ways. If the group is small, consider inviting everyone to join the initial planning sessions, where responsibilities are discussed and divided. If the group is large and better established, a slate of names can be submitted and voted on.

Often potential officers are concerned about not having enough energy or health to fulfill the job requirements. It helps to reassure them that the work load will be modest and that they can always resign. This is one reason why primary offices may have two people in each position, with the spouse automatically included if the patient is elected. This lessens the work load and allays concerns about being able to fulfill the office. It also encourages involvement of the (usually) more healthy spouse. A healthy spouse can be a vital member of the organization and should also be allowed to run for office. This process strengthens spousal relationships, as well as making your core working group larger. The members of the BOD will become the strongest advocates for the BBC and PR program, even after their term of office is completed.

Offices in the BOD

If the main offices for the BOD include two people for each position, there will be two cochairpersons, co–vice chairpersons, cosecretaries, and cotreasurers. The telephone chairperson, whose duties have already been discussed, should definitely be a member of the BOD. Another important member is someone who will keep track of birthdays and also send get well cards to group members. This member, or another, should be responsible for a short thank you note to the monthly guest speaker. A librarian can help start, and then keep track of, the lending library of medical books, audiocassettes, and videocassettes the group may wish to provide members.

A historian is responsible for scrapbooks and pictures to document the history of the group. If this task is left to the busy PR staff, the group is apt to be left with boxes of unidentified slides and pictures.

Someone who enjoys decorating for holidays and special events should hold an arts and crafts office. If the group decides to hold an annual holiday boutique, this is the person who would help organize it.

If the group is fortunate, someone will be willing to accept the office of editor and send out a monthly flyer or newsletter about BBC activities to all members. A social chairperson can help plan and organize group events.

All of these chairpersons can enlist the assistance of as many others on their committees as they wish. If people are left over and eager to participate, think of a title for them such as "at large." The more people actively participating, the more fun they have and the more active the organization. A health care professional, or PR staff member, should attend BOD meetings as an advisor.

Organization Name

Encourage the group to pick a name that has special meaning for them. BBC leaves a bit to be desired as a name that inspires feelings of group loyalty. Rather than having a name chosen by one person, or the BOD, get a slate of suggestions and vote on the choice. The winner should get some sort of prize, such as dinner for two donated by a local restaurant. Examples of a few names others have chosen for support groups include The PEP Pioneers, The Inspirations, The Breathsavers, The Senior Puffers, and The Wheezenpuffs.

Funding

Discourage dues for the BBC because the object is to include everyone as a member, regardless of income. A raffle at the monthly BBC meeting can be fun and also raise a little money. Raffle tickets should be inexpensive, such as five for a dollar. Raffle prizes can include donations of white elephants, home-baked goods, or homegrown fruits and vegetables, with perhaps a five-dollar bill as first prize. That amount of money will vary with the size of the group because it should come from raffle funds collected that day.

Encourage group involvement. Have one or two patients sell tickets, another pick the winning tickets out of a hat, while yet another reads off the winner by *name* rather than just by number. This activity may not guarantee much money, but valuable group interaction will result.

An annual holiday boutique can be a fund raiser. Depending on the group, a baked goods table, white elephant table, and other crafts can be considered. A raffle with three or four special prizes may be even more successful. These special prizes can be something handmade and donated by members of the group or gift certificates for dinners solicited from local restaurants. Local stores will sometimes donate gift baskets or gift certificates.

SOCIAL ACTIVITIES

The BOD can also plan other activities and social events during the year. The social events chairperson is in charge of generating ideas and organizing events. This is too large a task for one person, however, and needs the involvement of many in the group.

Holidays

An annual Christmas party is a must. If the group has a large enough treasury, the lunch or refreshments can be free. Be sure to decorate. Arrange early in the year for a local high school chorus to come and sing Christmas carols for (and with) the group. Bring a tape deck to play cassettes the rest of the time. Have a grab bag where everyone who brings in a gift gets to take one home. Try to get a spouse to dress up as Santa Claus and pass out candy canes. Although fun-loving patients may attempt this, the beard can cause feelings of suffocation. Have a big decorated box where toys and gifts for the needy can be collected. Be sure to take pictures for the group's albums.

Picnics

A summer picnic is another popular event and is easy to organize. Hot dogs and hamburgers can be barbecued, and, yes, patients on oxygen can do the barbecuing if they wish. Find a local park with easy access to parking and bathrooms. Get a head count of the number of people wishing to come, families included. Purchase paper plates, napkins, condiments, soft drinks, and other supplies at a discount store. Charge a minimal amount to cover expenses for the barbecue, potato salad, and other purchased food. Let those who wish to do so bring their favorite dish to share, then sit back and enjoy. A tape cassette for music, bingo with silly prizes, and a camera to record it all make for a fun afternoon.

General Guidelines for Other Events

If patients wish to attempt other events, start with something easy to organize and easy to arrange transportation for. An example would be a group meeting for lunch and then attending a matinee movie. Later, this can be expanded to something like an afternoon at a local dinner theater, a play, or even the circus. Tickets are purchased in advance, but everyone is responsible for their own transportation. For all activities:

- Plan ahead. This cannot be stressed often enough.
- Get suggestions from the patient group.
- Look for activities that will be low in physical stress.

- Aim for lighthearted fun, for example, a musical matinee with lunch rather than a museum tour with a lot of walking.
- Have a sign-up sheet. Get commitment on patient interest in the specific activity before proceeding with plans.
- Arrange end seats for those receiving oxygen or with canes.
- Make sure that stairs are limited and that bathroom access is easy.
- Book early to get the best seats.
- Group tickets, especially for the handicapped or seniors, are often discounted, especially if purchased in advance.
- Request a block of seats so that everyone can sit together.
- Request early seating to avoid standing in lines and to ensure leisurely entrance.
- A reminder call to participants before the trip is helpful. A volunteer can assist with this.

Refund Policy

Refunds can be a problem with a group that tends to get sick, but it *is* important to discourage the attendance of anyone who does not feel well. The group needs to feel safe in joining these excursions. Try to have a standby or waiting list. If refunds are not possible, the individual canceling needs to find his or her own replacements or pay for the already purchased tickets. If all else fails, suggest donating the tickets for use by someone who cannot afford the price or is hesitant to attempt something new.

Longer Group Trips

When ready to attempt longer group trips, the possibilities are numerous. General considerations for longer group trips are hospital policy and oxygen needs.

Hospital Policy

- Get permission from the medical director and a hospital administrator.
- The legal department may request written signed consents and physician approval.
- Clarify hospital policy for staff liability coverage.

Oxygen Needs[9]

- Know the patients' oxygen needs.
- Note the type of oxygen unit used by each patient.
- Make sure each patient has an adequate oxygen supply to last the trip as well as transportation time to and from home.
- Allow for delays and half-filled containers.
- Make sure your trip will not be to an altitude that will require extra oxygen.
- Make friends with the local oxygen suppliers. They may be persuaded to donate oxygen, or extra containers, for these trips.
- For longer trips, make sure to have oxygen waiting in patient rooms for your arrival. Payment should be worked out in advance. The local supplier may be of help with this.
- Make sure to have extra oxygen tubing, connectors, a wrench, and an oximeter.

Transportation

Bus

- Shop around. Deal with the manager. Don't be afraid to present your needs, such as a nonsmoking driver willing to help with patients and carryons; a bus with a restroom; a step stool for getting off and on the bus; and promptness.

- Have a checklist with the names of all patients to make sure everyone is on board before departure and on the return trip!
- Keep the patients' welfare in mind at all times. Let those receiving oxygen, or the most handicapped, board first.
- Provide beverages and snacks on a long trip. Include this in the cost of the ticket.
- Travel during daylight hours.
- Make sure everyone has transportation to and from the bus.
- Have costs include the tip for the driver.
- Make friends with senior bus drivers. They are a good source of valuable information.

Boats
Boats can be fun for short river cruises or harbor cruises.

- Ensure ease of access to the boat.
- Be aware that the boarding ramp is sometimes long or steep.
- Reserve seating on the main deck, if possible. Avoid climbing the steep stairs to upper decks.

Ships
Many travel agencies can now handle longer group cruises.[10] However, keep in mind the following:

- PR staff responsibility for patients remains.
- Verify oxygen acceptance by the cruise line well in advance.
- Verify oxygen delivery to the ship by your vendor well in advance.
- Start plans 9 months to 1 year in advance, taking into consideration the weather.
- Use this time as an incentive to get patients into a regular exercise program to increase fitness.
- Refer to the chapter on travel for other specifics.

Be a good customer. Appreciate the kindness and generosity of those who go the extra mile to make the trip a success. They always welcome a brief thank you note and often remember it the next time you book with them.

After PR graduation, many patients will be eager to attempt a long delayed trip. Although the PR program usually conducts a class on travel, the PR staff remains a good resource for patients about to embark on their own.

ENCOURAGING PATIENT INVOLVEMENT

Although this chapter deals with the social and recreational support of the patient, it is important to remember why this is considered to be so important. The goal is to help patients remain actively involved and maintain maximum fitness. With that in mind, remember that opportunities for patients to assume social responsibility should be considered along with offering them social support. Patients thrive on being able to help others rather than always being on the receiving end of assistance. Use volunteer assistance from patients as much as you possibly can. This really is part of their therapy.

Ask several graduates to greet and welcome each new group on the first day of the PR class. Encourage them to tell the new class how much PR helped enrich their lives. Encourage them also to occasionally drop by during later classes to say hello and offer support to the current class. On the *last* day of class, they may enjoy being asked to welcome the new graduates to the BBC with the presentation of a name tag along with a special invitation to the next BBC meeting.

At this first BBC meeting after graduation, new members can be introduced to the entire group by name and, if time permits, with a short biography. It is often surprising how many in the group will find that they have interests and backgrounds in common.

Other suggestions have been presented earlier on ways that patients can help at BBC meetings, such as acting as hosts or hostesses, taping the guest speaker, taking pictures, helping with the raffle, and writing thank you notes to the guest speaker.

Some patients enjoy taking part in research and feeling that they contribute to science, helping others with respiratory disease as they have been helped. Research participation may only mean taking part in a small study done by the PR staff. It can also be participation in a more formal and elaborate study done by a local university. If you have a nearby teaching hospital with a pulmonary division, check to see if they are doing anything that might be of interest to your group. The physicians there will be delighted to have potential access to a patient pool of volunteers and will reciprocate by providing speakers for your BBC meetings.

ENCOURAGING PHYSICAL ACTIVITY WHILE SOCIALIZING

One of the reasons to work so hard at the social support system of our patients is to keep them active and to help them maintain the physical fitness gains they have made during PR.[8] *Maintenance of these physical gains is essential.* Social and physical support are often interrelated. Many health care practitioners will testify that part of the success of a maintenance program is the group socialization that takes place at these sessions.

There is a lot to offer patients in addition to the *very* important maintenance exercise classes. This is *especially* important to remember if room for a maintenance exercise program is not available.

Check with the local YMCA or YWCA. Ask them to set aside the outside lane of the pool so that patients with oxygen can swim without getting tangled in their 50-ft oxygen tubing. Low-level exercise classes for patients with arthritis, also suitable for pulmonary patients, are offered in some areas. Community colleges are beginning to offer classes for pulmonary patients, and the local high school might be convinced to offer a slow dance class suitable for the respiratory impaired. And yes, patients receiving oxygen *can* dance.

At all of these classes, it is much easier for patients to participate in a group rather than struggling alone. Walking clubs can be formed in which the group meets once a week to walk together followed by lunch or a snack. Local parks, malls, and walking areas can be mapped out, complete with distances and bathroom locations.

Is an enclosed mall within driving distance of the BBC? Meeting with the mall manager might result in a formal arrangement between the mall and your walking group. It can be good publicity for both. Sometimes the mall can be opened an hour before the stores are opened. Perhaps they will agree to a measured walking route. The group may wish to make up cards that patients can fill out, on the honor system, and turn in as they complete set distances. Recognition can be given in various ways, such as a "wall of fame" with names and pictures on the wall of the PR gym.

Another idea that has had great success is a planned group walk to a destination across the country or to a special location. This is a simulated walk, of course, in which each 15 or 30 minutes of walking or bike riding can equal a mile. Mileage can be collected monthly from individual group members. The accumulated distances are plotted on a large map. This has the potential of becoming an elaborate project that generates much enthusiasm as well as the desired effect of an increase in the activity level of the group.

THE RESPIRATORY RALLY

A respiratory rally is the ultimate BBC meeting. The PEP Pioneers, of Torrance, CA, have been holding an annual rally for the past 20 years. Patients, family members, and the medical staff of hospitals and PR programs from the southern part of the state gather for a day of fun, fellowship, and education. Variations on this event now take place in other areas of the world with equal success. One example is Dr. Freddy Smeets of Belgium, who held his rally in a local castle!

Highlights of the day may include a well-known pulmonary physician as a speaker or a panel of speakers. A suggested requirement is that each speaker includes some jokes in their presentation. The rally should be *fun,* with everyone going home at the end of the day in high spirits.

Some form of physical activity is usually also part of a rally. In Torrance, it is the Pace Race, whereas other areas may have a 1-km or 1-mile walk. What is the Pace Race? It is a walk covering a measured distance short enough for anyone to cover without difficulty, such as a hospital parking lot or lawn. Each participant *estimates* the amount of time it will take to complete the course comfortably, without marked shortness of breath. The three who guess their time most accurately are the winners. Because distances are very short, these guesses are narrowed down to hundredths of a second, with an official race stopwatch marking the time. *Anyone* has the potential to come in first, including the most handicapped of patients. Everyone gets a certificate of participation in the race.

An annual rally can have 200 or 300 people attending. Plan carefully in advance for any large event to ensure that everything will run smoothly.

Rally, or Special Event, Timetable

9 Months to 1 Year in Advance

- Notify your medical director and hospital public relations department of your plans.
- Get their input and support.

Date

- When setting the date, avoid days that coincide with other events, such as the annual meetings of respiratory associations and national holidays.
- Remember to allow for the vagaries of the weather.
- Decide on the day of the week taking into consideration the physicians you hope to have attend.

Location

- Find an area with easy access that is large enough to hold the number of people that you anticipate attending.
- Ensure adequate bathrooms, kitchen facilities, sound system, and parking.
- Consider cost. A hospital auditorium will often work well. A cultural arts center or civic auditorium can sometimes be reserved at no cost, or minimal cost, for non-profit organizations.
- You are on your own on how to find a castle!

Theme

- Pick a catchy phrase such as "Humor for the Health of It," "Pioneer Days," "Breath of Spring," etc.
- Assign someone to be in charge of decorations, using the theme as the guide.
- Ask speakers to have topics appropriate to the theme.

Speakers

- The medical director of PR should be on the panel, introduce the panel, or be master of ceremonies.
- Although you may telephone the speakers you would like to have on your program, always follow up with a written letter repeating the date, time, topic, and length of time you wish them to speak.
- Most local physicians are happy to volunteer their time.
- If the speaker you wish is nationally known, or from out of the area, you need to reimburse him or her for expenses.
- Feel free to ask the physicians if they know a company that will cover their expenses and honorariums.

Vendors and Funding

- Industry support is vital in helping with expenses and honorariums.
- Some of the large companies may provide an educational grant.
- Contact all the drug representatives of companies producing the medications your patients use.
- Call all the home care companies in your area as well as the oxygen suppliers.
- Check with the respiratory department for the names of companies from which they make large purchases.
- Arrange for each contributing company to have a booth or table where they can exhibit their product and hand out literature, if they wish.
- The amount of money that can be requested from each company will depend on the size of the group that is expected to attend the event.
- Some vendors will explain what their budget limit is for an event or suggest a reasonable amount. They have an annual budget so it is important to get their commitment as early as possible.
- You often will have to follow through with a formal letter explaining the event and providing a tax ID number.

6 Months in Advance

Food

- If the event is to be held in the hospital, find out the policy of the dietary department. Do they want to provide the food or do they have a caterer whom they recommend?
- Find out what the charge is.
- If the hospital requires an outside caterer, box lunches are usually the easiest way to go.
- Have several vegetarian lunches.
- Remember that many of these patients have salt-restricted diets.
- Sometimes costs can be kept down by buying soft drinks and bottled water at a large discount store.
- Remember to provide snacks for volunteers arriving early.

Cost

- Add up the cost of the meeting area and speaker expenses, plus the cost of food and beverages for the projected number of participants.
- Remember that your volunteers will have free lunches.
- Add on another dollar or two for decorating expenses and entertainment.
- Deduct the amount of money pledged from participating vendors.

- Final cost for the day for each individual can range as high as $8 or $9 to being cost free for all participants.

Letters

- Send an initial letter to all PR programs in the area explaining what you have planned, along with specifics including the date, guest speakers, and an estimate of cost per ticket.
- Suggest that they contact local home care companies or drug representatives to see if their program can obtain sponsorship to help defray the costs of their bus or lunch.
- Assure them that anyone giving financial assistance to them will be provided with a display table at the rally.
- Send this letter to the hospital public relations department and to anyone else that you hope will attend.
- Send a copy to all the physicians in the area.

Entertainment

- Contact your hospital volunteer department for ideas.
- Request clowns or other forms of entertainment that they may be able to provide.
- Check other local agencies for volunteer talent.
- Have clowns greet the arriving buses and cars to create a festive mood.
- Piano players for background music or even patient groups with musical or comedic talents also can be of value.
- Remember that the object is to provide a fun-filled day!

Volunteer Help

- Put in an early request with the volunteer department of your hospital.
- Telephone the respiratory therapy or nursing school departments of your local college. They may wish to make attendance part of their curriculum and it may also lead to further interaction with them in the future.
- Do not forget to involve the patients and their families. The more involved they are the more they will enjoy themselves and the more creative they will become at turning this into an extravaganza.

Door Prizes

- Try to arrange to offer dinners for two from *chain* restaurants rather than from a local eatery if some participants are from outside the area.
- Send letters requesting donations of gift certificates to all the large chain restaurants.
- Gift baskets make excellent door prizes.
- Vendors will often provide a prize in addition to financial support.

Equipment

- Make a detailed checklist of *everything* that will be needed.
- Write down the date each item was ordered, as well as the date that each item is received.
- Now is the time to reserve things like helium for balloons, race timers from the local high school, linens, a piano, etc.

1 or 2 Months in Advance

- Step up publicity.
- Send letters to all participating hospitals.
- Request estimates of numbers planning to attend from each participating program. Don't forget to add in vendors and volunteers.
- Have each group keep track of their own patients.
- After payment has been received, promptly send admission raffle tickets and name tags to save time and confusion on the day of the rally.
- Note need for display tables for sponsoring vendors.

2 or 3 Days in Advance

- Confirm the participating number attending from any group that has not responded.
- Provide a final count to the caterer.
- Go over your checklist.
- Ensure a display table for each vendor.
- Assign duties to various individuals to avoid last-minute confusion.
- Make a *detailed* timed schedule of the final day's events.

This schedule may sound like overkill, but it is essential for a smoothly running event of the size about which we are talking. Also, by spreading the work out over a long period of time, it is possible to achieve an undertaking of this size while continuing the day-to-day activities of the PR program.

The Day of the Rally

- Arrive early, which is part of your detailed time schedule.
- With everything so well organized, all should be able to enjoy an event that will long be remembered by everyone who has the pleasure of being part of it.

IN SUMMARY

Although this chapter started out discussing the social and recreational support of the respiratory patient, it has expanded hopefully to show how this support naturally leads into exercise maintenance, self-sufficiency, and even increased community involvement. Social and recreational support of the patient may, at first glance, seem like a luxury and something of questionable value. In the grand scheme, however, it is vital to a patient group and can be woven into the continuum of care you establish for the well-being of your patients.

REFERENCES

1. California Thoracic Society Position Paper: The Principles of Pulmonary Rehabilitation. Tustin: California Thoracic Society, 1998.
2. ATS statement: standards for the diagnosis and care of patients with chronic obstructive pulmonary disease. Am J Respir Crit Care Med 1995; 152:S84(Part 2 of 2).
3. Ries AL. Position paper of the American Association of Cardiovascular and Pulmonary Rehabilita-tion: scientific basis of pulmonary rehabilitation. J Cardiopulm Rehabil 1990;10:418.
4. Ries AL, Carlin BW, Carrieri-Kohlman V, et al. Pulmonary rehabilitation: joint ACCP/AACVPR evidence-based guidelines. J Cardiopulm Reha-bil 1997;17:771.
5. Ries AL, Kaplan RM, Limberg TM, et al. Effects of pulmonary rehabilitation on physiologic and psychosocial outcomes in patients with chronic obstructive pulmonary disease. Ann Intern Med 1995;122:823–834.
6. Kaplin RM, Eakin EG, Ries AL. Psychosocial is-

sues in the rehabilitation of patients with chronic obstructive pulmonary disease. In: Casaburi R, Petty TL, eds. Principles and Practice of Pulmonary Rehabilitation. Philadelphia: WB Saunders, 1993.

7. Burns M. Travel hints for the person with COPD. In: Petty TL, Nett L, eds. Enjoying Life With Chronic Obstructive Lung Disease. 3rd ed. Cedar Grove, NJ: Laennec Publishing, 1995:125–133.

8. Burns MR. Continuing care programs. In: Casaburi R, Petty TL, eds. Principles and Practice of Pulmonary Rehabilitation. Philadelphia: WB Saunders, 1993:398–404.

9. Burns MR. Travel with oxygen. In: Tiep BL, ed. Portable Oxygen Including Oxygen-Conserving Devices. Spring Valley, NY: Futura Press, 1991: 421–436.

10. Burns M. Cruising with COPD. Am J Nurs 1987;87:479–482.

26 Sleep Disorders in Pulmonary Patients

Daniel O. Rodenstein

Professional Skills

Upon completion of this chapter, the reader will:

- Understand the sleep process in normal subjects
- Have an accurate idea of the physiologic consequences of sleep on the different systems of the organism, especially on the respiratory system
- Understand the special problems that sleep pose to the patient with pulmonary disorders
- Have an idea of some sleep-related diseases that may affect patients with pulmonary diseases

INTRODUCTION

Like any person, patients with pulmonary diseases go to sleep at least once a day. Although at first sight this is an obvious fact, sleeping is not always trivial. Indeed, sleep by itself represents a serious physiologic challenge for patients with chronic respiratory diseases, a challenge that many fail to manage well.

The pulmonary patient may experience serious problems during sleep on two accounts. First, sleep may have a primary deleterious effect on the pulmonary disease. Sleep may add the effect of specific sleep-related disorders to the basic pulmonary disease. This chapter reviews some basic notions about sleep, points out the influence of sleep physiology on the respiratory system in normal subjects and especially in patients with respiratory diseases, and describes some sleep-related diseases that may affect (like anybody else) patients with respiratory illness. The combined effect of these two types of disorders in a single individual may result in severe complications and even death.

SLEEP

Basic Facts

Although nobody knows the exact vital function of sleep, it is nonetheless true that after a number of hours of active wakefulness, people develop a feeling of tiredness and sleepiness. Keeping awake becomes more difficult, and finally the body enters a physiologic state different from wakefulness, known as sleep. The most obvious difference between wakefulness and sleep is that in the latter state the subject becomes "disconnected" from the external world. External stimuli (auditory, visual, and tactile) are ignored by the sleeping person, but this state of unresponsiveness is partial (i.e., stronger stimuli will induce an interruption of sleep) and spontaneously reversible: after several hours of sleep, the subject wakes up refreshed; sleepiness has vanished.

This cycle of events repeats itself with striking regularity about every 24 hours. In humans, sleepiness generally peaks in the late evening, and sleep occurs generally during the night. A second, less potent peak in sleepiness normally occurs after midday. Many people in the world respond to this weak sleepiness sensation in the form of a short period of sleep, known as siesta, whereas it is ignored by most people in the "developed" world.

Sleep may be viewed as a physiologic state that depends on a particular functional organization of the central nervous system. If the electrical activity of the cerebral cortex is examined by recording the electroencephalogram with surface electrodes, sleep is characterized (with respect to wakefulness) both by a slowing down of the frequency of the waves of the recordings and by an increase in the voltage amplitude of these electrical waves. As amplitude increases and frequency decreases progressively, sleep is defined as deeper (meaning, among other things, that the subject is less and less responsive to external and proprioceptive stimuli). In addition to the slowing frequency and increasing amplitude in the electroencephalogram, the eyeballs move slowly behind the closed eyelids, and the tonic activity of all skeletal muscles decrease progressively as sleep deepens. After a variable period of time in these stages, a new sleep state emerges: the electroencephalographic pattern has a higher frequency and lower voltage, like the one during wakefulness; the eyes show fast, coordinated movements, and the muscular tone is practically abolished, as if the subject was paralyzed. This sleep stage has been termed Rapid Eye Movement (REM) sleep, whereas the other type of sleep is accordingly known as non-REM sleep. The latter is usually divided in stages 1 to 4, depending on the particular frequency and voltage of the electrical waves.[1] Dreams are believed to occur almost exclusively in REM sleep.

The architecture of normal sleep varies with age. In the normal adult, sleep progresses from stage 1 to stage 4 non-REM sleep, and this is followed by a period of REM sleep. This succession is known as a sleep cycle and lasts for about 60 to 90 minutes. Four to seven cycles occur during a night. Stages 3 and 4 predominate in the first part of the night, whereas REM sleep predominates in the last half of the night (see Fig. 26-1). REM sleep is more prevalent in babies than later in life, whereas after age 50 to 60 years, it is common for stages 3 and 4 to nearly completely disappear.

Mechanisms of Sleep

Contrary to what may be believed, sleep is an active, not a passive, energy-dependent process. Sleep depends on active inhibition of neuronal activity in the brain. This active inhibition is initiated by neurons located in the preoptic area and around the lower brainstem reticular formation. Their action is to inhibit the excitatory waking neurons located in the reticular formation and other areas of the brainstem that are essential for the maintenance of the wake state. REM sleep seems to have a specific neuronal control, different from that of non-REM sleep. It is supposed that as wake goes on, sleep-promoting substances accumulate, increasing sleepiness until sleep state becomes evident. Sleep-promoting neurochemicals and cytokines have already been described (like serotonin or interleukin 1), but this area is only emerging at the present time.[2]

Physiologic Consequences of Sleep

As the responsiveness to external stimuli changes, so does the responsiveness to "internal" (proprioceptive) stimuli. In addition, sleep affects every physiologic system in the body. For instance, the heart rate decreases by about 5 to 10 beats/min with respect to the resting, supine, awake heart rate. This decrease is sleep specific and goes beyond the effects of posture and rest in wakefulness. Similarly, blood pressure decreases by about 10 mm Hg.[3] Kidney function changes too during sleep: glomerular filtration decreases, as do urine production and sodium excretion, whereas sodium and water resorption increase.[4] Salivary secretion stops at sleep onset, and the swallowing reflex is abolished during sleep.

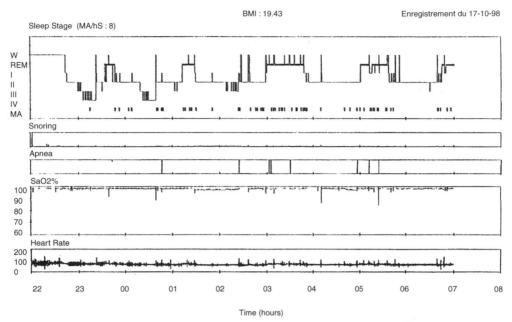

Figure 26-1. Schematic representation of a sleep recording in a normal individual. The *horizontal axis* represents time in hours. The graph starts at 22:00 hours and ends at 08:00 hours. The resolution of the graph is 30 seconds. Above the boxes are depicted the date of the recording (to the right), the body mass index (*BMI*) of the individual (center, in kilograms per squared meter), and the index of movement arousals per hour of sleep (*Ma/hS*). From top to bottom, the first box represents the hypnogram (schematic representation of the vigilance states). *W*, wakefulness; *REM*, Rapid Eye Movement sleep; *I, II, III,* and *IV,* the stages of non-REM or slow wave sleep; *MA,* movement arousal: each bar indicates that during that period of 30 seconds, a movement arousal has occurred. The second box represents snoring. The heights of the bars indicate the total noise recorded during that 30 seconds. The third box depicts apneas: each bar indicates that during that 30 seconds at least one apnea occurred. The fourth box represents arterial oxygen saturation (SaO_2%) measured transcutaneously with an oximeter. Each bar represents the mean $\pm$ 2 standard deviations of all measures recorded during that 30 seconds. The scale goes from 100 to 60% saturation. The last box represents heart rate, with the scale going from 200 to 0 beats/min. Again, each bar is the mean $\pm$ 2 standard deviations of all measurements performed during that 30 seconds. Note that in this normal, young female, sleep latency (the period from the start of the recording to the first sleep period) lasts for about 45 minutes. Five sleep cycles (a sleep cycle is the combination of stages of non-REM sleep followed by a period of REM sleep) occur during the night. Note that from time to time brief awakenings (return to wakefulness) and some movement arousals occur. Also note that stages 3 and 4 non-REM sleep predominate in the first half of the night, whereas REM sleep predominates in the second half of the night. No snoring and only a few apneas occur. Oxygen saturation remains high during the whole night. Note that both heart rate and heart rate variability decrease during sleep.

Peristaltic waves in the gastrointestinal system seem to slow down during sleep, although discrepancies are present between different gastrointestinal segments. Motor activity seems to be reduced much more consistently in the colon than in the esophagus. The endocrine system has tight connections with sleep and with the circadian rhythm. For instance, the secretion of growth hormone peaks during the first half of the sleeping time, synchronous with a period of stage 3 to 4 slow wave sleep.[5] About 80% of the daily secretion of growth hormone takes place during this sleep-related period. Cortisol secretion also peaks during the night, in fact during the early morning hours, and usually coincides with sleep.

However, cortisol secretion seems to be independent of sleep per se: even if a subject sleeps during the day and stays awake during the night, cortisol secretion will still peak in the early morning hours.[5] Prolactin secretion significantly increases during sleep, whereas thyroid-stimulating hormone levels are depressed during sleep.

Respiratory Consequences of Sleep

Minute ventilation decreases during sleep by about 10 to 15% beyond the supine awake basal volumes.[6] The decrease is mainly caused by a reduction in tidal volume, whereas average respiratory frequency remains similar in wakefulness and sleep.[7] However, frequency variability is strikingly reduced during non-REM sleep, where breathing becomes regular, especially during stages 3 and 4 non-REM sleep. In contrast, frequency is irregular during REM sleep, and the tidal volume variability also increases in this stage, perhaps in relation to the content of dreams (this has been frequently postulated but not demonstrated).

Blood gases also change during sleep. Arterial partial pressure of carbon dioxide ($PaCO_2$) increases by about 3 to 8 mm Hg, and arterial partial pressure of oxygen (PaO_2) decreases by about 2 to 5 mm Hg.[8] The various mechanisms causing these changes are complex and are briefly described here. Ventilation depends schematically on two different control systems: the metabolic controller and the volitional controller. The former adjusts ventilation so that the $PaCO_2$ value remains almost constant whatever the activity of the body. Thus, $PaCO_2$ is allowed to minimally fluctuate around a given value (the so-called set point, usually 39 mm Hg) by modifying ventilation as a function of the CO_2 production of the body so that CO_2 excretion matches CO_2 production. The volitional system attributes a higher hierarchy to the nonmetabolic roles of the respiratory system, overriding the metabolic controller. For instance, during speech or singing, it may be necessary to allow for enough expiratory time (i.e., time useful for speech) to reduce respiratory frequency to less than 4 to 5 breaths/min. This will result in CO_2 accumulation and increases in $PaCO_2$, but the metabolic controller will not react by increasing ventilation until the volitional task is finished. During sleep, ventilation is governed by the metabolic controller because the volitional controller is inhibited. As a consequence, the drive to breathe is reduced. Indeed, the set point of CO_2 is determined at least partly by a stimulation that depends on the wakefulness state, probably mediated by the volitional controller. Therefore, the "retreat" of this wakefulness drive to breathe will result in an increase in the set point of CO_2 and hence in a decrease in ventilation. The sleep CO_2 set point is around 42 to 45 mm Hg.[9]

Together with the sleep-related disappearance of the volitional control and of the wakefulness drive to breathe, the sensitivity of the metabolic respiratory controller to hypercapnia and probably also to hypoxia decreases.[10,11] The ventilatory responses to a resistive load are also decreased compared with wakefulness, a change with important physiologic consequences (see "Obstructive Sleep Apnea" section of this chapter). This means that during sleep, if the $PaCO_2$ increases, or if the PaO_2 decreases, the respiratory controller will react less briskly than in wakefulness so that the increase in ventilation in response to these stimuli will be less, and the correction of hypoxia and/or hypercapnia will be incomplete. Similarly, if the resistance to airflow increases, the response in terms of augmented efforts to breathe will be less than during wakefulness, meaning that ventilation will be less well defended, and thus will decrease during sleep. Whereas during wakefulness it would be maintained by the increased efforts of the respiratory pump.

Ventilation depends on the contraction of a series of skeletal muscles, usually referred to collectively as the respiratory pump. The muscle pump includes the diaphragm (the main respiratory muscle) and the intercostals and scaleni (accessory respiratory muscles), but also a series of muscles distributed along the upper airways, from the nose to the glottis. These muscles are activated with each inspiration in descending order so that the dilators of the nares are activated first and the diaphragm and intercostals last. As for all skeletal muscles, the tonic activity of these upper airway muscles decreases during sleep. In the nose, the reduction in the muscular activity of the dilator alae nasi (the muscles that dilate the nares when inspiratory airflow has to increase to slightly decrease nasal airflow resistance) has no important consequences. However, the reduction in the muscular activity of the muscles that constitute the walls of the pharynx results in a significant increase in total airway resistance to flow.[12] Indeed, the pharynx is the only portion of the upper airway that lacks rigid or semirigid structural support. The nose has bony walls, whereas the larynx has cartilaginous support, but the pharyngeal walls are just formed by muscles. Sleep decreases muscle tone, with two important consequences. First, the pharyngeal walls lose some rigidity, that is, the pharyngeal compliance increases. In other words, the walls become more floppy. Second, the cross-sectional area of the pharynx decreases, that is, anteroposterior and lateral diameters and the pharyngeal surface decreases. When a fluid flows through a tube, the resistance to flow depends on a series of parameters, the most important of which is the cross-sectional area of the tube. This is because the resistance is inversely proportional to the 4th power of the radius of the tube, whereas it is directly proportional to the simple length of the tube. This means, for instance, that if the tube doubles its length, resistance doubles. But if the tube radius is halved, the resistance increases 16 times. Thus, the decrease in pharyngeal cross-sectional area secondary to the sleep-related decrease in the muscle tone of its walls results in a 300 to 400% increase in total airflow resistance.[13]

This increase in resistance should immediately lead to a decrease in ventilation. Even during sleep, the metabolic controller will react to this impedance by increasing as much as possible (which is anyhow less than during wakefulness) the efforts to breathe of the respiratory pump muscles. This will in turn result in an increase in the negative pressure inside the thorax, transmitted through the airways to the airway opening (the nose and/or mouth). Indeed, the negative inspiratory pressure is the motor force causing inspiratory airflow. However, this enhanced negative inspiratory pressure will find a floppy tubing at the pharyngeal level, and instead of sucking air from the ambient inside the lungs, it will suck the pharyngeal walls inward, provoking a further reduction in pharyngeal surface and a further increase in pharyngeal resistance. In healthy people this leads to a new equilibrium, contributing to the sleep-related decrease in ventilation and to the increase in $PaCO_2$ and decrease in PaO_2.

The sleep-related generalized decrease in muscle tone also affects the respiratory pump muscles, sparing only the diaphragm (the diaphragm is a vital muscle that cannot be shut down even during sleep, a characteristic shared with the cardiac muscle). Hence, the activity of the intercostal muscles, the scaleni, and the pectoral muscles will decrease during sleep.[14] Again, this will have important ventilatory consequences. The contraction of the main respiratory muscle, the diaphragm, leads to an increase in the three diameters of the lower thoracic cage. The descent of the dome of the diaphragm increases the vertical dimension of the thorax. The upward lift given by the vertical costal fibers of the diaphragm to the lower ribs will result, because of the particular geometric form of the ribs, in an increase in the lateral and anteroposterior dimensions of the thorax. This latter effect is enhanced by the increased abdominal pressure (secondary to the descent of the diaphragmatic dome) pushing the lower ribs outward (the content of the thoracic segment covered by the lower ribs is the abdomen, not the lungs). The increase in the dimensions of the thorax creates the negative inspiratory pressure inside the thorax.[15] Curiously enough, this negative intrathoracic pressure will tend to draw the upper ribs inward, thus reducing the anteroposterior and lateral dimensions of the upper thorax and wasting the effects of the contraction of the diaphragm in distorting the rib cage rather than in inspiring ambient air into the lungs. This is usually avoided by the simultaneous contraction of the upper thorax accessory respiratory muscles, essentially the scaleni and upper ribs intercostals.

When the accessory respiratory muscles lose their activity during REM sleep, the diaphragm is almost left alone as the only contracting respiratory muscle, with a consequent decrease in the overall mechanical efficiency of the ventilatory pump. However, in a normal individual, tidal volume is still maintained because of the tight coupling between the upper and lower rib cage. In patients, alterations in this coupling have important detrimental implications, as will be discussed later.

Normally, when secretions accumulate in the bronchial tree because of hypersecretion, reduction in the clearing efficiency, or a combination of both factors, airway sensory receptors are stimulated. This results in the series of events characteristic of the cough reflex: rapid contraction of expiratory muscles against a closed glottis, followed by fast opening of the glottis and the production of high expiratory flows. The cough reflex is abolished during sleep, when secretions can accumulate in the bronchial tree. Only when the level of secretions is exceedingly high will cough occur. However, cough must be preceded by sleep interruption because cough is impossible during sleep. Therefore, for cough to proceed, first an awakening from sleep occurs, resulting in sleep disruption.

Figure 26-2 summarizes the main respiratory consequences of sleep.

Sleep Failure

Abnormal sleep generates a series of changes during wakefulness. In other words, sleep abnormalities are mainly perceived through their consequences during wakefulness. The consequences may range from minimal alterations in the quality of life to situations of severe lifestyle compromise for some persons. Sleep may be abnormal for different reasons, which can be schematically divided in three domains: abnormalities in sleep duration, sleep continuity, and sleep architecture.

Normal sleep duration varies among individuals, with an average daily duration of around 8 hours. Some normal people function well with only 3 to 4 hours of sleep per day, whereas others need close to 10 hours. Whatever the normal sleep duration needed by an individual, if this value is not achieved (sleep deprivation), the usual consequence is an increase in sleepiness during the following 24-hour cycle. This mild level of enhanced sleepiness can usually be easily tolerated. However, when sleep duration is significantly reduced for more than a couple of days, sleepiness begins to pose more serious problems and is less easily managed, especially during sedentary and routine activities.

Even if sleep duration is sufficient for a given individual, sleep function may be lost owing to sleep discontinuity (sleep fragmentation). This means that sleep is frequently

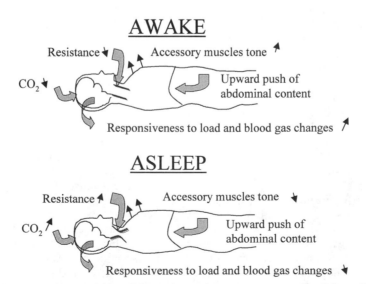

Figure 26-2. Schematic representation of the main respiratory consequences of sleep. For details, see the Respiratory Consequences of Sleep section. CO_2, carbon dioxide.

interrupted, either by complete awakenings or by arousal reactions. An arousal reaction is defined as a short duration (2–15 seconds) return to an electroencephalographic pattern characteristic of wake, interspersed in a sleep period (i.e., preceded and followed by a sleep pattern). Normally, 10 or so such episodes of arousals occur per hour of sleep.[16] Some believe they are important in allowing frequent changes in position and in this way avoid pressure sores. When sleep is abnormally fragmented, usually in excess of 20 to 25 arousals per hour, the daytime consequences are important.[17]

The last form of abnormal sleep is the loss of normal sleep architecture. This means decreased or absent deep (stages 3 and 4) non-REM sleep, decreased or absent REM sleep, or, on the contrary, excessive amounts of REM sleep that may alter the usual pattern in which REM sleep follows a more or less lengthy period of non-REM sleep. This kind of abnormality may have few consequences or may be manifested by severe daytime sleepiness.

The main chronic consequences of sleepiness are psychosocial and are characterized by a decrease in the capability for sustained attention, decreases in short-term memory, aggressiveness or its opposite, depression and disinterest, and cognitive dysfunction.[18] When these consequences are very serious, they may be mistaken for early dementia. When sleep deprivation and/or sleep fragmentation with a concomitant loss of normal sleep architecture are severe and long-standing, the degree of sleepiness may be so intense that short periods (2–5 seconds in duration) of electroencephalographic patterns typical of sleep, called microsleep periods, may intersperse during wakefulness so that during every minute of wakefulness some seconds of sleep always occur: the individual is never fully alert and awake.

SLEEP IN PATIENTS WITH RESPIRATORY DISEASES

Chronic Obstructive Pulmonary Disease

Patients with chronic bronchitis and emphysema may be seriously challenged during sleep. It is not at all infrequent to see deep falls in oxygen saturation during sleep in patients with borderline normal awake oxygen saturation owing to a variety of factors that have already been described. Patients decrease their ventilation during sleep for the same reasons that healthy people do: decrease in tidal volume resulting from the "dampened" wakefulness drive, with an increase in upper airway resistance, a decrease in the respiratory center reactivity to hypercapnia, hypoxia and resistive loading, and a decrease in the activity of the respiratory pump muscles. However, patients with chronic obstructive pulmonary diseases (COPD) manifest some specific features that add complexity to these factors.[19]

Oxygen is mainly transported in the blood attached to the hemoglobin, enclosed in the red blood cells. Depending on the PaO_2 dissolved in the blood in gaseous form, the hemoglobin molecule will incorporate more or less oxygen. When the hemoglobin carries all the oxygen it can incorporate, the hemoglobin is said to be fully saturated with oxygen, or 100% saturated. Lower levels of PaO_2 will result in the hemoglobin being less saturated. However, this relationship is not linear. When oxygen saturation is high (usually above 90%), the relationship is horizontal: large increases in PaO_2 result in small increases in oxygen saturation. Similarly, PaO_2 can significantly decrease without resulting in significant decreases in oxygen saturation. Around the level of 90% saturation (which corresponds roughly to a PaO_2 of 60 mm Hg), the relationship has an inflection point and becomes much more steep. Below this point, minimal changes in oxygen partial pressure result in larger changes in oxygen saturation. This has striking consequences in the oxygen saturation of patients with advanced COPD during sleep, who already during wakefulness have a PaO_2 close to 60 mm Hg. When these patients sleep, the resulting "normal" decrease in ventilation leads to a "normal" decrease in PaO_2 of about 5 mm Hg. However, because they are on the elbow of the hemoglobin dissociation curve, this small normal decline in

PaO_2 will result in a 5 to 10% loss in hemoglobin oxygen saturation, leading them to a nocturnal saturation level near 80%.

If patients with COPD have a significant degree of airflow obstruction, they usually have an increase in the physiologic dead space. Because during sleep the tidal volume decreases, and dead space does not significantly change, the proportion of the tidal volume that is wasted increases, leaving less effective tidal air for gas exchange. This may lead to a decrease in PaO_2 that is in excess of that of a normal individual, which, coupled with the fact that the patient is already on the steep part of the hemoglobin oxygen dissociation curve, results in large falls in oxygen saturation during sleep.

When COPD includes a significant component of emphysema, hyperinflation is common. Hyperinflation, characterized by an increase in total lung capacity, is accompanied by some noteworthy changes in the mechanics of the chest wall. The diaphragm is flattened and the ribs adopt an inspiratory, horizontal position. Thus, the vertical disposition of the costal fibers of the diaphragm is lost, and this impairs the ability of the diaphragm to exert an inspiratory action. As a consequence, the patient has to rely increasingly on his or her accessory respiratory muscles to maintain adequate ventilation during wakefulness. However, during sleep the activity of these accessory muscles is, normally, inhibited so that the patient is left, especially during REM sleep, with a lone and inefficient diaphragm. This leads to a striking reduction in ventilation during REM sleep periods, which, added to the previously mentioned factors, results in the typical deep falls in oxygen saturation (down to levels of 60% or less) during REM sleep. At the same time, hypercapnia develops or increases to levels above those of wakefulness.

The aggravation of hypoxemia and hypercapnia related to sleep is facilitated by the sleep-related decrease in the central ventilatory response to hypoxia and hypercapnia. Moreover, hypoxia is not a potent stimulus for awakening, and sleep may continue uninterrupted despite severe levels of hypoxemia. Of course, hypoxia will lead to increases in heart rate (to try to maintain oxygen delivery to the peripheral tissues), increases in pulmonary artery pressure, and a variety of other deleterious cardiovascular consequences, which by and large go unnoticed by the patient until late in the natural course of the disease, when the patient may develop signs and symptoms of cor pulmonale.

Obesity in these patients adds a particular problem that merits some comments. When an obese patient (particularly a patient with abdominal obesity) lies down, the abdominal contents displace cephalad, which pushes the diaphragm toward the rib cage. The craniocaudal diameter of the thorax is therefore reduced, and the functional residual capacity and the expiratory reserve volume decrease. This has two consequences: a decrease in the functional residual capacity and the closure of small airways in the more dependent parts of the lung, where blood perfusion in general is greater. Thus, a loss of functional alveolar units in the areas of good perfusion enhances the ventilation–perfusion mismatch already present in the lungs of these patients. This is perhaps the most important mechanism responsible for the decrease in PaO_2.[19]

In addition to these features, which are strictly related to sleeping per se, sleep continuity and duration may be impaired in patients with COPD. Chronic bronchitis is characterized by increased bronchial mucus secretion and an impaired bronchial clearance mechanism. Thus, these patients frequently wake up during the night to cough up the accumulated mucus (which may well take 30–60 minutes) and may have trouble returning to sleep. Indeed, cough represents an effort that worsens shortness of breath so that patients may need an aerosol with medication in the middle of the night. If all this happens after 4 hours of sleep, for instance, sleepiness will be decreased by the preceding sleep period, and falling back asleep may take longer. Hence, nocturnal total sleep time may be reduced even if the patients spend a normal amount of time in bed. Figure 26-3 shows data from a representative polysomnogram from a patient with COPD.

Finally, some of the medications these patients use may have deleterious effects on sleep. The β_2-agonists may provoke tachycardia and premature heart beats that can disturb sleep initiation if taken just before going to bed. Theophylline derivatives can also impair

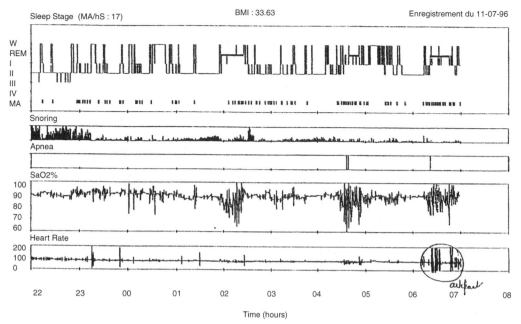

Figure 26-3. Schematic representation of a polysomnogram in a patient with COPD and moderate obesity. For abbreviations and symbols, see legend to Figure 1. Note first that sleep is not excessively fragmented (arousal index: 17 per hour), that only a few minutes of stage 3 non-REM sleep occur, and that stage 4 non-REM sleep is absent. Two periods of wakefulness (at 00:30 hours and 05:15 hours) occur owing to the need to cough and expectorate, in addition to several other short periods of wakefulness. The patient snores mildly but consistently throughout the night. Note that oxygen saturation is around 90% in wakefulness as well as in non-REM sleep but that during REM sleep it falls to 70% or less. The extreme variations in heart rate at the end of the night are a recording artefact.

sleep by increasing sleep latency (the time from lights off to the first minutes of sleep) and decreasing sleep efficiency (the ratio of total sleep time to the time in bed period).

Thus, patients with advanced COPD share with all other human beings the ventilatory challenges of sleep. However, because of their specific disease, they may fail to maintain adequate levels of ventilation during the night, whereas at the same time their disease will lead to inadequate sleep time, with the consequent daytime sleepiness and other symptoms owing to insufficient and unrefreshing sleep.

Restrictive Ventilatory Defects

Extrapulmonary Disorders

Extrapulmonary disorders are those that lead to respiratory failure in patients whose lungs are, basically, normal. These patients don't have airflow obstruction, or parenchymal abnormalities, yet are unable to breathe normally. The problem may arise in the skeleton (the best example is kyphoscoliosis); in the skeletal muscles, including the respiratory ones (e.g., all the myopathies like Duchenne muscular dystrophy); in the central neural system (as in spinal muscular atrophy or poliomyelitis); in the peripheral nerves (as in idiopathic diaphragmatic paralysis); in the neuromuscular junction (as in myasthenia gravis); or in the pleura (as in extended pleural fibrosis secondary to pleural tuberculosis).

The most important mechanism leading to sleep-related respiratory failure in these types of disorders is the weakness or the inefficient contractile properties of the respiratory muscles.[20] In kyphoscoliosis, for instance, the diaphragm may be normal but the deformation of the thoracic cage distorts its insertion points so that the net result is a loss in the inspiratory action of diaphragmatic contraction. In Duchenne muscular dystrophy, the primary defect is weakness of the muscles so that contraction force is decreased. Whatever the reason, the final result is hypoventilation, which is aggravated by sleep because of the additional loss of muscular activity linked to the sleep process. These patients hypoventilate during sleep, and their hypoventilation is even further aggravated during REM, when they lose the activity of the accessory muscles that have become "essential" muscles of respiration. As a consequence, the high levels of hypercapnia at the end of the night result in morning headaches. Hypoxia may be severe, with saturation levels below 60% for extended periods of the night. Nocturnal saturation abnormalities can be the first manifestation of progression of the disease and are worth monitoring as one follows these patients over time.

It is not unusual that REM sleep decreases first in these patients as disease progresses. As they enter REM sleep, ventilation falls dramatically, and after 1 to 2 minutes an arousal occurs, and patients go into non-REM sleep. Stages 3 and 4 non-REM sleep are less affected initially but may also decrease or even disappear totally afterwards. Sleep is then limited to stages 1 and 2 non-REM sleep, with a few minutes of REM sleep.

Patients generally complain of sleepiness, morning headaches, difficulties in concentrating, and even of severe dyspnea during the night awakenings. However, they don't usually volunteer these complaints unless specific questions are asked. Children may become aggressive, or school performances may deteriorate. The need for naps during the day may be the first symptom of severe sleep-related respiratory failure, itself heralding a progression of the disease that will lead to overt daytime respiratory failure. Figure 26-4 shows a typical example of a sleep recording in a patient with severe kyphoscoliosis.

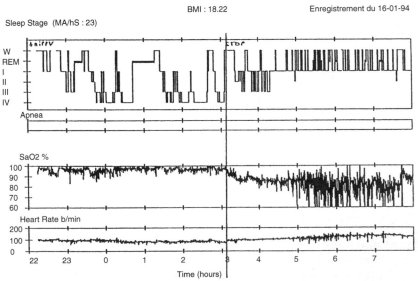

Figure 26-4. Schematic representation of a polysomnogram in a patient with severe kyphoscoliosis and respiratory failure. For abbreviations and symbols, see legend to Figure 1 (MAs are not shown on this record). During the first part of the night the patient is under noninvasive mechanical ventilation with a volumetric ventilator in the controlled mode using a nasal mask. At 03:00 hours the treatment is interrupted and the patient is allowed to go back to sleep breathing spontaneously. Note that during noninvasive ventilation, all sleep stages are present, sleep is stable, oxygen saturation stays above 95%, and heart rate decreases during sleep. After treatment interruption, sleep becomes fragmented, stage 4 non-REM sleep disappears, only a few minutes of REM sleep occurs, oxygen saturation is almost constantly below 85% (with frequent falls below 60%), and heart rate increases well beyond 100 beats/min.

Restrictive Pulmonary Disorders

Patients with pulmonary fibrosis and other restrictive pulmonary disorders behave like normal individuals during sleep, until the progression of their disease leads to the development of daytime hypoxemia in the range of a PaO_2 of 60 mm Hg. At this point, as in patients with obstructive conditions, and owing to the particular characteristics of the hemoglobin oxygen dissociation curve, further sleep-related decreases in ventilation will lead to impressive falls in nocturnal oxygen saturation. However, these patients will usually maintain the $PaCO_2$ at normal or below normal levels.[20]

Asthma

The existence of a specific entity labeled nocturnal asthma has been debated. Nocturnal asthma is characterized by episodes of shortness of breath and wheezing in the early morning hours, usually causing awakening, and subsiding after several minutes, sometimes after the expectoration of a variable quantity of thick phlegm. When the attacks become frequent they may impair total sleep duration (i.e., result in sleep deprivation) and lead to daytime sleepiness, a decrease in the ability to stay fully alert and to concentrate, and to a deterioration in cognitive functioning. Much research has been conducted on this particular topic. The conclusions seems to be that nocturnal asthma is nothing else than the nocturnal manifestations of poorly controlled bronchial asthma. Nevertheless, it is crucial to be aware of the existence of these nocturnal asthma attacks because they may be the initial sign that asthma is being poorly controlled and that a medication adjustment is needed. Nocturnal asthma symptoms may also imply that compliance with medication is less than optimal, which is a common occurrence in chronic diseases like asthma. Again, specific questions should be asked or the information about nocturnal attacks may go unnoticed.[21]

SPECIFIC SLEEP-RELATED DISORDERS THAT MAY AFFECT PULMONARY PATIENTS

Sleep disorders are too numerous and varied to be considered here at any length. However, some are worth mentioning as examples of the interaction between sleep disorders and pulmonary diseases, which sometimes may have deleterious consequences in particular patients.

Nocturnal Myoclonus

Nocturnal myoclonus or nocturnal restless legs syndrome is a common condition present in middle-aged and elder individuals. It consists of repetitive—every 20 to 30 seconds—contractions of lower limb muscles with a resulting leg jerk. These repetitive contractions occur in clusters of 30 minutes to 1 hour or more in duration, and two or three such episodes may be seen during a single night. They are generally present only during sleep, although some patients experience them during wakefulness. Patients may complain of leg "tiredness" at awakening, of nocturnal cramps, but they may also refer to disturbing excessive daytime sleepiness. This is because each lower limb muscle's contraction may (but does not necessarily) lead to a short arousal from sleep. This produces sleep fragmentation, with the consequent excessive daytime sleepiness, sensation of unrefreshing nocturnal sleep, and other psychosocial consequences of chronic sleep failure. If nocturnal myoclonus is present in a patient with pulmonary disease of enough severity to produce in itself an impairment in sleep quality and/or duration, the resulting daytime symptoms will aggravate an already stressful situation.

Obstructive Sleep Apnea Syndrome

Obstructive sleep apnea is characterized by the occurrence of multiple episodes of complete or almost complete upper airway occlusion during sleep. The floppy pharyngeal walls collapse inward, favored by the high negative inspiratory pressure. It follows a series of ineffective inspiratory efforts, of increasing intensity, as hypoxemia and hypercapnia develop. After 10 to 60 seconds in these asphyxic conditions, a reaction is elicited: an arousal from sleep, allowing for the opening of the pharynx, the resumption of breathing, and the correction of hypoxemia and hypercapnia. Whereas one such isolated episode is of no consequence, the occurrence of 20 to 70 episodes per hour of sleep for months or years results in a well-defined clinical entity known as obstructive sleep apnea syndrome.[22] Figure 26-5 shows a sleep recording in a patient with this syndrome.

A series of other phenomena take place in conjunction with the basic apnea-arousal mechanism. During apneas, partly owing to the decrease in the amplitude of lung expansion, a decrease in heart frequency occurs. Following the arousal reaction, a surge in sympathetic activity (both neural and hormonal) occurs, with an acceleration in heart frequency. In some patients, a typical bradycardia–tachycardia pattern emerges that can be recognized on a holter monitoring tracing. Simultaneously, alveolar hypoxia leads to pulmonary vasoconstriction and increases in pulmonary artery pressure. On the other hand, systemic arterial pressure decreases during apneas but increases after arousals, due to the sympathetic surge.[23] For reasons not fully understood, kidney function is altered, with an inversion in the normal biphasic urinary output: patients with obstructive sleep apnea increase the nocturnal diuresis and decrease the daytime one. As a consequence, nicturia is common and may be mistaken for early prostatic troubles.[24] Snoring, loud and

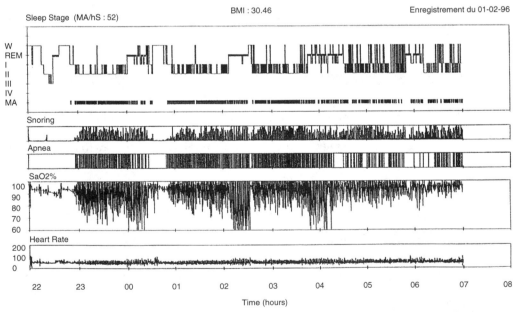

Figure 26-5. Schematic representation of a sleep recording in a patient with obstructive sleep apnea syndrome. For abbreviations and symbols, see legend to Figure 1. Note that sleep is abnormally fragmented (52 arousals per hour of sleep, nearly one arousal per minute) and that stages 3 and 4 non-REM sleep are almost absent. Snoring is of high intensity and constant throughout the night. Apneas are numerous, but their frequency decreases in the last quarter of the night. Apneas result in deep falls in oxygen saturation and in increases and decreases in heart rate. Note that in this moderately obese patient (BMI = 30.46 kg/m^2), REM sleep has a deleterious effect on oxygen saturation.

very disturbing for the bed partner, is almost constant in this disorder. Indeed, with each arousal, breathing resumes with high-frequency oscillations of the pharyngeal walls, producing the typical harsh sound known as snoring.

Patients with obstructive sleep apnea experience the full-blown array of clinical manifestations of sleep failure: excessive daytime sleepiness, unrefreshing sleep, morning headaches, morning sleep drunkenness (they need some time to get out of sleep and feel alert), intellectual deterioration, personality changes, and memory impairment. Impotence is frequently reported by males. The prevalence of this disorder is around 1 to 5% of the adult population, and it seems to be severe enough to require treatment in about 1%. Obstructive sleep apnea is favored by maleness, obesity, and a short mandibular bone. The typical patient is a rather overweight male in his 5th decade with a long-standing history of loud snoring. However, lean patients and women are not at all infrequent. Obstructive sleep apnea seems to be secondary to a reduction in pharyngeal cross-sectional surface, perhaps owing to fat apposition on the lateral pharyngeal walls, which is counterbalanced successfully during wakefulness by the increased activity of pharyngeal dilator muscles, mainly the genioglossus. The sleep-related decrease in the activity of these dilators "reveals" the structural pharyngeal narrowing, resulting in a high pharyngeal airflow resistance that leads to increased respiratory muscles pump efforts and to increases in the negative inspiratory pressures that favor the collapse of the floppy pharyngeal walls, finally resulting in complete or near complete pharyngeal occlusion and apnea.[25]

A subset of patients have a severe form of obstructive sleep apnea that is accompanied by signs of right heart failure, ankle edema, and pulmonary hypertension. Generally, these patients have at the same time obstructive sleep apnea syndrome and a coexisting lung disorder, most usually COPD, an especially dreadful combination. In a patient with a low awake level of PaO_2 owing to his or her lung disorder, sleep-related apneas will lead to extreme falls in PaO_2 (with the consequent rise in pulmonary artery pressure owing to pulmonary vasoconstriction) and in arterial oxygen saturation. Hypercapnia at the end of apneas will not be easily corrected during the few seconds of free breathing during the arousal reaction in a patient with impaired lung function, all the more so if the patient already has chronic daytime hypercapnia with a reduced ventilatory response. This will finally lead to the development of right heart failure and respiratory insufficiency.[26]

DIAGNOSTIC APPROACH TO SLEEP DISORDERS IN PULMONARY PATIENTS

Questions about sleep quality and symptoms of sleep failure should be periodically asked to patients with pulmonary diseases, especially when an obvious change occurs in their status that is not easily explainable by other factors. When poor sleep quality is suspected, or a rapid unexplained deterioration in the condition of the patient, a nocturnal oximetric recording is a useful initial screening test. If the oximetry result is strictly normal, either no special sleep-related disorder of respiration is present or the patient has not slept at all during that night (this is not an unusual occurrence). The next step is to repeat the oximetric recording (it is easily available, with little if any cost, and the devices are reliable). When the recording is abnormal, and typical of the sleep-related oximetric consequences of the disease of the patient, one may confidently conclude that the patient has sleep disorders. When doubts persist, or an atypical oximetric pattern is seen, one should proceed to a full night polysomnogram in a sleep center experienced in the management of patients with pulmonary diseases and in sleep-related breathing disorders. This is usually not necessary in COPD but may be worthwhile in patients with restrictive disorders of extrapulmonary origin.

THERAPEUTIC CONSIDERATIONS IN PULMONARY PATIENTS

As we have seen, sleep represents a formidable challenge for patients with severe respiratory disorders. Sleep worsens the consequences of the respiratory diseases, unraveling the fragility of the adaptive mechanisms developed to try to maintain normal blood gases. Is this enough to consider specific treatments for sleep periods in these patients? The answer is clearly yes for some patients, clearly no for others, and perhaps for still others.

Patients with restrictive extrapulmonary disorders and sleep-related hypoventilation benefit when they are treated with ventilatory assistance during sleep. This assistance may be in the form of noninvasive positive-pressure ventilation or invasive (usually via tracheostomy) mechanical ventilation. This allows for normal sleep, normalization of breathing during sleep, correction or near complete normalization of nocturnal and daytime blood gases, decreases in the need for hospital admissions, enhanced quality of life, and increased survival.[27]

In contrast, stable patients with COPD and sleep-related falls in oxygen saturation don't seem to benefit from ventilatory assistance. Of course, when long-term oxygen therapy (>15 h/d) is needed, night use of supplemental oxygen is mandatory; not only for practical reasons (the sleep period represents already a sizable part of the minimum 15 hours daily period) but also because sleep represents the portion of the day with the worst gas exchange condition. Sleep duration may be increased in these patients, and thus daytime symptoms of sleep failure decreased, by paying special attention to such issues as timing of administration of sleep-disturbing drugs, management of nocturnal secretions, and management of nocturnal shortness of breath with long-acting bronchodilators. In asthmatic patients, sleep may be improved with better control of the overall disease, with close follow-up of nocturnal attacks as a useful indication of suboptimal treatment.

In patients with a combination of diseases, it is important to adequately treat both conditions because a potentiating treatment effect seems to be present, as there is a potentiating effect in patients with coexisting sleep disorders and respiratory diseases.

Finally, a word of caution is needed concerning the use of "sleeping pills." Hypnotic and sedative drugs are among the most popular medications. They are frequently not considered as such by the patients, who frequently overuse them. For patients with respiratory diseases, sleeping pills have several undesirable effects that may in fact jeopardize the ability of these patients to breathe during sleep. Hypnotics and sedatives decrease minute ventilation, the tone of upper airway muscles, the arousal threshold of the brain, and the cough reflex threshold. These effects will worsen the sleep-related consequences of respiratory diseases. It is not uncommon that a borderline patient is precipitated into respiratory failure after the administration of hypnotics. A good example is the patient with COPD who has excessive mucus secretion that awakens him or her during the night. Frequently, patients will complain of awakening in the middle of the night, with subsequent difficulty in going back to sleep. This may be interpreted as insomnia and inadequately treated with hypnotics. The use of hypnotics and sedatives should be avoided in patients with severe respiratory diseases. The same holds true for alcohol, which has similar effects and should also be avoided in these patients.

CONCLUSIONS

Sleep, unavoidable as it is, represents a stressful period for patients with respiratory diseases. When the fragile equilibrium between the need to sleep and the need to breathe is altered, both abnormal breathing and abnormal sleep will occur. This will lead to the appearance of daytime symptoms that may greatly impair the ability of patients to enjoy life, an ability already hampered by respiratory symptoms. It is crucial to take due notice of these facts not only to avoid harming the patient but especially to realize that the disease has progressed to a stage in which the sleep challenge can no longer be adequately met by the failing respiratory system. Treatment optimization is then necessary, and the improvement of sleep-related symptoms may constitute the best indication of a successful intervention.

REFERENCES

1. Rechtschaffen A, Kales A. A manual of standardised terminology, techniques and scoring system for sleep stages of human subjects. Washington, DC: National Institutes of Health, 1968. Publication 204.
2. Krueger JM, Obál F Jr, Fang J. Why we sleep: a theoretical view of sleep function. Sleep Med Rev 1999;3:119–129.
3. Khatri IM, Fries ED. Haemodynamic changes during sleep. J Appl Physiol 1967;22:867–873.
4. Koopman MG, Koomen GCM, Krediet RT, et al. Circadian rhythm of glomerular filtration rate in normal individuals. Clin Sci 1989;77:105–111.
5. Van Cauter E, Plat L, Copinschi G. Interrelations between sleep and the somatotropic axis. Sleep 1998;21:553–556.
6. Krieger J. Breathing during sleep in normal subjects. In: Kryger MH, Roth T, Dement WC, eds. Principles and Practice of Sleep Medicine. Philadelphia: WB Saunders, 1994:217.
7. Stradling JR, Chadwick GA, Frew, AJ. Changes in ventilation and its components in normal subjects during sleep. Thorax 1985;40:364–370.
8. Bulow K. Respiration and wakefulness in man. Acta Physiol Scand 1963;59(Suppl 209):1–110.
9. Colrain IM, Trinder J, Fraser G. Ventilation during sleep onset in young adult females. Sleep 1990;13:491–501.
10. Gleeson K, Zwillich CW, White DP. Chemosensitivity and the ventilatory response to airflow obstruction during sleep. J Appl Physiol 1989; 67:1630–1637.
11. Douglas NJ, White DP, Weil JV. Hypoxic ventilatory response decreases during sleep in normal men. Am Rev Respir Dis 1982;125:286–289.
12. Remmers JE, Sauerland WJ, Anch AM. Pathogenesis of upper airway occlusion during sleep. J Appl Physiol 1978;44·931–938.
13. Hudgel DW, Hendrickx C, Hamilton HB. Characteristics of the upper airway pressure-flow relationship during sleep. J Appl Physiol 1988; 64:1930–1935.
14. Smith PE, Edwards RH, Calverley PM. Ventilation and breathing pattern during sleep in Duchenne muscular dystrophy. Chest 1989;96: 1346–1351.
15. De Troyer A, Estenne M. Coordination between rib cage muscles and diaphragm during quiet breathing in humans. J Appl Physiol 1984; 57:899–906.
16. Collard P, Dury M, Delguste P, et al. Movement arousals and sleep-related disordered breathing in adults. Am J Respir Crit Care Med 1996;154: 454–459.
17. Roehrs T, Merlotti L, Petrucelli N, et al. Experimental sleep fragmentation. Sleep 1994;17: 438–443.
18. Engelman H, Joffe D. Neuropsychological function in obstructive sleep apnoea. Sleep Med Rev 1999;31:59–78.
19. Folgering H, Vos P. Sleep and breathing in chronic obstructive pulmonary disease. Eur Respir Mon 1998;10:303–323.
20. Shneerson J. Sleep in neuromuscular and thoracic cage disorders. Eur Respir Mon 1998;10: 324–344.
21. Fitzpatrick MF, Jokic R. Nocturnal asthma. Eur Respir Mon 1998;10:285–302.
22. Krieger J. Clinical presentations of sleep apnoea. Eur Respir Mon 1998;10:75–105.
23. Hedner J, Grote L. Cardiovascular consequences of obstructive sleep apnoea. Eur Respir Mon 1998;10:227–265.
24. Rodenstein DO, d'Odemont JP, Pieters Th, et al. Diurnal and nocturnal diuresis and natriuresis in obstructive sleep apnea: effects of nasal continuous positive airway pressure therapy. Am Rev Respir Dis 1992;145:1367–1371.
25. Deegan PC, McNicholas WT. Pathophysiology of obstructive sleep apnoea. Eur Respir Mon 1998;10:28–62.
26. Chaouat A, Weitzenblum E, Krieger J, et al. Association of chronic obstructive pulmonary disease and obstructive sleep apnea syndrome. Am J Respir Crit Care Med 1995;151:82–86.
27. Hill NS. Noninvasive positive pressure ventilation in neuromuscular disease: enough is enough! Chest 1994;105:337–338.

27 The Role of Home Care

Susan L. McInturff
Patrick J. Dunne

▷ Professional Skills

Upon completion of this chapter, the reader will:

- Understand the reasons behind the shift of health care from the institutional setting to the home
- Identify patients who would benefit from and are candidates for home care
- Describe the role the respiratory therapist (RT) has in the patient's home care program
- Understand the types of respiratory home care equipment that are commonly used
- Grasp the importance of proper equipment selection for patients needing home oxygen
- Know the guidelines Medicare has for reimbursement of home oxygen therapy
- Understand how a patient is acuitized, follow-up care is established, and when the patient is ready for discharge from the home care program

An important aspect of a patient's comprehensive medical management takes place away from the physician's office, the acute care hospital, and the pulmonary rehabilitation classroom. It involves a multidisciplinary team that can provide continuity to the services of a pulmonary rehabilitation program, the physician's plan of care, or the hospital discharge plan. Home care is now considered an essential component of the short- and long-term treatment of the patient with pulmonary disease.

HOME CARE IN THE 1990s AND BEYOND

We have all seen the statistics: chronic obstructive pulmonary disease (COPD) in now the fourth most common cause of death in the United States and is the only major disease that is rising in prevalence and mortality.[1] It is estimated that up to 35 million Americans have COPD.[2] Pneumonia and influenza ranked as the sixth most common cause of death in 1995–1996.[3]

Pair these statistics with the fact that by the turn of this century, 35 million Americans will be aged 65 years and older.[2] Half of all health care expenditures will be consumed by this group.[4] The numbers of chronically ill Americans is expected to reach 148 million by the year 2030.[5] This is a staggering number of people who will be consuming health care.

With the advent of managed care and changes in Medicare reimbursement to reflect fixed payments for services based on diagnosis-related groups, health care providers are

495

looking for ways to limit the costs of providing that care. Hospitals are discharging patients much earlier in their course of care, often referred to as "quicker and sicker." These patients often have continued medical needs that were formerly met by keeping them in the hospital for several additional days, and in the case of patients requiring high technology such as assisted invasive ventilation, several additional months or longer. Other venues of health care are looking for ways to reduce the number of visits the patient makes to their facilities or uses their services.

What happens to patients who have continuing or ongoing medical needs or have been released from their inpatient program before they have all the information and skills they need to care for themselves? Home care is the answer to this question. Indeed, home care has been reported to be the fastest growing segment of health care today. Currently more than 20,000 providers of home care services exist.[6] Home care employment has more than doubled since 1988.[6]

A well-structured home care program will allow the continued treatment of the patient with nearly any type of health problem and with most of the therapeutic modalities available in the acute or long-term care setting. Intravenous therapy, wound care, oxygen and aerosol therapy, and invasive and noninvasive mechanical ventilation are all commonly performed in the patient's home. Home care also allows for ongoing assessment, education, and training of the patient. Home care can reinforce what a patient has been taught in a pulmonary rehabilitation program. For many patients, a good home care program is vital to their quality of life and long-term survival.

This chapter describes how to develop a comprehensive program for the home care patient and discusses the roles of the members of the home care team. It reviews the common types of home medical equipment (HME) that are used as well as reimbursement issues that are important to home care providers. The home visit, the plan of care, and determining when the patient is ready for discharge from the home care program are also discussed.

Benefits of Home Care

The goal of any outpatient treatment program is to perform a medical service outside the acute care facility. Home care permits these medical services to be rendered in the comfort and convenience of the patient's own home, which is also the least expensive site of care.[6,7] Home care allows for ongoing evaluation and treatment, which can identify emergent problems and often prevent a hospitalization, an emergency department or urgent care clinic visit, or a visit to the physician's office. For example, a nurse or RT performing a home visit may assess a patient and find that he or she has an increased cough, is now productive of purulent sputum, and has abnormal breath sounds and a fever. The nurse or RT can relay these symptoms to the patient's physician, who may then decide to treat the patient with antibiotic therapy without bringing him or her into the office. The nurse or RT performs a follow-up visit to evaluate the patient's response to therapy and compliance to the medication program.

The patient's home environment can enhance learning and provides a sense of control that is often lost in the acute care setting. Patients are happier at home and are more willing to cooperate with their medical program when they feel they have some control and input. Cancer patients have shown statistically significant improvement in their mental health and social dependency when receiving home care services.[8] Box 27-1 reviews some of the benefits of home care.

Candidates for Home Care

A large and varied population of patients exists who could be considered candidates for home care, most of them elderly and many of them inflicted with pulmonary disease.

Box 27-1. The Benefits of Home Care

Improves quality of life
Is cost-effective
Encourages self-management and independence
Allows for ongoing monitoring of patient response to treatment
Reduces the need for clinic visits, emergency department visits, and hospital
   admissions
Reduces risk of nosocomial infections
Improves mental health and social independence

Reprinted from McInturff SL, O'Donohue WJ. Respiratory care in the home and alternate
sites. In: Burton GC, Hodgkin JE, Ward JJ. Respiratory Care: A Guide to Clinical Practice.
4th ed. Philadelphia: Lippincott, 1997.

It has been estimated that 44% of all patients discharged from the hospital require posthospital medical or nursing care that cannot be provided by the family.[9] It has also been estimated that 20% of patients older than 65 years have functional and physical problems
that impair their ability to perform the essential activities of daily living.[9] Approximately
3.9 million Medicare beneficiaries were expected to receive home care services in
1997.[6]

Data from 1994 shows that pneumonia and COPD were among the top 10 diagnoses
of patients discharged to home care.[6] Asthma affects 14 to 15 million Americans and is
increasing in prevalence and mortality.[2] It is estimated that more than 40 million Americans
may be chronically ill with sleep-related disorders.[10] Many of these people have concomitant
or comorbid health conditions. These patient populations often require short- and/or
long-term home care; however, diagnosis alone does not make a patient a candidate for
home care. Box 27-2 reviews the types of patients who are considered potential candidates
for home care.

Box 27-2. Candidates for Home Care

Patients who are newly diagnosed with a disease and require education and
   training for that disease
Patients with the desire to be treated at home, particularly those with terminal
   illnesses
Patients who have had repeated hospitalizations
Patients with adequate family, caregivers, and financial resources
Patients with physical limitations
   Dyspnea that limits ADLs
   Ambulatory difficulties
   Difficulties with vision, speech, or hearing
Patients with functional impairments
   Cognitive disabilities
   Inability to perform ADLs
   Inability to monitor and administer medications and other treatments
Patients requiring medical devices that necessitate monitoring and maintenance

Adapted from McInturff SL, O'Donohue WJ. Respiratory care in the home and alternate sites. In:
Burton GC, Hodgkin JE, Ward JJ. Respiratory Care: A Guide to Clinical Practice. 4th ed.
Philadelphia: Lippincott, 1997.
ADLs, activities of daily living.

DELIVERY OF HOME CARE SERVICES

The delivery of home care services has many elements, and many personnel are involved in providing these services.

The Home Care Team

It has been shown that the use of multidisciplinary teams in patient care can improve quality of care and enhance patient satisfaction. The team provides continuity of care when transitioning from acute and skilled care to the home care setting. This team would include, as appropriate:

- The patient
- The patient's family
- Other caregivers
- The patient's physician(s)
- The hospital's discharge planner
- The home health agency, including nursing; physical, occupational, and speech therapy; and social services
- The hospital-based RT
- The home care RT
- The HME provider
- The insurance company's case manager or other liaison
- The pulmonary rehabilitation staff

Each member of the team has an integral function and purpose. For example, the discharge planner coordinates the predischarge activities of the other team members. The insurance case manager provides guidance as to the patient's health care benefits relative to the services required. The pulmonary rehabilitation staff provides recommendations as to the types of ongoing rehabilitation services the patient needs as well as a discharge plan. The HME company provides the equipment and related services the patient will need at home. The team members act cooperatively to help the patient achieve the goals established in the discharge plan.

Once the patient is discharged to a home care program, this team continues to evolve to reflect the patient's changing needs. The hospital staff would not remain on the team, but new members would most certainly be added. For example, a patient undergoing outpatient dialysis might now have a dialysis nurse on the team. A patient dying of lung cancer would have a hospice nurse and perhaps a hospice volunteer coordinator join the team. This team continues to customize its care to suit the patient's needs for the duration of the home care program.

The HME Provider

Once the physician has determined that the patient needs HME, the referral source (e.g., the discharge planner or pulmonary rehabilitation staff) will contact an HME provider to arrange for delivery of the equipment. The referral source must be prepared to provide specific information to the HME provider; Table 27-1 reviews the information the referral source should have in hand when making the referral.

Several factors must be considered when selecting an HME provider for the patient (if the patient has not already chosen one):

- Does the company provide service to the area in which the patient resides?
- Does the company have the equipment the patient needs?
- Does the company also carry any supplies or soft goods the patient needs?

Table 27-1. Information Required When Ordering Home Medical Equipment

Personal Information	Billing Information	Equipment Information
Name	Primary health insurance carrier	Type of equipment needed, including portability if home oxygen is being ordered
Physical address	Primary policy number	
Mailing address	Primary group number	
Telephone number	Billing address	Frequency of use
Date of birth	Billing telephone number, contact person	Hours of use
Social security number		Medications necessary
Height	Secondary health insurance carrier	Allergy status
Weight		Qualifying medical data (e.g., room air blood gas or oximetry results)
Next of kin	Secondary policy number	
Ordering physician	Secondary group number	
Primary physician	Billing address	Delivery location
Primary diagnosis	Billing telephone number, contact person	Delivery date, approximate time as appropriate
Secondary diagnosis		

- Will the company bill the patient's insurance for the equipment?
- Does the company provide 24-hour emergency service?
- Will the company deliver on weekends?
- Does the company charge for deliveries? For off-schedule or after-hours deliveries?
- Does the company have RTs or nurses on staff?

The HME provider may assist in determining what type of equipment the patient needs based on the information given by the referral source. For example, the referral source may request an aspirator for a child of school age. The provider, understanding that the patient attends school, might supply the child with a small, battery-powered machine in a carry bag instead of a heavy-duty stationary unit. If the physician desires a specific piece of equipment, such as a liquid oxygen system (LOX) instead of a concentrator, the provider cannot substitute any other type of oxygen equipment to reduce costs.

The HME provider has certain responsibilities to the patient. The provider is responsible for delivering the equipment in a timely manner, for example, oxygen equipment that has been ordered for a patient being discharged from the hospital should be delivered within a stated number of hours, not the next day. In fact, the oxygen equipment may need to be set up in the home before the patient arrives, and a portable system might need to be delivered to the patient's hospital room for use during transport home. The provider will also need to make arrangements with the patient to refill the oxygen as necessary.

The HME provider is responsible for the routine and ongoing maintenance of all equipment placed on rental to the patient. Such maintenance is performed at the time intervals recommended by the manufacturer or more frequently as needed. This service is performed at no charge to the patient if the equipment is rented. In the event that the equipment has been purchased, either privately by the patient or by the health insurance company, the patient must be informed of the required maintenance, the existence of any warranties, and whether a service contract is necessary. Many health insurance companies pay for service contracts as well as repairs on purchased equipment.

Depending on the type of respiratory equipment that is ordered, the HME provider will use a specially trained driver/technician to deliver and set up the equipment.[11] This practice varies by provider, but it is common for a technician to set up and teach patients to use oxygen equipment and compressor nebulizers. Some companies use technicians to set up equipment such as continuous positive airway pressure (CPAP) or apnea monitors, but this is not as common.

The Role of the Home Care RT

The primary duty of the home care RT is patient education and training.[12] Most home care RTs are employed by HME providers to teach patients how to correctly and safely use respiratory care equipment that has been prescribed by their physician. The education and training provided to the patient is not always a "one-time" service but rather continues as changes occur in the status of the patient. For example, a patient using home oxygen equipment might be instructed in its use during the initial setup, but it is discovered later that he or she does not remember how to clean the filter on the concentrator. The RT would then retrain the patient and encourage him or her to refer to the written instructions whenever uncertainty arises concerning any care instructions. Perhaps a couple of months later the patient is changed to a LOX; the RT would then instruct the patient in the use of this equipment.

The home care RT also provides education and training to the other members of the home care team. A patient using invasive mechanical ventilation may have a new caregiver that needs instruction on ventilator care. A home health nurse may need instruction about how to properly titrate a patient's oxygen flow using pulse oximetry. A patient's spouse may need training on proper technique for filling a portable liquid tank.

The RT also trains the patient and caregivers to perform many types of respiratory care procedures. Many of these care procedures are done similarly to how they are done in the acute care facility. The major differences are using clean technique instead of sterile technique when performing those procedures and reusing items that are normally considered "disposable," such as medication nebulizers and suction catheters.[13] Box 27-3 lists some of the respiratory care procedures that are done in the home care setting.

The RT's secondary responsibility is assessment. The RT evaluates many different elements of the patient's care. For example, the RT assesses the patient for retention of instructions on using the prescribed medical equipment or performing a respiratory care procedure. The RT would physically assess a patient with a new, congested cough. The RT evaluates a patient's compliance with his or her oxygen therapy prescription. Good assessment skills are essential to the home care RT.

The Home Visit

After receiving the referral, the home care RT will either set up the prescribed equipment or contact the patient, usually within the first 48 hours after the equipment has been set

Box 27-3. Respiratory Care Procedures Commonly Taught by the Home Care Respiratory Therapist

Tracheostomy tube and stoma care
Oral and endotracheal suctioning
Ventilator management
Oxygen administration
Nebulized medication administration
Peak flow monitoring
Infection control practices
Basic assessment (heart rate, blood pressure, chest auscultation in some instances, color)
Airway clearance techniques, postural drainage, and percussion
Breathing retraining, energy conservation

up by the driver/technician. This initial contact is usually done by telephone to assess the patient's understanding of the use of the equipment, and a home visit is scheduled.

The initial home visit accomplishes several things. It is used to evaluate the patient's knowledge of and ability to safely operate the prescribed equipment. It is used to train or evaluate the patient's ability to perform any related care procedures, that is, oral or tracheal suctioning or taking a nebulizer treatment. It is used to evaluate the appropriateness of the equipment and to determine whether it meets the patient's needs. It also establishes the patient's medical status. Elements of the initial visit should include:

- Patient evaluation, including relevant medical history and symptom profile
- Physical assessment, including identification of functional abilities and disabilities
- Evaluation of the patient's physical environment
- Evaluation of psychosocial issues
- Caregiver issues
- Need for ancillary services
- Equipment needs
- Financial resources

Patient Evaluation

The patient's current medical condition(s), chief complaint, and previous medical history should be obtained through direct interview or by interview with appropriate family members. This information can also be obtained from medical records when available. Smoking status and other pulmonary risk factors should be identified.[1,14,15] The patient should be questioned about their immunizations for influenza and pneumococcal pneumonia.[1] Symptom profile, medications, and alcohol use should also be identified.[16,17]

The patient's nutritional status should be evaluated because lung disease frequently contributes to undernutrition and dehydration.[18] Patients should be questioned as to current diet and eating habits as well as any problems they have in preparing meals. Patients receiving oxygen by nasal cannula often report a reduced sense of smell and taste, and elderly patients are known to have a decreased sense of smell, which can decrease appetite and contribute to malnutrition.[19]

Physical Assessment

This assessment includes routine vital signs, such as:

- Blood pressure
- Heart rate
- Respiratory rate
- Breath sounds
- Height and weight
- Temperature
- Inspection for cyanosis and clubbing
- Check for peripheral edema
- General appearance
- Blood oxygen levels by blood gas or pulse oximetry (when ordered by the physician)

The physical assessment of the patient should also identify any physical or functional limitations. Elderly patients frequently have sensory impairments that can inhibit their ability to care for themselves.[19] Decreased color discrimination can make it difficult for the patient to tell one colored pill from another. Up to 25% of elderly patients suffer from hearing loss, which reduces speech perception and comprehension; this can impair their ability to understand instructions. Overall sensory loss in the elderly contributes to impaired balance and coordination, decreased tactile sensation, and decreased response to pain.

Box 27-4. Psychosocial Issues That Are
Important to Evaluate

Patient's perception and acceptance of disease
Depression
Family dynamics, roles
Work history
Cultural issues, language barriers
Religious beliefs
Substance abuse by patient or family
Support system
Financial resources
Domestic violence, child abuse

Assessment of the Physical Environment

One of the first thing that must be determined when evaluating the patient's home environment is whether the patient is willing to allow home health care providers into the home. Some patients do not feel that they need home care services or do not like admitting outsiders into their home. Ultimately, the patient has the right to refuse these services.

The home must also be appropriate and conducive to care. For example, the home needs to have adequate electrical wiring to power any HME that uses electricity. The home must present no fire, safety, or health risks to the patient; it may be necessary to make adaptations to improve the home's safety and accessibility.[20]

Patients with an asthmatic component to their health problems need to have their homes evaluated for allergens and irritants that can trigger an asthma flare-up. Dust mites, mold, cigarette smoke, pet dander, the presence of household cleaners and many other factors can contribute to asthma symptoms.[21,22]

Space must be adequate to place all the necessary equipment and supplies, and appropriate facilities must be available to clean the equipment as required. The kitchen or laundry room might be used to clean equipment. The pantry might be used to store not only foodstuffs but also oxygen tubing or suction catheters as well.

The home's geographic location must also be considered. Patient needing HME may live in an area not serviced by an HME company or home health agency. They may live in a remote area where medical care is not easily accessed. In these situations, special arrangements need to be made for temporary placement in another home or care facility until the patient no longer requires home health care services.

Although it is ideal to evaluate the home for these potential problems before discharge from the hospital or pulmonary rehabilitation program, this does not always occur. Instead, personnel from the home health agency or HME provider may identify problems during the initial home visit. In that event, the home care personnel will work with the patient and his or her physician to facilitate the prescribed program within the confines of those problems.

Psychosocial Issues

Another important element is the psychosocial evaluation. Many issues can greatly enhance the success or failure of the home care program.[23-27] Box 27-4 reviews psychosocial issues that should be evaluated.

Caregiver Issues

Patients who are unable to perform their own medical care will need the assistance of caregivers. In fact, family caregivers provide 80 to 90% of all long-term home care services to family members.[2] Examples of other caregivers are:

- Immediate and extended family
- Friends
- Privately funded lay caregivers
- Home health aides or chore workers
- Home health nurses
- Volunteers (i.e., hospice)

Depending on the type and amount of care the patient requires, the patient must have an adequate number of people to provide that care. For example, a quadriplegic patient being mechanically ventilated would require around-the-clock assistance as well as a "backup" list of caregivers in the event someone is unable to work their allotted shift. A patient who only needs assistance with bathing may only need the assistance of a home health aide three times a week. Family and friends are frequently used for patients with only basic needs like assistance with cooking and cleaning. Family and friends are also frequently used to provide care for high-tech patients.

Regardless of the type of assistance needed, every caregiver must be evaluated to determine their appropriateness to provide that care. They must be evaluated for physical and functional disabilities just as the patient is evaluated. A caregiver, be it the patient's wife or the home health nurse, won't be adequate if he or she has a bad back and the patient needs assistance turning in bed. A caregiver with arthritic hands may not be capable of turning on or changing a regulator on an oxygen cylinder. A person with poor vision might not be able to read prescription labels or distinguish different medications.

The Need for Ancillary Services

Once the need for home care has been identified, referrals are made to the appropriate members of the home care team. One of the most beneficial aspects of home care is the opportunity for visits from a variety of specialty practitioners employed by the home health agency that receives the referral. During the discharge planning process or during the initial home visit by the home care RT or nurse, it may be determined that the patient needs the services of a physical or occupational therapist, for example. This therapist might be needed to assess the effectiveness of the prescribed exercise program or to train the patient in energy conservation techniques. They may work with the patient on performing activities of daily living or using a wheeled walker.

It may be determined that the patient needs not only nursing visits but also visits by a home health aide to assist the patient with bathing or a chore worker to help with cooking and cleaning. The psychosocial evaluation might reveal that the patient and family are having coping problems and would benefit from a visit by the home health agency's social worker. Box 27-5 lists the medical specialists typically available from a home health agency.

Box 27-5. Medical Specialists Employed by Home Health Agencies

Registered nurses	Physical therapists
Licensed vocational and practical nurses	Occupational therapists
Respiratory therapists[a]	Speech therapists
Nursing aides	Social workers

[a]Respiratory therapists (RTs) are not commonly employed by home health agencies because there is no direct payment for services rendered by RTs under many health insurance plans, particularly Medicare. Home health agencies may include the RT's wages in their overhead. Services rendered by RTs are often included in a home health agency's contract as negotiated with managed care organizations.

Equipment Needs

Patients with acute and chronic lung disease represent one of the largest population groups using HME, often also referred to as durable medical equipment. Depending on their medical condition and needs, a patient's physician may prescribe one or more pieces of equipment, ranging from walking aids, bathroom safety equipment, or nutritional support devices to oxygen equipment, aerosol administration devices, or invasive mechanical ventilation. Table 27-2 lists some common types of HME.

It is important to consider the HME provider when a patient needs equipment. All HME companies are not the same. Many specialize in respiratory care equipment, whereas others focus mainly on durable medical equipment. Some companies have RTs on staff, whereas others use specially trained driver/technicians to set up respiratory therapy equipment.

Financial Issues

A common misconception among health care professionals and lay people alike is that if a physician orders home care equipment or services, it must be covered by the patient's medical insurance. That is unfortunately not the case. It is essential to determine whether the patient's medical insurance includes that service or equipment as a benefit in the patient's particular plan. For example, Medicare, the federally funded insurance for people older than 65 years, has specific criteria the patient must meet to qualify for things like oxygen therapy equipment. Some equipment is not covered at all by Medicare, like bathroom safety equipment. Medicare and many other health insurance plans will cover equipment to treat obstructive sleep apnea but only if the patient has had an attended sleep study in a sleep laboratory. Some plans have a lifetime "cap" for specific services or equipment.

It should never be assumed that the patient is willing or able to pay for medical equipment or services in the event that they are not covered by their health insurance. Consider also how large a patient's copayment is; copayment amounts can be up to as much as 50% of the total monthly charge. Many health insurance plans, including Medicare, require a copayment of 20% of the allowed charges. Depending on the type and amounts of equipment or services needed, a patient's total copayment may be cost prohibitive.

The Home Care Plan

The purpose of all the assessments done during the initial visit is to use it to develop the home care plan. This plan is the comprehensive blueprint that identifies the patient's

Table 27-2. Common Types of Home Medical Equipment

Respiratory Care Equipment	Durable Medical Equipment
Oxygen therapy devices: stationary and portable systems	Walking aids: crutches, walkers, canes
Aerosol therapy devices: medication and large volume nebulizers, humidifiers	Wheelchairs: standard, lightweight, reclining, customized
Ventilatory assist devices: invasive and noninvasive mechanical ventilators, CPAP and bi-PAP devices, IPPB	Hospital beds and related aids: traction devices, trapezes, air flotation devices for decubitus prevention
Home diagnostic and monitoring equipment: apnea monitors, oximeters, sleep-recording devices, basic spirometry devices	Bathroom safety aids: commodes, bath or shower chairs, bath transfer benches, grab bars, hand-held shower attachments

CPAP, continuous positive airway pressure; biPAP, bilevel positive airway pressure; IPPB, intermittent positive-pressure breathing.

home care needs. It also identifies the services that are needed to meet those needs, as well as expected outcomes of those services. The plan incorporates both clinical and equipment monitoring.

A tool to aid the development of the home care plan is *acuity scoring*.[28] It uses weighted criteria against which the patient is compared and categorized. The patient's "score" dictates the type of follow-up care; for example, using one acuity scoring model, a higher score would indicate that the patient is poorly compliant, is medically unstable, and possesses a less than satisfactory understanding of how to use the home care equipment. This patient would need more monitoring and follow-up than would a patient who had a low score. Table 27-3 illustrates a type of acuity scoring.

Follow-up Care

Based on the home care plan and the patient's acuity score, the patient will be seen on a periodic basis by members of the home care team. The home care RT, in particular, will follow the patient to monitor the goals of care and adjust those goals as necessary. For example, the RT may need to do follow-up visits daily with a new oxygen client to titrate their oxygen flow rate during different activities. Once the titration is complete, the follow-up visit may be reduced to monthly to monitor the patient's progress with exercise tolerance. Acuity scoring is done during each follow-up visit to evaluate the patient's progress. The home care plan is then revised as indicated by changes in the patient's condition, psychosocial status, prognosis, and equipment needs and goals that are not achieved.[29,30]

A recent development in technology is now making it possible for follow-up care to be done by telemonitoring. Special computers and videophones allow the patient to measure vitals signs and transmit this information to the care provider. It is also possible for home oxygen providers to monitor oxygen equipment via computer link. The provider can check for contents, use time, and other equipment parameters at any time; the rationale for this type of telemonitoring is that it improves patient care through tighter equipment maintenance. It also potentially reduces the provider's service calls for complaints of equipment malfunction and empty tanks.

Discharging the Patient From Home Care Services

Most patients receiving clinical respiratory home care services will at some point likely be discharged from those services. Several areas need to be considered:

- Diagnosis
- The patient's ability to manage his or her own care
- The family's ability to manage the patient's care
- The patient's ability to independently manage activities of daily living
- The patient's acuity score
- The patient's ongoing equipment needs

The home care plan was used to establish specific goals related to the patient's care. Once those goals are met, the patient may no longer need the services of the RT. Regardless of this, the patient will continue to need equipment services as long as they continue to use any respiratory HME.

RESPIRATORY HME

As discussed, one of the major components of a home care program is the provision of medical equipment. Technology of HME has expanded greatly in the past 15 years to include many of the same technologies seen in acute care. It is not uncommon to see

Table 27-3. Example of Acuity Scoring[a]

Assessment Parameter, Point Value: Score 1–5	Best Case, Needs Little or No Monitoring, Modification = 1	Satisfactory but Needs Monitoring, Modification = 3	Worst Case, Needs Close Monitoring, Extensive Modification = 5
Patient's medical status	Medically stable	Recent exacerbation, hospital discharge	Medically complex, unstable
Physical abilities	No or mild physical impairments	Moderate physical impairments, needs some assistance	Severe physical impairments, needs assistance for all activities
Caregiver needs	Independent	Needs intermittent caregiver assistance	Needs caregivers around-the-clock
Physical environment	Safe, clean, suitable	Safe, needs minor modifications	Unsatisfactory, needs major modifications
Equipment needs	Low-tech, single piece (i.e., nebulizer, oxygen)	Low-tech, multiple pieces (i.e., nebulizer + oxygen, CPAP + oxygen)	High-tech (i.e., high flow oxygen, apnea monitor, ventilator)
Knowledge base	Good comprehension, performs skills as instructed	Fair comprehension, performs most skills as instructed, needs some review	Poor comprehension, cannot perform skills as instructed, needs assistance

CPAP, continuous positive airway pressure.

[a] Scoring Key: 6–13 points: follow-up in 1 mo to reassess, then quarterly; 14–24 points: follow-up in 2 to 4 wk to reassess, then monthly or quarterly as necessary; 25–30 points: follow-up in 1 wk (or sooner if necessary) to reassess, then in 2 to 4 wk as needed, then monthly.

home care patients who need invasive and noninvasive ventilatory support, intravenous pumps, enteral or parenteral nutrition therapy, or diagnostic testing. The challenge is in determining the most appropriate device to meet the patient's medical needs within the boundaries of the third-party payer's guidelines.

Oxygen Therapy Devices

Oxygen therapy has been proven to reduce mortality, reduce dyspnea, increase performance of activities of daily living, and improve quality of sleep and cognitive function in patients for whom it is medically indicated.[1] Patients with chronic lung disease and resultant chronic hypoxemia represent one of the largest population groups using home care equipment.

Three distinct types of stationary oxygen systems are used in home care:

- High-pressure cylinders
- Oxygen concentrators
- Liquid oxygen systems

Two distinct types of portable or ambulatory oxygen systems are used in home care:

- Small high-pressure cylinders
- Small liquid oxygen systems

High-Pressure Cylinders

The use of seamless steel or aluminum to contain gaseous oxygen under high pressure is the oldest and most reliable method of storing oxygen for subsequent administration. Oxygen is compressed to pressures of 2,200 to 2,400 psi (15,169 to 16,548 kPa) in cylinders of various sizes. The larger the cylinder, the more cubic feet (liters) of oxygen can be contained at the filling pressure of 2,200 psi (15,169 kPa). The most common sizes seen in the home are H or K tanks, containing 244 cubic feet (6,910 L); E tanks, containing 22 cubic feet; and D tanks, with 13 cubic feet.

The high-pressure stationary oxygen system has several advantages: no external power supply is required for operation; oxygen is not lost when the system is not in use; and it can also be used to power other pieces of respiratory equipment such as nebulizers, blenders, or ventilators. However, this type of stationary system has several disadvantages: each cylinder has a fixed capacity, necessitating frequent changes and refills, cylinders are heavy and are not easily moved; high-pressure oxygen cylinders pose a safety risk and must be properly secured; moderate hand strength is required to open valves and change regulators.

Stationary compressed oxygen tanks are rarely used as a patient's primary source of oxygen because of the limited amount of use time the tank has; for example, a patient receiving oxygen at 2 liters per minute (lpm) with continuous use would empty an H or K tank in less than 3 days. These tanks are instead used as a backup source of oxygen in the event that the primary source has failed in some way.

Oxygen Concentrators

An oxygen concentrator is an electrically powered device capable of separating oxygen from room air. A concentrator is boxlike and is about the size of an end table (Fig. 27-1). Oxygen concentrators use a molecular sieve of zeolite to absorb nitrogen from room air gas that is drawn into a compressor, pressurized to a relatively low level of 4 to 10 psi (27.6–69.0 kPa), and directed through the sieve bed. As the gas passes through the sieve bed, nitrogen is absorbed by the zeolite and the remaining oxygen is collected, concentrated, and passed through a flowmeter, where it is then delivered to the patient. Oxygen concentrators are capable of providing flow rates up to 6 lpm at concentrations of 85% or more. Generally, the lower the flow rate, the higher the oxygen concentration.

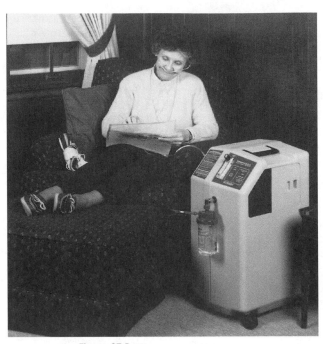

Figure 27-1. Oxygen concentrator.

Many concentrators have an oxygen concentration indicator that alerts the user should the concentration drop below an acceptable level.

Oxygen concentrators offer many advantages when used as a stationary oxygen system. The concentrator has the ability to provide oxygen without the need to be refilled. Concentrators are designed to run continuously, when properly maintained, and do so with minimum interruption. The console itself has an aesthetically pleasing appearance, and the patient or caregiver can easily operate the device. Concentrators have casters and weigh approximately 50 lb (22.5 kg), facilitating relocation throughout the home.

The use of oxygen concentrators has several disadvantages. A concentrator requires a source of electrical power (115 VAC) and, depending on the model, can consume up to 450 watts per hour. Any interruption in electrical power obviously renders the unit inoperable, which can be a problem if the patient lives in an area that experiences frequent power outages. The additional power usage will increase the patient's utility bill, and for some patients this is cost-prohibitive. Some utility companies offer special consideration and reduced rates for patients using electrically powered life support devices like concentrators. Concentrators produce extraneous noise in the range of 50 to 60 decibels, which some patients find bothersome, particularly at night. Concentrators also produce a moderate amount of heat that is exhausted into the room.

Because concentrators are low-pressure systems, they cannot be used to power other equipment like nebulizers or blenders. A concentrator is also a sophisticated piece of equipment and requires routine and periodic maintenance to ensure optimal performance. Patients are responsible for cleaning the foam intake filter on a weekly basis and for cleaning and disinfecting the humidifier if one is being used. They must also change the oxygen tubing and cannula as recommended by the provider. The HME provider is responsible for performing the preventive maintenance as recommended by the manufacturer.

A recent technological development offers some new advantages to the patient. A specially designed oxygen concentrator now allows the patient to fill small compressed oxygen cylinders from the concentrator.[31] The patient can actually use the concentrator while the cylinder is filling. The filling process is slow to prevent heat buildup; although this is an important safety feature, patients needs to understand that it *is* slow and anticipate their needs for a full cylinder well ahead of time. Depending on the size of the cylinder, fill time can be up to 8 hours.

Liquid Oxygen Systems

The third method of providing continuous oxygen therapy in the home is the LOX. Oxygen is stored in its liquid state at $-273°F$ ($-182.9°C$) in specially manufactured containers that are in essence sophisticated thermos bottles. These containers, called dewars, keep the oxygen in its liquid state and control the rate of evaporation through warming coils to provide sufficient gaseous oxygen for administration.

The primary advantage of the LOX is portability. Most stationary LOX dewars can be used to refill a smaller, lightweight version of the larger stationary unit. Figure 27-2 shows an example of a stationary LOX container with its smaller portable unit. Portable LOX containers, when filled with 1 to 2 lb (3.6 to 4.5 kg) of liquid oxygen, weigh approximately 10 to 12 lb and can provide continuous oxygen for up to 8 hours at a flow rate of 2 lpm. A portable LOX unit can be refilled from its stationary tank any number of times as long as the stationary tank contains an ample quantity of liquid oxygen, and the refilling procedure can be done by the patient.

Other favorable features associated with LOX systems include the availability of flow rates up to 15 lpm and that they operate without the need for electricity. Although the stationary tank needs to be refilled by the provider, it will last approximately 1 week with continuous use at 2 lpm. The stationary LOX tank can be placed on a roller base and moved around the home easily.

The LOX system is also quiet, producing only a small hissing sound from evaporation. This evaporation, however, is the biggest disadvantage to using the LOX. Simply stated, dewars are not capable of maintaining oxygen in the liquid state for an extended period. Under normal conditions, the amount of evaporation is controlled and immediately made available for administration. However, flow is occurring, as happens when the system is not being used, evaporation still occurs at a rate of approximately 250 L of gaseous oxygen every 12 hours. Warmer room temperatures and frequent transfilling of the portable tank

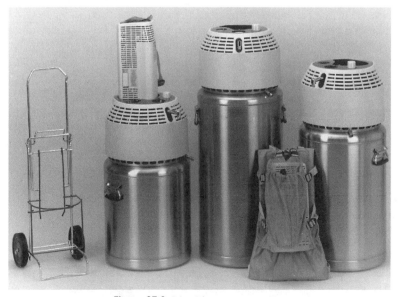

Figure 27-2. Liquid oxygen system.

cause the evaporative loss to be greater. The LOX not used for days may run dry solely through evaporative loss. The same applies to the portable LOX tank so that if a patient fills the portable tank the night before, the tank will have lost much of its contents by the next day.

Another disadvantage to the LOX is that oxygen in its liquid state is extremely cold and requires special handling. Gloves and protective eyewear must be worn by delivery personnel while filling the stationary tank to protect them from burns that occur when liquid oxygen comes in contact with skin. The tanks themselves are more costly for the HME provider to own and operate compared with the other oxygen delivery systems. Some patients find the portable tank transfilling procedure difficult and do not like noise created by the fill procedure. Patients must also be prepared to handle problems that can occur while filling the portable, such as freezing at the coupling of the portable and stationary tanks or overfilling or underfilling of the small tank.

A recent advancement in LOX technology is the low-loss container. Its enhanced insulation reduces evaporative loss common to stationary LOX tanks. The low-loss system is designed to be used *only* to fill a portable LOX tank. It has a content indicator like a traditional stationary tank but no flow control valve. Home oxygen providers are using the low-loss system in conjunction with an oxygen concentrator; the patient uses the concentrator as their stationary system and uses the low-loss system to fill a portable LOX tank. This combination reduces the number of deliveries the company needs to make to refill the stationary LOX tank or provide full compressed gas cylinders and provides the patient with the ultimate in portability. However, this approach to providing home oxygen does significantly increase the cost to the HME provider.

Portable and Ambulatory Oxygen Equipment
Contrary to what many patients think, they are not confined to their homes just because they use oxygen. Options are available that will allow them to be away from their stationary source of oxygen for several hours at a time. Small compressed oxygen cylinders and the portable LOX tank are the options, but determining which is the better option is complex.

Usually referred to as a portable oxygen system, it is important to categorize this equipment appropriately.[32] *Portable* oxygen equipment is small enough in size and weight to allow the patient to move it about, usually in a wheeled cart. *Ambulatory* systems are even smaller and lighter and can be carried on the body, usually by a shoulder carrying strap or in a bag. Box 27-6 outlines suggested criteria for selecting the most appropriate oxygen system for the patient. It may take some time before it can be decided which equipment is most appropriate. The patient's activities dictate their equipment needs, but the patient's activities may be limited when oxygen is first ordered for them. The home care RT will be able to identify the patient's changing needs during subsequent visits.

Oxygen-Conserving Devices
Oxygen-conserving devices are popular and useful additions to home oxygen therapy. Using either a passive reservoir system or electronic or pneumatic technology, these devices help extend the use time of a liquid or gaseous oxygen tank. They offer significant cost savings to the oxygen provider as well as a nice option for portability to the patient.[33]

Oxygen-conserving devices reduce the total amount of oxygen contents used in several ways. The reservoir system is a continuous flow device, but the oxygen flows into a reservoir where it is stored during the patient's expiratory phase. This allows a bolus of oxygen to be made available to the patient at the beginning of their next inhalation (Fig. 27-3). Although reservoir-type devices are continuous flow systems, they accomplish oxygenation goals at substantially lower flow rates than would otherwise be required using a conventional nasal cannula. For example, a reservoir device operating at 0.5 lpm can usually match the oxygenation levels attained with a conventional cannula at 2 lpm (assuming no increased demand exists for oxygen as during exertion). The major disadvantage to

Box 27-6. Suggested Criteria for Selecting the Most Appropriate Oxygen System
for the Patient

Stationary oxygen delivery system alone
   Patient is bed bound or unable to ambulate beyond the limits of a 50-foot
      length of tubing
   Patient requires nocturnal oxygen only
   Patient requires an oxygen source for a ventilator, continuous positive airway
      pressure, etc.
Stationary and portable oxygen delivery system (e.g., concentrator with E tank or
   liquid oxygen system)
   Continuous oxygen therapy is needed for a patient who only occasionally travels
      beyond the limits of a 50-foot length of tubing (e.g., occasional visits to the
      physician)
Stationary and ambulatory oxygen delivery system (e.g., concentrator with
   lightweight cylinders <10 lb or liquid oxygen system)
   Continuous oxygen therapy is needed for a patient who frequently travels
      beyond the limits of a 50-foot length of tubing (e.g., frequent trips outside
      the home for medical care, activities of daily living, recreation)

Adapted from McInturff SL, O'Donohue WJ. Respiratory care in the home and alternate sites.
In: Burton GC, Hodgkin JE, Ward JJ. Respiratory Care: A Guide to Clinical Practice. 4th ed.
Philadelphia: Lippincott, 1997.

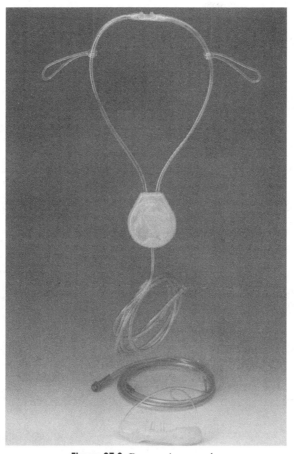

Figure 27-3. Reservoir cannula.

the reservoir-type nasal cannula is that it is rather unsightly to wear. Patients who dislike wearing a nasal cannula for cosmetic reasons would find this device even more unacceptable. For this reason and because other oxygen-conserving options are available, reservoir cannulas are seldom used.

Electronic and pneumatic oxygen-conserving devices are being widely used now. These devices work by pulsing small volumes of oxygen to the nasal cannula only during the first part of inspiration. These devices have been reported to reduce the amount of oxygen used by 50 to 75%.[33] Pulsed-dose conserving devices can be used on stationary, portable, and ambulatory oxygen systems and are suitable for use on either liquid or compressed oxygen tanks.

A disadvantage of using a pulsed-oxygen conserving device is that because it is delivered on demand, the patient will not receive oxygen should periodic interruptions occur in breathing, such as during sleep. Another concern is whether the patient will be adequately oxygenated during exertion; the patient's oxygen saturation should be monitored at rest and during exertion when they first start using a pulsed-dose conserving device. Careful patient and device selection is essential: it should meet the patient's physiological and ambulatory needs during all their activities.[34]

Oxygen-conserving devices have found their greatest acceptance when used to prolong the duration of ambulatory oxygen systems. When paired with a small aluminum cylinder, that is B, M6, or ML6, the conserving device makes for a lightweight ambulatory system (Fig. 27-4) that can last 10 hours or more. Using such a system greatly enhances a patient's sense of freedom. The drawback to this, however, is that these units are costly and not covered by many insurance companies, Medicare in particular. HME providers see the value added to both the patient and themselves by using these devices. Traditionally, a patient who is very active uses more oxygen and requires more frequent oxygen deliveries. With a conserving device, the patient can remain active and use less oxygen, thereby requiring less frequent deliveries, which is advantageous to the provider.

Transtracheal Oxygen Systems

The development of the transtracheal oxygen catheter in the 1980s occurred as a result of the desire to increase patient compliance when continuous oxygen therapy was ordered. Patients using traditional nasal oxygen tend to remove the cannula because of discomfort around the nares or ears or because they feel restricted or inconvenienced by it. Some patients refuse to use oxygen when they are in public because they are embarrassed by it.

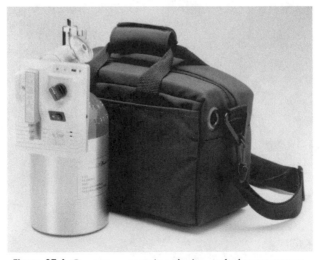

Figure 27-4. Oxygen-conserving device ambulatory system.

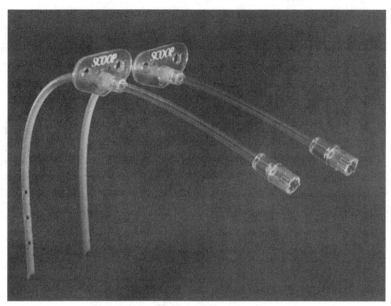

Figure 27-5. Transtracheal oxygen catheter.

It is also difficult to keep the nasal prongs in place during sleep, contributing to interrupted oxygen therapy and concomitant desaturation.

The transtracheal oxygen system is an invasive method of oxygen delivery. A small silastic catheter, approximately 20 cm long with a 9-French tract, is inserted into the trachea somewhere between the cricothyroid membrane and the notch of the manubrium (Fig. 27-5). The transtracheal catheter bypasses a considerable volume of anatomical deadspace (e.g., the hypopharynx), thereby reducing the amount of oxygen flow necessary to achieve the desired oxygenation. These flow rates, even though they are continuous, have been reported to be up to 50% less than with a conventional nasal cannula.[33]

The oxygen-conserving and aesthetic benefits of transtracheal oxygen therapy must be balanced with other aspects of a less desirable nature. Problems reported with its use include stoma site infection, stoma maintenance, inadvertent catheter displacement, kinking, and mucus plugs that adhere to the catheter. Other less prevalent complications include subcutaneous emphysema, mild hoarseness, and tract discomfort. Careful patient selection, training, and monitoring are essential, and if done so, these side effects can be significantly reduced.

Another consideration is the reimbursement of the transtracheal catheters. Many insurance companies, including Medicare, will not pay for transtracheal catheters. This is because they consider them to be in the same category as nasal cannulas, oxygen masks, and tubing, and these items are included in the rental fee they pay to the provider. Not every HME company is willing to provide these expensive catheters for which they receive no reimbursement.

Traveling With Oxygen

Many patients using oxygen admit that they feel tethered to their oxygen tank and that they cannot leave their home. We have described several portable and ambulatory systems that allow a patient to do just that, but what about the patient who wishes to travel? It is certainly possible to do long-distance traveling with oxygen. Car, train, bus, and commercial air travel can all be done by the patient with oxygen. It takes planning, however, and several details must be considered before traveling to ensure a safe and positive experience.

Healthy persons maintain an arterial partial pressure of oxygen (PaO_2) between 50 and 60 mm Hg at elevations of about 8,000 to 10,000 feet (2,440–3,050 m). Patients with COPD whose normal PaO_2 is 60 mm Hg have been shown to maintain PaO_2 levels in the 30 mm Hg range at these altitudes.[35] Consequently, it is important to carefully assess the patient for general health and to identify contraindications before attempting air travel. The normal response to hypoxemia is to increase ventilation, which may be difficult or impossible for a patient with severe pulmonary disease, making the patient unable to compensate for the resultant drop in blood oxygen level.

In-flight oxygen administration can assist the patient in managing this acute altitude stress. Most domestic airlines can supply oxygen at 2 to 4 lpm to patients requiring supplemental oxygen. They will not, however, allow patients to carry their own oxygen onboard, but they will allow the patient's empty oxygen cylinders to be checked as baggage. The airlines will not supply oxygen for use in the airport terminal, so it is advisable to have someone with the patient who can take the patient's oxygen equipment home once the patient has boarded the plane. It is also advisable to fly direct and have oxygen waiting at the arriving airport and at the traveler's ultimate destination. Airlines require a medical certificate from the patient's physician along with up to 2 weeks' advance notice. They also charge fees for this service for which the patient is responsible. The patient's oxygen provider can assist in making the necessary arrangements for onboard oxygen as well as for the delivery of oxygen equipment for use at the patient's travel destination.

Traveling by bus or train is also possible. The Greyhound bus line will allow a patient to bring a portable oxygen container on its buses, but the patient's stationary system cannot be checked as baggage. Prior arrangements need to be made to have oxygen available at the arriving bus terminal and the patient's final destination. Check ahead with private bus lines for their policies on traveling with oxygen. Patients traveling on AMTRAK can bring their stationary liquid tank or concentrator on board but they must travel in the nonsmoking sections of the train. If traveling with liquid oxygen, prior arrangements need to be made for having the tank refilled at the traveler's destination.

Travel by car is an easy way for a patient to make trips. Liquid oxygen tanks can be secured by a seat belt into the back seat of the car, but the patient will need assistance in placing it into the car, and great care must be taken when doing so. The stationary system must be removed from the car before filling the portable tank off of it, and both units must be kept upright at all times; allowing them to tip over will result in venting of the liquid oxygen, posing a safety hazard. The patient's oxygen provider can identify other oxygen suppliers along the patient's itinerary who can fill the stationary tank. It is essential that these locations be contacted before traveling because different suppliers carry different brands of equipment and all liquid systems are not compatible. Patients must also have a copy of their prescription available for these suppliers because the suppliers cannot legally provide oxygen without it.

Resources for the oxygen patient who wishes to travel are abundant. The American Association for Respiratory Care has developed an internet website specifically for such patients. This website, *Breathin' Easy Travel Guide,* is a comprehensive guide for oxygen suppliers and patients alike, and can be accessed at www.oxygen4travel.com.

Aerosol Therapy Devices

Many patients with chronic lung disease required inhaled medication therapy as part of the plan of treatment when they are discharged home. Several options are available: metered does inhalers (MDIs), compressor nebulizers, and bland aerosol delivery devices.

Metered Dose Inhalers

The MDI is a cost-effective, convenient, and routinely prescribed method of inhaled medication delivery. Its small size and ease of use make it the preferred method. It is ideal for the patient who attends school, works, or is otherwise away from home and needs to use inhaled medicine.

Technique is important when using an inhaler. It is necessary for the patient to inhale very slowly and actuate the MDI at the beginning of this inspiration. This can be a difficult skill for some patients to master, particularly for the patient who is extremely short of breath. Difficulty actuating the inhaler, and rapid, shallow inspiration are common. A valved holding chamber can make it easier for the patient to get a proper dose and is particularly recommended for older adults, younger children, and when inhaled cortico-steroids are used.[21]

Compressor Nebulizers

When a patient is unable to use an MDI, a compressor nebulizer is a relatively inexpensive and simple way for the patient to get inhaled medications. A compressor nebulizer is a small, oil-free machine that puts out approximately 10 lpm of flow to power medication nebulizers (Fig. 27-6A). A compressor nebulizer is usually powered by electricity, but battery-operated ones are also available at a substantially higher cost. Battery-operated compressors can be plugged into a cigarette lighter receptacle or run on its own internal battery (Fig. 27-6B). It is essential to check with the patient's medical insurance company to determine whether a battery-operated compressor nebulizer is a covered benefit because many will not cover this item.

Bland Aerosol Therapy

Bland aerosol therapy is most frequently used with home care patients having tracheosto-mies or laryngectomies for secretion control. This type of setup is composed of a large-volume nebulizer that is driven by an electrically powered high-output compressor. The aerosol is delivered through large-bore, usually disposable, tubing to a tracheostomy mask (Fig. 27-7). It can be heated or room temperature.

Whereas large-volume nebulizers are powered by oxygen with room air entrainment in the hospital, oxygen is bled into the circuit at the outlet of the nebulizer in the home care setting because the hospital can run the nebulizer on oxygen at 15 lpm; the equipment needed to provide oxygen at 15 lpm in the home is much more difficult to provide. Setup and maintenance of a high-output compressor with a nebulizer is not difficult for the patient or caregiver; however, a primary focus should be on cleaning the equipment and infection control.

Airway Clearance Devices

Adjuncts to therapy for patients needing secretion control include airway clearance devices. The most commonly prescribed device for this purpose is an *aspirator*. This device is used for oral and endotracheal suction. The aspirator can be either an electrically powered, heavy-duty type that is usually kept at the patient's bedside (Fig. 27-8), or a smaller, battery-operated version. The battery-operated aspirator is used most frequently for patients who leave the home for school, work, and recreational activities. It is also used as a backup to the heavy-duty type in the event of a power failure and when airway clearance is a critical issue.

Patients and caregivers are taught to perform the suctioning procedure, which for the most part is done as it is in the acute care setting. Clean technique and reuse of the suction catheters are the primary differences in the way this procedure is done in the home.[36]

Another common airway clearance device used in home care is the mechanical percus-sor. Similar to those used in the acute care setting, this is an electrically powered alternative to manual percussion and vibration. The patient and caregivers are taught proper position-ing techniques for optimal mobilization of secretions.

Manual cough assist devices such as the *flutter valve, mechanical exsufflator,* and *positive expiratory pressure* therapy are being used with increasing frequency in home care.

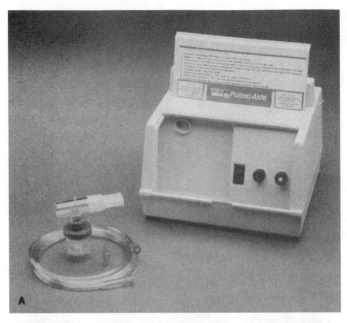

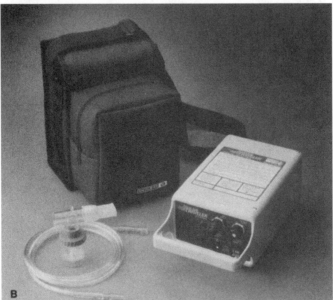

Figure 27-6. A. Compressor nebulizer. **B.** Battery-powered compressor nebulizer.

Many patients are taught to use these devices while in the acute care setting, and their use is part of the discharge plan. The home care RT can evaluate the patient's technique and compliance during home visits and retrain as necessary.

Ventilatory Assist Devices

Major advancements in the technology of HME give us the ability to treat patients with chronic respiratory insufficiency, ventilatory failure, and other breathing disorders. These devices are made to be "user friendly," allowing the home care RT to train the patient and other lay personnel to care for the ventilator-assisted individual.

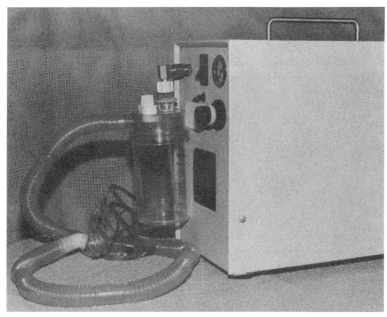

Figure 27-7. High-output compressor for bland aerosol administration.

Intermittent Positive-Pressure Breathing

Though not used frequently, intermittent positive-pressure breathing has its place in home care. It is used to treat chronic ventilatory insufficiency in patients with neuromuscular disorders such as muscular dystrophy and restrictive lung diseases such as kyphoscoliosis.[37,38]

The chief problem with using intermittent positive-pressure breathing at home is that these devices are no longer being manufactured. Home care providers must contend with using older equipment that if it fails may be impossible to repair. As an alternative, however,

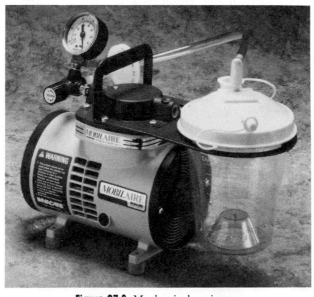

Figure 27-8. Mechanical aspirator.

a standard hospital-version intermittent positive-pressure breathing machine can be connected to a 50-psi air compressor used for bland aerosol therapy.

CPAP and Bilevel Therapy

Second to home oxygen therapy, CPAP and bilevel pressure therapy may be the next most common HME being used. It is used to treat obstructive sleep apnea, a condition wherein the patient's airway closes during sleep, causing snoring, oxygen deprivation, and sleep fragmentation. Patients with obstructive sleep apnea suffer from extreme daytime hypersomnolence, hypertension, and cardiac arrythmias. It is estimated that the incidence of sleep apnea in the general population is as much as 7%, and undiagnosed and untreated sleep disorders is a pandemic.[39,40]

CPAP therapy works by delivering pressurized airflow from a small blower at the bedside to a mask that the patient wears over the nose (and, infrequently, via a full-face mask). Figure 27-9 illustrates commonly used CPAP facial appliances. The air has been pressurized somewhere in the range of 5 to 15 cm H_2O or higher and acts as a "pneumatic splint," preventing the airway from closing off during sleep. Bilevel pressure therapy works the same way but gives the patient one pressure during inhalation and a lower pressure during exhalation. Bilevel pressure is useful when a patient has difficulty tolerating CPAP because it is easier to exhale. CPAP and bilevel therapy is the single most effective way to treat obstructive sleep apnea; surgical remedies, weight loss, oral appliances, and other methods have met with limited success.

The most difficult issue to be faced when starting a patient on CPAP or bilevel therapy is compliance. It takes a few weeks to adjust to the treatment, and many patients have difficulty tolerating a mask that is strapped onto the face. Proper mask fitting and patience are essential to ensuring the patient's success. Recent studies have reported improved compliance through the use of heated humidification inline.[41]

Home Mechanical Ventilation

The subject of home care would not be complete without a discussion of the management of patients using assisted ventilation. No longer are many of these patients kept in the hospital or long-term care facility. Although home ventilator care is complex, it is being done with increasing frequency. Proper patient selection, training, and follow-up care are essential to the success of a home ventilator program.[42,43] The reader is urged to refer to Chapters 21 and 22 of this book for comprehensive descriptions of mechanical ventilation performed in the United States and internationally.

Diagnostic and Monitoring Devices

Pulse Oximetry

Pulse oximeters are used routinely in the home care setting. They are used for "spot checks" as well as for titration and, for certain patients, continuous monitoring. Advances in technology have made them much easier to use, battery powered, and especially portable. Pulse oximetry must only be done by order of the patient's physician.

As convenient as they are, pulse oximeters do have drawbacks. Readings can be inaccurate under certain conditions, and the RT and patient must be aware of those conditions. For example, poor perfusion at the probe site can cause lower than expected readings; this is encountered often with the elderly patient with cold hands or the patient with diabetes who has poor peripheral circulation. Warming the patient's hand will result in more accurate readings.

Excessive movement at the probe site can prevent the oximeter from reading at all or can make the heart rate inaccurately high. Excessive ambient light interferes with the function of the sensor and so no reading will be taken; this is important to remember when trying to titrate a patient's ambulatory oxygen needs by taking them out for a walk on a sunny day. Low batteries can also give low readings.

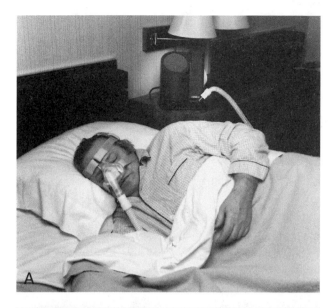

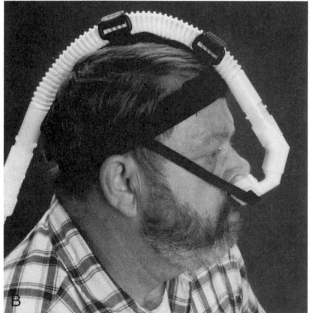

Figure 27-9. A. CPAP mask. **B.** Nasal pillows used with CPAP.

One of the biggest drawbacks to home oximetry is the dependence the patient and family have on it. The patient may experience benign momentary changes in oxygen saturation that can throw patients and families into a panic. It is important that they understand that the oximetry readings are only a small part of the patient's medical picture and should be used in conjunction with other aspects of the patient's condition, like heart rate, respiratory rate, and color.

Cardiorespiratory Monitoring

This type of monitoring is done primarily on at-risk infants suffering from apnea of prematurity, apnea of infancy, or apparent life-threatening events.[44] The devices are small, lightweight, and monitor heart rate, apnea duration, and equipment failures. Cardiorespiratory monitors do not prevent apnea events from occurring but will alert the parent or caregivers to them.

Patient selection is an important issue. Parents must be capable of using the equipment properly and must be instructed on proper response to all alarms. They must be trained in infant CPR and must also know how to troubleshoot equipment problems. Cardiorespiratory monitoring is not indicated for normal infants, and neither is routine monitoring of preterm infants.

Sleep-Recording Devices

It is now possible to perform a limited sleep study in the comfort of the patient's own bed. Portable sleep-recording devices are being used with increasing frequency to confirm a suspected diagnosis of obstructive sleep apnea. They present the patient with an alternative to the formal polysomnogram performed in a traditional sleep disorders center.

Portable sleep-recording devices usually measure airflow, snoring, oxygen saturation, heart rate, and body position. They do not record neurological data and are not intended to diagnose other types of sleep disorders.

REIMBURSEMENT ISSUES

We have referred to medical insurance and reimbursement issues repeatedly in this chapter and for good reason. A good home care program for a patient cannot be established without reimbursement for the equipment and/or services rendered. It is vital to establish which aspects of the patient's home care needs are reimbursable before initiation of these services. Patients and their families are seldom willing or able to accept the financial burden of HME and home care services. For example, on finding out that they do not qualify under Medicare's criteria for home oxygen, many patients refuse the equipment if they have to pay for it themselves. Although a patient with severe obstructive sleep apnea needs a CPAP device, he or she may not want it if it turns out that medical equipment is not a benefit of his or her health insurance policy, even though his or her apnea is considered critical.

It is important for the referral source, the home care provider, and the patient to understand how reimbursement works. Managed care, Medicare, health maintenance organizations, preferred or participating providers—it can all be confusing, particularly to beneficiaries, our patients.

Medicare

Medicare, a federally funded health insurance program, is probably the most commonly billed insurance company. Its beneficiaries include people aged 65 years and older and people who have been 100% medically disabled for 2 consecutive years. (This is why a 30-year-old quadriplegic patient on a mechanical ventilator can be covered by Medicare.) Medicare has two distinct parts: Part A, funded by payroll taxes, covers hospitalization, skilled nursing facility care, and home health and hospice care; Part B, a voluntary supplement to Part A paid in part by the beneficiary in monthly premiums, covers things like doctors' services, outpatient clinical laboratory services, and HME.[45]

Medicare has specific coverage guidelines for items like oxygen equipment, hospital beds, electric wheelchairs, etc. It is important to understand that although the patient's physician orders a piece of equipment or a service for him or her, it does not mean that it is automatically covered by Medicare. Medicare does not cover some commonly used items, like grab bars and other bathroom safety aids, at all.

Medicaid

Medicaid is a jointly funded federal and state medical assistance program for the economically disadvantaged. It serves low-income mothers and children for acute and ambulatory medical services; nonelderly disabled persons who use health insurance services and long-term care; and low-income elderly people who use it as a supplement to their Medicare benefits.[45] As with Medicare, Medicaid has specific coverage guidelines, and it cannot be assumed that Medicaid will pay for something because the physician has ordered it.

Private Commercial Insurance

Private commercial health insurance is another source of reimbursement for home care services. Employers as part of their employee benefits package frequently provide it. Private insurance is also purchased individually by the consumer. In either case, the beneficiary pays premiums. Benefits and coverage vary widely among the different types of commercial insurance plans. Many follow Medicare's criteria for defining their coverage; however, policy coverage varies for each beneficiary, so it is essential to verify coverage before providing the service.

Managed Care

Managed care has drastically changed the way medical care is administered. Its primary objective is to control the cost of health care through rigorous management of the use of health care resources. Some managed care organizations provide services directly, whereas others enter into contracts with health care providers to obtain these services at greatly reduced rates. Some require preauthorization, others require that the primary physician be the "gatekeeper" for all the services a patient needs. Managed care is, at the very least, complex, and the patient, the referral source, and the provider should contact the managed care organization to verify coverage issues.

Documentation of Medical Necessity

A prescription for equipment or services that are included as a benefit of a patient's health insurance plan does not automatically guarantee that it will be reimbursed. For example, a prescription stating "home oxygen at 2 lpm prn shortness of breath" would not qualify for Medicare payment of home oxygen services although Medicare pays for home oxygen. Third-party payers, especially Medicare, require justification that services are medically necessary and reasonable. Insurance carriers will only pay for the services the patient has been shown to medically need, not for what is convenient to the patient or family and not necessarily what the patient or physician may desire. Common requirements for documenting medical necessity are:

- Diagnosis(es)
- Prognosis
- Length of need
- Height, weight
- Place of service
- Results of medical tests (i.e., sleep study, blood gas, or oximetry)
- Goals of treatment
- Other treatments tried that have been unsuccessful

The physician must be concise when writing a prescription or completing a certificate of medical necessity and should avoid ambiguous verbiage like "PRN" or "for emergency use." Neither Medicare nor Medicaid will pay for medical equipment or services when prescribed in that manner. Instead, the specific use times, such as "during sleep" or "during exercise" should be indicated.

Obtaining reimbursement for home oxygen equipment is more complicated than for other types of home care equipment. Medicare has specific and rigid coverage criteria. They also require the patient's physician to complete a special certificate of medical necessity to document that the patient has met that criteria. Box 27-7 reviews Medicare's coverage criteria for home oxygen.

Reimbursement for Respiratory Therapy Services

Much discussion has been given to the home care team and the professional services provided by the various professionals on the team. Medicare and most other insurers do provide nursing care as part of their covered benefits, as well as those of physical, occupational, and speech therapists. Social workers, home health aides, and other paid caregivers are reimbursed as well.

Unfortunately, however, services provided by RTs in the home are still not covered by Medicare or by many other insurance plans. Medicaid reimbursement for RTs varies by state, and services are often limited when they are covered. Managed care presents the greatest hope for the home care RT because medical equipment providers and home health agencies negotiate their services into contracts with individual managed care plans.[46] Despite the lack of reimbursement for RTs, most HME providers have them on staff to work with and follow their pulmonary patients.

Box 27-7. Medicare Coverage Criteria for Home Oxygen

A. Continuous long-term oxygen therapy when
1. PaO_2 ≤55 mm Hg or SaO_2 ≤88%, or
2. PaO_2 56–59 mm Hg or SaO_2 89%, with
    a. Edema owing to congestive heart failure, or
    b. Evidence of pulmonary hypertension or cor pulmonale, or
    c. Elevated hematocrit ≥56
3. ABGs or SaO_2 by pulse oximetry obtained following optimal medical management
4. ABGs or SaO_2 by pulse oximetry obtained either with the patient in a chronic stable state as an outpatient or within 2 days prior to discharge from an inpatient facility to home
5. Repeat ABGs or pulse oximetry 3 mo after initial certification when
    a. Initial PaO_2 ≥56 mm Hg or SaO_2 89%, or
    b. The physician's initial estimated length of need was 1–3 mo
6. Certificate of medical necessity and prescription for oxygen therapy have been completed by the physician
7. Revised certificate of medical necessity when the oxygen prescription changes (i.e., flow rate, hours of use, change in equipment)
B. Oxygen with exercise when
1. SaO_2 ≤88% or PaO_2 ≤55 mm Hg during exercise, while resting PaO_2 ≥56 mm Hg or SaO_2 89% and
2. Demonstration of improvement in hypoxemia that was evidenced when the patient exercised while breathing supplemental oxygen
C. Nocturnal oxygen when
1. SaO_2 ≤88% or PaO_2 ≤56 mm Hg evidenced during sleep, with SaO_2 ≥89% or PaO_2 ≥56 mm Hg during the day, or
2. A decrease in PaO_2 >10 mm Hg or desaturation of >5% associated with nocturnal restlessness, insomnia, or other physical or mental impairments attributable to nocturnal hypoxemia

PaO_2, partial pressure of oxygen; SaO_2, arterial oxygen percent saturation; ABGs, arterial blood gases.

SUMMARY

The need for home care services in the immediate and long-term future is not expected to diminish. Rather, as previously stated, several forces are at work that will actually spur home care services to even greater utilization levels than ever before. Moreover, it is inevitable that technological advances will add yet another impetus to home care, as procedures and techniques once thought to be the exclusive domain of the hospital become feasible for in-home application.

However, reimbursement issues will continue to be the primary challenge facing home care providers, those prescribing home care services, and ultimately those receiving home care services. In this regard, it will be essential that archaic and nonsensical coverage-payment guidelines be abandoned and replaced with reimbursement strategies that accurately reflect the complexity and related expense of appropriately prescribed and provided home care services. The irony is that "appropriately prescribed and provided home care services" represents a significant and proven cost-effective alternative to more costly institutional care. And, home care has repeatedly been identified by consumers as being preferable to institutional care.

Hopefully, public and private health care policy makers will soon see the tremendous benefits and value that high-quality home care can offer the nation's beleaguered health care system. In the interim, home care providers will continue to be challenged by uncertain and confusing policies, with the successful ones continuing to reinvent themselves as the US health care system continues its own structural evolution.

REFERENCES

1. The National Lung Health Education Program Executive Committee. Strategies in preserving lung health and preventing COPD and associated diseases. Respir Care 1998;3:185.
2. Spratt G. The role of the home care respiratory therapist. AARC Home Care Bull 1999; July/August:2.
3. Pneumococcal and influenza vaccination levels among adults aged ≥65 years; United States, 1995. MMWR Morb Mortal Wkly Rep 1997; 39:913.
4. AARC Videoconference helps RTs prepare for future health care changes. AARC Times 1995; 19(11):64.
5. Cathcart M. Managed care: wringing more out of each health care dollar. AARC Times 1996; 20(12):1.
6. Just the facts: data tell the home care story. AARC Home Care Bull 1998;Nov/Dec.
7. Dunne PJ. Demographics and financial impact of home respiratory care. Respir Care 1994;4:309.
8. McCorkle R, Jepson C, Malone D, et al. The impact of posthospital care on patients with cancer. Res Nurs Health 1994;4:243.
9. Home Care Advisory Panel. Guidelines for the Medical Management of the Home Care Patient. Chicago: American Medical Association, 1992.
10. Bunch D. RTs find opportunities in sleep diagnostics and monitoring. AARC Times 1995;6:18.
11. Malloy N. Home care 101: tips for ensuring properly trained HME delivery personnel. Adv Manage Respir Care 1998;November:26.
12. Dunne PJ. The role of the respiratory care practitioner in home care. NBRC Horizons 1992; 18:4.
13. McInturff SL. Proceed with caution. Adv Manage Respir Care 1999;October:24.
14. Smoking cessation: clinical practice guideline 18. Washington, DC: Agency for Health Care Policy and Research, 1996. AHCPR publication 96-0692.
15. Krider SJ. Interviewing and respiratory history. In: Wilkins RL, Krider SJ, Sheldon RL, eds. Clinical Assessment in Respiratory Care. 3rd ed. St. Louis: CV Mosby, 1995.
16. McInturff SL. Assessment of the home care patient. In: Wilkins RL, Krider SJ, Sheldon RL, eds. Clinical Assessment in Respiratory Care. 4th ed. St. Louis: CV Mosby, in press.
17. Selection and team assessment of the pulmonary rehabilitation candidate. In: American Association of Cardiovascular and Pulmonary Rehabilitation: Guidelines for Pulmonary Rehabilitation Programs. Champaign, IL: Human Kinetics, 1993.
18. Epley D. Nutritional assessment in home care patients. Home Care Provider 1999;4(3):102.
19. Larsen PD, Hazen SE, Hoot Martin JL. Assessment and management of sensory loss in elderly patients. AORN J 1997;65(2):432.
20. Salmen JPS. The Do-able Renewable Home: Making Your Home Fit Your Needs. Washington, DC: American Association of Retired Persons, 1994.
21. Guidelines for the diagnosis and management of asthma: expert panel report 2. Washington, DC: National Heart, Lung, and Blood Institute, 1997. NIH publication 97–4051.

22. Mitchell T. The great indoors. RT 1998;June/July:39.

23. Thorson JA. Coming of age: affective disorders and older persons. AARC Times 1998;November:16.

24. Adkins CL. Healthcare in the melting pot. Adv Providers Post-Acute Care 1998;December:33.

25. Dean PR. Personal perception of chronic illness. Home Care Provider 1999;April:54.

26. Davidhizar R, Shearer RA. Helping elderly clients adjust to change and loss. Home Care Provider 1999;August:147.

27. Lacey M. Recognizing patterns of child abuse in the home. Home Care Provider 1998;December:319.

28. Koens J. Respiratory report card: acuity scoring for home oxygen care scores one for patient assessment. Adv Manage Respir Care 1999;5:63.

29. Dunne PJ, McInturff SL. The home visit. In: Dunne PJ, McInturff SL, eds. Respiratory Home Care: The Essentials. Philadelphia: FA Davis, 1998.

30. Gourley D. Care planning. AARC Home Care Bull 1999;March/April:3.

31. Olson K. A win-win situation. RT 1998;June/July:59.

32. McInturff SL, O'Donohue WJ. Respiratory care in the home and alternate sites. In: Burton GC, Hodgkin JE, Ward JJ, eds. Respiratory Care: A Guide to Clinical Practice. 4th ed. Philadelphia: Lippincott, 1997.

33. Hoffman LA. Novel strategies for delivering oxygen: reservoir cannula, demand flow, and transtracheal oxygen administration. Respir Care 1994;4:363.

34. Sclafani J. Pulse oxygen delivery systems: which system is best for which patient? AARC Times 1998;October:12.

35. Gong H. Advising pulmonary patients about commercial air travel. J Respir Dis 1990;2:484.

36. Home Care Focus Group. AARC clinical practice guideline: suctioning of the patient in the home care setting. Respir Care 1999;1:99.

37. Bach JR. Pulmonary rehabilitation considerations of Duchenne muscular dystrophy: the prolongation of life by respiratory muscle aids. Crit Rev Phys Rehabil Med 1992;3:239.

38. Aerosol Therapy Guidelines Committee. AARC clinical practice guideline: intermittent positive pressure breathing. Respir Care 1993;12:1189.

39. Yang KL. Sleep and sleep-disordered breathing. In: Dantzker DR, MacIntyre NR, Bakow ED, eds. Comprehensive Respiratory Care. Philadelphia: WB Saunders, 1995:804.

40. Dement WC. Bridging the knowledge gap. RT 1999;June/July:29.

41. Massie CA, Hart RW, Peralez K, et al. Effects of humidification on nasal symptoms and compliance in sleep apnea patients using continuous positive airway pressure. Chest 1999;2:403.

42. Make BJ, Hill NS, Goldberg Al, et al. Mechanical ventilation beyond the intensive care unit. Chest 1998;5:289s.

43. Home Care Focus Group. AARC clinical practice guideline: invasive mechanical ventilation in the home. Respir Care 1995;40:1313.

44. McDonald J, McInturff SL, McIntyre C. Pediatric respiratory home care. In: Dunne PJ, McInturff SL, eds. Respiratory Home Care: The Essentials. Philadelphia: FA Davis, 1998.

45. Shaw Miller L, Dunne PJ. Reimbursement. In: Dunne PJ, McInturff SL, eds. Respiratory Home Care: The Essentials. Philadelphia: FA Davis, 1998.

46. Marshall G. The evolving role of RTs in the home setting. RT 1999;April/May:13.

28 Travel for the Patient With Respiratory Disease

Bruce P. Krieger

◎ Professional Skills

Upon completion of this chapter, the reader will:

- Describe the etiology of altitude-related hypoxemia
- Evaluate whether patients will require supplemental oxygen when they fly
- Prepare a plan to help technology-dependent patients travel safely

INTRODUCTION

During the past 4 decades, air and sea travel has expanded from a relatively exclusive few to more than 500 million domestic airline passengers and millions more enjoying luxury cruises throughout the world.[1] These passengers include individuals with chronic pulmonary disease, many of whom require special equipment such as medications, supplemental oxygen (O_2), and mechanical ventilators. As one O_2-dependent patient remarked, being tethered to a tank need not be the same as chained to an anchor.[2] Advances in technology, such as lightweight O_2 systems and portable mechanical ventilators, have allowed patients more freedom to experience meaningful trips. O_2 concentrators and mechanical ventilators are now portable enough to fit in staterooms and hotel rooms.[3] Coupled with these advances in technology, pulmonary rehabilitation programs have emphasized the goal of maintaining as normal a life pattern as possible,[4] including traveling for leisure and business.

Travel for the technology-dependent patient with pulmonary disease can pose vexing problems. Airline travel requires exposure to a physiologically hostile environment because of the occurrence of hypobaric hypoxia as well as other adverse environmental changes.[1] Therefore, the travel industry has had to adapt to passenger needs within the restraint that their prime concern is to provide safe transportation for the public while maintaining a high standard of service that is economically feasible.[5] This chapter explores the physiologic effects of hypobaric hypoxia on healthy individuals as well as those with cardiopulmonary disease. It emphasizes the pretravel evaluation of the traveler and provides recommendations on how to procure appropriate medical needs during travel.

EFFECTS OF HYPOBARIC HYPOXIA

Physiology

Traveling by commercial aircraft poses complex problems for the patient with pulmonary or cardiopulmonary disease because of the occurrence of hypobaric hypoxia in flight. The etiology of hypobaric hypoxia is best understood by a review of the alveolar gas equation

Box 28-1. Alveolar Gas Equation

$$PAO_2 = (P_B - P_{H_2O})FiO_2 - PaCO_2/R$$

PAO_2, alveolar partial pressure of oxygen (O_2) (in milliliters of mercury); P_B, barometric pressure; P_{H_2O}, water vapor tension (47 mm Hg); FiO_2, fraction (%) of inspired O_2; $PaCO_2$, arterial partial pressure of carbon dioxide (in millimeters of mercury); R, respiratory exchange coefficient; (CO_2 production/O_2 consumption).

(Box 28-1).[6] Alveolar partial pressure of oxygen (PAO_2) is directly related to barometric pressure (P_B). PAO_2 determines arterial partial pressure of oxygen (PaO_2) based on the alveolar minus arterial gradient [$P(A-a)O_2$] for the individual patient. Subjects with pulmonary disease frequently have widened $P(A-a)O_2$ gradients, resulting in abnormal oxygen tension. At an altitude of 8000 ft, which is equivalent to Sun Valley, Idaho,[7] or the lowest P_B allowed in a commercial aircraft (564 mm Hg), the PaO_2 in healthy individuals is approximately 60 mm Hg, which corresponds to an arterial oxygen percent saturation (SaO_2) of approximately 90% (Fig. 28-1). However, in a patient with a $P(A-a)O_2$ gradient of 20 mm Hg, the PaO_2 is predicted to be approximately 50 mm Hg, with a corresponding SaO_2 of 85%. It is in this range of the oxyhemoglobin dissociation curve that small changes in PaO_2 can translate to significant decreases in SaO_2 and therefore oxygen delivery (DO_2) (Box 28-2).

The ceiling of air under which we reside at sea level is equal to 1 atm absolute, which is equivalent to 760 mm Hg or 14.70 psi. As altitude increases, P_B decreases, which results in lower partial pressure of inspired oxygen (PiO_2). For each 1000 ft of elevation, PiO_2 decreases by approximately 5 mm Hg.[8] Table 28-1 displays the gas pressures under hypobaric conditions for altitudes that are encountered by the traveling public. For exam-

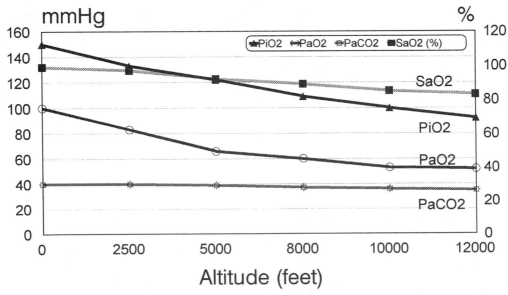

Figure 28-1. Arterial gas tensions at increasing altitude. Partial pressure of inspired oxygen (PiO_2), arterial partial pressure of oxygen (PaO_2), and arterial partial pressure of carbon dioxide ($PaCO_2$) are measured in millimeters of mercury (vertical axis on the left). Arterial oxygen percent saturation (SaO_2) is depicted as a percentage (vertical axis on the right). (From Krieger BP. Travel for the technology-dependent patient with lung disease. Clin Pulm Med 1995;2:1–29; and Hecht H. A sea-level view of altitude problems. Am J Med 1971;50:703–708.)

Box 28-2. DO_2 Equation

$$DO_2 = CO \times CaO_2$$

DO_2, oxygen (O_2) delivery; CO, cardiac output (heart rate $\times$ stroke volume); CaO_2, arterial O_2 content (Hgb $\times$ 1.34 $\times$ SaO_2 + [0.0031][PaO_2]); Hgb, hemoglobin (in grams); SaO_2, arterial O_2 percent saturation; PaO_2, arterial partial pressure of O_2 (in millimeters of mercury).

ple, in-cabin altitude is usually maintained between 5000 and 8000 ft, whereas visitors to Santa Fe, New Mexico, are exposed to an altitude of 10,000 ft. Other commonly visited destinations that are at moderate or high altitudes are depicted in Figure 28-2. At the ultimate altitude obtainable by humans while breathing ambient air (Mount Everest), the PiO_2 is only approximately one-third that of sea level, resulting in a PiO_2 of 43 mm Hg and a PaO_2 of 28 mm Hg, which corresponds to an SaO_2 of 70% despite extreme hypocarbia (end tidal CO_2 = 7.5 mm Hg).[9]

At moderate or high elevations, the inspired gas density is decreased, which is thought to be the reason for the improved midexpiratory flow rates that have been reported at altitude.[10] Associated with the decreased gas density, however, is the possibility of expansion of enclosed gases according to Boyle's Law ($P \times V = K$, where P = pressure, V = volume, and K = constant). At 5000 ft, an enclosed gas volume is estimated to be approximately 20% greater than at sea level, whereas at 8000 ft an approximately 40% expansion occurs. Recently, a patient with a giant intrapulmonary bronchogenic cyst experienced a fatal air embolus on a commercial aircraft.[11] The authors hypothesized that the cyst enlarged and ruptured as predicted by Boyle's Law, which allowed air to enter the systemic circulation. Although barotrauma in commercial aviation records is rare, other cases of air embolism and pneumothoraces have been reported.[12,13]

Table 28-1. Gas Pressures Under Hypobaric Conditions

Altitude (ft)	Ambient Pressure			
	ATA	psi	B_P	PiO_2
0	1	14.70	760	150
5,000	0.83	12.19	630	122
6,000	0.80	11.76	608	118
8,000	0.74	10.91	564	109
10,000	0.69	10.12	523	100
12,000	0.64	9.34	483	92

From Hultgren H. High Altitude Medicine. Stanford, CA: Hultgren Publications, 1997:3, 9; and de la Hoz RE, Krieger BP. Dysbarism. In: Rom WN, ed. Environmental and Occupational Medicine. 3rd ed. Philadelphia: Lippincott-Raven Publishers, 1998:1359–1375.
ATA, atmosphere absolute; psi, pounds per square inch; B_P, barometric pressure (in milliliters of mercury); PiO_2, partial pressure of inspired oxygen (in milliliters of mercury) corrected for water pressure (47 mm Hg).

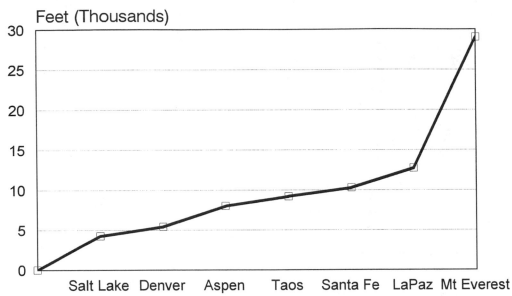

Figure 28-2. Altitudes of popular travel destinations. The in-cabin P_B on commercial aircraft is the equivalent of that between Denver and Aspen's altitude (5000–8000 ft). (From Hultgren H. High Altitude Medicine. Stanford, CA: Hultgren Publications, 1997:3, 9.)

Acute Pulmonocardiac Responses to Hypobaric Hypoxia in Healthy Individuals

Although "hypoxia" and "hypoxemia" are often used interchangeably, in physiologic terms they are distinctly different.[14,15] Understanding this distinction is integral to comprehending how individuals acutely adapt to hypobaric hypoxia. Hypoxemia is defined as a decrease in the oxygenation of blood as measured by PaO_2 or as SaO_2, whereas hypoxia is defined as a decrease in DO_2 to the tissues. Therefore, hypoxemia can occur without hypoxia (such as at moderate to high altitude) if an appropriate cardiac response to desaturated blood occurs. As can be seen in the DO_2 equation (see Box 28-2), a decrease in SaO_2 will result in a decrease in arterial oxygen content. However, DO_2 can be maintained by a compensatory increase in cardiac output (CO).

As the PaO_2 decreases to less than 60 mm Hg, the peripheral hypoxemia-mediated chemoreceptors in the carotid bodies are stimulated, which results in hyperventilation.[16,17,18] The increase in minute ventilation is caused more by an increase in tidal volume than by changes in breathing frequency.[19] This results in hypocarbia and respiratory alkalosis, which may partially suppress the hypoxic drive,[10,16] but also results in an elevation in PaO_2 and therefore PaO_2. In addition, the $P(A-a)O_2$ gradient is narrowed, even in patients with chronic obstructive pulmonary disease (COPD).[19,20]

The acute ventilatory response to hypobaric hypoxia has been shown to be blunted by the ingestion of alcoholic beverages. Roeggla et al.[21] demonstrated that when healthy individuals ingested the equivalent of 1 L of beer, no significant changes in PaO_2 or $PaCO_2$ occurred at an altitude of 5061 ft. However, when the same amount of alcohol was consumed at 9840 ft in these 10 volunteers, the median PaO_2 decreased from 69.0 to 64.0 mm Hg ($P < .01$) and the median $PaCO_2$ increased from 32.5 to 34.0 mm Hg ($P < .01$). This blunted response to the acute effects of hypobaric hypoxia are similar to what has been reported when individuals ingested diazepam.[21] Although this may not be deleterious in healthy individuals, patients with diseases that lower their baseline oxygenation may be more severely affected.

When hyperventilation becomes inadequate in preventing further decrements in SaO_2

and arterial oxygen content, the cardiovascular system responds by increasing CO. The increase in CO offsets the decrease in arterial oxygen content, and DO_2 is preserved. An early study[22] performed under isocarbic conditions ascribed the hypoxemia-induced increase in CO to reflexive tachycardia without an associated increase in stroke volume. However, a study done in our lab[23] under hypoxic, hypocarbic conditions using noninvasive measurements of stroke volume, CO, tidal volume, and SaO_2 showed statistically significant increases in heart rate, stroke volume, and CO in 10 healthy men subjected to lower concentrations of inspired O_2.

Acute Pulmonocardiac Responses to Hypobaric Hypoxemia in Patients With Pulmonary Disease

A few investigators have studied how outpatients with COPD acutely adapt to altitude. Graham and Houston[19] exposed 18 men with nonhypoxemic COPD who had a mean forced expiratory volume in one second (FEV_1)/forced vital capacity (FVC) ratio of 33% and a mean FEV_1 of 0.97 L to an altitude equivalent to 8000 ft at rest and during exercise and compared the changes with the same degree of activity at sea level (Fig. 28-3). Subjectively, the patients complained of mild fatigue and insomnia. Although the minute ventilation at rest did not change between sea level and altitude, it was significantly increased during exercise at altitude (17% higher, $P < .05$). PaO_2 was significantly lower at altitude, but this reached statistical significance only with exercise. Interestingly, the $P(A-a)O_2$ gradient narrowed at altitude because of hypocarbia. Respiratory rate, pulse rate, and dead space ratio (V_D/tidal volume) did not change significantly at rest or with exercise at altitude. Dyspnea was not a major complaint even when patients with COPD had a PaO_2 as low as 40 mm Hg.[20,24] One explanation for this lack of dyspnea may be adaptation by these subjects to hypoxemia that they regularly experience at sea level, especially during sleep.

The cardiovascular responses to altitude noted by Graham and Houston[19] were similar

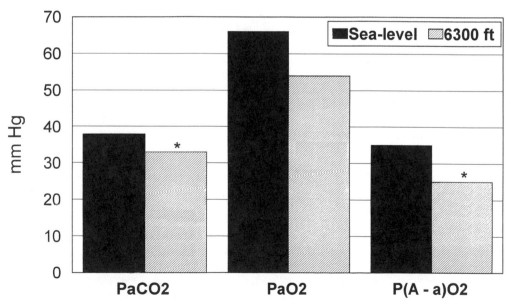

Figure 28-3. Arterial blood gas values at rest and at 6300 ft in eight patients with COPD. *$P < .05$ compared with measurements at sea level. $PaCO_2$, arterial partial pressure of carbon dioxide; PaO_2, arterial partial pressure of oxygen; $P(A-a)O_2$, alveolar minus arterial gradient. (Data from Graham WGB, Houston CS. Short-term adaptation to moderate altitude: patients with obstructive lung disease. JAMA 1978:240:1491–1494.)

to those in a study performed by Berg and colleagues.[25] They exposed eight men with nonhypoxemic COPD (mean PaO_2 = 72 mm Hg, mean FEV_1 = 0.97 L) to the equivalent of 8000 ft. No significant changes between sea level and altitude were noted for arterial pressure, heart rate, cardiac ectopy, or pulsus paradox until supplemental O_2 was administered at altitude. After O_2 was begun, pulse pressure diminished, blood pressure declined, and pulsus paradox reduced. It was hypothesized that the administration of O_2 resulted in decreased intrathoracic pressure swings because of a decrease in work of breathing. However, no measurements of oxygenation were recorded in the study to compare with the work of Graham and Houston. Other studies have also noted that patients report that it "is easier to breathe" at altitude, perhaps because of reduced gas density.[26]

Hypoxemia causes an acute increase in pulmonary arterial pressure mainly because of precapillary vasoconstriction,[27] although the compensatory increase in CO also contributes slightly. This response is not lost in patients with primary pulmonary hypertension.[28] Therefore, in patients with significant pulmonary hypertension, ascent to even moderate altitudes may result in an increase in pulmonary vascular resistance resulting in acute right heart strain, which could be fatal. In addition, the rise in pulmonary arterial pressure may suddenly open a patent foramen ovale, resulting in worsening hypoxemia owing to an acute right to left shunt.[29,30]

Theoretically, hypobaric-induced hypoxemia and the associated hyperventilation and compensatory increase in CO could predispose susceptible persons to myocardial ischemia. However, a study of almost 100 visitors (mean age, 70 years) to Vail, Colorado (8200 ft), showed no electrocardiographic signs of myocardial ischemia.[31] Even so, travelers who have a predisposition to cardiac dysrhythmias may experience an increase in their arrhythmia when at moderate altitude.[32]

Effect of Hypobaric Hypoxia on Sleep

Cheyne-Stokes respirations were noted by climbers in the 19th century at altitudes less than 12,000 ft.[33] Cheyne-Stokes respiration consists of a progressive and repetitive crescendo–decrescendo pattern of breathing in which hyperpnea and tachypnea is followed by bradypnea, hypopnea, and usually short apneas. This cycle then repeats throughout the night.[34] During the hyperventilatory phase of Cheyne-Stokes respirations, pulse oximetry recordings show a decrease in oxygen saturation. This nocturnal desaturation is believed to be the underlying mechanism for acute mountain sickness, which is experienced by 25% of travelers to moderate altitudes.[35] Acetazolamide moderates the O_2 desaturation during periodic breathing by inducing a metabolic acidosis and compensatory hyperventilation.[36] Acetazolamide has been recommended to prevent acute mountain sickness when traveling to altitudes of 8000 ft or higher.[37,38]

AIR TRAVEL

Aircraft Cabin Conditions

A common misconception by the general public and health care personnel is that commercial aircraft cabins are pressurized to sea level.[16,18,20,39,40,41] In actuality, aircraft cabins are maintained at a pressure relative to the aircraft's altitude, which can range from 20,000 to 40,000 ft. Cabin pressure is regulated by a series of outlet valves that maintain the cabin pressure between 7.5 and 8.7 psi greater than the outside environment; the exact pressure differential differs for each type of aircraft. For example, the differential in an L-1011 aircraft between the ambient pressure and the cabin is approximately 8.4 psi.[8] At an altitude of 40,000 ft, the outside P_B is 2.72 psi (140 mm Hg).[39] Therefore, the cabin pressure would be equivalent to 11.12 psi (8.4 + 2.72), which equals approximately 575 mm Hg or the equivalent altitude of Aspen, Colorado (see Fig. 28-2). At this altitude, the PiO_2 is approximately 110 mm Hg (see Fig. 28-1), which corresponds to a PaO_2 in healthy individuals of approximately 60 mm Hg.

In a comparison of 204 commercial aircraft, Cottrell[8] calculated the median cabin altitude to be 6,214 ft, with a range up to 8,915 ft. During the study, cruising altitude ranged from 10,000 to 60,000 ft, with higher altitudes (mean, 7004 ft) being obtained for older aircraft compared with newer planes (mean, 5280 ft). The largest cabin-atmospheric differential was obtained by the supersonic Concord (10.7 psi), which is necessary because of the craft's high cruising altitude (>40,000 ft). According to Federal Aviation Administration requirements, the cabin altitude pressure is required to be maintained at less than 8,000 ft unless temporary diversions are required to avoid inclement weather.[18] As noted earlier in the section describing adaptations to hypobaric hypoxia, the resistance to airflow at altitude is slightly decreased, thus resulting in an increase in peak expiratory flow rate.[10] However, other conditions that are unique to airline cabins may worsen the status of patients with pulmonary disease.[15,42] Cabin humidity and temperature are usually low, which may result in the drying of secretions and the ineffective expectoration of sputum. In addition, if a flight allows cigarette smoking, carbon monoxide will be recirculated,[43] which may worsen oxygen desaturation in patients who are on the steep portion of the oxyhemoglobin dissociation curve.[17] Boyle's Law[44] predicts that hyperinflation may worsen at altitude in patients with bullous lung disease if they have areas with extremely prolonged time constant (resistance × compliance). If a bullous overexpands, this could compromise lung function by encroaching on adjacent lung tissue[45] as well by causing hyperinflation and worsening diaphragmatic function.[46]

Newer aircraft recirculate more in-cabin air as a means of saving fuel. Although not unique to the pulmonary patient, this enclosed environment can promote exposure to aerosolized pathogens such as atypical bacteria, viruses, and granulomatous organisms. A well-documented case report of multidrug-resistant *Mycobacterium tuberculosis* being transmitted to passengers and crew during a long international flight was recently published.[47]

Another factor to consider on airplane flights is the prolonged immobilization of the patient. This increases the risk for developing deep venous thrombosis and subsequently pulmonary thromboembolic disease.[48,49] Cases of pulmonary embolism have been reported both on disembarkation and a few days after long trips. This is especially important in the traveling patient with pulmonary disease who may be predisposed to hypercoagulability because of older age and underlying chronic disease states. A report of sudden death occurring during airflights noted that 18% were caused by pulmonary thromboembolic disease.[48] Women who had a history of deep venous thrombosis and were older than 40 years were at higher risk.[48]

In-flight Medical Incidents

Because airlines are only required to report in-flight deaths, the reported numbers of in-flight medical emergencies probably represents an underestimation.[50] Statistics from the Seattle-Tacoma Airport indicate that the frequency of medical occurrences were 1/39,600 inbound passengers,[51] whereas foreign carriers reported an incident of 1/13,000 to 21,000 passengers.[52] However, for patients who have disabilities that were reported to the airlines preflight, the incidence of a medical occurrence during flight was 1/350 passengers.[52] Although the incidence seems low, it translates into at least two emergency calls per day from inbound flights to the Seattle-Tacoma Airport and an estimated incidence of 3,000 in-flight medical emergencies annually on domestic airlines.[53]

The most common respiratory complaint encountered in flight is dyspnea. As expected, this is more frequent in passengers with known obstructive lung disease.[51] However, cardiovascular, neurologic, and gastrointestinal tract complaints are more common than respiratory complaints according to reported statistics.[18,52,53–55] The most frequent cause of death reported on commercial aircraft is cardiac, and frequently the afflicted passenger has no known preexisting conditions. The estimated incidence of this is 1 per 3 to 10 million passengers.[50,52]

Medical Evaluation Before Flying

Although respiratory complaints are only the fourth leading cause of medical incidents in flight, pulmonary diseases are the most common reason for preflight medical evaluations.[15] In one study of 233 passengers referred to a major domestic airline's private advisory service for preflight clearance during a 3-month period in 1991,[18] two-thirds of the diagnoses were of a pulmonary nature, including COPD (39%), lung cancer (7%), pre–lung transplant (2%), and other respiratory diagnoses (20%). Before mobilized jet ways were used to board and disembark from commercial aircraft, the routine way of determining whether a patient was medically cleared to fly was whether he or she could walk up the set of stairs to the aircraft's entrance way.[40,56] Since then, multiple physiologic and clinical parameters have been evaluated to assess passengers' fitness to fly, including the presence of hypoxemia or hypercarbia, dyspnea on minimal exertion, abnormal pulmonary function tests, pulmonary hypertension, or unstable cardiac conditions.[5,24] With the recognition that hypobaric hypoxia is the major physiologic stress while flying, attention has focused on being able to predict in-flight oxygenation.[8,15,56] Therefore, the most pragmatic recommendation concerning who should be evaluated before commercial airflight is to screen patients who have a predicted PaO_2 of less than 50 mm Hg at altitude (5000–8000 ft).[18,24,57–59] For an ambulatory patient with COPD who is not hypercarbic, a PaO_2 greater than or equal to 72 mm Hg recorded at sea level should be adequate to safely fly in commercial aircraft.[57] However, complicating conditions such as cardiac disease, anemia, active bronchospasm, pulmonary hypertension, or bullous lung disease may compromise patients with COPD even if the PaO_2 is 72 mm Hg or higher.[15] In addition, patients with active sinusitis or otitis media may not be able to equilibrate their inner ear and be distressed because of this.[44] A more dangerous situation occurs in patients who have recently undergone abdominal surgery because of the possibility of wound dehiscence owing to expansion of gas within the gastrointestinal tract as predicted by Boyle's Law.[5,44] Similarly, patients who have had thoracic surgery or a pneumothorax within 3 weeks may be at risk when flying.[5]

Since the early 1980s, various studies have made efforts to predict in-flight oxygenation. One of the first studies to measure the PaO_2 during flight was undertaken by Schwartz et al.[20] In this study, 13 patients with COPD had arterial blood gases measured at rest at sea level and then again while flying in an unpressurized cabin at 5412 and 7380 ft. In addition, they were exposed to 17.2% O_2 mixture at rest and with light exercise at sea level. All the patients had an FEV_1/FVC ratio less than or equal to 50% and no evidence of restrictive lung disease, ischemic heart disease, or cerebral vascular disease. They all had PaO_2 greater than or equal to 55 mm Hg at rest while on room air at sea level. This study found that the patients' PaO_2 decreased from 68.0 ± 0.3 mm Hg (mean ± 1 SD) to 51.0 ± 9.1 mm Hg at 5412 ft and further declined to 44.7 ± 8.7 mm Hg at 7380 ft. There was only a weak correlation between the PaO_2 measured a few weeks before the flight at sea level and the in-flight PaO_2, whereas a PaO_2 measured within 2 hours of flight had a better predictive value for estimating the in-flight PaO_2. The part of the study in which the patients breathed a fraction of inspired oxygen (FiO_2) of 17.2% showed a strong correlation with in-flight PaO_2 at 5412 ft (52.5 ± 9.6 mm Hg vs. 51.0 ± 9.1 mm Hg). In a subsequent letter to the editor,[60] the same authors recommended that breathing an FiO_2 of 15% O_2 at sea level would predict in-flight oxygenation at a cabin altitude of 8000 ft.

During the same year that Schwartz et al.[20] published their data on unpressurized in-flight oxygenation, Gong et al.[24] proposed the acronym "hypoxia-altitude simulation test" (HAST) to describe the use of hypoxic gas mixtures to predict oxygenation at altitude.[57] This acronym has subsequently been termed the "high-altitude simulation test" to better

Table 28-2. High-Altitude
Simulation Test

Simulated Altitude		
feet	meters	FiO$_2$(%)
0	0	20.9
5,000	1,524	17.1
8,000	2,438	15.1
10,000	3,048	13.9

FiO$_2$, fraction of inspired oxygen.

describe its purpose to patients and their families.[15] The HAST is relatively easy to perform and requires only a premixed hypoxic (O_2 plus nitrogen) gas mixture (or an O_2 blender), a pulse oximeter (or arterial blood gas analyzer), an electrocardiogram, and a mouthpiece with a nose clip (or a tight-fitting mask with the least amount of dead space possible). By using lower concentrations of O_2 (Table 28-2), hypobaric hypoxia is simulated. As originally described, steady-state conditions were assumed to be attained within 15 minutes, at which time the patient was asked to walk in place to simulate having to ambulate around the cabin of an aircraft.[15,20,57] Recent confirmation of the accuracy of HAST was provided by a group from Australia who measured oxygenation in a hypobaric chamber and with the HAST.[61] They found that the HAST accurately predicted hypobaric hypoxemia at altitudes of 6000 and 8000 ft and that steady-state conditions were met within 5 minutes both in healthy individuals and in patients with COPD. They also noted a significant reduction in PaO$_2$ with light exercise, thus confirming the need for simulated walking during the HAST. However, the HAST does not reproduce the other in-cabin changes that occur at altitude such as the lower air density, lower P$_B$, and reduced humidity.[15]

Other investigators have developed regression equations to predict PaO$_2$ at altitude by evaluating patients with COPD in hypobaric chambers.[40,62] Dillard et al.[63] recommended that the FEV$_1$ be incorporated into these equations to improve the accuracy, although others have questioned whether the added expense and inconvenience is justified.[64] These equations are listed in Box 28-3. As mentioned previously, the patient with normoxic COPD who is in a stable state and has a recent PaO$_2$ greater than or equal to 72 mm Hg does not necessarily need to be screened unless other concomitant conditions exist.

Box 28-3. Regression Equations for Predicting PaO$_2$
at Altitude

Patients with chronic obstructive pulmonary disease:

(a) $22.8 - 2.74(x) + 0.68(y)$

(b) $0.453(y) + (0.386)(FEV_1\% \text{ predicted}) + 2.44$

Patients with restrictive lung disease:

(a) $25.0 - 3.12(x) + 0.62(y)$

PaO$_2$, arterial partial pressure of oxygen (O_2); x, altitude (in thousands of feet); y, PaO$_2$ (in milliliters of mercury) at sea level; FEV$_1$% predicted, forced expiratory volume in 1 second (relative to predicted normal).

Testing with HAST has advantages over prediction equations,[15,56] including (*a*) allowing the patient to subjectively experience the sensation of hypoxemia; (*b*) allowing prediction of oxygenation during light exercise, such as walking around the cabin; and (*c*) allowing the evaluation of patients regardless of the etiology of pulmonary disease or whether concomitant diseases (cardiac, hematologic, cerebrovascular, or psychologic) are present to affect the patient's subjective and objective response to a simulated cabin environment. The HAST also permits adjustment of supplemental O_2 to meet the requirement of the patient under hypoxemic conditions.

A recent article showed that the addition of 2 L/min of supplemental O_2 in an enclosed environment with an FiO_2 of 15% was adequate to return the pulse oximetry to values obtained while breathing ambient air at sea level ($FiO_2 = 21\%$).[65] Three groups of 10 patients each were studied including healthy individuals, patients with restrictive lung disease, and patients with obstructive lung disease. However, only 2 patients had resting pulse oximetry at sea level of less than 92%, and both of these were in patients with obstructive lung disease. Still, the study provides a guideline as to how much supplemental O_2 may be necessary for patients to maintain adequate in-flight oxygenation when arrangements have to be made without the availability of a HAST.

Because hypoxia can adversely affect other medical conditions, screening of the traveler also needs to include a detailed history of possible cardiovascular problems and anemia (especially sickle cell disease and sickle cell β thalassemia).[66] Patients with recent cerebral infarction may develop worsening of their neurologic deficits because of cerebral hypoxia. As mentioned earlier, recent thoracic surgery or pneumothorax are relative contraindications to fly because of the potential expansion of enclosed gas according to Boyle's Law.[5]

Planning Air Travel for Pulmonary Patients

Planning for air travel with supplemental O_2 requires preparation by the patient well ahead of takeoff.[2,67] Although most major domestic and international airlines allow O_2 to be used in the flights, many of the smaller airlines and regional carriers will not accept passengers with supplemental O_2.[2,15] No domestic carrier allows a passenger to use their own O_2 tank. Rather, they require that the airline supplies the source of O_2. Liter flow is 2 to 8 L/min via face mask and/or cannula.[2,56,67] Some carriers will contact the patient's personal physician directly, whereas others only require a letter. The fee for the supplemental O_2 varies and is based on the number of flight segments. In addition, the carriers will not supply O_2 while on the ground so that if the patient requires supplemental O_2 at rest or when in an airport at altitude, these arrangements have to be made separately. If transportation (such as a wheelchair) between flight segments or to ground transportation is necessary, then arrangements are required before takeoff. Recent publications have listed the differences between air carriers, although these policies frequently change.[24,59,67–69] Therefore, the traveler will always need to make arrangements at least 48 hours ahead of time for domestic airlines and as long as a week before traveling on an international carrier.

Other arrangements are required before embarkation. Seat selection should ideally be at the front of the aircraft or near a lavatory. Nonstop flights are preferable for convenience and to limit the extra cost of using O_2, which is based on a per-segment charge. Furthermore, it is advisable to travel during normal business hours in case any equipment fails or a need arises for changes that might occur because of flight plan alterations.[2,67]

Before even contacting the air carrier, however, the patient should have a detailed evaluation by their treating physician. Recommendations can be based on previous experience or may require a HAST test or other estimation of O_2 requirements. The physician should supply the patient with a brief summary of their medical history, medication requirements, O_2 requirements, stability to travel, and a list of physicians en route and at their final destinations who they may contact in case of emergencies.[15,67] In addition, airports have emergency physicians available, and their names and numbers can be provided before travel by the travel agent. Some travel agencies specialize in arranging for trips for patients with medical problems and can be helpful, especially for international trips.[2]

Any patient traveling with O_2 will need to have a companion who is able to help with their equipment and their medications. Some international carriers require that an extra seat be purchased in lieu of a charge for O_2. Most carriers will allow empty O_2 tanks to be checked as luggage. Because of recent in-flight O_2 generator–related disasters, these restrictions are becoming much more stringent. Patients should carry all their medications on board as well as packing duplicates in their luggage.[56,67] Moreover, they should bring tape, scissors, extra tubing, cannulas, and adapters, especially if they use an O_2-conserving device.[15] Along with their medications, the traveler should have a copy of all medical information as well as their advanced directives, and these directives need to be understood by their traveling companion.

On the day of departure, the patient should be well rested and void before boarding the plane. Simple measures such as not overeating and avoiding sedatives, alcohol, caffeine (which may cause diuresis), and tight-fitting clothing should be taken. Also, on flights longer than 1 to 2 hours, patients should stand up and exercise their leg muscles periodically to avoid the risk of deep venous thrombosis.

Most of these arrangements need to be organized by the patient. Therefore, the patient should have either experience with traveling with O_2 or a knowledgeable travel agent. Most travelers should obtain extra trip cancellation insurance and medical air transport insurance, especially if traveling outside their home country. Although seemingly arduous, these arrangements can be done relatively expediently by the experienced traveler.[2]

Medical-Legal Aspects of Traveling With Medical Equipment

The prime concern of any carrier is to provide safe transportation for its passengers. Therefore, it is considered reasonable for an air carrier to refuse passage to passengers who they feel are not medically fit to travel by air.[5]

When a passenger is stricken in flight, it is common for airline personnel to ask for the assistance of any physician who may be on board in the role of a "good samaritan."[52,59] A survey of 577 in-flight deaths noted that in 43% of cases, on-board physicians offered medical assistance.[50] However, one survey of 42 physicians who responded to in-flight emergencies found a certain degree of reservation about volunteering their services mainly because the physicians felt that emergency care was outside their field of expertise.[70] Other concerns included medical-legal implications, which vary widely among countries.[52] For example, in the British and American legal systems, no legal obligation for a physician to provide aid to a stranger exists, whereas some European countries consider it a criminal offense if assistance is not rendered by a physician even if that physician is not "qualified" to provide the required medical services. Moreover, even qualified physicians may not be knowledgeable about the various physiologic changes that could affect diagnosis and treatment while at altitude.[52] Furthermore, no consensus exists as to whether a physician should be reimbursed for services rendered, as publicized by a recent legal battle occurring in London.[71] Many physicians noted that their services were not acknowledged and that no effort was made to deal with their ambivalence, especially when an afflicted passenger dies while under their emergent care.[52,59,72] However, most physicians face difficult decisions on a daily basis and should be psychologically prepared to respond appropriately.[15]

Since 1986, domestic airline carriers have been required by the Federal Aviation Administration to carry a medical kit that contains a sphygmomanometer, a stethoscope, an oropharyngeal airway, and various medications (epinephrine, diphenhydramine, 50% dextrose, and nitroglycerin tablets) along with an instruction book.[53] Although not a Federal Aviation Administration requirement, some major domestic carriers are now equipped with cardiac defibrillators and have trained their personnel in the proper use of these defibrillators along with basic and advanced life support methods. These changes have been popularized by incidents in which journalists have written that passengers could have been saved if such equipment had been available. The exact impact of this equipment, both favorable and harmful, has yet to be determined.[52,53] This is especially pertinent given the extremely low incidence of fatal medical emergencies that occur in flight.[50,53]

TRAVEL AT SEA LEVEL FOR THE TECHNOLOGY-DEPENDENT PULMONARY PATIENT

Cruise Ships

Although the cruise industry does not have a uniform policy, most cruise lines allow patients to bring their own equipment on board, including O_2 concentrators, without charging a fee.[67] Some actually rent O_2 concentrators when cruising is done internationally. Usually more than 4 weeks' advance notice is required before departure. Although allowing patients to bring their own equipment eliminates one of the problems of traveling, frequently the patient needs to fly to the cruise ship and therefore will still need to deal with the airline industry.

If the patient requires continuous supplemental O_2 and/or portable O_2 when ambulating, adequate equipment needs to be prearranged for excursions away from their concentrator. Therefore, the patient needs to contact his or her O_2 vendor along with the cruise line to be certain that tanks can be refilled and that the O_2 supplier will be open when the ship is docked.[2]

When booking a cruise, patients need to work closely with their travel agent. A detailed letter should be sent to the cruise line with an expected response confirming the date and destination of the cruise, the cabin number, the equipment that is going to be brought on board, the electrical requirements of such equipment, the portable equipment that will be used, the wheelchair that will be required, and the electrical supply for any electrical equipment that may be necessary (such as a nebulizer, a nasal continuous positive airway pressure machine, a percussor, or a suction device).[2] In addition, the astute cruiser may want to ask whether the cabin has been newly painted or carpeted before sailing because this may adversely affect the patient. Last, the letter needs to contain the name and telephone number of the O_2 supplier at home so that further details can be worked out and to ask for confirmation that all arrangements have been made.

The problem of hypobaric hypoxia will not be encountered when cruising because travel is occurring at sea level. However, travel sickness may occur, which could adversely affect the overall medical status of the patient. Appropriate steps can be taken to prevent this. However, many medications used to prevent sea sickness have cardiovascular and drying side effects that need to be discussed with the patient's physician before departure. The patient should also request a cabin near an elevator and in a nonsmoking area of the ship. Most large cruise ships have medical personnel on board for assistance. However, most carriers are foreign and therefore the qualifications of health care personnel can vary, as can the quality and presence of advanced medical equipment.[73] More recently, cruise ship lines have begun to associate themselves with medical advisory teams that can be reached via satellite to help diagnose and treat patients. This is made easier if patients provide a summary of their medical history, medications, and advance directives.

The United States Coast Guard has a hazardous material branch (202.267.1577), as does the Department of Transportation under the regulation DOT-E 9856 (202.366.4535), for more specific questions about cruising with O_2.[67]

Travel by Private Auto

Patients who require supplemental O_2 as well as other medical technology frequently opt to travel by private car or recreational vehicle.[15] Large-volume tanks can be secured in the back seat or in an appropriately designed auto or recreational vehicle. In the latter, O_2 concentrators can also be used. It is advisable that a backup, portable system is available in case of vehicle breakdown or accidents. Patients need to make arrangement with O_2

suppliers so that refills can be obtained throughout the trip. Therefore, travel should be done during usual business hours.[2] In addition, patients and their companions need to be warned against allowing tanks to overheat when left in the trunk or the back of a vehicle and to be certain that inflammable materials are not in close proximity to O_2 tanks. Not only are O_2 concentrators convenient for recreational vehicles, they can also be moved to most motel and hotel rooms. If travel is going to take the patient to higher altitudes, adjustments need to be made in the O_2 flow, and this needs to be discussed with their physician before departure.

Travel by Bus and Rail

Most long-distance bus carriers and commercial railroads allow passengers to travel with their own portable O_2 containers and frequently with O_2 concentrators for longer trips.[67] As with other forms of transportation, arrangements need to be made with the carrier before departure. In addition, request for a seat in a nonsmoking area of the bus or train should be sought in advance. Each carrier has limits as to how many O_2 containers can be stowed as baggage. It is advised that an extra supply of O_2 be available to the traveler and that they are familiar with how to have their equipment serviced (in case of an unexpected problem).

TRAVELING WITH ADVANCED MEDICAL TECHNOLOGY

Increasing numbers of patients now rely on portable mechanical ventilator support for use at home either on a continuous or a nocturnal basis. A growing number of patients rely on a noninvasive method of full or partial mechanical ventilator support.[3] Similar to the requirements for portable O_2, policies concerning the use of mechanical ventilators on aircraft and on ships vary with each carrier. Usually, a portable ventilator is allowed in flight but must be able to fit under the seat in front of the traveler and be powered by a dry- or gel-cell battery.[67,74] Some European carriers have electrical hookup; even so, it is best to have a battery backup, especially if the patient is dependent on assisted ventilation. Similarly, noninvasive mechanical ventilator support devices, such as bilevel positive airway pressure devices, may require electrical adapters or batteries. One recent study showed that the accuracy of the delivered tidal volume and flow rates of mechanical ventilators, including continuous positive airway pressure units, may be altered by the lower P_B encountered at altitude.[75] The lower density of gas at altitude alters the system's ability to make the appropriate calculation of pressure. Therefore, adjustments for this need to be considered before air flight. Similarly, because of Boyle's Law, the cuffs of endotracheal or tracheostomy tubes will expand if filled with air in flight, which could be dangerous to the patient. An alternative is to use saline to inflate the cuff while at altitude.[76]

Recently, reports have emerged describing the use of commercial aircraft to transport patients with advanced lung disease to medical centers for lung transplantation or pulmonary thromboendarterectomy.[76,77] These flights will require six to nine seats in the plane so that the patient's gurney can be placed above the seat and adequate room is available for the accompanying medical personnel, usually a critical care nurse and physician.[76] Because of the lower P_B in flight, intravenous solutions need to be regulated by battery-powered pumps to ensure proper delivery of medication if this is critical to the patient's hemodynamic status. In addition, the delivered FiO_2 will need to be adjusted either before or during flight with noninvasive monitors (pulse oximetry) and/or end tidal carbon dioxide monitors. It should be noted, however, that some air carriers do not allow the use of suction equipment on board because it may interfere with the aircraft navigational system. Furthermore, detailed calculations will be necessary so that enough portable O_2 is available, especially on longer flights. Even though these medically complicated patients can be safely transported on commercial aircraft,[76,77] it is usually advisable that a qualified air ambulance service transport these patients when feasible.

ACKNOWLEDGMENT

I greatly appreciate the secretarial support of Ms. Alina Tomas and the financial support of the BERTH ABESS Pulmonary Research Fund.

REFERENCES

1. Harding RM, Mills FJ. Medical aspects of airline operations, I: health and hygiene. BMJ 1983; 286:2049–2051.
2. Petersen P. Good If Not Great Travel With Oxygen. Charlotte, NC: Raven Publishers, 1996.
3. Make J, Hill NS, Goldberg AI, et al. Mechanical ventilation beyond the intensive care unit. Chest 1998;113(Suppl):289S–244S.
4. Rodrigues JC, Ilowite JS. Pulmonary rehabilitation in the elderly patient. Clin Chest Med 1993;14:429–436.
5. Mills FJ, Harding RM: Fitness to travel by air, I: physiological considerations BMJ 1983;286: 1269–1271.
6. Weinberger SE. Principals of Pulmonary Medicine. Philadelphia, PA: WB Saunders, 1992:16.
7. Hultgren H. High Altitude Medicine. Stanford, CA: Hultgren Publications, 1997:3, 9.
8. Cottrell JJ. Altitude exposure during aircraft flight: flying higher. Chest 1988;92:81–84.
9. West J, Hackett P, Maret K, et al. Pulmonary gas exchange on the summit of Mt. Everest. J Appl Physiol 1983; 55:678–687.
10. Coates G, Gray G, Mansell A, et al. Changes in lung volume, lung density, and distribution of ventilation during hypobaric decompression. J Appl Physiol 1979;46:752–755.
11. Zaugg M, Kaplan V, Widmer U, et al. Fatal air embolism in an airplane passenger with a giant intrapulmonary bronchogenic cyst. Am J Respir Crit Care Med 1998;157:1686–1689.
12. Neidmart P, Suter PM. Pulmonary bulla and sudden death in a young aeroplane passenger. Intensive Care Med 1985;11:45–47.
13. Gil HS, Stetz FK, Chong K, et al. Nonresolving spontaneous pneumothorax in a 38-year-old woman. Chest 1996;110:835–837.
14. Block ER. In: Fishman AP, ed. Update: Pulmonary Diseases and Disorders. New York: McGraw-Hill, 1982:349–365.
15. Krieger BP. Travel for the technology-dependent patient with lung disease. Clin Pulm Med 1995;2:1–29.
16. Lenfant C, Sullivan K. Adaptation to high altitude. N Engl J Med 1971;284:1298–1309.
17. Harding RM, Mills FJ. Problems of altitude, I: hypoxia and hyperventilation. BMJ 1983;286: 1408–1410.
18. Gong H. Air travel and oxygen therapy in cardiopulmonary patients. Chest 1992;101;1104–1113.
19. Graham WGB, Houston CS. Short-term adaptation to moderate altitude: patients with obstructive lung disease. JAMA 1978:240:1491–1494.
20. Schwartz JS, Bencowitz H, Moser KM. Air travel hypoxemia with chronic obstructive pulmonary disease. Ann Intern Med 1984;100:473–477.
21. Roeggla G, Roeggla H, Roeggla M, et al. Effect of alcohol on acute ventilatory adaptation to mild hypoxia at moderate altitude. Ann Intern Med 1995;122:925–927.
22. Phillips BA, McConnell JW, Smith MD. The effects of hypoxemia on cardiac output: a dose-response curve. Chest 1988;93:471–475.
23. Sackner MA, Hoffman RA, Stroh D, et al. Thoracocardiography: part 1—noninvasive measurement of changes in stroke volume comparison to thermodilution. Chest 1991;99:613–622.
24. Gong H. Advising COPD patients about commercial air travel. J Respir Dis 1984;5:28–39.
25. Berg BW, Dillard TA, Derderian SS, et al. Hemodynamic effects of altitude exposure and oxygen administration in chronic obstructive pulmonary disease. Am J Med 1993;94:407–412.
26. Christopherson JK, Hlasita MD. Pulmonary gas exchange during altered gas density breathing. J Appl Physiol 1982;52:221–225.
27. Marshall C, Marshall B. Site and sensitivity of hypoxia pulmonary vasoconstriction. J Appl Physiol 1983;55:711–716.
28. Hultgren H. High Altitude Medicine. Stanford, CA: Hultgren Publications, 1997:475.
29. Wilmshurst PT, Byrne JC, Webb-Peploe MM. Relation between interstitial shunts and decompression sickness in divers. Lancet 1989;2:1302–1306.
30. Moon RE, Camporesi EM, Kisslo JA. Patent foramen ovale and decompression sickness in divers. Lancet 1989;1:513–514.
31. Yaron M, Alexander J, Hultgren H. Low risk of myocardial ischemia in the elderly at moderate altitude. J Wilderness Med 1995;6:20–28.
32. Hultgren H. High Altitude Medicine. Stanford, CA: Hultgren Publications, 1997:429.
33. Mosso A. Life of Man on the High Alps. London: Fisher Unwin, 1989:44.
34. West JB, Peters RM, Aksner G, et al. Nocturnal periodic-breathing at altitudes of 6,300 and 8,050 m. J Appl Physiol 1986;61:280–287.
35. Honigman B, Theis MK, Koziol-McLain J, et al. Acute mountain sickness in a general tourist population at moderate altitudes. Ann Intern Med 1993;118:587–592.
36. Larson EB, Roach RC, Schoene RB. Acute mountain sickness and acetazolamide: clinical efficiency and effect on ventilation. JAMA 1982;248: 328–332.
37. Cain SM, Dunn JE. Low doses of acetazolamide to aid accommodation of men to altitude. J Appl Physiol 1966;21:1195–2000.
38. Birmingham Medical Research Expeditionary So-

ciety Mountain Sickness Group. Acetazolamide in the control of acute mountain sickness. Lancet 1981;1:180–183.

39. Liebman J, Lucas R, Moss A, et al. Airline travel for children with chronic pulmonary disease. Pediatrics 1976;57:408–410.

40. Shillito FH, Tomashefski JF, Ashe WF. The exposure of ambulatory patients to moderate altitudes. Aerosp Med 1963;Sept:850–857.

41. Gong H. Air travel and patients with chronic obstructive pulmonary disease [editorial]. Ann Intern Med 1984;100:595–597.

42. Latimer KM, O'Byrne PM, Morris MM, et al. Bronchoconstriction stimulated by airway cooling. Ann Rev Respir Dis 1983;128:440–443.

43. Mattson ME, Boyd G, Byar D, et al. Passive smoking on commercial airline flights. JAMA 1989; 261:867–872.

44. de la Hoz RE, Krieger BP. Dysbarism. In: Rom WN, ed. Environmental and Occupational Medicine. 3rd ed. Philadelphia: Lippincott-Raven Publishers, 1998:1359–1375.

45. Wade JF, Mortenson R, Irvin CG. Physiologic evaluation of bullous emphysema. Chest 1991; 100:1151–1154.

46. Travaline JM, Addonizio P, Criner GJ. Effort of bullectomy on diaphragm strength. Am J Respir Crit Care Med 1995;152:1697–1701.

47. Kenyon TA, Valway SE, Ihle WW, et al. Transmission of multidrug-resistant *Mycobacterium tuberculosis* during a long airplane flight. N Engl J Med 1996;334:933–938.

48. Cruickshank J, Gorlin R, Jennett B. Air travel and thrombotic episodes: the economy class syndrome. Lancet 1988;2:497–498.

49. Ferrari E, Chevallier T, Chapelier A, et al. Travel as a risk factor for venous thromboembolic disease: a case-control study. Chest 1999;115:440–444.

50. Cummins RO, Chapman PJC, Chamberlain DA, et al. In-flight deaths during commercial air travel: how big is the problem? JAMA 1988;259:1983–1988.

51. Cummins RO, Schubach JA. Frequency and types of medical emergencies among commercial air travelers. JAMA 1989;261:1295–1299.

52. Mills FJ, Harding RM. Medical emergencies in the air, I: incidence and legal aspects. BMJ 1983;286:1131–1132.

53. Cottrell JJ, Callaghan JT, Kohn GM, et al. In-flight emergencies: one year of experience with the enhanced medical kit. JAMA 1989;262:1653–1656.

54. Speizer C, Rennie CJ III, Breton H. Prevalence of in-flight medical emergencies on commercial airlines. Ann Emerg Med 1989;18:26–29.

55. Skjenna OW, Evans JF, Moore MS, et al. Helping patients travel by air. CMAJ 1991;144:287–293.

56. Krieger BP. Oxygen in the air. Emerg Med 1997;29:77–82.

57. Gong H, Tashkin DP, Lee EY, et al. Hypoxia-altitude simulation test. Am Rev Respir Dis 1984;130:980–986.

58. Bjorkman BA, Selecky PA. High-altitude simulation at rest and exercise to determine oxygen therapy needs in hypoxemic patients during airplane travel: a community hospital experience [abstract]. Chest 1988;94(Suppl):31S.

59. AMA Commission on Emergency Medical Service. Medical aspects of transportation aboard commercial aircraft. JAMA 1982;247:1007–1011.

60. Schwartz J. Hypoxemia during air travel [letter]. Ann Intern Med 190;112:147–148.

61. Naughton MT, Rochford PD, Pretto JJ, et al. Is normobaric simulation of hypobaric hypoxia accurate in chronic airflow limitation? Am J Respir Crit Care Med 1995;152:1956–1960.

62. Dillard TA, Berg BW, Rajagopal KR, et al. Hypoxemia during air travel in patients with chronic obstructive pulmonary disease. Ann Intern Med 1989;111:362–367.

63. Dillard TA, Rosenberg AP, Berg BW. Hypoxemia during altitude exposure: a meta-analysis of chronic obstructive pulmonary disease. Chest 1993;103:422–425.

64. Apte NM, Karnad DR. Altitude hypoxemia and the arterial-to-alveolar oxygen ratio [letter]. Ann Intern Med 1990;112:547–548.

65. Cramer D, Ward S, Geddes P. Assessment of oxygen supplementation during air travel. Thorax 1996;51:202–203.

66. Green RL, Huntsman RG, Serjeant GR. Sickle-cell and altitude. BMJ 1971;4:593–595.

67. Stoller JK. Travel for the technology-dependent individual. Respir Care 1994;39:347–362.

68. Gong H. Air travel and altitude in hypoxemic patients. Pulm Perspect 1989;6:8–12.

69. American Association for Respiratory Care (AARC). Requirements for Traveling With Oxygen. Dallas: AARC, 1992.

70. Hays MB. Physicians and airline medical emergencies. Aviat Space Environ Med 1977;48:468–470.

71. Goldsmith C. Is there a doctor on the plane? yes, if he can bring his bill pad. *Wall Street Journal.* October 8, 1998:B1.

72. Wakeford R. Death in the clouds. BMJ 1986; 293:1642–1643.

73. Perrin W. Cruise ships and medical care. Condé Nast Traveler 1994;Dec:37–46.

74. Lifecare. Heading south this winter? tips for traveling with a ventilator. In: Alert: New Ideas in Respiratory Care. Lafayette, CO: Lifecare, Nov/Dec 1993.

75. Fromm R, Varon J, Lechin AE, et al. CPAP machine performance and altitude. Chest 1995; 108:1577–1580.

76. Wachtel AS, Allen HN, Lewis HI. Aeromedical transport of the mechanically ventilated patients. J Intensive Care Med 1997;12:310–315.

77. Kramer MR, Jakobson DJ, Springer C, et al. The safety of air transportation of patient with advanced lung disease: experience with 21 patients requiring lung transplantation or pulmonary thromboendarterectomy. Chest 1995;12:310–315.

29 Marketing of Pulmonary Rehabilitation

Roberta N. Clarke

◗ Professional Skills

Upon completion of this chapter, the reader will:

- Understand that marketing is based on the concept of relationships and exchanges
- Recognize the four classic ways of viewing the exchange process: the production concept, the product concept, the sales concept, and the marketing concept
- Develop and prepare outcome measures for your pulmonary rehabilitation program, allowing the use of the resulting outcome measures in the program's marketing
- Identify the desired market behaviors for a marketing exchange to occur
- Perform a competitive analysis through the following activities: call for promotional materials, visit the competitor websites, "blind shop" your competitors, market research, if the budget of the program allows it, and map out where your competitors are located
- Understand the tools of marketing strategy, which is the marketing mix: product/service, price, place, and promotion
- Periodically adjust the pulmonary rehabilitation program marketing strategy to reflect the changing marketplace

The marketing of pulmonary rehabilitation is, as marketing is throughout most of the health care field, misunderstood and oversimplified. Too often, it is equated only with advertising, promotion, public relations, and communications. In this circumstance, an example of the focus of marketing commonly is: What should we put in our brochure? How can we get the hospital to advertise our pulmonary rehabilitation program? And, most recently, should our pulmonary rehabilitation program have a website?

Unfortunately, these questions neglect consideration of more significant issues such activities raise, such as whether the market that one is targeting is even receptive to reading a brochure; whether the information in the brochure is relevant for the market receiving it; and whether the market might be better reached through broadcast media, direct selling efforts, websites, clinical journal articles, or other forms of communication. Even more important, the focus on communication fails to address whether the product or service (for our purposes, a pulmonary rehabilitation program) offering is attractive to the market regardless of the form of communication used, whether price is a barrier to usage of the offering, whether potential patients are being referred by those in a position to provide access to the pulmonary rehabilitation program, and whether the hours and location of the service prove to be barriers to usage of the service. Most important, the focus on communication and promotion do not ask the essential question: Does the product or service offering provide a recognized benefit to the market?

Those who are more knowledgeable about marketing at least recognize the need to include market research and marketing intelligence in a broad definition of marketing; without these, one cannot fathom the complexities, attitudes, and motivations of the market to which one is directing one's efforts. A truly informed understanding of marketing requires a recognition of the complete set of marketing mix tools as the foundation of marketing strategy, plus some comprehension of consumer behavior, market segmentation, competitive analysis, product/service line issues, service marketing, brand management, marketing evaluation, and social marketing. This cannot all be covered in this one chapter. For more in-depth coverage, see Kotler[1] or Clarke and Kotler.[2]

MARKETING RELATIONSHIPS AND THE EXCHANGE OF BENEFITS

Marketing is based on the concept of exchange: the seller provides a benefit to the buyer and the buyer in exchange provides a benefit to the seller through the purchase of the seller's product or service. For example, a car dealer provides a benefit to his customer through the sale of a car; the core benefit is personal transportation for the customer. Secondary benefits to the customer purchasing the car might be social status (as the customer might brag to his friends about his new Mercedes), safety (with the inclusion in the car of front and side airbags and ABS brakes), and ease in finding one's way to new locations through the use of the global positioning system in the new car. In exchange, the car dealer receives a monetary benefit from the sales exchange from the payment of money that the customer makes to the dealer.

Without the mutual exchange of benefits, it is unlikely that an exchange will happen. To receive a benefit, each party has to give something up to provide a benefit to the other party. If either the seller or the customer does not see a benefit in the exchange, then that party lacks the motivation to engage in an exchange transaction. For example, pulmonary rehabilitation programs benefit from physician referrals of patients because, with each new patient, the programs receive reimbursement and increased program size (in terms of numbers of patients). If, however, a physician does not believe that a pulmonary rehabilitation program is able to significantly improve his or her patient's current or prospective quality of life or health status, then little benefit is perceived by the physician (and thus by the patient) in referring the patient to the pulmonary rehabilitation program. As a result, the exchange will not happen.

Marketing invests not only in creating exchanges but also in creating relationships between sellers and customers. A relationship, in marketing terms, is a long-term stream of exchanges between a seller and a customer. The purpose of marketing is not merely to make a single exchange take place but to provide a benefit that is so significant that the customer, in anticipation of receiving future significant benefits, will want to engage in a continuing set of exchanges. Therefore, marketing should appropriately direct its resources not merely to attracting new customers but also to keeping and serving its existing customers so that they will return to engage in future exchanges (follow-up and maintenance exercise programs). It is the failure to recognize the value of keeping existing customers in long-term relationships that misguides many health care organizations to spend most of their marketing resources on attracting new customers, when the real potential for growth comes from attracting more business from existing customers.

A pulmonary rehabilitation program, often placed within a hospital or sometimes within a closed-panel managed care plan, has a limited set of physicians from which it can expect to gain referrals. If it attracts only one or two patient referrals from each potential referring physician, then it cannot grow beyond that initial base of referrals. It has not developed the long-term relationship with its physician customers (in this case, referring customers). What the program should seek is a continuing stream of referrals (exchanges) from those physicians who have referred to the pulmonary rehabilitation program in the past. Marketing efforts should be guided by the answers to the following questions:

> Who has referred to the program in the past?
> Are they continuing to refer patients to the program? If not, why not? (This requires market research to find the answer.)
> Do you think that you are capturing all of each physician's pulmonary rehabilitation referrals or only some of them?
> If only some of them, what types of referrals are you losing and why? (Again, this will require further market research.)

Once a program has the answers to these questions, it can attempt to remedy the problems causing referral sources to divert their referrals elsewhere or to discontinue referring potential pulmonary rehabilitation patients to anyone. For example, suppose market research uncovers physicians who state that they prefer to send their patients to a neighboring pulmonary rehabilitation program because that pulmonary rehabilitation program has weekend and evening hours. The marketing effort then must either respond by expanding the hours of service or must accept the fact that it has placed itself at a competitive disadvantage by maintaining more limited hours of service. This limitation is likely to allow the competing program to continue to attract these physicians' referrals and to maintain with them a long-term relationship. The way to address this marketing problem then is to make operational changes (expanded hours) rather than to consider more promotion or advertising, neither of which will address the identified operational problem.

Conventional marketing wisdom now holds that it costs five times as much to capture a new customer as it does to keep one. Promotion, advertising, health fairs, and websites (updated, well-maintained websites as opposed to static websites that are rarely revisited) are expensive to fund and, interactive websites aside, are usually directed toward capturing new customers. More value can be achieved through directing one's resources to keeping existing customers by serving them well and by providing them with the benefits they seek so that they will continue to give you business. The patient referred by a new referring physician does not necessarily bring in more revenue dollars than does the patient referred by a physician who has referred many times before. But there is a cost to promoting to the new physician, to explaining the benefits the program provides, the program characteristics, the types of program components and services provided, and so on. Although, clearly, some marketing funds need to be directed to promotion and capturing new business, more resources than in the past must be dedicated to better serving those who already do business with you.

THE PRODUCTION, PRODUCT, SALES, AND MARKETING CONCEPTS

In the exchange between the seller and the customer, marketers focus their efforts on different parts of the exchanges, usually with differing results. There are four classic ways of viewing the exchange process: the production concept, the product concept, the sales concept, and the marketing concept (Fig. 29-1; Box 29-1). We will briefly cover each of them, beginning with the production and product concepts, and see how they apply to pulmonary rehabilitation.

The Production Concept

The production concept focuses on the organizational capabilities allowing the efficient production of products and services, using the resources one already has or contemplates having in the near future. This concept assumes that marketing of the products or services is a given, that production is the primary management function to be performed, and that the market will necessarily want that which has been produced. Other than ensuring that the product or service is available and, owing to efficient production, within a price range that is affordable by the market, marketing plays little role in this exchange.

The Product Concept

The product concept may be viewed as a subset of the production process. The product concept again focuses on the existing resources of the organization, as does the production concept, but the high quality of the products or services that result from those resources

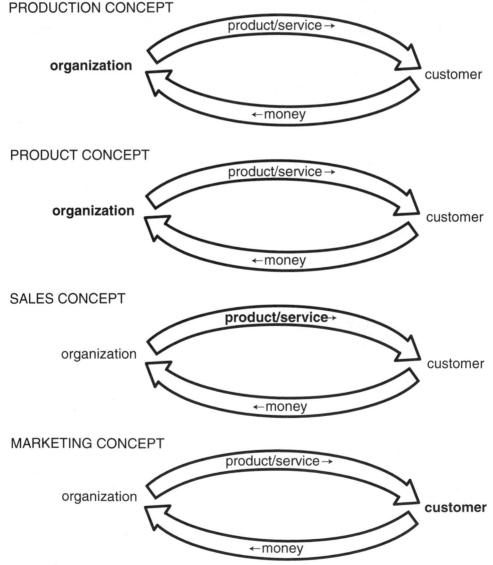

Figure 29-1. Production, product, sales, and marketing concepts. Bolded words indicate the focus of the marketing effort in each marketing concept.

Box 29-1. Marketing Orientation

Production concept
Product concept
Sales concept
Marketing concept—this is the best orientation

becomes the focus rather than the efficiency of production. This concept assumes that people will buy the products or services because of their high quality. Health care organizations have often operated by this concept owing to the assumptions that (*a*) high quality is the most important factor in the purchase of health care services and that (*b*) the marketplace is able to distinguish between varying levels of quality in health care.

Of course, given the numerous attempts of health care professionals to measure health care quality in the past decade, none of which has been accepted as definitive, it seems that no one has yet been able to define quality in the health care field. The National Forum for Health Care Quality Measurement and Reporting, an outgrowth of the President's Commission on Consumer Protection and Quality, was formed specifically to try to unify the many definitions of health care quality being put forth by such respected organizations as the JCAHO (Joint Commission on Accreditation of Healthcare Organizations), NCQA (National Committee for Quality Assurance), AMAP (American Medical Accreditation Program), FACCT (Foundation for Accountability), Quality of Health Care in America Project (part of the National Academy of Science's Institute of Medicine), and Consumer Coalition of Quality Health Care. The American Association of Cardiovascular and Pulmonary Rehabilitation Guidelines for Pulmonary Rehabilitation Programs,[3] the Official Statement of the American Thoracic Society: Pulmonary Rehabilitation 1999,[4] and Pulmonary Rehabilitation Joint ACCP/AACVPR Evidence-Based Guidelines[5] all are attempting to identify and define quality, but no universal agreement exists on how to adapt the guidelines to fit the specific pulmonary condition (e.g., restrictive lung disease). Moreover, none of these guidelines have systematically tested the patient perspective of quality through market research, using the 36-Item Short Form Health Survey or other market research tools, to test for customer satisfaction, so quality from the customer perspective remains unaddressed.

With no agreement on what constitutes quality in health care, all health care organizations, including pulmonary rehabilitation programs, have felt free to claim that they have high-quality health care. But, from a marketing standpoint, this provides no advantage to the health care organization because (*a*) few in the marketplace believe these claims given the ubiquitousness of the claim, (*b*) the claim provides no differentiation for a health care organization because it is likely that the organization's competitors are making the same claims, and (*c*) the organization itself may be deceived into viewing itself as high quality based on statements made to the marketplace. If so, it is not allowing itself to pursue the necessary discipline of examining its quality on a regular and systematic basis so as to engage in continuous quality improvement, which might in fact then place the organization in the position of having a service offering that is differentiated, at least for a period of time, by its quality. And this still leaves the question of what exactly is quality?

The Sales Concept

The sales concept focuses not on producing the product or service (whether of highest presumed quality or not) but on selling it. Whereas the first two concepts expect that demand is greater than or at least equal to supply, the sales concept comes into play when demand is less than supply (i.e., there are more units of service available than there are people who want to buy the service). Under these conditions, many organizations assume that it is necessary to stimulate demand, whether for the generic service or for the particular brand or provider of service. Stimulation of demand usually takes the form of advertising, promotion, and selling; it is from the sales concept that marketing derived negative aspects of its reputation (for hard sell, deceptive advertising, and gimmicky promotion).

Although it is not wrong to engage in advertising and promotion—in fact, it is necessary to promotes one's offering to the market if the market is to recognize that a benefit is being offered—it is poor marketing if that is the primary focus of marketing. The presumption of the sales concept is that if the customer only knew about the product or service offering, or if only the organization could attract attention to the offering through some unusual or interesting promotion, the customer would then buy it. However, similar to the production concept and the product concept, the sales concept does not explore whether the offering provides benefits to the customer. It unthinkingly assumes the benefits to be there and thus identifies the most important task to be that of raising awareness and comprehension of and preference for the product or service offering. In this vein, a pulmonary rehabilitation program manager who sighs "if the physicians only remembered we were here so that they would refer," or "if we could only get the hospital to give us a larger advertising budget, we could send out more brochures or advertise on local TV," but does not think to ask "are we providing a benefit to our various markets?" is a manager who is engaging in the sales concept.

The Marketing Concept

The marketing concept requires that the seller or organization producing the offering begin its marketing strategy by focusing on the market, not on the production of the product or service, not on the provider's view of quality of the product or service, and not on selling the product or service. The marketing concept is the focus within the exchange concept that marketing should take; whenever the marketing function and marketing strategy begins by serving the needs of something other than the marketplace, whether that be the seller, the insurer, the regulator, or the payer, it is destined not to be successful.

Table 29-1. Marketing Wants and Needs in Pulmonary Rehabilitation

Market	Pulmonary Rehabilitation Program Wants From Market	Market Wants From Pulmonary Rehabilitation Program
Physicians	Referrals of patients	Better health status and quality of life for the referred patient, best presented as outcomes and patient satisfaction data
	Earlier referral of patients before end-stage disease	A satisfied patient (a referral that does not reflect badly on the physician)
Patients	Self-referral	Better health status and quality of life
	Patient behavior to reflect recommendations of the pulmonary rehabilitation program (compliance)	A program that is convenient, easy to use/attend, and reimbursed
Payers, employers	Protocols that send patients to pulmonary rehabilitation programs when there is pulmonary disease, coverage of the full range of components/services provided by pulmonary rehabilitation programs	Friendly and empathetic staff, cost savings, proven efficacy, best presented as outcomes data

Employing the marketing concept, although the desired ideal of good marketing, is easier said than done. The marketing concept begins with determining what the market needs and wants; this, however, first requires identifying who the market is. In truth, most marketing efforts have more than one market. Health care providers certainly would consider the patients to be one of their markets. Referring physicians or other referring clinicians may also be a market. Managed care organizations and insurers are another market, as are employers, and so on. Once the seller's markets have been identified, the seller must determine what benefits each market wants and, in turn, what it wants from each market. Different markets are likely to want different benefits from the seller, and the seller may want different benefits from each market.

In the case of pulmonary rehabilitation programs, one might expect what is shown in Table 29-1.

USING OUTCOME MEASURES TO IMPLEMENT THE MARKETING CONCEPT

Implementing the marketing concept requires that the seller provide at least some of the benefits desired by the market, enough benefits to be competitive or to convince the market to take action. If one takes the payer, employer, and physician markets, it becomes easy to see why it might be difficult to market pulmonary rehabilitation programs to them. Payers and employers want cost savings and proven efficacy, presented in the form of research-based outcomes data. Physicians too want outcomes data; some physicians (increasing in number over time) are also sensitive to cost savings. The key marketing question then becomes: can pulmonary rehabilitation programs produce the desired outcome data for these markets?

Brian Carlin (1998)[6] notes in an article regarding outcomes measurement in pulmonary rehabilitation that the biochemical outcome measures that "may be the most accurate markers of how a person responds, at a cellular level, to rehabilitation therapy . . . have been the least studied of all of the outcome components of (the clinical) domain" (p 119), to include physiologic, dyspnea, and resource utilization components. One reason for this is the invasive procedures needed to collect the data from blood sampling draws to muscle biopsies. He goes on to say, regarding another outcome measurement, of physiologic measures of lung function (lung volumes and flow rates) before and after receiving pulmonary rehabilitation: "It has been shown, however, that lung volumes and flow rates do not change following pulmonary rehabilitation therapy" (p 119).[6] Yet this physiologic measure has served well in asthma and in determining the effects of lung surgery. The limitations of using pulmonary function measurement in outcomes is that it poorly correlates with dyspnea, health status, or health care utilization of the pulmonary patient (American Thoracic Society 1999 Pulmonary Rehabilitation Statement). Carlin[6] added, regarding resource utilization (another outcome measure): "Although measurement of these components is important, many of the studies involving pulmonary rehabilitation were not performed within the realm of the current health care environment (managed care, health maintenance organization). Such outcome measures are of great importance and must continue to be assessed in this ever-changing health care environment" (p 121).

Although pulmonary rehabilitation programs have produced positive outcome documentation (such as lower extremity training improving exercise tolerance and being recommended as part of pulmonary rehabilitation and the symptom of dyspnea improving with pulmonary rehabilitation), continued scientific research is needed to document many of the other components of a comprehensive pulmonary rehabilitation program, that is, rehabilitation of the non–chronic obstructive pulmonary disease and pediatric patient, should cigarette smokers be enrolled in pulmonary rehabilitation programs, what is the best type of upper extremity exercise, etc.[5] Programs cannot merely cite anecdotal evidence regarding the benefits of pulmonary rehabilitation. Supportive anecdotes may please those working in pulmonary rehabilitation programs, but the plural of anecdotes is not data; data are what most of the key markets need to be convinced of the value of the exchange.

Studies documenting positive outcomes and/or cost savings must be done or the exchanges desired by the pulmonary rehabilitation programs with the payer and employer markets will not likely happen. Moreover, because physicians are increasingly relying on protocols laid down by payers, and as physicians become more sensitive to issues of health care cost and outcomes, they too will require the same studies if they are to see the exchange (between the pulmonary rehabilitation programs and themselves) as beneficial. As Carlin notes, "it must be shown that a certain intervention actually benefits a patient . . . the assessment of outcomes is, and will be ever more so, an indicator of the overall effectiveness of comprehensive pulmonary rehabilitation" (p 124).[6]

The various markets desire many other benefits besides outcomes. Physicians want not only demonstrably good outcomes for the patients whom they refer, they also want programs that the patients like so that the patients will not return to complain to the referring physician. Patients want convenient hours and locations, easy-to-follow instructions, reimbursed services, and friendly and empathetic staff, in addition to wanting a better quality of life for themselves. Sophisticated marketers identify all the significant benefits sought by the market(s) and then attempt to deliver as many as are necessary to make the desired exchanges happen.

IDENTIFYING THE DESIRED MARKET BEHAVIORS

The marketing exchange requires not only that the seller produce desired benefits for the market but that the seller identify and develop a strategy to elicit the desired behaviors from the market. Take the physician market, for example. Pulmonary rehabilitation programs not only want physicians to refer patients to the programs but to refer them before they reach end-stage disease status. Pulmonary rehabilitation programs are not unique in this request.

Rheumatologists have also, for years, requested that primary care physicians refer, early in the onset of the disease, patients who begin to suffer the ills of arthritis. In the early stages, arthritis can be treated before permanent damage to the joints is done. The longer the delay in receiving proper treatment (which is often beyond the scope of that delivered by primary care physicians), the greater the chance of irreparable damage. Unfortunately, it is common for primary care physicians to try to treat the early stages of arthritis themselves, resorting to referring the patient to a rheumatologist only when the patient's pain and functional loss are beyond what the primary care physician believes he or she can treat. By this point, permanent arthritis-caused damage is likely to have occurred.

If the various behaviors desired by the seller from the market can be identified, then strategies can be developed that can attempt to elicit these behaviors. For example, realizing that some primary care physicians might not know that they should be referring a patient with arthritis to a specialist early in the onset of the disease, the professional association representing rheumatologists developed a clear list of symptoms that identified when a patient needed to be referred to a rheumatologic specialist. This list was distributed to primary care physicians throughout the country. In addition, an analysis of the marketing exchange with payers uncovered the need for research that would demonstrate that a patient who was referred early in the onset of the disease to a rheumatologist would end up costing the payer less than a patient who remained with the primary care physician. Without this research to demonstrate either better outcomes or greater cost-effectiveness of rheumatologic specialist intervention, and given the propensity of managed care organizations to have primary care physicians assume responsibility for treating patients who might in earlier years have otherwise seen specialists, the successful marketing of rheumatology physicians could not have happened.

Without clear thinking about what one wants from the market, it is likely that strategic action will be poorly directed. Merely to say that pulmonary rehabilitation programs want physician referrals and self-referrals (from patients) is not sufficient to give guidance for marketing strategy. Referrals will not be approved in a managed care environment unless the managed care organization is willing to cover the referral. Moreover, many insurers have guidelines and protocols that spell out when a referral is allowed, for what specific services a referral is allowed, how much service (in terms of time, number of visits, and so on), and to which providers. Thus, the behavior desired from the physicians and patients must, in many cases, be tied directly to the behaviors wanted from the insurers and managed care organizations: the coverage of comprehensive pulmonary rehabilitation, the provision to physicians of guidelines and protocols that encourage appropriate referral to pulmonary rehabilitation programs, and, for each pulmonary rehabilitation program, a contract with the insurers and managed care organizations. As noted previously, some of this can be achieved only with cost and/or outcome data that show to the insurers and managed care organizations the benefits of using pulmonary rehabilitation programs.

COMPETITIVE ANALYSIS

A central component of marketing is a competitive analysis. Historically, in the health care field, providers did not openly acknowledge competition. Hospitals talked of their service areas as if they had a divine right to serve the people living in that service area. Willingness to recognize competition has progressed unevenly in the United States; the Northeast region of the country still maintains some "gentlemen's agreements" between competing health care organizations, whereas on the West Coast the gloves have clearly come off and many health care organizations are openly battling it out for market share.

Regardless of where a program is located, save for rural areas where few health care providers of any type practice owing to sparse populations, pulmonary rehabilitation programs face competition. Many face direct competition in the form of other pulmonary rehabilitation programs in the same setting (e.g., hospital-based pulmonary rehabilitation programs competing with other hospital-based pulmonary rehabilitation programs). Other competition includes rehabilitation hospitals, comprehensive outpatient rehabilitation facilities (CORFs), home health agencies, and physician office–based pulmonary rehabilitation programs. In addition, some of these programs may raise the bar in competition by providing services in locations convenient for the patient, such as local senior centers where the elderly congregate for weekly bridge games, and at home or on-site, as part of their overall service to the patient. And then there are non–pulmonary rehabilitation competitors providing a component of pulmonary rehabilitation, such as stop smoking seminars.

It is typical of most organizations that they underestimate their competitors, dismiss the quality and strengths of the competitors, and, as a result, are unprepared to respond to the competition. It is never comforting to learn that your competitors are performing equal to or better than you are, whether it be in terms of reputation, patient-perceived quality of service, hours of service, location, customer service orientation, or other aspects of service. Nonetheless, this is valuable information to have. If you know what your competition is doing, it allows you either to replicate their strengths, so that you will no longer be at a competitive disadvantage, or at least to recognize the need to respond, whether by imitation of their strengths or by developing a distinctive competence for your own program. Ignorance of the competition invites being blind sided by their successful efforts. Ignoring the competition does not make the competition disappear; it merely gives them leeway to develop and pursue new strategies that may take yet more business away from your program before you have time to respond.

Therefore, it is important, as a part of a sophisticated marketing function, to systematically identify and assess what the competition is doing. A pulmonary rehabilitation program

Box 29-2. Ways of Systematically Identifying and Assessing
the Competition

> Request promotional literature from the competition
> Visit competitor websites
> "Blind shop" competitors
> Conduct market research
> Map out the location of competitors, including their range of services

could follow several activities, on a yearly or routine basis, that may help keep track of the activities of those whose success is likely to lessen the success of their own program (Box 29-2).

Call the Competition and Ask for Promotional Literature

Call competitors (at least once a year) as if you were a pulmonary rehabilitation patient and ask for them to send any promotional literature they may have. This lets you see not only what the competitors are claiming they do, what services they provide, and so on, but it gives you a sense of the quality of promotional materials they provide versus what you provide. If you have a willing physician who is not identified with your program, you might also have the physician ask for (physician-oriented) promotional material to see if the promotion directed to the physician market differs from that directed toward patients.

Visit Competitor Websites

Visit competitor websites and look for the same type of information as you would look for in the written promotion described above. Also, visit websites that pulmonary patients are likely to frequent (ask them which sites they visit). See if any of your competitors are linked into these websites; visit chat groups on these websites frequently as they often offer enormous insights into what patients are saying about their pulmonary providers, the care they receive, and what treatments work for them.

"Blind Shop" Your Competitors

It is possible that you can "blind shop" your competitors (i.e., visit and use your competitors' services as if you were a patient to see the level of convenience, customer service, speed, quality of service, and so on that they provide); this is difficult because you need a person with pulmonary disease (except for programs such as stop smoking programs). However, blind shopping can be enormously valuable in educating your program about how competing programs provide service. Just as the flight experience can vary dramatically from airline to airline (Southwest Airline personnel are in costume handing out candy on Halloween, whereas some other airlines barely muster a Merry Christmas on Christmas Day), so can the service experience in health care settings. These are experiential differences that can be recognized only through the experience itself. However, these experiences are often one of the key determinants of customer satisfaction.

Conduct Market Research

Market research with referring and nonreferring physicians is recommended if it is within the budget of the pulmonary rehabilitation program. Although referring physicians can identify what they—and their patients—like and dislike about your program, they are the physicians who are the most satisfied because they are still referring to your program. (This of course may not be the case if the physicians are captive and can refer only to your program because of insurance/managed care rules for the patient or to the employment conditions of the physician.) Physicians who do not refer to your program presumably are referring elsewhere and can tell you how the competing programs perform, their strengths and weaknesses, and what it would take in the way of program changes for you to attract their referrals away from the competition. Or, alternatively, nonreferring physicians are not referring to any pulmonary rehabilitation program because they are either unaware of the programs or they do not believe that pulmonary rehabilitation programs provide significant benefits to them or their patients. (This is where positive outcome data could help market a pulmonary rehabilitation program.)

Determine the Location of Your Competitors, Including the Range of Services

Map out where your competitors are located, including the range of services provided by each. Sometimes, what is not evident in discussion becomes evident when visually mapped out. This includes mapping out individual providers who are not in similar organizational settings (such as hospitals) who provide competing services, as well as nondirect competitors (such as the for-profit smoking cessation competitors) who may compete on a service-specific basis. It also includes accounting for disease management programs in areas such as asthma, which may have sessions offered in facilities that do not have a direct competitor. Some disease management programs will be hard to represent on a map because they are largely delivered through the mail, telephone reminders, group meetings in a variety of locations, and so on. Because many disease management programs (in asthma) are offered not by traditional pulmonary rehabilitation programs or hospitals but by pharmaceutical companies and national disease management companies, they will not necessarily be captured on a map, but their presence as competitors must be represented. Otherwise, it is possible to ignore them temporarily as competitors; however, these large competitors have the resources to outspend local programs. They may in the future represent potential joint venture partnerships and deserve ongoing attention. Collaboration with competitors is possible simultaneously when competing with them; for example, competing providers sometimes join forces so that they represent a larger piece of business when sitting down to negotiate with managed care plans.

The value of competitor information is that it guides both proactive and reactive marketing strategy. Unless a field is unchanging, one will see some competitors surge ahead while others fall behind. In the current environment, pulmonary rehabilitation programs that devote attention to evidence-based medicine, to more rigorous screening of patients (owing to insurers' and employers' concerns), to the use of science and empirical data to drive pulmonary rehabilitation practice and the design of pulmonary rehabilitation programs, and to non–outcome-related benefits sought by physicians and patients are likely to be the ones in the forefront.

THE TOOLS OF MARKETING STRATEGY: THE MARKETING MIX

The basic tools of marketing strategy are the marketing mix: product or service, price, place, and promotion. The four components should be viewed as a jigsaw puzzle: the puzzle is not complete unless all four pieces are put in place and fit with each other.

As an example of the need for them to mesh well with each other, consider the possibility of marketing another professional service: legal services. A law firm seeking to position itself as a top-notch, high-quality law firm (product or service) would need to charge high fees (price), be located in an upscale office building (place), and promote itself in ways that suggest quality (holding a once a year invitation-only golf tournament for its professional staff and clients at a prestigious country club) (promotion). Imagine if instead it located itself in a decaying area in a building that was dirty and dingy (place) and advertised itself on the basis of price ("10 hours or more of legal staff time: $99.99 an hour") (promotion and price). Clearly, the latter strategy is a recipe for disaster.

The tools themselves are self-explanatory. However, some useful comments can be made about each as they apply to pulmonary rehabilitation programs.

Product or Service

Healthcare providers produce and provide services. Services are (*a*) intangible, meaning that the service itself cannot be touched, tasted, felt, and so on; however, the people who deliver the service are tangible as is the location in which the service is delivered; (*b*) perishable, meaning they cannot be stored once they are produced, so when a patient fails to show up for an appointment, the service scheduled for that time is lost forever; (*c*) variable, meaning that one group counseling session may differ dramatically from another—they vary; and (*d*) inseparable, meaning that the service cannot be separated from the person who provides it, and the customer generally also must be present, so he or she too is inseparable from the service provider. The marketing implications of being a service—from staff recruitment and training to scheduling and appointment systems to cleaning schedules for the facilities in which the services are delivered—are too enormous to cover here. A good explanation of service marketing is provided in Heskett et al.[7]

Pulmonary rehabilitation programs comprise a variety of services, referred to by marketers as a product or service line. The service lines in pulmonary rehabilitation programs will differ somewhat. However, if they differ significantly, this can cause confusion in the marketplace. Individual chiropractors may provide different services in their offices, for example. Some provide only spinal manipulation; others offer not only spinal manipulation but promote themselves as alternatives to primary care physicians, stating that they are able to diagnose and treat most common forms of illness. As a result, a person looking for a new chiropractor does not know what the new chiropractor he or she is visiting is likely to offer in the way of services before his or her visit; the patient may be expecting only spinal manipulation when instead the chiropractor takes his blood pressure and initiates a series of diagnostic tests unrelated to spinal manipulation.

Occupational therapists suffer from the same problem. Some occupational therapists are dedicated to restoring function sufficient to allow the individual to return to work. Others spend most of their time in skilled nursing facilities, with people who will never return to work, to maintain the residents in the skilled nursing facility at their highest level of functioning. Some occupational therapists spend much of their time developing and providing training to patients on technological and mechanical devices that are designed to improve functioning; others use little in the way of technological and product support. As a result, when one asks an occupational therapist: "What do you do?" the answer may vary significantly according to whom you ask because of the breadth of patient population serviced, the facility where service is provided, and the range of services offered.

In a more limited manner, the same problem may manifest itself with pulmonary rehabilitation. Medicare provides no national standards as of 1999 for what pulmonary rehabilitation services are covered. Some pulmonary rehabilitation specialists and programs view the practice of pulmonary rehabilitation as focusing largely on end-stage or significant pulmonary disease. In contrast, others view the service line as equally divided between prevention, where disease has not been evident yet, and treatment. Some pulmonary rehabilitation programs accept smokers as patients, with the hope that their intervention will get the smoker to stop smoking. Other pulmonary rehabilitation programs are unwilling to admit smokers into their programs as patients at all.

This is a marketing problem because not only do pulmonary rehabilitation programs have to market themselves but the profession as a whole has to market itself. If the profession does not speak with a unified voice, it is that much harder to get a message across because multiple and conflicting messages may be reaching the marketplace. Physicians may not know fully for what diseases, stage of disease, or type of therapy they can refer a patient to a pulmonary rehabilitation program and for what they should refer elsewhere. Insurers are often accused of trying to provide coverage only for the minimum necessary.

They may be justified in covering less rather than more of the service line, adopting the statements put forth by those pulmonary rehabilitation specialists who support only the most limited definition of what a pulmonary rehabilitation program does. And nonpulmonary competitors can use the division in the profession to position themselves against pulmonary rehabilitation programs by saying "even the pulmonary rehabilitation specialists themselves say they do not provide prevention services." Although this is a marketing problem that one pulmonary rehabilitation program by itself is unable to address, it is a problem that conceivably affects all pulmonary rehabilitation programs and needs to be addressed on a professionwide basis.

And again, the claim that pulmonary rehabilitation specialists can and should provide prevention services will not receive wide approval from buyers (insurers, managed care organizations, employers) and referrers unless research supports the claim. Although everyone agrees that prevention, especially smoking cessation, is important, that in no way suggests that pulmonary rehabilitation programs are the mechanism best suited to provide these prevention services. As stated before, cost and outcome data—evidence that pulmonary rehabilitation programs are better able to get smokers to stop smoking for the long term than are their non–pulmonary rehabilitation program competitors—are the best arguments to use in marketing to purchasers, if in fact this is the decision that the profession wishes to make. This ultimately devolves into a service line decision: what services do pulmonary rehabilitation programs provide?

Price

Many prices are to be considered because in health care, where many reimbursers have many different contracts with a variety of service providers, everyone rarely pays the same price for a specified service. Moreover, even when an insurer, managed care organization, Medicare, or other source pays for the services of a pulmonary rehabilitation program, the patient still incurs out-of-pocket costs (deductibles, uncovered services in the service line, etc.). The nonmonetary costs include the discomfort and fear of developing dyspnea with exercise or of having an arterial blood gas taken, the dehumanization that occurs every time a patient has to put on a hospital gown (which, as one patient stated in a focus group interview, made him feel like a concentration camp prisoner, stuck in the same uniform as all the others around him), the waiting to be seen, and so on. The larger pricing challenge may be the internal price to the system in a capitated environment (which speaks to cost efficiencies, reengineering processes to cut costs), but the nonmonetary pricing issues are significant enough to create marketing problems if ignored.

Place

The three aspects to the concept of place are geographic access, time access, and promotional access.

Geographic Access

Geographic access relates to such issues as distance the patient must travel to reach the program, difficulties in parking at the facility, lack of public transportation that is modified to serve the handicapped, and the ease with which the patient can reach the program once he or she arrives at the facility. (Does it require a long walk? Are there stairs? Is the signage directing the patient to the program area clear?) Of the three types of access issues that pulmonary rehabilitation programs face, geographic access is probably best addressed.

Time Access

Time access speaks to the hours and days of service availability, not only in terms of the time when the pulmonary rehabilitation specialists are on site at the program but also available on the telephone to answer questions, to help with medication concerns, and so on. And increasingly, with interactive websites becoming more common, the availability of information over the web is an access problem—if the expectations are that your program should have a well-designed website where information is easily accessible.

Promotional Access

Promotional access is the least well-understood access issue from a conceptual standpoint. Consider that one could promote a pulmonary rehabilitation program either by sending out a professional representative to seek referrals of patients from physicians or, alternatively, by advertising in local newspapers, in community centers serving seniors, on television, and on websites directed to the lay public seeking self-referrals (not that these are mutually exclusive but that they are distinctly different ways of promoting a pulmonary rehabilitation program). The first example (seeking referrals from physicians) is called a push strategy; it relies on what is essentially personal selling on the part of the physician or pulmonary rehabilitation specialist to make the patient aware of and convince the patient to attend the pulmonary rehabilitation program. Historically, professional service organizations (hospitals, law firms, dental practices, physician practices) relied on the push strategy. In the past 2 decades, the norms against advertising have broken down, however, allowing more health care organizations to engage in a pull strategy, where the organization advertises and promotes itself in the public media with no involvement of personal selling.

Push Strategy

The advantages of a push strategy are that the costs are usually less than that of a pull strategy (although health care organizations usually spend so little on promotion relative to other industries that even push strategies are insensibly underfunded). Personal recommendation by an "expert" through the use of the push strategy will also usually outweigh any amount of advertising and impersonal promotion; it is unlikely that a patient will say "my physician told me I should go to the Smith Hospital pulmonary rehabilitation program, but I liked the advertising of the Jones Hospital pulmonary rehabilitation program. I think I'll go there." The disadvantages of the push strategy are that (*a*) the "experts" may know enough to make informed judgments *and* one of those judgments may be that *your* pulmonary rehabilitation program is not as high quality as another pulmonary rehabilitation program; selling alone will not suffice; and (*b*) you have no control over what the "expert" will say. Referrers are not paid (and it is illegal to pay them—that is called a kickback) and are free to say and recommend what they want.

Pull Strategy

A pull strategy, on the other hand, can give more control over the content of the message to the pulmonary rehabilitation program. The program can decide exactly what it wants to say and how it wants to say it in advertising, in brochures, on websites, and so on. However, the disadvantages to a pull strategy are significant. First, many in the health care field are still somewhat uncomfortable with the advertising of health care services. Physicians, who are counted on for referral may be especially unlikely to appreciate aggressive advertising campaigns if the advertising strikes them in any way as unprofessional. Yet, a strategy of playing it safe by producing low-key promotional campaigns that will not offend may backfire because the campaigns may be so low key that they do not attract the attention of the market and therefore do not attract patients to the program.

Equally important as a disadvantage, pull campaigns are very expensive. It is the rare health care provider organization that is willing to commit the funds necessary to a pull campaign to make it effective. The alternative of committing whatever funds are available—but completely inadequate—to a pull campaign is wasteful. A critical mass of advertising is necessary merely to create awareness of a brand name (e.g., the Saint Elsewhere Pulmonary Rehabilitation Program) without necessarily conveying a message (e.g., we have expanded evening hours of service). Given the small size of most pulmonary rehabilitation programs, it is not probable that such funds as are necessary would be made available for a successful pull strategy.

Promotion

One need not be astute to recognize that the discussion of promotional access overlaps directly with the marketing tool of promotion. They are intertwined and often indistinguishable. Therefore, what has been discussed previously can be applied in this section directly. The tendency to look at marketing and see only the promotional aspects of it is prevalent throughout the health care field; it is a common mistake and should be avoided by starting the discussion of the promotional aspects of the strategy by first asking: Who is the target for the promotion and advertising? What benefits do we have to offer them? How are we going to present these benefits to them? Are the benefits offered through the use (or purchase or referral or whatever) of our services competitive with other services offered to the same market? Will the target market have access to our promotion? How will we measure their response to our promotion and/or advertising? Failure of a pulmonary rehabilitation program to address advertising and promotion in this manner will likely result in unsuccessful promotion.

Some time-honored promotional practices of pulmonary rehabilitation programs may fare well, looking through the eyeglass provided by these questions. For example, inservices directed toward community groups such as the American Lung Association would seem to be a good tactic for promotional purposes. On the other hand, investment in National Pulmonary Rehabilitation Week may not provide a good payoff. Although pulmonary rehabilitation specialists and program graduates may find this week to be positive, it is not clear that others do.

By example, consider another group in the health care field that has its special week: National Nursing Home Week. Did you know there even was a National Nursing Home Week? If so, did you know when it was? Did it change your behavior? That is, did it make it more likely that you would recommend nursing homes to patients or friends? Did it increase the overall brand equity of nursing homes in general? Do you really care about National Nursing Home Week? Almost certainly, the answer is "no," as a small study of the value of the week to the nursing home industry showed.

Now ask these same questions of someone other than a pulmonary rehabilitation specialist (and the specialist's relatives, program graduates, and family members) about National Pulmonary Rehabilitation Week. Again, the answer is likely to be "no." No special reason exists to promote heavily in that one week that which must be promoted year round if demand for pulmonary rehabilitation programs is to remain high year round. The focus on the one week is probably a result of there being inadequate funds to promote year round as opposed to National Pulmonary Rehabilitation Week being developed as a well-grounded promotional strategy. In reality, it is better, when funds are limited, to undertake only a few promotional activities and to do those few well rather than to try to undertake many, all underfunded, and do all of them poorly. This could be a vindication of National Pulmonary Rehabilitation Week, if that is in fact what happens. It is best to reexamine every promotional and advertising dollar and ask the strategic questions noted previously.

SUMMARY

In a highly competitive environment, it is no longer appropriate to ask if one should market one's program's services. By making the services available, one is already engaging in marketing. The key issues then become designing marketing strategies with an eye to developing long-term relationships with one's customers, not merely seeking short-term exchanges with each customer or referral source. In addition, pulmonary rehabilitation programs must seek to act by the marketing concept rather than the production, product, or sales concepts, none of which provide the desired focus on the marketplace. A third point is the recognition that, in today's health care field, the singularly most important benefit sought by the many markets with which pulmonary rehabilitation programs deal may be documented outcomes, supported by solid research. Marketing requires also that pulmonary rehabilitation programs identify not only what the various markets want from pulmonary rehabilitation programs but also what exact behaviors the pulmonary rehabilitation programs' marketing efforts are intended to elicit from the various markets.

Furthermore, good marketing requires a competitive analysis. Few pulmonary rehabilitation programs operate today without competition. In light of that, and recognizing that no one likes to acknowledge their competition, especially if the competitors might be outperforming one's own pulmonary rehabilitation program, the failure to carry out a competitive analysis represents nothing short of bad management and bad marketing. Good marketing strategy development involves using the tools of the marketing mix: product or service, price, place, and promotion. These tools must all fit together like a jigsaw puzzle or the marketing strategy will be flawed. As opposed to the commonly held view of marketing as a few brochures, a celebration of National Pulmonary Rehabilitation Week, and some advertising, marketing is an analytically based function that systematically collects data, analyzes it, and periodically adjusts the marketing strategy to reflect the changing marketplace.

REFERENCES

1. Kotler P. Marketing Management. 9th ed. Englewood Cliffs, NJ: Prentice Hall, 1998.
2. Clarke R, Kotler P. Marketing for Health Care Organizations. 2nd ed. Englewood Cliffs, NJ: Prentice Hall, 2000.
3. American Association of Cardiovascular and Pulmonary Rehabilitation. Guidelines for Pulmonary Rehabilitation Programs. 2nd ed. Champaign, IL: Human Kinetics, 1998:1–248.
4. American Thoracic Society. Pulmonary rehabilitation—1999: official statement of the American Thoracic Society adopted by the ATS board of directors, November 1998. Am J Respir Crit Care Med 1999;159:1666–1682.
5. Ries AL, et al., The ACCP/AACVPR Pulmonary Rehabilitation Guidelines Panel. Pulmonary rehabilitation: joint ACCP/AACVPR evidence-based guidelines. J Cardiopulm Rehabil 1997;17:371–405.
6. Carlin BW. Outcome measurement in pulmonary rehabilitation. Resp Care Clinics of North America. Pulm Rehab 1998;4(1):113–127.
7. Heskett J, Sasser E, Hart C. Service Breakthroughs: Changing the Rules of the Game. New York: Free Press, 1990.

30 Reimbursement for Pulmonary Rehabilitation

Lia Shaw Miller
Gerilynn L. Connors

Professional Skills

Upon completion of this chapter, the reader will:

- Trace the evolution of health care insurance from the 18th century to the 21st century
- Identify the sources of health care financing and programs that represent each type
- Describe the Medicare program, its components, coverage, and claims processing mechanism
- Identify the dominant forms of managed care and compare and contrast their characteristics
- Understand the specific requirements for pulmonary rehabilitation treatment documentation
- List the Medicare noncovered services and how they impact your program's documentation
- Develop a pulmonary rehabilitation patient medical record keeping method that meets your program's goals to document outcomes and be used for benchmarking
- State the similarities in health care around the world in terms of economics and standards of care

HISTORICAL PERSPECTIVE

Historically, the demand for health insurance originated in the breakdown of a household economy, as families depended on the employment of the primary wage earner for income and on the services of physicians and hospitals for medical treatment. Illness caused an interruption in the flow of income to a household, causing economic hardship. The need for health insurance in the United States was more than a private problem. The strain of the rising cost of health care imposed on society as a whole generated great debate in the politics of health insurance in the early 1900s and continues to do so today as we move into the 21st century.

Before the enactment of the Medicare and Medicaid programs, health care was financed through private commercial insurance or was paid for privately. As far back as 1798 Congress created a system of compulsory hospital insurance for merchant seamen. This, however, was an unusual step to protect a group that was vital to foreign commerce.[1,2] As early as 1900, a few states became involved with workmen's compensation laws, and by 1920 these laws were accepted by 42 states. Cash payments for a worker's time lost from the job because of injury or illness was the first benefit, later followed by coverage for health care and rehabilitation services.

Box 30-1. A Chronological Development of Health Insurance in the United States

1798	The federal government established a limited system of compulsory hospital insurance for merchant seaman
1904	The Socialist political party is first to endorse health insurance
1912	Theodore Roosevelt's Bull Moose party platform supports national health insurance
1920	Forty-two states enact workers' compensation laws
1929	The first private hospital insurance established at Baylor University Hospital
1929	Rural farmer's health cooperative established in Elk City, Oklahoma, by physician Michael Shadid; it is one of the first prepaid health plans in the United States
1930s	Blue Cross plan first organized financial protection to its subscribers
1935	Social Security Act passes, calling for equal access to health care
1939	California and Michigan medical societies organize the first Blue Shield plans providing coverage for physician services
1942	Kaiser Permanente Medical Care Program established in Northern California and the Vancouver-Portland region
1948	Unions negotiate health insurance benefits for members and the Internal Revenue Service allows premiums as a business expense for employers and nontaxable income for employees
1949	The Truman administration introduces a bill for comprehensive and universal health care coverage; caused great debate in the legislature for the next 16 years
1965	Congress establishes Medicare and Medicaid as amendments to the Social Security Act
1965	Medicare supplement insurance, "Medigap," policies are developed to fill the gaps and supplement the benefits and coverage Medicare provides
1969	State and local Physician Review Organizations (PROs) and Certificate of Need (CON) laws established as a mechanism to review quality of care and public need for services as a way of controlling costs
1972	Medicare program expands to include coverage for the disabled and individuals with end-stage renal disease
1973	Congress enacts the Health Maintenance Organization Act of 1973 (PL 93-222)
1977	Medicare leaves the Social Security Administration to be administered by the Health Care Financing Administration (HCFA), an agency within the US Department of Health and Human Services (DHHS)
1978	The HCFA develops a new system for uniform hospital reporting to enhance quality and uniformity
1982	Comprehensive Outpatient Rehabilitation Facility (CORF) regulations established
1983	Diagnosis Related Groups (DRGs) phased in for hospital admissions based on 467 DRGs, a prospective payment system (PPS) to control costs
1986	Omnibus Reconciliation Act gives states the option to expand Medicaid coverage as it pertains to respiratory care services for home ventilator–dependent individuals
1988	Medicare Catastrophic Coverage Act expands Medicare benefits, but because of the nation's budget deficit, it is repealed
1990	Congress expands Medicare coverage for low-income working disabled persons with the Qualified Disabled and Working Individual (QDWI) program
1991	More than 34 million elderly and disabled people enrolled in Medicare, costing more than $104 billion
1992	By order of Congress, the variety of MedSup policies is reduced to 10 standardized policies, A–J, offering specific and identical benefits for each plan
1996	Health Insurance Portability and Accountability Act of 1996 (NIPAA) passes, designed to protect health insurance coverage for workers and their families when they change or lose jobs
1997	Population of Medicare beneficiaries consists of 33.7 million elderly and 5.0 million nonelderly persons, costing more than $208 billion
1997	Balanced Budget Act of 1997 (BBA) signed into law, thereby achieving the target Medicare savings of $115 billion in fiscal years 1998–2002
1999	National public education campaign around Medicare occurs, implementing the largest peacetime education program the federal government has ever undertaken

The Medicare and Medicaid programs evolved during a 53-year period, starting with Theodore Roosevelt's Bull Moose party platform in 1912. The Bull Moose party platform first promoted the ideal of having national health insurance.[1,3] Then, in 1935, when the Social Security Act was passed, Congress submitted bills that called for equal access to health care because the major source of health care financing was provided by not-for-profit, prepayment, or commercial insurance plans. During the Truman administration, in 1949, a bill was introduced calling for comprehensive and universal health care coverage. This domestic legislation was stalled in Congress for years because of political squabbles debating whether it was politically feasible and whether it should be narrowed in scope. Congress feared that this general medical insurance plan would be a "giveaway" program independent of need that would help the "well-off" American, cause a glut of demand for services beyond the supply capacity, and create excessive federal control of physicians, leading to Socialism in America. Truman's advisors narrowed the eligibility of the plan to persons 65 years and older who had contributed to a Social Security program during their past employment. Intense debate occurred over some form of national health insurance from 1949 to 1965, when at last the Medicare and Medicaid laws were finally passed under the guidance of the Kennedy and Johnson administrations. The laws were amendments to the Social Security Act, which incorporated proposals from three sources: the Johnson administration to limit coverage of hospital and nursing home care financed through Social Security; the American Medical Association plan for "elder care" providing comprehensive benefits, but with limited eligibility; and the Republican Byrne proposal, which was not compulsory and covered physician services and drugs. The Byrne proposal was also financed by general federal revenues instead of Social Security.[4] The great complexity between governmental process and social policy is evident in the health insurance arena. The chronological development of health insurance in the United States is shown in Box 30-1.

SOURCES OF HEALTH CARE FINANCING

In the United States, the financing of health care services originates from three basic sources: (*a*) federal and state governmental health insurance programs, (*b*) nongovernmental health insurance programs, and (*c*) private pay. A further explanation of the different sources for reimbursement is shown in Box 30-2. Payment of health care services is made by third-party payers or by the patient. A third-party payer is an organization (e.g., a

Box 30-2. Sources of Health Care Financing

Nongovernmental health insurance programs
  Private/commercial health insurance plans
  Managed care organizations
  Medicare Supplement/Medigap plans
Federal and state health insurance programs
  Medicare
  Medicaid
  Hill-Burton Program
  Comprehensive Outpatient Rehabilitation Facility
  Veterans Health Administration program
  Civilian Health and Medical Program of the Uniformed Services (CHAMPUS)/
    TRICARE
  Federal Employees Health Benefit (FEHB) program
Casualty insurance program
  Workers' compensation, related to accidents on the job

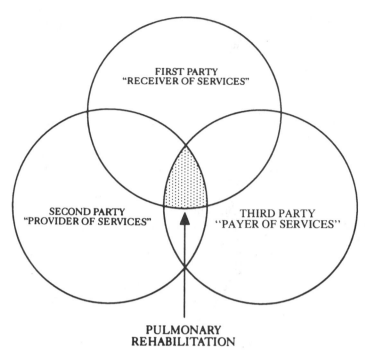

FIRST PARTY
"RECEIVER OF SERVICES"

SECOND PARTY
"PROVIDER OF SERVICES"

THIRD PARTY
"PAYER OF SERVICES"

PULMONARY
REHABILITATION

Figure 30-1. The correlation of insurance terminology to pulmonary rehabilitation is necessary for effective communication with the insurance industry and for program reimbursement. Pulmonary rehabilitation involves first-, second-, and third-party involvement, with each party having a specific function as it relates to pulmonary rehabilitation. Understanding the party function is essential to ensure reimbursement for the program.

commercial insurance company) that pays or insures medical/health expenses on behalf of its beneficiaries, members, or clients. Therefore, the patient receiving the medical service is considered the first party, the provider of the medical service is considered the second party, and the organization paying for the medical service is the third party (Fig. 30-1).

NONGOVERNMENTAL HEALTH INSURANCE PROGRAMS

Private Health Insurance Programs

Private health insurance programs are a method of redistributing the financial risk associated with major illnesses from individuals to collectives mediated by commercial insurance companies. Private insurers underwrite the coverage without becoming involved in the delivery system. Insurance was developed to protect people from economic hardships. The social reform movement of 1915 to 1920 argued that health insurance would relieve poverty caused by sickness by distributing the uneven wage losses and medical costs that individual families experienced. I.M. Rubinow, a leading authority on social insurance who was both a physician and an actuary as well as a Socialist, saw health insurance as the means to sever the vicious cycle of disease and poverty.[2] Health insurance would prevent the families of the sick from becoming destitute and thereby prevent further sickness. The first private insurance was established at Baylor University Hospital in 1929 and was called a prepaid plan. The university hospital agreed to provide 1500 schoolteachers up to 21 days of hospital care a year for $6.00 per person.[1,2] When the Depression occurred in the 1930s, the financial insecurity of the nation's voluntary hospitals was exposed and hospitals began to turn to insurance as a way to remain solvent. The first organization to develop financial protection for its subscribers against economic loss by hospitalization was the Blue Cross program. At the time, payment for services was negotiated between the hospital and the plans. Then, in 1939, the California State Medical Society organized the first Blue Shield plan, covering comprehensive medical and surgical services during hospitalization for a premium of $1.70 per month.[1] In the same year, the medical society in Michigan also organized a prepayment plan.[2] Blue Cross and Blue Shield plans were multiplying rapidly, as were the number of plan subscribers. In 1948, the Supreme Court ruled that unions could negotiate health insurance benefits for their members. The Internal Revenue Service ruled that health insurance premiums paid by employers were considered a business expense and premiums paid by employees were not taxable income. These changes caused such an explosion in subscribers during the years that by 1978, approximately 83 million people had Blue Cross coverage and about 70 million people had Blue Shield coverage. Commercial insurances that were either mutual (owned by policyholders) or stock (outside ownership) also entered the health insurance market, offering insurance for a variety of personal risks. More than 700 commercial insurance companies wrote most of the health insurance policies in 1978.[5] Between 1993 and 1997 the proportion of the population younger than 65 years with private health insurance remained stable at 70 to 71%. Approximately 92% of private coverage was obtained through a current or former employer or union in 1997.[6]

Managed Care

The concept of managed care in the United States as we know it today is an outgrowth of the private sector and dates back to the late 1920s. The vision of Michael Shadid, a local physician in Elk City, Oklahoma, was the first attempt to reorganize medical care on a prepaid, comprehensive basis. In 1929 he established a rural farmer's cooperative health plan in a community of 6000, selling membership subscriptions to local farmers to raise money for a new hospital and to establish annual dues to cover the costs of care.[2] In 1934, the medical staff of the cooperative consisted of four new specialists and a dentist and was supported by 600 family memberships. Managed care continued to evolve with the establishment of the Ross-Loos Clinic in Los Angeles, the creation of two physicians, Donald Ross and H. Clifford Loos. The clinic was originally designed to provide comprehensive medical services to employees of the Los Angeles Department of Water. By 1935, the Ross-Loos Clinic had grown to include other employee groups, mostly from governmental agencies, enrolling more than 12,000 workers.

Between 1930 and 1960 numerous other major prepaid group practice plans emerged, including the Group Health Association in Washington, DC, in 1937, the Kaiser Permanente Medical Care Program in 1942, the Group Health Cooperative of Seattle in 1947. Despite the opposition such programs experienced from organized medicine, they also experienced significant success in attracting enrollees.

In early 1970, the term health maintenance organization (HMO) was given to prepaid group practice plans to emphasize the focus on health promotion and prevention, thus making HMOs more attractive. Paul M. Ellwood, Jr, a Minneapolis physician, is responsible for introducing the term (HMO) that we associate most frequently with managed care today. The growth of managed care increased significantly when Congress enacted the HMO Act of 1973 (PL 93-222). The legislation provided grants and loans to develop new HMOs. To qualify for funding, an HMO had to offer specific basic services and charge premiums based on "community"-wide health care costs.

The concept of managed care is more often discussed than it is defined. This may be because managed care is used in many ways and eludes clear definitions. Partially, this may be because managed care refers to both programs that coordinate, rationalize, and direct the delivery of care without being risk based, and it also refers to care managed by organizations that assume full financial risk for the care managed. As managed care has evolved in the past few decades, so has its own unique vocabulary and accompanying acronym list. See Box 30-3 for a glossary of terms. It is essential to recognize that not all

Box 30-3. Glossary of Managed Care Terms

Ambulatory Patient Classification (APC): A prospective payment system for the outpatient, ambulatory care provided in hospital ambulatory surgery, emergency department, and outpatient clinic settings. APCs provide an incentive for health care providers to become more efficient. Payment is set in advance based on the diagnostic and treatment classification system.

Approved Charge: The maximum fee that a third-party payer (insurer organization) will use in reimbursing providers for a given service.

Assignment: The method of Medicare reimbursement whereby a physician or supplier agrees to accept the amount approved by the Medicare carrier as total payment for covered services. The physician or supplier submits the claim on behalf of the beneficiary and is paid directly.

Beneficiary: Individual who is using or eligible to use insurance benefits, including health insurance benefits, under an insurance contract.

Capitation: A payment system whereby managed care plans pay health care providers a negotiated fixed dollar amount, usually monthly, for providing services to a plan member (per capita). Providers are not reimbursed for services that exceed the fixed amount.

Carrier: A commercial health insurance company that contracts with the Health Care Financing Administration (HCFA) to process claims for Medicare Part B services.

CHAMPUS: The Civilian Health and Medical Program of the Uniformed Services is a government program that provides hospital and medical services to active-duty and retired Armed Services personnel younger than 65 years and their eligible dependents.

Coordination of Benefits (COB): The provision and procedures used by insurers to avoid duplicate payment when a person is covered by two or more health insurance plans. Coordination determines which insurance is the primary payer.

Copayment: A specified dollar amount or percentage of health care costs that the beneficiary is required to pay for health care services.

Physicians' Current Procedural Terminology (CPT): A list of identifying codes for reporting medical services and procedures performed by physicians and other health care professionals. The industry standard for reporting of physician procedures and services.

Durable Medical Equipment (DME): Medical equipment that must be able to withstand repeated use, is not disposable, is used to serve a medical purpose, is generally not useful to a person in the absence of sickness or injury, and is appropriate for use in the home.

Diagnosis Related Groups (DRGs): Payment categories for inpatient hospital services based on principal diagnosis, secondary diagnosis, surgical procedures, age, sex, and presence of complications. Financing mechanism used under Medicare's prospective payment system (PPS) and selected other providers whereby reimbursement to hospitals is made at a set rate.

End-Stage Renal Disease (ESRD): A medical condition in which a person's kidneys no longer function, requiring the individual to receive dialysis or a kidney transplant to sustain his or her life.

Explanation of Medicare Benefits (EOMB): The statement that informs beneficiaries and physicians about what action was taken by the carrier in processing the Medicare claim. The notice includes information for both parties about their appeal rights and liability for the cost of services.

Fee-for-Service (FFS): A payment system in which an amount is reimbursed for each encounter or service provided. Payment is made retrospectively or after the fact.

Fiscal Intermediary (FI): A private health insurance organization under contract with the HCFA to process Medicare Part A claims.

Gatekeeper: A primary care physician responsible for overseeing and coordinating all aspects of a patient's care under managed care plans.

Box 30-3 (*Continued*)

Health Insurance Claim (HIC) Number: The unique alphanumeric Medicare entitlement number assigned to a Medicare beneficiary that appears on the Medicare card.

Health Maintenance Organization (HMO): An organization that provides a comprehensive range of health benefits to an individual for a prepaid fee. An HMO contracts with health care providers, physicians, hospitals, and other health professionals, and members are required to use participating providers for all health services.

Indemnity: Traditional insurance programs that pay a fixed amount for covered services received. Generally referred to as fee-for-service programs.

Independent Practice Association (IPA): A health maintenance organization (HMO) delivery model in which the managed care organization contracts with a physician organization, which, in turn, contracts with individual physicians. The physicians are members of the IPA, an independent legal entity, but maintain their own separate offices and identities. The HMO reimburses the IPA on a capitated basis. Physicians are compensated by the IPA on a per capita fee schedule or fee-for-service basis.

International Classification of Diseases, 9th Edition, Clinical Modification (ICD-9-CM): Coding system of diagnoses required on all bills submitted for Medicare payment and most other third-party payers.

Medigap: A Medicare supplement policy designed to provide coverage for Medicare deductibles and coinsurance; some policies provide additional benefits. Policies must conform to 1 of 10 standard packages of benefits, referred to as A through J.

Medicare Summary Notice (MSN): The notice that informs beneficiaries and physicians about what action was taken by the carrier in processing the Medicare claim. Replaces the older Explanation of Medicare Benefits (EOMB).

Participating Physician: A physician who agrees in advance and in writing to accept assignment for all Medicare claims.

Preauthorization: A method of monitoring and controlling utilization by evaluating the need for medical service before it is performed.

Prospective Payment System (PPS): The standardized payment system implemented in 1983 by Medicare to help manage health care reimbursement whereby the incentive for hospitals to deliver unnecessary care is eliminated. Under the PPS, hospitals are paid fixed amounts based on the principal diagnosis (DRGs) for each Medicare hospital stay.

managed care is the same, no two managed care plans are exactly alike, and acquiring a working knowledge of the language allows one to comfortably navigate the system. For the purposes of this section we will state that managed care refers, in general, to efforts to coordinate, account for, and direct the use of services to achieve desired access, services, and outcomes while containing costs. Furthermore, risk-based managed care describes care from organizations that provide or contract to provide health care in broad specified areas for a defined population for a predetermined prepaid fee. In addition, managed care organizations (MCOs) take on the financial risk to deliver the services for the predetermined fee. MCOs use various cost-controlling techniques.

Managed care differs from conventional health insurance in that the MCO either provides the services directly or enters into contracts to provide them. In contrast, a commercial insurer underwrites the coverage without becoming involved in the delivery system. Managed care combines the responsibility for paying for a specifically defined set of health services with an active component of cost control related to providing those services and at the same time attempting to control the quality of and access to those services. A broad range of care and services in the acute care setting (hospital care, physician care, outpatient ancillary services, and prescription medications) is offered by the MCO. The benefits are defined in advance along with any payments that the member of the plan will be responsible for as copayments or deductibles. In this definition the MCO receives a fixed sum of money to pay for the benefits in the plan for the population of enrollees. This fixed sum of money may be composed of premiums paid by the enrollees, capitation payments made on behalf of the enrollees from a third party, or a combination of both.

The primary objective of managed care is control of health care expenditures through stringent management of health care resources. However, this characteristic no longer exclusively distinguishes managed care from other private health insurance plans. Increasingly, health insurers are using strategies such as preauthorization for services, copayments, and physician gatekeeping, to manage the use of health care resources, thereby trimming costs.

MCOs are typically classified into two dominant forms: (*a*) HMOs and (*b*) preferred provider organizations (PPOs). An HMO is a prepaid health plan delivering comprehensive care to members through designated providers. HMOs combine insurer and providers into one entity. Enrollees choose a primary care physician to coordinate their care (i.e., a gatekeeper). PPOs are entities through which employer health benefit plans and health insurance carriers contract to purchase health care for beneficiaries. Typically, PPOs offer the flexibility for beneficiaries to use non-PPO providers. In exchange for this freedom of choice is usually substantial deductibles and/or copayments that apply to care from non-PPO providers.

A third form of managed care is the exclusive provider organization, a variation of the PPO with characteristics of an HMO. Beneficiaries are limited to using specific providers and hospitals, and exclusive provider organizations may use gatekeeper approaches similar to HMOs for authorizing specialty services. As shown in Table 30-1, enrollment in exclusive provider organizations is not as common as HMOs and PPOs.

HMOs come in three major forms:

1. Group Model HMO: Contracts with independent multispecialty physician groups to provide all physician services to the HMO's members. Physicians receive a per-member payment or capitation.
2. Staff Model HMO: Employs salaried physicians and other health professionals who provide care solely for members of one HMO.
3. Independent Practice Association (IPA) HMO: An HMO contracts directly with associations of independent physicians and hospitals to provide the total health care for a defined number of members in a defined geographic area. Physicians maintain their own separate offices and identities. HMOs typically compensate their IPAs on an all-inclusive physician capitation basis to provide services to the

Table 30-1. 1999 Managed Care Enrollment in the United States

Type	Enrollment, in millions
Preferred provider organization	89.1
Health maintenance organization	79.3
Exclusive provider organization	13.0
Total	181.4

Adapted from Managed Care On-Line wwebsite. Available at:
http://www.mcareol.com/factshts/factnati.htm. Accessed March 16, 2000.

members; the IPA in turn can compensate its participating physicians on either a fee-for-service (FFS) basis or some combination of FFS and primary care capitation. Generally, primary care physicians are paid on a capitation basis and specialists are paid on an FFS basis.

HMOs in direct response to consumer resistance to joining traditional HMOs, and the desire to attract more customers, developed a hybrid program called a point of service HMO. Point of service HMOs allow members to seek care from nonparticipating physicians or hospitals for an additional premium. Use of nonparticipating providers is much more costly, with high deductibles and copays.

MCOs use a variety of methods to compensate providers. The primary ways MCOs share financial risk with physicians involves some combination of capitation, prepayment, and FFS withholds. Capitation entails the payment of a predetermined per-member fee paid at predetermined intervals for all covered services regardless of the level of utilization. Depending on the form of HMO, the arrangement can be either two or three tiered. The two-tiered payment structure exists when the HMO pays the capitation fees directly to the individual physician or small group practices without the payment passing through the IPA. A three-tiered payment structure has the additional administrative layer for processing the capitations. In the three-tiered arrangement the IPA becomes the middle tier.[7] MCOs may also withhold a portion of FFS payments to form pools of money from which reimbursement for specialty services are drawn, and surplus funds may be returned to individual physicians. Physicians who participate in PPOs receive compensation on a reduced FFS basis rather than on a shared financial risk.[6]

As the competitive climate has intensified, hospitals and their medical staffs have formed joint venture companies to create new managed care products. The provider-sponsored organization arrangement pools resources to create a range of services that can be marketed directly as an HMO or offered as a package to existing HMOs.

Cost containment in health care is one of the biggest challenges this nation is facing in the 21st century. Emerging trends that are eroding insurance coverage of all types are resulting in Americans lacking insurance and becoming underinsured. Rising premium costs, a reduction or cap on outpatient pharmaceutical benefits, and the loss of Medicaid coverage due to welfare reform are fast becoming a widespread problem.[8] Managed care has changed the way in which health care is financed by changing the incentives in the health care system. Stringent utilization review and economic disincentives for physicians and hospitals are resulting in denial of care and shifting the cost to the patient. In some cases the physicians provide the care, knowing they will never be reimbursed for it. Opponents of managed care argue that providers of care can only make a profit by providing less care. Through managed care a repolarization in health care is emerging. In managed care, providers profit by providing only the services absolutely necessary in treating patients and by maintaining the health of its members. Opponents of FFS argue that there is less incentive to keep people healthy because providers profit when people are sick and use health care services.

In theory, managed care can succeed by lowering costs for individual services and/ or improving the efficiency of services provided to treat a specific illness. Higher cost subsequent care may be avoided by using preventive measures and providing more effective care early on. In addition, by the substitution of less costly modes of care (e.g., outpatient instead of inpatient surgery), it may achieve the same result at a lower cost.

Pulmonary rehabilitation program directors will need to spend time researching and acquainting themselves with the HMOs, PPOs, and IPAs in their geographic area to effectively work within the managed care network. If your facility has a managed care contract coordinator, communicating with that individual is important. A working knowledge of the procedure for obtaining preauthorization for pulmonary rehabilitation treatment with each plan will be critical to enrolling patients in your program. Learning the mechanics of insurances of all types is a basic skill that should be mastered.

Medicare Supplement

The federal "Medicare Act," passed in 1965 and effective in 1966, was never intended to cover all health care services. As a result of this gap in coverage, the Medicare supplemental insurance policy was developed. In 1999, approximately 84% of Medicare beneficiaries were enrolled in the traditional Medicare program.[9] In addition, many beneficiaries purchased private insurance, commonly know as a Medigap policy. This type of supplement policy was designed to fill in some of the gaps created by Part A and Part B deductibles, copays, and noncovered services that the beneficiary is responsible for but that Medicare does not pay. Some policies offer coverage of services that the Medicare program does not, such as partial coverage for prescription medication. Until 1992, there were dozens of different Medicare supplement policies. This made it difficult to compare policies and prices. In 1992, by order of Congress, companies were prohibited from marketing and selling any Medicare supplement that did not conform to 1 of 10 standard packages of benefits, designated as Plans A through J. The 10 standard plans do not apply to Minnesota, Massachusetts, and Wisconsin because these states had alternative Medigap standardization programs in effect before the federal legislation was enacted.[10] With traditional Medicare and Medigap coverage, little restriction is placed on choice of doctor or hospital or on access to specialists, procedures, or diagnostic tests as long as the providers are Medicare approved and the services are covered by Medicare. Another source of Medicare supplemental insurance is the employer group insurance for retirees. Some private employer group insurance plans can be continued after retirement. Retirement plans provided by employers or unions are not subject to the rules that apply to Medigap policies, and special rules may apply. The options available to supplement Medicare can be confusing to the patient and the program director. An excellent resource for consumer information is the state Information, Counseling, and Assistance Program. Information, Counseling, and Assistance Program offices can provide Medicare beneficiaries with insurance information and answer questions. The Health Care Financing Administration (HCFA) makes grants to states for health insurance advisory services programs. To locate the telephone number of the Information, Counseling, and Assistance Program office nearest you, contact the state insurance department or Medicare.

FEDERAL AND STATE HEALTH INSURANCE PROGRAMS

Medicare

Medicare, established by Congress in 1965, is the federal health insurance program for people 65 years or older, people younger than 65 years with disabilities, people with end-stage renal disease, and certain otherwise noncovered aged persons who elect to buy into Medicare. The Medicare Act is known as Title XVIII of the Social Security Act. When Medicare was implemented in 1966, the program covered persons 65 years and older. In 1972, the program was expanded to cover persons who are entitled to Social Security or Railroad Retirement disability benefits for at least 24 months, persons with end-stage renal disease, and certain otherwise noncovered aged persons. The intent of Medicare's architects was to provide the elderly and the disabled with a program that would help to decrease their out-of-pocket costs for medically necessary health service. Medicare, however, is neither a comprehensive health care system nor cost free; many health care services are not covered, and Medicare beneficiaries are required to share the costs of such coverage. Less than half of the elderly's total health care spending is covered by Medicare. On average, the elderly spend a fifth of their household income for health services and premiums.[9]

The concern over the spiraling cost of health care in the Medicare program and the acknowledgment that the former approaches to controlling the cost of health care were not effective triggered development of the prospective payment system (PPS). Medicare's PPS dramatically changed the way hospitals were paid. Effective October 1, 1983, Medicare began to phase in payment rates for hospital admissions based on 467 diagnosis related groups (currently nearly 500 diagnosis related groups are established), thus changing Medicare from a cost system to a price system.[11-14] Under the PPS, Medicare no longer reimbursed hospitals on a retrospective, cost-based formula but instead reimbursed them at a predetermined amount, per admission, based on the patient's diagnosis within a diagnosis related group for providing whatever medical care is required during that patient's inpatient hospital stay. In some instances the payment received may be less than the hospital's actual costs, and in other cases it may be more. The bottom line is that the hospital absorbed the loss or profited from the predetermined payment schedule.

As part of the Balanced Budget Act (BBA) of 1997, Congress mandated changes to the Medicare program that direct the HCFA to replace Medicare's cost-based reimbursement method with more restrictive prospective payment methods that apply to postdischarge services, the fastest-growing component of Medicare in the 1990s.[15] Services that will be paid under the new PPS include skilled nursing facilities, hospital outpatient department services, inpatient rehabilitation services, and home health care. Ambulatory patient categories, similar to diagnosis related groups for hospital inpatient reimbursement, have been developed so that services classified within each group are comparable clinically and with respect to the use of resources. Payment for services is predetermined based on an ambulatory patient category diagnosis and treatment classification system.[16] Relative payment rates for covered hospital outpatient department services using 1996 hospital claims and cost report data have been established as specified in the law. The BBA further mandated that various adjustments to payments be established as necessary to ensure equitable payments under the system.[16] Medicare's change from a retrospective payment system to a PPS is a significant effort to control rapidly increasing outpatient costs. It is expected that other third-party insurers, including state Medicaid programs, will eventually adopt a similar payment structure. It is unclear at this time where hospital outpatient pulmonary rehabilitation services fit into the new PPS and what ambulatory patient categories will be used for reimbursement.

The HCFA was granted a postponement of the January 1999 implementation of the PPS for hospital outpatient services to accomplish its Year 2000 computer conversion. A notice of the anticipated implementation date will be published in the Federal Register at least 90 days in advance of the implementation date. As of March 8, 2000, no notice was published.[17]

In 1998 the Medicare program insured about 39 million people (34 million elderly and 5 million disabled enrollees). Before enactment of the Medicare program, less than half of all elderly Americans had health insurance. In 1999 Medicare covered virtually everyone 65 years and older. Medicare beneficiaries make up one in seven Americans, and this proportion is projected to grow to one in five by 2030, when the number of beneficiaries will exceed 76 million.[9]

The overall responsibility for the administration of the Medicare program is held by the US Department of Health and Human Services (DHHS) with the assistance of the Social Security Administration. The HCFA is a federal agency within the DHHS and has the primary responsibility for the Medicare and Medicaid programs, two national health care programs that benefit approximately 75 million Americans. The HCFA, along with the Health Resources and Services Administration, also runs the Children's Health Insurance Program, a program that is projected to cover approximately 10 million uninsured children in the United States. Since creation of the HCFA in 1977, its spending on behalf of Medicare beneficiaries has increased by a factor of almost 10 (from $21.5 billion in 1977 to $214.6 billion in 1997), and the number of individuals eligible for Medicare has grown from 26 million to approximately 39 million in 1999.[18] A summary of the relationship and responsibilities of the DHHS to the HCFA and the Social Security Administration is shown in Table 30-2.

Table 30-2. The Administration of Medicare

Federal Agencies Department of Health and Human Services	
Health Care Financing Administration	**Social Security Administration**
Defines Medicare benefits	Processes Medicare applications
Policy formulation and guidelines	Determines eligibility/entitlement
Sets Medicare rates	Maintains master beneficiary record
Administers Medicare program	Issues Medicare card
Contracts for claims payment	Provides public information
Intermediaries and carriers	

Medicare Coverage

Medicare consists of two separate parts: (*a*) Part A, Hospital Insurance, and (*b*) Part B, Supplementary Medical Insurance. As part of the BBA of 1997, Congress enacted dramatic changes to the Medicare program. These changes are all part of the new Medicare "Part C," also known as "Medicare + Choice." Beneficiaries must have Part A and Part B to enroll in a Part C plan.

The financing of Medicare Part A is primarily through a mandatory payroll tax, and most individuals 65 years and older are automatically entitled to Medicare because they are eligible for Social Security or Railroad Retirement benefits. Most all employees and self-employed workers in the United States work in employment covered by the Medicare Hospital Insurance program and pay Federal Insurance Contributions Act or Self-Employment Contributions Act taxes on earnings. The Federal Insurance Contributions Act tax rate is 1.45% of all earnings, without limit, paid by both employers and employees (2.9% total). For the self-employed, the tax rate is 2.90% of all earnings without limit. The Part A trust fund receives additional income from several sources, including a portion of the income taxes levied on Social Security benefits paid to high-income earners, premiums from individuals who are not otherwise eligible for the program and enroll voluntarily, general funds reimbursements of the cost of certain other uninsured individuals, and interest earnings on the invested assets of the trust fund.[15] The Medicare Part B program is a voluntary supplementary medical insurance program and is financed (25%) through premium payments ($45.50 per month in 2000) and through contributions (75%) from general revenue of the US Treasury. Ninety-five percent of all Part A beneficiaries enroll in Part B.[9] The financing of the Medicare Part C program, Medicare + Choice, is complex and is determined by which plan is chosen. The funding for Medicare + Choice primarily comes from the Part A and Part B trust funds in proportion to the relative weights of Part A and Part B benefits to the total benefits paid by the Medicare program.[9]

The Medicare Part A program covers inpatient hospital services, skilled nursing facility benefits, home health care visits following a hospital or skilled nursing facility stay, and hospice care. Medicare Part B covers physician and outpatient hospital services (e.g., pulmonary rehabilitation), home health care visits not covered under Part A, annual mammography and other cancer screening, and other services such as laboratory procedures and durable medical equipment. Both Part A and Part B Medicare have deductibles and copayments. A description of coverage for Medicare Part A and Part B is shown in Table 30-3.

An increasing number of Medicare beneficiaries receive their health care through HMOs. In 1997, the national rate of enrollment in managed care plans for persons 65 years and older was 12%. The highest levels of enrollment are in the West. In 1997, 38% of Medicare beneficiaries in California were enrolled in HMOs compared with 34% in

Arizona, 22% in Florida, 13% in New York, and 2% in Indiana.[6] As part of the BBA, Congress enacted dramatic changes to the Medicare program. These changes are all part of the newly created Medicare + Choice, Part C of Medicare. Medicare Part C opens a whole new range of options for Medicare beneficiaries to receive benefits and is intended to increase beneficiary participation in HMOs and other private plans. The BBA, in addition to expanding the types of plans that can contract with Medicare, changed the way plans are paid to encourage more plans to participate throughout the nation, especially in rural areas. The common element in all of the Medicare + Choice plans is that the plans contracting with Medicare will receive a fixed monthly amount for each enrolled beneficiary. In any geographic area, this amount, generally known as the capitation rate, will be the same regardless of which Medicare + Choice plan a beneficiary chooses.

In addition, the new law requires that beginning January 1, 2000, the HCFA adjusts payments to plans to more accurately reflect the actual health status of beneficiaries. Options under the new program include HMOs; provider-sponsored organizations; PPOs; private FFS plans; and, on a limited basis, medical savings accounts (tax free) that are combined with high-deductible catastrophic plans.

The 1999 Medicare reform proposal introduced by President Clinton calls for the "modernization and strengthening of Medicare into the 21st century." Medicare as it exists today does not include all of the necessary coverage to ensure high-quality health care for the millions of seniors and disabled beneficiaries that depend on the program. A key issue addressed in the proposal, where the current Medicare program falls short, is

Table 30-3. Explanation of Medicare Coverage

Part A, Intermediaries, Hospital Insurance (2000 deductible: $776)	Part B, Carriers, Medical Insurance (2000 premium: $45.50; annual deductible: $100)
Hospitalization: semiprivate room and board, general nursing, and other hospital services and supplies	Medical expenses: doctors' services, inpatient and outpatient medical and surgical services and supplies, diagnostic tests, and ambulatory surgery Center facility fees for approved procedures and durable medical equipment; also covers outpatient physical and occupational therapy and mental health services
Skilled nursing facility care: semiprivate room and board, skilled nursing and rehabilitative services, and supplies	Clinical laboratory service: blood tests, urinalyses, and more
Home health care: part-time skilled nursing care, physical therapy, speech language therapy, home health aid services, and durable medical equipment	Home health care: part-time skilled care, home health aid services, durable medical equipment when supplied by a home health agency while getting Medicare-covered home health care, and other supplies and services
Hospice care: medical and support services from a Medicare-approved hospice, drugs for symptom management, and support services for the terminally ill	Outpatient hospital services: services for the diagnosis or treatment of an illness or injury (e.g., pulmonary rehabilitation)[a]
Blood: when furnished at a hospital or skilled nursing facility during a covered stay	Blood: pints of blood needed as an outpatient or as part of a Part B–covered service CORF

[a] All hospital outpatient department service claims, including pulmonary rehabilitation, are processed by intermediaries, not carriers.

access to affordable prescription drugs. Included in the Clinton administration's reform proposal is the creation of a voluntary Medicare Part D prescription drug benefit that would be affordable and available to all beneficiaries. The financing of this benefit will be a critical factor in the debate taking place in Congress to reach a bipartisan agreement.[19]

Medicare Claims Processing

The processing of Medicare claims is handled by nongovernment, private organizations or agencies (e.g., a commercial insurance company) that contract to serve as the fiscal agent between health care providers (e.g., hospitals and physicians) and the federal government. These private contractors process claims locally for Medicare Part A and Part B and are known as intermediaries and carriers.

Medicare intermediaries process Part A claims for institutional services including inpatient hospital services, skilled nursing facilities, home health agencies, hospice services, and hospital outpatient claims for Medicare Part B, which includes pulmonary rehabilitation. Medicare carriers process Part B claims for services by physicians and medical suppliers, including durable medical equipment and ambulance services. A summary of the responsibilities of intermediaries and carriers is shown in Table 30-4. The focus of this section is on fiscal intermediaries.

A fiscal intermediary is usually assigned to a hospital and, generally speaking, is a function of geographics. Intermediaries have evolved into state-oriented agencies. For example, an intermediary may service the entire country but may establish regions with designated personnel to handle all claims within that region. Program directors should know who their intermediary is. The intermediary must follow policies established by the HCFA; however, the HCFA has given intermediaries latitude to interpret general policy statements broadly or specifically. In response to the absence of a national pulmonary rehabilitation coverage policy for outpatient pulmonary rehabilitation, fiscal intermediaries have taken on the task, with the HCFA's approval, of developing local medical review policies, which are Medicare reimbursement policies created at the local level by fiscal

Table 30-4. Summary of the Responsibilities of Fiscal Intermediaries and Carriers

Intermediaries	Carriers
Determine costs and reimbursement rates	Determine charges allowed by Medicare
Maintain records	Maintain quality of performance records
Establish controls	Assist in fraud and abuse investigations
Safeguard against fraud and abuse or excessive use	Assist both suppliers and beneficiaries as needed
Conduct reviews and audits	Process claims: services by physicians and medical equipment suppliers (i.e., durable medical equipment and ambulance services)
Process claims: inpatient hospital; skilled nursing facilities; home health agencies; hospice services; and all hospital outpatient claims for Medicare part B, including pulmonary rehabilitation	
Make payments to providers for services	Make payments to physicians and suppliers for services
Assist both providers and beneficiaries as needed	

intermediaries and/or carriers. According to the American Association for Respiratory Care, intermediaries in Alabama, Arkansas, California, Florida, New York, Ohio, Pennsylvania, and Virginia either have developed or are in the final phases of developing local medical review policies on pulmonary rehabilitation.[20] At this time, most states' intermediaries do not have specific pulmonary rehabilitation reimbursement guidelines, local medical review policies, established. Without specific reimbursement policy statements, the intermediary may search for a document on a general level and apply it as a rationale for the decision to pay or deny payment. In some instances, if no specific policy exists for an intermediary justifying reimbursement, the absence of policy may be the reason for denial. Yet, another intermediary, given the same scenario, may provide reimbursement simply because reimbursement is not specifically prohibited. As a result, different intermediaries, all using the same manual, have varying policies regarding reimbursement for pulmonary rehabilitation programs, creating significant discrepancies from one state to another.

National organizations, including the American Association of Cardiovascular and Pulmonary Rehabilitation, the American Association for Respiratory Care, the American College of Chest Physicians, the American Thoracic Society, and the National Association for Medical Direction of Respiratory Care, are all working closely with the HCFA regarding development of a national coverage policy for pulmonary rehabilitation. The drafting of guidelines is focused solely on coverage because of the policy process within the HCFA at this time. The major provisions in the BBA of 1997 that applied to traditional Medicare coverage reduced its growth. With this in mind, it is clear that the HCFA does not want a policy that will widen the eligibility criteria for Medicare beneficiaries, thus increasing Medicare costs significantly. On the other side of the discussion, the pulmonary community wants to ensure that there is a scope of services available to those who would benefit the greatest from pulmonary rehabilitation programs.[21]

With the seemingly endless changes occurring in health care, numerous opportunities are available for the pulmonary rehabilitation program director and team members to promote legislation regarding pulmonary rehabilitation and respiratory care. Program directors' participation in the political process can benefit programs. Joining your state's organization if you are not already a member is the first step. Joining national organizations such as the American Association of Cardiovascular and Pulmonary Rehabilitation and the American Association for Respiratory Care is the next step. Get to know who your local legislators are. Making the connection at whatever level, state and/or national, is critical to becoming informed, being involved, and making your concerns be known. At a time when the Medicare program has undergone the greatest reform since its enactment more than 30 years ago and managed care continues to gain a stronger foothold and have an ever-increasing presence in both the public and private sectors, allied health professionals have an unprecedented opportunity to empower themselves through getting involved in the legislative process.

Medicaid

Medicaid is a federal-state entitlement program for low-income Americans. The Medicaid program was enacted in 1965, at the same time as Medicare, under Title XIX of the Social Security Act. The program pays for medical assistance for certain vulnerable and needy individuals and families with low incomes and resources. Medicaid is jointly funded by the federal and state governments. The federal government makes federal matching funds available to states for the costs they incur in paying health care providers for providing covered services to eligible recipients. State participation is voluntary, and, since 1982, forty-nine states have chosen to participate. In Arizona, a federal assistance program, under a waiver of some basic federal requirements, is available as an alternative to Medicaid. Medicaid programs are also operational in the District of Columbia, Puerto Rico, the Virgin Islands, Guam, American Samoa, and the Northern Mariana Islands.

Three basic groups of low-income people are eligible for Medicaid: (*a*) low-income parents and children who use Medicaid for acute and ambulatory services; (*b*) low-income elderly persons who use Medicaid to receive assistance with their Medicare premiums, copayments, and deductibles as well as nursing home and prescription drug costs; and (*c*) disabled persons who use Medicaid for acute and long-term care services.

Each state, within broad national guidelines established by federal statues, regulations, and policies, is allowed to (*a*) establish its own eligibility standards, (*b*) develop provider payment policies, and (*c*) determine benefits. As a result of this flexibility allowed to states under federal Medicaid guidelines, considerable variation can be seen in services provided from state to state.[15,22] However, the scope of services provided by states' Medicaid plans must include certain basic services to receive federal matching funds. A list of basic services covered under the Medicaid program is seen in Box 30-4. Administration of Medicaid is carried out by state Medicaid agencies.

In 1986 the Omnibus Budget Reconciliation Act gave states the option of expanding the Medicaid program to include services for ventilator-dependent individuals. Medicaid will often pay for home care items that are not covered by other third-party payers, such as Medicare. For tracheostomy or ostomy care patients who require supplies, Medicaid may pay for those necessary supplies.

The Medicaid program is the single largest source of federal funds to the states. Of the $271.3 billion federal grant-in-aid dollars issued to the states in 1999, 40% is estimated to be federal Medicaid funds. In 1997, Medicaid covered 40.6 million Americans. Ten percent (4.1 million) of these were elderly, 17% (6.8 million) were disabled, about 52% (21 million) were children, and approximately 8.6 million (21%) were adults in families with children.[22]

As the cost of Medicaid continues to increase, the growth of managed care systems as an alternative to the traditional FFS system in Medicaid will be closely monitored for its effectiveness in cost savings. With the Congressional Budget Office estimating that the federal government will spend $107 billion on Medicaid in fiscal year 1999 and $159 billion in fiscal year 2004, managed care is expected to have an ever-increasing presence in governmental insurance programs.[22]

Box 30-4. Basic and Optional Services Under the Medicaid Program[a]

Minimum services that states *must* cover:
  Hospital care (inpatient and outpatient)
  Nursing home care
  Physician services
  Laboratory and x-ray services
  Immunizations and other early periodic screening, diagnostic, and treatment
    services for children
  Family planning services
  Federally qualified health center and rural health clinic services
  Nurse midwife and nurse practitioner services
Optional services that states *may* cover:
  Prescription drugs
  Institutional care for individuals with mental retardation
  Home- and community-based care for the frail elderly, including case
    management
  Personal care and other community-based services for individuals with
    disabilities
  Dental and vision care for adults

[a] States that participate in the Medicaid program must cover a minimum set of benefits. States have the option of covering additional services that qualify for federal matching funds as well.

Hill-Burton Program

In 1946 Congress passed Public Law 79-725, under Title VI of the Public Health Service Act, the Hospital Survey and Construction Act, more commonly known as the Hill-Burton Act. The law initially was created to provide federal grants to modernize hospitals that had become obsolete during the Depression and World War II (1929–1945). Title XVI of the Public Health Service Act, an amendment to the Hill-Burton Program, was enacted in 1975 and established federal grants, loan guarantees, and interest subsidies for health care facilities. A facility that receives grant funds or assistance under the Hill-Burton Program must provide a reasonable volume of services to persons unable to pay and make their services available to all persons residing in the facility's area in return for the funds. The free or low-cost medical services are extended to those persons who are *uninsured* and *underinsured* and *meet eligibility criteria.* The US DHHS is responsible for administering the program. The Division of Facilities Compliance and Recovery, under the DHHS, is responsible for day-to-day management of the program to ensure that obligated facilities provide free or reduced-cost medical services. The Division will also assist eligible persons in obtaining free medical care.[23,24]

Facilities are allowed to choose which services it will provide at no or reduced cost and are required to provide a specified amount of uncompensated care as outlined in its Allocation Plan. The services are published by the facility in a written notice provided to all persons requesting uncompensated services in the facility. Eligibility for services is based on a person's family size and income. Individuals may qualify if their income falls within the poverty guidelines, as published in the Federal Register each year. Your hospital admissions, business, or patient accounts office will be able to assist the uninsured or underinsured pulmonary rehabilitation candidate with eligibility determination.

Comprehensive Outpatient Rehabilitation Facility

A comprehensive outpatient rehabilitation facility (CORF) is a Medicare-certified health care facility that is defined as:

> *a nonresidential facility that is established and operated exclusively for the purpose of providing diagnostic, therapeutic, and restorative services to outpatients for the rehabilitation of injured, disabled, or sick persons, at a single fixed location, by and under the supervision of a physician (Code of Federal Regulations 42: Section 485.51).*[25–27]

CORFs are required to provide at least physical therapy and social services and to either contract with or employ a medical director. Additional CORF services are occupational therapy, speech-language pathology, respiratory therapy, psychological services, orthotic and prosthetic device services, nursing care services, drugs and biologicals, and durable medical equipment. In the federal regulations, respiratory therapy services are defined as (Section 410.100 [3e]) "services for the assessment, diagnostic evaluation, treatment, management, and monitoring of patients with deficiencies or abnormalities of cardiopulmonary function." These services include:

1. Application of techniques for support of oxygenation and ventilation of the patient and for pulmonary rehabilitation.
2. Therapeutic use and monitoring of gases, mists, and aerosols and related equipment.
3. Bronchial hygiene therapy.
4. Pulmonary rehabilitation techniques, such as exercise conditioning, breathing retraining, and patient education in the management of respiratory problems.
5. Diagnostic tests to be evaluated by a physician, such as pulmonary function tests, spirometry, and blood gas analysis.
6. Periodic assessment of chronically ill patients and their need for respiratory therapy.

Several requirements must be met for respiratory therapy services to be covered as CORF services. First, a physician must refer the individual to the facility and must also certify that the individual needs skilled rehabilitation services. In addition, a comprehensive and interdisciplinary assessment must be conducted on each patient admitted to the CORF, and a plan of care, with measurable objectives, must be established. Second, all services must be provided while the individual is under a physician's care, and they must be furnished on site at the CORF, except for the home evaluation visit. The plan of care must be reviewed and updated at least every 60 days by the interdisciplinary team, and the physician must certify or recertify that the plan is being followed, that the patient is making progress, and that the treatment is having no harmful effects on the patient.

One of the advantages of a CORF-based pulmonary rehabilitation program is that services continue to be reimbursed under Medicare Part B on an adjusted cost basis or applicable fee schedule under the new provisions of the BBA. The provisions of the BBA of 1997 have, however, created uncertainty for reimbursement of other outpatient therapy services. The BBA of 1997 incorporates a revised payment cap of $1500 per year on specific outpatient rehabilitation services furnished by a CORF (does not apply to therapists in independent practice). The payment cap includes $1500 on occupational therapy and $1500 on physical and speech therapy, combined. No limit has been imposed on respiratory therapy.[28]

Veterans Health Administration Benefits

The Veterans Administration (VA) provides inpatient and outpatient services, including preventive and primary care. These include diagnostic and treatment services, rehabilitation, mental health and substance abuse treatment, home health, respite and hospice care, and drugs in conjunction with VA treatment to eligible veterans enrolled in the VA health care system. In 1996, the Veterans Health Care Eligibility Act (Public Law 104-262) was enacted and requires that veterans must be enrolled to receive care at VA medical facilities.

The new system has seven priority groups ranging from group 1 for veterans with service-connected conditions rated 50% or more disabling to group 7 for veterans with nonservice-connected or 0% disabilities with income and net worth above a certain limit who agree to pay specified copayments. Veterans are assigned to a priority group when they enroll.

Enrollees in the VA health care system pay no monthly premium for VA care. When a veteran uses services a copayment may be required depending on their VA eligibility rating (priority group). If a veteran has a priority group 1 rating he or she will receive treatment at no cost. All other copayment responsibilities are set by law and depend on the individual's income.

Enrollment is valid for 1 year and is reviewed and renewed automatically each year depending on the priority group and available funds and resources. If the VA cannot renew the veteran's enrollment for the following year, the veteran will be notified in writing 60 days before enrollment expires. The VA recommends that if a veteran has Medicare or Medicaid that he or she keep the coverage for flexibility in the future.[29]

The VA health care system is in the process of changing from a hospital-based system of care to a more effective and economical health care system based on primary and ambulatory care. To accomplish this goal, community-based outpatient clinics are being established nationwide. The clinics are located in existing government facilities or in private health care facilities under contract with the VA.[29]

The VA facilities are inconsistent when it comes to offering pulmonary rehabilitation services. No written policies or guidelines are available regarding referral or reimbursement of pulmonary rehabilitation for VA patients. Each VA facility has the authority to decide whether to offer a pulmonary rehabilitation program. In many instances it is difficult to find space, supplies, and staffing for a potential program. VA patients interested in pulmonary rehabilitation should contact their local county VA service office.

Civilian Health and Medical Program of the Uniformed Services/TRICARE

The Civilian Health and Medical Program of the Uniformed Services (CHAMPUS), now called TRICARE, is a regionally managed health care program for active-duty and retired members of the uniformed services younger than 65 years, their families, and their survivors.[30] Military personnel separating from military service (not retiring) are no longer eligible for coverage under TRICARE/CHAMPUS. Retired military personnel 65 years or older receive Medicare benefits. In response to the need for controlling the ever-increasing costs of health care, and the overcrowded military hospital and clinics, the Department of Defense developed the TRICARE program in the early 1980s. The CHAMPUS/TRICARE program offers eligible beneficiaries three options for their health care. (*a*) TRICARE Prime, an HMO option in which military treatment facilities are the principal source of health care, referral to specialty care using a network of military and civilian providers; (*b*) TRICARE Extra, a PPO option that uses a civilian health care network and military facilities on a space-available basis; and (*c*) TRICARE Standard, an FFS program option (new name for old CHAMPUS program). CHAMPUS/TRICARE has specific requirements for documentation of services provided for reimbursement to occur. Contact the regional administrator in your area for specific rules.[31]

Federal Employees Health Benefits

Government employees—civil service workers—have numerous health insurance plans available to them. Managed care plans and FFS plan options are generally available. Each plan will have its own outline of coverage that specifies benefits, copays, and deductibles. Federal employees should contact their human resources office or the health plan directly to determine applicable coverage for pulmonary rehabilitation.

CASUALTY INSURANCE

Workers' Compensation Program

Workers' compensation is a state-regulated insurance program that pays medical bills and some lost wages for an employee who sustains a work-related injury or disease.[32] Each state determines the coverage limits available to this patient group. The Occupational Safety and Health Administration (OSHA) requires screening spirometry of workers at work sites with potential occupational respiratory hazards to avoid a disastrous health outcome and liability. It is possible for a patient, because of a work-related injury (i.e., federal black lung benefits), to have Medicare as a secondary payer to Workers' compensation. Workers' compensation is an area of reimbursement for the pulmonary rehabilitation director to investigate further.

DOCUMENTATION FOR REIMBURSEMENT

Pulmonary rehabilitation reimbursement in the 21st century is a dynamic arena in which regulatory changes occur rapidly. To optimize the revenue for pulmonary rehabilitation, the program director/coordinator/team leader must be familiar with the facility's business office and contracting department, where decisions are made with regard to negotiating contracts and reimbursement.[33] A business office representative and the facility contracting specialist should be invited to be on your pulmonary rehabilitation team. The liaison developed with these departments will expand the pulmonary rehabilitation program's understanding and exposure to the constantly changing reimbursement field from managed care to Medicare. Uniformity in handling and reimbursing pulmonary rehabilitation claims is not consistent in the United States. What is known are the do's and don'ts of Medicare. Because other third-party payers will often follow the rules set by Medicare, it is helpful to clearly understand those rules.

Human error can cause reimbursement nightmares as it pertains to a patient's billing claim, medical record, and rehabilitation program documentation. A claim denial by a third-party payer may be due to technical errors as it relates to program documentation, the billing office bill submission, or the medical records department chart completeness.[34] The golden rule for documentation does not exist, but specific guidelines apply. Some third-party payers have developed policy statements for reimbursement of pulmonary rehabilitation services. As a program director, one must determine if such a document exists in your state or region. Where no policy is available, collaboration with other local program directors to extend your expertise and offer assistance to the third-party payer in developing such a document may be a positive opportunity to help set the standards. Understanding the current third-party payer guidelines for reimbursement of your interdisciplinary team home departments, such as respiratory therapy, physical therapy, and occupational therapy services, may also be helpful in understanding the current trends for reimbursement and how changes or directives seen in those disciplines may also impact the pulmonary rehabilitation program.

Medicare Documentation Requirements

Medicare requires that documentation reflect an individualized, skilled needs evaluation within the interdisciplinary team's scope of practice, license, and expertise.[34] Initial patient evaluations must identify the problems, develop a specific plan of treatment, and set concrete goals. All documentation must demonstrate the clinical rationale for the skilled intervention. The documentation must reflect medical necessity to continue pulmonary rehabilitation as a skilled service. See Box 30-5 for pulmonary rehabilitation treatment documentation requirements.

The program documentation must match the itemized bill (UB92) for date of service and duration of treatment. The documentation must refer to patient outcomes. The documentation must cover the following areas: treatments must be ordered by a physician; qualify as a covered service or policy benefit; be reasonable and necessary for the diagnosis and/or treatment of the pulmonary illness; be consistent with the nature and severity of the individual's symptoms and diagnosis; be reasonable in terms of procedure/modality, amount, frequency, and duration of treatment; be accepted by the professional community as being safe and effective treatment for the purpose used; be a level of complexity that the services can be rendered only by a skilled clinician; and be delivered by qualified health professionals in accordance with state and federal regulations; also, the pulmonary

Box 30-5. Pulmonary Rehabilitation Treatment Documentation Requirements

Physician order for therapy
Individualized and showing medical necessity
Interdisciplinary teams work in their scope of practice in accordance with state and federal regulations
Initial assessment must identify the problems
Plan of treatment must be specific and show need for skilled level of intervention
Goals must be specific to promote recovery, restore function, and be measurable
Treatment is reasonable, necessary, and clinically based for the diagnosis and procedure
Treatment is accepted by the professional community as safe and effective for the diagnosis and evidence based

Box 30-6. Medicare Noncovered Services

Nonindividualized treatment, education, and training
Routine psychological screening and/or routine psychological therapy
Duplication of services between occupational, physical, and respiratory therapy and
   nursing
Treatment that exceeds the patient's needs for the identified condition
Routine, nonskilled, and/or maintenance care
Repetitive services for chronic baseline conditions
Plateau in patient's progress toward goals
Inability to sustain gains
No overall improvement
Generalized exercise
Poor rehabilitation potential exists with the patient
Treatment that is not reasonable and necessary because of lack of significant
   objective findings in preliminary pulmonary diagnosic testing
Routine follow-up visits
Viewing of films or videotapes, listening to audiotapes, completing interactive
   computer programs
Any supervised or independent technology-based instruction
Exercise equipment or supplies
Biofeedback services for relaxation
Nutritional counseling
Social services
Team and/or family conferences
Documentation time
Discharge summaries
Educational materials such as books, etc.

rehabilitation services must not exceed the patient's particular pulmonary rehabilitation needs, must promote recovery, must restore function, and must ensure safety affected by the illness or injury, have an expectation that there will be measurable improvement of the patient's condition in a reasonable and generally predictable period of time, and demonstrate practical improvement. To optimize program reimbursement under Medicare guidelines, a clear understanding of what is *not* covered is also important. These noncovered services should never show up on the patients UB92 or in documentation. See Box 30-6 for the Medicare list of noncovered services.

Reasons for Medicare denial may include providing known noncovered services to the patient, the patient is expected to spontaneously return to his or her previous level of function without skilled therapeutic intervention, treatment is for maintenance of a chronic baseline condition, treatment is to merely maintain a functional level, patients with acute and or unstable disease, patients incapable of participating in pulmonary rehabilitation because of mental or physical limitations, documentation does not support measurable benefit, and including patients are unable or unwilling to benefit from the treatment.

Billing for pulmonary rehabilitation charges must follow Medicare guidelines: charges are itemized to reflect the date of service, revenue code, and current procedural terminology codes and units, and each treatment procedure or modality billed must match the documentation in the daily therapy notes by date and units. The patient's bill is submitted on an itemized UB92.

The Patient's Medical Record

The patient's record in a pulmonary rehabilitation program requires specific documentation that is significant, concise, to the point, and use standardized terms.[35] Handwritten notes or computer-generated notes will facilitate the data entry of pertinent patient information.

Each institution will have general rules that govern medical record keeping. Check with your medical records department for the specifications. One must systematically collect and document patient data. The patient record improves communication and continuity of care among the interdisciplinary team members.[36] The pulmonary rehabilitation chart is the only means the program has to prove that they are providing appropriate care and meeting established standards. No matter how frustrating we think charting may be, is must be done, so make it as simple, straightforward, and specific as possible, easy to follow and read. The pulmonary rehabilitation patient's medical record is an information-intensive document. One must also not forget that the chart is a legal document that can be sent into court.

The pulmonary rehabilitation progress note is the repository of medical facts and critical thinking pertaining to the pulmonary patient. It must be concise, a vehicle of communication about the patient's condition to those who access the health record. The progress notes must be readable, easily understood, complete, accurate, and completed in black ink.[37] The interdisciplinary team's documentation must be flexible enough to logically convey what happened during the therapy, the chain of events occurring during the treatment session, as well as guaranteeing full accountability for the documented material, and clearly documenting who recorded the information, and when it was recorded.[38]

Computers in the health care setting are standard, and the interdisciplinary team should become familiar with the hospital computer information systems available, and how integration of the patient's record and test results can be accessed through the computer system to make documentation more efficient.[39] Computerized patient records support patient-focused care by points of documentation that give the interdisciplinary team greater time with the patient through reduced manual and clerical activities.[40] The handwritten medical record can only be used by one person, at one location, at one time and is often poorly organized and illegible; data retrieval for outcome documentation is time-consuming. Moving from the handwritten pathway to the automated system will be an important transition to a computerized interdisciplinary documentation system.[40] The use of computers may allow the development, quantitative perspective, and realization of the virtual patient record. The virtual patient record is the documentation of all health-relevant data that accumulates during a person's lifetime at the touch of a finger using the age of networked computers.[41] To assist pulmonary rehabilitation programs with patient documentation, computer voice recognition programs are available.[42] It is not a 22nd century idea but is available now. You can communicate with your computer in the most natural way—by speaking. You talk to your computer and the words appear immediately on the screen in your document. The program also has a vocabulary builder to personalize both the vocabulary and language model to match your writing style and how you dictate. So the specialized language of pulmonary rehabilitation can be built into your program for recognition accuracy. The countless charting hours in time and money saved may outweigh the cost of the software program. This program is also available in other languages, including British English, French, German, Italian, Spanish, and Dutch.[42]

Three basic methods are used for patient record keeping: the traditional chart, the problem-oriented medical record (POMR), and computer documentation.[35,37,38] The traditional chart (block chart or source-oriented record) is divided into specific areas of blocks. These blocks may include the admission sheet, physician order sheet, progress notes, history and physical examination, medication sheet, medical test reports, care plans, and discharge summaries. This format is easy to record but makes it more difficult to follow a specific problem/event.

The POMR, known as the Weed system after its developer, is one format of documentation. It is used to systematically gather clinical data, formulate an assessment, and select an appropriate treatment plan and record changes made to the original treatment plan. POMR consists of four basic components: the database, problem list, progress notes, and plan. The exact format each of these components takes varies between institutions. In the pulmonary rehabilitation POMR chart, the database includes past medical records, assessments done by the interdisciplinary team, and diagnostic test results. The database builds the baseline for the individualized program. The problem list will be the target areas/deficits found in the evaluation process that interferes with the pulmonary patient's physical/psychological health and ability to function. The problem list is dynamic, with the deletion and addition of problems as indicated. Goals and outcome data are developed from the problem list and supported by the progress note. The progress notes of the medical record chart may be narrative or written in the soaping format which entails subjective, objective, assessment, and plan documentation. Soaping systematically reviews one health problem. The subjective information is obtained from the pulmonary rehabilitation patient, a family member, or a significant other. The objective information is based on the interdisciplinary team's assessment of the patient, observations, and test results as measured, factually described, or collected. The assessment is the analysis/critical thinking of the patient's problems as found during the subjective and objective gathering phase. The plan of action consists of the steps to be taken to address, treat, and resolve the problems. The implementation occurs under the plan and is the actual administration of the specific treatment. Evaluation occurs through the collection of measurable data as to the patient's response to the intervention, and revision addresses any changes made to the original treatment plan based on the evaluation.

Patient documentation requires critical thinking on the part of the interdisciplinary team members.[37] Critical thinking is defined as "the process of purposeful, self-regulatory judgment. This process gives reasoned consideration to evidence, contexts, conceptualizations, methods and criteria."[43] The future of patient documentation may become a blueprint, a critical pathway alternative because good documentation is the cornerstone of quality data.[44] Medical records are documents that can travel from the courtroom to the hospital to the team conference. We must always remember that medical records are the witnesses whose memory never dies, an indelible defense if the documentation is precise and meticulous.[36]

Accrediting agencies (the Joint Commission on Accreditation of Healthcare Organizations [JCAHO]), payers (Medicare, MCOs, Blue Cross, etc.), and providers (integrated delivery systems) mandate documentation of outcomes. It is helpful for the program to use accepted, standardized tools for outcome evaluations. See Chapter 20 on Outcomes. The faces of accrediting agencies may also be changing. ISO 9000 is an international quality system used in manufacturing that may be working its way into the health care arena.[45] The ISO 9000 sets high standards, employers know it and trust it, and it may be less expensive than the JCAHO. We may see the ISO 9000 become an alternative or a complement to the JCAHO. Hospitals, home health agencies, skilled nursing facilities, rehabilitation and long-term care hospitals, and home medical equipment providers are not the only organizations evaluated through accreditation. Two organizations that accredit managed care plans are the National Committee for Quality Assurance and the JCAHO. Accreditation is the process by which an organization recognizes a program of study or meets predetermined standards.[46]

Benchmarking is one form of documenting outcomes. Benchmarking in pulmonary rehabilitation is the comparison of value indicators with high-performing organizations. "The goal of benchmarking is to identify outstanding performance regarding cost-effectiveness, quality of life, and best practices in relation to Pulmonary Rehabilitation interventions."[43] It is clearly understood that patient documentation that leads to outcome analysis entails critical thinking on the part of the interdisciplinary team. The cognitive skills the interdisciplinary team must use in critical thinking are interpretation, analysis, evaluation, inference, explanation, and self-regulation. It is interesting to note that the scientific method uses these skills as well. Self-regulation refers to the practitioner's ability to competently, efficiently, and promptly adapt and modify to changes in pulmonary rehabilitation clinical practice. The pulmonary rehabilitation specialist must continually assess quality improvement outcomes and evidence-based outcomes to modify the pulmonary rehabilitation program to the patient's individual needs.

The 1997 Balanced Budget Act carried many demands for data reporting and documentation because of capitated payment in managed care plans in accordance with the health status of the enrollees and the implementation of prospective payment for home health agencies, skilled nursing facilities, rehabilitation, and long-term care hospitals. When changes occur in the reimbursement method it also demands supporting documentation to justify payment and may necessitate complete overhauls of facility information systems throughout the health care industry.

The *International Classification of Diseases, 9th Revision, Clinical Modification* (*ICD-9-CM*) has been the standard reporting of diagnosis and institutional procedures for almost 2 decades. Improving the health terminology systems in the United States with guidelines, criteria selection, and public policy implication is never ending. The current *ICD-9-CM* classification groups patients in broad categories that do not allow for the development of refined guidelines or the comparison of patient outcomes or benchmarks. To improve this reporting system one proposal works with the standards community to develop a framework for integration of clinical terminology that is practical for use in the patient care area, process management, outcome analysis, and decision support.[47] Because of an international treaty, the United States moved in 1999 to the updated 10th edition (*ICD-10*) for tabulations of mortality. The clinical modifications of the 10th edition, *ICD-10-CM,* replaces the older book for reporting of diagnoses. This new edition has thousands of improved codes, and the HCFA has funded the development of a procedure coding system (PCS) for the *ICD-10* (*ICD-10-PCS*). The PCS represents body systems, operations, body parts, approaches, and devices. The new codes do not resemble the American Medical Association Current Procedural Terminology codes that the HCFA now requires physicians and other disciplines to use in coding services. The new reporting system, based on *ICD-10-CM* and *ICD-10 PCS,* will require extensive training of physicians and other providers with substantial changes in the facilities information systems. The HCFA uses coding and documentation not only to determine the level of payment but for monitoring the quality of care and for creating performance profiles.

HEALTH CARE AROUND THE WORLD

The information on health care around the world is not intended as an all-inclusive list of international countries, their health care systems, insurance, or reform issues. The purpose is to show our similarities and to allow us to understand the need for international collaboration in pulmonary rehabilitation,[48–58] making our differences our strengths. In fact, in reviewing the international health care literature, "reform of the reform" is the norm. It is comforting to know that the United States is not alone in our plight for a health care system of equity, quality, completeness, and cost effectiveness. See Section VI, International Approach to Pulmonary Rehabilitation, for specific information on Canada, Europe, Japan, the Philippines, and South America.

When one reviews the health care systems of the world and their reimbursement it is difficult to compare each country because of differences in statistical methods used and because each government uses different criteria to define health care costs. The pulmonary rehabilitation reimbursement dilemma of the United States has also been seen in Europe and Tokyo.[57] The structure of the pulmonary rehabilitation programs and diseases admitted to the program are also varied as a result of cultural differences, the countries' medical insurance systems, and target diseases.[57]

It is the intent of this section to provide a glance into health care around the globe, showing the differences and at the same time the similarities. Health care reform crosses international borders. Not one country is spared this ongoing dilemma to reduce health care spending and improve health care standards.

Australia

Australia,[59-62] like the United States, is a federation of states. It provides universal access to health care, keeping its total health care spending to about 8.5% of the gross domestic product. Coronary heart disease continues to be the biggest killer in indigenous Australians, who have one of the highest prevalence rates of noninsulin-dependent diabetes mellitus in the world. In secondary schools, student smoking has not decreased as much as in adults, and obesity continues to increase. A literature review of rehabilitative interventions for chronic obstructive pulmonary disease (COPD) patients show an emphasis on community-based programs for pulmonary rehabilitation because the program in the community can address the specific needs of the population, be a cost-benefit, and be flexible in delivery.

Australia, although bordered by oceans is influenced by the global health care trends—no one is denied its influence. The trends in Australia's health care system show increases in health care spending, increases in cost of hospital and other institutionalized care and health insurance. Other reasons for increases in Australian health care costs are the aging population and use of sophisticated and expensive equipment. Care is shifting from the hospital to the home/community, an increase is being seen in the continuum of care programs, health care networks are being established, the focus is on quality, and unfortunately the focus is on treatment rather than prevention. The health care dynamics in Australia are changing.

Brazil

The Brazilian[63] health care system provides health care for all as a result of government mandates. Health care is at a crisis because of the heavy demand and lack of funding, which results in coverage going to only a few. The heavy demand of health care has seen the private, managed care plans emerge. The future of reform will be interesting.

Canada

The 1999 budget for Canada had changes to increase health care, improve the health of Canadians, and improve health research. The government of Canada provides funding to the provincial and territorial health systems through the Canada Health and Social Transfer program. The system provides insured hospital and medical care services to all eligible Canadian residents.[64] Health care reform[65] has seen Canada's provincial Medicare system cut inpatient care and community service and, in 9 of 10 province's hospitals, have consolidated under regional authorities. The integration of services across the continuum of care has not been successful in any of the provinces. An assessment of the Health Program Guidelines in Canada was done to determine strategic effectiveness, operational efficiency, and perceived needs.[66]

Canada believes that research is the cornerstone of quality health, as seen in its existing programs. To better facilitate health research the government is developing the Canadian Institutes of Health Research,[67] an agency of the federal government reporting to Parliament through the Minister of Health. A multidisciplinary approach emphasizing integration, not separation, and collaboration to health questions research would be carried out. Under the Canadian Institutes of Health Research, institutes would be created that would reflect Canada's health priorities. Just a few of the institutes that may be created are respiratory diseases, clinical evaluation, aging, and women's health. The pulmonary rehabilitation specialist must carefully follow the institutes to determine how the pulmonary patient population of Canada[68,69] may benefit from the health priorities set.

See Table 30-5 to understand where Canadian health costs are and how they compare with the international arena.[70]

Asthma deaths and hospitalizations have increased. In students aged 5 to 19 years surveyed, more than 13% currently had asthma, and asthma accounts for one-quarter of school absenteeism. COPD is the fifth most common cause of death in North America

Table 30-5. 1994 Data on Health Care Spending in Canada and Japan

Country	Health Expenditure as a Proportion of GDP	Nominal Spending per Capita, US $
Canada	9.9% GDP on health care (Rank 3 of 29)	$1824 per capita (Rank 14)
Japan	7% GDP on health care (Rank 22)	$2614 per capita (Rank 3)

GDP, gross domestic product.

today and is the only leading cause of death that is rising in prevalence. In 1990 and 1991 Canada spent $62.2 million on hospital costs owing to emphysema and chronic bronchitis; approximately 6000 people died of COPD during the same period. From 1988 to 1989 direct medical costs of adult asthma were an estimated $393 million annually. Including indirect costs owing to time lost at work and disability, the costs rise to $591 million annually. An average of 58 asthma-related deaths per year occurred during the 1980s. The Canadian Lung Association[71] has a page of recommendations for the management of COPD from preventive medication to coping strategies.

China

China[72] no longer has universal free basic health care. Health care responsibility is given to the provincial and county governments, with health care providers having considerable financial independence. A fee-for-service system is one of the payment mechanisms used. Because of the reform an inequity of access to services with inefficient use of resources has occurred. Knowledge of the problems exists, and solutions are being worked on. It is stated that China has not seen a decline of the health status of the population because of the reforms secondary to improved socioeconomic conditions and continued emphasis on prevention.

There exists a wide variation of coverage for health care benefits among urban Chinese workers. Out-of-pocket medical expenditures are present and could reach as high as 25% of a worker's annual income. Chinese businesses are experiencing financial burdens in providing medical benefits to workers.[73]

Since 1992 health care reform has been addressed in China.[74] The emphasis has been on cost recovery, profit making, diversification of services, and development of alternative financing strategies for health care services provided in the public sector. Medical cost inflation has occurred; cooperative medicine in the rural areas has been dismantled because of reform, with other changes also occurring.

Finland

COPD constitutes a national health problem not only in the United States but also in Finland.[54] Data from the Finnish National Hospital Discharge Register and the Register of Deaths was compared with different treatment practices. It was noted that random clinical trials are needed to determine standards of care. The results did show that medications and easy access to treatment resulted in improved survival rates of asthmatics and COPD patients. It is time for pulmonary rehabilitation to become part of the standard of care for pulmonary patients in Finland.

France

France,[75] as other countries, has been taking a sharp axe if not a guillotine to decrease its public expenditure. Health care services, which are mandatory and universal, are targeted because it was considered an extravagant program, allowing the citizens of France to consult as many doctors as they wanted as often as they wanted. French physicians have not experienced the cutbacks seen by their colleagues elsewhere. Health reform is on the block with the health care system now undergoing its biggest reform since 1945. Most of the French population is covered by three major national health insurance funds. The largest national health insurance fund covering only salaried workers is the Caisse Nationale d'Assurance Maladie des Travailleurs Salaries, which is financed by compulsory contributions from all wage earners and employers. The public has the opportunity to subscribe to private insurance simultaneously with the national health insurance, and most of the French do. The national health insurance is funded by social security contributions from working people, and with fluctuations in economic activity, health care deficits loom. The French government is reforming the rules and regulations of all involved in the health care system, from doctors to administrators. Reform is looking to improve the quality and safety of health care services, not only to reduce the cost. The government is doing this by evaluating clinical outcomes and patient satisfaction. The French people have a multilevel concept of health that includes not only the absence of disease but the avoidance of health risks and prevention of illness. The expensive coverage of this type of health has caused the need for reform. France is following epidemiological data on infectious disease but has included other areas such as chronic bronchitis. This is an exciting time for pulmonary rehabilitation specialists in France to show the government that pulmonary rehabilitation addresses this multilevel concept. France has been very involved with organizing consensus conferences and publishing clinical practice guidelines whose goal is to "systematically develop statements to assist practitioner and patient decisions about appropriate health care for specific clinical circumstances".[75]

Germany

The German[76,77] health care system has been divided into inpatient and ambulatory care sectors, and this has caused a fragmented system of care delivery. Now health care reforms have started to change this. In the inpatient setting, funding no longer is through per diem charges but a prospective payment system, permitting ambulatory surgery and care services to be offered in the inpatient settings. Reform has not yielded substantial cost savings at this time.

The German Medical Association has rejected cost-cutting reforms of the health system for fear that health care will be rationed and quality will be compromised. The government plans to create a fine-tuned system of referring general practitioners to limit direct access to specialists. Those patients who use the general practitioner will have their health insurance fees reduced. Severe criticisms of the reforms from health professionals grow.

Great Britain

Great Britain[78–81] has a National Health Service of socialized medicine that is experiencing rumblings of reform. The system needs modernization, from the building of new health care facilities (37 new hospitals planned) to remodeling the old. The government has put money into this project. Another reform idea is to consolidate services so duplication is not present. A 24-hour hotline for health-related questions, called NHS Direct, is currently serving 40% of the United Kingdom (Great Britain, Scotland, Wales, and Northern Ireland), with expansion to 100%. The hospital medical professional recruitment is aiming at improving pay and working conditions. An information technology program to integrate all health care facilities is under way. National standards of care, called National Service Frameworks, are developing white papers on treatment models for specific service or care groups. The goal is to introduce one white paper a year, with coronary heart disease and mental health to be developed first. The standards will measure compliance and outcomes. This is an opportunity to be used by the pulmonary rehabilitation community to advise and assist in the development of white papers for pulmonary disease treatment models. A trend is occurring in the United Kingdom for the citizens to use private insurance and private hospitals. The private sector has more modern treatment options available, and it takes less time to see the physician. At this time there are no laws mandating quality of care in the private sector, so the citizen must be the judge. The wait list in the National Health Service is being limited to an individual to spend no more than 18 months on the list. When one looks at the statistic that as of September 1999 the total number of people on the hospital wait list was 1,091,535, one can see the dilemma. The outpatient waiting list is more than 13 weeks. A recent health care professional vacancy survey found, as of March 1999, the following vacancies: 15,000 nurses, 1000 dental and medical consultants, and 2500 allied professionals (physical, occupational, and radiology technologist).

Movement toward a more patient-centered service less dominated by institutions is the goal of a 10-year reform program. The government introduced 481 primary care groups in England, each consisting of 50 general practitioners covering 100,000 people. This replaces the two-tier system that only allowed more than half of all budget-holding general practitioners to buy community and hospital care. The goal is to create a primary care–led service in which general practitioners would have significant control over hospital budgets. The goal of the British government is to make the National Health Service the best possible, offering quality care, available care, and new consumer-focused services.

Greece

Health care reform in Greece[82] started in 1983 when a National Health System was started by the state. Reform objectives include the expansion of the health sector, improved equity, and the state being totally responsible for health care delivery. During the past 10 years, reform results have proved a public-private mix in financing and delivery in favor of the private sector. In fact, the Greek health system is the most "privatized" program among the European countries. Reasons why health reform failed to meet its objectives were the enforcement of full-time and exclusive hospital employment for doctors, no private hospital expansion allowed, and the private sector being able to introduce new health technology faster. Reform of the reform was voted for in 1997 to address the shortcomings of the 1983 reform.

Israel

Israel's health minister has reported that the health system faces financial collapse.[83] The government has proposed to increase treasury contributions, to increase supplemental payments from the Israel residents, and to increase the global tax. The Israel Medical Association has spoken out against charging for a visit to the doctor. On average, Israelis consult physicians more than 10 times a year. National health insurance laws were implemented in 1995. Changes caused by health care reform have taken place in the provision of health services by Israel's sick funds and how these services are financed. It is a health care system with dynamic changes and challenges ahead.

Italy

In 1978 Italy reformed their health care system to a universal system covering all citizens.[84] Ever since, reformists have tried to change the system, giving more financial and managerial responsibilities to the regions. Reform challenges continue.

Now reform is taking the centrally planned, vertically integrated National Health Service into a market-oriented system.[85] Public funders will contract directly with individual providers. The ultimate goal of the reform is to guarantee universal coverage (not yet attained with the 1978 reform), secure global spending limits, promote efficiency in the delivery of care, and enhance responsiveness to consumers. Monitoring the impact of the reform on the health care system will be necessary.

A study done by the Universita degli Studi, Napoli, was published in 1997 that evaluated 52 COPD patients treated with a personalized rehabilitation program joining traditional techniques of rehabilitation and an exercise training program.[86] Data collected on the patients included the 12-minute walk and pulmonary function tests. The results of the study showed an improvement in the fitness level of COPD patients with exercise training that was maintained at 1-year follow-up.

Japan

The Japanese health care system is undergoing major changes.[87–89] Japan's medical care is financed through a pluralistic social insurance system.[87] The system has mandatory enrollment based on employment or residence. The premiums for the insurance are proportional to income. A dramatic increase in medical insurance fees for salaried workers occurred in 1997, also increasing the contribution to the medical bills. Japan's system is similar to that of Germany. Japan's medical care is egalitarian, advocating the doctrine of equal political, economic, and legal rights for all citizens. Many cross-subsidization's are seen among plans. Once a person is in the plan, no opportunity is available for them to opt out by buying private insurance. The elderly are subsidized by the young plus budget subsidies and income-proportional premiums. Regardless of the multiple insurers, all payments to providers flow through a national fee schedule. In a national fee schedule any new procedure becomes automatically available to everyone and is very expensive. Reform efforts continue addressing the problems of a fee schedule system. Expensive high technology is often curtailed by the fee schedule. In Japan the fee schedule is revised every 2 years from recommendations made by the Central Social Health Insurance Council, an advisory committee of the Minister of Health and Welfare in Japan. Different from the public sector, academic hospitals get direct subsidies from the government or university budgets for capital and possible operating expenses. The person needing health care has the freedom of choice to choose any physician or hospital, and physicians decide themselves about appropriate treatments. The payment system is based on the review and reimbursement, keeping administrative costs down. It has been noted that medical costs in Japan are about half those in the United States for both payers and providers. Hospitals in Japan (except government and university hospitals) started from solo practice, family businesses. The for-profit, investor-owned hospital in Japan is prohibited. A lack of nursing homes exist in Japan, resulting in a high hospital admission rate of people 65 years and older, and about one-third of them have been hospitalized for more than a year. The age, length of stay, and diagnosis of this aged population make for an ideal setting for aggressive pulmonary rehabilitation. In the year 2000, Japan will have a greater proportion of its people older than 65 years; therefore, the government is proposing public insurance for long-term care, covering care in the home and in public and private nursing homes.

The government is promoting home treatment and, again, outpatient pulmonary rehabilitation is needed. Medications are dispensed through physicians in private practice (80%) and by hospitals (89%).[87] This policy evolved from the legacy of Chinese medicine that had no formal separation between pharmacist and physician. Income is generated through the dispensing of medications. This reimbursement practice is being phased out, thereby depriving hospitals of their principal source of cash.[90]

A program in Japan to combat cancer does focus on preventive measures and a nationwide cancer information network.[89] Following this program closely may allow for a pulmonary network and prevention measures that may overlap. Pulmonary rehabilitation is a discipline seen in Japan, but its approach differs from that in the United States.[57,91] Reimbursement for pulmonary rehabilitation is at a rate of 35% of that provided for cardiac rehabilitation. Pulmonary rehabilitation in the current medical insurance system in Japan is not specialized but categorized together with rehabilitation for cerebrovascular disorders and bone fractures.[57]

A 1-year follow-up of pulmonary rehabilitation patients with emphysema looked at 12 patients who participated in an inpatient pulmonary rehabilitation program.[92] The study included follow-up 1 year after discharge. The recommendations were for the development of a maintenance program to help patients retain the benefits of pulmonary rehabilitation long term.

The Netherlands

A study was reported in 1996 on the benefits of outpatient pulmonary rehabilitation with 64 asthma and COPD patients.[93] Data collection included spirometry, bicycle ergometry, walking distance, and the Questionnaire for Asthma and COPD, which measures quality of life, compliance within therapy, ability to cope, and social support. Positive results were more dramatic in patients with asthma or mild COPD, with some improvement seen in severe COPD patients. This published article documents the need to emphasize prevention and earlier intervention of the pulmonary rehabilitation principles in patients with lung disease.

Long-term oxygen therapy is established in the scientific community to increase survival in hypoxemic patients with COPD, resulting in oxygen being prescribed for at least 15 hours a day in many European countries. A survey was designed to evaluate the oxygen clients of the largest oxygen company in The Netherlands. The conclusion was that in a selected group of long-term oxygen patients with COPD, both oxygen prescription and usage were often inadequate. This was found to be especially true when the oxygen prescription was written by a non–chest physician.[94] Striving for a standard of care for pulmonary patients is an international goal that erases borders, cultural differences, and language barriers. The United States is not alone.

New Zealand

New Zealand[95] has a tradition of private provision of primary health care. The current four regions of New Zealand's health authority are being merged into one body, centralized and separated from the Ministry of Health. This new central body will be purchasing from the private sector and allow private-sector involvement in Crown Health Enterprises. To cap expenditures the regional health authorities have done budget holding, which is seen as the first step toward managed care arrangements. The reform of the health care system is unclear as public discontent grows. Health reform is not the only issue that spans the continents, but evaluation of outcomes in pulmonary rehabilitation have been documented in Auckland, New Zealand, that are positive.[96] This reinforces that pulmonary rehabilitation is the standard of care for pulmonary patients.

Russia

The collapse of the Soviet Union in 1991 led Russia to replace the system of socialized medicine by a system of health insurance involved in the decentralization of health services.[97,98] A nationwide system of obligatory medical insurance was adopted by the Russian Federation in 1993 (Compulsory Health Insurance System). The goal was to target a source of funding for health care and to stop the decline in health outcomes. Today the Russian health care system has shifted from a national health system characterized by highly centralized management and control to a decentralized but fragmented multitude of state systems. The state systems are centralized at the local level and are run by local administrations with limited government experience. The government's role is not well defined, which risks the disintegration of the national system. The reform will continue to see challenges and change.

Spain

In 1998 a study of asthma was undertaken in Spain to evaluate the morbidity and mortality of asthma. In Spain, the incidence of asthma has increased, resulting in a substantial increase in the economic impact of this condition.[99] Total direct and indirect expenses were determined for asthma patients in a northern area of Spain for a 1-year period. The asthma was classified according to the 1992 International Consensus Report on Diagnosis and Treatment of Asthma of mild, moderate, and severe. Results are an estimated average, with the total annual asthma cost in US dollars of $2879 per patient, with $1336 for mild asthma, $2407 for moderate asthma, and $6393 for severe asthma. Indirect costs were reported to be twice as high as direct costs for all levels of severity. The cost of asthma was high and increased with the severity of the disease. The goal is to develop optimal intervention strategies for all levels of asthma severity to impact the rising morbidity and mortality associated with asthma in Spain. It is critical for pulmonary rehabilitation specialists to become involved with developing and implementing the intervention strategies for asthma.

Switzerland

Health care premiums increased significantly in Switzerland from 20% to 50% in 1996.[100] The goal was a countrywide flat rate for essential medical care, but this is not being realized. Sickness insurance payments are alleviated by subsidies through the federal and cantonal (territorial districts in Sweden) authorities. Reform is occurring in the government programs with some new laws replacing laws dating to 1911. It is interesting to note that in a published review article on pulmonary rehabilitation from Switzerland, the standard of care for the COPD patient was pulmonary rehabilitation.[101]

Taiwan

A study of 13 COPD patients who participated in a multidisciplinary pulmonary rehabilitation program was conducted.[102] Evaluation of pulmonary function, exercise capacity, and 6-minute walk distance was done. The results showed that patients with moderately severe COPD can improve exercise capacity, subjective symptoms, and quality of life through pulmonary rehabilitation. Another international study is needed to collaborate pulmonary rehabilitation as a standard of care for patients with pulmonary disease.

SUMMARY

The evolution of health insurance in the United States since the 1700s has been very dynamic and noncomplacent. The rising cost of health care has impacted society, creating great political debates. The sources of health care financing have had changing faces over the centuries, from nongovernmental health insurance programs to federal and state health insurance programs to casualty insurance.

The intent of this chapter is to provide a framework to build on in the process of learning and understanding the financing of health care and ultimately the reimbursement of pulmonary rehabilitation. As we enter the 21st century, this nation is faced with the challenges of the financing and management of health care for the growing number of Americans who rely on both public and private health insurance programs for protection. Managed care will clearly play a key role in cost containment for governmental and private health insurance programs with its increasing penetration into both sectors and its ongoing development of cost-control strategies well into the 21st century. The changes under the Balanced Budget Act of 1997 will extend the life of the Medicare Trust Fund and reduce Medicare spending, in addition to the Medicare + Choice options increasing beneficiary participation in managed care plans. The growth of managed care in the Medicare program by the year 2009 is expected to reach 14 million, accounting for approximately one-third (31%) of the Medicare population.[9] Managed care is here to stay, and learning how to navigate the system is critical to pulmonary rehabilitation program survival. It is up to the pulmonary rehabilitation director and medical director to educate managed care organizations and other third-party payers about the benefits of a comprehensive pulmonary rehabilitation program.[33]

The need for accurate documentation for outcomes, benchmarking, and reimbursement cannot be over emphasized. The e-commerce highway will drive the pulmonary rehabilitation program documentation to the next level. It will be an exciting ride and one with which we must keep up. The realization of the virtual patient record through networked computers is in our future. We need to collaborate with our colleagues throughout the world to improve the standard of care for our pulmonary patient and make our differences our strengths.[48,58,103,104] The evidence-based practice of pulmonary rehabilitation must become a standard in the pulmonary health care network. Through collaboration with our colleagues, we must shift the focus of our programs from treatment to prevention, ultimately impacting our patients' quality of life and our country's economy.

REFERENCES

1. LeBrun P, Miller JM, Raichel TM. Financing for health education services in the United States. Prepared by Blue Cross and Blue Shield Association per HHS Contract 200-79-0916, 1980.
2. Starr P. The Social Transformation of American Medicine. New York: Basic Books, 1982:198–363.
3. Mittelmann M. Rehabilitation issues from an insurer's viewpoint: past, present, future. Arch Phys Med Rehabil 1980;61:587.
4. Guccione AA. Needs of the elderly and the politics of health care. Phys Ther 1988;68:1386.
5. Simmock P, Bauer DW. Reimbursement issues in diabetes. Diabetes Care 1984;7:291.
6. Kramarow E, Lentzner H, Rooks R, et al. Health and Aging Chart Book, United States 1999. Hyattsville, MD: National Center for Health Statistics, 1999.
7. Bodenheimer T, Grumback K. Reimbursing physicians and hospitals: health care policy: a clinical approach. JAMA 1994;272:971–977.
8. Kuttner R. The American health care system: health insurance coverage. N Engl J Med Health Policy Rep 1999;340:153–158.
9. Henry J. Kaiser Family Foundation. The Medicare Program: Medicare at a Glance. Menlo Park, CA: Henry J. Kaiser Family Foundation, 1999.
10. Health Care Financing Administration. Guide to health insurance for people with Medicare. Washington, DC: US Department of Health and Human Services, 1997. HCFA publication 02110.
11. Ellis RP, McGurie TG. Insurance principles and the design of prospective payment systems. J Health Econ 1988;7:215.
12. Fetter RB, Freeman JL, Mullin RL. DRGs: how they evolved and are changing the way hospitals are managed. Pathologist 1985;Jun:17.
13. Russell LB, Manning CL. The effect of prospective payment on Medicare expenditures. N Engl J Med 1989;320:439.
14. Dore D. Effect of the Medicare prospective payment system on the utilization of physical therapy. Phys Ther 1987;67:964.
15. Waid M. Brief Summaries of Medicare and Medicaid Title XVIII and Title XIX of the Social Security Act. Hyattsville, MD: Health Care Financing Administration, DHHS, 1998.
16. Balanced Budget Act of 1997, PL105-33, HR 2015, Senate and House of Representatives of the United States of America. Washington, DC: GPO, 1997:195–196.
17. Implementation update. Available at: http://www.hcfa.gov. Accessed March 13, 2000.
18. Iglehart J. The American health care system: Medicare. N Engl J Med 1999;340:4.
19. Families USA Foundation. Key features of "Medicare Reform" proposals. Available at: http://www.familiesusa.org. Accessed October 6, 1999.
20. AARC Continuing Care and Rehabilitation Bulletin. Dallas, TX: AARC, Nov/Dec 1998.
21. Porte P. News from the hill. News and Views of AACVPR 1999. Middleton, WI 1999;13:3.
22. Henry J. Kaiser Family Foundation, Kaiser Commission on Medicaid Basics. Medicaid: A Primer, an Introduction and Overview. Washington, D.C.: Kaiser Commission, 1999.
23. Health Resources and Services Administration, Department of Health and Human Services Office of Special Programs. Frequently asked questions by consumers about receiving Hill Burton or free or reduced cost care. Available at: http://158.72.83.8/osp/dfcr/obtain CONSFAQ.htm.
24. Health Resources and Services Administration (HRSA). The Hill-Burton Free Care Program. Available at: http://www.hcfa.gov. Accessed October 28, 1999.
25. Porte P. Legislation and respiratory rehabilitation. Respir Care 1983;28:1498.
26. Comprehensive outpatient rehabilitation facility. Federal Register 1986;51(220):41332.
27. Comprehensive outpatient rehabilitation facility: rules and regulations. Federal Register 1982; 47(241):56282.
28. O'Sullivan J, Franco C, Fuchs B, et al. Medicare Provisions in the Balanced Budget Act of 1997 (BBA 97, P.L. 105-33): CRS Report for Congress. Bethesda, MD: Penny Press, 1997:17–29.
29. Department of Veterans Affairs (VA). Veterans

health administration. Available at: http://www.va.gov. Accessed October 28, 1999.

30. Military Health System website. TRICARE information: the history of CHAMPUS and its evolving role in TRICARE. Available at: http://www.tricare.osd.mil. Accessed October 28, 1999.

31. Military Health System website. What is TRICARE? Available at: http://www.tricare.osd.mil. Accessed October 28, 1999.

32. Health Care Financing Administration. Guide to Third Party Liability. Rockville, MD: US Department of Health and Human Services, 1980; 421;311–368.

33. Limberg T. How does pulmonary rehabilitation survive in a managed care market? Respir Care Clin N Am 1998;4:1.

34. Beytas LJ, Connors GL. Organization and Management of a pulmonary rehabilitation program. In: Hodgkin JE, Connors GL, Bell CW, eds. Pulmonary Rehabilitation: Guidelines to Success. 2nd ed. Philadelphia: Lippincott, 1993; 562–586.

35. Scanlan CL. Patient safety, communication, and record-keeping. In: Scanlan CL, Wilkins RL, Stroller JK ed. Egan's Fundamentals of Respiratory Care. 7th ed. St. Louis: Mosby, 1999: 33–37.

36. Nisonson I. The medical record. Bull Am Coll Surg 1991;76(9):24–26.

37. Des Jardins T, Burton GG. Recording skills: the basis for data collection, organization, assessment skills (critical thinking), and treatment plans. In: Clinical Manifestations and Assessment of Respiratory Disease. 3rd ed. St. Louis: Mosby, 1995:141–151.

38. Aghili H, Mushlin RA, Williams RM, Rose JS. Progress notes model. Proc AMIA Annu Fall Symp 1997:12–16.

39. Gardner RM, Elliott CG, Greenway L. The computer for charting and monitoring. In: Kacmarek RM, Hess D, Stroller JK, eds. Monitoring in Respiratory Care. St. Louis: Mosby, 1993:565–585.

40. Glassman KS, Kelly J. Facilitating care management through computerized clinical pathways. Top Health Inf Manage 1998;19(2):70–78.

41. Mohr JR. A quantitative perspective on the virtual patient record (VPR) and its realization. Medinfo 1998;9(Pt 1):21–25.

42. Dragon Systems website. Available at: http://www.dragonsystems.com. Accessed February 19, 2000.

43. Wood KJ. Critical Thinking: Cases in Respiratory Care. Philadelphia: F.A. Davis, 1998:5.

44. Stegall GC. Blueprints: a critical pathway alternative. Hosp Case Manag 1998;6(5):95–98.

45. Moore LM. High standards: ISO 9000 comes to health care. Trustee 1999;52(2):10–14.

46. Iezzoni LI. The demand for documentation for Medicare payment [editorial]. N Engl J Med 1999;341(5).

47. Chute CG, Cohn SP, Campbell JR. A framework for comprehensive health terminology systems in the United States: development guidelines, criteria for selection, and public policy impli-cations: ANSI Healthcare Informatics Standards Board Vocabulary Working Group and the Computer-Based Patient Records Institute Working Groups on Codes and Structures. J Am Med Inform Assoc 1998;5(6):503–510.

48. Guidelines for the management of chronic obstructive pulmonary disease. S Afr Med J 1998; 88(9):999–1002,1004,1006–1010.

49. Thoonen BP, van Schayck CP, van Weel C, et al. Present and future management of asthma and COPD: proceedings from WONCA1998. Fam Pract 1999;16(3):313–315.

50. Villiger B. Rehabilitation in COPD. Ther Umsch 1999;56:131–135.

51. Proceedings of the 3rd International Conference on Advances in Pulmonary Rehabilitation and Management of Chronic Respiratory Failure, Florence, Italy, March 11-14, 1998. Monaldi Arch Chest Dis 1999;54:55–97.

52. Albalak R, Frisancho AR, Keeler GJ. Domestic biomass fuel combustion and chronic bronchitis in two rural Bolivian villages. Thorax 1999;54: 1004–1008.

53. Donelan K, Blendon RJ, Schoen C, Davis K, Binns K. The cost of health system change: public discontent in five nations. Health Aff (Millwood) 1999;18(3):206–216.

54. Tuuponen T, Keistinen T, Kivela SL. Regional differences in long-term mortality among hospital-treated asthma and COPD patients. Scand J Soc Med 1997;25(4):238–242.

55. Hupkens CL, van den Berg J, van der Zee J. National health interview surveys in Europe: an overview. Health Policy 1999;47(2):145–168.

56. Health Shield website. Available at: http://www.healthshield.co.uk/index.htm. Accessed November 4, 1999.

57. Kida D, Jinno S, Nomura K, Uamodo K, Katsura H, Kudoh S. Pulmonary Rehabilitation Program Survey in North America, Europe, and Tokyo. J Cardiopulm Rehabil 1998;18:301–308.

58. Smeets F. Proposal for a European COPD network. Lung 1990;168(Suppl):509–513.

59. Harrigan P. Australia reports on health priorities. Lancet 1997;350:793.

60. Hall J. Incremental change in the Australian health care system. Health Aff (Millwood) 1999; 18(3):95–110.

61. Schoo AM. A literature review of rehabilitative interventions for chronic obstructive pulmonary disease patients. Aust Health Rev 1997;20(3): 120–132.

62. Farrell M. Trends in the global health care environment: the developed countries. Contemp Nurse 1998;7(4):180–189.

63. Hensley S. Brazilian healthcare at a crossroads: private sector flourishes as the government's program buckles under heavy demand, lack of funding. Mod Healthc 1999;29(20):34–36, 38.

64. Davies BJ. Canada's health system. Croat Med J 1999;40(2):280–286.

65. Naylor CD. Health care in Canada: incrementalism under fiscal duress. Health Aff (Millwood) 1999;18(3):9–26.

66. Caro DH. A comprehensive assessment of Canadian health program guidelines: international

health system implication. World Hosp 1993; 29(1):5–13.

67. Health Canada Online website. Available at: http://www.hc-sc.gc.ca/english/. Accessed November 10, 1999.

68. Lacasse Y, Brooks D, Goldstein RS. Trends in the epidemiology of COPD in Canada, 1980 to 1995, and rehabilitation. Chest 1999;116(2): 306–313.

69. Brooks D, Lacasse Y, Goldstein RS. Pulmonary rehabilitation programs in Canada: national survey. Can Respir J 1999;6(1):55–63.

70. Deber R, Swan B. Canadian health expenditures: where do we really stand internationally? CMAJ 1999;160(12):1730–1734.

71. Canadian Lung Association website. Available at: http://www.lung.ca. Accessed November 10, 1999.

72. Hesketh T, Zhu WX. Health in China: the healthcare market. BMJ 1997;314:1616–1618.

73. Hu TW, Ong M, Lin ZH, Li E. The effects of economic reform on health insurance and the financial burden for urban workers in China. Health Econ 1999;8(4):309–321.

74. Wong VC, Chiu SW. Health-care reforms in the People's Republic of China: strategies and social implications. J Manag Med 1998;12(4-5): 270–286.

75. Country profile: France. Lancet 1997:349:7.

76. Busse R, Schwartz FW. Financing reforms in the German hospital sector: from full cost cover principle to prospective case fees. Med Care 1997;35(Suppl 10):OS40–OS49.

77. Durand de Bousingen D. German health-care reform put on the agenda. Lancet 1999;353: 2048.

78. Varnell M. New life for Britain's National Health Service. Adv Respir Care Pract 1999;Sept 27: 20.

79. Dean M. Labour's health reform begins. Lancet 1999;353:1163.

80. Milewa T. Health for all and British health policy: a comment on the quest for "healthy public policy." J Manag Med 1996;10:59–64.

81. Shekelle P, Roland M. Measuring quality in the NHS: lessons from across the Atlantic. Lancet 1998;352:163–164.

82. Liaropoulos LL, Kaitelidou D. Changing the public-private mix: an assessment of the health reforms in Greece. Health Care Anal 1998; 6(4):277–285.

83. Bentur N, Berg A, Gross R, Chinitz D. Health system reform and the elderly: the case of Israel. J Aging Soc Policy 1998;10(2):85–104.

84. Vicarelli, Mallet JO. Italy: a national health service with a tumultuous history. Cah Sociol Demogr Med 1999;39(1):5–23.

85. Taroni F, Guerra R, D'Ambrosio MG. The health care reform in Italy: transition or turmoil. J Health Hum Serv Adm 1998;20(4):396–422.

86. Caputi M, Meoli I, Manna M, Speranza A, Esposito V, Marsico SA. Proposal of a thoraco-

pulmonary rehabilitation program in patients with chronic obstructive pulmonary disease. Minerva Med 1997;88(7-8):293–298.

87. Ikegami N, Campbell JC. Medical care in Japan. N Engl J Med 1995;333:1295.

88. Goo M. In Japan, health care is the issue. Nieman Reports 1997;51(1):54.

89. Ross C. A move for Japanese health reform. Lancet 1994;343:721.

90. Under the knife. Economist, September 12, 1997;344:65.

91. Hirata K, Okamoto T, Shiraishi S, Ohtsuda T. The efficacy and practice of exercise training in patients with chronic obstructive pulmonary disease (COPD): in process citation. Nippon Rinsho 1999;57(9):2041–2045.

92. Inoue M, Ohtsu I, Tomioka S, et al. One year follow-up of pulmonary rehabilitation patients with pulmonary emphysema: physiological outcome. Nihon Kokyuki Gakkai Zasshi 1998; 36(9):7.

93. Bruinings AL, Bauer H, Mensen EA, Willems L. Good results of outpatient pulmonary rehabilitation: 2-year experience in the Rijnland Zeehospitium in Katwijk. Ned Tijdschr Geneeskd 1996;140(29):150.

94. Kampelmacher MJ, Van Kesteren RG, Alsbach GP, et al. Prescription and usage of long-term oxygen therapy in patients with chronic obstructive pulmonary disease in The Netherlands. Respir Med 1999;98:46–51.

95. Coney S. Business as usual for New Zealand's health care. Lancet 1997;349:37.

96. Young P, Dewse M, Fergusson W, Kolbe J. Improvements in outcomes for chronic obstructive pulmonary disease (COPD) attributable to pulmonary rehabilitation. Aust N Z J Med 1999; 29(1):59–65.

97. Chernichovsky D, Potapchik E. Genuine federalism in the Russian health care system: changing roles of government. J Health Polit Policy Law 1999;24(1):115–144.

98. Field MG. Reflections on a painful transition: from socialized to insurance medicine in Russia. Croat Med J 1999;40(2):202–209.

99. Serra-Batlles J, Plaza V, Morejon E, Comella A, Brugues J. Costs of asthma according to the degree of severity. Eur Respir J 1998;12(6): 1322–1326.

100. New health charges shock for swiss. Lancet 1995;346:2.

101. Villiger B. Rehabilitation in COPD. Ther Umsch 1999;56(3):131–135.

102. Lin MC, Liaw MY, Huang CC, Tsai YH. A multidisciplinary pulmonary rehabilitation program for patients with moderately severe chronic obstructive pulmonary disease. J Formos Med Assoc 1997;96(11):869–873.

103. De Muralt B, Fitting JW. Respiratory Rehabilitation. Schweiz Med Wochenschr 1992;122(37): 1347–1351.

104. Barandun J. Value and costs of pulmonary rehabilitation. Schweiz Rundsch Med Prax 1997; 86(50):1979–1983.

31 Physical Medicine Interventions and Rehabilitation of Patients With Neuromuscular Weakness

John R. Bach

⟫ Professional Skills

Upon completion of this chapter, the reader will:

- Discuss the hazards of oxygen therapy for patients with alveolar hypoventilation
- Evaluate three styles of the negative-pressure ("body") ventilators with respect to efficacy and practicality
- Describe the three noninvasive positive-pressure techniques of assisted ventilation with respect to efficacy and comfort
- Describe the technique of glossopharyngeal breathing (GPB), indications for its use, and methods for evaluating efficacy
- Discuss the manual and mechanical methods of assisted coughing
- Discuss the clinical indications for the use of noninvasive methods of respiratory assistance as alternatives to tracheostomy

INTRODUCTION

Respiratory complications are the most common cause of morbidity and mortality for patients with neuromuscular disease. Respiratory complications result from the progressive inspiratory and expiratory muscle weakness inherent in these conditions. Even for neuromuscular conditions that seem to be static, senescent loss of myoneural tissues and, for children, normal growth can create a progressive worsening of the clinical picture. Thus, even patients with conditions like postpoliomyelitis, spinal cord injury, and spinal muscular atrophy (SMA)[1] can eventually require inspiratory and expiratory (respiratory) muscle assistance. Impaired lung growth, spinal deformity, decreased lung compliance, concomitant obstructive sleep apnea, sedative and oxygen administration, and malnutrition or

591

obesity can all decrease the ability of already weakened inspiratory muscles to maintain adequate alveolar ventilation. Inspiratory muscle function, like expiratory muscle function, is also important for clearing airway secretions. Eventually, either carbon dioxide (CO_2) narcosis or acute respiratory failure occur because of the inability of the respiratory muscles to generate an effective cough, usually during intercurrent upper respiratory tract infections (chest colds).

THE NEUROMUSCULAR CONDITIONS

Patients with lung disease have primarily oxygenation impairment and can benefit from supplemental oxygen administration. Patients with neuromuscular conditions have primarily ventilatory impairment and need assistance for respiratory muscle function. Their evaluation and management is distinctly different from that of patients with oxygenation impairment. Physical medicine interventions are used to facilitate breathing, coughing, and physical functioning for patients with these conditions (Box 31-1).

The progressive neuromuscular diseases include myopathies, generalized neuropathies, and motor neuron diseases. Patients with some central nervous system disorders, skeletal deformities, morbid obesity, and myelopathies such as high-level tetraplegia caused by spinal cord injury and even some patients with severe respiratory impairment caused by intrinsic or obstructive pulmonary disease also need to be treated by similar principles. Description of all of these disorders is beyond the scope of this chapter, but the interested reader can find good references elsewhere.[2,3] However, the same evaluation and management principles apply to all the listed conditions.

THE REHABILITATION TEAM AND PATIENT MANAGEMENT STAGES

Episodes of acute respiratory failure are often avoidable for patients with neuromuscular disease.[4] However, in a recent survey of neuromuscular disease clinics it was found that for most of their patients, this is often overlooked.[5] Likewise, many nonrespiratory management aspects are little understood by most physicians treating patients with neuromuscular disease.[6] Many patients with the conditions listed in Box 31-1 use ventilators for most of their lives. Thus, it is important for the physician who manages their ventilatory insufficiency to be aware of more than only the ventilator management options. The treating physician also needs some understanding of the evaluation of neuromuscular, musculoskeletal, cognitive, and cardiac aspects of care as well as the management of functional deficits.

In addition to orthopedic, chest physician, and physical medicine specialists, the treatment team usually includes physical, occupation, and respiratory therapists and possibly a nutritionist, psychologist, and social worker. The physical and occupational therapists provide and train the care providers in performing joint mobilization to maximize articular range of motion and perform exercises to increase the strength of muscles with greater than antigravity strength and to increase endurance, coordination, balance, functional mobility, and transfer capabilities. They also train the patient in energy conservation, offer assistive devices and orthoses to minimize fatigue and support articulations, and train the patient and caregivers in personal care activities. Occupational therapists also train the patient in the use of environmental control systems and robotics for upper extremity activities of daily living. The therapist evaluates the home and suggests modifications to eliminate barriers and assesses the patient's wheelchair needs. Either the occupational therapist or the respiratory therapist can fabricate and fit custom interfaces and strap retention systems for the noninvasive delivery of intermittent positive-pressure ventilation (IPPV).

Box 31-1. Neuromusculoskeletal and Medical Conditions Amenable to Physical
Medicine Interventions

Myopathies
  Muscular dystrophies
    Dystrophinopathies—Duchenne and Becker dystrophies
    Other muscular dystrophies—limb-girdle, Emery-Dreifuss, facioscapulohumeral,
      congenital, childhood autosomal recessive, and myotonic dystrophy and/or
      other myopathies
  Non-dystrophy myopathies
    Congenital, such as nemaline, spheroid body, and fiber-type disproportion
    Metaboliclike, such as maltase deficiency
    Mitochondrial, such as Kearns-Sayre syndrome
    Inflammatory, such as polymyositis
    Mixed connective-tissue disease
    Myopathies of systemic disease, such as carcinomatous myopathy, cachexia/
      anorexia nervosa, medication associated
    Myoneural junction disease, such as myasthenia gravis
Peripheral neurological disorders
  Motor neuron diseases
    Spinal muscular atrophies
    Poliomyelitis
    Amyotrophic lateral sclerosis
Myelopathies of rheumatoid, infectious, spondylitic, vascular, traumatic, or
  idiopathic etiology
Neuropathies
  Hereditary sensory motor neuropathies
  Phrenic neuropathies—associated with cardiac hypothermia, surgical or other
    trauma, radiation, phrenic
  Electrostimulation, familial, paraneoplastic or infectious etiology, and with lupus
    erythematosus
  Tetraplegia associated with pancuronium bromide, botulism
  Guillain-Barrè syndrome
Central nervous system disorders
  Multiple sclerosis
  Disorders of supraspinal tone such as Friedreich's ataxia
Sleep-disordered breathing, including obesity hypoventilation; central and
  congenital hypoventilation syndromes; and hypoventilation associated with
  diabetic microangiopathy, familial dysautonomia, or Down's syndrome
Skeletal pathology such as kyphoscoliosis, osteogenesis imperfecta, and rigid spine
  syndrome
Hypercapnic instrinsic or obstructive lung disease

A respiratory therapist who is trained in the use of noninvasive respiratory muscle aids is essential to maintain patients free of respiratory complications and tracheostomy, as well as for safe decannulation and transition of individuals from ventilatory support via a translaryngeal or tracheostomy tube to using only noninvasive aids. The respiratory therapist trains the patient, family, and medical staff in assisted coughing techniques, noninvasive IPPV, insufflator–exsufflators, and other respiratory interventions. He or she trains in oximetry feedback to guide in the use of these devices, and sets up the home mechanical ventilation program. The therapist must be familiar with and be able to prepare different IPPV interfaces and instruct in their use. In addition, a specifically trained respiratory therapist must be available at all times to evaluate equipment difficulties and resolve technical problems. In monitoring the efficacy of the home respiratory management program, his or her participation and communication with the managing physician is vital for its success and the successful management of intercurrent chest colds without hospitalization.

The prosthetist–orthotist can design, fabricate, and fit orthodontic bite plates and construct custom acrylic low-profile nasal and oronasal interfaces for noninvasive IPPV.[7] With the many nasal interfaces on the market, including custom-molded varieties like the SEFAM interface (SEFAM kit, available from Respironics Inc, Murrysville, PA), the prosthetist–orthotist is less often needed.

The rehabilitation nurse is often the principal trainer in personal hygiene, skin care, and adaptive equipment for activities of daily living.

The speech-language pathologist evaluates verbal function and communication and provides vocal reeducation or augmentative communication. He or she evaluates for dysphagia, performs methylene blue swallowing tests, assists in barium swallow video fluoroscopic evaluations, provides appropriate family education, and assists in cognitive retraining. The speech-language pathologist can also help in training the patient to learn to use the soft palate to seal off the nasopharynx for successful use of mouthpiece IPPV.

The psychologist evaluates cognitive and affective functioning. This includes the evaluation of judgment, perception, memory, and coping mechanisms. He or she helps the patient and family develop effective coping skills.

The social worker evaluates disposition options, financial and community resources, and possible lifestyle changes to accommodate residual disabilities.

The vocational counselor evaluates vocational interests, experience, aptitudes, skills, and opportunities. He or she prepares a program for improving marketable skills, facilitates communication between the patient and employment and training agencies, and counsels potential employers. Many 24-hour ventilator users with no extremity function are gainfully employed.[8]

Loss of lean body mass is a common problem for patients with neuromuscular respiratory muscle dysfunction. In fact, malnutrition and weight loss are independent and significant determinants of morbidity and mortality for people with pulmonary impairment, whether owing to intrinsic lung disease or respiratory muscle dysfunction. Weight loss to a mean total body weight of 70 lb occurs for patients with Duchenne muscular dystrophy at the point of requiring ventilator use. The nutritionist is important for assessing caloric intake and guiding nutrient intake under the limitations imposed by bulbar muscle dysfunction and ventilator use. Other key team members include the recreation therapist and dentist. They are asked to participate as the need arises.

It is important to consider patients with neuromuscular disease in three management stages (Box 31-2). The reader is referred to other sources for the comprehensive management of the first two stages for which the medical and rehabilitation team is intensively involved.[9] This chapter emphasizes the interventions that are needed to prolong survival and optimize quality of life for patients in the stage of prolonged survival.

RESPIRATORY MUSCLE AIDS

The respiratory muscles can be aided by manually or mechanically applying forces to the body or intermittent pressure to the airway. The devices that act on the body include negative-pressure body ventilators (NPBVs), which assist respiratory muscles by intermittently creating subatmospheric pressure around the thorax and abdomen, and body ventilators, which apply force to the body to mechanically displace respiratory muscles. Positive-pressure ventilators can assist inspiratory muscle function, and manual abdominal thrusts and mechanical exsufflation assist expiratory muscle function. Certain blowers deliver continuous positive airway pressure (CPAP). CPAP splints open the airway but does not in itself assist respiratory muscle function and will no longer be considered here.

Most Common Errors

Misinterpretation of Symptoms
Whereas the symptoms of hypoxia are commonly recognized and can include dyspnea, cognitive changes, and anxiety, the symptoms of hypercapnia are often ignored. They can

Box 31-2. Key Management Interventions for Neuromuscular Disease Stages

General diagnostic and management considerations
    Early diagnosis for family planning
    Counseling to prevent counterproductive family psychodynamics, to educate
        concerning future therapeutic options, and to encourage goal-oriented
        activities and future planning
    Management of nutritional, gastrointestinal, and swallowing difficulties
    Monitoring for and prevention of cardiac complications
Ambulatory stage
    Early use of supportive physical and occupational therapy, orthopedic surgery,
        and possibly splinting to maintain orthopedic integrity, ambulation, and
        pulmonary compliance
Wheelchair-dependent stage
    Facilitation of independence in activities of daily living
    Prevention or correction of back deformity
    Maintenance of limb range of motion and pulmonary compliance
The stage of prolonged survival
    Facilitation of patient self-direction and care provider management
    Facilitation of functional independence with assistive devices
    Use of noninvasive respiratory muscle aids to maintain normal alveolar
        ventilation and clear airway secretions

include fatigue; dyspnea; morning headaches; drowsiness; difficulties with sleep, swallowing, speech, and concentration; frequent nightmares; irritability; anxiety; impaired intellectual function; and depression. Although people with either ventilatory impairment or lung disease with oxygenation impairment complain of shortness of breath when walking, wheelchair users with ventilation impairment rarely complain of shortness of breath despite severe hypercapnia and impending respiratory failure. Instead, they complain of anxiety and inability to fall asleep. Many orthopneic patients have little or no ability to breathe without ventilatory assistance when fully supine. This can be because of a disproportionate degree of diaphragm weakness compared with that of the accessory inspiratory muscles. Instead of providing respiratory muscle aids to permit sleep and prevent respiratory failure, emergency department physicians tend to treat these symptoms as though they are from oxygenation impairment or congestive heart failure, a frequent source of confusion.

For small children with neuromuscular disease, the initial signs of nocturnal underventilation might just be frequent arousals from sleep. This is often mistaken for the simple need to be turned, or it may be considered normal. Children with SMA type 1 develop pectus excavatum and extremely attenuated lung growth unless they benefit from nocturnal noninvasive IPPV.

Inadequate Pulmonary Function Studies
People with neuromuscular conditions are routinely sent for a comprehensive battery of pulmonary function tests. However, because people with neuromuscular conditions rarely have significant concomitant lung disease, most of these tests are of little benefit, and the ones that can be helpful are not among those usually done.

Failure to Appropriately Monitor Sleep
Polysomnography is only warranted for patients with relatively normal respiratory muscle function who present with symptoms of sleep-disordered breathing. Polysomnography indicates the presence of central and obstructive apnea. It does not indicate that symptoms are caused by underventilation secondary to inspiratory muscle weakness. To diagnose and treat the latter, the tests described in the Patient Evaluation section must be obtained.

Overreliance on Arterial Blood Gases

Arterial blood gas analyses are not warranted for the routine monitoring of patients with neuromuscular disease. The required information can be obtained using end tidal CO_2 measurements, oxyhemoglobin percent saturation (SaO_2) monitoring, and venous blood sampling for bicarbonate levels.

Treatment for Oxygenation Rather Than for Ventilation Impairment

The treatment of patients with oxygenation impairment typically includes supplemental oxygen, bronchodilators, and chest physical therapy. For people with chronic lung disease, oxygen therapy can prolong life. However, for people with primarily ventilatory impairment, oxygen therapy exacerbates hypercapnia and its symptoms and increases the risk of respiratory complications and respiratory failure.[10] Emergency department physicians tend to manage patients with neuromuscular disease by administering oxygen, bronchodilators, and often mild sedatives to "help the patient sleep." When the sedatives and oxygen exacerbate underventilation and exacerbate respiratory failure, the patients undergo translaryngeal intubation and then tracheotomy when ventilator weaning is delayed. Intubation and tracheostomy should be unnecessary for most patients managed with respiratory muscle aids. Bronchodilators, too, must be used with caution because they can exacerbate tachycardia in myopathic patients who may already have clinically apparent cardiomyopathy. Furthermore, instead of overemphasizing the effort-intensive use of chest percussion, people with weak respiratory muscles need to have their cough flows normalized by the use of inspiratory and expiratory muscle aids. Chest percussion and postural drainage should not be used for well patients or anyone without productive airway secretions.

Intubation and Tracheostomy Paradigm Paralysis

Many physicians suffer from intubation and tracheostomy paradigm paralysis.[11] The paradigm is that people who cannot breathe need ventilators and ventilation must be delivered and airway secretions must be eliminated via invasive tubes. Nevertheless, much controversy remains over when to institute "mechanical ventilation." In reality, about 90% of episodes of respiratory failure occur during chest colds because of inability of respiratory muscles (mostly expiratory muscles) to cough out airway secretions.[10] Intubation or tracheostomy is rarely needed for ventilatory support, even for patients with no measurable vital capacity (VC) provided that they have sufficient bulbar muscle function with which to generate greater than 160 L/min of assisted peak cough flows (PCFs).[12] Essentially, they need sufficient bulbar muscle function with which to speak. Like inspiratory muscles, expiratory muscles can be assisted to increase PCFs and eliminate airway secretions, but the use of noninvasive methods is contrary to the treatment paradigms that physicians spent so much time learning.

INSPIRATORY MUSCLE AIDS

Body Ventilators

The NPBVs intermittently create subatmospheric pressure around the thorax and abdomen to assist or support the inspiratory effort.[13] They include tank ventilators like the iron lung, Porta-lung, chest shell ventilator, and wrap-style ventilators (Fig. 31-1). NPBVs are suitable for overnight ventilatory support and can often adequately ventilate neuromuscular patients with little or no VC despite the frequent nocturnal occurrence of transient oxyhemoglobin desaturations caused by apparent episodes of airway collapse.[14] Most patients, however, eventually have to be switched to the more effective noninvasive IPPV methods for daytime and nocturnal support.[15]

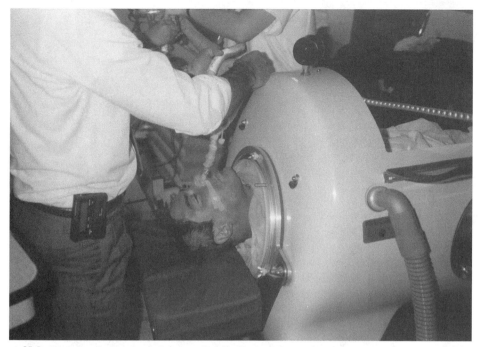

Figure 31-1. High-level spinal cord–injured individual with no ventilator-free breathing ability supported by the Porta-Lung NPBV so that he could be extubated and safely transitioned to noninvasive IPPV.

Body ventilators that act directly on the body include the rocking bed and the intermittent abdominal-pressure ventilator (IAPV). The rocking bed (J. H. Emerson Co, Cambridge, MA) rocks the patient at an arc of 15 to 30°. Gravity cyclically displaces the abdominal contents, causing diaphragmatic excursion to assist ventilation. This device is generally not as effective as NPBVs or noninvasive IPPV.

The IAPV (Exsufflation Belt, Respironics Inc, Murrysville, PA) consists of an elastic inflatable bladder incorporated within an abdominal corset worn beneath the patient's outer clothing (Fig. 31-2). The sac is intermittently inflated by a positive-pressure ventilator. Bladder action moves the diaphragm upward, causing a forced exsufflation. During bladder deflation the abdominal contents and diaphragm fall to the resting position, and inspiration occurs passively. A trunk angle of 30° or more from the horizontal is necessary for it to be effective. If the patient has any inspiratory capacity or is capable of GPB, he or she can add the autonomous tidal volume to the mechanically assisted inspiration. The IAPV generally augments tidal volumes by about 300 mL, but volumes as high as 1200 mL have been reported.[16] Patients with less than 1 hour of ventilator-free breathing ability often prefer to use the IAPV when sitting rather than the noninvasive methods of IPPV.[16] The IAPV is often inadequate in the presence of scoliosis or obesity.

Noninvasive IPPV

When positive-pressure ventilators became widely available in the United States in 1956, many necessarily recumbent body ventilator users with little or no measurable VC refused to undergo tracheotomy to use IPPV and, thereby, to facilitate their mobility outside the body ventilator. Many of these patients, however, learned how to receive IPPV via a mouthpiece held between their lips and teeth. Others learned how to have the mouthpiece fixed near the mouth by either a metal clamp attached to the wheelchair or fixed onto the controls that operate the motorized wheelchair (sip and puff, chin control, etc.)

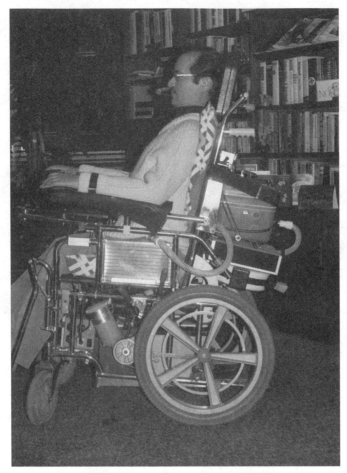

Figure 31-2. Positive-pressure ventilator mounted on a motorized wheelchair and driving an IAPV that is being worn under the patient's clothing.

(Fig. 31-3). They used the mouthpiece for IPPV as necessary[17] and were thus freed from their body ventilators during daytime hours.

Dr. Augusta Alba recognized that patients would occasionally nap while sitting in their wheelchairs using mouthpiece IPPV without the mouthpiece falling out of their mouths.[18] By 1964 many patients in one center had left their body ventilators to use up to 24-hour mouthpiece IPPV.[15] Ultimately, several hundred patients relied on this technique alone or in combination with body ventilators for up to 24-hour ventilatory support for 40 years or more before nasal IPPV was described.[13] Orthodontic bite plates and custom shells were fabricated to increase comfort and efficacy and eliminate the risk of orthodontic deformity with long-term use.

With the advent of the lipseal (Malincrodt, Pleasanton, CA) (Fig. 31-4) in 1972, mouthpiece IPPV could be delivered during sleep with less air (insufflation) leakage out of the mouth and with little risk of the mouthpiece falling out of the mouth. In 1978, portable volume ventilators became available with the option of producing regular deep insufflation (sighs) and with safety alarms and other features.[18]

Mouthpiece and nasal IPPV are open systems that rely in large part on central nervous system reflexes to prevent excessive insufflation leakage during sleep.[19] Ventilator alarms are generally unnecessary when using these systems because many patients can learn GPB and use the SaO_2 alarms of oximeters. The SaO_2 alarms can also be useful for feedback, as will be described, and for monitoring the nocturnal efficacy of noninvasive IPPV.[15]

In 1982, as an alternative to mouthpiece IPPV for "resting" the inspiratory muscles of French muscular dystrophy patients, DeLaubier, Rideau, and Bach delivered IPPV via urinary drainage catheters positioned into the nostrils.[18] In 1984, nasal CPAP masks became commercially available in the United States and were first used as interfaces for delivering nasal IPPV.[20–22] Nasal interfaces are now commercially available from Respironics (Murrysville, PA), Healthdyne (Minneapolis, MN), Malincrodt Inc (Pleasanton, CA), and ResCare Inc (San Diego, CA). Each design applies pressure differently to the nose and paranasal area. Because it is impossible to predict which model will be preferred by any particular patient, several must be tried. Many patients use different styles on alternate nights to vary skin contact pressure. These difficulties can also be alleviated by the preparation of custom-molded nasal interfaces.[7]

Also in 1984, nasal IPPV was first used for 24-hour ventilatory support for a multiple sclerosis patient with a VC of 100 mL and no ventilator-free breathing ability.[20] Nasal IPPV can be effective in providing long-term as well as acute ventilatory support for patients with little or no VC.[20] Because patients generally prefer mouthpiece IPPV or use of the IAPV during daytime hours, nasal IPPV is most practical only for nocturnal use.[16] Daytime nasal IPPV is indicated for those who cannot retain a mouthpiece[23] because of oral muscle weakness or inadequate jaw opening or when neck movement is insufficient

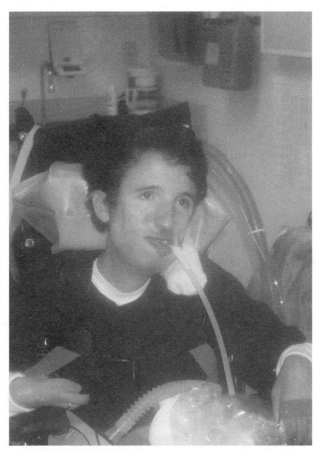

Figure 31-3. Twenty-four–hour ventilator user with Duchenne muscular dystrophy receiving IPPV via a mouthpiece while in a motorized wheelchair.

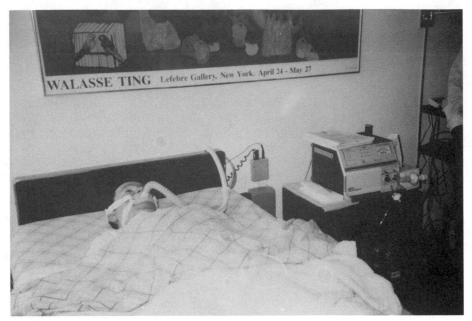

Figure 31-4. Patient with no measurable VC using mouthpiece IPPV with lipseal retention for nocturnal ventilatory support.

to grab a mouthpiece. Twenty-four–hour nasal IPPV can, nevertheless, be a viable alternative to tracheostomy even for some patients with severe lip and oropharyngeal muscle weakness.

Oral–nasal interfaces were described for long-term supported ventilation in 1989.[18] These interfaces used strap retention systems like those for mouthpiece and nasal IPPV. Respironics Inc. and Healthdyne recently released new oral–nasal interfaces. However, because effective ventilatory support can usually be provided by either nasal or mouthpiece IPPV or, when necessary, by mouthpiece IPPV with the nose plugged by cotton pledgets and tape, strap-retained oral–nasal interfaces have not been widely used.

Strapless oral–nasal interfaces with bite-plate retention have been used in Europe since 1985. These interfaces not only provide an essentially airtight seal for the delivery of IPPV, but simple tongue thrust is adequate to expel them.[7] The bite-plate retention is also important for patients living alone who are unable to independently don straps.[7]

Cough Versus Airway Suctioning

Tracheal suctioning causes irritation, increases secretions, may be accompanied by severe hypoxia, and is at best effective in clearing only superficial airway secretions. Routine tracheal suctioning misses mucous plugs adherent between the tube and the tracheal wall and misses the left main stem bronchus 54 to 92% of the time.[24] This at least in part accounts for the fact that 70% of pneumonias occur in the left lung.[24] Furthermore, attempts at suctioning airway secretions via the nose or mouth are poorly tolerated and rarely effective. Noninvasive IPPV cannot be effective indefinitely for patients with generalized muscle weakness without effective use of expiratory muscle aids at least during intercurrent chest colds,[25] following general anesthesia, and during other periods of bronchial hypersecretion.

A normal cough requires a precough inspiration or insufflation to about 85 to 90% of total lung capacity.[26] Glottic closure follows for about 0.2 seconds, and sufficient intrathoracic pressure is generated to obtain PCF over 6 L/sec on glottic opening.[27] Total expiratory volume during normal coughing is about 2.3 to 2.5 L.[26]

Decreases in VC, bulbar muscle dysfunction, and abdominal muscle weakness result in decreased PCFs. These flows are further diminished after general anesthesia and during respiratory tract infections because of fatigue, temporary weakening of inspiratory and expiratory muscles,[28] and bronchial mucus plugging. The attainment of adequate PCFs is critical for preventing pulmonary complications and respiratory failure.[4]

Manually Assisted Coughing

Techniques of manually assisted coughing involve different hand and arm placements for expiratory cycle thrusts (Fig. 31-5). For patients with less than 1.5 L of VC, flows are increased by preceding the assisted exsufflation with a deep insufflation.[29] A manual resuscitator, a portable volume ventilator, or an In-exsufflator (J. H. Emerson Co, Cambridge, MA) is used to deliver the deep insufflation. Manually assisted coughing requires a cooperative patient, good coordination between the patient and the care provider, and adequate physical effort and often frequent application by the caregiver. It is often less effective in the presence of severe scoliosis, and certain techniques must be performed with caution when the rib cage is osteoporotic. Manually assisted coughing remains greatly underused. When inadequate, mechanical insufflation–exsufflation can be lifesaving.

Mechanical Insufflation-Exsufflation

In 1951 Barach et al.[30] described mechanical exsufflation. He used a vacuum cleaner motor with a 5-inch solenoid valve attachment to an iron lung portal. At peak negative pressure in the tank, the valve opened, triggering an exsufflation as intratank pressure became atmospheric in 0.06 seconds.[30] An additional increase in exsufflation flow was obtained by timing an abdominal compression to valve opening.[31] Investigators reported that the use of these techniques "completely replaced bronchoscopy as a means of keeping the airway clear of thick tenacious secretions." Another "patient would have required bronchoscopy or reopening of the tracheotomy if the exsufflator had not been successful in clearing the airway."[30]

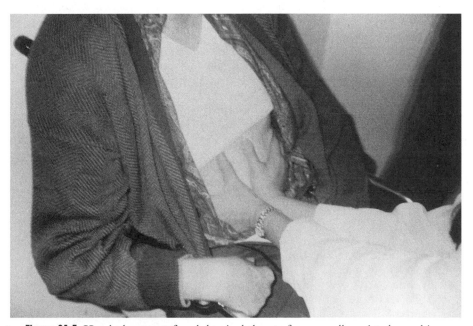

Figure 31-5. Hand placement for abdominal thrusts for manually assisted coughing.

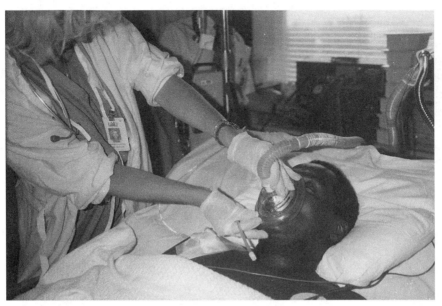

Figure 31-6. Mechanical insufflation–exsufflation delivered to a patient with muscular dystrophy.

In 1953 various portable devices, the best known of which was the Cof-flator (OEM Co, Norwalk, CT),[32] became available to deliver mechanical insufflation–exsufflation directly to the airway via a mouthpiece, mask, or endotracheal tube.[32,33] Insufflation and exsufflation pressures were independently adjusted for comfort and efficacy. The Cof-flator consisted of a two-stage axial compressor that inflated the lungs with positive pressures, usually to about 40 to 60 cm H_2O. The pressure in the upper respiratory tract was then dropped to 40 to 60 cm H_2O below atmosphere in 0.02 seconds. The negative pressure was usually maintained for 2 to 3 seconds.[34,35] The Cof-flator went off the market in the mid-1960s, when tracheostomy and tracheal suctioning and bronchoscopy became the standards for airway secretion management.

In February of 1993, the J. H. Emerson Co (Cambridge, MA) released a mechanical insufflator-exsufflator (In-exsufflator) into the American market. It operates like the Cof-flator except that cycling between positive and negative pressure can be adjusted manually as well as automatically (Fig. 31-6). The manual cycling feature facilitates caregiver–patient coordination of inspiration and expiration with the patient's insufflation and exsufflation but requires an additional hand for an abdominal thrust or if one hand is inadequate to affix the mask. One possible treatment alternative consists of applying about five cycles of insufflation and exsufflation through the oral–nasal mask, translaryngeal or tracheostomy tube, followed by a brief period of normal breathing or ventilator use to avoid hyperventilation. Five or more treatments are given in one sitting, and the treatments are repeated until no further secretions are expulsed and any mucous plug–associated oxyhemoglobin desaturation is reversed. Treatments can be required as frequently as every 10 minutes during chest colds. An abdominal thrust applied during the exsufflation cycle further increases PCF and airway mucus expulsion.[29] Although no medications are usually required for its use by ventilator users with neuromuscular conditions, liquefaction of sputum using heated aerosol treatments can facilitate exsufflation when secretions are inspissated.

Pulmonary flow rates, VC, and SaO_2, when abnormal, improve immediately with clearing of mucous plugs by mechanical insufflation–exsufflation.[29] An increase in VC of 15 to 42% was noted immediately after treatment in 67 patients with "obstructive dyspnea" and a 55% increase in VC was noted after mechanical insufflation–exsufflation in patients with neuromuscular conditions.[34] We have observed up to 400% improvement in VC and normalization of SaO_2 as mechanical insufflation–exsufflation eliminates mucous plugs for acutely ill ventilator-assisted neuromuscular patients.[29]

No reports of damaging side effects have been disclosed in more than 6000 treatments in 400 patients using mechanical insufflation–exsufflation, many of whom had primarily lung disease.[36] Consistent with this is the fact that in more than 650 patient-years and hundreds of applications by our neuromuscular ventilator users, no episodes of pneumothorax, aspiration of gastric contents, or other complications were observed as a result of mechanical insufflation–exsufflation. Borborygmus and abdominal distension are infrequent and are eliminated by decreasing insufflation pressures. The absence of any decrease and, indeed, the consistent increase in forced expiratory flows in the immediate postexsufflation period indicate that no sustained airway collapse results from mechanical insufflation–exsufflation.[29]

Patient Evaluation

People with neuromuscular conditions need to be evaluated regularly for inspiratory and expiratory muscle weakness. The VC, maximum insufflation capacity (MIC), maximum glossopharyngeal single breath capacity (GPmaxSBC), PCF, assisted PCF, end tidal CO_2, and oximetry are monitored.

A simple spirometer is used to measure VC and MIC. The VC is measured in the sitting, supine, and side-lying positions and, for those who use spinal braces, with the braces on and off. A well-fitting body jacket can increase the VC, whereas a poorly fitting one can decrease it. The MIC is determined by insufflating the lungs, either by delivering one deep insufflation or by teaching the patient to "air stack" (hold with a closed glottis) consecutively delivered volumes. Insufflation can be delivered via a mouthpiece, nosepiece (Fig. 31-7), or oral–nasal interface and is provided by a manual resuscitator, portable volume ventilator, or In-exsufflator (see Fig. 31-6). In addition, GPB can often be used to independently provide maximal insufflation, and the GPmaxSBC is determined.

GPB involves the use of the glottis to capture boluses of air and draw them into the lungs. GPB is essentially air stacking gulps of air. Each glossopharyngeal breath consists of 6 to 9 gulps of 60 to 200 mL each. During the training period the efficiency of GPB

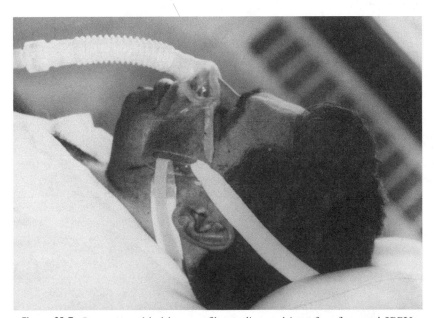

Figure 31-7. Custom-molded low-profile acrylic nasal interface for nasal IPPV.

is monitored by measuring the milliliters of air per gulp, gulps per breath, and breaths per minute that are exhaled into a spirometer. The GPmaxSBC determination usually requires 15 to 20 gulps.

The PCFs are measured via peak flow meter. First, unassisted PCFs are measured by having the person cough as forcefully as possible through the peak flow meter. Then, if the VC is less than 1500 mL the patient is insufflated to the MIC and then again asked to cough forcefully through the flow meter as an abdominal thrust is timed to the glottic opening. This is assisted PCF, which is often 2 to 10 times greater than unassisted PCF. If the person is too weak to grab a mouthpiece and cough through it, an oral–nasal interface is used.

The SaO_2 and end tidal CO_2 are measured. If symptoms of hypoventilation are present, if the VC in the supine position is at least 30% less than when sitting or the person requires two or more pillows to fall asleep, if the VC is less than about 40% of predicted normal in any position, if the end tidal CO_2 levels indicate diurnal hypoventilation (are $\geq$44 mm Hg), or if daytime SaO_2 decreases below 95% without the suspicion of lung disease or mucus plugging, sleep is monitored by oximetry. An oximeter with a printer that averages data by the hour is used (Ohmeda #3760, Louisville, KY). The Ohmeda oximeter gives the percentage of time that the SaO_2 is below 90%, 85%, 80%, and 70% and the low and mean SaO_2 values for each hour and for the night.

Goals: Oximetry Feedback Protocol and GPB

Because respiratory failure results from hypoventilation or, more frequently, inadequate PCFs, and because cough volumes of greater than 2 L are required to maximize PCFs, the clinical goals are to provide multiple daily maximal insufflation to maximize MIC, to maintain normal alveolar ventilation around the clock, and to maximize PCFs.

Thrice daily maximal insufflation with a manual resuscitator are prescribed before the VC decreases below 50% of predicted normal and improvements in MIC are monitored. Patients who complain of symptoms of hypoventilation—typically fatigue, morning headaches, daytime drowsiness, difficulty concentrating, and sleep disturbances, especially when mean nocturnal SaO_2 is less than 94%—are offered nocturnal nasal or lipseal IPPV and are provided with the interfaces with which they are most comfortable. When assisted PCFs decrease below 270 L/m and the VC is less than 1500 mL, patients are instructed in assisted coughing with maximal insufflation and in mechanical insufflation–exsufflation with concomitant abdominal thrusts and are provided with an oximeter as well as with less than 2-hour access to a portable volume ventilator and an In-exsufflator (J. H. Emerson Co, Cambridge, MA). Infants with SMA type 1 are provided with high-span bilevel positive airway pressure to promote lung growth, ease nocturnal breathing difficulty, and prevent pectus excavatum. In general, inspiratory/expiratory positive airway pressure spans of 15 to 20/3 are used for children with SMA type 1. Older children and adults, if initially using bilevel positive airway pressure, are switched from it to the use of portable volume ventilators for noninvasive IPPV to permit independence in air stacking.

The oximeter is used for feedback to the patient and care provider. Desaturation below 95% is almost always caused by lung underventilation if the person is not receiving noninvasive IPPV, does not have airway secretion encumberment, and has a VC below 40% of predicted normal. When hypoventilation and airway mucus are not appropriately managed, desaturation can eventually result from the development of lung disease, most commonly atelectasis and pneumonia, which often result in respiratory failure. People who do not have oximeters in the home before developing a chest cold usually wait too long to seek help and by the time they call the physician, their SaO_2 is already very low and pneumonia may already be present. Thus, an oximeter is prescribed once the assisted PCFs decrease below 270 L/m because at this level patients are at high risk of respiratory failure during chest colds or other episodes of bronchial mucous plugging.[4]

GPB can provide an individual with weak inspiratory muscles and little or no measurable VC with normal ventilation. In addition, it ensures perfect safety when the patient is not using a ventilator or in the event of mechanical ventilator failure.[37] Although potentially extremely useful, GPB is rarely taught because few health care professionals are familiar with the technique. GPB is also rarely useful in the presence of an indwelling tracheostomy tube. It cannot be used when the tube is uncapped as it is during tracheostomy IPPV. Even when capped, the gulped air tends to leak around the outer walls of the tube and out the tracheostomy site as airway volumes and pressures increase during the air stacking process of GPB. The safety and versatility afforded by effective GPB are key reasons to eliminate tracheostomy in favor of noninvasive inspiratory and expiratory aids.

Intrapulmonary Percussive Ventilation

Based on the principles of high-frequency jet ventilation, the Bird Corp (Exeter, UK) developed an internal airway percussor. This hand-held device delivers 30-mL sine wave oscillations through a mouthpiece. In general, tracheobronchial clearance can be improved by combining chest physiotherapy with high-frequency oscillation.[38] The Percussionator, Impulsator, and Spanker respirators (Percussionaire Corp, Sandpoint, ID) can deliver aerosolized medications while providing high-flow minibursts of air to the lungs at a rate of 2 to 7 Hz. Although no studies have demonstrated efficacy or need for this device in people with primarily ventilatory impairment, it seems reasonable that pulsating the airway might inch secretions out of alveoli and terminal bronchioles into larger airways, from where they can be expelled by forced exsufflation and manually assisted coughing.

VENTILATOR STYLE PREFERENCE: TRACHEOSTOMY IPPV VERSUS NONINVASIVE PHYSICAL MEDICINE ALTERNATIVES

From a population of 695 ventilator users, we surveyed those with greater than 1 month of experience in the use of both tracheostomy and noninvasive methods to compare their ventilator use preferences. They were divided into two groups: the 111 ventilator users initially managed by noninvasive IPPV and subsequently switched to tracheostomy IPPV (group 1) and the 59 ventilator users switched from tracheostomy IPPV to noninvasive aids (group 2).[39] The ventilator users in both groups preferred the noninvasive methods overall. This was also true for individual aspects such as appearance, convenience, comfort, security, facilitation of speech, swallowing, and sleep. In fact, the 59 patients in group 2 unanimously preferred using noninvasive IPPV overall. Thirty-five percent of the tracheostomy IPPV users expressed the desire to return to noninvasive aids, whereas none of the patients using noninvasive aids wished to switch back to tracheostomy IPPV.

EMPLOYMENT

Six hundred nineteen ventilator users with neuromuscular conditions were surveyed for their employment and marital status and satisfaction with life.[8] The 313 males had a mean age of 46.5 years, and the 306 females had a mean age of 52.2 years. About 38% were gainfully employed despite essentially continuous ventilator use and lack of extremity function. The occupations of the 242 ventilator users in descending order of frequency were accounting/banking, social work/counseling, small business ownership, teaching, engineering and science, corporate business administration, journalism, computers, law, college professorship, art, insurance, sales, investment brokerage and financial analysis, real estate, medicine, architecture, administration (other), sales, speech-language pathology, and the priesthood. In addition, ventilator users reported being students, housewives, and active volunteers for various philanthropic causes.

MARRIAGE/DIVORCE

One hundred eighty-six of 621 ventilator users who undertook the same survey, 97 males and 89 females, were married before requiring ventilatory support and remained married and living with their spouses. Another 20% of ventilator users who were single before requiring ventilator use married for the first time after becoming ventilator users. About 16.2% of the ventilator users who were married before the onset of ventilator dependence were divorced subsequently and have not remarried during a mean of 22.7 years of ventilator use.[8] This group became ventilator users at the mean age of 28 years. For comparison, the general nondisabled population has a divorce rate of 30% for people married at the mean age of 28 years.

LIFE SATISFACTION

When asked to indicate how satisfied they were with their lives by circling a number from 1 to 7 where 1 is very dissatisfied and 7 is very satisfied, the 615 individuals who responded had a mean score of 5.1. Two hundred forty-two nondisabled health care professionals reported 5.33 ± 1.20 for satisfaction with their own lives.

When asked how activities of daily living–dependent, ventilator-dependent individuals would respond to this question, however, the health care professionals' mean estimate of the ventilator users' responses was 2.42 ± 1.37. This was significantly worse than the ventilator users' actual responses $(P < .0001)$.[8]

Differences also existed between individuals using noninvasive ventilatory aids and those using tracheostomy IPPV. The noninvasive group was older than the tracheostomy group (50 vs. 45.8 years, $P < .001$), had significantly less upper limb function, and used ventilatory support for fewer hours per day (15.5 vs. 17.7 h/d, $P < .05$) but for more years (22 vs. 17 years, $P < .005$). The tracheostomy IPPV group, however, had a mean satisfaction index of 4.68 as opposed to 5.04 for the noninvasive group $(P < .05)$.[8]

This study demonstrated the extent to which health care professionals underestimate severely disabled, ventilator-assisted individuals' satisfaction with life. This is important because physicians' assessment of patients' quality of life, and the relative desirability of certain types of existence, determine the likelihood of individuals receiving life-sustaining interventions. Physicians consider patients' quality of life more often to support decisions to withhold therapy than to support decisions to use mechanical ventilation. This may be further seen in the fact that mouthpiece IPPV is introduced to individuals with neuromuscular disease in only a few Jerry Lewis Muscular Dystrophy Association Clinics in the United States.[1] Some clinicians have gone so far as to say "The use of chronic assisted ventilation should be avoided." Others consider the long-term use of assisted ventilation for individuals with Duchenne muscular dystrophy to be "most controversial" and an issue that "raises enormous ethical difficulties."[5]

ETHICS

Purtilo[40] observed that most discussions of ventilator use has focused on the critically ill patient maintained by tracheostomy IPPV in intensive care units. She pointed out that this has "fostered misconceptions and stereotypes" regarding other appropriate uses of ventilators. There is, likewise, great potential for "misunderstanding of the ethical issues involved in treating patients whose chronic maintenance depends on either positive or negative long-term ventilator support." Informed decisions about ethically and financially complex matters such as long-term ventilator use should be made by examining the life satisfaction of competent individuals who have already chosen these options. Most severely disabled ventilator users with neuromuscular disease are satisfied with their lives despite the inability to achieve many of the "usual" goals associated with quality of life in the physically able population. Their principal life satisfaction derives from social relationships, the reorganization of goals, and from their immediate home environment. Self-directed individuals, once properly informed, should be treated as competent to make decisions regarding their welfare. Paternalism on the part of health care professionals undermines the goals of rehabilitation.

In addition to reducing cost, the use of noninvasive respiratory muscle aids can provide effective long-term ventilatory support 24 hours a day; can help avoid acute pulmonary morbidity, hospitalization, intubation, and premature death; and is greatly preferred over invasive alternatives.[39] Furthermore, the use of these methods eliminates the ethical considerations concerning suicide by withdrawal of ventilatory support because users of noninvasive methods are not passively attached to a respirator but actively control their lung ventilation. The individual's personal sense of controlling his or her life is also enhanced by using these methods.

Purtilo[40] summed up an article on ethical issues concerning the management of ventilator users by saying that misconceptions about the undesirability of "'going on a respirator' have far-reaching negative effects for persons now happily being supported on a respirator, and mitigate the positive effects it could have for some types of chronically impaired persons whose quality of life also could be enhanced by the use of a ventilator." Freed[41] stressed the importance of professionals not imposing their own concepts, values, and judgments onto the disabled person. Clinicians should be cognizant of their inability to gauge disabled patients' life satisfaction and potential for social and vocational productivity. They should also refrain from allowing inaccurate and unwarranted judgment of subjective factors associated with quality of life in the general population affect patient management decisions.

ABBREVIATIONS

CO_2—carbon dioxide
CPAP—continuous positive airway pressure
GPB—glossopharyngeal breathing
IAPV—intermittent abdominal-pressure ventilator
IPPV—intermittent positive-pressure ventilation
MIC—maximum insufflation capacity
NPBV—negative-pressure body ventilator
PCF—peak cough flows
SaO_2—oxyhemoglobin saturation
VC—vital capacity

REFERENCES

1. Bach JR, Wang TG. Noninvasive long-term ventilatory support for individuals with spinal muscular atrophy and functional bulbar musculature. Arch Phys Med Rehabil 1995;76:213–217.
2. Younger DS, ed. Paralysis: part 1. Semin Neurol 1991;13:241–315.
3. Younger DS, ed. Paralytic syndromes: part II. Semin Neurol 1991;13:319–379.
4. Bach JR, Ishikawa Y, Kim H. Prevention of pulmonary morbidity for patients with Duchenne muscular dystrophy. Chest 1997;112:1024–1028.
5. Bach JR. Ventilator use by muscular dystrophy association patients: an update. Arch Phys Med Rehabil 1992;73:179–183.
6. Bach JR. Standards of care in Muscular Dystrophy Association clinics. J Neurol Rehab 1992;6:67–73.
7. McDermott I, Bach JR, Parker C, et al. Custom-fabricated interfaces for intermittent positive pressure ventilation. Int J Prosthodontics 1989;2:224–233.
8. Bach JR, Barnett V. Psychosocial, vocational, quality of life and ethical issues In: Bach JR, ed. Pulmonary Rehabilitation: The Obstructive and Paralytic Conditions. Philadelphia: Hanley & Belfus, 1996:395–411.

9. Bach JR. Guide to the Understanding and Management of Neuromuscular Disease. Philadelphia: Hanley & Belfus, 1999:1–165.

10. Bach JR, Rajaraman R, Ballanger F, et al. Neuromuscular ventilatory insufficiency: the effect of home mechanical ventilator use vs. oxygen therapy on pneumonia and hospitalization rates. Am J Phys Med Rehabil 1998;77:8–19.

11. Bach JR. Do you suffer from intubation and tracheostomy paradigm paralysis? Respir Intervent 1993;93:3, 13.

12. Bach JR, Saporito LR. Criteria for extubation and tracheostomy tube removal for patients with ventilatory failure: a different approach to weaning. Chest 1996;110:1566–1571.

13. Bach JR. Update and perspectives on noninvasive respiratory muscle aids: part 1—the inspiratory muscle aids. Chest 1994;105:1230–1240.

14. Bach JR, Penek J. Obstructive sleep apnea complicating negative pressure ventilatory support in patients with chronic paralytic/restrictive ventilatory dysfunction. Chest 1991;99:1386–1393.

15. Bach JR, Alba AS, Bohatiuk G, et al. Mouth intermittent positive pressure ventilation in the management of post-polio respiratory insufficiency. Chest 1987;91:859–864.

16. Bach JR, Alba AS. Total ventilatory support by the intermittent abdominal pressure ventilator. Chest 1991;99:630–636.

17. Bach JR, Alba AS, Saporito LR. Intermittent positive pressure ventilation via the mouth as an alternative to tracheostomy for 257 ventilator users. Chest 1993;103:174–182.

18. Bach JR. A historical perspective on the use of noninvasive ventilatory support alternatives. Respir Care Clin N Am 1996;22:161–181.

19. Bach JR, Robert D, Leger P, et al. Sleep fragmentation in kyphoscoliotic individuals with alveolar hypoventilation treated by nasal IPPV. Chest 1995;107:1552–1558.

20. Bach JR, Alba AS, Mosher R, et al. Intermittent positive pressure ventilation via nasal access in the management of respiratory insufficiency. Chest 1987;92:168–170.

21. Ellis ER, Bye PTP, Bruderer JW, et al. Treatment of respiratory failure during sleep in patients with neuromuscular disease, positive-pressure ventilation through a nose mask. Am Rev Respir Dis 1987;135:148–152.

22. Kerby GR, Mayer LS, Pingleton SK. Nocturnal positive pressure ventilation via nasal mask. Am Rev Respir Dis 1987;135:738–740.

23. Bach JR, Alba AS. Management of chronic alveolar hypoventilation by nasal ventilation. Chest 1990;97:52–57.

24. Fishburn MJ, Marino RJ, Ditunno JF. Atelectasis and pneumonia in acute spinal cord injury. Arch Phys Med Rehabil 1990;71:197–200.

25. Bach JR. Update and perspectives on noninvasive respiratory muscle aids: part 2—the expiratory muscle aids. Chest 1994;105:1538–1544.

26. Leith DE. Cough. In: Brain JD, Proctor D, Reid L, eds. Lung Biology in Health and Disease: Respiratory Defense Mechanisms, Part 2. New York: Marcel Dekker, 1977:545–592.

27. Fugl-Meyer AR, Grimby G. Ventilatory function in tetraplegic patients. Scand J Rehab Med 1971;3:151–160.

28. Mier-Jedrzejowicz A, Brophy C, Green M. Respiratory muscle weakness during upper respiratory tract infections. Am Rev Respir Dis 1988;138:5–7.

29. Bach JR. Mechanical insufflation-exsufflation comparison of peak expiratory flows with manually assisted and unassisted coughing techniques. Chest 1993;104:1553–1562.

30. Barach AL, Beck GJ, Bickerman HA, et al. Mechanical coughing: studies on physical methods of producing high velocity flow rates during the expiratory cycle. Trans Am Physicians 1951;64:360–363.

31. Barach AL, Beck GJ, Bickerman HA, et al. Physical methods simulating mechanisms of the human cough. J Appl Physiol 1952;5:85–91.

32. The OEM Cof-flator Portable Cough Machine. St Louis, MO: Shampaine Industries.

33. Segal MS, Salomon A, Herschfus JA. Alternating positive-negative pressures in mechanical respiration (the cycling valve device employing air pressures). Dis Chest 1954;25:640–648.

34. Barach AL, Beck GJ, Smith RH. Mechanical production of expiratory flow rates surpassing the capacity of human coughing. Am J Med Sci 1953;226:241–248.

35. Bickerman HA. Exsufflation with negative pressure: elimination of radiopaque material and foreign bodies from bronchi of anesthetized dogs. Arch Intern Med 1954;93:698–704.

36. Barach AL. The application of pressure, including exsufflation, in pulmonary emphysema. Am J Surg 1955; 89:372–382.

37. Bach JR, Alba AS. Noninvasive options for ventilatory support of the traumatic high level quadriplegic. Chest 1990;98:613–619.

38. George RJD, Geddes DM. High frequency oscillations and mucociliary transport. Biomed Pharmacother 1989;43:25–30.

39. Bach JR. A comparison of long-term ventilatory support alternatives from the perspective of the patient and care giver. Chest 1993;104:1702–1706.

40. Purtilo RB. Ethical Issues in the treatment of chronic ventilator-dependent patients. Arch Phys Med Rehabil 1986;67:718–721.

41. Freed MM. Quality of life: the physician's dilemma. Arch Phys Med Rehabil 1984;65:109–111.

32 Rehabilitation in Non-COPD Lung Disease

Richard S. Novitch

▷ Professional Skills

Upon completion of this chapter, the reader will:

- Appreciate that the predominant cause of respiratory-related disability is caused by chronic obstructive pulmonary disease (COPD) and that COPD data provide a useful framework for evaluating rehabilitation in non-COPD illness
- Understand that the multidisciplinary approach to pulmonary rehabilitation applies to all patients and that the benefits of pulmonary rehabilitation are not unique to COPD
- Appreciate that referrals to an inpatient pulmonary rehabilitation setting are "physiologically blind" and that a significant amount of postacute inpatient care is given to patients with respiratory disorders
- Appreciate the spectrum of deficits in patients undergoing pulmonary rehabilitation and understand how rehabilitation programs are designed to address these problems
- Review outcomes of studies performed in patients with non-COPD and interstitial lung disease (ILD)
- Be familiar with data reflecting functional outcomes after pulmonary rehabilitation in COPD and non-COPD patients
- Be familiar with current thinking regarding rehabilitation in COPD versus non-COPD illness and understand that any bias regarding the utility of pulmonary rehabilitation in this population is not supported by the data

INTRODUCTION

It is impossible to discuss pulmonary rehabilitation in lung diseases other than COPD without a tightly integrated discussion of COPD rehabilitation. There is no such thing as a pulmonary rehabilitation program for nonobstructive lung diseases alone. There are simply not enough referrals to justify this type of activity. (Similarly, a large body of literature does not exist about pulmonary rehabilitation in nonobstructive lung diseases.) Most patients who present with disability as a result of chronic lung disease have COPD. It has been estimated that the total number of cases of all the ILDs is about 3 to 5% the total number of cases of COPD in the population.[1]

Pulmonary rehabilitation has been practiced by physicians and associated health care professionals for more than 100 years in various forms. During this time, the field has changed to fit the needs of the patients it serves and the afflictions that plague them. The initial practice of pulmonary rehabilitation was geared for patients with nonobstructive lung disease. This has changed as the epidemiology of lung disease in our society has changed. It is impossible to have a lengthy discussion about pulmonary rehabilitation today without mentioning COPD. However, the number of non-COPD patients receiving some sort of pulmonary rehabilitation inflates if one includes all the patients with intrinsic restrictive parenchymal diseases, asthma, cystic fibrosis, chest wall and neuromuscular disorders, and the status postpneumonia/respiratory failure/adult respiratory distress syndrome group. Professionals in the fields of pulmonary medicine; nursing; respiratory, physical, and occupational therapy; and exercise physiology and sports medicine have used the expanded knowledge base available to them from treating COPD patients to meet needs of patients with nonobstructive lung disease. Pulmonary rehabilitation, therefore, attempts to meet the needs that exist among respiratory patients for an enhanced quality of life in three basic arenas: (*a*) disability as a result of chronic and progressive intrinsic lung disease (*b*) living with chronic respiratory insufficiency, and (*c*) survival and recovery from critical (respiratory) illness.

For the sake of discussion, it is useful to divide the history of pulmonary rehabilitation into three eras defined by the epidemiologic changes in lung disease that have taken place during the past century. The first era, of course, is defined by the application of modern medical therapy and the use of mechanical ventilation for restrictive disorders such as tuberculosis and polio. The second era centers on the emergence of COPD as the preeminent respiratory disorder of adults in the second half of the 20th century. The third era, the one we have just entered, will be defined as the one that began with the publication of the American College of Chest Physicians/American Association of Cardiovascular and Pulmonary Rehabilitation[2] and American Thoracic Society[3] position papers supporting the utility and efficacy of pulmonary rehabilitation using evidence-based medicine and the inclusion of pulmonary rehabilitation as standard care in the National Emphysema Treatment Trial (NETT) study.

The third era of pulmonary rehabilitation, which we are now entering, is perhaps less exciting than the first era, during which pioneers in this field first applied multidisciplinary care to patients in an empiric manner, and the second era, when rigorous testing of these therapies was first undertaken. This third era of pulmonary rehabilitation will be characterized by the broad application of standardized care, whose scientific foundation has undergone rigorous testing and peer review, to an aging population suffering from an increasingly broad array of idiopathic, iatrogenic, environmental, and lifestyle-induced lung disease. The nature of these disorders will span the range from obstructive to restrictive and from chronic to postacute. Undoubtedly, the increasing prevalence of chronic lung disease in our society will drive an increase in demand for availability of pulmonary rehabilitation services as well as a better understanding of its role in the care of patients with respiratory impairment chronically and acutely.

THE GOALS OF PULMONARY REHABILITATION

The goals of pulmonary rehabilitation are exactly the same as those of rehabilitation involving functional impairment arising from any other organ system. The function of the injured organ, in this case pulmonary function, will not be affected. The goal of rehabilitation, therefore, is to provide a structured, supportive environment where the patient can reverse the reversible factors in pulmonary disability and develop physical and cognitive coping skills to assist in maximizing recovery. In this sense, pulmonary rehabilitation holds the same types of goals in all its domains, from the intensive care unit to the outpatient clinic and among a variety of diagnoses.

Our goal in pulmonary rehabilitation is to allow our patients to work toward exploring the boundaries that ventilatory limitation places on them from physical, cognitive, and emotional perspectives. One great disadvantage that many of our patients have concerning rehabilitation is advanced age. Most patients with chronic lung disease are older, and many have never had to cope with chronic illness in the past. Not only are these patients experiencing difficulty after suffering a loss of exercise capacity, but they are also suffering from losses that occur with advanced age, such as the loss of work, the death of a spouse, an empty nest, and the loss of friends as well as the physical isolation that accompanies respiratory impairment.

OUR SPECIAL INTEREST IN PULMONARY REHABILITATION FOR NONOBSTRUCTIVE LUNG DISEASE

Our special interest in pulmonary rehabilitation in lung diseases other than COPD originates from the location of our practice in an acute rehabilitation hospital. Our institution's mission in this setting is to facilitate the discharge of patients from acute care and to provide acute rehabilitative services to a broad constellation of patients in various disease categories, including pulmonary, cardiac, orthopedics, and neurology. In this sense, the pulmonary referrals that we receive are "physiologically blind." Our experience in pulmonary rehabilitation, therefore, reflects a broad variety of diagnoses and different etiologies of ventilatory impairment. This niche is the exception rather than the norm among groups with an academic or clinical interest in pulmonary rehabilitation. Most pulmonary rehabilitation services are delivered in an ambulatory setting to patients with COPD who are stable or recovering from acute illness. Most published studies focus on pulmonary rehabilitation in COPD as opposed to other respiratory illnesses. However, a significant amount of work is being performed in clinical rehabilitation in postacute and ambulatory care in patients with other respiratory diagnoses. It may or may not be called pulmonary rehabilitation and may encompass isolated patients with unusual diagnoses mixed in with a larger population of patients with COPD or cardiac disease or in a general rehabilitation setting. Pulmonary rehabilitation in non-COPD illness may also include patients in chronic respiratory failure who are stable or weaning, asthma, cystic fibrosis, and pre- or postlung transplantation. The group of clinicians that may find our work most applicable might be those treating patients in an inpatient postacute care setting such as a weaning unit or an acute or subacute rehabilitation facility.

Our experience with an eclectic population is that pulmonary rehabilitation has as much to offer to patients with ventilatory limitation from other causes as it does in COPD. From a clinical point of view, there seem to be more similarities than dissimilarities in rehabilitating COPD versus non-COPD patients. This seems to be the case across the symptom complex that our patients experience: dyspnea, exercise intolerance, activities of daily living (ADLs), emotional/cognitive (anxiety/depression/coping), and response to rehabilitation and handicap.

The dissimilarities between rehabilitation of COPD and non-COPD illness seem to lie in the domain where the natural history of the particular diagnosis dramatically impacts the clinical course. The disorder that comes to mind most prominently where this is the case is ILD. Few patients with ILD are referred for rehabilitation. In our experience, however, these patients seem to have similar outcomes in the rehabilitation program. Unfortunately, because patients with lung disease tend to maintain life quality despite significant physiologic impairment, both COPD and ILD patients tend to be referred with advanced disease. Therefore, it seems that in the perirehabilitative period, patients with ILD tend to do more poorly because of the aggressive nature of their underlying illness, especially when severe hypoxemia and pulmonary hypertension are present.

PULMONARY REHABILITATION OF THE PATIENT WITHOUT COPD

Program Overview

The past decade has brought numerous changes in the health care system that have also changed the role of pulmonary rehabilitation. Our focus in the past had been on pulmonary rehabilitation for patients with COPD in the acute rehabilitation hospital setting and the outpatient setting. However, as our experience broadened and we developed positive outcomes, our referrers widened the scope of patients referred to our program. Our intuition was that the structure of the rehabilitation program was of no unique benefit to patients with COPD as opposed to other lung diseases. This belief was fostered by the location of our practice within a general rehabilitation setting as opposed to a strict cardiopulmonary environment.

Exercise Reconditioning

Our motto in this setting of very debilitated patients with very severe airway obstruction became "pulmonary rehabilitation is more than just treadmills." Our belief was that most of the improvement in rehabilitation in the presence of severe physiologic impairment was correlated to improvement unrelated to true aerobic "conditioning." Our model of improvement is composed of two discrete effects of pulmonary rehabilitation. The first effect is called the "rehabilitation effect." It describes the phenomenon whereby patients became more encouraged and more efficient (i.e., less minute ventilation for a particular amount of work). The second effect, more difficult and perhaps, in many patients, impossible to achieve, is a true "training effect." This second and more desirable effect, layered on the rehabilitation effect, was achievable by only a subset of the entire population. Only patients able to achieve a threshold of high-intensity exercise in addition to the anaerobic threshold perhaps could attain higher levels of oxygen uptake and superior outcomes from exercise reconditioning. This notion was fostered by works by Casaburi and others[4-7] that showed that attainment of the anaerobic threshold during exercise in the COPD population seemed unrelated to pulmonary function. This model of pulmonary rehabilitation, which remains hypothetical, could account for both the gains made by an elderly, debilitated population with very severe airway obstruction or those unable to achieve a physiologic training effect, as well as superior gains made by those able to achieve the anaerobic threshold. Empirically, we thought that patients with physiologic impairment from restrictive diseases would also benefit from the rehabilitation effect. This model could also account for beneficial outcomes in rehabilitation for patients with asthma, cystic fibrosis, and neuromuscular respiratory failure.[8-13]

Upper Body Activity and Unsupported Arm Exercise

The state of the art in pulmonary rehabilitation has been that patients receive multidisciplinary treatment.[14] The primary focus of treatment is exercise, but attention is also given to improving ADLs, dyspnea control, education, and diagnostic evaluation and treatment for comorbidity such as malnutrition or mood disorders. The central role of exercise in pulmonary rehabilitation has been well established.[15] Our view of the non-COPD population is that the negative impact that restrictive ventilatory limitation imposes on quality of life and mobility is just as prevalent in non-COPD lung disease as it is in COPD.

Patients with COPD have difficulty with a variety of life activities that usually involve the recruitment of accessory muscles of respiration. The difficulty that patients with lung disease experience in performing unsupported arm activity associated with ADLs is well documented. These activities remove shoulder girdle support that optimizes length–tension relationships in muscle groups in the neck, back, and thoracic cage. Early accessory muscle recruitment is a result of hyperinflation, diaphragmatic shortening, and diaphragmatic muscle weakness. This phenomenon can be observed in the physiology laboratory as paradoxical change in esophageal and gastric balloon pressures throughout the respiratory cycle during unsupported arm exercise.[16]

Clinically, we have documented the deleterious impact of COPD on ADLs. Patients with COPD have difficulty with the various ADLs that they perform in their home as well as test in our institution. The types of ADLs that we examine include upper and lower body dressing; safety and ease of surface to surface transfers in the bed, bath, and car; and dependence in toileting, bathing, and grooming.

Many inpatient rehabilitation facilities in the United States and Canada use the Functional Independence Measure (FIM) to gauge the caregiver needs of their patients and to document the effect of rehabilitation as an outcomes measure.[17] This scale was originally intended for the neurologically impaired, but its use has broadened. However, many researchers and clinicians involved in pulmonary rehabilitation have not embraced its use because it neglects many of the disease-specific aspects of lung disease, such as dyspnea, that are so prominent in disability arising from COPD.

We have collected data that documents this type of impairment in the COPD and non-COPD population. Although the impairment scores across the board are not as low on the pulmonary service as on the neurology service, a general impairment is still seen in the ADL FIM scores and a positive outcome after rehabilitation. The impact on ADL in non-COPD lung disease seems to be as great on the ADL FIM of patients with COPD. The outcome scores are indicative of a positive response to treatment as well. No studies of unsupported arm exercise in non-COPD lung disease exist, but it is reasonable to assume that increased demands on the diaphragm and early accessory muscle recruitment are the most likely mechanism.

Cognition and Mood Disorders in Pulmonary Rehabilitation

Any clinician involved in pulmonary rehabilitation is acutely aware of the high rate of anxiety and depression in a population with chronic severe lung disease. Several studies of the prevalence of mood disorders and anxiety in COPD have been performed.[18] These studies have proposed models to account for the generation of depressed mood and anxiety. Dyspnea is implicated as having a central role in a vicious cycle that leads to inactivity and deconditioning, resulting in further dyspnea and depression. Impairment in memory and cognition have been described in patients with severe COPD.[19] The mechanism of brain dysfunction is not well known but is probably related to ischemic injury. Ischemic brain injury in areas associated with "Executive Function" have been implicated as a cause of depression and lack of motivation refractory to treatment in the geriatric population.[20] Clinically, disorders of adjustment, anxiety, and depression seem as prevalent in non-COPD lung disease as in COPD.

Pulmonary rehabilitation by itself has been demonstrated to have an ameliorative effect on some depressed patients with COPD.[21] However, surprisingly few data are available on a systematic approach to the treatment of affective disorders in chronic lung disease or chronic respiratory failure other than descriptive studies.

RESULTS OF PULMONARY REHABILITATION IN NON-COPD LUNG DISEASE

The frequency at which patients with non-COPD lung disease are admitted to our multidisciplinary inpatient rehabilitation program has increased from approximately 10% during a 5-year period in the 1980s to about 20% today. This reflects the changing nature of our referral pattern, paralleling the changing needs of the hospitals and pulmonologists who represent our referral base. Whereas in the past we admitted more chronic stable patients with COPD, from the hospital and the home, our role is now facilitating the discharge of patients with acute pulmonary illness from intrinsic lung disease or as a result of medical complications.

A retrospective analysis of the outcome of patients with nonobstructive lung diseases at the Burke Rehabilitation Hospital during a rehabilitation program was performed by Foster and Thomas.[22] Patients with nonobstructive lung disease participated in the same inpatient multidisciplinary rehabilitation program as patients with COPD. The length of stay was approximately 4 weeks for both groups. Box 32-1 lists the various diagnoses encountered among the study patients. Patients in this group presented with intrinsic parenchymal disease as well as thoracic wall disorders, neuromuscular disease, and resolving acute diseases such as pneumonia and adult respiratory distress syndrome. The pulmonary function data obtained from the study patients who were compared with COPD patients can be seen in Table 32-1.

The outcome variable that was used was the 6-minute walk distance performed at the time of admission to the hospital and at the time of discharge. The 32 non-COPD patients had an initial 6-minute walk distance of 276 ± 219 feet. The increase in ambulation distance at the end of the study was 574 ± 367 feet, with a gain of 298 ± 290 feet from rehabilitation. The results attributable to the rehabilitation program were similar for the non-COPD study patients compared with the COPD controls. Typically, the average 6-minute admission walk distance for our COPD patients is in the 300 to 400 foot range, and the "average" patient can expect their walk distance to approximately double. The average forced expiratory volume in 1 second for COPD patients in this study was 0.65 ± 0.28 L, and they about doubled their initial walk distances on discharge. These clinical results have remained consistent throughout the years among several studies we have performed. However, with shorter elapsed times before patients arrive after their initial admission to acute care as well as shorter lengths of stay, we have noted a decrease in admission and discharge 6-minute walk distances. The results of this study are in Table 32-2.

Box 32-1. Summary of Diagnoses of Non-COPD Patients Admitted for Rehabilitation

Fibrothorax
Bronchiectasis
Neuromuscular disease
Interstitial lung disease
   Sarcoidosis
   Idiopathic pulmonary fibrosis
   Radiation fibrosis
   Scleroderma
Chest wall deformity
   Kyphoscoliosis
   Postpolio syndrome
   Thoracoplasty
Diaphragmatic paralysis
   Postcoronary artery bypass graft
   Postthoracotomy
Postlung resection
   Lobectomy
   Pneumonectomy
   Bronchopleural (cutaneous) fistula
Postrespiratory failure
   Pneumonia
   ARDS

COPD, chronic obstructive pulmonary disease; ARDS, adult respiratory distress syndrome.

Table 32-1. Admission Pulmonary Function Test Values for COPD and Non-COPD Patients[a]

	COPD	(% Predicted)	Non-COPD	(% Predicted)
No. of Patients	317		32	
FVC (L)	1.58 ± 0.62	(47 ± 16)	1.20 ± 0.45	(39 ± 16)
FEV$_1$ (L)	0.65 ± 0.28	(29 ± 12)	0.88 ± 0.35	(41 ± 22)
FEV$_1$/FVC (%)	42 ± 10		75 ± 14	
Pi$_{max}$ (cm H$_2$O)	38 ± 17	(44 ± 18)	39 ± 22	(41 ± 24)
Pe$_{max}$ (cm H$_2$O)	51 ± 28	(31 ± 15)	43 ± 23	(27 ± 13)
pH	7.42 ± 0.04		7.41 ± 0.03	
PCO$_2$ (mm Hg)	44 ± 8		43 ± 8	
PO$_2$ (mm Hg)	63 ± 14		67 ± 12	

Adapted with permission from Foster S, Thomas HM III. Pulmonary rehabilitation in lung disease other than chronic obstructive pulmonary disease. Am Rev Respir Dis 1990;141:602–603. COPD, chronic obstructive pulmonary disease; FVC, forced vital capacity; FEV$_1$, forced expiratory volume in 1 second; Pi$_{max}$, maximum inspiratory pressure; Pe$_{max}$, maximum expiratory pressure; PCO$_2$, partial pressure of carbon dioxide; PO$_2$, partial pressure of oxygen.
[a]Values are mean $\pm$ SD.

PULMONARY REHABILITATION IN ILD

A dearth of published studies are available looking at pulmonary rehabilitation for patients with ILD. Our impression has been that despite the comparable results that we have obtained in treating these patients, the referral rate for patients with COPD remains higher than ILD because of a general pessimism about these illnesses. The long-term prognosis for patients with ILD is generally poor and the degree of physiologic impairment is advanced when these patients present to clinical attention. Patients with idiopathic pulmonary fibrosis have limited long-term survival and little hope for improvement once their illness has become disabling. This usually coincides with arterial hypoxemia and pulmonary hypertension.

However, we have been surprised at how well our patients with ILD and idiopathic pulmonary fibrosis have responded to pulmonary rehabilitation. These patients are also encouraged to hear that positive outcome data are available regarding pulmonary rehabilitation in their disorder. Of course, these patients are reminded that pulmonary rehabilita-

Table 32-2. Ambulation Distances on a 6-Minute Walk Test in COPD and Non-COPD Patients

	No. of Patients	6-min Walk Distance, mean $\pm$ SD, ft		
		Admission	Discharge	Change
COPD	317	380 ± 313	751 ± 562	371 ± 419
Non-COPD	32	276 ± 219	574 ± 367	298 ± 290
COPD vs. non-COPD		$P = .06$	$P = .08$	$P = .30$

Adapted with permission from Foster S, Thomas HM III. Pulmonary rehabilitation in lung disease other than chronic obstructive pulmonary disease. Am Rev Respir Dis 1990;141:601–604. COPD, chronic obstructive pulmonary disease.

Table 32-3. Diagnoses of Patients Admitted for Pulmonary Rehabilitation, January 1, 1990, to September 30, 1994

Diagnosis	No. of Patients
COPD	628
Pulmonary fibrosis	26
Status postrespiratory failure	15
Asthma	12
Diaphragmatic paralysis	11
Status postthoracoplasty	10
Kyphoscoliosis	10
Obesity-hypoventilation	4
Neuromuscular disease	4
Bronchiectasis	4
Miscellaneous	27
Total	751

With permission from Novitch RS, Thomas HM III. Pulmonary rehabilitation in chronic interstitial disease. In: Fishman AP, ed. Pulmonary Rehabilitation. New York: Marcel Dekker, 1996:683–700.
COPD, chronic obstructive pulmonary disease

tion is only about improving function and not about improving lung physiology or the disease outcome.

When clinicians make decisions regarding candidacy for rehabilitation in ILD, I believe that the underlying assumption about these patients is that they are performing at the maximum level allowed by their physiologic derangement. That is to say, the belief is that their physical performance is so tightly correlated to their capacity for exercise that there is no room for improvement. Conversely, my sense is that when most clinicians view a patient with COPD they believe that because of the insidious, slowly progressive nature of this illness that plenty of reasons always exist (e.g., depression, malnutrition) for patients to underperform. Therefore, almost all patients with COPD must be good candidates for

Table 32-4. Diagnoses of Pulmonary Rehabilitation Patients With Interstitial Lung Disease

Diagnosis	No. of Patients
Idiopathic pulmonary fibrosis	17
Scleroderma	2
Sarcoidosis	4
Radiation fibrosis	1
Desquamative interstitial pneumonitis	2
Total	26

With permission from Novitch RS, Thomas HM III. Pulmonary rehabilitation in chronic interstitial disease. In: Fishman AP, ed. Pulmonary Rehabilitation. New York: Marcel Dekker, 1996:683–700.

Table 32-5. Pulmonary Function Test Values in 23 Patients With Interstitial Lung Disease

	Mean ± SD[a]	% Predicted
FVC (L)	1.67 ± 0.78	50 ± 21
FEV$_1$ (L)	1.39 ± 0.56	53 ± 20
FEV$_1$/FVC (%)	81 ± 14	
MVV (LPM)	66 ± 32	64 ± 25
Pe$_{max}$ (cm H$_2$O)	77 ± 33	51 ± 18
Pi$_{max}$ (cm H$_2$O)	56 ± 22	65 ± 20
DLCO (mL/mm Hg/min)	7.7 ± 3.0	37 ± 16 (n = 7)
pH	7.44 ± 0.04	
PCO$_2$ (torr)	40 ± 6	
PO$_2$ (torr)	63 ± 19	

[a]Except where indicated, values are the means of the 23 patients who completed the rehabilitation program.

With permission from Novitch RS, Thomas HM III. Pulmonary rehabilitation in chronic interstitial disease. In: Fishman AP, ed. Pulmonary Rehabilitation. New York: Marcel Dekker, 1996:683–700.

FVC, forced vital capacity; FEV$_1$, forced expiratory volume in 1 second; MVV, maximal voluntary ventilation; Pe$_{max}$, maximum expiratory pressure; Pi$_{max}$, maximum inspiratory pressure; DLCO, diffusion capacity of carbon dioxide; PCO$_2$, partial pressure of carbon dioxide; PO$_2$, partial pressure of oxygen.

pulmonary rehabilitation, whereas patients with ILD may always be considered as having little to gain.

The opposite of this notion, however, is what has been clinically apparent to us. Novitch and Thomas[23] reported a retrospective series of 26 patients admitted for inpatient pulmonary rehabilitation in a 45-month period between 1990 and 1994. The percentage of patients with nonobstructive lung diseases treated during that period was 14.4%. The number of patients with ILD was 26, or 3.46% of the total 751 patients viewed in this analysis. A breakdown of the pulmonary patients treated at Burke Rehabilitation Hospital during this study is in Table 32-3. Of the 26 patients with ILD evaluated retrospectively, 17 presented with idiopathic pulmonary fibrosis (Table 32-4).

Patients who were included in this study successfully completed the rehabilitation program. Pulmonary function data on the 23 patients qualifying for analysis revealed a mean forced vital capacity of 50% predicted, a forced expiratory volume in 1 second of 53% predicted, a diffusion capacity of carbon dioxide of 37% predicted, and a mean arterial partial pressure of oxygen of 63 mm Hg (Table 32-5).

The main outcome measure was the 6-minute walk distance performed at the time of admission and discharge to the rehabilitation program. The results of this group are in Table 32-6. Significant gains were seen across the spectrum of physical activity. The patients doubled their 6-minute walk distance and number of stairs ascended and improved their times in continuous upper and lower body ergometry. These data suggest that patients with ILD benefited from the same type of pulmonary rehabilitation program and in the same magnitude that our COPD patients have historically experienced.

FUNCTIONAL IMPROVEMENT AFTER PULMONARY REHABILITATION

We use the FIM for measuring outcome in all of our inpatient rehabilitation programs. This instrument consists of 18 domains of functional activity that describe a person's

Table 32-6. Results of Pulmonary Mean ± SD Rehabilitation in Patients With Interstitial Lung Disease[a]

Activity	Admission	Discharge	P
6-min walk test, ft	315 ± 348	719 ± 537	.0001
No. of stairs climbed	12 ± 11	24 ± 19	.0004
Bicycle ergometry, min	8.3 ± 4.7	12.2 ± 4.7	.025
Arm ergometry, min	5.9 ± 3.3	22.2 ± 34.3	.038

[a]Values are the means ± SD for the 23 patients who completed the rehabilitation program.
With permission from Novitch RS, Thomas HM III. Pulmonary rehabilitation in chronic interstitial disease. In: Fishman AP, ed. Pulmonary Rehabilitation. New York: Marcel Dekker, 1996:683–700.

ability to care for himself or herself and to live independently. The domains include independence in self-care, surface to surface transfers, locomotion, and communication. The FIM data are collected and submitted for tabulation, summarization, and benchmarking.

The FIM is a useful instrument in evaluating the effects and outcome of inpatient rehabilitation. It is disease independent and attempts to describe an individual's caregiver needs independent of exercise performance. Patients receive a score from 1, total dependence, to 7, total independence, in 18 specific attributes grouped into 3 general domains: ADLs, mobility, and cognition.

We have completed a pilot study retrospectively reviewing the performance of 514 patients with COPD and 132 patients (20.4%) with non-COPD diagnoses admitted to our pulmonary rehabilitation unit at the Burke Rehabilitation Hospital from January 1, 1996 through February 28, 1999. Our aim was to see whether the FIM score could characterize not only the diminution in walk distance but also in an objective measure of their quality of life. The other objective was to see whether this instrument could capture the objective improvement in both motor and ADL domains. We found that both groups, COPD and non-COPD, improved their 6-minute walk distances and motor and ADL FIM scores by similar magnitudes. We believe that further study is required to validate these data for the COPD population as it relates to the 6-minute walk test and maximal oxygen consumption. We believe the FIM might be an especially useful tool as an outcome measure for patients in non-COPD illnesses such as neuromuscular respiratory failure, where functional gains occur outside the domain of maximal exercise performance.

SUMMARY

Pulmonary rehabilitation is entering an era of maturity in which academicians will focus their research on finding the best evidence-based methods of delivering care and clinicians will be faced with an aging population requiring pulmonary rehabilitation services. Our experience in caring for and studying the effects of pulmonary rehabilitation in non-COPD lung disease is that this "restricted" minority has as much to gain as the "obstructed" majority. This seems to be true in terms of both mobility and capacity to perform functional activity. These data support the notion that pulmonary rehabilitation is of no unique benefit to patients with COPD.

A significant amount of investigation remains to be done to explore the physiologic generation of disability in chronic lung disease and the best modalities to address these deficits. A bias seems to exist against referring patients with chronic interstitial diseases that may be based on a working knowledge of the natural history of these illnesses and a nihilism surrounding prospects for recovery. However, there certainly seems to be a role for rehabilitation in these diseases, and no surgeon would allow a potential recipient to eschew a preoperative rehabilitation in preparation for lung transplantation. Most importantly, further prospective studies are needed regarding outcomes for non-COPD patients undergoing pulmonary rehabilitation.

REFERENCES

1. Coultas DB, Zumwalt RE, Black WC, et al. The epidemiology of interstitial lung diseases. Am J Respir Crit Care Med 1994;150:967–972.
2. Ries AL, Carlin BW, Carrieri-Kohlman V, et al. Pulmonary rehabilitation: joint ACCP/AACVPR evidence-based guidelines. Chest 1997;112:1363–1396.
3. Larreu SC, ZuWallach R. Pulmonary rehabilitation—1999: ATS position paper. Am J Respir Crit Care Med 1999;159:1666–1682.
4. Casaburi R, Storer TW, Ben-Dov I, et al. Effect of endurance training on possible determinants of VO_2 during heavy exercise. J Appl Physiol 1987;62:199–207.
5. Casaburi R, Patessio A, Ioli F, et al. Reductions in exercise lactic acidosis and ventilation as a result of exercise training in patients with obstructive lung disease. Am Rev Respir Dis 1991;143:9–18.
6. Wasserman K, Sue DY, Casaburi R, et al. Selection criteria for exercise training in pulmonary rehabilitation. Eur Respir J 1989;2(Suppl 7):604S–610S.
7. Casaburi R, Wasserman K, Patessio A, et al. A new perspective in pulmonary rehabilitation: anaerobic threshold as a discriminant in training. Eur Respir J 1989;2(Suppl 7):618S–623S.
8. Gallefoss F, Bakke PS, Kjaersgaard PK. Quality of life assessment after patient education in a randomized controlled study on asthma and chronic obstructive pulmonary disease. Am J Respir Crit Care Med 1999;159:812–817.
9. Boulet LP, Boutin H, Cote J, et al. Evaluation of an asthma self-management education program. J Asthma 1995;32(3):199–206.
10. Cambach W, Wagenaar RC, Koelman TW, et. al. The long-term effects of pulmonary rehabilitation in patients with asthma and chronic obstructive pulmonary disease: a research synthesis. Arch Phys Med Rehabil 1999;80(1):103–111.
11. Emtner M, Finne M, Stalenheim G. A 3-year follow-up of asthmatic patients participating in a 10-week rehabilitation program with emphasis on physical training. Arch Phys Med Rehabil 1998;79(5):539–544.
12. Abd AG, Braun NMT, Baskin MI, et al. Diaphragmatic dysfunction after open heart surgery: treatment with a rocking bed. Ann Intern Med 1989;111:881–886.
13. Goldstein RS, Avendano MA, De Rosie J, et al. Intermittent positive-pressure ventilation via a nasal mask in patients with restrictive ventilatory failure. Chest 1990;97:80s.
14. Fishman DB, Petty TL. Physical, symptomatic and psychological improvement in patients receiving comprehensive care for chronic airways obstruction. J Chronic Dis 1971;24:775–785.
15. Lacasse Y, Wong E, Guyatt GH, et. al. Meta-analysis of respiratory rehabilitation in chronic obstructive pulmonary disease. Lancet 1996;348:1115–1119.
16. Martinez FJ, Courser JI, Celli BR. Respiratory response to arm elevation in patients with chronic airflow obstruction. Am Rev Respir Dis 1991;143:476–480.
17. Uniform Data System for Medical Rehabilitation. Buffalo, NY: UB Foundation Activities, 1996.
18. Light RW, Merrill EJ, Despars JA, et al. Prevalence of depression and anxiety in patients with COPD: relationship to functional capacity. Chest 1985;87:35–38.
19. Grant I, Heaton RK, McSweeney AJ, et al. Neuropsychologic findings in hypoxemic chronic obstructive pulmonary disease. Arch Intern Med 1982;142:1470–1476.
20. Kalayan B, Alexopoulos GS. Prefrontal dysfunction and treatment response in geriatric depression. Arch Gen Psychiatry 1999;56(8):713–718.
21. Emery CF, Leatherman NE, Burker EJ, et al. Psychological outcomes of a pulmonary rehabilitation program. Chest 1991;100(3):613–617.
22. Foster S, Thomas HM III. Pulmonary rehabilitation in lung disease other than chronic obstructive pulmonary disease. Am Rev Respir Dis 1990;141:601–604.
23. Novitch RS, Thomas HM III. Pulmonary rehabilitation in chronic interstitial disease. In: Fishman AP, ed. Pulmonary Rehabilitation. New York: Marcel Dekker, 1996:683–700.

33 Rehabilitation for the Pediatric Patient with Pulmonary Disease

Kathy Lee Bishop-Lindsay
G. Scott Lea

▷ Professional Skills

Upon completion of this chapter, the reader will be able to:

- Provide an overview of pathophysiology of each disease and the impact on rehabilitation
- Apply theories and definitions of rehabilitation to the individual with a pediatric pulmonary disease
- Discuss barriers to growth and development of the individual and name at least one strategy to overcome these barriers
- Discuss precautions to establishing an exercise prescription in this patient population

This chapter presents an adaptation of the principles of pulmonary rehabilitation, which have been modified and applied to the pediatric pulmonary population.[1] In pediatric pulmonary rehabilitation, the child is rehabilitated to his or her highest potential of medical, mental, emotional, social, developmental, and vocational level (Box 33-1). This chapter includes a discussion of asthma, cystic fibrosis (CF), bronchopulmonary dysplasia (BPD), neuromuscular diseases, and scoliosis.

The objectives of the chapter are to describe a clinical overview of each disease, to discuss the pathophysiology of the disease, and to define rehabilitation theories and practice in the pediatric pulmonary population. Considerations of disease severity, oxygenation, limitations in ventilation owing to secretions and musculoskeletal pump deficits, responses to exercises, and exercise testing and prescriptions are also discussed. The most common chronic and restrictive lung diseases, both inherited and acquired, are presented in this chapter.

OBSTRUCTIVE AND RESTRICTIVE LUNG DISORDERS

Technically, all pulmonary diseases can be categorized according to the primary functional abnormality produced.[2] Obstructive lung diseases produce obstruction to airflow. The hindrance to airflow may be in upper, lower, or both airways. The other major disease category, restrictive lung diseases, includes diseases that affect the chest wall and lung parenchyma and produce reductions in lung volumes.[3,4] Restrictive lung disease results from a variety of disorders, including skeletal/thoracic abnormalities such as scoliosis and neuromuscular diseases such as muscular dystrophy.[2,3] Some diseases, CF, for example, may have both obstructive and restrictive clinical features as the primary disease progresses and lung tissue is destroyed.

Box 33-1. Suggested Goals of Pediatric Pulmonary Rehabilitation[8,15,16,21,37]

Psychosocial
- Improve self-esteem
- Enable the patient or family/caregiver to independently perform medical care
- Minimize the impact of the disease on the daily activity and lifestyle of the patient/family/caregiver
- Decrease complaints of shortness of breath
- Teach the individual self-monitoring skills for safe play and exercise
- Decrease fear of the individual and family/caregiver to allow participation in play and exercise
- Allow the child to participate in a play activity with peers

Knowledge
- Increase knowledge of disease
- Identify signs and symptoms of exacerbation and plan for appropriate medical care
- Instruct in proper use and administration of medications
- Promote adherence with plan of care
- Teach family/caregiver safe and effective home manual ventilation techniques
- Increase knowledge/application of techniques to improve airflow
- Independent in pursed-lips breathing
- Teach individual/family/caregiver to be independent with effective cough or assisted cough
- Increase knowledge and practice of relaxation techniques

Medical
- Improve secretion clearance techniques
- Improve ventilation and perfusion matching
- Develop effective coughing techniques and breath control
- Improve and help normalize growth and development where possible
- Independent and safe/effective home suctioning techniques
- Decrease episodes of exacerbations, bronchospasm, and hospitalizations
- Independent in airway clearance technique

Exercise
- Increase endurance and activity level
- Improve trunk range of motion and efficiency
- Decrease complaints of shortness of breath with a specific activity
- Improve distance walked on a 6-minute walk test
- Improve heart rate response, respiratory rate, rating of perceived exertion, and level of dyspnea for a given activity or exercise

Asthma

Any clinician who has listened to the prolonged exhalation of a patient with asthma in the emergency department knows that asthma is an obstructive disease. Most respiratory diseases in children are obstructive, and asthma is the most common. The prevalence rate has increased 72% from 1982 to 1994.[5] Asthma is the leading cause for absence from work and school. Mortality rates for asthma have also increased, and more than 5000 people in the United States die from this disease each year.[6]

Despite the discouraging statistical trend, a great deal of progress has been made. Changes in the clinical setting have resulted from a better understanding of the disease process and the role of inflammation. New medications and delivery systems are being developed. The revised "Practical Guide for the Diagnosis and Management of Asthma" was completed in 1997 and is being put into practice as a user-friendly teaching tool.[6,7]

Asthma is defined primarily as a chronic inflammatory disorder of the airways. Inflammation is present even during periods without symptoms. Inflammation results from a variety of factors, including viral infections, inhaled allergens, and environmental factors. Recurrent episodes of airway inflammation result in diffuse airway obstruction. The obstruction produces characteristics of wheezing, shortness of breath, chest tightness, and cough. Coughing typically occurs at night and in the early morning and often wakes the patient. This inflammatory process causes the already hyperresponsive airway to be even more sensitive to stimuli.

Exercise can provoke symptoms in 80% of people with asthma.[8] Exercise-induced asthma produces bronchospasm, which usually peaks 5 to 10 minutes after stopping exercise and resolves within 60 minutes.[6] Symptoms include a reduction in exercise capacity, chest tightness, dyspnea, wheezing, and coughing during or after exercise. The primary stimulants in exercise-induced asthma may be cooling and drying of the airways caused by increased minute ventilation during exercise.[9] The severity of the episode is affected by type, duration, and intensity of exercise. Temperature and time since previous exercise are factors in symptom development.[9] Exercising in cold, dry air causes more problems than exercising in warm, humid air. Swimming is less likely to produce symptoms than is running. Sports or activities with intermittent, short periods of activity are least likely to cause symptoms. Pretreatment with a β_2-agonist or anti-inflammatory such as cromolyn or nedocromil can prevent exercise from triggering asthma symptoms.[6] A 6- to 10-minute warm-up may eliminate the need for pretreatment with medications.

Medical

The primary goals of asthma management include the prevention of acute exacerbations and minimizing chronic symptoms. Other important objectives include maintaining a normal activity level, optimizing lung function, and avoiding side effects. Part of the treatment plan should be directed at reducing exposure to allergens or triggers and should include environmental control. Environmental control aims to reduce or remove such triggers as tobacco smoke, dust mites, animal dander, cockroaches, mold, dust, and pollen.[6]

The new medical management guidelines and recent advances in medications provide the best opportunity yet for control of asthma symptoms. Maintenance therapy begins with an anti-inflammatory medication and adds a bronchodilator as needed. Advances in medications include a new category of anti-inflammatory agents, leukotrien modifiers, which may eliminate or reduce the need for steroids.[6,9,10] For those unable to use metered dose inhalers effectively, steroids and bronchodilators are available in powdered forms. Long-acting bronchodilators are available in tablet form. An anticholinergic broncho-dilator is available for use with the more common β_2 bronchodilators. These new anticho-linergic bronchodilators can also be used separate from the β_2 medication for individuals who do not respond to them. Short-acting β_2 medications are now used as rescue inhalers for relief of symptoms.[6,9]

Rehabilitation Program

Asthma rehabilitation programs aim to promote self-management and improve quality of life. Patient or caregiver education is one tool in achieving self-management. Objectives of education are described in Box 33-2. The patient must be taught to assess his or her respiratory status. The measurement of peak flow helps to assess respiratory status, determining interventions required, and evaluating response to therapy. The most critical aspect of self-management, however, is the most difficult to control: motivation and adherence with the plan of care. The establishment of individualized and mutually agreed

Box 33-2. Asthma Rehabilitation: Objectives of Education[8,9]

After completing an asthma rehabilitation program, the participant will be able to discuss:

General description of asthma and patient triggers

Medications, including purpose, dosage, frequency, and administration technique

Self-assessment, including use of peak flow meter

Control removal of environmental triggers

Daily maintenance plan (including plans for school or daycare)

Plan for acute exacerbation (when to increase therapy and when to call a physician)

Identification and removal of medical barriers

on goals encourages compliance. However, the episodic nature of asthma, with relatively long periods of stability, discourages adherence with a plan of care.

When poorly controlled, asthma interferes with the daily life of the individual and the family. Days are missed from school and work. The family lifestyle is changed. Patients and families experience fear, frustration, and anger. Well-meaning parents may discourage their child from physical activity because of fear of an attack. Children with asthma may feel that they cannot compete with other children in athletic activities or may accommodate their illness by avoiding strenuous exercise. This may result in reduced self-esteem and a pattern of inactivity and deconditioning.

Exercise Program

Multiple studies have attempted to evaluate the effect of exercise on children with asthma. The results have been inconclusive and have not identified the ideal exercise program for children with asthma. However, the results have demonstrated that children with asthma can safely participate in an exercise program. We do not need research to appreciate the need for physical activity in the normal growth and development of a child. Beneficial effects of exercise programs include improved cardiopulmonary fitness, increased exercise tolerance, increased oxygen consumption, and decreased resting heart rate.

Children can be taught to perform relaxed diaphragmatic breathing and effective coughing techniques. Teaching children requires creative thinking and the use of age-appropriate techniques. If learned and practiced often, relaxed diaphragmatic breathing can help prevent or lessen the severity of an attack. Used in conjunction with pursed-lips exhalation, the respiratory rate is decreased and the child may feel less anxious. Learning to recognize early asthma symptoms is important for the proper use of relaxation and breathing exercises.

Rehabilitation for children with asthma should not be so regimented. Play is important in development and growth and can help incorporate exercise into a normal lifestyle. Children, especially adolescents, rebel against formal, structured methods that do not allow "play." With proper medical management, children should be able to participate in any exercise, including competitive sports. Athletes with asthma have competed successfully in a variety of sports, including ice skating and track.[8] The goal of medical and rehabilitative care should be to enable the child to participate in whatever activity is desired without limitations or experiencing symptoms.

Cystic Fibrosis

Medical

CF is the leading genetic cause of death for Caucasian children in the United States.[4,11–15] Approximately 30,000 individuals are affected with CF, with upward of a thousand new cases being diagnosed each year.[11,14] CF occurs in 1 of every 3,300 live births.[11] The good news is that the median survival age is now 31 years.[11] The defective gene was identified nearly a decade ago, but the intervention of gene therapy to eradicate the disease and its sequelae remains elusive to researchers.[11] The defect in the sodium and chloride channels in epithelial cells leads to changes in multiple organ systems.[11,14] The primary cause of death is from pulmonary complications.[14,16] Thick, tenacious secretions block airways and provide a prime breeding area for infections.[11,16] The combination of persistent secretions, chronic infection, and inflammation results in obstruction, leading to declines in oxygenation and eventually impacting exercise tolerance. Early diagnosis, intervention, and prevention are the foundations for care of the individual with CF.[17] Use of anti-inflammatory medications antibiotics, pancreatic replacement enzymes, airway clearance, exercise, and nutritional supplements are key elements of medical treatment.[14] Newer medications such as ibuprofen, dornase alfa (Pulmozyme), and inhaled tobramycin (TOBI) are aimed at reducing airway inflammation, thinning secretions, and treating infections, respectively.[11,14]

Airway Clearance Techniques

Airway clearance is a crucial component to a rehabilitation program for the patient with CF.[12,14–19] Secretions need to be mobilized and expectorated to optimize ventilation and perfusion matching during exercise.[12] Airway clearance techniques (Box 33-3) improve secretion mobilization, ventilation, oxygenation, and chest wall and cough mechanics. The gold standard for airway clearance until recently has been chest physical therapy consisting of percussion, vibration, and bronchial drainage.[18,19] Newer techniques have been developed that have been shown to be as effective in clearing mucus and preserving pulmonary function as the gold standard.[18,20] Choosing the best airway clearance technique for a patient is tantamount for success of this facet of the overall care program. Developing an individualized airway clearance program incorporates medical history, clinical presentation, severity of illness, cost and efficacy of devices, availability of assistance, needs of the patient and the family, cognitive level, age, and time constraints.[18] Thomas and colleagues[20] performed a meta-analysis of research studies comparing airway clearance techniques used during the past 27 years. A combination of traditional (gold standard) therapy and exercise was more effective in improving forced expiratory volume in 1 second compared with only traditional treatment. No significant differences were found among the other techniques analyzed. Patients may benefit from a combination treatment, but the only consensus at this time is that airway clearance must be done at least once a day and should be increased during an exacerbation.[14]

Exercise Program

An ideal rehabilitation program should have components of airway clearance, endurance activities, flexibility training, postural exercises, and weight training.[14,16] Exercise is not only beneficial as an adjunct to airway clearance but as a way to improve self-esteem, endurance, and flexibility and to build or maintain muscle mass; exercise is also hypothesized to slow progression of osteoporosis.[15,16,21,22] A standard exercise prescription (Box 33-4) consists of mode (device or type of exercise to be performed, i.e., walking, cycling, basketball), duration (length of time for exercise), frequency (number of times per day or week), and intensity (the level at which the exercise is performed, usually measured in heart rate or oxygen consumption).[13,14,23]

A thorough evaluation of the individual should be performed before initiating an exercise program.[12,14,15,21] Oxygen saturation should be evaluated at rest and during exercise in all patients with CF to evaluate hypoxemia.[12] A musculoskeletal screen to evaluate posture, flexibility, and strength is important to isolate specific needs of the individual.[15] A functional test such as a 6-minute walk test, which is standardized and easily repeatable, is a good clinical tool to use to evaluate oxygen saturation and hemodynamic response to a normal activity.[12,23,24] Suggestions then can be made regarding use of supplemental oxygen for a home exercise program. Monitoring heart rate, rating of perceived exertion, respiratory rate, and blood pressure during the timed walk test help the clinician to formulate an exercise prescription for the patient. Rating of perceived exertion is a subjective measure of work.[21,25] Scales ranging from 6 to 20 and 0 to 10 are used to estimate a

---

Box 33-3. Alternative Airway Clearance Techniques

Chest physiotherapy	Active cycle of breathing
Percussion, vibration, shaking, bronchial drainage	Positive expiratory pressure
	Mask, mouthpiece, oscillating PEP
Forced expiratory technique	Mechanical percussors/vibrators
High-frequency chest wall oscillations/ high-frequency chest compression	Autogenic drainage
	Intrapulmonary percussive ventilation

Adapted from Hardy KA. A review of airway clearance: new techniques, indications, and recommendations. Resp Care 1994;39(5):440–452.

Box 33-4. Suggested Components of an Exercise Prescription[12,14,25,55]

Mode

Tricycle, bicycle, swimming, tennis, crab
    soccer, basketball, wheelchair basketball,
    aerobic dancing, jogging, running,
    walking, climbing, wheelbarrow racing,
    cross-country skiing, skating, weight
    lifting, elastic bands, step aerobics,
    snowshoeing, etc.

Frequency

4–5 times per week; in some cases the
    individual is only able to perform short
    bouts of exercise (<5–10 continuous
    minutes; progress first to 2–3 times a day
    and then increase duration as above)

Duration

Progress to 20–30 continuous minutes of
    "aerobic" activity (may take 6–8 wk to
    progress to that level if untrained)

Intensity

70–85% heart rate range of peak heart rate
    from exercise tolerance test
11–15 (6–20 scale) or 3–5 (0–10 scale) on
    Borg Rating of Perceived Exertion Scale
0–1 on Dyspnea Levels Scale (No. of breaths
    to count to 15 in an 8-second period,
    score 0–4)

Precautions

- All activity/exercise should be age appropriate
- Be aware of growth plate development in planning activity/exercise
- Undergo a thorough medical examination before starting any exercise program
  (include oxygen saturation at rest, with activity, and recovery)
- Supplemental oxygen should be used per physician order (should be determined
  from results of exercise tolerance test)
- No exercise/play should cause any level of pain
- History of osteoporosis
- Evaluate sudden rib pain/soreness (even with a cough)
- Allow extra fluids for hydration
- Allow extra calories in meal plan for exercise/play
- Check blood glucose levels if diabetic
- Avoid exercise/vigorous play just before or immediately after a meal
- Avoid heat and extreme temperatures and high-pollution times of day
- Choose an activity that will be enjoyable and can be done throughout the year
- Ensure adequate rest, watch for signs/symptoms of fatigue
- Watch for decline in activity/play level
- Use metered dose inhalers before exercise if indicated by previous symptoms
- Airway clearance regimen should be incorporated into program
- Allow a warm-up (5–10 minutes) and cool down (5–10 minutes) to avoid an
  increase in bronchospasm and musculoskeletal injury
- Practice good hand washing (2 minutes) and cleaning of equipment
- Limit vigorous play/exercise with an exacerbation
- Alert the individual/parent/caregiver that a decline in activity level with a
  change of symptoms should be reported to the health care team
- Watch for complaints of increased dyspnea or shortness of breath
- Give the individual choices of programs to keep activities fun and improve
  adherence
- Reevaluate the program and hemodynamic responses to activity to adjust the
  program

level of work as a measure of intensity. A child or adolescent may not be able to find a pulse to check for a target heart rate. Using a simple scale that correlates with a measure of exercise intensity like heart rate may be easier for the child to understand. Measuring the number of coughs and secretions expectorated during the walk test help to assess efficacy of the present airway clearance program and how the patient handles secretions with exercise. All of this information will help establish the level of intensity for the home exercise program. Last, bronchodilators may be useful before initiation of exercise to improve airflow in some patients with reactive airways.[12]

Orenstein and colleagues[26] exercised patients 3 times a week at 70 to 85% of the patient's maximal attainable heart rate while jogging or walking for a 3-month test period. Improvements were shown in endurance, ventilatory muscle endurance, and peak oxygen consumption. The control group did not participate in the structured exercise program and had a significant decline in the forced expiratory volume in 1 second. Their results suggest that exercise tolerance and cardiorespiratory fitness could be improved with this method of training for patients with CF. A study by Keens and his colleagues[27] used two different modalities to train respiratory muscles. Subjects performed specific ventilatory muscle training or participated in upper body activities such as swimming and canoeing. Pulmonary function did not improve significantly, but ventilatory muscle endurance increased by 56% with both modalities for patients with CF. Nixon and associates[28] studied the prognostic effect of exercise testing in patients with CF for 8 years. The conclusions of the study suggested that level of fitness was directly related to prognosis even when gender and disease severity was taken into consideration. These studies reinforce that some form of aerobic exercise is beneficial and needs to be a component of any exercise prescription for a patient with CF.

Strauss and his colleagues[29] performed a study that used weight training for a 3-month period using a graded intensity. Muscle strength increased and residual volume along with the ratio of residual volume to total lung capacity and total lung capacity all decreased. The researchers were unclear as to why these components of pulmonary function tests improved. Improving expiratory muscle strength may have played a role. To what extent weight training will benefit patients with CF is still unknown and needs further research.

Precautions

Weight loss is a fear and an excuse for not exercising expressed by many adolescents and young adults with CF. Conversely, female patients fear weight gain or even development of muscle bulk. These two fears alone may impact adherence to the program. Proper nutrition, caloric intake, and supplementation should be part of the foundation to an exercise program for an individual with CF.[14] Working with the team members should put these fears to rest. Every effort should be made to present a well thought out approach to best serve the individual. Parents of younger children should be included in the plan especially if the meal plan and use of enzymes will be changed. During an exacerbation, calorie needs may increase, but exercise and activity levels should decrease to accommodate the illness.

Patients who have diabetes as a comorbidity should have their blood glucose evaluated for responsiveness to a given activity.[30] Preparations for snacks and appropriate supplements to avoid hypoglycemia are important. Time of day of exercise in conjunction with type and intensity of exercise may be crucial if insulin is used for glucose management. Avoiding exercise or play when the glucose level is falling, such as before a meal, or when the insulin dose is peaking will help prevent hypoglycemic episodes.[31]

Osteopenia is a medical concern for all members of the team taking care of the individual with CF.[22] Multiple factors result in bone demineralization and eventual osteoporosis in patients. Nutrition status, growth and development, vitamins, and absorption of vitamins play roles in the cascade of events leading to bone demineralization. Many studies in the last few years have demonstrated that patients with CF before lung transplantation have significant bone loss and osteoporosis per dual-energy radiograph absorptiometry.[32] The exact etiology is multifactorial, but the impact on rehabilitation and activities of daily living may be limiting. Pain from vertebral fractures may limit chest physical therapy and hinder coughing and secretion mobilization as well as prevent the child from participating in play activities.

A clinician should always remember to give the individual choices to keep the activities fun and improve adherence. Standard precautions and infection control should be used if patients are to exercise or play in a shared space for the safety of all clients. Appropriate hemodynamic parameters, including oxygen saturation at rest and during exercise, heart rate, and rating of perceived exertion, are key to setting a safe and progressive exercise program. Proper breathing-controlled techniques in combination with airway clearance before and after an activity may allow the child to participate in any type of exercise. Many school-aged children with CF express that they have a fear of coughing in front of their friends. Teaching the child or young adolescent pursed-lips breathing, controlled coughing, or huffing will help improve airflow, decrease respiratory rate, and limit paroxysmal coughing. These small changes may help them fit in with their peers. Making the child with CF feel that he or she can fit in to participate in play activities or sports will allow them to build confidence and self-esteem. Exercise will then become an enjoyable activity and not something thought of as a necessity.

Bronchopulmonary Dysplasia

In 1966 Northway described a new clinical condition, BPD.[33] Newborn infants receiving positive-pressure ventilation and high concentrations of oxygen developed secondary pulmonary injury. No single cause is responsible for the condition. Instead, it is a result of the cumulative effect of several factors, including pulmonary immaturity, high oxygen concentrations, positive-pressure ventilation with high airway pressure, and duration of exposure.

Clinically, BPD is characterized by tachypnea, retractions, crackles, wheezing, hypoxemia, and hypercarbia. Anatomically, alveolar structure is abnormal.[34] Fibrosis of alveolar septa is evident, with areas of hyperinflation adjacent to areas of atelectasis. Interstitial edema and thickening of the alveolar basement membrane are present. Mucosal hyperplasia reduces the lumen of small airways. In addition, excessive production of mucus and compromise of mucociliary transport occur. Frequently, large airways are involved, manifested as tracheomalacia or bronchomalacia. Pulmonary artery hypertension is commonly present, and cor pulmonale may occur in severely affected children.

These anatomic abnormalities have physiologic impacts.[34] Pulmonary fibrosis and interstitial edema decrease lung compliance. Resistance to airflow is increased by narrowing of the airway lumen and the presence of excess mucus. Minute ventilation is usually increased secondary to an increase in respiratory rate. However, tidal volume is usually decreased, resulting in increased dead space ventilation. The end result of the changes is increased work of breathing.

The clinical severity of BPD varies from thriving infants with minimum oxygen requirements to the infant with chronic respiratory failure dependent on mechanical ventilation via tracheostomy. Chronic respiratory disease results from damage to lung parenchyma and airways. Acute distress may result from upper or lower respiratory infections or from exacerbation of BPD itself. An exacerbation of BPD is similar to an asthma exacerbation. In fact, most children with BPD also have reactive airway disease.

Neurologic sequelae are common, occurring in 30% of affected infants.[35] These sequelae range from a major handicap to learning disabilities. Premature infants on mechanical ventilation are at risk for intraventricular and subdural hemorrhage. Many of them have also survived critical periods of instability with periods of hypoxemia. Developmental delays often result from prolonged stays in the intensive care unit and hospital. The intensive care unit environment has far too many negative experiences, and the entire hospital environment has far too few positive experiences to promote development in a challenged infant.

Medical

Children with BPD often have little pulmonary reserve, and medical management can be a delicate balancing act. Diuretics, bronchodilators, and anti-inflammatory medications are used to reduce airway resistance and work of breathing.[33] Diuretic therapy often leads to electrolyte imbalances requiring supplements. Antibiotics, including aerosolized medications, are given to treat infections.

Children with BPD and tracheobronchial malacia are especially difficult to manage. A congenital abnormality of the cartilage in the airway results in a weakened area that collapses and narrows the airway, particularly on forced exhalation.[36] These children can go into severe respiratory distress when agitated or stressed, or even by straining while stooling. In severe cases, the child may be sedated to avoid episodes of distress. Positive end-expiratory pressure may also be effective in preventing airway collapse. Infants with BPD who are hypoxic on room air receive supplemental oxygen. Chronic hypoxia can cause pulmonary hypertension and cor pulmonale.[36] Oxygenation should be monitored and oxygen weaned as tolerated, avoiding hypoxemia during sleep and exertion, such as when feeding.

The child with severe BPD may require mechanical ventilation via tracheostomy. Growth, muscle strength, and ability to wean from ventilation depend on adequate nutrition. Calorie requirements are high, estimated to be 25 to 50% higher than for a healthy child owing to increased work of breathing.[37] Fluid restrictions and feeding disorders often result in inadequate caloric intake. Enteral feeding may be required to supplement oral intake. When reducing ventilatory support, the child must be carefully observed. Failure to tolerate weaning can be demonstrated in a variety of subtle ways: a decrease in oral feeding, slowed weight gain or weight loss, or change in social interaction. The needs of the child and family can determine the goals of weaning. Even a short period of freedom from mechanical ventilation can make a tremendous impact on the life of a family.

Parents of a child with BPD at home learn common sense precautions: avoid exposure to crowds and to people with colds and respiratory infections. Viral respiratory infections, frequently respiratory syncytial virus in the fall and winter months, can be devastating. Setbacks in weaning owing to increased work of breathing often results from a respiratory syncytial virus infection. Immunization for respiratory syncytial virus should be administered to each child. Routine immunizations must also be kept up to date. Hospitalization is also to be avoided whenever possible because of risk of exposure to other infections.[36]

Physical Rehabilitation

Long-term outcomes of patients with BPD are difficult to predict. Pulmonary function studies are abnormal for many years in children recovering from BPD.[34] Many of them also have reactive airway disease. However, these children are generally able to participate in all the normal childhood activities. Developmental potential is more uncertain. Frequently, cognitive and motor function are impaired.[37] However, it is difficult to differentiate developmental delay from neurologic damage, and these children can make surprising progress in a rehabilitation program. A study by Buschbacher[38] revealed that 70 to 80% of ventilator-dependent patients with BPD can be weaned from a ventilator. Even when weaning and decannulation are not possible, ventilator support can often be reduced and these children can learn to speak and feed orally and interact with their environment.

The ideal goal for these children is a safe discharge home. For some children this means discharge home on ventilatory support. For other children, discharge home is not an option. Wherever the location, each child deserves to be in a program or environment that will allow them to fulfill their potential.

Exercise Program

Infants with BPD present with a diversity of clinical needs that are best handled by a multidisciplinary team emphasizing growth and development. Interdisciplinary goals require teamwork at the bedside. The speech pathologist and respiratory therapist work together to help the trached child learn to vocalize. The child life specielist and physical therapist develop a list of play activities to address motor deficits. The respiratory therapist works with physical therapy to make the child as mobile as possible and monitors the patient during activities. Treatment is directed toward two goals: preventing further harm, either neurologic or pulmonary, and promoting growth, both physical and developmental.

Children receiving ventilatory support need to be carefully monitored when active or stressed. Acceptable ranges for carbon dioxide, oxygen saturation, respiratory rate, and heart rate should be set based on an individual status. Because some children have an elevated respiratory and heart rate at rest, ranges given as activity guidelines in textbooks do not always apply to these patients. The tracheostomy tube must be protected and the child monitored for signs of hypoxemia and respiratory distress. Measurements of oxygen saturation must be combined with clinical assessments. End tidal carbon dioxide levels should be measured before and after exercise. If necessary, ventilatory support can be increased during periods of increased activity. Even patients who no longer require supplemental oxygen should be monitored for hypoxemia during exercise.

Therapies may be prescribed to address specific motor impairments or for areas of developmental delay. However, for infants and children, play is exercise therapy. Therapeutic play sessions, including interdisciplinary sessions with occupational, physical, and speech therapies, are an important part of rehabilitation. These children need every opportunity to explore and interact with their environment and other people. Rather than prescribe specific activities, efforts should be directed toward removing barriers to physical activity. The child should be as mobile as possible. Simplify the equipment required for care. If the child will tolerate one, use a portable ventilator. Improved mobility will help the therapist provide more effective therapies. Rehabilitation programs for children with BPD can promote growth and development, reduce the time required for weaning from mechanical ventilation, and shorten the discharge process.[39]

RESTRICTIVE LUNG DISORDERS

Neuromuscular Disease

Medical
Neuromuscular disorders, degenerative muscle diseases, and paralytic syndromes involving the chest wall will limit the volume of air inhaled with a given breath, thereby affecting pulmonary function.[16,40–42] The ability to coordinate muscle movement to perform inspiration and forced expiration may be impaired in any of these diseases.[40] This limitation may be slow and progressive or abrupt, as in a traumatic accident. Cerebral palsy, muscular dystrophy, and Down's syndrome are diseases in which the musculoskeletal deficits have profound implications on the pulmonary system.[17] Musculoskeletal changes from muscle weakness, muscle imbalance, or muscle tone (either high tone in the case of cerebral palsy or low tone in the case of Down's syndrome) may result in scoliotic changes in the rib cage, further restricting air movement.[17,41,43] A pulmonary rehabilitation program for these patients must focus not only on enhancing movement and coordination of the thorax and shoulder girdle but on an effective cough.[4] An effective cough that mobilizes and clears secretions is key to prevention of pulmonary complications.[17]

Duchenne Muscular Dystrophy

Duchenne muscular dystrophy (DMD) is an inherited disease affecting males.[40,41,44] The disease leads to progressive loss of muscle control, tone, and function.[40,43] The ability to cough and clear secretions will become impaired.[4,40,45,46] Prevention of infection and secretion retention are keys to avoiding respiratory distress and eventual failure requiring mechanical ventilation.[41] The primary cause of death for patients with DMD is respiratory failure.[47,48] Education for parents, caregivers, and patients on recognizing signs and symptoms of decline in the respiratory system are also important to delay pulmonary compromise.[45] Any change in sleep pattern, vivid nightmares or dreams, morning headaches, confusion, or increasing level of fatigue may be signs of carbon dioxide retention and the need for medical intervention.[49] Myocardial damage has been reported in greater than 90% of patients with DMD.[41,44,50] Precautions should include evaluation of both the cardiac and the pulmonary system before initiating an exercise program in this patient population.

Exercise Program

Simple diaphragmatic breathing exercises, stacking of breaths with or without manual assistance, are major components of a program for these individuals.[4,45] Inspiratory muscle training can play a role in improving force and endurance of the respiratory muscles in patients with neuromuscular disease.[51] Efficacy of inspiratory muscle training is limited by disease progression and type of training regimen used. Standard chest physiotherapy, breathing exercises, and intermittent positive-pressure breathing have been shown to improve pulmonary function during a 3-month study in patients with DMD. Improved efficiency in diaphragmatic breathing patterns was demonstrated in these patients. Wanke and associates[52] studied inspiratory muscle training for patients with DMD. The results of the training persisted for longer than 6 months in certain patients in the study. They concluded that this type of training is useful in the early stages of the disease.

An individual treatment plan and ongoing reassessment of the plan is important to meet that patient's needs. The individual's level of disease severity and progression will limit progress with the exercise program. Functional activities such as walking may initially be part of the rehabilitation program, but once the child progresses to a wheelchair the goals of the program will shift more toward maintaining posture, flexibility, and enhancement of cough.[43] The use of abdominal binders is recommended as strength decreases to help with positioning the diaphragm in a more advantageous position.[4] A decline in activity level, increased shortness of breath, or complaints of tiredness are signals from the patient about fatigue. In a degenerative type of disorder, this is not a desired outcome. Alert the family, caregiver, and patient to these signals to slow down or even stop the pulmonary rehabilitation program and contact the team for assistance.

Scoliosis

Medical and Exercise Program

Scoliosis can be idiopathic or from spinal deformities developed from muscle weakness, imbalance in muscle tone, and denervation.[4,40,45] Treatment for scoliosis ranges from conservative to surgical intervention depending on the age of the patient, the severity of the curve, the progressive nature of the deformity, and the underlying etiology.[40] Exercise and its role in the treatment of scoliosis is controversial. Some studies have shown no benefit from exercise, but a recent study by Weiss and colleagues[53] demonstrated relatively no progression in curve angle with treatment of physiotherapy only. Athanasopoulos and colleagues[54] did not look at curve progression in their study. They were able to demonstrate improvements in pulmonary function and aerobic work during a 2-month training period of endurance exercise.

Pulmonary function, ventilation and perfusion matching, and risk for pulmonary complications should be considerations when planning a program for an individual with scoliosis no matter what the etiology.[40,45] Effective cough, airflow, and volume of air movement are key components to any program for a patient with a restrictive lung disorder.[45] Teaching positions to improve ventilation and chest expansion and instructing ways to strengthen and enhance respiratory muscle endurance will help with secretion mobilization, cough, and prevention of atelectasis.[4] The ability to stack breaths to enhance air volume for cough and development of an exercise plan to enhance chest wall movement and conditioning should not be overlooked. The patient's breathing pattern may be shallow and rapid at rest and during exercise owing to the length tension relationship of the respiratory muscles from the change in the angle of the thorax.[24] The heart rate may also be elevated at rest owing to these abnormalities in the pulmonary system. Hemodynamic parameters for the exercise program should therefore include a dyspnea scale and a scale to rate perceived exertion. Teaching signs and symptoms of fatigue and decline in activity should also be included in the overall plan.

Five important respiratory diseases in children have been presented relative to the pathology and the effect of this on activity or exercise. An assessment of the child's disease process, clinical presentation, home needs, and self-desires are critical to the design of an effective rehabilitation program. Such a program would promote not only growth and development, but self-worth and enjoyment. The disease process has already made the child unique, and in most cases the last thing the child wants outside of the hospital is to stand out. To be like his or her peers and joining in on play, sports, and other activities are vital. The team must identify needs and precautions, focus educational efforts so as not to overwhelm the child or family, and design something that will be fun and at the same time beneficial for the child.

REFERENCES

1. Connors G, Hilling L, eds. Guidelines for Pulmonary Rehabilitation Programs: American Association of Cardiovascular & Pulmonary Rehabilitation. 2nd ed. Champaign, IL: Human Kinetics, 1998.
2. Scanlin C, Rupple G, El-Gandy A. Synopsis of cardiopulmonary diseases. In: Scanlin C, ed. Egan's Fundamentals of Respiratory Care. 6th ed. Philadelphia: Mosby, 1995.
3. West JB. Pulmonary Pathophysiology: The Essentials. 3rd ed. Baltimore: Williams & Wilkins, 1987.
4. DeCesare JA, Graybill-Tucker CA, Gould AL. Physical therapy for the child with respiratory dysfunction. In: Irwin S, Tecklin J, eds. Cardiopulmonary Physical Therapy. 3rd ed. St. Louis: Mosby-Year Book, 1995.
5. Welsh K, Magnusson M, Napoli L. Asthma clinical pathway: an interdisciplinary approach to implementation in the inpatient setting. Pediatr Nurs 1999;23(1):79–87.
6. Practical Guide for the Diagnosis and Management of Asthma. Bethesda MD: National Heart, Lung and Blood Institute, 1997. NIH publication 97-4053.
7. Lockey R. The basic principles of asthma management today. J Respir Dis 1998;Suppl 19(3): S7–S13.
8. Magee C. Asthma. In: Campbell SK, Vander Linden DW, Palisano RJ, eds. Physical Therapy for Children. Philadelphia: WB Saunders, 1995.
9. Expert Panel Report 2: Guidelines for the diagnosis and management of asthma: National Asthma Education and Prevention Program. Bethesda, MD: NHLBI Information Center, February 1997.
10. Geller E, ed. Respiratory pharmaceutical reference. Adv Manage Respir Care. 1997;6(9): 53–65.
11. Facts about cystic fibrosis. http://www.cff.org/factsabo.htm.
12. Nixon PA. Cystic fibrosis. In: ACSM's Exercise Management for Persons With Chronic Diseases and Disabilities. Champaign, IL: Human Kinetics, 1997.
13. Orenstein DM, Nixon PA. Patients with cystic fibrosis. In: Franklin BA, Gordon S, Timmis GC, eds. Exercise in Modern Medicine. Baltimore: Williams & Wilkins, 1989.
14. Orenstein DM, Noyes BE. Cystic fibrosis. In: Casaburi R, Petty TL, eds. Principles and Practice of Pulmonary Rehabilitation. Philadelphia: WB Saunders, 1993.
15. Tecklin JS. Physical therapy for children with chronic lung disease. PT 1981;61(12):1774–1782.
16. Watchie J. Cardiopulmonary Physical Therapy: A Clinical Manual. Philadelphia: WB Saunders, 1995.
17. Moerchen VA, Crane LD. The Neonatal and Pediatric Patient. In: Frownfelter DL, Dean E, eds. Principles and Practice of Cardiopulmonary Physical Therapy. 3rd ed. Chicago: Mosby-Year Book, 1996.
18. Hardy KA. A review of airway clearance: new techniques, indications, and recommendations. Respir Care 1994;39(5):440–452.
19. Downs AM. Physiological basis for airway clearance techniques. In: Frownfelter DL, Dean E, eds. Principles and Practice of Cardiopulmonary Physical Therapy. 3rd ed. Chicago: Mosby-Year Book, 1996.
20. Thomas J, Cook DJ, Brooks D. Chest physical therapy management of patients with cystic fibrosis: a meta-analysis. Am J Respir Crit Care Med 1995;151(3 pt 1):846–850.
21. Dean E, Frownfelter D. Chronic primary cardiopulmonary dysfunction. In: Frownfelter DL, Dean E, eds. Principles and Practice of Cardiopulmonary Physical Therapy. 3rd ed. Chicago: Mosby-Year Book, 1996.
22. Bachrach LK. Osteopenia in cystic fibrosis: symposium session. Pediatr Pulm 1997;Suppl 14: 200–201.

23. Krug PG. Exercise testing and training: secondary cardiopulmonary dysfunction. In: Frownfelter DL, Dean E, eds. Principles and Practice of Cardiopulmonary Physical Therapy. 3rd ed. Chicago: Mosby-Year Book, 1996.

24. Darbee J, Cerny F. Exercise testing and exercise conditioning for children with lung dysfunction. In: Irwin S, Tecklin J, eds. Cardiopulmonary Physical Therapy. 3rd ed. St Louis: Mosby-Year Book, 1995.

25. Downs AM. Clinical application of airway clearance techniques. In: Frownfelter DL, Dean E, eds. Principles and Practice of Cardiopulmonary Physical Therapy. 3rd ed. Chicago: Mosby-Year Book, 1996.

26. Orenstein DM, Franklin BA, Doershuk CF, et al. Exercise conditioning and cardiopulmonary fitness in cystic fibrosis: the effects of a three-month supervised running program. Chest 1981;80(4):392–398.

27. Keens TG, Krastins IR, Wannamaker EM, et al. Ventilatory muscle endurance training in normal subjects and patients with cystic fibrosis. Am Rev Respir Dis 1977;116(5):853–860.

28. Nixon PA, Orenstein DM, Kelsey SF, et al. The prognostic value of exercise testing in patients with cystic fibrosis. N Engl J Med 1992;327(25):1785–1788.

29. Strauss GD, Osher A, Wang CI, et al. Variable weight training in cystic fibrosis. Chest 1987;92(2):273–276.

30. Pfeifer T. Diabetes in cystic fibrosis. Clin Pediatr 1992;Nov:682–687.

31. Nettles AT, Weinhandl J. Diabetes secondary to cystic fibrosis: an increasing clinical problem. Diabetes Educ 1990;16(6):478–482.

32. Aris R, Neuringer I, Weiner M, et al. Severe osteoporosis in patients with cystic fibrosis before and after lung transplantation. Pediatr Pulm 1995; Suppl 12:258.

33. Barrington KJ, Finer N. Treatment of bronchopulmonary dysplasia. In: Goldsmith J, Spitzer A, eds. Clin Perinatol 1998;25(1):177–197.

34. Boyle K, Baker V, Cassaday C. Neonatal pulmonary disorders. In: Barhart S, Czervinske M, eds. Perinatal and Pediatric Respiratory Care. Philadelphia: WB Saunders, 1995.

35. Williams JL, Cumming JA. Bronchopulmonary dysplasia. Thorac Imaging 1986;1(4):16–24.

36. Groothuis JR, Louch GK, Van Eman C. Outpatient management of the preterm infant. J Respir Care Pract 1996;9(4):69–73.

37. Kelly M. Children with ventilator dependence. In: Campbell SK, Vander Linden DW, Palisano RJ, eds. Physical Therapy for Children. Philadelphia: WB Saunders, 1995.

38. Buschbacher R. Outcomes and problems in pediatric pulmonary rehabilitation. Am J Phys Med Rehabil 1995;74(4):287–293.

39. Buschbacher R, Tsangaris M, Shay T. Rehab and bronchopulmonary dysplasias. J Respir Care Pract 1996;9(4):75–77.

40. Clough P. Restrictive lung dysfunction. In: Hillegass EA, Sadowsky HS, eds. Essentials of Cardiopulmonary Physical Therapy. Philadelphia: WB Saunders, 1994.

41. Bach JR. Neuromuscular and skeletal disorders leading to global alveolar hypoventilation. In: Bach JR, ed. Pulmonary Rehabilitation: The Obstructive and Paralytic Conditions. Philadelphia: Hanley & Belfus, 1996.

42. Adkins HV. Improvement of breathing ability in children with respiratory muscle paralysis. PT 1968;48:577–581.

43. Bach JR. Pulmonary rehabilitation in musculoskeletal disorders. In: Fishman AP, ed. Pulmonary Rehabilitation. New York: Marcel Dekker, 1996.

44. Bar-Or O. Muscular dystrophy. In: ACSM's Exercise Management for Persons With Chronic Diseases and Disabilities. Champaign, IL: Human Kinetics, 1997.

45. Dean E, Frownfelter D. Chronic secondary cardiopulmonary dysfunction. In: Frownfelter DL, Dean E, eds. Principles and Practice of Cardiopulmonary Physical Therapy. 3rd ed. Chicago: Mosby-Year Book, 1996.

46. Bach JR. Conventional approaches to managing neuromuscular ventilatory failure. In: Bach JR, ed. Pulmonary Rehabilitation: The Obstructive and Paralytic Conditions. Philadelphia: Hanley & Belfus, 1996.

47. Bach JR, Ishikawa Y, Kim H. Prevention of pulmonary morbidity for patients with Duchenne muscular dystrophy. Chest 1997;112:1024–1028.

48. De Troyer A, Estenne M. Neuromuscular disorders. In: Fishman AP, ed. Pulmonary Rehabilitation. New York: Marcel Dekker, 1996.

49. MDA/Publications/Quest 5-5/Breathe Easy: Options for Respiratory Care: http://www.mdausa.org/publications/Quest/q55breathe2.html.

50. Siegel IM. Pulmonary problems in Duchenne muscular dystrophy: diagnosis, prophylaxis, and treatment. Phys Ther 1975;55(2):160–162.

51. McCool FD, Tzelepis GE. Inspiratory muscle training in the patient with neuromuscular disease. Phys Ther 1995;75(11):1006–1014.

52. Wanke T, Toifl K, Merkle M, et al. Inspiratory muscle training in patients with Duchenne muscular dystrophy. Chest 1994;105(2):475–482.

53. Weiss HR, Lohschmidt K, el-Obeidi N, et al. Preliminary results and worst-case analysis of inpatient scoliosis rehabilitation. Pediatr Rehabil 1997;1(1):35–40.

54. Athanasopoulos S, Paxinos T, Tasafantakis E, et al. The effect of aerobic training in girls with idiopathic scoliosis. Scand J Med Sci Sports 1999;9(1):36–40.

55. Temes WC. Cardiac rehabilitation. In: Hillegass EA, Sadowsky HS, eds. Essentials of Cardiopulmonary Physical Therapy. Philadelphia: WB Saunders, 1994.

34

The Canadian Perspective

Roger Goldstein
Dina Brooks

⟫ Professional Skills

Upon completion of this chapter, the reader will:

- Discuss characteristics of pulmonary rehabilitation in Canada
- Discuss differences between pulmonary rehabilitation programs in Canada and the United States

INTRODUCTION

Pulmonary rehabilitation is an interdisciplinary approach to the management of individuals with chronic respiratory conditions and their families.[1] The goals of pulmonary rehabilitation include achieving and maintaining the individual's maximum level of independence and functioning in the community, thereby improving their health-related quality of life (HRQL).

The benefits of pulmonary rehabilitation for those with chronic airflow obstruction have become clearer as a result of well-designed randomized controlled trials. A recent meta-analysis of pulmonary rehabilitation for individuals with chronic obstructive pulmonary disease (COPD)[2] included 14 randomized controlled trials in which rehabilitation was compared with usual community care. More than 400 patients were included. The authors noted that rehabilitation resulted in clinically important improvements in dyspnea and in mastery.

A subsequent systematic overview examined the effectiveness of components of pulmonary rehabilitation in COPD, including exercise intensity, upper versus lower limb training, inspiratory muscle training, breathing exercises, education, and psychosocial support.[3] Although both exercise training and psychosocial support improved functional exercise capacity as well as HRQL, the influence of education was less clear because few studies of education had been undertaken. Similar conclusions were reported in the evidence-based guidelines of the joint American College of Chest Physicians (ACCP)/ American Association of Cardiovascular and Pulmonary Rehabilitation (AACVPR) Pulmonary Rehabilitation Guidelines Panel.[4]

In this chapter, we comment on pulmonary rehabilitation in Canada in terms of program availability, content, staffing, and the use of outcome measures. Much of the information has been derived from a recent collaborative Canadian Thoracic Society/ Canadian Physiotherapy Cardiorespiratory Society questionnaire that was circulated to all Canadian rehabilitation programs.[5]

CANADIAN GUIDELINES FOR PULMONARY REHABILITATION

Although several useful publications describing the influence of rehabilitation have been authored by Canadians,[2,3,6] no specifically Canadian clinical practice guidelines or consensus statements on pulmonary rehabilitation exist. However, a section on rehabilitation is included in the Canadian guidelines for the assessment and management of COPD.[7] An exercise-based rehabilitation program is advocated for individuals with limited exercise tolerance provided that rehabilitation is understood to be part of the comprehensive management of COPD as opposed to an isolated management approach. Thus, patients should be clinically stable, should have reasonable expectations, and should be able to communicate clearly. When present, associated medical conditions should be well controlled. The other components of management, such as smoking cessation, appropriate vaccination, optimal bronchodilator prescription, and judicious use of oxygen, all play a role that complements the effects of rehabilitation. Indeed, some clinicians would include these components as part of the rehabilitation of individuals with chronic airflow limitation.

Walking on a treadmill or cycling for at least 20 to 30 minutes 3 times per week often forms the core of the program. This is blended with leisure walking, interval training, and upper limb training. Ultimately, a home-based program is designed and practiced under supervision with the aim of encouraging a lifestyle that will include regular exercise. Other components of rehabilitation, such as breathing retraining, energy conservation education, and psychosocial support, are used as required.

EPIDEMIOLOGY OF COPD IN CANADA

Individuals with COPD constitute by far the most common diagnostic category among those participating in Canadian programs. COPD is characterized by progressive and incompletely reversible airflow limitation and includes chronic bronchitis, emphysema, and combinations of the above.[7] In the late 1980s, COPD was the fifth leading cause of mortality in North America, and its prevalence was increasing.[8] Information specific to Canada was derived from the Canadian National Mortality Database. These data reflected a leveling of mortality from COPD among men but a steady increase among women.[9] More recently, the epidemiology of COPD in Canada between 1980 and 1995 has been described.[10] It was estimated that 750,000 Canadians had chronic bronchitis or emphysema diagnosed by a health professional (prevalence rate: aged 55–64 years, 4.7%; 65–74 years, 5.4%; ≥75 years, 8.3%). Although the age-standardized mortality rate remained stable throughout this period in men(~45/100,000 population), it doubled in women (8.3/100,000 in 1980 to 17.3/100,000 in 1995). For the period 1984–1993, COPD was the fourth leading cause of mortality among male Canadians 65 years and older and the fourth most common cause of hospitalization. Among women 65 years and older COPD was the seventh leading cause of death and the sixth most frequent cause of hospitalization.

Thus, COPD represents a major health issue in Canada and will likely remain so for decades.[10] Although the distribution of those likely to benefit from rehabilitation (moderate or severe COPD) is not known, it may be assumed that given the relatively late clinical presentation of this condition, they compose at least 30% of those diagnosed as having COPD. Based on a recent survey of pulmonary rehabilitation programs in Canada,[5] approximately 4500 individuals in all diagnostic categories could receive pulmonary rehabilitation in a given year. This represents 0.6% of all patients with COPD, a situation likely to be representative of many countries. It indicates the need for careful consideration as to how wider access to the effective components of rehabilitation might best be organized by those who deliver health care and those responsible for its resource allocation.

CHARACTERISTICS OF PULMONARY REHABILITATION PROGRAMS IN CANADA

Until recently there was no comprehensive information on pulmonary rehabilitation programs in Canada. In the United States, the American Association for Respiratory Care and the AACVPR have reported on the content and format of American pulmonary rehabilitation programs.[11-13] In June 1996, we surveyed all pulmonary rehabilitation programs in Canada[14] that could be identified by our rehabilitation network, which included physician and nonphysician health professionals, as well as provincial lung associations. The survey was undertaken to characterize programs in terms of their size, duration, components, staffing, and outcome measures.

The survey instrument was designed after a detailed review of the literature on pulmonary rehabilitation, a review of other questionnaires,[11-13] and expert opinion. The response rate of 86% suggests that the information provided represented a fairly comprehensive view of Canadian pulmonary rehabilitation programs.

Program Setting and Characteristics

A total of 44 programs were offered in Canada by 36 facilities. Most of these programs were in the larger, more populated Canadian provinces (mainly Ontario, British Columbia, and Quebec).

There were four times as many outpatient programs as there were inpatient programs. Most facilities (97%) offered outpatient rehabilitation, whereas 22% also offered an inpatient program. This finding is in keeping with the active encouragement of community-based programs as part of the Canadian health care strategy. Even in the absence of formal comparison studies between inpatient and outpatient programs, evidence shows that both approaches result in improvements in functional exercise capacity and HRQL among patients with COPD.[6,15,16] In a prospective randomized controlled trial of inpatient pulmonary rehabilitation, Goldstein et al.[6] identified clinically important and statistically significant improvements in exercise tolerance and functional status among the rehabilitation group compared with individuals who received conventional community care. Similarly, Ries and colleagues[15] evaluated the influence of outpatient-based rehabilitation on exercise tolerance and functional status among a similar population and identified improvements in exercise performance and symptoms in patients with moderate to severe COPD. Because the outcome measures used differed between these two studies, it was difficult to compare the effectiveness of the two approaches. However, Wijkstra and colleagues[16] used outcome measures similar to those used by Goldstein et al.[6] to study community-based respiratory rehabilitation, allowing some comparison between these two studies. It suggests that the magnitude of the improvements were similar between the two programs.

The modality of rehabilitation has important cost implications. Assuming that the magnitude of the improvement is consistently similar, those eligible will be directed toward outpatient management or home care rehabilitation, both of which have been found to be beneficial in improving exercise capacity, dyspnea, and measures of leg effort.[17] For those too impaired for frequent travel or with associated medical or psychosocial conditions, inpatient rehabilitation continues to provide a more intensively supervised alternative.

Follow-up after discharge from pulmonary rehabilitation was available in 86% of the programs in Canada and consisted of periodic assessment (100%) as well as support groups (68%) and supervised exercise sessions (63%). Important issues such as the benefits of the initial phase of rehabilitation and the added benefits of follow-up remain unresolved. For how long and at what intensity will follow-up enhance or maintain the improvements achieved during the intensive phase of rehabilitation? The answers to these questions also have important clinical and economic implications. Clearly, it is desirable to maintain or enhance the benefits in HRQL and functional exercise capacity at the lowest level of resource allocation. Although poor self-management practices and lack of adherence to treatment protocols after discharge from respiratory rehabilitation have a negative impact on the maintenance of improvements gained through respiratory rehabilitation,[15] few studies have addressed the influence of follow-up on compliance with treatment or maintenance of function. With time, a reduction in patient compliance results in a gradual loss of the benefit of respiratory rehabilitation.[15] The influence of the various compliance-enhancing methods on maintaining the benefits of respiratory rehabilitation remains to be defined.[18]

Program Size, Length, and Frequency

Canadian respiratory rehabilitation programs (inpatient and outpatient) enroll 12 patients (range, 2–48) at any given time for a duration of 7.5 weeks (range, 1–19). Outpatient programs enroll 13 patients (range, 5–48) for a duration of 8.3 weeks (range, 2–26), and inpatient programs enroll 9 patients (range, 2–26) for a duration of 4.6 weeks (range, 1–8). Adding the estimated maximum number of individuals that each program could accommodate in a year, approximately 4569 individuals with chronic respiratory conditions could receive pulmonary rehabilitation in Canada each year.

There are no clear guidelines on the length of pulmonary rehabilitation programs required to maximize effectiveness. The results of the meta-analysis[2] strongly support pulmonary rehabilitation that includes at least 4 weeks of exercise training. A posthoc analysis based on these results showed a significant difference between the programs of 6 months' duration and the other programs in terms of the improvement in distance walked in 6 minutes. However, because these findings were data driven, they should be interpreted cautiously, and further randomized trials are needed to establish the minimum length of an effective pulmonary rehabilitation program.

Type and Source of Patients

The most commonly represented diagnostic group in pulmonary rehabilitation programs in Canada is patients with COPD, who were included in 100% of programs. Other groups included those with restrictive conditions (93%), adults with asthma (82%), those pre- or postlung volume reduction surgery (64%), those pre- or postlung transplant surgery (45%), adults with cystic fibrosis (46%), and patients who were mechanically ventilated (18%). Most programs (80%) accepted patients who were still smoking.

Although the efficacy of pulmonary rehabilitation has been rigorously examined only among individuals with COPD, rehabilitation is offered to many individuals with chronic respiratory conditions as well as those involved with lung transplantation or lung volume reduction surgery.[19] As recommended by the ACCP/AACVPR Pulmonary Rehabilitation Guidelines Panel,[4] pulmonary rehabilitation should be considered for any individual with stable disease of the respiratory system provided that realistic goals are set.

Program Content

More than 90% of programs (inpatient and outpatient) in Canada included breathing retraining, education, exercise, and upper extremity training. More than 80% of the programs included relaxation, psychosocial support, and nutrition. The other components were activities of daily living (73%), inspiratory muscle training (39%), and smoking cessation (32%). It is interesting to note the low percentage of facilities that included smoking cessation as a component of their program, although more than 80% included smokers.

Thus, our program contents are consistent with the evidence in support of particular interventions[3,4] in that they include exercise training as well as upper extremity strength and endurance training. Although the evidence as to the effectiveness of patient education and psychosocial support remains equivocal, most programs follow expert opinion and include educational and psychosocial support as part of their program.

Educational topics that are usually addressed in Canadian programs are shown in Table 34-1. Medication use and inhaler techniques were the topics most frequently addressed. Sexuality was the topic least frequently addressed.

Program Staffing

The application of a multidisciplinary team, which is frequently used in rehabilitation in Canada, has carried over to pulmonary rehabilitation. All programs included physical therapists. Physicians, nurses, occupational therapists, respiratory therapists, and dietitians are part of all inpatient programs, but less than 70% of outpatient programs had these team members. Other members of the team who participated on a part-time basis included pharmacists, social workers, psychologists, recreational therapists, exercise physiologists, and chaplaincy services. The medical director was a respirologist (69%) or an internist (14%). The program manger was most often a physical therapist.

In a National Institutes of Health–sponsored workshop on pulmonary rehabilitation research,[1] the participants recognized the need to define the optimal size and composition of the pulmonary rehabilitation team. We are not aware of published work that evaluates the composition or training of rehabilitation professionals, and a formal continuing education program for pulmonary rehabilitation health care professionals does not exist.

Measures and Testing Performed

Measures of pulmonary function, exercise, and chest radiographs were included in most Canadian programs (91%, 50%, and 50%, respectively). Almost all programs (98%) also included a measure of functional exercise capacity—usually a 6- or 12-minute walking test. Of note, most programs (71%) measured HRQL, the Chronic Respiratory Questionnaire being the most frequently used (19 programs), followed by the Medical Outcomes Study 36-Item Short Form Health Survey.

The inclusion of measures of HRQL in addition to the usual outcome measures for

Table 34-1. Educational Topics That Are Usually Addressed in Canadian Pulmonary Rehabilitation Programs

Topic	Facilities That Include this Topic (%)
Use of inhalers	94
Medications	94
Relaxation/panic control	92
Oxygen therapy	92
Energy conservation	92
Nutrition	89
Activities of daily living	86
Signs of infection	83
Strengthening exercises	83
Aerobic exercise	81
Breathing exercises	78
Indoor and outdoor pollution	72
Travel	67
Sexuality	47

pulmonary rehabilitation reflects the gradual evolution of this field away from anecdotes of success toward valid reproducible and more meaningful measures essential to the design of clinical trials. Given the weak correlations between measures of exercise and HRQL, the former should not be used as a surrogate measure for the latter, but rather HRQL must be measured directly.[20] It was therefore exciting to note the number of Canadian programs that have adopted a measure of HRQL as a primary outcome following rehabilitation.

COMPARISON BETWEEN CANADIAN AND AMERICAN PROGRAMS

Canadian rehabilitation programs are similar to those in the United States in terms of the patients enrolled and their program components.[13] They differ substantially in their staffing and in their use of outcome measures. In both countries, the predominant diagnostic groupings are COPD, asthma, and restrictive conditions (e.g., pulmonary fibrosis, kyphoscoliosis, and neuromuscular conditions). Educational contents are similar, with sexuality being the topic least covered in each case. Whereas only 49% of programs in the United States include physical therapists, they are present in 100% of Canadian programs. Other staffing is similar, with physicians, respiratory therapists, and dietitians being involved in more than 70% of both programs. Functional exercise capacity is measured routinely in less than 40% of the programs in the United States, whereas it is a primary outcome in 100% of Canadian programs. Pulmonary function tests and electrocardiograms were the most frequently performed tests in programs in the United States (80% and 67%, respectively).

SUMMARY

Pulmonary rehabilitation in Canada is well established, with many programs that are both multidisciplinary and multidimensional, incorporating exercise, education, and psychosocial support. Outcome measures include both HRQL and functional exercise capacity. This reflects the Canadian emphasis on the scientific basis of respiratory rehabilitation. Currently available programs are only able to service a small percentage of those who might benefit from them. Therefore, alternative approaches such as home or community-based programs will be required if pulmonary rehabilitation is to become more widespread.

REFERENCES

1. Fishman AP. Pulmonary rehabilitation research. Am J Respir Crit Care Med 1994;149:825–833.
2. Lacasse Y, Goldstein RS, Wong E, et al. Meta-analysis of respiratory rehabilitation in chronic obstructive pulmonary disease. Lancet 1996;348:1115–1119.
3. Lacasse Y, Guyatt GH, Goldstein RS. The components of a respiratory rehabilitation program: a systematic overview. Chest 1997;111:1077–1088.
4. ACCP/AACVPR Pulmonary Rehabilitation Guidelines Panel. Pulmonary rehabilitation: joint ACCP/AACVPR evidence-based guidelines. Chest 1997;112:1363–1396.
5. Brooks D, Lacasse Y, Goldstein RS. Pulmonary rehabilitation programs in Canada: national survey. Can Respir J 1999;6(1):55–63.
6. Goldstein RS, Gort EH, Stubbing D, et al. Randomized controlled trial of respiratory rehabilitation. Lancet 1994;344:1394–1397.
7. Canadian Thoracic Society Workshop Group. Guidelines for the assessment and management of chronic obstructive pulmonary disease. CMAJ 1992;147:420–428.
8. Feinlieb M, Rosenberg HM, Collins JG, et al. Trends in COPD morbidity and mortality in the United States. Am Rev Respir Dis 1989;140:S9–S18.
9. Mafreda J, Mao Y, Litven W. Morbidity and mortality from chronic obstructive pulmonary disease. Am Rev Respir Dis 1989;140:S19–S26.
10. Lacasse Y, Brooks D, Goldstein RS. Trends in the epidemiology of chronic obstructive pulmonary disease in Canada, 1980–95. Chest 1999;116:306–313.

11. Bickford LS, Hodgkin JE. National pulmonary rehabilitation. Respir Care 1988;33:1030–1043.
12. Bickford LS, Hodgkin JE. National pulmonary rehabilitation. J Cardiopulm Rehabil 1988;8:473–491.
13. Bickford LS, Hodgkin JE, McInturff SL. National pulmonary rehabilitation survey update. J Cardiopulm Rehabil 1995;15:406–411.
14. Brooks D, Lacasse Y, Goldstein RS. Pulmonary rehabilitation programs in Canada: a national survey. Can Respir J 1999;6:55–63.
15. Ries AL, Kaplan RM, Limberg TM, et al. Effects of pulmonary rehabilitation on physiologic and psychosocial outcomes in patients with chronic obstructive pulmonary disease. Ann Intern Med 1995;122:823–832.
16. Wijkstra PJ, TenVergert EM, van Altena R, et al. Long term benefits of rehabilitation at home on quality of life and exercise tolerance in patients with chronic obstructive pulmonary disease. Thorax 1995;50:824–828.
17. Strijbos JH, Postma DS, van Altena R, et al. A comparison between outpatient hospital based pulmonary rehabilitation program and a home-care pulmonary rehabilitation program in patients with COPD: a follow-up of 18 months. Chest 1996;109;366–372.
18. Guyatt GH, Berman LB, Townsend M. Long-term outcome after respiratory rehabilitation. CMAJ 1987;137:1089–1095.
19. Fishman AP, ed. Pulmonary Rehabilitation: Lung Biology in Health and Disease. New York: Marcel Dekker, 1996;91.
20. Jones PW, Quirk FH, Baveystock CM, et al. A self-complete measure of health status for chronic airflow limitation: the St. George's Respiratory Questionnaire. Am Rev Respir Dis 1992;145:1321–1327.

35 The European Perspective

Nicolino Ambrosino

⊘ Professional Skills

Upon completion of this chapter, the reader will:

- Discuss characteristics of pulmonary rehabilitation (PR) in Europe
- Discuss differences between PR programs in Europe and North America

INTRODUCTION

To provide a European perspective of PR is difficult, as we need to remember that the political union of the different western European countries is still in progress. Health service policies are different. Although most function under public supervision, the modalities of reimbursement range from totally private to mainly public. In addition, only a few European universities and teaching hospitals include specific training in PR as part of their curricula. Therefore, this chapter includes statements of the only "European" institution dealing with PR, that is, the European Respiratory Society (ERS). In 1992, a report of the ERS Rehabilitation and Chronic Care Scientific Group stated that "the task for the 1990's will be an extensive multidisciplinary application of scientific principles."[1] In this perspective, the empiric approach followed in the previous 30 years has been certainly followed by evidence-based therapeutic principles.[2–5] European researchers have contributed to clarify the clinical and physiologic effects of comprehensive PR programs and the individual components of such programs.

THE THEORY

Definition

According to that report,[1] the aims of PR should be "to restore patients to an independent, productive and satisfying life and prevent further clinical deterioration to the maximum extent compatible with the state of the disease," a definition that somehow attributes to PR an effect on the natural history of the disease.

Most recently, an official European definition of PR has been given by the ERS Task Force Position Paper.[6] This definition states: "Pulmonary rehabilitation is a process which systematically uses scientifically based diagnostic management and evaluation options, to achieve the optimal daily functioning and health-related quality of life (HRQL) of individual patients suffering from impairment and disability due to chronic respiratory disease, as measured by clinically and/or physiologically relevant outcome measures." This definition does not seem very different from the definition developed by the National Institutes of Health Workshop on Pulmonary Rehabilitation Research.[7] "Pulmonary Rehabilitation is a multidimensional continuum of services directed to persons with pulmonary disease and their families, usually by an interdisciplinary team of specialists, with the goal of achieving and maintaining the individual's maximum level of independence and function-

Box 35-1. Pulmonary Rehabilitation Components Recommended by the European Respiratory Society Task Force Position Paper

Optimal medical treatment
Smoking cessation
Exercise training
Arm exercise
Gymnastic exercise
Respiratory muscle training and rest
Breathing retraining
Chest physiotherapy
Education of the patient and family
Psychologic aspects and support
Long-term oxygen therapy
Home mechanical ventilation
Nutrition therapy
Nursing care

Data from ERS Task Force Position Paper: selection criteria and programs for pulmonary rehabilitation in COPD patients. Eur Respir J 1997;10:744–757.

ing in the community." Nevertheless, when we examine the individual components of rehabilitation, some differences appear. They mainly relate to the comprehensive treatment of patients with respiratory diseases.

Components

In the recent joint American College of Chest Physicians/American Association of Cardiovascular and Pulmonary Rehabilitation (ACCP/AACVPR) evidence-based guidelines for PR,[5] the four individual components highlighted included lower extremity training, upper extremity training, ventilatory muscle training, and psychosocial/behavioral intervention. In contrast, the PR components recommended by the ERS Task Force[6] are many more (14 in total), as shown in Box 35-1.

Certain therapeutic components have been the subject of particular research efforts in Europe. The physiologic effects of less well-accepted components, such as breathing retraining, is one such area.[8–11] Indeed, although breathing retraining is included as a component of the PR programs by the European Task Force Position Paper,[6] the specific recommendation is not too dissimilar to that of the ACCP/AACVPR: "Breathing Retraining cannot be routinely recommended." Another area where the European authors have provided significant insight is the use of noninvasive mechanical ventilation during exercise to help train the most severely disabled patients with lung disease.[12,13] Peripheral muscle training has also been specifically addressed by European studies,[14] and, in general, the findings and recommendations are in agreement with those of the North American guidelines.

The European perspective of PR includes a larger number of therapeutic components than does the North American perspective. Indeed, as shown in Box 35-1, some topics are closely linked to the concept of long-term chronic care. The ERS working group responsible for the report[6] is the Rehabilitation and Chronic Care Working Group. For example, a recent study on the improvement in survival in chronic obstructive pulmonary disease (COPD) patients following nutritional replacement (an area not usually within the domain of PR in North America) comes from a well-known European PR group.[15]

It is worth noting that in Europe, institutions primarily devoted to PR have developed the intermediate care units designed to treat acute or chronic respiratory failure (mainly by noninvasive mechanical ventilation) and to manage patients with difficult weaning from mechanical ventilation.[16-18] This difference in programmatic concepts, in turn, leads to issues related to differences in patient selection.

Eligibility Criteria

The recommendation of the ERS Task Force Position Paper[6] is that almost all COPD patients may be incorporated into a PR program, including one or more of the various forms of therapy included in Box 35-1. The program can be completed in an inpatient or outpatient program or even at home.[19-21] In the report, the indication for home oxygen therapy and mechanical ventilation is reserved for the most severe patients.[22,23] Age and degree of airway obstruction are not considered to be exclusion criteria.[24] The only contraindications for participation in a rehabilitation program are (*a*) lack of motivation and compliance of the patient and (*b*) presence of any disease process that interferes with PR, such as terminal cancer.[24]

Smoking abstinence represents another controversial area. Although the ERS Task Force Position Paper[6] reports that "optimal therapy should be conducted on nonsmoking patients or patients actively involved in a smoking cessation program," no clear, firm statement has been made that actual smokers should not be admitted to a PR program. Indeed, across Europe a wide range of opinions and behaviors exist, mostly linked to local or even individual habits, in general the Mediterranean countries being more "lenient" than the Northern ones.

Box 35-2 shows the indications for a PR program. The inclusion of acute or chronic respiratory failure is not surprising in light of the previously mentioned concept of PR as a continuum of therapy along the natural disease history of patients with respiratory diseases. Indeed, although few countries in Europe have adopted the North American concept of the respiratory therapist (with the role of direct care and management of ventilators and ventilated patients), physiotherapists are often involved in the treatment of acute ON chronic respiratory failure in COPD, or neuromuscular patients by means of noninvasive ventilation.[8,25] These professionals are considered extremely important in other classical rehabilitation procedures, such as postural drainage, passive or active training of limb and respiratory muscles, prolonged weaning, etc. The use of comprehensive PR in lung transplantation has also been documented in Europe.[26] Likewise, some of the most interesting studies of the benefits of PR in bronchial asthma, especially using high-intensity physical training like swimming, have been conducted in Europe.[27-30]

Box 35-2. Indications for Pulmonary Rehabilitation Generally Accepted in Europe

Chronic obstructive pulmonary disease
Bronchial asthma
Cystic fibrosis
Bronchiectasis
Chronic respiratory insufficiency from any cause
Acute ON chronic respiratory insufficiency
Neuromuscular and chest wall diseases
Pulmonary fibrosis, pneumoconiosis, and other interstitial diseases
Preabdominal and postabdominal and thoracic surgical procedures, including
    cardiovascular and lung volume resection surgery
Sleep-related disorders of breathing
Lung transplantation

Rehabilitation Program Location

According to the ERS Task Force Position Paper,[6] a well-based rationale exists for inpatient PR. In-hospital treatment allows comprehensive diurnal assessment and treatment of the individual patient with disabling lung disease outside of the habitual home environment. This may help better stabilize or reverse health-related physiopathologic or psychopathologic aspects. Assessment and treatment during inpatient programs should focus not only on obvious impairments and handicaps but also on more hidden aspects of the disease known to affect the HRQL. Based on these assumptions, some selection criteria have been formulated for inpatient programs.[6] They are shown in Box 35-3.

Inpatient rehabilitation facilitates training of the most severely disabled patients, e.g., those with supplemental oxygen or those receiving noninvasive mechanical ventilation.[31] Different short- and long-term studies have reported on the outcomes of inpatient versus outpatient treatment from different European centers. In general, they provide support for the argument that different patients may require different programs, depending on issues that do not only relate to the specific component of PR.[32-34]

According to the ERS Task Force Position Paper,[6] the specific aim of outpatient rehabilitation programs are to alleviate dyspnea, to increase exercise tolerance, to educate patients, to improve HRQL, and to ensure a long-term commitment to regular physical activity. The selection criteria for outpatient programs are shown in Box 35-4.

The outpatient setting of a PR program is frequently used in Europe, and the beneficial results have been widely reported.[35,36] The allocation either to an outpatient setting or to a home rehabilitation program has been based on the severity of disease and of dyspnea.[35] Home- and community-based PR programs have been used in COPD and asthmatic patients, with favorable outcomes.[36,37] Using a unique combination of modes, we have recently reported the results of an outpatient day-hospital–based PR program in COPD patients and asthmatics.[38] The patients were referred by general practitioners or by respiratory physicians. The program included the optimization of pharmacologic treatment, three 3-hour sessions per week for 8 to 10 weeks, that consisted of (*a*) supervised incremental exercise to achieve 30 minutes of continuous cycling at 50 to 70% of the maximal load achieved on an incremental cycloergometer exercise test carried out at admission; (*b*) abdominal and upper and lower limb muscle activities, including lifting progressively increasing light weights, shoulder and full arm circling, and other exercises using the protocol developed by Clark et al.[14]; (*c*) patient and family education, including education sessions that were diagnosis specific (e.g., for COPD, it focused on maintaining smoking abstinence; for asthma, it concentrated on environmental control, importance of inhaled

Box 35-3. Selection Criteria for Inpatient Programs According to the European Respiratory Society Task Force Position Paper

Need for an integrated 24-h supervised monitoring management plan, including training, teaching of coping skills, and other aspects of daily life functioning
Behavioral intervention to correct psychosocial problems
Need for specific intervention strategies, such as nutritional therapy
Participation in preoperative and postoperative rehabilitation programs
Post–intensive care patients with either disabling respiratory problems or weaning failure after acute respiratory support
Identification and assessment of patients for long-term oxygen therapy or long-term home mechanical ventilation
Logistic aspects when outpatient rehabilitation is not available and the traveling distance does not allow the patient to participate in intensive rehabilitation

Data from ERS Task Force Position Paper: selection criteria and programs for pulmonary rehabilitation in COPD patients. Eur Respir J 1997;10:744–757.

Box 35-4. Selection Criteria for Outpatient Programs
According to the European Respiratory Society
Task Force Position Paper

Patients in a stable state of moderate to severe disease
Capable of maintaining an independent lifestyle
No major psychologic problems
Absence of nonpulmonary disease

Data from ERS Task Force Position Paper: selection criteria and programs
for pulmonary rehabilitation in COPD patients. Eur Respir J
1997;10:744–757.

steroids, etc.); and (*d*) nutritional programs and psychosocial counseling, when appropriate. A multidisciplinary team consisting of chest physicians, nurses, physical therapists, dietitians, and psychologists provided the overall care. If desired, patients could rest in dedicated beds and were provided with balanced meals at the hospital facilities. After discharge from the program, patients were encouraged to perform daily life activities, but neither structured exercise programs nor periodical hospital visits were prescribed. The only follow-up visits were 6 and 12 months after discharge. During these visits, a physiologic evaluation was performed and outcome measures were reassessed. This outpatient day-hospital–based program improved exercise tolerance, dyspnea, and quality of life and reduced hospital admissions during the posttreatment year. Although after 1 year the benefits in exercise tolerance were lost, at least more than half of all patients still reported improvements in their HRQL.[38] In comparison to the 2 years before treatment, in the year following the program (at a daily cost per patient of 131 Euros or US$153), hospital admissions per patient (at a daily cost per patient of 260 Euros, US$300) significantly decreased from 0.9 ± 0.8 and 0.9 ± 0.7 in the 2 years preceding treatment to 0.03 ± 0.2.[38] A similar decrease was documented in the number of exacerbations per year requiring systemic steroids.[38] This novel approach successfully incorporated the benefits of in-hospital close supervision (with its intrinsic benefits) with those of home care (with its cost-saving effect).

The ERS Task Force Position Paper[6] defines home care as any supportive or therapeutic measure provided in the home setting by health care professionals, including physicians, nurses, respiratory therapists, occupational therapists, speech therapists, physiotherapists, social workers,nutritionists, psychiatric services, and personnel of medical equipment manufacturers. A well-structured home care program should provide treatment, with most of the therapeutic modalities available in the hospital setting. It allows continued education and a postdischarge follow-up. The primary tasks of home care rehabilitation according to the ERS Task Force are shown in Box 35-5. In addition, the patient's eligibility criteria for respiratory home care are shown in Box 35-6.

The ERS Task Force recommendation[6] is that "home care in the setting of pulmonary rehabilitation is more an adjunct measure during out-patient programs, or after in-patient programs for 'fine tuning and outcome observation' than an appropriate substitute to formal rehabilitation." Notwithstanding these limitations, several European studies have focused on the effectiveness of PR programs completed at home. An old British study[39] had shown that a simple training scheme administered from a hospital clinic or a family doctor's office was safe, feasible, and of benefit to patients with chronic bronchitis. Likewise, home exercise training programs have been successfully implemented in patients with cystic fibrosis.[40] The European trials have shown beneficial effects on exercise tolerance and HRQL in COPD patients.[41–43] In some cases, the results were similar to those observed with outpatient hospital-based PR programs.[44]

Outcome Measures

Proper evaluation of potential patients is the keystone of a successful PR program.[45] The so-called functional approach, which related impairment (the physiologic deficit), disability (total effect of impairment on the patient's life), and handicap (the social disadvantages) to the comprehensive program of care, is one approach. It is useful to not only monitor the patient's functional status, but it also enables the rehabilitation team to set and achieve goals and to ultimately improve the quality of a patient's life.

The ERS recommendations[6] for the individual PR program include the following minimum measurements: the 6-minute walk test as an indirect measure of exercise capacity; the baseline and transitional dyspnea index, the modified Medical Research Council scale, or the Oxygen Cost Diagram to rate dyspnea; and the St George Respiratory Questionnaire or the Chronic Respiratory Disease Questionnaire to assess quality of life.[46–49] This is in line with the recent North American PR joint AACP/AACVPR evidence-based guidelines.[5]

Currently in Europe, a division of opinion exists between researchers and practitioners regarding the appropriate outcomes to be measured. Many practitioners claim that rehabilitation needs to be made as simple and as practical as possible so it can develop widespread acceptance. Their concern is that complex measurements will become a barrier to their widespread use, especially if the measures proposed for evaluation are too technically or administratively demanding.[50] In line with this "minimalist" trend is the increasing use of the incremental shuttle walk test.[51] Measurements of ventilatory, circulatory, and metabolic adaptations to exercise during protocols "in the field," such as walking or stair climbing or upper limb exercise, should be encouraged, particularly in severely limited patients. Abnormalities observed in the field are likely to reflect more closely symptoms and limitations referred by the patients during daily life activities.

Laboratory tests such as cycle ergometry, however, remain the gold standard to assess a patient's maximal exercise tolerance. By using an incremental exercise protocol, as currently recommended by the ERS Task Force,[52] it is possible to have a good indicator of factors that eventually limit exercise tolerance and identify the work rates that the patient can tolerate easily (moderate) or sustain with difficulty (heavy). The integration of information obtained with protocols in the laboratory and in the field represent the best way to address questions relative to the patient's ability to sustain specific tasks. Walking tests have been proposed for assessing exercise tolerance in severely disabled

Box 35-5. Primary Tasks of Home Care Rehabilitation According to the European Respiratory Society Task Force

Support of the patient in the adjustment of recommended therapeutic measures to the individual housing and social situation of the patient

Support of the patient and his or her family in maintenance of technical devices and troubleshooting in case of dysfunction

Involvement and training of relatives, friends, and neighbors in supportive measures to promote independence of the patient from third-party services and to strengthen social contacts

Reinforcement of patient adherence to therapeutic regimens and intervention in the case of deteriorating compliance

Intervention during episodes of acute exacerbations of the underlying pulmonary disease process

Maintenance and further development of skills and functional improvements gained during the rehabilitation process

Assessment of success of measures prescribed and function capabilities of the patient after adequate time intervals

Data from ERS Task Force Position Paper: selection criteria and programs for pulmonary rehabilitation in COPD patients. Eur Respir J 1997;10:744–757.

Box 35-6. Patients Eligible for Respiratory Home Care

Newly diagnosed and first-time hospitalized patients with handicaps who are not
  eligible for rehabilitation programs after discharge from acute care hospitals
Patients discharged with new respiratory equipment
Patients with recurrent exacerbations and repeated hospitalizations
Patients with ongoing exacerbations treated by the physician at home
Anxious, confused, and forgetful patients
Patients after formal inpatient or outpatient rehabilitation programs
End-stage terminal patients who want to stay at home

patients. This information, obtainable with the shuttle test, may be considered of greater value compared with other unpaced walking tests, particularly if ventilatory and metabolic measurements are recorded.[53]

THE PRACTICE

Compared with the ERS Task Force Position Paper,[6] the real situation of PR in the continent is confusing. The European data reported in this chapter are based on a Japanese study comparing the organization and content of PR programs of North America, Europe, and Japan.[54] These data must be considered with caution because different institutions had to answer a questionnaire not tailored to the ERS position.

Between December 1994 and February 1995 the survey was conducted among 67 European institutions from 14 countries: Belgium, 10; Denmark, 4; Finland, 3; France, 13; Germany, 5; Great Britain, 2; Hungary, 2; Italy, 9; The Netherlands, 2; Norway, 1; Poland, 1; Spain, 3; Sweden, 4; and Switzerland, 8. The response rate to the 13-item questionnaire was 40%.

PR programs were offered by 74% of responding hospitals in Europe. PR team members involved in those programs were as follows: physiotherapists in 61%, respiratory physiotherapists in 63%, nurses in 78%, dietitians in 51%, social workers in 53%, occupational therapists in 22%, physicians in 20%, and psychologists in 16%. The same was true for North American institutions except that the occupational therapists were much less involved in Europe. Occupational therapy (OT) was present in only half of the European programs compared with North American (United States + Canada). In addition, it is worth noting that differences exist among different countries in Europe. For instance, in Italy, a physiotherapist, the same professional with a single degree represents respiratory physiotherapy and occupational therapy. The team leader was a medical doctor in 78% of programs. In no institution was the leader a nurse.[54]

Most PR programs in North America were outpatient in nature (98%), whereas both outpatient and inpatient programs were adopted in Europe (65% and 55% of the programs, respectively). There are two possible reasons for this difference. One relates to the difference in reimbursement. Reimbursement may be a significant problem in North America, where a heavier burden of medical cost is placed on patients receiving PR than in Europe. For instance, the previously mentioned day-hospital–based PR program[38] had a daily cost about half that of the same program performed on an inpatient basis.

In Europe, a cohort style (a group of patients attending classes together), with a small average number of patient per class (9.6 ± 11.0), was reported by 69% of the programs. Another 30% of institutions adopted both a class style and a person-to-person style. The average age of the patients was 57 ± 12 years. The types of lung disease of these patients were mainly emphysema (90%) and bronchitis (80%). These proportions differed from those in North America in that sequel of tuberculosis and brochiectasis were more common in Europe.[54]

The survey offers insight as to the prevalence of the different components reported by the different programs. They included education in 86%, medication optimization in 90%, breathing retraining in 80%, oxygen adjustment in 78%, walking in 61%, activities of daily living in 28%, nutrition in 55%, upper and lower extremity exercise in 61%, relaxation in 65%, psychosocial support in 59%, family education in 33%, pulmonary hygiene in 59%, cycle ergometry in 45%, smoking cessation in 69%, treadmill in 33%, and respiratory muscle training in 49%. Interestingly, cycle ergometry and treadmill taken together were available in less than 80% of European programs. Because it is likely that both exercise systems coexist in the same institutions, the likely proportion with the gold standard exercise systems is certainly smaller. The message is that not all institutions performing PR have an exercise training program that complies with the recent PR joint ACCP/AACVPR evidence-based guidelines.[5] The data indicate that cycle ergometry, treadmill, and upper and lower extremity exercise taken together are underrepresented in Europe compared with North America. Likewise, activities of daily living and family education also seem underused compared with in North America.

The survey also provides insight as to the problems faced by PR programs, including limited reimbursement (43%), lack of staff (31%), problems with equipment and space (24%), too time consuming (41%), lack of hospital recognition (6%), and patient acceptance (20%). Interestingly, European institutions complained less about reimbursement than did the North American counterpart.[54]

Finally, the survey provided insight as to the lack of postrehabilitation follow-up. A follow-up support group was included in 24% of the programs, additional exercise classes in 31%, a patient club in 35%, a newsletter in 16%, and recreations in 10%. Certainly, more emphasis on follow-up activities is needed.

Outcome Measures

Subsequently, the same authors[55] sent a questionnaire to all the hospitals that had replied to the previous one.[54] These data have been presented as an abstract at the 1997 annual ATS meeting and were kindly sent to me by Dr. K. Kida (e-mail, 13 January 1999).

The survey instrument consisted of a 13-item questionnaire sent by mail in December 1995 to 101 institutions, 50 in North America and 51 in Europe. Responses were collected by mail or facsimile through the end of February 1996. Among the 101 institutions surveyed, the response rates were 38% (19/50) and 41% (21/51) for North America and Europe, respectively, and included 10 countries in Europe and 14 states in North America. Responses from Canada were included in North America. European institutions included

Box 35-7. Medical Tests Reported in Pulmonary Rehabilitation European Institutions

Prebronchodilator and postbronchodilator spirometry (100%)
Lung volumes (95%)
DLCO (71%)
Arterial blood gases (95%)
Chest roentgenogram (90%)
Electrocardiogram (90%)
Complete blood cell count (90%)
Chemistry panel (90%)

Data from Nomura K, Kida K, and the Project Team. Assessment of pulmonary rehabilitation programs (PRP): data from a survey conducted in North America and Europe. Am J Respir Crit Care Med 1997;155(Suppl 4):A453.
DLCO, diffusion capacity for carbon monoxide.

Box 35-8. Methods of Evaluating Outcome Reported
in European Institutions

Prerehabilitation and postrehabilitation walking distance (57%)
Prepulmonary and postpulmonary stress test (52%)
Review of patient home exercise training logs (24%)
Strength measurement (14%)
Flexibility and posture (5%)
Performance on training (43%)
Dyspnea level (57%)
Cough, sputum, or wheezing (62%)
Weight change (38%)
Psychologic test (24%)
Changes in activities of daily living (19%)
Knowledge test (9%)
Respiratory exacerbations (29%)
Frequency and duration of hospitalizations (52%)
Frequency of emergency department visits (33%)

Data from Nomura K, Kida K, and the Project Team. Assessment of pulmonary rehabilitation programs (PRP): data from a survey conducted in North America and Europe. Am J Respir Crit Care Med 1997;155(Suppl 4):A453.

4 from Belgium and Germany; 3 from Switzerland; 2 from Italy, Sweden, and The Netherlands; and 1 from Hungary, Norway, Poland, and Spain.

Patients underwent a rapid initial assessment, without differences between Europe and North America. The methods of assessment were as follows: patient interview by the medical staff (67%), a questionnaire filled in by the patient himself or herself (23%), or both methods (10%); vital signs (90%); breathing sounds (86%); breathing pattern (67%); right-sided heart function (76%); body weight (90%); body height (90%); and body mass index (43%).

Dyspnea was assessed by the Borg scale in 57%; visual analogue scale (VAS) was used by 19%. Other scales, such as the Medical Research Council, < Oxygen Cost Diagram, and baseline and transitional dyspnea index were used less frequently. In addition, psychosocial function was assessed with HRQL in 29%; depression in 19%; stress in 14%, and coping style in 14.3%. Nutritional assessment was performed in approximately 80% of the European institutions.

Exercise tolerance was assessed by means of 6-minute walk distance in 48%, ergometer in 71%, and treadmill in 33%. Activities of daily living were evaluated by means of upper extremity evaluation in only 9.5% of programs, daily activities in 71%, frequency of going out in 57%; willingness to perform independently in 48%, and change in living environment in 52%. The conventional medical tests and outcome measurements performed in Europe are shown in Boxes 35-7 and 35-8, respectively.[55]

The first survey[54] indicated that a major target disease for PR is COPD. The results of the second survey[55] suggested that there were some major differences between Europe and North America in the way patients are assessed for PR programs:

• Assessment is performed during a short time period in North America compared with Europe
• HRQL assessment was performed at much higher rates in North America than in Europe
• Nutritional assessment was performed more frequently in Europe
• Changes in activities of daily living were used more frequently in North America, whereas number of hospitalizations was used more in Europe[38]

From these data, the authors conclude that the assessment system reflects program content, size of the institution, and the medical insurance system in Europe and North America.[55]

Finally, in 1996 a survey of PR programs in Italy was completed by sending a questionnaire to all members of the Italian Association of Hospital Pneumologists. The results were published in the official journal of the society.[56] Fifty-nine percent of the institutions claimed to have PR programs. There is a geographical difference, with more programs in the North than in the South. In addition, the overall organization of individual programs differed among different institutions. In only half of the institutions was the program under the supervision of a respiratory specialist. Even though diseases are said to be treated according to international guidelines, exercise training is performed less than expected, and outcome measurement relies more on conventional physiopathologic assessments than on specific requirements.

SUMMARY

In conclusion, Europe has provided strong scientific support for clinical and physiologic research in PR. Differences in organization of PR programs among different countries reflect differences in the national health systems, health care organization, politics, and history. The ERS is the unifying institution in this field. The ERS Task Force Position Paper[6] reflects the summary of the different characteristics of PR programs in different countries. As a whole, the European idea of PR revolves around the concept of comprehensive chronic care of the patient which includes a wide spectrum of patients, from those with minimal symptoms to the most severely disabled. In this, it differs from the North American idea of PR,[5,7] in which emphasis is placed on the treatment of patients in the middle of that spectrum. Although precise information regarding the reality in different countries is still lacking, a recent survey suggests that differences exist between North America and Europe. Besides patient selection, they relate to location of the program (inpatient, outpatient, or home), individual components of programs, and outcome measures. In addition, studies focusing on the cost/benefit, cost/efficacy, and cost/utility ratios of European PR programs are lacking. It is likely that with the constant exchange of concepts and ideas, these differences will become less apparent. After all, our goal is one and the same: to help patients achieve their maximal function.

REFERENCES

1. Donner CF, Howard P. Pulmonary rehabilitation in chronic obstructive pulmonary disease (COPD) with recommendations for its use. Eur Respir J 1992;5:266–275.
2. Goldstein RS, Gort EH, Stubbing D, et al. Randomized controlled trial of respiratory rehabilitation. Lancet 1994;344:1394–1397.
3. Ries AI, Kaplan RM, Limberg TM, et al. Effects of pulmonary rehabilitation on physiologic and psychosocial outcomes in patients with chronic obstructive pulmonary disease. Ann Intern Med 1995;122:823–832.
4. Lacasse Y, Wong E, Guyatt GH, et al. Meta-analysis of respiratory rehabilitation in chronic obstructive pulmonary disease. Lancet 1996;348:1115–1119.
5. ACCP/AACVPR. Pulmonary rehabilitation: joint ACCP/AACVPR evidence-based guidelines. Chest 1997;112:1363–1396.
6. ERS Task Force Position Paper: selection criteria and programs for pulmonary rehabilitation in COPD patients. Eur Respir J 1997;10:744–757.
7. NIH workshop summary: pulmonary rehabilitation research. Am J Respir Crit Care Med 1994;149:825–833.
8. Ambrosino N, Paggiaro PL, Macchi M, et al. A study of short-term effect of rehabilitative therapy in chronic obstructive pulmonary disease. Respiration 1981;41:40–44.
9. Willeput R, Vauchaudez JP, Lender D, et al. Thoracoabdominal motion during chest physiotherapy in patients affected by chronic obstructive lung disease. Respiration 1983;44:204–214.
10. Gosselink RAAM, Wagenaar RC, Rijswijk H, et al. Diaphragmatic breathing reduces efficiency of breathing in patients with chronic obstructive pulmonary disease. Am J Respir Crit Care Med 1995;151:1136–1142.
11. Vitacca M, Clini E, Bianchi L, et al. Acute effects of deep diaphragmatic breathing in COPD pa-

tients with chronic respiratory insufficiency. Eur Respir J 1998;11:408–415.

12. Keilty SEJ, Ponte J, Fleming TA, et al. Effect of inspiratory pressure support on exercise tolerance and breathlessness in patients with severe stable chronic obstructive pulmonary disease. Thorax 1994;49:990–994.

13. Bianchi L, Foglio K, Pagani M, et al. Effects of proportional assist ventilation on exercise tolerance in COPD patients with chronic hypercapnia. Eur Respir J 1998;11:422–427.

14. Clark CJ, Cochrane L, Mackay E. Low intensity peripheral muscle conditioning improves exercise tolerance and breathlessness in COPD. Eur Respir J 1996;9:2590–2596.

15. Schols MWJ, Slangen J, Volovics L, et al. Weight loss is a reversible factor in the prognosis of chronic obstructive pulmonary disease. Am J Respir Crit Care Med 1998;157:1791–1797.

16. Nava S, Confalonieri M, Rampulla C. Intermediate respiratory intensive care in Europe: a European perspective. Thorax 1998;53:798–802.

17. Nava S, Ambrosino N, Clini E, et al. Non-invasive mechanical ventilation in the weaning of patients with respiratory failure due to chronic obstructive pulmonary disease: a randomized study. Ann Intern Med 1998;28:721–728.

18. Nava S. Rehabilitation of patients admitted to a respiratory intensive care unit. Arch Phys Med Rehabil 1998;79:849–854.

19. Donner CF, Braghiroli A, Lusuardi M. Selection criteria for pulmonary rehabilitation. Eur Respir Rev 1991;1:472–474.

20. Ambrosino N, Vitacca M, Rampulla C. Standards for rehabilitative strategies in respiratory disease. Monaldi Arch Chest Dis 1995;50:293–318.

21. Clark CJ. Setting up a pulmonary rehabilitation programme. In: Muir JF, Pierson DJ, eds. Pulmonary Rehabilitation in Chronic Respiratory Insufficiency. Thorax 1994(1);49:270–278.

22. Zielinkski J, Sliwinski P. Indications for and methods for long-term oxygen therapy (LTOT). Eur Respir Rev 1991;1:536–540.

23. Muir JF. Home mechanical ventilation in patients with chronic obstructive pulmonary disease. Eur Respir Rev 1991;1:550–562.

24. Ambrosino N, Foglio K. Selection criteria for pulmonary rehabilitation. Respir Med 1996;90: 317–322.

25. Nava S, Evangelisti I, Rampulla C, et al. Human and financial costs of noninvasive mechanical ventilation in patients affected by COPD and acute respiratory failure. Chest 1997;111:1631–1638.

26. Stiebellehner L, Quittan M, End A, et al. Aerobic endurance training program improves exercise performance in lung transplant recipients. Chest 1998;113:906–912.

27. Cochrane L, Clark C. Benefits and problems of a physical training programme for asthmatic patients. Thorax 1990;45:345–351.

28. Varray AL, Mercier JG, Terral CM, et al. Individualized aerobic and high intensity training for asthmatic children in an exercise readaptation program: is training always helpful for better adaptation to exercise? Chest 1991;99:579–586.

29. Ambrosino N, Meriggi A. Chest physiotherapy in asthma. Eur Respir Rev 1993;3:353–356.

30. Emtner M, Herala M, Stalenheim G. High-intensity physical training in adults with asthma: a 10-week rehabilitation program. Chest 1996;109: 323–330.

31. Rooyackers JM, Dekhuizen RNP, Van Herwaarden CLA, et al. Training with supplemental oxygen in patients with COPD and hypoxaemia at peak exercise. Eur Respir J 1997;10:1278–1284.

32. Ketelaars CAJ, Huyer Abu-Saad H, Schlosser MAG, et al. Long-term outcome of pulmonary rehabilitation in patients with COPD. Chest 1997;112:363–369.

33. Vallet G, Ahmaidi S, Serres I, et al. Comparison of two training programs in chronic airway limitation patients: standardized versus individualized protocols. Eur Respir J 1997;10:114–122.

34. Buchi S, Villiger B, Sensky T, et al. Psychosocial predictors of long-term success of in-patient pulmonary rehabilitation of patients with COPD. Eur Respir J 1997;10:1272–1277.

35. Wedzicha JA, Bestall JC, Garrod R, et al. Randomized controlled trial of pulmonary rehabilitation in severe chronic obstructive pulmonary disease patients, stratified with the MRC dyspnea scale. Eur Respir J 1998;12:363–369.

36. Cambach W, Chadwick-Straver RVM, Wagenaar RC, et al. The effects of a community-based pulmonary rehabilitation programme on exercise tolerance and quality of life: a randomized controlled trial. Eur Respir J 1997;10:104–113.

37. Bendstrup KE, Ingemann Jensen J, Holm S, et al. Out-patient rehabilitation improves activities of daily living, quality of life and exercise tolerance in chronic obstructive pulmonary disease. Eur Respir J 1997;10:2801–2806.

38. Foglio K, Bianchi L, Bruletti G, et al. Long-term effectiveness of pulmonary rehabilitation in patients with chronic airway obstruction (CAO). Eur Respir J 1999;13:125–132.

39. McGavin CR, Gupta SP, Lloyd EI, et al. Physical rehabilitation for the chronic bronchitic: results of a controlled trial of exercises in the home. Thorax 1977;32:307–311.

40. de Jong W, Grevink RG, Roorda RJ, et al. Effect of a home exercise training program in patients with cystic fibrosis. Chest 1994;105:463–468.

41. Wijkstra PJ, Van Altena R, Kraan J, et al. Quality of life in patients with chronic obstructive pulmonary disease improves after rehabilitation at home. Eur Respir J 1994;7:269–273.

42. Wijkstra PJ, TenVergert EM, Van Altena R, et al. Long term benefits of rehabilitation at home on quality of life and exercise tolerance in patients with chronic obstructive pulmonary disease. Thorax 1995;50:824–828.

43. Wijkstra PJ, van der Mark TW, Kraan J, et al. Effects of home rehabilitation on physical performance in patients with chronic obstructive pulmonary disease (COPD). Eur Respir J 1996;9: 104–110.

44. Strijbos JH, Postma DS, Van Altena R, et al. A comparison between an outpatient hospital-based pulmonary rehabilitation program and a home-care pulmonary rehabilitation program in patients

with COPD: a follow-up of 18 months. Chest 1996;109:366–372.

45. Ambrosino N, Clini E. Evaluation in pulmonary rehabilitation. Respir Med 1996;90:395–400.

46. Butland RJA, Pang J, Gross ER, et al. Two, six and 12 minute walking tests in respiratory disease. BMJ 1982;284:1607–1608.

47. Mahler D, Guyatt GH, Jones PW. Clinical measurement of dyspnea. In: Maher D, ed. Dyspnea. New York: Marcel Dekker, 1998:149–198.

48. Jones PW, Quirk FH, Baveystock CM, et al. A self-complete measure of health status for chronic airflow limitation. Am Rev Respir Dis 1992; 145:1321–1327.

49. Guyatt GH, Berman LB, Townsend M, et al. A measure of quality of life for clinical trials in chronic lung disease. Thorax 1987;42:773–778.

50. Ambrosino N. Field tests in pulmonary disease [editorial]. Thorax 1999;54:191–193.

51. Sing SJ, Morgan MDL, Scott S, et al. Development of a shuttle walking test of disability in patients with chronic airflow obstruction. Thorax 1992;47:1019–1024.

52. ERS Task Force. Clinical exercise testing with reference in lung diseases: indications, standardization and interpretation strategies. Eur Respir J 1997;10:2662–2689.

53. Forte S, Carlone S, Onorati P, et al. Shuttle test vs 6-minute walking test in the evaluation of exercise tolerance in COPD patients. Eur Respir J 1997; 10:177S.

54. Kida K, Jinno S, Nomura K, et al. Pulmonary rehabilitation program survey in North America, Europe and Tokyo. J Cardiopulm Rehabil 1998; 18:301–308.

55. Nomura K, Kida K, and the Project Team. Assessment of pulmonary rehabilitation programs (PRP): data from a survey conducted in North America and Europe. Am J Respir Crit Care Med 1997;155(Suppl 4):A453.

56. Foglio K, Bagnato A, Pagani M, et al. L'applicazione di programmi di riabilitazione respiratoria nella realtà pneumologica italiana: una indagine conoscitiva del Gruppo di Studio "Riabilitazione Respiratoria" dell'AIPO. Rass Patol App Resp 1998;13:150–155.

36 The Japanese Perspective

Kozui Kida

⊳ Professional Skills

Upon completion of this chapter, the reader will:

- Discuss characteristics of pulmonary rehabilitation in Japan
- Discuss differences among pulmonary rehabilitation programs (PRPs) in Japan, Europe, and the United States

In 1995, both the American Thoracic Society and the European Respiratory Society published statements dealing with standards for the diagnosis and care of patients with chronic obstructive pulmonary disease (COPD).[1,2] Many of the case components used in PRPs were discussed in these statements. Characteristics of PRPs determined by a national survey in the United States were reported in 1988,[3] and resurvey data were reported in 1995.[4] The data indicated that marked variations exist in the structure of PRPs among institutions responding to the surveys.[3,4] On the other hand, in Japan the concept of pulmonary rehabilitation has a history of only a few decades, and the major disease target has been primary lung tuberculosis and its sequelae.[5] Physiotherapy, including postural drainage, breathing retraining, and exercise training, is prescribed most frequently, and a physiotherapist joins the PRP team in many cases.[5] It seems that a comprehensive approach with a well-organized and tailored program administrated by a medical team is uncommon in Japan.[6]

CHARACTERISTICS OF COPD IN JAPAN

The pathophysiology of COPD patients in Japan might differ from that of patients in other countries, especially North America, for two reasons.[7] First, COPD patients in Japan tend to be older than those in North America, where the peak prevalence is observed in the sixth decade of life.[8] According to a 1998 government report,[9] the prevalence of COPD in Japan is estimated to be only 14.3/100,000 in men and 2.4/100,000 in women in the sixth decade of life; it then sharply increases in the seventh decade of life to 97.5 and 18.7/100,000 in men and women, respectively. The prevalence continues to rise for both men and women with advancing age.[9]

The greater prevalence of emphysema in a much older age group in Japan than in North America might lead to the inclusion of large numbers of patients showing a deterioration in their activities of daily living or the frail elderly. This may be the reason that the major limiting factor, "lack of basic physical strength," is so common (47.7%) among Japanese patients in PRPs.[10] This might be owing to the relative lack of nursing homes and the provision of very low-cost medical care for the elderly. Thus, many private hospitals become de facto long-term care facilities.[11]

Second, pathologically determined emphysema was found to be frequently complicated by primary tuberculosis and its sequelae in an autopsy series of approximately 4000 patients, 29.6% in men and 16.0% in women,[12] suggesting that restrictive ventilatory disorders are superimposed on airflow obstruction by emphysema. These possible dissimilarities in both the pathophysiology and age distribution of the patient population in Japan compared with North America and Europe may contribute to several specific problems for PRPs in Japan.[10]

SURVEY OF PRPs IN TOKYO

We report the results of a survey of PRPs in North America and Europe and provide the first report of the results of a survey of PRP in Tokyo.[10]

PRPs were available at 56% of hospitals in North America and 74% in Europe but at only 20% of hospitals in Tokyo. Most PRPs were conducted in an outpatient setting in

Table 36-1. Comparison of Pulmonary Rehabilitation Program Content in North America, Europe, and Tokyo

| Content Item | Program (%) | | | P Value | | |
	North America (n = 50)	Europe (n = 51)	Tokyo (n = 202)	North America vs. Europe	North America vs. Tokyo	Europe vs. Tokyo
Education about pulmonary disease	98	86	20	<.05	<.0001	<.0001
Medication	92	90	20	NS	<.0001	<.0001
Breathing re-training	90	80	47	NS	<.0001	<.0001
Oxygen	86	78	84	NS	NS	NS
Walking	86	61	39	<.005	<.0001	<.005
ADLs	84	28	20	.000	<.0001	NS
Nutrition	84	55	36	<.005	<.0001	<.05
Upper and lower extremity exercise	82	61	24	<.05	<.0001	<.0001
Relaxation	78	65	13	NS	<.0001	<.0001
Psychosocial support	78	59	1	<.05	<.0001	<.0001
Family education	76	33	20	.000	<.0001	<.05
Pulmonary hygiene	74	59	42	NS	<.0001	<.05
Bicycle ergometer	72	45	6	<.01	<.0001	<.0001
Smoking cessation	70	69	66	NS	NS	NS
Treadmill	68	33	6	<.01	<.0001	<.0001
Respiratory muscle training	58	49	47	NS	NS	NS

Adapted from Kida K, Jinno S, Nomura K, et al. Pulmonary rehabilitation program survey in North America, Europe, and Tokyo. J Cardiopulm Rehabil 1998;18:301.
NS, not significant; ADLs, activities of daily living.

North America (98%), whereas both outpatient and inpatient programs were adopted in Europe (55% inpatient and 65% outpatient). The types of lung disease referred to PRPs were mainly COPD in both North America and Europe, although these accounted for only 34% of referrals in Tokyo; however, referrals for primary tuberculosis sequelae ($P = .028$) and bronchiectasis ($P = .021$) were more common in Europe, similar to the situation in Tokyo.

The following PRP items were available at significantly higher rates in North America than in Europe: family education, psychologic support, nutritional instruction, treadmill, ergo-bicycle, walking training, and increasing the activities of daily living; most of these items were unavailable in Tokyo (Table 36-1). From these data, we conclude that PRPs in North America are more multidimensionally oriented. Target diseases differ among North America, Europe, and Tokyo, however. PRPs in Tokyo differed from those in North America and Europe and were poorly programmed. Problems arising in PRPs in the three regions include lack of manpower and insufficient reimbursement.

PERSPECTIVES IN JAPAN

These possible dissimilarities in both the pathophysiology and age distribution of the patient population in Japan from those in North America and Europe may contribute to several specific problems with PRPs in Japan (Table 36-2).[13]

First, the high prevalence of poorly motivated patients (79.5%) is a major problem for PRPs in the Tokyo district. One reason is that a proper assessment system or selection method for patients referred to PRPs is lacking. An initial assessment for PRP is essential and indicated as an important factor[14] for enhancing program effectiveness, leading to time savings and cost-effectiveness. In particular, an assessment of cognition is needed for patients of advanced age. The Mini-Mental State Examination is the most commonly used method and has been extensively validated.[15] Another possible reason for poorly motivated patients is insufficient information about the long-term effects of PRPs. This is likely owing to inadequate education of the PRP staff about comprehensive PRPs.

Table 36-2. Problems for Hospitals With Pulmonary Rehabilitation Programs in Tokyo

Questionnaire Item	Program (%) (N = 45)
Manpower	71
Reimbursement	51
Staff education	47
Equipment	44
Time availability	44
Techniques	36
Continuity	36
Lack of education materials	22
Lack of acceptance by hospital	16
Lack of acceptance by other staff	11

Adapted from Kida K, Jinno S, Nomura K, et al. Pulmonary rehabilitation program survey in North America, Europe, and Tokyo. J Cardiopulm Rehabil 1998;18:301.

Second, PRPs in the Tokyo district remain mostly directed only to oxygen therapy (84.2%); long-term oxygen therapy is a universal component of PRPs.[16-18] The prevalence of other components of most comprehensive PRPs remains low compared with in North America and Europe (see Table 36-1).[10] To carry out the systematic and comprehensive programs typical in North America or Europe, a qualified and specialized medical staff is essential, a component still lacking in Japan. A system for registering respiratory therapists began only in 1996; however, this registry is still considered insufficient because candidates are selected only by a written examination among general nurses, physiotherapists, and clinical engineers working in a clinical field, not those specializing in respiratory therapy. For a proper program together with a specialized medical team, it is expected that improvements in items to increase exercise tolerance and self-management; to increase compliance concerning medication and medical equipment, such as oxygen use; and to further an understanding of the disease condition, even in frail elderly patients, are necessary.[19]

Third, it is interesting to see that the problems that arise in PRPs are similar to those in North America and Europe[10] despite the differences in socioeconomic background, medical service, and medical insurance among countries[20]; manpower (71.1%), charges and reimbursement (51.1%), staff education (46.7%), and time consumption (44.4%) were problems for hospitals. The reimbursement for pulmonary rehabilitation seems to be inadequately low because the recent medical insurance system in Japan[20] provides reimbursement for pulmonary rehabilitation at a rate of only about 35% of that provided for cardiac rehabilitation. Furthermore, pulmonary rehabilitation is not specialized and is categorized together with rehabilitation for cerebrovascular disorders or bone fractures.[20]

SUMMARY

Pulmonary rehabilitation in Japan remains undeveloped and reflects the greater prevalence of lung tuberculosis and its sequelae. Pulmonary rehabilitation has not targeted COPD as it has in North America; however, the prevalence of COPD in Japan will increase sharply because of higher smoking rates. Thus, pulmonary rehabilitation needs to advance in comprehensive and multidimensional aspects with a team approach. From this viewpoint, proper reimbursement will be essential to maintain qualified comprehensive pulmonary rehabilitation in the future.

REFERENCES

1. American Thoracic Society statement: standards for the diagnosis and care of patients with chronic obstructive pulmonary disease. Am J Respir Crit Care Med 1995;152(2 Pt 2): S77–S120.
2. European Respiratory Society. Consensus statement: optimal assessment and management of chronic obstructive pulmonary disease. Eur Respir J 1995;8:1398–1420.
3. Bickford LS, Hodgkin JE. National pulmonary rehabilitation survey. J Cardiopulm Rehabil 1988; 8:473–491.
4. Bickford LS, Hodgkin JE, McInturff SL. National pulmonary rehabilitation survey: update. J Cardiopulm Rehabil 1995;15:406–411.
5. Haga T. Pulmonary rehabilitation. In: Kitamoto O, ed. Pulmonary Tuberculosis, Internal Medicine Series No. 7. Tokyo: Nankodo, 1972:247–259.
6. Haga T. Pulmonary rehabilitation in chronic respiratory insufficiency. In: Haga T, Uemura T, Koga R, et al., eds. Cardio- and Pulmonary Disability and Elderly: Series of Rehabilitation Medicine No. 21. Tokyo: Ishiyaku-Syuppan, 1983: 53–118.
7. Thurlbeck WM. Pathology of chronic airflow obstruction. In: Cherniack NS, ed. Chronic Obstructive Pulmonary Disease. Philadelphia: WB Saunders, 1991:3–20.
8. Higgins MW, Thom T. Incidence, prevalence, and mortality: intra- and intercountry differences. In: Hensley MJ, Saunders NA, eds. Clinical Epidemiology of Chronic Obstructive Pulmonary Disease. New York: Marcel Dekker, 1989:23–43.
9. Mortality statistics. J Health Welfare Stat 1998; 45:408–418.
10. Kida K, Jinno S, Nomura K, et al. Pulmonary rehabilitation program survey in North America, Europe, and Tokyo. J Cardiopulm Rehabil 1998; 18:301–308.
11. Ikegami N, Fries BE, Takagi Y, et al. Applying RUG-III in Japanese long-term care facilities. Gerontologist 1994;34:628–639.

12. Jinno S, Kida K, Ootubo K. Epidemiology of emphysema: analysis by autopsy in a series of elderly patients. Jpn J Thorac Dis 1994;32:193–199.

13. Williams TF, Cooney LM Jr. Principles of rehabilitation in older persons. In: Hazzard WR, Bierman EL, Blass JP, et al., eds. Principles of Geriatric Medicine and Gerontology. 3rd ed. New York: McGraw-Hill, 1994:343–348.

14. Connors GL, Hilling LR, Morris KV. Assessment of the pulmonary rehabilitation candidate. In: Hodgkin JE, Connors GL, Bell CW, eds. Pulmonary Rehabilitation: Guidelines to Success. 2nd ed. Philadelphia: JB Lippincott, 1993:50–71.

15. Folstein MF, Folstein SE, Mc Hugh PR. "Minimental state": a practical method for grading the cognitive state of patients for the clinician. J Psychiatr Res 1975;12:189–198.

16. Hodgkin JE. Pulmonary rehabilitation: definition and essential components. In: Hodgkin JE, Connors GL, Bell CW, eds. Pulmonary Rehabilitation: Guidelines to Success. 2nd ed. Philadelphia: JB Lippincott, 1993:1–14.

17. Fishman AP. Pulmonary rehabilitation: from empiricism to science. In: Fishman AP, ed. Pulmonary Rehabilitation. New York: Marcel Dekker, 1996:15–31.

18. Hodgkin JE. Benefits and the future of pulmonary rehabilitation. In: Hodgkin JE, Connors GL, Bell CW, eds. Pulmonary Rehabilitation: Guidelines to Success. 2nd ed. Philadelphia: JB Lippincott, 1993:587–604.

19. NIH workshop summary: pulmonary rehabilitation research. Am J Respir Crit Care Med 1994; 149:825–833.

20. Ando H, ed. Guideline for the Reimbursement of Medical Insurance in Japan. Tokyo: Igakutusinsya, 1996.

37 The Latin American Perspective

José R. Jardim
Aquiles A. Camelier
Denise Miki

⬡ Professional Skills

Upon completion of this chapter, the reader will understand:

- Pulmonary rehabilitation has shown steady and increased growth in Latin America
- Most rehabilitation centers comprise multidisciplinary teams, including pulmonologists, chest physiotherapists, dietitians, and others
- The rehabilitation centers are related to public institutions, and no reimbursement policy is offered either by private insurance or by public health in most countries
- Most centers have a comprehensive program, including lower and upper extremities training and educational and psychosocial sessions; specific respiratory muscle training is not emphasized
- All centers include some evaluation at the beginning and end of the programs, mainly using the 6-minute walk test and/or a simple incremental test on the treadmill or cycloergometer; evaluation of upper extremity performance or respiratory muscle strength is less common
- There is a growing concern in doing research among the various centers

Latin America includes 17 countries composing portions of North America (Mexico), Central America (Guatemala, Nicaragua, Honduras, Panama, Costa Rica, and San Salvador), and South America (Venezuela, Colombia, Peru, Ecuador, Chile, Bolivia, Paraguay, Uruguay, Argentina, and Brazil). The 450 million Latin Americans basically speak two languages: Portuguese in Brazil (160 million people) and Spanish (290 million) in all the other countries. Some similarity is seen between both languages, making communication possible among these countries. Two other countries in the region have Spanish as their native language but are located in the Caribbean—Cuba and the Dominican Republic. A third Caribbean country speaks Spanish, Puerto Rico, but it is politically linked to the United States as an associate state.

From an economic standpoint, wide variation is seen among the Latin American countries; the same is also true concerning the scientific development and the health care systems.

For decades, scientific relations among Latin American respirologists were rather uncommon, with stronger connections with the United States, Canada, and Western Europe than among themselves. The development of the Central America and Caribbean

Table 37-1. Number of Pulmonary
Rehabilitation Centers
in Latin America in 1998
(N = 28)

Country	Number
Brazil	15
Argentina	3
Mexico	3
Uruguay	2
Colombia	2
Chile	1
Venezuela	1
Peru	1

Respiratory Federation, the Latin American Thoracic Association,[1] and a society of pediatricians specializing in respiratory diseases has increased the frequency of regional international meetings and the circulation of regional periodicals.

Pulmonary rehabilitation is a rather new field in Latin America. The first center opened less than 15 years ago in Santiago, Chile. Currently, approximately 28 rehabilitation centers operate in the region, inhomogeneously distributed (Table 37-1). Brazil has led the creation of new programs in the past few years, with most of them based on the experience of the first program opened in 1993 at the Federal University of Sao Paulo (UNIFESP).[2]

The data in this chapter are based on information obtained through a 45-question survey sent to 19 pulmonary rehabilitation centers throughout Latin America. Since completion of the survey, we have learned of 6 more centers, which brings the total certified number to 25. Thus, we believe that the information provided in this chapter reflects the actual reality of Latin America on this particular topic.

This survey was aimed at outpatient programs only. The lack of any comment related to inpatient rehabilitation does not necessarily mean that this kind of program is not available in Latin America, but it is difficult to provide information with any degree of accuracy.

Sixty-two percent of the centers keep some degree of relation to another rehabilitation program in the same country, whereas a little more than half of the groups (53%) maintain a special relationship with a foreign rehabilitation program. Half of the centers are also used for cardiac rehabilitation.

REIMBURSEMENT

By and large, the rehabilitation centers are located in and run by public institutions (60%), mostly universities, and the patients are charged no fee. In most countries, no adopted reimbursement policy is available from either the public health system or private insurance companies despite the fact that motor rehabilitation has been recognized as an essential component in the treatment of musculoskeletal diseases and has been reimbursed for a long time. This clearly shows the urgent need for local studies specifically designed to evaluate the cost-effectiveness of pulmonary rehabilitation.

A few centers run either entirely private programs or programs on a partial-time basis, charging US$220 to 300 monthly for a three times a week program.

TEAM COMPONENTS

Most rehabilitation centers in Latin America are composed of multidisciplinary teams. The number of members varies among the different centers, but on average they involve pulmonologists, chest physiotherapists, and dietitians. Nurses, cardiologists, and occupational therapists were reported by 37% of the programs and psychologists by 21%. Only two centers reported the presence of an exercise physiologist. Usually larger teams are seen in places where academic and research work is being carried out, such as at National Institute of Respiratory Diseases (INER) (Mexico) and UNIFESP (Sao Paulo, Brazil), which have teams of 12 to 15 persons.

PATIENT POPULATION

Despite the large number of smokers in Latin America (around 35% of the adult population), only a few centers (UNIFESP/BR and INER) offer the help of a smoking cessation clinic to their patients. Recently, in an international conference (ATS, San Diego, CA, 1999) it was debated whether a smoker could be accepted in a rehabilitation program. Twelve (63%) of the Latin American centers do not allow smokers to join their programs, and would accept them only after they have quit smoking for at least 3 months.[3]

Most patients entering pulmonary rehabilitation programs in Latin America are referred by lung specialists, a smaller percentage by thoracic surgeons, and a few by general practitioners. These numbers probably reflect the lack of knowledge of the general medical population concerning the beneficial effects of this new therapeutic approach.

This lack of knowledge is also corroborated by the fact that most patients enrolled in the programs already suffer from very severe disease, with airflow obstruction below 40% predicted. Some patients are already hypercapnic, and most are severely hypoxemic. Moderate chronic obstructive pulmonary disease (COPD) patients have only been trained in four centers (21%). The lack of local specific guidelines for rehabilitation may offer the best explanation for the low referral of patients with less severe respiratory impairment.

All centers are specifically working with COPD patients. Some of them manifest some experience working with patients with diseases other than COPD, like interstitial pulmonary fibrosis and chronic asthma. Few centers have seen patients with neuromuscular disease and cystic fibrosis. Two centers have had children in their programs, but, as far as we know, Latin America has no formal pediatric rehabilitation centers.

INITIAL EVALUATION

Practically all centers complete an initial clinical and physiotherapeutic assessment. Only 40% of the programs include in the assessment a maximal ergometry test to evaluate the pulmonary and cardiovascular exercise response. If we consider that most patients referred to a rehabilitation center are elderly and that training is accomplished with a high load, it might be that those patients not subjected to an initial maximal test are being submitted to an unnecessary risk.

In an evaluation of 100 COPD patients undergoing a maximal cycloergometer test limited by symptoms at UNIFESP/BR, approximately 30% of them had one of the following alterations: hypertension, chest pain, electrocardiographic abnormalities, extra systoles, and others. Fortunately, those changes were not severe and, after appropriate treatment, only a small group could not join the rehabilitation program. This points out the benefit of a screening exercise because it may help optimize a patient's treatment.

A simple nutritional evaluation is undertaken in most of the centers, but in some of them research has been conducted on this matter.[4] Anabolic steroids are not routinely prescribed. Interestingly, 28% of patients are receiving oral corticosteroids and 45% are receiving inhaled steroids.[5,6] Approximately 20% of patients are on continuous oxygen therapy. Some centers supply their patients with oxygen during the training sessions.[7]

PROGRAM COMPONENTS

Duration

In Latin America, approximately 40% of the programs are run for 3 months, 5% for 1 month, and 5% for 4 months; the other 50% stated a different duration from the aforementioned ones but they did not specify the duration of their programs. Patients usually exercise three times a week (73%) or sometimes twice a week (31%); in just one program (5%) exercise is on a daily basis. In 75% of the centers the exercise sessions last 60 to 120 minutes. Forty-four percent of patients required supplemental oxygen during exercise, most by nasal catheter.

Lower Extremity Exercise

All centers (100%) include lower extremity exercise in their programs, using either a treadmill (79%) and/or a cycloergometer (68%). The treadmill load is set just with speed changes in half of the programs. The other half use a combination of speed and inclination changes. The load for training is based on an incremental test and is calculated at 80% of the maximum load achieved in 53% of the programs. In 16% of the programs the exercise is performed at 70% of the maximum oxygen consumption; just one program trains their patients at the cardiac frequency measured at the anaerobic threshold level. Most centers calculate the load by more than one method. Half of the programs allow 1 month for the patients to get used to this high load. With a few exceptions, the exercise is usually carried out in a patient group as opposed to individually.

Upper Extremity Exercise

Approximately 90% of the Latin American programs routinely associate upper extremity exercise with their general conditioning training. Weights are used in 84% of the centers, and in more than half of them (58%) exercises are done with diagonal movements; however, it is not clear whether the proprioceptive technique is being used. Other methods cited include the use of dowels (32%), arm cycloergometers (16%), and elastic bands (11%). One center reported no use of upper extremity exercise.

Respiratory Muscle Training

Six programs (32%) routinely include respiratory muscle training, and five (26%) prescribe this modality of exercise only when respiratory muscle weakness was thought to be an important component of the dyspnea. Five centers (32%) never include respiratory muscle training in their programs. Training is conducted using pressure-limited devices (inspiratory threshold trainer), with a pressure load varying between 10 and 80% of the maximal inspiratory pressure.[8–11] A global pulmonary rehabilitation program without specific respiratory muscle training is able to increase ventilatory muscle strength in patients with COPD.[12] Just one center has included active diaphragmatic exercise in its routine program. An association has been shown between impaired lung function and changes in ultrastructure of the human diaphragm. One study shows that the muscle adapts at a subcellular level in the face of loads imposed by COPD.[13] Currently, no centers have reported submitting COPD patients to respiratory muscle rest with negative pressure ventilation.[14]

After the end of the full rehabilitation program, the patients are encouraged to continue exercising at home. In 30% of the centers the patients return once or twice a week for maintenance sessions. The prescription for home exercise is based on the patient's exercise load at the end of the formal program.

EDUCATIONAL SESSIONS

Education is part of the pulmonary rehabilitation program in all centers (100%). The educational program usually comprises a 30- to 60-minute class once a week focusing on emphysema/bronchitis, nutrition, pharmacotherapy, exercise, relaxation, and oxygen therapy. Simple reading material is used in 73% of the centers, videos are available in 32% of the programs, and other methods are used in 50% of the centers.

Thus, most centers use two or more methods to educate patients. An obligatory participation of the family in the educational program is reported by most centers (63%). In some, no family commitment is included in the program (21%). In 21% of the centers the families are invited and it is up to them to decide their level of participation. Forty-two percent of the centers have one discussion per week, and the remaining groups have two to three discussions a week.

OUTCOME MEASUREMENTS

All centers (100%) include the 6-minute walk test in their evaluation as a measure of exercise performance, and two centers (10%) also complete the 12-minute walk test; only one center (5%) uses the shuttle test. Measurements of ventilatory and metabolic response to exercise are recorded in eight centers, five of them on a cycloergometer and three on a treadmill. A simple incremental test on either cycloergometer or treadmill is completed by 60% of the programs. Besides the maximal test, half of the programs include a symptom-limited endurance test with a submaximal load. Despite the fact that almost all centers (90%) include exercise for the upper extremity in their programs, only 40% of them evaluate their patients with an incremental test to calculate the exercise load.

Maximal inspiratory and expiratory pressures are measured in 63% of the programs. Health-related quality of life is assessed in 13 centers (68%) by either the St. George's Respiratory Questionnaire (n = 8) or the Chronic Respiratory Disease Questionnaire (n = 5). To the best of our knowledge, the St. George's Respiratory Questionnaire has been validated only in Brazil[15] and Mexico, and the Chronic Respiratory Disease Questionnaire has not been validated in any country in Latin America. It is interesting that although only 21% of the programs reported inclusion of a psychologist on their teams, 37% of them require patients to answer depression and anxiety questionnaires. It has been shown at the UNIFESP that 40% of their COPD patients scored low enough on the Beck Questionnaire to be diagnosed as having depression, and 80% had anxiety or anxiety trait.[16] Little is known about the use of the information obtained.

Oxygen saturation is measured by means of pulse oximetry during activities of daily living in seven centers (37%). By and large, these activities include the most common ones, such as walking on a flat surface, simulations of changing clothes or taking a shower, combing the hair, and others. Moderate to severe COPD patients, when performing simple activities such as sweeping the floor, cleaning the blackboard, lifting pots, and replacing lamps, have high oxygen uptake (45 to 58% maximal peak oxygen uptake), which may explain the tiredness reported by them during simple activities involving the upper limbs. Their minute ventilation over maximum ventilatory ventilation (VE/MVV) is high (55 to 63%), which leads them to a high level of perceived dyspnea.[17]

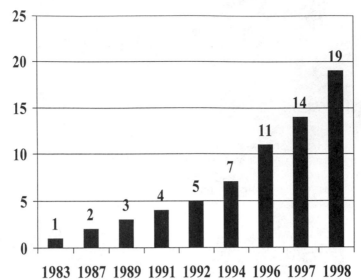

Figure 37-1. Cumulative frequency of opening of new pulmonary rehabilitation centers in Latin America.

In conclusion, there is every reason to be optimistic. It is true that the development of formal programs of pulmonary rehabilitation has been relatively slow in Latin America and has lagged behind that in other parts of the developed world. But it is also true that progressive growth is extending throughout Latin America (Fig. 37-1). The degree of development varies according to the region, but it is encouraging that several centers have published original data and contributed to the advancement of this important area of pulmonary therapy. We firmly believe that with the increase in regional communications and the development of a common journal, this important area will see a great leap during the next decade.

REFERENCES

1. Jardim J. ALAT: A Thoracic Association for Latin America. Respir Care Matters 1997;2:8–9.
2. Neder JA, Jardim J, Cendon SP, et al. Maximal and submaximal exercise responses in COPD patients submitted to a comprehensive pulmonary rehabilitation program. Am J Respir Crit Care Med 1996;153(4):A172.
3. Herrera-Kiengelher LL, Caloca JV, Ponce MPC, et al. Conecimento sobre tabaquismo en escolares de primaria: impacto de una platica educativa. Rev Inst Nat Enf Resp Mex 1998;11:36–42.
4. Sachs A, Lerario MC, Wasjberg M, et al. Vitamin C intake in chronic obstructive pulmonary disease elderly patients in Sao Paulo, Brazil. Am J Respir Crit Care Med 1996;153(4):A168.
5. Jardim J, Ferreira IM, Sachs S. Nutrition, anabolic steroids and growth hormone. Phys Med Rehabil Clin N Am 1996;7(2):253–75.
6. Ferreira IM, Verreschi IT, Nery LE, et al. The influence of 6 months of oral anabolic steroids on body mass and respiratory muscles in undernourished COPD patients. Chest 1998;114:19–28.
7. Cendon SP, Gondim H, Ferreira IM, et al. The influence of breathing 4 L/min of oxygen on exercise performance in chronic obstructive pulmonary disease. Am J Respir Crit Care Med 1996; 153(4):A780.
8. Montes de Oca M, Celli BR, Rassulo J. Progress of respiratory muscle dysfunction in patients with severe chronic obstructive disease. Arch Bronconeumol 1997;33(11):561–565.
9. Lisboa C, Munoz V, Beroiza T, et al. Inspiratory muscle training in chronic airflow limitation: comparison of two different training loads with a threshold device. Eur Respir J 1994;7(7):1266–1274.
10. Villafranca C, Borzone G, Leiva A, et al. Effect of inspiratory muscle training with an intermediate load on inspiratory power output in COPD. Eur Respir J 1998;11(1):28–33.
11. Lisboa C, Borzone G. Ventilatory muscle training. In: Cherniack NS, Altosa MD, Homma I, eds. Rehabilitation of the Patient With Respiratory Disease. New York: McGraw-Hill, 1999:519–528.
12. Dal Corso S, Mayer A, Salerno P, et al. A nonspecific rehabilitation program increases respiratory

muscle strength in patients with bronchial obstructive disease. Am J Respir Crit Care Med 1997;155(4):A918.

13. Orozco-Levi M, Gea J, Lloreta J, et al. Structural adaptations of diaphragm in patients with chronic obstructive pulmonary disease (COPD). Rev Colomb Neumol 1997;9:15–26.

14. Gutierrez M, Beroiza MT, Contreras G, et al. Weekly cuirass ventilation improves arterial blood gases in chronic airflow limitation patients. Am Rev Respir Crit Care Med 1988;138:617.

15. Souza TC, Jardim JR, Jones P. Validity of the St. George Respiratory Questionnaire in chronic obstructive pulmonary disease in Brazil. Eur Respir J 1999;14:238S.

16. Bernardes de Souza C, Bogossian M, Jardim JR, et al. Depression and anxiety: two important aspects in patients with chronic obstructive pulmonary disease (COPD). Am J Respir Crit Care Med 1996;153(4):A783.

17. Velloso M, Silva AC, Cendon S, et al. Analysis of metabolic and ventilatory parameters during the activities of daily living (ADL) in patients with chronic obstructive pulmonary disease (COPD) and normal subjects. Am J Respir Crit Care Med 1999;159:A586.

38 The Philippine Perspective

Percival Punzal

▷ Professional Skills

Upon completion of this chapter, the reader will:

- Describe how pulmonary rehabilitation programs are conducted in the Philippines
- Compare similarities and differences of local rehabilitation programs with those of programs in other countries
- Define the present and future prospects of pulmonary rehabilitation in the country

Chronic obstructive pulmonary disease (COPD) is the seventh leading cause of mortality in the Philippines.[1] The experience of local pulmonologists and general practitioners taking care of these patients demonstrates the profound impact of this progressively debilitating disease. Active smoking has been cited as the most important cause.[2] More than half of the patients are older than 60 years at the onset of disease, with more men affected than women.[2]

Despite the improvement of pharmacotherapy in recent decades, Filipino COPD patients, like their counterparts in other countries, were able to achieve only partial and temporary relief of symptoms. This is perhaps the most significant reason for the establishment of pulmonary rehabilitation programs in the country, starting in the early 1990s. Three medical institutions in Metro Manila—the Philippine Heart Center, the Lung Center of the Philippines, and Philippine General Hospital—have multidisciplinary pulmonary rehabilitation programs.

MAJOR OBJECTIVES OF PULMONARY REHABILITATION PROGRAMS

These programs are established means of enhancing medical therapy to alleviate symptoms of patients with chronic lung diseases.[3-9] The major objectives of the program are to:

1. Enable the patients and family members to acquire knowledge about their disease
2. Restore patients to their highest level of independent function
3. Improve exercise tolerance
4. Reduce the number of exacerbations and consequent hospital confinements
5. Improve their quality of life

The specific goals for a given patient may vary depending on the degree of disability, and those individualized goals are set during admission to the program.

PATIENT SELECTION

Patients are admitted to the program through a referral system. More commonly, these are individuals who are diagnosed as having COPD (emphysema and chronic bronchitis), bronchial asthma, or bronchiectasis based on clinical diagnosis confirmed by history, physical examination, spirometry, and chest roentgenogram. They are noted to have disabilities varying from moderate to severe. It is essential that they are stable for at least 2 weeks while following an acceptable medical regimen. Likewise, no acute or chronic conditions should be present that would contraindicate participation in the exercise program.

The "ideal patient" is somebody who is disabled by the disease but not incapacitated and has the proper motivation to complete the program.

Prerehabilitation assessment is accomplished by:

1. Initial interview using questionnaires assessing the patient's social background and medical history
2. Shortness of Breath Questionnaires[10]
3. Baseline tests of lung function and exercise tolerance using arterial blood gas determination, spirometric studies, the 6-minute walk test,[11] and an incremental symptom-limited treadmill exercise test[12]

PROGRAM STRUCTURE

The organization and structure of pulmonary rehabilitation programs in the Philippines varies in the different centers, but the basic components are essentially the same. All are done on an outpatient basis with a duration of 4 to 8 weeks (1 or 2 d/wk). The approach is multidisciplinary, involving medical and allied health workers from various areas of expertise. At the Philippine Heart Center the 8-week program is divided into three phases:

Phase 1 (week 1) is composed of evaluation of the patient's pulmonary status and functional capacity, educational sessions on pulmonary pathophysiology as they relate to chronic lung diseases, and planning of an exercise program.

Phase 2 (weeks 2–4) is composed of twice weekly sessions on both education and exercise. Topics included in the discussions are options in medical treatment and concepts of respiratory care, among other things. Patients meet with a psychiatrist for an hour of group support weekly.

Phase 3 (weeks 5–8) consists of once weekly sessions involving exercise, education reinforcement, and group support meetings. This is concluded by the graduation day, which is considered the most special day of pulmonary rehabilitation and is devoted to social activities to "celebrate" the patients' completion of the program.

After finishing the course, patients are reevaluated using identical protocols (6-minute walk test and treadmill exercise testing) to assess the improvement of exercise capacity. Their shortness of breath in relation to specific activities is reexamined using the same set of standardized questionnaires.

MEMBERS OF THE REHABILITATION TEAM

The staff works under the supervision of the head of the pulmonary and critical care division of the institution. The *program director* is a pulmonary physician with special interest and training in pulmonary rehabilitation. He is the administrator, educator, and research coordinator. His responsibilities include program development, revision, and management. The *assistant program director* is also a pulmonary physician trained in pulmonary rehabilitation who assists the program director in the development, supervision, and marketing of the program. He takes over the function of the program director when necessity arises. *Pulmonary fellows in training* are active members of the rehabilitation team. They are trained to assist in the initial evaluation of patients, perform the exercise tests, and act as facilitators during discussions. The *psychiatrist* provides a venue for patients to cope with their disease by helping them develop appropriate skills. The *respiratory therapist* conducts the initial interview, pulmonary function, and exercise tests used for evaluating patients before and after rehabilitation. He or she also acts as an educator on strategies for improving patients' disabilities and trains the patient and family members in the proper techniques of breathing, respiratory care, and use of pulmonary devices. Likewise, he or she facilitates communication between the patient, his or her family, and the rehabilitation team. The *physical therapist* provides warm-up and upper body exercises to strengthen muscles. Emphasis is made on the coordination of breathing and body movements. The *nutritionist* evaluates the dietary requirements of patients and recommends appropriate food and supplements. The *social worker* discusses monetary assistance to patients who could not afford the program's financial requirements.

COMPONENTS OF THE PROGRAM

Education

Patient education is a central component of pulmonary rehabilitation.[13] Patients are provided with a cordial and informal classroom atmosphere by the members of the rehabilitation team. Lectures and discussions with the help of visual aids, slides, and videotapes are conducted by the staff in the simplest and clearest terms possible. Patients are encouraged to be active participants through questions and comments during the discussions. Here, they learn the nature of their diseases and the available forms of therapy. Open and honest discussions have proven to be most helpful, especially the one on the natural course of the disease. Other topics include proper use of oxygen, "hows and whys" of exercise, hows and whys of medications, proper use of various drug delivery systems, energy-saving and breathing techniques, postural drainage, chest physiotherapy, relaxation and travel, prevention of infections, early recognition of acute symptoms and appropriate emergency measures. Nutritional counseling is done individually in one session.

Sexual counseling is another important part of the program. It is done usually in a group discussion. When necessary, questions are dealt with privately with the patient and his or her partner. It has been previously noted that intimacy is especially important to patients with chronic lung disease because it is a powerful antidote to the depression that most patients feel.[14] Recommendations are made in terms of preparations and precautions that both partners should know if they intend to engage in the activity.

The session on smoking cessation is considered to be one of the most important meetings. Although most of the patients quit smoking years before they are admitted in the program, a few of the patients enrolled are current smokers. Family members and acquaintances who smoke are also invited to join a discussion in which the emphasis is on the hazardous effects of smoking and techniques on how to quit the habit.

Many patients have depression and anxiety.[15,16] Group support sessions[17] are conducted so that patients will learn how to deal with the lifestyle changes imposed by the chronic lung disease. Two potential problematic areas are how they view themselves and how they relate to others. Discussions with the psychiatrist help them develop coping mechanisms. Great importance is placed on adequate family support.

Exercise Training Program

Patients who enter the program are deconditioned. This is the reason why exercise programs for both upper and lower extremities are recommended.[18–21] Lower body exercise training involves supervised walking on a treadmill during the scheduled visits. It is started at a level that patients can sustain for several minutes. At home, they are encouraged to continue this exercise daily at a walking pace that approximates their sustained treadmill speed. Training levels are subsequently increased during the supervised sessions, and training continues at intensity levels that represent high percentages of their maximum exercise tolerance.[12] The goal is to have them walk continuously for 30 minutes. All patients are instructed to keep exercise diaries to monitor their progress. Any untoward symptoms occurring during exercise are documented.

Upper body exercise training is composed of prescribed arm exercises and upper body cycle ergometry. The arm exercises are done in three sets with six repetitions daily. Initially, they are performed without hand weights. Subsequently, light hand weights (1–2 lb) were added as tolerated. Cycle ergometry is performed initially without resistive load for 15 minutes. The load is subsequently added during the following sessions.

Filipinos are generally known as "natural lovers of dances." Many of our patients were dance enthusiasts in their younger years, and this is the reason for the incorporation of dancing as a form of exercise. Of course the beat has to be relatively slow to allow them to do the movements for 10 minutes.

Supplemental oxygen is used as necessary for both upper and lower body exercises to maintain an oxygen saturation level of 90% or higher during exercise. The modified Borg Scale[22] is used to quantify the degree of shortness of breath and fatigue after the exercises.

FINANCIAL CONSIDERATIONS

Unlike in other countries where the program is paid for by health maintenance organizations or government reimbursements, patients in the Philippines pay for the program by using their own personal resources. If they cannot afford the cost, they are evaluated by social workers for financial assistance.

THE FUTURE OF PULMONARY REHABILITATION IN THE PHILIPPINES

Pulmonary rehabilitation in the Philippines is in its infancy compared with other similar programs in developed countries. This is true if one considers the number of medical institutions with trained personnel who can conduct the program, the number of patients who benefit from it, and the acceptance by the medical community as a whole. Lately, however, a gradual surge of interest has occurred among physicians and allied health workers to work for the establishment of their own programs. Efforts are now being geared toward improving health care delivery for patients with chronic lung diseases, preventing exacerbations/hospital confinements, and improving their functional capacity as well as quality of life through a comprehensive and multidisciplinary approach.

ACKNOWLEDGMENT

The author thanks Dr Teresita de Guia, head of the Pulmonary and Critical Care Division—Philippine Heart Center, for her comments and suggestions in the preparation of the article.

REFERENCES

1. National Advisory Committee. National Health Plan–Department of Health. Manila, Philippines, 1995.
2. Punzal PA. COPD Council Survey on chronic obstructive pulmonary disease in the Metro Manila. Philippine College of Chest Physicians, 1994.
3. Blanco ME, Punzal PA, Koh AT, et al. Pulmonary rehabilitation: a multidisciplinary program for Filipino COPD patients. Phil J Chest Dis 1993;1:3.
4. Guzman AV, Punzal PA, Koh AT, et al. Long term follow-up of patients with COPD in a comprehensive pulmonary rehabilitation program. Phil Heart Center J 1997;4:37.
5. Chua JQ, Punzal PA, Koh AT, et al. Long term benefits of pulmonary rehabilitation in the exercise capacity and shortness of breath of patients with chronic obstructive pulmonary disease. Phil Heart Center J 1997;4:82.
6. American Thoracic Society. Standards for the diagnosis and care of patients with chronic obstructive pulmonary disease (COPD). Am J Respir Crit Care Med 1995;152:S77.
7. Siafakas NM, Vermeire P, Pride MB. Optimal assessment and management of chronic obstructive pulmonary disease (COPD): European Respiratory Society Task Force. Eur Respir J 1995;8: 1398.
8. Ries AL. Position paper of the American Association of Cardiovascular and Pulmonary Rehabilitation: scientific basis of pulmonary rehabilitation. J Cardiopulm Rehabil 1990;10:418.
9. Casaburi R, Petty TL. Principles and Practice of Pulmonary Rehabilitation. Philadelphia: WB Saunders, 1993.
10. Eakin EG, Resnikoff PM, Prewitt LM, et al. Validation of a new dyspnea questionnaire, UCSD Shortness of Breath Questionnaire. Chest 1998;113:619–624.
11. Guyatt GH, Thompson PJ, Berman LB. How should we measure function in patients with chronic heart and lung diseases? J Chronic Dis 1985;38:517.
12. Punzal PA, Ries AL, Kaplan RM, et al. Maximum intensity exercise training in patients with chronic obstructive pulmonary disease. Chest 1990;100: 618.
13. ACCP/AACVPR Pulmonary Rehabilitation Guidelines Panel. Pulmonary rehabilitation: joint ACCP/ACCVPR evidence-based guidelines. Chest 1997;112:1363.
14. Kravetz HM, Pheatt N. Sexuality in the pulmonary patient. In: Hodgkin JE, ed. Pulmonary Rehabilitation: Guidelines to Success. 2nd ed. Philadelphia: JB Lippincott, 1993.
15. Light RW, Merrill EJ, Despars JA. Prevalence of depression and anxiety in patients with COPD. Chest 1985;87:35.
16. Borak J, Sliwinski P, Piasecki Z. Psychological status of COPD patients on long term oxygen therapy. Eur Respir J 1991;4:59.
17. Emery CF, Leatherman NE, Burker EJ. Psychological outcomes of a pulmonary rehabilitation program. Chest 1991;100:613.
18. Belman MJ. Exercise in patients with chronic obstructive pulmonary disease. Thorax 1993;48: 936.
19. Celli BR. Pulmonary rehabilitation in patients with COPD. Am J Respir Crit Care Med 1995; 152:861.
20. Ries AL, Ellis B, Hawkins RW. Upper extremity exercise training in chronic obstructive pulmonary disease. Chest 1988;93:688.
21. Lake FR, Henderson K, Briffa T. Upper-limb and lower-limb exercise training in patients with chronic airflow obstruction. Chest 1990;97:1077.
22. Borg GAV. Psychophysical bases of perceived exertion. Med Sci Sports Exerc 1982;14:377.

39 The USA Perspective

Gerilynn L. Connors
Jeanne E. Ruff

⬡ Professional Skills

Upon completion of this chapter, the reader will:

- Explain the significance of statistics in the fight to prevent and treat chronic lung disease
- Describe the essential components of pulmonary rehabilitation
- Understand how prevention should be integrated into each essential component of pulmonary rehabilitation
- List the conditions appropriate for pulmonary rehabilitation besides chronic obstructive pulmonary disease (COPD)
- Discuss the management issues to be addressed when orchestrating a pulmonary rehabilitation program
- State the role outcomes/benchmarking has in a pulmonary rehabilitation program

EPIDEMIOLOGY IN THE UNITED STATES

Pulmonary rehabilitation programs have evolved and grown during the past several decades in the United States in response to the increase in patients with chronic lung disease. One in seven deaths are attributable to lung disease, with more than 30 million people in the United States living with chronic lung diseases such as asthma, emphysema, and chronic bronchitis.[1] COPD increased 60% from 1982 to 1995, with an estimated 16.4 million Americans afflicted.[2] In fact, COPD and allied conditions rank fourth among the leading causes of death in the United States.[3] Lung cancer is also a devastating disease that negatively impacts the lives of those afflicted and the economy. Pulmonary rehabilitation may be an option for these individuals.[4] Lung cancer is the leading cause of cancer mortality in both men and women in the United States, with an estimated 158,900 deaths in 1999, which is 28% of all cancer deaths. Mortality has been increasing since the 1930s.[5] Lung cancer has been the leading cause of cancer deaths in men since the early 1950s. In 1987, lung cancer surpassed breast cancer to become the leading cause of cancer deaths in women.[5] In 1999, it is estimated that there will be 171,600 new cases of lung cancer, a 28% increase in the incidence between 1973 and 1996. Of the hospital discharges attributed to cancer in 1996, 11.6% were attributed to lung cancer, the highest among all malignant neoplasms.[5]

Asthma affects an estimated 17 million Americans, with increases in the prevalence and mortality rates during the past decade.[6] The estimated number of American lives affected with a deficiency of a protein known as α_1-antitrypsin, which results in an inherited form of emphysema, is 50,000 to 100,000.[7]

In 1996 the total estimated US health expenditure was $1035.1 billion, an average annual increase of 4.4% from the previous year.[8] The cost of chronic lung disease both economic and personal is staggering. To lessen this burden, pulmonary rehabilitation must become the "standard of care" for the treatment and prevention of chronic lung disease, not just an "alternative of care."

COLLABORATION OF PULMONARY REHABILITATION PRACTICES

In response to the increase in the prevalence of the patient population serviced by pulmonary rehabilitation and the scientific studies documenting consistent benefits, professional organizations have acknowledged the value of the practice of pulmonary rehabilitation. In 1993, the American Association of Cardiovascular and Pulmonary Rehabilitation (AACVPR) published the first national guidelines for pulmonary rehabilitation programs. In 1998, the AACVPR released the second edition of the national guidelines.[9] In 1995 the American Thoracic Society (ATS) published a statement on the assessment and treatment of patients with COPD that included pulmonary rehabilitation in the treatment plan.[10] In 1999, the ATS published a second official statement on pulmonary rehabilitation owing to the efficacy and scientific foundation of pulmonary rehabilitation being firmly established.[11] The first ATS position statement on pulmonary rehabilitation was published in 1981. The American College of Chest Physicians and the AACVPR in 1997 coauthored an evidence-based practice guideline supporting the value of pulmonary rehabilitation.[12] In 1994, the National Institutes of Health Consensus Conference on Pulmonary Rehabilitation published the workshop summary, which also included a definition of the process of pulmonary rehabilitation.[13]

This recognition of the practice of pulmonary rehabilitation was also noted by the Medical Advisory Panel of the National Blue Cross Blue Shield Association in 1996, declaring this service as a "reasonable technology" for patients with chronic obstructive pulmonary disease.[14] Medicare intermediaries in certain states across the United States have developed specific guidelines for pulmonary rehabilitation programs. Continued collaboration with national organizations[15] and our colleagues across the world will bring pulmonary rehabilitation into the 21st century as an integral part of the clinical management, health maintenance, and disease prevention of people with chronic pulmonary disease.

CONDITIONS APPROPRIATE FOR PULMONARY REHABILITATION

COPD patients account for most patients entering and participating in pulmonary rehabilitation programs. This is traditional, but we must go beyond our comfort zone and expand the program options to other conditions as well.[4,9,16-21] Tobacco smoking is the main cause of COPD, and encouragement and support from the pulmonary rehabilitation program to terminate this addiction is important and critical. Awareness of risk factors and identification of at-risk populations are areas that the rehabilitation program should become involved with. As rehabilitation experts, we must expand the application of pulmonary rehabilitation to other chronic lung conditions.[9,16] In fact, although neuromuscular disorders and thoracic wall deformities are incurable, supportive treatment to improve the patient's quality of life is used. This supportive treatment should consider pulmonary rehabilitation as a standard of care to meet the patient's individual needs.[17] The optimal age for intervention and types of treatment for cystic fibrosis are being studied.[18] Cystic fibrosis is a disease for which pulmonary rehabilitation is very appropriate. Box 39-1 lists various patient conditions appropriate for pulmonary rehabilitation. These patients will challenge the pulmonary rehabilitation specialist beyond the continuum of traditional care. The components of a comprehensive pulmonary rehabilitation program (assessment, patient training, exercise, psychosocial intervention, and follow-up) will be the same for

Box 39-1. Traditional and Nontraditional Conditions
Appropriate for Pulmonary Rehabilitation

Obstructive disorders
  Asthma
  Asthmatic bronchitis
  Chronic bronchitis
  Emphysema
  Chronic obstructive pulmonary disease
  Bronchiectasis
  Cystic fibrosis
  Bronchiolitis obliterans
Restrictive disorders
  Interstitial fibrosis
  Rheumatoid lung disease
  Lung disorders secondary to collagen-vascular disease
  Occupational lung disease
  Environmental lung disease
  Sarcoidosis
  Kyphoscoliosis
  Spondylitis
  Parkinson's disease
  Postpolio syndrome
  Amyotrophic lateral sclerosis
  Diaphragm dysfunction
  Multiple sclerosis
Other disorders
  Nicotine addiction
  Lung cancer
  Primary pulmonary hypertension
  Postthoracic surgery
  Lung transplantation pre/post
  Lung volume reduction surgery pre/post
  Ventilator dependency
  Pediatric patients with pulmonary disease
  Morbid obesity
  Sleep apnea
  Primary tuberculosis

these patients, but modification of the program components is vital to address the specific needs of the patients. It means redesigning the pulmonary rehabilitation program for disease specification. The key to successful patient outcomes is individualization of the program to the patient's needs. Innovative strategies for each component of pulmonary rehabilitation will need to be developed and enhanced for the nontraditional diseases. The continuum of care for chronic pulmonary disease begins at birth and ends with death. Pulmonary rehabilitation must become integrated into this continuum of care for earlier detection and prevention of pulmonary disease and for the nontraditional conditions.

THE INTERDISCIPLINARY TEAM IN PULMONARY REHABILITATION

In the United States we have the privilege of working with an interdisciplinary team of health care specialist in pulmonary rehabilitation. Members of each specialty use their expertise to assess, treat, and follow-up the patient in the program as appropriate.[9] See

Box 39-2 for an extensive list of the interdisciplinary team members of a pulmonary rehabilitation program.

Not every member of the interdisciplinary team will assess the patient, but if a specific patient deficit is evaluated, then the appropriate specialist intervenes. Every pulmonary rehabilitation program in the United States must have a medical director.[9] This physician must have special training and knowledge (pulmonary function, exercise testing, acute and chronic pulmonary medicine, treatment of lung disease, and a special interest and belief in pulmonary rehabilitation) of the pulmonary patient population we serve. The medical director acts as an administrator, diagnostician, clinician, educator, research coordinator, and a source of knowledge for the team. The medical director acts as a liaison between the interdisciplinary team, the patient, and the patient's primary care physician. A designated program coordinator/director/team leader will manage the program. The individual should be a health care professional with clinical experience and expertise in the care of patients with pulmonary disease. The coordinator must understand the philosophy and goals of pulmonary rehabilitation. The program coordinator works under the guidance and supervision of the program medical director. The coordinator is responsible for the "ABCs" of the pulmonary rehabilitation program. The role may encompass program development, management, marketing, and education. The coordinator will function as a liaison with the team, facilitator of the patient's total treatment program, leader, educator, and communicator.

The need for other team members to evaluate the patient will be determined from the initial patient assessment and deficiencies noted. The composition of the interdisciplinary team will depend on the facility resources and patients' needs. Not every patient

---

Box 39-2. Interdisciplinary Team Members of a Pulmonary Rehabilitation Program[a]

Patient
Primary care physician
Medical director
Program coordinator/director/team leader
Respiratory therapist or technician
Registered or licensed vocational nurse
Physical therapist
Occupational therapist
Exercise physiologist
Dietitian
Social worker
Clinical psychologist
Social worker
Psychiatrist
Chaplain or pastoral care associate
Speech therapist
Physiatrist
Recreational therapist
Pulmonary function technologist
Patient graduate volunteers
Home care personnel
Business office representative
Vocational rehabilitation counselor

[a]Not every member of the interdisciplinary team may be involved with the patient. It depends on the individual patient assessment.

requires all of the interdisciplinary services mentioned in Box 39-2, but the services should be available if required. Each interdisciplinary team member must possess the knowledge and skills to assess, treat, train/educate, reevaluate, document, and determine home recommendations for the pulmonary patient. Program strength and success is based on the unique talents, traits, and dedication of the interdisciplinary team. Pulmonary rehabilitation is a "team effort" not a "one-person operation."

ESSENTIAL COMPONENTS OF A COMPREHENSIVE PULMONARY REHABILITATION PROGRAM

From the various published guidelines emerges a consensus regarding certain essential components to be included in pulmonary rehabilitation programs across the United States.[22,23] These components are assessment, patient training, exercise therapy, psychosocial intervention, and follow-up, with prevention incorporated into every component.[9] Patient goals and objectives are established during each component, which reinforces the foundation of the program (Fig. 39-1). Pulmonary rehabilitation is not just an exercise or education program. It is an individualized program that meets the special needs of each pulmonary patient through assessment, patient training, exercise, psychosocial intervention, and follow-up.

Prevention

The essential components of pulmonary rehabilitation must also incorporate preventive strategies, including health education that addresses risk factors, behavioral changes that decrease the risk of disease, and efforts to slow the deterioration and complications of the disease and to avoid or lessen disability.

The treatment of chronic lung disease must be directed toward preventive treatment strategies with the goals of improving patients' symptoms, function, and quality of life.[24–26] Smoking is responsible for 82% of patients diagnosed with COPD.[7] Nicotine intervention should be an integral part of every pulmonary rehabilitation program. Understanding the personal and economic impact of the symptoms of cough and shortness of breath emphasizes the need for earlier intervention, not just treatment of pulmonary disease. In fact, the top 20 reasons given by patients for physicians' office visits in 1996 ranked cough as the fourth principal reason for the visit.[27] The top 20 reasons given by patients for emergency department visits in 1996 ranked shortness of breath as the sixth principal reason for the visit and cough as the eighth.[28] The onset of COPD is very insidious, developing over 20 to 30 years. During this time the patient experiences a long asymptomatic period during which early detection of lung disease is critical. Any person with a history of smoking; a family history of lung disease; occupational or environmental exposures; and the symptoms

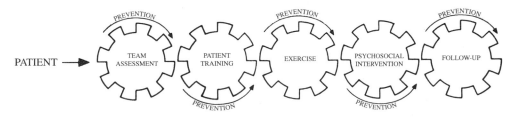

Figure 39-1. The essential components of pulmonary rehabilitation are very specific. Once the initial assessment is completed, the foundation of the patient's individualized program is developed. Prevention should be integrated into every component. Training or exercise also does not constitute a pulmonary rehabilitation program.

of chronic cough, mucus production, shortness of breath, or high blood pressure should always be given a spirometry test as advocated by the National Lung Health Education Program.[25] The spirometry test is the best assessment tool available to determine the health or disease status of a person's lungs.[26,29] "Test your lungs, know your numbers" is the motto of the National Lung Health Education Program. An interpretation tool to use with the spirometry test is "lung age."[30] The lung age interpretation is compared with the person's chronological age to give an objective picture of the individual's premature aging of his or her lungs. It is a wonderful tool to assist with prevention and improve treatment compliance. In 1979, Macklem and Permutt stated[31]:

> *"In considering the simplicity of determination of FEV$_1$ and its potential use in detecting individuals who are headed toward serious trouble at a time when intervention might have prevented a disastrous outcome, it is interesting to explore the reasons why the spirometer has not achieved a position comparable to the clinical thermometer, the sphygmomanometer, the ophthalmoscope, the chest x-ray and the electrocardiogram."*

Now is the time to be aggressive in disease prevention leading to improved quality of life. The medical community has known the scientific basis of the spirometry test for years—it is time we use it. See Chapter 18 for a detailed discussion on prevention. Prevention must be incorporated into each component of pulmonary rehabilitation if our goal is to improve the patient's quality of life and outcomes.

Assessment

The cornerstone of the pulmonary rehabilitation program is patient assessment. The process begins with a patient interview, along with documentation of the medical history, and diagnostic tests. Symptom evaluation, physical, nutritional, and activities of daily living are also evaluated. The assessment continues with an educational, exercise, and psychosocial assessment and, finally, individualized patient goals. The actual forms used for the documentation of the assessments vary from program to program.

The medical history[9] is one of the first steps in the assessment process. Most information is gathered from the patient's medical record, which can be found in inpatient records, or from the primary care or specialist's office records, along with a patient interview. The medical history typically includes comorbidities, respiratory history, family history of pulmonary disease, active medical problems, other medical and surgical histories, all current medications, allergies and drug intolerances, smoking history, risk factors, environmental exposures, vocational status, substance abuse history, goals, and supportive care needs.

Diagnostic tests complement the medical history and assist in the proper diagnosis of the rehabilitation candidate.[9] A clinical assessment alone is insufficient to detect, diagnose, or characterize lung disease. The diagnostic tests assist in developing a specific plan of care to include medication use and prescriptions for exercise therapy. Box 39-3 lists the most common diagnostic tests recommended for the initial assessment of the pulmonary rehabilitation candidate.

It is important to understand the patient's symptom history. Symptom assessment[9] includes dyspnea, cough, sputum production and fatigue, breath sounds, chest pain, hemoptysis, postnasal drainage, reflux, heartburn, edema, and dysphagia, which are common in pulmonary patients. These symptoms are typically assessed with regards to onset, location, quantity, frequency, and duration and are often included in the clinical documentation for outcomes and medical necessity for payment authorization. In fact, dyspnea, a common symptom reported by pulmonary patients, can be improved with pulmonary rehabilitation.[32]

Physical assessment[9] includes measuring and evaluating vital signs, use of accessory muscles of respiration, breathing pattern, chest examination, finger clubbing, arterial

Box 39-3. Medical Tests Recommended for the Initial Assessment of the Pulmonary Rehabilitation Candidate[a]

Prebonchodilator and postbronchodilator spirometry
Diffusing capacity
Lung volume study
Resting electrocardiogram
Resting arterial blood gases
Arterial oxygen saturation by pulse oximetry at rest and with activity
Posterior/anterior and lateral chest radiography
Complete blood cell count
Blood chemistry profile
Theophylline level (if applicable)
Exercise test with cutaneous oximetry and/or arterial blood gases

[a]It is generally recommended not to repeat the testing if done within the 3 months before starting a rehabilitation program, if the patient was stable, or as determined by the pulmonary rehabilitation medical director.

oxygen saturation measurements with pulse oximetry at rest and during activity, edema, and other signs of heart failure.[33] Nutritional assessment[9] is important in pulmonary rehabilitation because maintaining adequate nutrition is a problem in 50% of patients hospitalized with COPD, and poor nutritional status is a significant predictor of mortality.[34,35] The minimal measurements of a nutritional assessment include height, weight, body mass index, recent weight changes, fluid intake, chemistry profile, and alcohol consumption. It is suggested to have the resource of a dietitian or nutritionist available should the patient's nutritional assessment warrant further follow-up.

Educational, exercise, activities of daily living, and psychosocial evaluations complete the pulmonary rehabilitation assessment process. The educational assessment[9] evaluates the patient's knowledge of the disease and treatment program. Based on the evaluation, teaching strategies emphasizing collaborative self-management can be developed for the patient. The hospital accreditation body—the Joint Commission on Accreditation of Healthcare Organizations (JCAHO)—requires documentation of the patient's education plans, comprehension of learning, cultural diversity, language, hearing and vision interventions, and individualization and prioritization of learning needs. For this to occur, an educational assessment must be done.

To develop a safe exercise training program, the minimum exercise test performed is a 6- or 12-minute walk test, but an exercise tolerance test, or a metabolic exercise tolerance test with gas exchange, may also be appropriate. The type of exercise testing varies from program to program in the United States. This variation is driven by program objectives, individual patient status and goals, available resources, questions identified in the initial assessment process, and cost. No single testing protocol has been clearly established.

The exercise evaluation[9] is important in determining the oxygen needs during pulmonary rehabilitation and the patient's current level of functional capacity. Physical limitations, orthopedic issues, transferring abilities, and cardiac function are determined during the exercise assessment (see Box 39-4). See Chapter 12 for a detailed explanation of exercise assessment.

Activities of daily living assessment[9] includes areas of upper extremity strength, proper breathing techniques with daily activities, energy conservation techniques, food procurement and preparation, leisure impairment, sexual dysfunction, and the need for adaptive equipment. A functional task performance and work environment assessment may also be needed. See Chapter 13 for a detailed discussion of occupational therapy for the pulmonary patient.

Psychosocial assessment[9] addresses several patient areas: perception of quality of life,

Box 39-4. Key Components of an
Exercise Assessment

Physical limitations
Orthopedic problems
Breathing pattern abnormalities
Dyspnea level
Chest mobility issues
Medications prescribed, both oral and inhaled
Gait abnormalities
Transferring abilities
Exercise tolerance
Oxygen needs
Cardiac status
Exercise modifications

ability to adjust to the disease, motivation levels, emotional distress, substance abuse, cognitive impairment, interpersonal conflict, other psychopathology, significant neuropsychological impairment, coping style, and sexual dysfunction. In many pulmonary rehabilitation programs, specific outcome tools aid in addressing this assessment component. The interdisciplinary health care professionals who make up the pulmonary rehabilitation team also provide valuable resource information to meet this assessment need.

The assessment process is the foundation from which patient and program goals are developed and outcome measurements are tracked. As stated earlier, a review of the patient's medical records from the primary care physician or pulmonologist can provide a summary and overview of the past history and assessment requirements. Documentation of these assessments to include specific outcome tools are part of the patient's medical record in pulmonary rehabilitation. The ongoing assessment of the patient by the interdisciplinary team sets the strong foundation for an individualized and comprehensive pulmonary rehabilitation program. Assessment is the precursor to patient training, exercise, psychosocial intervention, and follow-up. Assessment is also critical to prevent and detect the early onset of lung disease when intervention may prevent a disastrous outcome.

Patient Training

The goals of training/education of patients with chronic lung disease and their significant others is for patients to understand their underlying pulmonary disorder and the principles of collaborative self-management. This enables patients to be active participants in their health care and improves compliance with the treatment program. See Chapter 6 for a detailed explanation of patient education. The program content covered in the rehabilitation program depends on the patient's individual needs and diagnosis.[9] A sample of topics covered in patient training are listed in Box 39-5.

Exercise Training

The exercise assessment is critical to obtain a baseline of patient function and to develop an exercise prescription, which includes a target heart rate, an oxygen prescription (to maintain an oxygen saturation level of $\geq 90\%$), and ratings of perceived exertion and dyspnea. The exercise prescription also includes upper and lower extremity training, strength training, respiratory muscle training, and a home exercise program. See Chapters 10, 11, and 12 for a detailed explanation of exercise training.

The ongoing exercise support and follow-up of patients who have completed a pulmonary rehabilitation program is a home exercise prescription. Tracking patients into a maintenance exercise program has increased significantly during the past several years. Although some patients may choose to continue the exercise therapy on their own, or in

Box 39-5. Program Content for a Pulmonary
Rehabilitation Program

Normal anatomy and physiology of the lungs
Pathophysiology of pulmonary disease
Medical test understanding
Breathing retraining
Bronchial hygiene
Medication use
Exercise principles
Energy conservation and activities of daily living
Respiratory care modalities and equipment
Collaborative self-management
Nutrition
Psychosocial issues
Ethical issues

an unsupervised setting, periodic follow-up checks by way of a telephone call or written correspondence can be helpful in complying with the lifestyle changes. A written individualized home exercise program is particularly important for this group of patients (see Box 39-6).

The exercise follow-up in either method (i.e., a supervised setting or self-directed) provides for ongoing interaction between the pulmonary rehabilitation staff, the patient, and the participant's primary care physician. Sending updated reports regarding the participant's progress and compliance with the home-based exercise program, and additional information gathered from follow-up activities and questionnaires, are methods of ensuring the relationship with the pulmonary rehabilitation team and in particular with the referring physician(s).

Psychosocial Intervention

Psychosocial intervention[9] is incorporated throughout the program in understanding the patient's medical and psychosocial stressors in their life as a result of their chronic pulmonary disease. The clinical interpretation and integration of the psychological evaluation is needed to avoid an underdiagnosis or misdiagnosis. An example is the common signs of depression (insomnia, loss of appetite, decreased energy, dysphoria, etc.), which can be directly associated with hypoxemia secondary to the pulmonary disease and not a primary diagnosis of depression. In specific cases, patient referrals to a psychologist or psychiatrist may be indicated. The type of psychosocial interventions may be one-on-one or group format. The support system developed by a program is important and may include crisis management, patient advocacy, resource acquisition, and active listening. Family members

Box 39-6. Components of a Home Exercise Program

Self-monitoring guidelines for a target heart rate, heart rate range,
    and appropriate dyspnea levels
Exercise frequency, duration, mode, and intensity
Warm-up and cool-down
Instruction on completing the exercise log
Prebronchodilator medication instructions
Breathing techniques with exercise
Exercise intervals when appropriate
Exercise advice during exacerbations
Relaxation techniques

Box 39-7. Follow-up Options for Pulmonary Rehabilitation

Maintenance exercise classes
Physician's office visits
Communicating with the primary care physician on the patient's progress
Support/emotional groups
Continuing educational meetings
Caregiver support groups such as Well Spouse
Program graduate's telephone tree
Social events
Program newsletters
Greeting cards for birthday, get well, sympathy, and "just because"
Graduate volunteering in the pulmonary rehabilitation program
Community groups such as the American Lung Association Better Breathers' Club
Telephone follow-up
Home visits
"Tune-up," reevaluation programs for graduates
Observance of National Pulmonary Rehabilitation Week
Home health referral
Vocational rehabilitation

and significant others should be encouraged to participate in the pulmonary rehabilitation program. The pulmonary patient may experience anger, hostility, depression, stress, lack of assertiveness, and anxiety. Modifying lifestyles through newly learned disease management and prevention skills is critical to prevent relapse and facilitate adaptive coping. Relaxation and stress management training is useful in reducing anxiety and depression. The evaluation, acknowledgement, and treatment of psychosocial disorders must be integrated into the comprehensive treatment plan. The pulmonary patient must be very courageous as he or she confronts the enormous challenges associated with living with chronic pulmonary disease. If the interdisciplinary team fails to detect the presence of significant psychosocial pathology, the patient will fail. Psychosocial intervention can be critical.

Follow-up

No matter how elaborate a pulmonary rehabilitation program is, if it does not incorporate a follow-up component, the benefits and program compliance will be in jeopardy. It is not conceivable to expect a patient to follow through with the multitude of home recommendations on discharge from the program unless follow-up is instituted. In the inpatient care setting, when a patient is admitted to the hospital, the goal is to work toward discharge. In the rehabilitation setting, when a patient enters a pulmonary rehabilitation program, the goal is to immediately begin working on the follow-up program for the patient. Success the patient has achieved in the program will not stand alone and must be supported on discharge with follow-up. Maintenance exercise is just one form of program follow-up.[36,37] Follow-up options vary among institutions, as listed in Box 39-7.

Rehabilitation is an ongoing process that requires long-term follow-up of months to years. Relationships and lifestyle changes are started in rehabilitation, and the nurturing that continues after program graduation will result in positive patient outcomes.

NATIONAL EMPHYSEMA TREATMENT TRIAL (NETT)

Renewed interest in the surgical excision of lung tissue from patients with diffuse emphysema and hyperinflation occurred in the United States during the 1990s. The original

Box 39-8. National Emphysema Treatment Trial Comprehensive Pulmonary Rehabilitation Model

Medical diagnostic evaluation and management
Exercise assessment and training (stretching, endurance, strength training, lower extremity, flexibility, upper extremity, strength, and a daily home exercise program)
Skills/education evaluation and training
Psychosocial assessment, counseling, and treatment
Nutritional assessment and treatment
Long-term rehabilitation follow-up

surgical procedure was described by Brantigan in the 1950s but was plagued with a high mortality rate and limited sustained clinical benefit. This surgery, which is referred to as lung volume reduction surgery (LVRS), has resulted in some patients experiencing significant improvements in dyspnea, breathing mechanics, lung function, inspiratory muscle strength, maximal walk distance, and self-selected walking velocity.[38,39] Questions from the medical community and Medicare were raised about the indications, selection criteria, complication rate, and long-term benefits of LVRS. This prompted Medicare to suspend funding for the operation in December 1995 and request additional research to determine the specific indications for the surgery, the efficacy of LVRS, and which patients are most likely to benefit from the procedure. The result is the NETT prospective collaborative clinical research study, which is cosponsored by the HCFA and the National Institutes of Health. In this study, the HCFA recognized pulmonary rehabilitation as the standard of care for the patient study groups involved. The comprehensive pulmonary rehabilitation model in the NETT includes the components shown in Box 39-8.

PROGRAM MANAGEMENT

Program management starts with understanding the customer or patient population that will be serviced by pulmonary rehabilitation. Typically this begins with an account of the number of patient admissions in your facility by diagnosis, determination of who would be eligible for pulmonary rehabilitation, and the pulmonary medicine volumes/service potential. Next to drive program management is the reimbursement status, from which revenue projections are based. As with any service line development, expenses must be offset by a revenue source. The planning of sound financial controls and solid financial projections are necessary for a successful program. However, revenue projections can be challenging because of the changing regulatory controls imposed by third-party payers in the United States. Efforts are under way to encourage and support the development of standardized reimbursement codes specifically for pulmonary rehabilitation services. Until this is completed, however, variations will continue among states and programs as to how pulmonary rehabilitation services are charged and the levels of reimbursement.

Pulmonary rehabilitation programs in the United States have typically been hospital based, in the respiratory therapy department or, as is now common, as part of a cardiovascular and pulmonary rehabilitation department. The latter is in response to the need for diversification and cross training to maintain adequate revenue sources and to reduce duplication of staff and equipment. In addition to hospital-based programs, clinics and comprehensive outpatient rehabilitation facilities are also considerations. The key factors in site selection are accessibility for patients, safe environmental conditions, and appropriate medical and emergency supervision. See Box 39-9 for location options for pulmonary rehabilitation programs.

The facilities and equipment used in pulmonary rehabilitation programs must meet state, federal, and JCAHO safety code standards. Box 39-10 provides a list of facility considerations for pulmonary rehabilitation programs.

Regardless of the facility design and equipment, the most important aspect to any successful pulmonary rehabilitation program is the interdisciplinary team, which projects confidence, enthusiasm, and a positive attitude in meeting the goals and objectives of pulmonary rehabilitation.

Participants in a pulmonary rehabilitation program are typically in small groups or on a one-on-one basis. In a 1995 national US survey of pulmonary rehabilitation programs, the average group size was nine; the mean program length was 9 weeks for 2 hours per day, 2.5 days per week, for a total program time of 45 hours.[40] It is difficult to set specific guidelines for scheduling purposes; however, a typical program in the United States may include[9] 30 to 50 hours over a 4- to 12-week period, 2 to 4 hours per day, meeting 2 to 3 days per week including the components of assessment, training/education, psychosocial intervention, and exercise.

The pulmonary rehabilitation policy and procedure manual defines the rules for the program operations. It provides a narrative description of the program services and is needed for JCAHO compliance. See Box 39-11 for a sample of contents for the pulmonary rehabilitation policy and procedure manual.

In addition to outlining the unique aspects of the pulmonary rehabilitation program, the policy and procedure manual should also include the administrative policies of the patient's rights, organizational ethics, the management of information, infection surveillance and universal precautions monitoring, safety management, and the annual departmental educational initiatives. The new employee orientation process that ensures adequate clinical training and competencies would also be part of the policy and procedure manual for pulmonary rehabilitation.

Box 39-9. Location Options for Pulmonary Rehabilitation Programs

Inpatient care
    Acute care during hospitalization
    Transitional care unit
    Rehabilitation hospital
Outpatient care
    Outpatient hospital setting
    Physician office
    Clinic setting
    Skilled nursing facility
    Subacute care facility
    Long-term care facility
    Residential outpatient facility
    Comprehensive outpatient rehabilitation facility
    Share facility with other rehabilitation programs (cardiac, etc.)
Alternative sites
    Storefront
    Home resident
    Fitness center or spa
    Wellness center
    Senior citizen center
    Local high school or community college
    Adult education center
    Places of worship
    Club meeting halls

Box 39-10. Facility Considerations for Pulmonary Rehabilitation Programs

Physical ground
  Adequate and convenient parking, including handicapped accessibility
  Elevator access, not only stairs
  Safety hazards
Program location
  Easy access to water/drinking source
  Rest rooms, including handicapped access, alarms
  Education classroom: size, emotion of environment, access, and ventilation
  Exercise facility: space, ventilation, and safety
  Clinical assessment locations
  Administrative services location
    Confidentiality of patient records
    Patient privacy
    Displayed copy of the Patient's Bill of Rights
    Emergency supplies (i.e., oxygen source, delivery apparatus, resuscitation
      mask, first aid supplies, and bronchodilator medications)
  Oxygen source, delivery apparatus, and monitoring device for oxygen
    saturation
  Storage space for equipment
  Hand washing facilities
Environmental issues
  Optimal light, temperature, and ventilation control
  Avoidance of chemical odors, scented perfumes, etc.
  Hazardous material requirements

Adapted from American Association of Cardiovascular and Pulmonary Rehabilitation. Program management. In: Guidelines for Pulmonary Rehabilitation Programs. 2nd ed. Champaign, IL: Human Kinetics, 1998.

Box 39-11. Sample of Contents for the Pulmonary Rehabilitation Policy
          and Procedure Manual

Mission statement
Patient's Bill of Rights
Criteria for patient selection and admission into the program
Process of assessment
Outline of the basic components of pulmonary rehabilitation
Hours of operations
Preentrance medical testing, exercise testing protocols, and postprogram test
  evaluations
Physician standing orders
Emergency procedure: cardiac arrest, disaster
Equipment utilization
Documentation requirements
Staffing requirements, based on a competency-based job description
Continuous quality improvement plans/outcome measurements/benchmarking
Administrative policies
Medicare rules pertaining to facility/exercise area
Facility requirements: exercise, education, administration, clinical, and rest room
  alarms
Security
Safety practices

The JCAHO is a centralized, US governmental monitoring body responsible for standard setting and voluntary accreditation of hospitals, long-term/subacute care facilities, outpatient clinics, and home care agencies. The JCAHO develops and publishes standards, skills check, and is the most important US accrediting organization in health care. The JCAHO was formed in 1951 by the American College of Surgeons, the American Hospital Association, and the American Medical Association. In 1999, the JCAHO co-sponsored a world symposium on improving health care worldwide through accreditation. Discussion topics of the symposium were as follows: Can universal quality standards be used? What influence does health care financing have on the delivery of high-quality health care? Should the health system reform be legislated and rely on the private sector? Can an accreditation system that includes professional credentialing and evidence-based practice improve health care outcomes?[41] The symposium summary stated that greater emphasis is on accountability in the United States and worldwide, which has triggered growth within the internal (organizational) quality management program and external (cross-organizational) benchmarking arena with comparative data, accreditation, or certification. Collaboration will continue to drive the quality of patient care, and the pulmonary rehabilitation program manager must be informed about these issues.

A significant component of effective program management is the tracking of clinical outcomes (JCAHO requirement) and partaking in benchmarking activities.[42–45] Outcome measurements have been addressed in Chapter 20. Benchmarking and quality improvement go hand in hand. In the past, benchmarking relied on more subjective identification of "leaders in the field." Achievable benchmark of care (ABC) is now determined by measuring and analyzing performance on process-of-care indicators.[46] Important characteristics for benchmarking are able to measure level of excellence; are demonstrable and attainable; and are derived from data in an objective, reproducible, and predetermined fashion; therefore, providers with high performance are selected to define a level of excellence, but the number of cases are carefully taken into consideration.

Benchmarking is the systematic process of searching and identifying the best practice of delivering a service and then implementing those practices that will lead to superior performance.[47] It is evaluating how pulmonary rehabilitation is delivered by different programs, and then comparing similar outcome data between programs on work processes. Examples may include referral practices, testing data, length of time in pulmonary rehabilitation, or staffing practices. The data are then evaluated to determine whether the work practice resulting in a best performance program is applicable and can be implemented in a program of lesser performance. Data gathering is necessary to have a basis from which program operations can be judged objectively and to see where improvements are necessary, which will lead to an enhanced competitive status in the market place. The key elements for benchmarking to be effective are in Box 39-12.

Box 39-12. Key Elements of Benchmarking

Determine what processes are to be defined in the benchmarking initiative
Understand your own process in detail
Determine the benchmarking project scope
Choose relevant, common, and consistent measurements or data
Study programs that reflect best practice as based on the data
Judge whether the proposed work practices are appropriate to your program and should be adopted
Plan and implement the new practices
Measure the effects of the new work practice to see if the change had an impact on performance

THE AACVPR PROGRAM CERTIFICATION

The impetus to develop a national program certification process came from the membership of the AACVPR.[48] It was believed that a standard should be developed to which pulmonary rehabilitation programs in the United States could compare/benchmark themselves. The national certification is based on the following documents:

- AACVPR Guidelines for Pulmonary Rehabilitation Programs, 2nd ed[9]
- AACVPR Clinical Competency Guidelines for Pulmonary Rehabilitation Professionals[49]
- AACVPR Outcomes Committee. Outcome Measurement in Cardiac and Pulmonary Rehabilitation[50]

It is hoped that the certification process will lead to programs being "certified" and that the process will strengthen the commitment of programs to comply with the standards, as recommended by the AACVPR.

The first program certification process began in the fall of 1998. A total of 291 applications were submitted for review, which included both pulmonary and cardiac rehabilitation programs. The recommendations of the National Program Oversight Committee with the approval of the AACVPR Board of Directors granted 254 programs certification in 1999, of which 96 were pulmonary rehabilitation programs. The certification is valid for 3 years. The application process for program certification is annual.

The feedback from the membership of the AACVPR and other professionals in the field of pulmonary rehabilitation has been positive. Most AACVPR state affiliates were involved in the process, which indicated their commitment to this new initiative. Initial concerns regarding program certification existed, such as the time commitment for programs applying and the state committees reviewing the application requirements; liability issues relative to the state's involvement; impact on the program's competition should a program become certified and another program in the same geographic area not become certified; and, finally, how the certification process might influence reimbursement. These questions have not been fully answered because of the newness of the process, and in specific circumstances they are a nonissue. It is believed that the future of program certification will grow strong and be strengthened by committing to the national standards as outlined by AACVPR. Furthermore, the practice of pulmonary rehabilitation will be enhanced throughout the United States.

CONCLUSION

As pulmonary rehabilitation specialists, we are constantly striving for excellence to bring the evidence-based practice of pulmonary rehabilitation to the patient populations we serve. We must expand beyond the traditional COPD program admission into the "other" chronic lung conditions. To have a personal and economic global impact we must incorporate prevention into each component of a comprehensive pulmonary rehabilitation program. These essential components are assessment, patient training, exercise, psychosocial intervention, and follow-up. Collaboration with our colleagues around the world will bring a new energy and optimism into pulmonary rehabilitation.

REFERENCES

1. American Lung Association. Diseases A to Z. Available at: http://www.lungusa.org/diseases/lungchronic.html. Accessed January 24, 2000.
2. Trends in chronic bronchitis and emphysema: morbidity and mortality: epidemiology and statistics unit, November 1999. Available at: http://www.lungusa.org. Accessed January 24, 2000.
3. Ten leading causes of death in the United States for 1998. Vol 47. Washington, DC: US National Center for Health Statistics, US Dept of Health and Human Services, 1999. National Vital Statistics Report No. 22.
4. Sassi-Dambron D. Pulmonary rehabilitation after treatment for lung cancer: a pilot study. Continuing Care Rehabil Bull 1999;Sept/Oct:3.
5. Trends in lung cancer morbidity and mortality: epidemiology and statistics unit, December 1999. Available at: http://www.lungusa.org/diseases/lungchronic.html. Accessed January 24, 2000.
6. Trends in asthma morbidity and mortality: epidemiology and statistics unit, November 1999. Available at: http://www.lungusa.org/diseases/lungchronic.html. Accessed January 24, 2000.
7. American Lung Association. Emphysema. Available at: http://www.lungusa.org/diseases/lungchronic.html. Accessed January 24, 2000.
8. US health expenditures, 1965-1996: health, United States, 1998. In: The World Almanac and Book of Facts. Primedia, NJ: National Center for Health Statistics, US Dept of Health and Human Services, 1999.
9. American Association of Cardiovascular and Pulmonary Rehabilitation. Guidelines for Pulmonary Rehabilitation Programs. 2nd ed. Champaign, IL: Human Kinetics, 1998.
10. American Thoracic Society. Standards for the diagnosis and care of patients with chronic obstructive pulmonary disease (COPD) and asthma. Am J Respir Crit Care Med 1995;152:577-121.
11. American Thoracic Society Medical Section of the American Lung Association. Pulmonary rehabilitation—1999. Am J Respir Crit Care Med 1999; 159:1666-1682.
12. Pulmonary rehabilitation: joint ACCP/AACVPR evidence-based guidelines. Chest 1997;112: 1363-1396.
13. Fishman AP. NIH workshop summary: pulmonary rehabilitation research. Am J Respir Crit Care Med 1994;149:825-833.
14. Medical Advisory Panel Letter, National Blue Cross and Blue Shield Association. How to Inform Payers and Influence Payment for Cardiac and Pulmonary Rehabilitation Services. Middleton, WI: American Association of Cardiovascular and Pulmonary Rehabilitation, 1999.
15. Asakura K. Collaboration of national organizations and the legislative means to advance pulmonary rehabilitation. Respir Care Clin N Am 1998; 4:173-182.
16. Fishman AP, ed. Pulmonary Rehabilitation: Lung Biology in Health and Disease. Vol 91. New York: Marcel Dekker, 1996.
17. Shneerson JM. Rehabilitation in neuromuscular disorders and thoracic wall deformities. Monaldi Arch Chest Dis 1998;53(4):415-418.
18. Koch C, McKenzie SG, Kaplowitz H, et al. International practice patterns by age and severity of lung disease in cystic fibrosis: data from the Epidemiologic Registry of Cystic Fibrosis (ERCF). Pediatr Pulmonol 1997;24(2):147-154.
19. Foster S, Thomas HM III. Pulmonary rehabilitation in lung disease other than chronic obstructive pulmonary disease. Am Rev Respir Dis 1990; 141(3):601-604.
20. Stice KA, Cunningham CA. Pulmonary rehabilitation with respiratory complications of postpolio syndrome. Rehabil Nurs 1995;21(1):37-42.
21. Kozui K, Satoru J, Koichiro N, et al. Pulmonary Rehabilitation Program Survey in North America, Europe, and Tokyo. J Cardiopulm Rehabil 1998; 18:301-308.
22. Celli BR. Standards for the optimal management of COPD: a summary. Chest 1998;113(Suppl 4):283S-287S.
23. Mahler DA. Pulmonary rehabilitation. Chest 1998;113(Suppl 4):263S-268S.
24. Ferguson GT. Management of COPD: early identification and active intervention are crucial. Postgrad Med 1998;103(4):129-134, 136-141.
25. The National Lung Health Education Program Executive Committee. Strategies in preserving lung health and preventing COPD and associated diseases: the National Lung Health Education Program (NLHEP). Chest 1998;113(Suppl): 123S-155S.
26. Connors GL, Hilling L. Prevention, not just treatment. Respir Care Clin N Am 1998;4:1-12.
27. Top 20 reasons given by patient for physician's office visits, 1996. In: The World Almanac and Book of Facts. Primedia, NJ: National Center for Health Statistics, US Dept of Health and Human Services, 1999.
28. Top 20 reasons given by patients for emergency room visits, 1996. In: The World Almanac and Book of Facts. Primedia, NJ: National Center for Health Statistics, US Dept of Health and Human Services, 1999.
29. Petty TL. Pulmonary rehabilitation: where we've been and where we should be going. Presented at the Ninth Annual Meeting of the American Association of Cardiovascular and Pulmonary Rehabilitation, Portland, OR, October 1994.
30. Morris JF, Temple W. Spirometric "lung age" estimates for motivating smoking cessation. Prev Med 1985;14:655-662.
31. Macklem PR, Permutt S. The Lung in Transition Between Health and Disease. New York: Marcel Dekker, 1979.
32. Mahler DA, Havel A. Clinical measurement of dyspnea. In: Dyspnea. Mahler DA, ed. Mount Kesco, NY: Futura, 1996:75-100.
33. Pierson DJ, Wilkins RL. Clinical skills in respiratory care. In: Pierson DJ, Kacmarek RM, eds. Foundation of Respiratory Care. New York: Churchill Livingstone, 1992:431-455.
34. Donahoe M. Nutritional aspects of lung disease. Respir Care Clin N Am 1998;4:85-112.
35. Gray-Donald K, et al. Nutritional status and mor-

tality in chronic obstructive pulmonary disease. Am J Respir Crit Care Med 1996;153:961–966.

36. Garvey C. Maintenance exercise for pulmonary patients. Continuing Care Rehabil Bull 1999; May/June:3–4.

37. Grosbois JM, Lamblin C, Lemaire B, et al. Long term benefits of exercise maintenance after outpatient rehabilitation program in patients with chronic obstructive pulmonary disease. J Cardiopulm Rehabil 1999;19:2160–225.

38. Cooper JD, et al. Bilateral pneumectomy (volume reduction) for chronic obstructive pulmonary disease. J Thorac Cardiovasc Surg 1995;109:106–119.

39. Sciurba FC, et al. Improvements in pulmonary function and elastic recoil after lung volume reduction surgery. N Engl J Med 1996;334:1095–1099.

40. Bickford LS, Hodgkin JE, MacIntruff SC. National Pulmonary Rehabilitation Survey: update. J Cardiopulm Rehabil 1995;15:406–411.

41. Ente BH. Joint Commission World Symposium on Improving Health Care Through Accreditation. Jt. Comm J Qual Improv 1999;25:602–613.

42. Jungbauer JS, Fuller B. Feasibility of a multi-state outcomes program for cardiopulmonary rehabilitation. J Cardiopulm Rehabil 1999;19(6):352–359.

43. Consortium of Health Systems. Health systems consortium puts benchmarking online. Data Strateg Benchmarks 1999;3(6):87–89.

44. Moralis M. Benchmarking web sites. Hosp Q 1998;1(3):80–82.

45. The 1998 benchmarking guide. Available at: http://www.amhpi.com/hhn/doc16428.htm. Accessed January 24, 2000.

46. Weissman NW, Allison JJ, Kiefe Cl, et al. Achievable benchmarks of care: the ABCs of benchmarking. J Eval Clin Pract 1999;5(3):269–281.

47. Bogan C, English M. Benchmarking for Best Practice. New York: McGraw-Hill Inc, 1994.

48. American Association of Cardiovascular and Pulmonary Rehabilitation web site. Available at: http://www.aacvpr.org. Accessed February 2, 2000.

49. Pulmonary Clinical Competencies Working Group of the American Association of Cardiovascular and Pulmonary Rehabilitation. Clinical competency guidelines for pulmonary rehabilitation professionals. J Cardiopulm Rehabil 1995; 15:173–178.

50. AACVPR Outcomes Committee. Outcome measurement in cardiac and pulmonary rehabilitation. J Cardiopulm Rehabil 1995;15:394–405.

40 Benefits and the Future of Pulmonary Rehabilitation

John E. Hodgkin

⬭ Professional Skills

Upon completion of this chapter, the reader will be able to:

- Describe the reported benefits to those patients who participate in a pulmonary rehabilitation program
- Discuss the benefits of the individual components of care used for those with chronic lung disease
- List issues of concern in pulmonary rehabilitation that still need to be resolved or clarified

As emphasized in the preceding chapters, pulmonary rehabilitation requires the use of many individually tailored treatment modalities and a management system that can be used to help the patient achieve and maintain the highest functional capacity possible. Box 40-1 outlines the components of a pulmonary rehabilitation program. Many benefits have been reported by pulmonary rehabilitation programs using these components of care.[1-6] The overall benefits reported for pulmonary rehabilitation programs, the demonstrated benefits for each individual component of care, and the future of pulmonary rehabilitation are discussed in this chapter.

OVERALL BENEFITS OF PULMONARY REHABILITATION

A summary of benefits reported through the use of the pulmonary rehabilitation modalities described in this book is shown in Box 40-2. Many patients achieve reduction in respiratory symptoms, reversal of anxiety and depression, and improvement in their sense of control over their status.[7-9] All programs have reported an enhanced ability, for most patients, to carry out activities of daily living,[10-21] improved exercise ability,[22-65] better quality of life,[10-21,47,50,51,63,66-73] and decreased dyspnea.[4,47,49,62-64,68,74-76] Some patients are able to continue or return to gainful employment.[10,13,48,49,51,69,77-80] All of the randomized controlled trials of pulmonary rehabilitation (seven to date) have reported benefits from the programs (Table 40-1).[47-51,68,69,75]

A reduction in the number of days of hospitalization required by patients with chronic obstructive pulmonary disease (COPD) following pulmonary rehabilitation has been reported.[8,15,20,78,79,81-90] Patients at Loma Linda University Medical Center had a reduction

Box 40-1. Components of Pulmonary Rehabilitation

General
    Patient and family education
    Proper nutrition, including weight control
    Avoidance of smoking and other inhaled irritants
    Avoidance of infection (e.g., immunization)
    Proper environment
    Adequate hydration
Medications
    Bronchodilators
    Expectorants
    Antimicrobials
    Corticosteroids
    Cromolyn sodium/nedocromil sodium
    Leukotriene antagonists/inhibitors
    Diuretics
    Psychopharmacologic agents
Respiratory therapy techniques
    Aerosol therapy
    Oxygen therapy
    Home use of ventilators
Physical therapy modalities
    Relaxation training
    Breathing retraining
    Chest percussion and postural drainage
    Deliberate coughing and expectoration
Exercise conditioning
Occupational therapy
    Evaluate activities of daily living
    Outline energy-conserving maneuvers
Psychosocial rehabilitation
Vocational rehabilitation

from approximately 19 days of hospitalization in the year before the pulmonary rehabilitation program to slightly more than 6 days of hospitalization in the year after completion of the program.[81] This trend continued for the 8 years for which follow-up data were available.[81] Some might suggest that this reduction in days of hospitalization simply reflects the deaths of the sickest patients during the initial years of follow-up, leaving healthier patients toward the end. However, the curve for hospital days required during the 8-year period for only those patients still surviving at the end of 8 years was similar to the curve reflecting data for all of the patients (Fig. 40-1). This decrease in hospital days obviously

Box 40-2. Demonstrated Benefits of Pulmonary Rehabilitation

Reduction in dyspnea
Reversal of anxiety and depression
Improved mastery (sense of control) over status
Enhanced ability to carry out activities of daily living
Increased exercise ability
Better quality of life
Reduction in hospital days required
Prolongation of life in selected patients (i.e., use of continuous oxygen in patients with severe hypoxemia)

Table 40-1. Randomized Controlled Trials of Pulmonary Rehabilitation

Study	Study Design	Patients (No.)	Patient Characteristics	Outcomes
Goldstein et al., 1994[50]	8 wk of inpatient rehabilitation followed by 16 wk of partially supervised home training vs. control group given conventional care	89	Treatment group mean age, 66 y; FEV$_1$, 35% predicted	Treatment group had significant increases (37.9 m) in 6MWD and submaximal cycle endurance time (4.7 min) and significant improvements in dyspnea, emotion, and mastery components of the CRDQ and dyspnea as measured by the TDI (+2.7 units).
Reardon et al., 1994[75]	6 wk of comprehensive outpatient rehabilitation vs. untreated control group	20	Treatment group mean age, 66 y; FEV$_1$, 35% predicted	No significant change in maximal exercise testing in either group; rehabilitation patients had significantly lower exertional dyspnea during exercise testing and lower overall dyspnea as measured by the TDI
Ries et al., 1995[47]	8 wk of comprehensive outpatient rehabilitation vs. educational control group	119	Treatment group mean age, 61.5 y; FEV$_1$, 1.21 L	Significant postrehabilitation improvement in $\dot{V}O_2$max and treadmill endurance time and decreased exertional and overall dyspnea; no significant postrehabilitation change in HRQL (Quality of Well-Being score), number of hospital days, or survival
Wijkstra et al., 1994[68] and 1996[48]	12 wk of home-based multidisciplinary rehabilitation vs. untreated control group	43	Treatment group mean age, 64 y; mean FEV$_1$, 44% predicted	Treatment group showed a significant increase in work rate, $\dot{V}O_2$max, and 6MWD (438–447 m) and decreases in exertional dyspnea and inspiratory muscle work rate during incremental cycle exercise testing; HRQL (CRDQ) increased significantly in the treatment group
Strijbos et al., 1996[49]	12 wk of hospital-based outpatient vs. 12 wk of home rehabilitation vs. untreated control group followup, 18 mo	45	Treatment group mean ages 61.2 and 60.0 y; FEV$_1$, 40.4 and 45.5% predicted in outpatient and home rehabilitation groups	Both outpatient and home-based rehabilitation groups had increases in maximal cycle work level and 4MWD and decreases in exertional dyspnea compared with the control group; gains made in the outpatient group tended to peak after formal rehabilitation then gradually decline; those in home-based rehabilitation tended to gradually increase during the 18-mo observation period
Bendstrup et al., 1997[51]	12 wk of hospital-based outpatient rehabilitation vs. untreated control group	32	Treatment group mean age, 64 y; mean FEV$_1$, 1.02 L	At 12 and 24 wk, the treatment group had a significant increase in 6MWD (113 vs. 21 m) and activities of daily living higher than the control group; CRDQ scores were significantly higher at 24 wk
Wedzicha et al., 1998[69]	8 wk of exercise and education vs. education alone; hospital or home based depending on level of dyspnea	126	Mean ages ranged from 69 to 73 y; mean FEV$_1$, 36 to 38% predicted	In the group with moderate dyspnea (n = 66), exercise training and education led to improvement in the shuttle walking distance and health status compared with education alone; exercise ability and health status did not significantly change in either group with severe dyspnea

FEV$_1$, forced expiratory volume in 1 second; 6MWD, 6-min walk distance; CRDQ, Chronic Respiratory Disease Questionnaire; TDI, Transitional Dyspnea Index; $\dot{V}O_2$max, maximal oxygen consumption; HRQL, health-related quality of life.
With permission from Official Statement of the American Thoracic Society: pulmonary rehabilitation—1999. Am J Respir Crit Care Med 1999;159:1666.

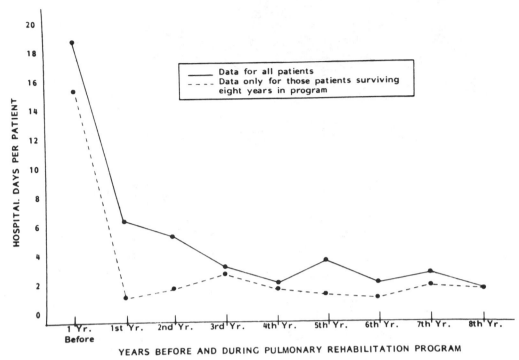

Figure 40-1. Analysis of hospital days before and during a pulmonary rehabilitation program, Loma Linda University Medical Center.

can result in a substantial reduction in cost by helping the patient function more adequately in an outpatient setting.

Although the decrement in forced expiratory volume in 1 second (FEV_1) for a normal population is estimated to be 20 to 30 mL/y,[91,92] the reported decrement for patients with COPD ranges from 40 to 80 mL/y.[93–100] No study yet reported has shown a significant alteration in the mean rate of decrease in the FEV_1 in COPD patients with significant respiratory impairment.

It is commonly stated that no evidence exists that pulmonary rehabilitation for patients with COPD improves survival. Although it is clear that oxygen therapy significantly improves survival in COPD patients who are seriously hypoxemic,[101,102] many believe that the other aspects of care commonly used in these persons do not significantly prolong life. However, some reports suggest that pulmonary rehabilitation can lead to improved survival.

In a study comparing 252 rehabilitated COPD patients with 50 control subjects selected from an outpatient clinic, Haas and Cardon[13] reported 5-year mortality rates from respiratory failure of 22% in rehabilitated patients compared with 42% in control subjects.

In a study by Petty and associates,[93] 182 COPD patients (mean FEV_1, 0.94 L) were accepted for pulmonary rehabilitation between 1966 and 1968. Survival at 5 years was 41% and at 10 years was 17%. Patients who participated in this program in Denver had significantly improved survival at 2.5 years compared with the only other study of COPD patients residing at a similar high altitude (i.e., the Veterans Administration Cooperative Study by Renzetti and coworkers).[99] Survival at 2.5 years in the study by Petty et al. was 67% compared with 50% in the Veterans Administration Cooperative Study. Petty et al. also reported slightly better survival in patients participating in their pulmonary rehabilitation program compared with matched control patients who received ordinary care in the same community.[103]

In a report by Hodgkin and associates,[104,105] patients (mean FEV_1, 1.53 L) participating in a university hospital pulmonary rehabilitation program showed significantly better long-term survival than in most previous reports (i.e., 5-year survival was 86% and 10-year survival was 64%). Patients in this study had chronic bronchitis and/or emphysema (patients with evidence of asthma were excluded). Of particular note is that pulmonary function was less impaired in these patients than in those studied by Burrows et al.,[106] Postma et al.,[98,107] and Petty et al.[93] In an attempt to compare patients from this pulmonary rehabilitation program with those of like severity getting "ordinary care" but not participating in a formal pulmonary rehabilitation program, patients with an FEV_1 above 1.24 L from this study were compared with patients with a similar level of pulmonary impairment from the Burrows and Earle Chicago study.[94] Patients from the pulmonary rehabilitation program of Hodgkin and associates with an FEV_1 greater than 1.24 L had a significantly better survival rate at 2 to 7 years of follow-up than did patients with similar impairment in the Burrows and Earle study. The authors point out that the improved survival rate in the group, as a whole, was probably because the patients entering this study had milder disease. However, they also suggested that the good comprehensive respiratory care, including careful follow-up, they received through the pulmonary rehabilitation program might also be responsible for some of the improved survival compared with that in earlier studies.

Sneider and colleagues[87] reported the experience of patients participating in their pulmonary rehabilitation program between 1976 and 1987. During this time, 1592 patients were evaluated; however, only 212 patients (mean FEV_1, 1.19 L) completed the entire pulmonary rehabilitation program. Patients with a reactive airway disease component were not specifically excluded from this study population. Survival at 5 and 10 years was 86% and 66%, respectively. Of particular interest was the comparison performed by Sneider and associates of their 212 patients completing the pulmonary rehabilitation program with the 921 patients with similar impairment who did not complete the rehabilitation program and with a group of 100 randomly selected patients with similar pulmonary impairment who died of COPD at the same hospital during a 10-year period.[87] Five- and 10-year survival was significantly better in those completing the full pulmonary rehabilitation program than in the other two groups from the same community and cared for at the same hospital.

Burns and coauthors[108] reported the results of patients (mean FEV_1, 0.97 L) completing a pulmonary rehabilitation program between 1977 and 1987. Subjects in this study had emphysema and/or chronic bronchitis. Survival figures from this study were better than those in the Burrows Chicago study.[106] Survival in the Burrows Chicago study (200 COPD patients with a mean FEV_1 of 1.04 L) was 52% at 5 years and 23% at 10 years compared with 58% at 5 years and 32% at 10 years in the Burns and associates study.

One of the largest studies to suggest that good comprehensive care may improve survival in patients with COPD is the National Institutes of Health Intermittent Positive-Pressure Breathing (NIH/IPPB) trial.[109,110] In this study, a definite effort was made to exclude asthmatics and include only those patients with typical COPD (985 patients with a mean FEV_1 of 1.03 L). The age and level of pulmonary impairment was similar to those of subjects in the Burrows Chicago study.[106] A comparison of patients from the NIH/IPPB study was made with those from the Burrows Chicago group. Survival was similar in patients with the least obstruction (postbronchodilator FEV_1 above 42.5% of predicted) but, as shown in Figure 40-2, in more obstructed patients, was greater in the NIH/IPPB patients than in the Burrows Chicago group. The most obvious potential explanation for this would seem to be that the Burrows group did not exclude hypoxemic patients, as was done in the NIH/IPPB study. The first 3 years of the Burrows study preceded the widespread use of home oxygen therapy, which was given to patients in the NIH/IPPB study who became significantly hypoxemic during the study. This is a reasonable explanation for survival differences among patients with the most severe obstruction (FEV_1, <30.5% of predicted); 22% of the NIH/IPPB patients in this category eventually received

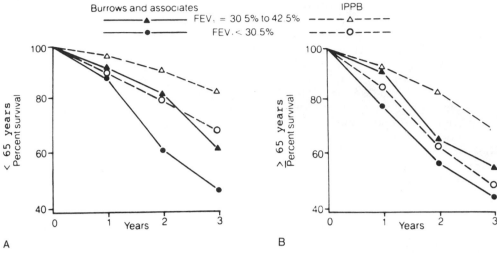

Figure 40-2. Comparison of survival in the National Institutes of Health Intermittent Positive-Pressure Breathing (*IPPB*) trial (*open symbols*) with that of patients in the Burrows Chicago study (*closed symbols*). **A.** Patients younger than 65 years at the start of the studies. **B.** Patients 65 years of age and older. *Circles,* patients with a baseline postbronchodilator forced expiratory volume in 1 second (*FEV₁*) of less than 30.5% predicted; *triangles,* patients with a baseline postbronchodilator FEV_1 of 30.5 to 42.5% predicted. (Reprinted with permission from Anthonisen NR, Wright EC, Hodgkin JE, et al. Prognosis in chronic obstructive pulmonary disease. Am Rev Respir Dis 1986;133:14–20.)

home oxygen therapy. However, only 12% of the less-obstructed patients (FEV_1, 30.5–42.5% of predicted) in the NIH/IPPB study received home oxygen, so this is not likely to account for mortality differences between these two groups. It is certainly possible that survival was better in the NIH/IPPB patients because of the careful assessment, education, and intense follow-up (i.e., good comprehensive respiratory care) they received as being part of a clinical trial.

One randomized controlled trial compared the effect of a pulmonary rehabilitation program with a group education program in 119 patients with COPD.[47] Survival at 6 years was slightly better in the group participating in the comprehensive pulmonary rehabilitation program, that is, 67%, compared with 56% for the education-only group. This difference, however, was not statistically significant, possibly because of the lack of power, that is, not enough individuals enrolled in the study to detect a significant survival advantage.

The factors that affect survival in patients with COPD have been reviewed.[111] The patient's postbronchodilator FEV_1 and age have been reported to be the best predictors of survival.[110,111] It seems logical that if one is to achieve a significant reduction in the rate of respiratory function deterioration and definite prolongation of life, the principles of pulmonary rehabilitation discussed in this book must be applied earlier in the course of the disease rather than waiting until severe, irreversible impairment of function is present.

A Joint Committee of the American College of Chest Physicians and the American Association of Cardiovascular and Pulmonary Rehabilitation developed a report reviewing the scientific literature dealing with pulmonary rehabilitation in patients with COPD.[5] The report reviewed the scientific basis for pulmonary rehabilitation in patients with COPD, in whom most of the research in this area has been conducted. The document reviewed therapeutic components in pulmonary rehabilitation including lower extremity training, upper extremity training, ventilatory muscle training, and psychosocial/behavioral interventions. Health outcome topics reviewed included psychosocial/behavioral

Table 40-2. Summary of Recommendations and Evidence Grades for Pulmonary Rehabilitation Guidelines for Patients With COPD

Component/Outcome	Recommendations	Grade
Lower extremity training	Lower extremity training improves exercise tolerance and is recommended as part of pulmonary rehabilitation	A
Upper extremity training	Strength and endurance training improves arm function; arm exercises should be included in pulmonary rehabilitation	B
Ventilatory muscle training	Scientific evidence does not support the routine use of VMT in pulmonary rehabilitation; it may be considered in selected patients with decreased respiratory muscle strength and breathlessness	B
Psychosocial, behavioral, and educational components and outcomes	Evidence does not support the benefits of short-term psychosocial interventions as single therapeutic modalities; longer-term interventions may be beneficial; expert opinion supports inclusion of educational and psychosocial intervention components in pulmonary rehabilitation	C
Dyspnea	Pulmonary rehabilitation improves the symptom of dyspnea	A
Quality of life	Pulmonary rehabilitation improves health-related quality of life	B
Health care utilization	Pulmonary rehabilitation has reduced the number of hospitalizations and days of hospitalization	B
Survival	Pulmonary rehabilitation may improve survival	C

With permission from Pulmonary rehabilitation: joint ACCP/AACVPR evidence-based guidelines. Chest 1997;112:1363.
COPD, chronic obstructive pulmonary disease; VMT, ventilatory muscle training.

measures, dyspnea, quality of life, health care utilization, and survival. The committee assigned a letter grade designating the overall strength of the scientific evidence for each of the recommendations made. The following rating scale was used: A, scientific evidence provided by well-designed, well-conducted, controlled trials (randomized and nonrandomized) with statistically significant results that consistently support the guideline recommendation; B, scientific evidence provided by observational studies or by controlled trials with less consistent results to support the guideline recommendation; C, expert opinion that supports the guideline recommendation because the available scientific evidence did not present consistent results or because controlled trials were lacking. See Table 40-2 for a summary of recommendations and evidence grades in this document.

BENEFITS OF INDIVIDUAL COMPONENTS OF CARE

General Care

Although few data have been published relating to the value of education for respiratory patients, teaching patients about their disease process and its treatment is an integral part of pulmonary rehabilitation (see Chapter 6).[112,113] A pulmonary rehabilitation knowledge test has been developed and validated.[114] Education of COPD patients can indeed improve their knowledge of the disease.[113,115]

A careful evaluation of nutritional factors and diet patterns can be of major help to patients with COPD. In obese patients, a weight-reduction program can lessen the work of breathing, resulting in reduced dyspnea. A high-protein diet, with multiple small feedings, can help prevent or reverse weight loss. Adequate protein in the diet may help reverse the diminished respiratory muscle strength observed in poorly nourished individuals.[116] Proper nutrition may help patients resist respiratory infections[117] and may help restore the ventilatory response to hypoxemia[118] and hypercapnia[119] in severely mal-nourished individuals. Reduced body weight has been reported to be a predictor of survival, independent of the FEV_1.[120-122] Currently, data are insufficient to determine whether adequate nutrition support in undernourished patients with COPD can significantly alter their survival. However, studies suggest that further clinical research to help answer this question is justifiable.[121,123,124] (See Chapter 14 for further information regarding nutrition support.)

Cessation of smoking is fundamental to achieving subjective and objective improvement. Stopping smoking generally results in an improved appetite, decreased dyspnea, a reduction in cough and sputum, and improved pulmonary function.[125,126] Smoking has been shown to increase the risk of getting an influenza infection.[127] The Lung Health Study[128] demonstrated that patients with mild degrees of airway obstruction had improvements in their FEV_1 and a slower rate of decline compared with patients who continued to smoke. One of the most impressive studies to show that stopping smoking can improve survival in COPD patients was that reported by Postma and Sluiter[107] (Fig. 40-3). (For a comprehensive discussion of smoking cessation, see Chapter 15.)

Influenza vaccinations, yearly, and a pneumococcal vaccine help reduce the risk from these specific infections. It has recently been recommended that the pneumococcal vaccina-

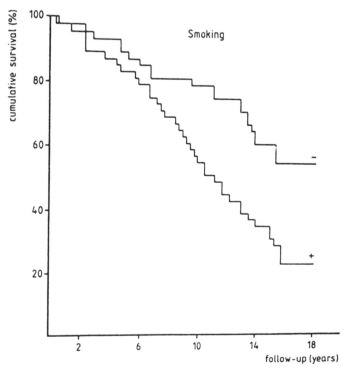

Figure 40-3. Cumulative survival curves of continuing smokers (+) and ex-smokers (−). (Reprinted with permission from Postma DS, Sluiter HJ. Prognosis of chronic obstructive pulmonary disease: the Dutch experience. Am Rev Respir Dis 1989;140:S100.)

tion be repeated in individuals older than 65 years if it has been more than 5 years since their initial vaccination.[129] Because dehydration can thicken sputum, promote atelectasis, and drop cardiac output, adequate hydration should be promoted.

Medications

Almost all patients benefit from a consistent program of medications, as described in Chapter 7. On the other hand, all these agents have significant side effects and, when not used appropriately, can lead to a worsening of the patient's conditions. Bronchodilators not only help relieve bronchospasm but also can enhance mucociliary clearance. Antimicrobial agents limit the airway irritation and inflammation that result from bacterial respiratory infections. Corticosteroids lessen airway inflammation and the adverse effects of allergy; in addition, they facilitate bronchodilator action. Two nonsteroidal anti-inflammatory medications, cromolyn sodium and nedocromil sodium, available for inhalation, and several leukotriene antagonists, available in oral form, can reduce the need for corticosteroids in patients with bronchial asthma. Digitalis is useful for patients with left ventricular failure, and diuretics are beneficial for the fluid retention of left ventricular decompensation and cor pulmonale. Proper use of psychopharmacologic agents can significantly improve some COPD patients' ability to function effectively.

Respiratory Therapy Techniques

Aerosol Therapy

Various devices have been used to aerosolize bronchodilators, corticosteroids, nonsteroidal anti-inflammatory agents, mucolytic agents, bland mist, and antimicrobials. Although little support exists for aerosolization of the latter three agents, clearly inhalation of bronchodilators and the anti-inflammatory medications are of tremendous benefit. Inhalation of a sympathomimetic medication accomplishes faster bronchodilation, with fewer systemic side effects, than oral ingestion or parenteral administration of the same agent. Inhalation of corticosteroids accomplishes much of the anti-inflammatory effect while significantly reducing the risk of systemic side effects. (See Chapter 8 for a discussion of aerosol therapy.)

Oxygen Therapy

Supplemental oxygen has clearly been shown to lessen the adverse effects of significant hypoxemia, such as pulmonary hypertension, polycythemia, and neuropsychologic dysfunction, in COPD patients. Specifically, patients with an arterial partial pressure of oxygen of 55 mm Hg or less on room air (oxygen saturation $\leq$88%) or less than 60 mm Hg (oxygen saturation <90%) and evidence of polycythemia or right-sided heart dysfunction, when stable, have achieved a significant prolongation of life with continuous oxygen compared with nocturnal oxygen only.[101,102] Patients who develop significant hypoxemia during exercise testing can improve their exercise tolerance by using supplemental oxygen during exercise training.[22,130–134] Nocturnal oxygen is beneficial for patients with sleep apnea or arrhythmias resulting from nocturnal hypoxemia.[135–137] Use of supplemental oxygen in patients with severe hypoxemia can result in a survival rate similar to that of patients with similar levels of impairment (i.e., FEV_1) but without severe hypoxemia (Fig. 40-4).[110] (See Chapter 9 for the latest concepts regarding oxygen therapy.)

Assistance With Mechanical Ventilation

Although IPPB therapy was used for many years in patients with pulmonary disorders, no evidence suggests that in outpatients with chronic disease such therapy has any advantage over less expensive and simpler methods of aerosol therapy, such as cartridge inhalers or compressor nebulizers. The National Heart, Lung, and Blood Institute–sponsored study comparing IPPB devices with compressor nebulizers in outpatients with COPD

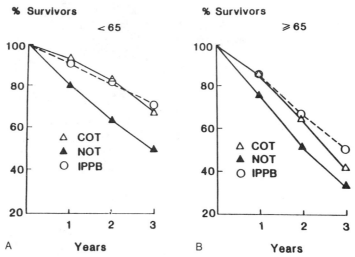

Figure 40-4. Comparison of survival in the National Institutes of Health Intermittent Positive-Pressure Breathing (*IPPB*) and NOTT trials. All patients had a baseline FEV_1 of less than 30% predicted. **A.** Data from patients younger than 65 years at the beginning of the studies. **B.** Patients 65 years of age and older. *Circles,* patients in the IPPB trial; *open triangles,* hypoxemic patients receiving continuous oxygen therapy (*COT*); *closed triangles,* hypoxemic patients receiving 12 hours of nocturnal oxygen therapy (*NOT*). (Reprinted with permission from Anthonisen NR, Wright EC, Hodgkin JE, et al. Prognosis in chronic obstructive pulmonary disease. Am Rev Respir Dis 1986;133:14–20.)

showed no difference in morbidity or mortality between patients in the two groups.[109] This evaluation in 985 patients did not demonstrate any role for periodic IPPB treatments in outpatients with COPD. Noninvasive ventilation, nasal or oral, and ventilation via a tracheotomy tube may be useful in patients with chronic respiratory failure (see Chapters 21 and 22).

Physical Therapy Modalities

Relaxation Training

Relaxation techniques, such as biofeedback or listening to soothing music, can help anxious patients reduce fear and tension and may be useful for persons with the high-fear–high-anxiety personality type[138,139]; however, long-term benefits from these brief interventions have not been demonstrated.[6] Some relaxation exercises, such as contracting and then relaxing skeletal muscle groups, can help reduce dyspnea and anxiety in patients with COPD.[140] Other demonstrated benefits include a slowing of the respiratory rate and heart rate, as well as lowering oxygen consumption.[141,142]

Breathing Retraining

Training patients with COPD to slow their respiratory rate with a prolonged exhalation (with or without the use of pursed lips) helps control dyspnea and results in improved ventilation, increased tidal volume, decreased respiratory rate, and a reduced alveolar–arterial oxygen difference.[143–148] Such a breathing pattern not only helps relieve dyspnea but can improve the ability to exercise and carry out activities of daily living. The benefits of pursed-lips breathing are often discovered by patients before instruction from health care providers. A couple of reports describe an increase in breathlessness with pursed-lips breathing in COPD patients at rest[149] and during exercise.[150] An early study reported benefit from diaphragmatic breathing[151]; however, recent studies have questioned the value of this technique in COPD patients.[152–154]

An improvement in respiratory muscle strength and endurance can be accomplished through voluntary normocapnic hyperpnea[155-159] and inspiratory resistive loading.[160] Although ventilatory muscle endurance training can result in improved exercise capacity in some COPD patients,[158-161] evidence is not yet available that respiratory muscle training adds to the improved quality of life or enhanced activity level that can be achieved through exercise training using the lower or upper extremities.[5]

Deliberate Cough, Chest Percussion, and Postural Drainage

Teaching patients how to cough properly can result in more effective expectoration. The forced expiration technique for coughing has been recommended for expectorating sputum.[162,163] Postural drainage, when accompanied by chest percussion or vibration, has also been recommended to help clear secretions from obstructed airways. Positive expiratory pressure therapy has been advocated as an adjunct for individuals who have difficulty expectorating airway secretions.[164,165] A comprehensive review of chest physical therapy was recently published.[166] In the outpatient setting, postural drainage should be reserved for patients with large amounts of sputum (i.e., >30 mL/d).[167] No evidence is available that postural drainage is beneficial in COPD patients with smaller amounts of sputum during acute exacerbations of COPD[168] or in those with uncomplicated pneumonia.[169] (See Chapter 12 for a review of chest physical therapy.)

Exercise Conditioning

Exercise training should be an essential component of any pulmonary rehabilitation program. Many studies have reported an enhanced exercise level following such general conditioning exercises as walking, bicycle riding, and swimming.[22-65]

One of the greatest benefits of exercise conditioning is to allow patients to do more work for any given oxygen consumption. In effect, patients become more efficient, and increased muscular strength and endurance enable them to accomplish more. As a result, the patients can better tolerate daily activities. Although exercise training has little effect on pulmonary function, it has been shown to improve sleep, appetite, and tolerance of dyspnea. Studies demonstrate that COPD patients can exercise at a considerably higher percentage of their maximal exercise capacity than had originally been recommended.[58,170-172] Exercise training above the anaerobic threshold has been reported to achieve more benefit than training at a lower intensity level in COPD patients who can exercise to a high enough intensity to reach an anaerobic threshold.[52,53,65,173] Adding upper extremity exercise training to traditional lower extremity training is recommended for COPD patients.[5,61,174-178] (See Chapters 10 and 11 for a comprehensive discussion concerning a proper approach to exercise training in patients with respiratory disease.)

Occupational Therapy

An occupational therapy evaluation will help identify short- and long-term reasonable goals for the patient, will disclose tasks important for the patient that are precluded by functional limitations, and will reveal patterns of daily activities in which energy can be conserved for other productive and worthwhile activities. A home visit will often disclose unexpected architectural barriers and often leads to significant improvement in the patient's ability to function in his or her real world (see Chapter 13).

Psychosocial Rehabilitation

Patients disabled from COPD commonly exhibit emotional reactions, such as depression, fear, anxiety, hostility, and denial, all of which impair functional capacity.[7] Psychotherapy, sometimes requiring a psychologist or psychiatrist, and the appropriate use of psychopharmacologic agents can help such patients better cope with their disease process (see Chapter 16). Sexual dysfunction is often a crucial obstacle to overall rehabilitation and should be addressed positively (see Chapter 17). The attitudes transmitted by the entire rehabilitation team and the interactions among the patients themselves contribute significantly to the psychologic rehabilitation of the patients.

Vocational Rehabilitation

Although some individuals will be able to continue working in their current occupations, many others will need to either quit their jobs or to alter the type of work performed. A proper evaluation and categorization of the patient's capacities are important for successful rehabilitation. The goals of vocational and functional rehabilitation may vary after careful evaluation of the patient. Possible goals include:

- Returning the patient to the job he or she is holding
- Returning the patient to the same occupational field or plant but in a different job or location
- Changing the occupational field to a totally different one in which the patient can use previous training or existing skills
- Job retraining and reemployment
- Entering the patient in a sheltered workshop program
- Retraining the individual in daily self-care with an eye to conservation of effort and efficiency of motion[179]

When a patient is employed in an unhealthy environment, or if further progression of disease is anticipated and continued employment therefore unlikely, it may be desirable to train the patient for a sedentary occupation in anticipation of the future course of the disease.

Lung Surgery

Lung transplantation in patients with serious lung impairment can clearly improve a patient's level of activity and length of life.[180] The role of pulmonary rehabilitation with and without lung volume reduction surgery in COPD patients is being assessed currently in a multicenter National Heart, Lung, and Blood Institute trial.[181] Pulmonary rehabilitation should be used routinely, preoperatively, in patients scheduled for lung transplantation.[182] (See Chapter 23 for a discussion of surgical intervention in patients with COPD.)

FUTURE CHALLENGES OF PULMONARY REHABILITATION

Although no slowing of the rate of pulmonary function deterioration has been shown, reports of improvement in survival through pulmonary rehabilitation were reviewed earlier in this chapter. Clearly, instituting a comprehensive respiratory care program earlier in the course of a patient's disease will provide more potential for favorably altering the course of the disease.

Unfortunately, only 20 to 35% of participants in most smoking cessation programs quit permanently. An enhanced effort needs to be directed toward the prevention of respiratory diseases rather than waiting until significant respiratory impairment has occurred to begin instituting therapy.

Visiting nurse associations and such socially oriented service programs as Meals on Wheels and Homemakers exist in many locations; however, the establishment of such services in every community would substantially enhance the ability for pulmonary rehabilitation programs to provide adequate support.

The evidence that pulmonary patients reap psychologic, psychosocial, or behavior benefits from pulmonary rehabilitation is weak. Well-controlled studies using validated measures of psychologic and behavior functioning are needed. A standardized and accepted tool for assessing quality of life changes in patients with respiratory disease would be beneficial.

Each member of the pulmonary rehabilitation team needs to be aware of the factors that can lead to failure of rehabilitation so that the potential for success can be optimized. Reasons for failure include lack of competent and dedicated medical supervision, inclusion of inappropriate patients, lack of individualization so that the very sick and the nearly well get the same treatment, poor communication with referring physicians, lack of objective documentation, excessive commercialization, poor organization of the program, lack of personal access between the patients and the program on an ongoing basis, failure to establish realistic goals, and lack of flexibility in the therapeutic offerings.

One of the major limitations continues to be the failure of many primary care physicians to refer their pulmonary patients for rehabilitation. Teams must redouble their efforts to familiarize these physicians with the benefits of rehabilitation.

The problem of inadequate reimbursement for pulmonary rehabilitation, in some areas, needs to be resolved. Third-party payers must be educated about the cost savings (e.g., reduction in hospital days) that can be achieved through pulmonary rehabilitation. More information regarding the impact on health care resources needs to be collected in this era of "managed care."

Steps should be taken to ensure that the special needs and problems of respiratory patients are incorporated into the curricula of allied health schools, including nursing, respiratory therapy, physical therapy, occupational therapy, and dietetics. Psychologists, psychiatrists, chaplains, social workers, and others involved in counseling patients and their families need to be knowledgeable about the special needs of respiratory patients to fully meet their needs.

The routine use of spirometry in the office can assist in identifying respiratory disease before clinical signs and symptoms appear. Decreasing the number of persons who smoke remains the key to a major reduction in disability from respiratory disease.

The optimal duration of a pulmonary rehabilitation program has not yet been determined. The role of ongoing maintenance programs to help maintain the benefits achieved from pulmonary rehabilitation programs needs to be clarified.

The value of pulmonary rehabilitation in patients with chronic respiratory impairment owing to diseases other than COPD and asthma has been reported, but more data would help clarify the specific components of pulmonary rehabilitation that are needed in these individuals.

REFERENCES

1. Official statement of the American Thoracic Society: pulmonary rehabilitation. Am Rev Respir Dis 1981;124:663.
2. Ries AL. Position paper of the American Association of Cardiovascular and Pulmonary Rehabilitation: scientific basis of pulmonary rehabilitation. J Cardiopulm Rehabil 1990;10:418.
3. Hodgkin JE. Benefits of pulmonary rehabilitation. In: Fishman AP, ed. Pulmonary Rehabilitation. New York: Marcel Dekker, 1996:33.
4. Lacasse Y, Wong E, Guyatt GH, et al. Meta-analysis of respiratory rehabilitation in chronic obstructive pulmonary disease. Lancet 1996; 348:1115.
5. Pulmonary rehabilitation: joint ACCP/ AACVPR evidence-based guidelines. Chest 1997;112:1363.
6. Official statement of the American Thoracic Society: pulmonary rehabilitation—1999. Am J Respir Crit Care Med 1999;159:1666.
7. Dudley DL, Glaser EM, Jorgenson BN, et al. Psychosocial concomitants to rehabilitation in chronic obstructive pulmonary disease. Chest 1980;77:413, 544, 677.
8. Agle DP, Baum GL, Chester EH, et al. Multidiscipline treatment of chronic pulmonary insufficiency: 1, psychologic aspects of rehabilitation. Psychosom Med 1973;35:41.
9. Fishman DB, Petty TL. Physical, symptomatic, and psychological improvement in patients receiving comprehensive care for chronic airway obstruction. J Chronic Dis 1971;24:775.
10. Kass I, Dyksterhuis JE. The Nebraska COPD Rehabilitation Project: a program to identify the factors involved in the rehabilitation of patients with chronic obstructive pulmonary disease: a multidisciplinary study of 140 patients. Omaha:

University of Nebraska, 1971. Final Report, Social and Rehabilitation Service, DHEW Project RD-2517-m.

11. Daughton DM, Fix AJ, Kass I, et al. Physiological-intellectual components of rehabilitation success in patients with chronic obstructive pulmonary disease (COPD). J Chronic Dis 1979;32:405.

12. Miller WF, Taylor HF, Pierce AK. Rehabilitation of the disabled patient with chronic bronchitis and pulmonary emphysema. Am J Public Health 1963;53(suppl):18.

13. Haas A, Cardon H. Rehabilitation in chronic obstructive pulmonary disease: a five-year study of 252 male patients. Med Clin North Am 1969;53:593.

14. Cherniack RM, Handford RG, Svanhill E. Home care of chronic respiratory disease. JAMA 1969;208:821.

15. Petty TL, Nett LM, Finigan MM, et al. A comprehensive care program for chronic airway obstruction: methods and preliminary evaluation of symptomatic and functional improvement. Ann Intern Med 1969;70:1109.

16. Kimbel P, Kaplan AS, Alkalay I, et al. An in-hospital program for rehabilitation of patients with chronic obstructive pulmonary disease. Chest 1971;60(suppl):6S.

17. Shapiro BA, Vostinak-Foley E, Hamilton BB, et al. Rehabilitation in chronic obstructive pulmonary disease: a two-year prospective study. Respir Care 1977;22:1045.

18. White B, Andrews JL Jr, Mogan JJ, et al. Pulmonary rehabilitation in an ambulatory group practice setting. Med Clin North Am 1979;63:379.

19. Krumholz RA. Pulmonary outpatient rehabilitation: a four-year follow-up. Ohio State Med J 1973;69:680.

20. Moser RM. Rehabilitation of the COPD patient: lesson 40 in weekly update: pulmonary medicine. Princeton, NJ: Biomedia, 1979.

21. Balchum OJ. Rehabilitation in chronic obstructive pulmonary disease. Arch Environ Health 1968;16:614.

22. Pierce AK, Paez PN, Miller WF. Exercise therapy with the aid of a portable oxygen supply in patients with emphysema. Am Rev Respir Dis 1965;91:653.

23. Miller WF. Rehabilitation of patients with chronic obstructive lung disease. Med Clin North Am 1967;51:349.

24. Woolf CR, Suero JT. Alterations in lung mechanics and gas exchange following training in chronic obstructive lung disease. Dis Chest 1969;55:37.

25. Bass H, Whitcomb JF, Forman R. Exercise training: therapy for patients with chronic obstructive pulmonary disease. Chest 1970;57:116.

26. Nicholas JJ, Gilbert R, Gabe R, et al. Evaluation of an exercise therapy program for patients with chronic obstructive pulmonary disease. Am Rev Respir Dis 1970;102:1.

27. Rusk HA. Pulmonary problems. In: Rehabilitation Medicine. 3rd ed. St. Louis: CV Mosby, 1971.

28. Woolf CR. A rehabilitation program for improving exercise tolerance of patients with chronic lung disease. CMAJ 1972;106:1289.

29. Wasserman K, Whipp BJ. Exercise physiology in health and disease. Am Rev Respir Dis 1973;112:219.

30. Degre S, Sergysels R, Messin R, et al. Hemodynamic responses to physical training in patients with chronic lung disease. Am Rev Respir Dis 1974;110:395.

31. Alpert JS, Bass H, Szucs MM, et al. Effects of physical training on hemodynamics and pulmonary function at rest and during exercise in patients with chronic obstructive pulmonary disease. Chest 1974;66:647.

32. Brundin A. Physical training in severe chronic obstructive lung disease. Scand J Respir Dis 1974;55:25.

33. Shepard RJ. Exercise and chronic obstructive lung disease. Exerc Sport Sci Rev 1976;4:263.

34. McGavin CR, Gupta SP, Lloyd EL, et al. Physical rehabilitation of chronic bronchitis: results of a controlled trial of exercises in the home. Thorax 1977;32:307.

35. Chester EH, Belman MJ, Bahler RC, et al. Multidisciplinary treatment of chronic pulmonary insufficiency: 3. The effect of physical training on cardiopulmonary performance in patients with chronic obstructive pulmonary disease. Chest 1977;72:695.

36. Schrijen F, Jezek V. Haemodynamic variables during repeated exercise in chronic lung disease. Clin Sci Mol Med 1978;55:485.

37. Unger KM, Moser KM, Hansen P. Selection of an exercise program for patients with chronic obstructive pulmonary disease. Heart Lung 1980;9:68.

38. Sinclair DJM, Ingram CG. Controlled trial of supervised exercise training in chronic bronchitis. BMJ 1980;280:519.

39. Cockcroft AE, Saunders MT, Berry G. Randomized controlled trial of rehabilitation in chronic respiratory disability. Thorax 1981;36:200.

40. Hughes RL, Davison R. Limitations of exercise reconditioning in COLD. Chest 1983;83:241.

41. Tydeman DE, Chandler AR, Graveling BM, et al. An investigation into the effects of exercise tolerance training on patients with chronic airways obstruction. Physiotherapy 1984;70:261.

42. Holle RHO, Williams DV, Vandree JC, et al. Increased muscle efficiency and sustained benefits in an outpatient community hospital–based pulmonary rehabilitation program. Chest 1988;94:1161.

43. Carter R, Nicotra B, Clark L, et al. Exercise conditioning in the rehabilitation of patients with chronic obstructive pulmonary disease. Arch Phys Med Rehabil 1988;69:118.

44. Mall RW, Medeiros M. Objective evaluation of results of a pulmonary rehabilitation program in a community hospital. Chest 1988;94:1156.

45. Busch AJ, McClements JD. Effects of a supervised home exercise program on patients with severe chronic obstructive pulmonary disease. Phys Ther 1988;68:469.

46. Strijbos JH, Koeter GH, Meinesz AF. Home care rehabilitation and perception of dyspnea in

chronic obstructive pulmonary disease (COPD) patients. Chest 1990;97:1095.

47. Ries AL, Kaplan RM, Limberg TM, et al. Effects of pulmonary rehabilitation on physiologic and psychosocial outcomes in patients with chronic obstructive pulmonary disease. Ann Intern Med 1995;122:823.

48. Wijkstra PJ, Van der Mark TW, Kraan J, et al. Effects of home rehabilitation on physical performance in patients with chronic obstructive pulmonary disease (COPD). Eur Respir J 1996; 9:104.

49. Strijbos JH, Postma DS, Van Altena R, et al. A comparison between an outpatient hospital-based pulmonary rehabilitation program and a home-care pulmonary rehabilitation program in patients with COPD. Chest 1996;109:366.

50. Goldstein RS, Gort EH, Stubbing D, et al. Randomised controlled trial of respiratory rehabilitation. Lancet 1994;344:1394.

51. Bendstrup KE, Ingemann Jensen J, Holm S, et al. Out-patient rehabilitation improves activities of daily living, quality of life and exercise tolerance in chronic obstructive pulmonary disease. Eur Respir J 1997;10:2801.

52. Casaburi R, Patessio A, Ioli F, et al. Reductions in exercise lactic acidosis and ventilation as a result of exercise training in patients with obstructive lung disease. Am Rev Respir Dis 1991; 143:9.

53. Casaburi R, Wasserman K, Patessio A, et al. A new perspective in pulmonary rehabilitation: anaerobic threshold as a discriminant in training. Eur Respir J 1989;2:618s.

54. Maltais F, Leblanc P, Simard C, et al. Skeletal muscle adaptation to endurance training in patients with chronic obstructive pulmonary disease. Am J Respir Crit Care Med 1996;154:442.

55. Maltais F, Leblanc P, Jobin J, et al. Intensity of training and physiologic adaptation in patients with chronic obstructive pulmonary disease. Am J Respir Crit Care Med 1997;155:555.

56. Casaburi R, Porszasz J, Burns MR, et al. Physiologic benefits of exercise training in rehabilitation of patients with severe chronic obstructive pulmonary disease. Am J Respir Crit Care Med 1997;155:1541.

57. Horowitz MB, Littenberg B, Mahler DA. Dyspnea ratings for prescribing exercise intensity in patients with COPD. Chest 1996;109:1169.

58. Punzal PA, Ries AL, Kaplan RM, et al. Maximum intensity exercise training in patients with chronic obstructive pulmonary disease. Chest 1991;100:618.

59. Cooper CB. Determining the role of exercise in patients with chronic pulmonary disease. Med Sci Sports Exerc 1995;27:147.

60. Celli BR. Pulmonary rehabilitation in patients with COPD. Am J Respir Crit Care Med 1995; 152:861.

61. Lake FR, Henderson K, Briffa T, et al. Upper-limb and lower-limb exercise training in patients with chronic airflow obstruction. Chest 1990; 97:1077.

62. Reardon J, Awad E, Normandin E, et al. The effect of comprehensive outpatient pulmonary rehabilitation on dyspnea. Chest 1994;105: 1046.

63. Grosbois J-M, Lamblin C, Lemaire B, et al. Long-term benefits of exercise maintenance after outpatient rehabilitation program in patients with chronic obstructive pulmonary disease. J Cardiopulm Rehabil 1999;19:216.

64. O'Donnell DE, McGuire M, Samis L, et al. The impact of exercise reconditioning on breathlessness in severe chronic airflow limitation. Am J Respir Crit Care Med 1995;152:2005.

65. Casaburi R. Mechanisms of the reduced ventilatory requirement as a result of exercise training. Eur Respir Rev 1995;5:42.

66. Atkins CJ, Kaplan RM, Timms RM, et al. Behavioral exercise programs in the management of chronic obstructive pulmonary disease. J Consult Clin Psychol 1984;52:591.

67. Guyatt GH, German LB, Townsend M. Long-term outcome after respiratory rehabilitation. CMAJ 1987;137:1089.

68. Wijkstra PJ, Van Altena R, Krann J, et al. Quality of life in patients with chronic obstructive pulmonary disease improves after rehabilitation at home. Eur Respir J 1994;7:269.

69. Wedzicha JA, Bestall JC, Garrod R, et al. Randomized controlled trial of pulmonary rehabilitation in severe chronic obstructive pulmonary disease patients, stratified with the MRC dyspnoea scale. Eur Respir J 1998;12:363.

70. Wijkstra PJ. Pulmonary rehabilitation at home (editorial). Thorax 1996;51:117.

71. Guyatt GH, Berman LB, Towsend M. Long-term outcome after respiratory rehabilitation. CMAJ 1987;137:1089.

72. Vale F, Reardon JZ, ZuWallack RL. The long-term benefits of outpatient pulmonary rehabilitation on exercise endurance and quality of life. Chest 1993;103:42.

73. Reardon J, Patel K, ZuWallack RL. Improvement in quality of life is unrelated to improvement in exercise endurance after outpatient pulmonary rehabilitation. J Cardiopulm Rehabil 1993;13:51.

74. Strijbos JH, Sluiter HJ, Postma DS, et al. Objective and subjective performance indicators in COPD. Eur Respir J 1989;2:666.

75. Reardon J, Awad E, Normandin E, et al. The effect of comprehensive outpatient pulmonary rehabilitation on dyspnea. Chest 1994;105: 1046.

76. American Thoracic Society. Dyspnea: mechanisms, assessment, and management: a consensus statement. Am J Respir Crit Care Med 1999; 159:321.

77. Petty TL, MacIlroy ER, Swigert MA, et al. Chronic airway obstruction, respiratory insufficiency, and gainful employment. Arch Environ Health 1970;21:71.

78. Lustig FM, Haas A, Castillo R. Clinical and rehabilitation regime in patients with chronic obstructive pulmonary disease. Arch Phys Med Rehabil 1972;53:315.

79. Kass I, Dyksterhuis JE, Rubin H, et al. Correlation of psychophysiological variables with vocational rehabilitation outcome in patients with

chronic obstructive pulmonary disease. Chest 1975;67:433.

80. Fix AJ, Daughton D, Kass I, et al. Personality traits affecting vocational rehabilitation success in patients with chronic obstructive pulmonary disease. Psychol Rep 1978;43:939.

81. Burton GG, Gee G, Hodgkin JE, et al. Respiratory care warrants studies for cost-effectiveness. Hospitals 1975;49:61.

82. Hudson LD, Tyler ML, Petty TL. Hospitalization needs during an outpatient rehabilitation program for severe chronic airway obstruction. Chest 1976;70:606.

83. Lertzman MM, Cherniack RM. Rehabilitation of patients with chronic obstructive pulmonary disease. Am Rev Respir Dis 1976;114:1145.

84. Jensen PS. Risk, protective factors, and supportive interventions in chronic airway obstruction. Arch Gen Psychiatry 1983;40:1203.

85. Johnson HR, Tanzi F, Balcham OJ, et al. Inpatient comprehensive pulmonary rehabilitation in severe COPD. Respir Ther 1980;May/June:15.

86. Nichol J, Hodgkin JE, Connors G, et al. Strategies for developing a cost-effective pulmonary rehabilitation program. Respir Care 1983;28:1451.

87. Sneider R, O'Malley JA, Kahn M. Trends in pulmonary rehabilitation at Eisenhower Medical Center: an 11-years' experience (1976-1987). In: Hodgkin JE, ed. Pulmonary rehabilitation symposium. J Cardiopulm Rehabil 1988;8:453.

88. Lewis D, Bell SK. Pulmonary rehabilitation, psychosocial adjustment and use of healthcare services. Rehabil Nurs 1995;20:102.

89. Sahn SA, Nett LM, Pett TL. Ten-year follow-up of a comprehensive rehabilitation program for severe COPD. Chest 1980;77(suppl):311.

90. Wright RW, Larsen DF, Monie RG, et al. Benefits of a community-hospital pulmonary rehabilitation program. Respir Care 1983;28:1474.

91. Ferris BG Jr, Anderson DO, Zickmantel R. Prediction values for screening tests of pulmonary function. Am Rev Respir Dis 1965;91:252.

92. Kory RC, Callahan R, Boren HG, et al. Veterans Administration—Army cooperative study of pulmonary function: 1. Clinical spirometry in normal men. Am J Med 1961;30:243.

93. Petty TL, Sahn SA, Nett LM. Ten-year follow-up of a comprehensive rehabilitation program for severe COPD. Chest 1980;77(suppl):311.

94. Burrows B, Earle RH. Course and prognosis of chronic obstructive lung disease. N Engl J Med 1969;280:397.

95. Boushy SF, Thompson HK, North LB, et al. Prognosis in chronic obstructive pulmonary disease. Am Rev Respir Dis 1973;108:1373.

96. Diener CF, Burrows B. Further observations on the course and prognosis of chronic obstructive lung disease. Am Rev Respir Dis 1975;111:719.

97. Emergil C, Sobol BJ. Long-term course of chronic obstructive pulmonary disease: a new view of the mode of functional deterioration. Am J Med 1971;51:504.

98. Postma DS, Burema J, Gimeno F, et al. Prognosis in severe chronic obstructive pulmonary disease. Am Rev Respir Dis 1979;119:357.

99. Renzetti AD Jr, McClement JH, Litt BD. The Veterans Administration Cooperative Study of pulmonary function: III. Mortality in relation to respiratory function in chronic obstructive pulmonary disease. Am J Med 1966;41:115.

100. Davis AL, McClement JH. The course and prognosis of chronic obstructive pulmonary disease. In: Current research in chronic respiratory disease: Proceedings of the 11th Aspen emphysema conference. Arlington, VA: DHEW, 1968:219.

101. Medical Research Council Working Party. Long-term domiciliary oxygen therapy in chronic hypoxic cor pulmonale complicating chronic bronchitis and emphysema. Lancet 1981;1:681.

102. Nocturnal Oxygen Therapy Trial Group. Continuous or nocturnal oxygen therapy in hypoxemic chronic obstructive pulmonary disease: a clinical trial. Ann Intern Med 1980;93:391.

103. Petty TL. Pulmonary rehabilitation. Am Rev Respir Dis 1979;122(suppl):159.

104. Bebout DE, Hodgkin JE, Zorn EG, et al. Clinical and physiological outcomes of a university-hospital pulmonary rehabilitation program. Respir Care 1983;28:1468.

105. Hodgkin JE, Branscomb BV, Anholm JD, et al. Benefits, limitations and the future of pulmonary rehabilitation. In: Hodgkin JE, Zorn EG, Connors GL, eds. Pulmonary Rehabilitation: Guidelines to Success. Boston: Butterworth, 1984.

106. Burrows B, Traver GA, Cline MG. Predictors of mortality in chronic obstructive pulmonary disease. Am Rev Respir Dis 1979;119:895.

107. Postma DS, Sluiter HJ. Prognosis of chronic obstructive pulmonary disease: the Dutch experience. Am Rev Respir Dis 1989;140(suppl):S100.

108. Burns MR, Sherman B, Madison R, et al. Pulmonary rehabilitation outcome. J Respir Care Pract 1989;2:25.

109. Intermittent Positive-Pressure Breathing Trial Group. Intermittent positive-pressure breathing therapy of chronic obstructive pulmonary disease. Ann Intern Med 1983;99:612.

110. Anthonisen NR, Wright EC, Hodgkin JE, et al. Prognosis in chronic obstructive pulmonary disease. Am Rev Respir Dis 1986;133:14.

111. Hodgkin JE. Prognosis in chronic obstructive pulmonary disease. In: Hodgkin JE, ed. Chronic Obstructive Pulmonary Disease. Clin Chest Med 1990;11(3):555.

112. Gilmartin ME. Patient and family education. Clin Chest Med 1986;7:619.

113. Neish CM, Hopp JW. The role of education in pulmonary rehabilitation. In: Hodgkin JE, ed. Pulmonary Rehabilitation Symposium. J Cardiopulm Rehabil 1988;11:439.

114. Hopp JW, Lee JW, Hills R. Development and validation of a pulmonary rehabilitation knowledge test. J Cardiopulm Rehabil 1989;7:273.

115. Ashikaga T, Vacek PM, Lewis SO. Evaluation of a community-based education program for individuals with chronic obstructive pulmonary disease. J Rehabil Res Dev 1980;46:23.

116. Arora NS, Rochester DF. Respiratory muscle strength and maximal voluntary ventilation in

undernourished patients. Am Rev Respir Dis 1981;126:5.

117. Wilson DO, Rogers RM, Hoffman RM. Nutrition and chronic lung disease: state of the art. Am Rev Respir Dis 1985;132:1347.

118. Doekel RC Jr, Zwillich CW, Scoggin CH, et al. Clinical semistarvation: depression of hypoxic ventilatory response. N Engl J Med 1976; 295:358.

119. Askanazi J, Weissman C, La Sala PA, et al. Effect of protein intake on ventilatory drive. Anesthesiology 1984;60:106.

120. Wilson DO, Rogers RM, Wright EC, et al. Body weight in chronic obstructive pulmonary disease: the National Institutes of Health Intermittent Positive Pressure Breathing Trial. Am Rev Respir Dis 1989;139:1435.

121. Schols AMWJ, Slangen J, Volovics L, et al. Weight loss is a reversible factor in the prognosis of chronic obstructive pulmonary disease. Am J Respir Crit Care Med 1998;157:1791.

122. Gray-Donald K, Gibbons L, Shapiro SH, et al. Nutritional status and mortality in chronic obstructive pulmonary disease. Am J Respir Crit Care Med 1996;153:961.

123. Wilson DO, Rogers RM, Pennock BE, et al. Nutritional intervention in malnourished emphysema patients. Am Rev Respir Dis 1985; 131(part 2):61.

124. Efthimiou J, Fleming J, Gomes C, et al. The effect of supplementary oral nutrition in poorly nourished patients with chronic obstructive pulmonary disease. Am Rev Respir Dis 1988; 137:1075.

125. Buist AS, Nagy JM, Sexton GJ. Effect of smoking cessation on pulmonary function: a 30-month follow-up to two smoking cessation clinics. Am Rev Respir Dis 1979;120:953.

126. Camilli AE, Burrows B, Knudson RJ, et al. Longitudinal changes in forced expiratory volume in one second in adults. Am Rev Respir Dis 1987; 135:794.

127. Kark JD, Legiush M, Rannon L. Cigarette smoking as a risk factor for epidemic A (HI,NI) influenza in young men. N Engl J Med 1982; 307:1042.

128. Anthonisen NR, Connett JE, Kiley JP, et al. Effects of smoking intervention and the use of an inhaled anticholinergic bronchodilator on the rate of decline of FEV_1: the Lung Health Study. JAMA 1994;272:1497.

129. Butler JC, Shapiro ED, Carlone GM. Pneumococcal vaccines: history, current status, and future directions. Am J Med 1999;107:69S.

130. Barach AL. Ambulatory oxygen therapy: oxygen inhalation at home and out of doors. Dis Chest 1959;35:229.

131. Bradley BL, Garner AE, Billiu D, et al. Oxygen-assisted exercise in chronic obstructive lung disease: the effect on exercise capacity and arterial blood gas tensions. Am Rev Respir Dis 1978; 118:239.

132. Cotes JE, Gilson JC. Effect of oxygen on exercise ability in chronic respiratory insufficiency. Lancet 1956;1:872.

133. Leggett RJE, Flenley DC. Portable oxygen and exercise tolerance in patients with chronic hypoxic cor pulmonale. BMJ 1977;2:84.

134. Stein DA, Bradley BL, Miller WC. Mechanisms of oxygen effects on exercise in patients with chronic obstructive pulmonary disease. Chest 1982;81:6.

135. Kearley R, Wynne JW, Block AJ, et al. The effect of low flow oxygen on sleep disordered breathing and oxygen saturation. Chest 1980;78:682.

136. Tirlapur VG, Mir MA. Nocturnal hypoxemia and associated electrocardiographic changes in patients with chronic obstructive pulmonary disease. N Engl J Med 1982;306:125.

137. Tiep BL. Long-term home oxygen therapy. In: Hodgkin JE, ed. Chronic obstructive pulmonary disease. Clin Chest Med 1990;11:505.

138. Sexton DL. Relaxation techniques and biofeedback. In: Hodgkin JE, Petty TL, eds. Chronic Obstructive Pulmonary Disease: Current Concepts. Philadelphia: WB Saunders, 1987:99.

139. Gift AG, Moore T, Soeken K. Relaxation to reduce dyspnea and anxiety in COPD patients. Nurs Res 1992;41:242.

140. Renfroe KL. Effect of progressive relaxation on dyspnea and anxiety in patients with chronic obstructive pulmonary disease. Heart Lung 1988; 17:408.

141. Benson H. The Relaxation Response. New York: Morrow, 1975.

142. Benson H, Kotch JB, Crassweller KD. The relaxation response: a bridge between psychiatry and medicine. Med Clin North Am 1977;61:929.

143. Mueller RE, Petty TL, Filley GF. Ventilation and arterial blood gas changes induced by pursed lip breathing. J Appl Physiol 1970;28:784.

144. Motley HL. The effects of slow deep breathing on the blood gas exchange in emphysema. Am Rev Respir Dis 1963;88:484.

145. Paul G, Eldridge F, Mitchell J, et al. Some effects of slowing respiration rate in chronic emphysema and bronchitis. J Appl Physiol 1966; 21:877.

146. Sergysels R, Willeput R, Lenders D, et al. Low frequency breathing at rest and during exercise in severe chronic obstructive bronchitis. Thorax 1979;34:536.

147. Thoman RL, Stoker GL, Ross JC. The efficacy of pursed-lips breathing in patients with chronic obstructive pulmonary disease. Am Rev Respir Dis 1966;93:100.

148. Tiep BL, Burns M, Kao D, et al. Pursed lips breathing training using ear oximetry. Chest 1986;90:218.

149. Breslin EH, Ugalde V, Bonekat HW, et al. Abdominal muscle recruitment during pursed lip breathing in COPD (abstract). Am J Respir Crit Care Med 1996;153:A128.

150. Spahija J, de Marchie M, Grassino A. Pursed-lips breathing during exercises increases dyspnea (abstract). Am Rev Respir Dis 1993;147:A729.

151. Miller WF. A physiologic evaluation of the effects of diaphragmatic breathing training in patients with chronic pulmonary emphysema. Am J Med 1954;17:471.

152. Willeput R, Vachaudez JP, Lenders D, et al. Thoracoabdominal motion during chest physio-

therapy in patients affected by chronic obstructive lung disease. Respiration 1983;44:204.

153. Vitacca M, Clini E, Bianchi L, et al. Acute effects of deep diaphragmatic breathing in COPD patients with chronic respiratory insufficiency. Eur Respir J 1998;11:408.

154. Gosselink RAAM, Wagenaar RC, Sargeant AJ, et al. Diaphragmatic breathing reduces efficiency of breathing in chronic obstructive pulmonary disease. Am J Respir Crit Care Med 1995;151:1136.

155. Leith DE, Bradley ME. Ventilatory muscle strength and endurance training. J Appl Physiol 1976;41:508.

156. Peress L, McClean P, Woolf C, et al. Respiratory muscle training in severe chronic obstructive pulmonary disease. Am Rev Respir Dis 1979;119(4, part 2):157.

157. Celli BR. Respiratory muscle function. Clin Chest Med 1986;7:567.

158. Pardy RL, Reid WD, Belman MJ. Respiratory muscle training. Clin Chest Med 1988;9(2):287.

159. Belman MJ, Mittman D, Weir R. Ventilatory muscle training improves exercise capacity in chronic obstructive pulmonary disease patients. Am Rev Respir Dis 1980;121:273.

160. Pardy RL, Rivington RN, Despas PJ, et al. The effects of inspiratory muscle training on exercise performance in chronic airflow limitation. Am Rev Respir Dis 1981;123:426.

161. Larson JL, Kim MJ, Sharp JT, et al. Inspiratory muscle training with a pressure threshold breathing device in patient with chronic obstructive pulmonary disease. Am Rev Respir Dis 1988;138:689.

162. Pryor JA, Webber BA, Hodson ME, et al. Evaluation of the forced expiration technique as an adjunct to postural drainage in treatment of cystic fibrosis. BMJ 1979;2:417.

163. Sutton PP, Parker RA, Webber BA, et al. Assessment of the forced expiration technique, postural drainage and directed coughing in chest physiotherapy. Eur J Respir Dis 1983;64:62.

164. Mahlmeister MJ, Fink JB, Hoffman GL, et al. Positive-expiratory-pressure mask therapy: theoretical and practical considerations and a review of the literature. Respir Care 1991;36:1218.

165. AARC Clinical Practice Guideline: use of positive airway pressure adjuncts to bronchial hygiene therapy. Respir Care 1993;38:516.

166. Sobush DC, Hilling L, Southorn PA. Bronchial hygiene therapy. In: Burton GG, Hodgkin JE, Ward JJ. eds. Respiratory Care: A Guide to Clinical Practice. 4th ed. Philadelphia: JB Lippincott, 1997:501.

167. Murray JF. The ketch-up bottle method. N Engl J Med 1979;300:1155.

168. Anthonisen P, Riis P, Sogaard-Andersen T. The value of lung physiotherapy in the treatment of acute exacerbations in chronic bronchitis. Acta Med Scand 1964;175:715.

169. Graham WGB, Bradley GA. Efficacy of chest physiotherapy and intermittent positive-pressure breathing in the resolution of pneumonia. N Engl J Med 1978;299:624.

170. Hodgkin JE, Litzau KL. Exercise training target heart rates in chronic obstructive pulmonary disease. Chest 1988;94:30S.

171. Ries AL, Archibald CJ. Endurance exercise training at maximal targets in patients with chronic obstructive pulmonary disease. J Cardiopulm Rehabil 1987;7:594.

172. Carter R, Nicotra B, Clark L, et al. Exercise conditioning in the rehabilitation of patients with chronic obstructive pulmonary disease. Arch Phys Med Rehabil 1988;69:118.

173. Wasserman K, Sue DY, Casaburi R, et al. Selection criteria for exercise training in pulmonary rehabilitation. Eur Respir J 1989;2(Suppl 7):604S.

174. Celli BR, Rassulo J, Make BJ. Dyssynchronous breathing during arm but not leg exercise in patients with chronic airflow obstruction. N Engl J Med 1986;314:1485.

175. Ries AL, Ellis B, Hawkins RW. Upper extremity exercise training in chronic obstructive pulmonary disease. Chest 1988;93:688.

176. Ellis B, Ries AL. Upper extremity exercise training in pulmonary rehabilitation. J Cardiopulm Rehabil 1991;11:227.

177. Martinez FJ, Vogel PD, Dupont DN, et al. Supported arm exercise vs unsupported arm exercise in the rehabilitation of patients with severe chronic airflow obstruction. Chest 1993;103:1397.

178. Couser JI, Martinez FJ, Celli BR. Pulmonary rehabilitation that includes arm exercises reduces metabolic and ventilatory requirements for simple arm elevation. Chest 1993;103:37.

179. Matzen RV. Vocational rehabilitation: the culmination of physical reconditioning. Chest 1971;60(Suppl):21S.

180. Trulock EP, Egan TM, Kouchoukos NT, et al. Single lung transplant for severe chronic obstructive pulmonary disease. Chest 1989;96:738.

181. Weinmann GC, Hyatt R. Evaluation and research in lung volume reduction surgery. Am J Respir Crit Care Med 1996;154:1913.

182. Goldstein RS, Hall MJ. Pulmonary rehabilitation before and after lung transplantation. In: Fishman AP, ed. Pulmonary Rehabilitation. New York: Marcel Dekker, 1996:739.

Index

Pages numbers set in *italics* denote figures; those followed by a t denote tables; those followed by a b denote boxes.